SECOND EDITION

CLINICAL MEDICAL ASSISTING

A Professional, Field Smart Approach to the Workplace

Michelle E. Heller

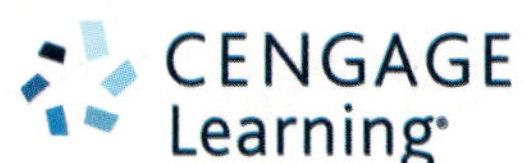

Clinical Medical Assisting: A Professional, Field Smart Approach to the Workplace, Second Edition
Michelle E. Heller

SVP, GM Skills & Global Product Management: Dawn Gerrain

Product Director: Matthew Seeley

Product Team Manager: Stephen Smith

Senior Director, Development: Marah Bellegarde

Product Development Manager: Juliet Steiner

Senior Content Developer: Lauren Whalen

Product Assistant: Mark Turner

Vice President, Marketing Services: Jennifer Ann Baker

Marketing Manager: Jessica Cipperly

Senior Production Director: Wendy Troeger

Production Director: Andrew Crouth

Content Project Manager: Thomas Heffernan

Senior Art Director: Jack Pendleton

Manager, Digital Production: Jamilynne Myers

Media Producer: Virginia Harrison

Cover image(s): © stevecoleimages/Getty Images

Library of Congress Control Number: 2015953061

ISBN: 978-1-305-11086-1

Cengage Learning
20 Channel Center Street
Boston, MA 02210
USA

Cengage Learning is a leading provider of customized learning solutions with employees residing in nearly 40 different countries and sales in more than 125 countries around the world. Find your local representative at **www.cengage.com**

Cengage Learning products are represented in Canada by Nelson Education, Ltd.

To learn more about Cengage Learning Solutions, visit **www.cengage.com**

Purchase any of our products at your local college store or at our preferred online store **www.cengagebrain.com**

Notice to the Reader

Publisher does not warrant or guarantee any of the products described herein or perform any independent analysis in connection with any of the product information contained herein. Publisher does not assume, and expressly disclaims, any obligation to obtain and include information other than that provided to it by the manufacturer. The reader is expressly warned to consider and adopt all safety precautions that might be indicated by the activities described herein and to avoid all potential hazards. By following the instructions contained herein, the reader willingly assumes all risks in connection with such instructions. The publisher makes no representations or warranties of any kind, including but not limited to, the warranties of fitness for particular purpose or merchantability, nor are any such representations implied with respect to the material set forth herein, and the publisher takes no responsibility with respect to such material. The publisher shall not be liable for any special, consequential, or exemplary damages resulting, in whole or part, from the readers' use of, or reliance upon, this material.

Printed in the United States of America
Print Number: 01 Print Year: 2015

Above all, I dedicate this book to God—for through Him all things are possible

Special Dedication: I dedicate this book to the memory of Lyn Veach and Lyn's children, Chris and Kelly. Lyn, my former coauthor, died during the early stages of development of this edition. Lyn's words still live on in the pages of this text. Lyn was one of the first graduates of the very first medical assisting program in Columbus, Ohio, paving the way for those that followed. Later, Lyn went on to get her degree in medical technology. Lyn spent several years preparing students to follow in her footsteps. Her love for students was matched by their love for her. I miss her kindness and her special gift of humor.

Michelle Heller

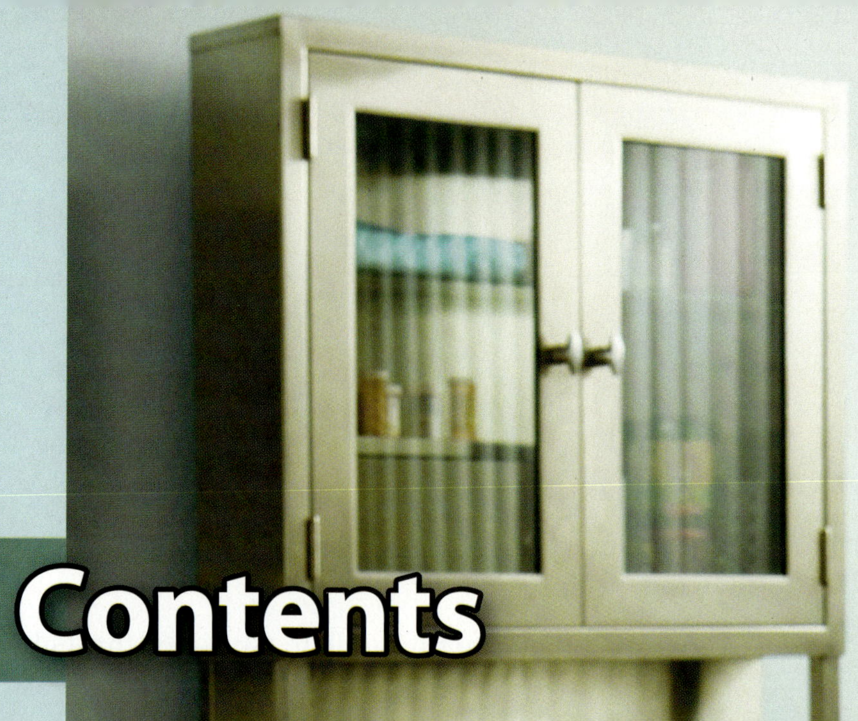

Contents

List of Procedures xxii
Preface xxv
About the Authors xxx
Acknowledgments xxxi

CHAPTER 1 Journey to Professionalism 1

- Professionalism and the Clinical Medical Assistant 3
  - A High Degree of Professionalism 5
  - Scope of Practice and Standard of Care 6
  - Patients' Bill of Rights 7
  - Ethics and Morals 7
- Developing Your Professional Persona 7
- The Keys to Your Professionalism Journey 8
  - Key #1: Professional Communication 8
  - Key #2: Performing as a Team Member (Collaboration) 12
  - Key #3: Engagement 12
  - Key #4: Accountability 15
  - Key #5: Respect 16
  - Key #6: Problem-solving 17
  - Key #7: Mindfulness 17
  - Key #8: Adaptability 18
- Time Management Principles 19
- Developing Professionalism Skills 20

CHAPTER 2 **Clinical Trends in Health Care** 28

- **Patient Protection and Affordable Care Act** 30
  - Reforming Health Care 30
  - Pay for Performance Organizations 31
  - Patient-Centered Approach 32
  - Pay for Coordination Organizations 32
- **The Role of Information Technology in Newer Health Care Delivery Models** 35
- **The Medical Assistant's Role in New Delivery Models** 36

CHAPTER 3 **The Complete Medical Record and Electronic Charting** 39

- **The Medical Record** 41
  - Electronic Medical Records 42
- **Important Uses of the Medical Record** 45
- **Medical Records Formats** 45
  - Source-Oriented Medical Record (SOMR) 45
  - Problem-Oriented Medical Record (POMR) 45
  - Combining Formats 48
- **Creating a Paper Chart** 48
  - Maintaining the Medical Record 48
- **Contents of the Medical Record** 48
  - Administrative Information in a Medical Record 49
  - Clinical Information in a Medical Record 49
- **EHR Responsibilities for the Medical Assistant** 61
  - Checking Electronic Tasks 61
  - Checking Clinical Today or Equivalent in Another EHR 61
- **Laws That Affect the Medical Record** 62
  - HITECH Act 62
  - The Health Insurance Portability and Accountability Act of 1996 (HIPAA) 62
  - Meaningful Use 63
- **Sharing Protected Information with Other Health Care Professionals** 66
  - Fees Associated with Copying of Medical Records 66
  - Retention of Medical Records 67
  - Disposal of Medical Records 67
  - Confidentiality 67
  - Electronic Access Audit/Activity Log 67

CHAPTER 4 **Fundamentals of Documentation** 72

- **Guidelines for Documenting in the Patient's Chart** 75
  - Documenting for Legal Success 75
  - General Guidelines for Documenting in the Patient's Medical Record 76
  - The Use of Medical Abbreviations in Chart Entries 79
  - Documenting Chief Complaints and Progress Notes 79

Documenting Laboratory Procedures 79
Documenting In-Office Procedures 81
Documenting Medications 82
Documenting Prescriptions 83
Documenting Patient Education Sessions 86
Documenting Telephone Calls 88
Identifying Critical Information for Scheduling Outside Procedures 88

■ **Making Corrections or Addendums to Chart Notes 92**

■ **Compose Professional Correspondence Using Electronic Technology 92**

CHAPTER 5 **Conducting a Patient Screening 99**

■ **The Communication Cycle 102**

■ **Therapeutic Communication 102**
The Use of Nonverbal Communication or Body Language 103

■ **Incorporating Effective Interviewing Techniques 103**
Effective Questioning Techniques 103
Ineffective Questioning Techniques 103
Effective Listening Techniques 103

■ **The Screening Process 105**
Greeting Stage 105
Performance of Height, Weight, and Vital Signs 106
Medication Reconciliation 106
Drug Allergies 106
Obtaining the Chief Complaint and History of Present Illness 106

■ **The Role of the Medical Assistant in History Collection 108**

■ **Tools Used to Collect Medical History Information 109**

■ **The Comprehensive Medical History 111**
Personal Medical History 111
Family Medical History 112
Social History 113
Depression Screening 114
Preventive Care Section 114
Concluding the Interview 115

CHAPTER 6 **Assisting Patients with Special Needs 120**

■ **Legal Issues and the Special Needs Patient 123**
Laws for the Hearing Impaired Patient 123
Laws Assisting the Visually Impaired Patient 124
Accessible Design Standards for Persons with Physical Disabilities 125
Laws for Non-English-Speaking Patients 125

■ **Working with Patients with Special Needs 126**
Diversity in Health Care 126
Barriers to Communication and Techniques to Overcome 126
Working with Visually Impaired Patients 130

Working with Hearing Impaired and Deaf Patients 132
Working with Pediatric Patients 139
Working with Physically Disabled Patients 141
Working with Patients Who Have Intellectual Disabilities 142

CHAPTER 7 **Health Coaching and Patient Navigation** 152

- **Population Management** 155
- **What Is Health Coaching?** 155
  - Resources 156
  - Demonstrate Respect for Individual Diversity 157
  - Patient Concerns 157
  - Self-Boundaries 158
- **Focus of Health Coaching** 158
  - Office Policies 158
  - Hygienic Practices 158
  - Health Maintenance and Disease Prevention 159
  - Osteoporosis Screening and Bone Density Scan 164
  - Pre- and Post-Op Care Instructions 164
  - Provide Support for Terminally Ill Patients 164
  - Recognition of Substance Abuse 165
  - Domestic Violence Screening and Detection 165
- **The Role of the Patient Navigator or Advocate** 166
  - Resource Information 166
  - Transition of Care 168

CHAPTER 8 **Principles of Infection Control** 177

- **Medical Abbreviation Review** 180
- **The Infection Process** 180
- **The Infection Cycle** 180
  - Infectious (Causative) Agents 180
  - Reservoir 182
  - Portal of Exit 182
  - Means of Transmission 183
  - Portal of Entry 183
  - Susceptible Host 183
- **Environmental Requirements for Microorganisms** 183
- **Stages of Infection** 185
  - Invasion and Multiplication Stage 185
  - Incubation Stage 185
  - Prodromal Stage 185
  - Acute Stage 185
  - Declining Stage 185
  - Convalescent Stage 185
- **The Body's Natural Defenses** 185
  - The Process of Inflammation 186
  - The Immune System 186
  - The Immune Response 186

Types of Immunity 186
Immunizations 187
Types of Vaccines 187

■ **Infection Control** **187**
Medical Asepsis 188
Surgical Asepsis 189

■ **Universal Blood and Body Fluid Precautions** **189**
Standard Precautions 189
The Biohazard Label 190
Transmission-Based Precautions 191

■ **Bloodborne Diseases** **193**
HIV/AIDS 193
Hepatitis 194

■ **OSHA Regulations** **194**
Bloodborne Pathogen Standard 194
Blood, Body Fluids, and OPIM 195
Exposure Determination 195
Exposure Control Plan 195
Regulated Waste 197

■ **Exposure to Hazardous Chemicals** **199**
OSHA'S Chemical Hygiene Plan 199

■ **Safeguards in the Educational Environment** **201**

CHAPTER 9

Sterilization Procedures, Instrument Identification, and Surgical Supplies 210

■ **Asepsis** **213**

■ **Sanitization, Disinfection, and Sterilization** **213**
Sanitization Procedures 213
Disinfection Procedures 214
Sterilization Techniques 216

■ **Types of Instruments Used in Minor Surgery** **220**
Identifying the Parts of a Surgical Instrument 220
Categories of Instruments 222

■ **Solutions and Supplies Used for Minor Surgeries** **229**
Common Solutions Used in Minor Surgery 229
Common Supplies Used in Minor Surgery 230
Common Anesthetics Used in Minor Surgery 232
Suture Materials and Other Supplies to Close the Skin 232

■ **Suture and Staple Removal** **235**

CHAPTER 10

Assisting with Minor Office Surgeries and Wound Care Procedures 249

■ **Developing a Sterile Conscience** 252

■ **Patient Safety Considerations** 252

■ **Types of Procedures Performed in the Medical Office/Tray Setups** 252

Procedures That Require No Special Equipment 253
Procedures That Require the Use of Special Equipment, Lasers, or Chemicals 253

■ **Preparing for Office Surgeries 256**
Setup Procedures 256
Once the Patient Enters the Surgical Suite 257

■ **Performing a Surgical Handwash and Applying Surgical Attire 262**

■ **Assisting the Physician before and during the Procedure 263**
Pre-Procedure Tasks 263
During the Procedure 264
At the Conclusion of the Surgery 264

■ **Wound Care 264**
Stages of Wound Healing 264
Today's Wound Care Philosophy 265
Types of Dressings 266
Types of Bandage Material 267
Wound Care Alternatives 268

CHAPTER 11 **Vital Signs and Measurements 290**

■ **Introduction to the Patient 293**
Screening the Patient 293
The Patient Intake 293

■ **Height and Weight 293**
BMI or Body Fat Percentage 293

■ **Vital Signs 295**
Temperature 295
Pulse 300
Respiration 302
Blood Pressure 304
Electronic Vital Signs 307
Pain Assessment 307
Pulse Oximetry 307

CHAPTER 12 **The Physical Exam 324**

■ **Age-Specific Exams 327**

■ **The Examination Room 327**
Preparation of the Exam Room 327
Instruments for Examination 328

■ **Patient Preparation 331**

■ **Patient Positioning and Draping 331**

■ **Patient Assessment 332**
Completing the Visit 337

CHAPTER 13 **Eye and Ear Exams and Procedures 347**

■ **Eye and Ear Snapshot 350**
Eye Anatomy 350
Ear Anatomy 350

■ Eye and Ear Abbreviation Review 352
■ Eye and Ear In-Office and Telephone Screening Tips 352
■ Common Diseases or Conditions of the Eyes 352
Cataracts 352
Macular Degeneration 352
Conjunctivitis 352
Corneal Abrasion 353
■ Common Diseases and Disorders of the Ears 353
Neurosensory Hearing Loss 353
Conductive Hearing Loss 353
Cerumen Impaction 356
Ear Infections 356
■ Featured Eye Procedures 356
Visual Acuity Testing 356
Eye Instillation 360
Eye Irrigation 360
■ Common Eye Medications 361
■ Featured Ear Procedures 361
Hearing Acuity 361
Speech and Word Recognition 363
Ear Instillation 364
Ear Irrigation 364
Miscellaneous Ear Procedures 364
■ Common Ear Medications 365
■ Common Lab Tests That Coincide with Ear Disorders 365
Ear Culture 365

CHAPTER 14 Cardiovascular Exams and Procedures 379

■ Cardiovascular System Snapshot 382
Heart Anatomy 382
Blood Vessels 383
Cardiovascular Physiology 384
Cardiac Conduction System 384
■ Cardiovascular Abbreviation Review 385
■ Cardiovascular In-Office and Telephone Screening Tips 385
■ Common Cardiovascular Diseases 385
Cardiac Arrhythmias 386
Coronary Artery Disease 387
Other Cardiovascular Conditions 390
■ Featured Cardiovascular Procedures 390
Electrocardiograms 391
Holter Monitor 400
Miscellaneous Cardiovascular Procedures 401
■ Common Cardiovascular Treatments and Medications 403
■ Common Lab Tests That Coincide with Cardiovascular Disorders 403

CHAPTER 15 Pulmonary Examinations and Procedures 414

- **Respiratory System Snapshot** 417
  - Lung Anatomy 417
  - Pulmonary Physiology 417
- **Pulmonary Abbreviation Review** 419
- **Respiratory In-Office Screening and Telephone Screening Tips** 419
- **Common Respiratory Diseases** 419
  - Contagious Infections 419
  - Tuberculosis 420
  - Lung Cancer 421
  - Emphysema 422
- **Featured Pulmonary Procedures** 425
  - Pulmonary Function Testing 425
  - Peak Flow Testing 426
  - Pulse Oximetry Testing 427
  - Sputum Collection 428
  - Miscellaneous Pulmonary Procedures 428
- **Common Pulmonary Treatments and Medications** 430
  - Nebulizers 430
  - Inhalers 430
  - Oxygen Administration 431
- **Common Lab Tests That Coincide with Respiratory Disorders** 432

CHAPTER 16 Gastrointestinal Exams and Procedures 444

- **Digestive System Snapshot** 447
  - Types of Digestion 447
  - Accessory Glands of the Gastrointestinal System 448
- **Gastrointestinal Abbreviation Review** 448
- **Gastrointestinal In-Office and Telephone Screening Tips** 448
- **Common Gastrointestinal Diseases** 449
  - Gastroesophageal Reflux Disease (GERD) 449
  - Ulcerative Colitis and Crohn's Disease 449
  - Cirrhosis 449
  - Colorectal Cancer 450
  - Other Gastrointestinal Conditions 452
- **Featured Gastrointestinal Procedures** 452
  - Rectal Exams 453
  - Fecal Occult Blood Testing 454
  - Sigmoidoscopy 455
  - Miscellaneous Gastrointestinal Procedures 456
- **Common Gastrointestinal Treatments and Medications** 456
- **Common Lab Tests That Coincide with Gastrointestinal Disorders** 456

CHAPTER 17 Women's Health Issues: Obstetrics and Gynecology 468

■ **Female Reproductive System Snapshot** 470
- Ovaries 470
- Fallopian Tubes 471
- Uterus 471
- Vagina 472
- The Menstrual Cycle 472
- Menopause 473

■ **Obstetric and Gynecologic Abbreviation Review** 476

■ **Gynecologic In-Office and Telephone Screening Tips** 476

■ **Common Obstetric and Gynecologic Diseases** 476
- Vulvodynia 476
- Vaginitis 476
- Uterine Fibroids 476
- Breast Cancer 477
- Other Common Obstetric and Gynecologic Diseases 477

■ **Featured Gynecologic Procedures** 480
- Gynecological Exam 480
- Medical Assistant's Responsibility during a Pap and Pelvic Exam 485
- Pelvic Exam for Women Who Have Vaginal Symptoms 487
- Mammography 487
- Miscellaneous Gynecologic Procedures 487

■ **Common Gynecologic Treatments and Medications** 488

■ **Common Lab Tests That Coincide with Women's Health Issues** 488

■ **Featured Obstetric Procedures** 488
- The Initial or First Prenatal Exam 489
- Return Prenatal Visits 491
- Miscellaneous Prenatal Diagnostic Tests and Procedures 492

■ **Common Obstetric Treatments** 494

■ **Common Lab Tests That Coincide with Pregnancy** 494

■ **Labor and Delivery** 494

■ **Postnatal or Postpartum Period** 496
- Six-Week Postpartum Visit 496

CHAPTER 18 Urology and Male Reproductive Exams and Procedures 507

■ **Urological and Male Reproductive System Snapshot** 510
- The Urinary System 510
- The Male Reproductive System 510

■ **Urological Abbreviation Review** 511

■ **Urinary System In-Office and Telephone Screening Tips** 512

■ **Male Reproductive System In-Office and Telephone Screening Tips** 513

■ **Common Urological Diseases and Conditions** 513
- Urinary Tract Infection (UTI) 513
- Overactive Bladder (OAB) 513

Renal Calculi (Kidney Stones) 514
Erectile Dysfunction (ED) 514
Benign Prostatic Hypertrophy (BPH) 514
Testicular Cancer 515

■ **Provider Examination** **515**

■ **Featured Urological Procedures** **517**
Urinary Catheterization 517
Diagnostic Testing 518
Intravenous Pyelogram (IVP) 519
Percutaneous Suprapubic Bladder Aspiration 519
Transrectal Ultrasound (TRUS) 520
Vasography 520

■ **Common Surgical Procedures for Male Reproductive Organs** **520**
Vasectomy 520
Transurethral Resection of the Prostate (TURP) 520
Circumcision 521

■ **Common Urological Treatments and Medications** **521**
Kidney Stone Treatments 521
Urethral Dilatation 521
Dialysis 521
Kidney Transplant 523
Common Urological Medications 523

■ **Common Lab Tests That Coincide with Urological Disorders** **523**

CHAPTER 19 **Other Specialty Procedures** **528**

■ **Introduction** **530**

■ **Allergy Specialty** **530**
Types and Causes of Allergies 530
Common Allergy Diagnostic Tests 534
Allergy Treatments 536

■ **Anti-aging Procedures** **537**
Anti-aging Treatments 537
The Role of the Medical Assistant in Assisting with Anti-aging Procedures 539

■ **Complementary and Alternative Medicine (CAM)** **539**
Description and Purpose of CAM 539
Provider Concerns 539
Types of CAM 540

CHAPTER 20 **Diet and Nutrition** **549**

■ **The Digestive Process** **552**

■ **Nutrition Abbreviations Review** **552**

■ **Nutrients** **553**
Fiber, Electrolytes, and Metabolism 553
Function of Vitamins and Minerals in the Body 554

■ **Nutrition through the Life Cycle** **554**
Infancy (The First Year of Life) 554
Childhood (Ages 1 to 10) 554

Adolescence (Ages 10 to 19) 554
Adult (Age 20+) 555
Seniors 555

■ **Planning a Healthy Diet** **555**
Reading Food Labels 555
Health Benefits of the Food Groups 555
Nutritional Guidelines 555

■ **Educating Patients about Good Nutrition** **558**
■ **Exercise for Weight Maintenance** **560**
■ **Nutrition Screening and Assessment** **562**
■ **Obesity** **562**
Health Effects of Obesity 562

■ **Weight Loss Diets** **563**
■ **Bariatric Surgery** **563**
■ **Special Diets** **563**
■ **Eating Disorders** **564**
Anorexia Nervosa 564
Bulimia Nervosa 564
Compulsive Overeating 564
Night Eating Syndrome 564

■ **Foodborne Illnesses** **564**

CHAPTER 21

Evaluation and Care of the Pediatric Patient 571

■ **Pediatric Age Classifications** **574**
■ **Age-Appropriate Communication** **574**
■ **Infant/Toddler Measurements** **575**
Height/Length 575
Weight 577
Circumferences 577
Pediatric Vital Signs 578

■ **Pediatric Development** **579**
Motor Development 579
Sensory Development 580
Language Development 580

■ **Visual and Hearing Screenings** **581**
Visual 581
Auditory 581

■ **Immunizations** **581**
Schedules 581
Controversies 581

■ **Pediatric Injections** **585**
Reducing Pain during Immunizations 585
Intranasal Route for Giving Immunizations 586

■ **Newborn Screenings** **586**
■ **Circumcision** **586**

■ **Adolescent Care** 587
Height and Weight 587
Puberty 588
Sports and Athletics 588
■ **Behavioral and Mental Health Issues** 588
Depression 588
Eating Disorders 589
Abuse 589
Suicide 589

CHAPTER 22 **Orthopedics, Rehabilitation, and Physical Therapy** 600

■ **Musculoskeletal System Snapshot** 602
■ **Musculoskeletal Abbreviation Review** 606
■ **Musculoskeletal In-Office and Telephone Screening Tips** 606
■ **Common Orthopedic Conditions** 607
Strain 607
Sprain 607
Dislocation 607
Fracture 607
Osteoporosis 609
Other Orthopedic Conditions 610
■ **Featured Orthopedic Procedures** 611
Assisting with the Orthopedic Exam 611
Application of Immobilization Devices 611
Ambulatory Assistive Devices 613
Common Exams Using Diagnostic Imaging 617
■ **Common Orthopedic Treatments** 617
Surgical Procedures 617
Rehabilitation 618
Arthritis Treatments 621
Exercises 621
■ **Common Orthopedic Medications** 623
■ **Common Diagnostic Tests That Coincide with Orthopedic Disorders** 623

CHAPTER 23 **Fundamentals of the Medical Laboratory** 640

■ **Rationale for Laboratory Tests** 643
■ **Laboratory Regulations** 643
Clinical Laboratory Improvement Amendment (CLIA ’88) 643
Testing Categories 644
■ **Implications of Clia ’88 for the Medical Assistant** 646
■ **Other Accreditation Options for POLs** 646
■ **Classifications of Laboratories** 646
■ **Laboratory Departments** 646
■ **Quality Assurance** 648
Quality Control 648
Test Logs 649

Orientation of Personnel 650
Maintenance Checks on All Equipment and Instruments 650
Required Calibration of Instruments 650
Temperature Checks 650
Proficiency Testing 650
Reference Ranges 651
■ **Safety in the Laboratory** **651**
■ **Hazards** **651**
■ **Processing Requests for Laboratory Tests** **652**
The Laboratory Requisition Form 652
■ **Preparing the Patient for Laboratory Testing** **655**
■ **General Guidelines for Specimen Collection, Handling, and Transport** **655**
Specimen Collection 655
Preserving Specimens 655
Sources of Contamination 656
■ **The Laboratory Report** **656**
Abnormal or Panic Test Values 657
■ **Flow Sheets** **658**
■ **The Microscope** **658**
Parts of the Microscope 658
Care and Maintenance 659
■ **The Centrifuge** **659**
Operating the Centrifuge 660

CHAPTER 24 **Blood Collection Techniques** **671**

■ **Why Do We Collect Blood?** **673**
■ **Venipuncture** **674**
Equipment and Supplies 674
■ **Vacuum Tube System** **677**
Multisample Needles 677
Holders and Adapters 677
Vacuum Tubes 678
■ **Winged Infusion (Butterfly) System** **680**
■ **Blood Collection Tray** **681**
■ **Performing the Venipuncture** **682**
Assembling Equipment and Supplies 682
Identifying the Patient 682
Positioning the Patient 682
Selecting the Site 683
■ **Specimen Collection by the Syringe Method** **684**
■ **Specimen Collection by the Vacuum Tube Method** **685**
■ **Specimen Collection by the Butterfly Method** **685**
■ **Patient Response and Complications** **685**
■ **The Failed Venipuncture** **685**
■ **Criteria for Specimen Rejection** **686**
Improper Labeling of Specimen Tubes 687
Use of Incorrect Specimen Tubes 687
Incorrect Collection Time 687

Incorrect Specimen Handling 688
Hemolyzed and Lipemic Specimens 688
■ **The Capillary Puncture** **688**
Equipment 688
Common Sites for Collection 689
Preparing the Site 689
Collecting the Specimen 689
Order of Draw 689
■ **General Guidelines for Specimen Handling** **690**
■ **Drawing Blood Cultures** **690**

CHAPTER 25 **Urinalysis** **705**
■ **Urinalysis Medical Terms and Abbreviation Review** **708**
■ **Composition of Urine** **708**
■ **Specimen Collection** **708**
General Collection Guidelines 708
Urine Specimen Containers 709
Methods of Collection 709
Types of Urine Specimens 710
■ **Quality Control** **711**
■ **Routine Urinalysis** **712**
Physical Examination 712
Chemical Urinalysis 714
■ **Microscopic Examination** **718**

CHAPTER 26 **Hematology and Coagulation Studies** **738**
■ **Medical Abbreviation Review** **741**
■ **Hematopoiesis** **741**
■ **Blood Components** **741**
Serum and Plasma 741
Erythrocytes 741
Leukocytes 742
Thrombocytes 743
■ **Coagulation** **743**
■ **Basic Hematology Studies** **743**
■ **The Complete Blood Count (CBC)** **744**
Red Blood Cell Count 744
White Blood Cell Count 744
Platelet Count 745
Hemoglobin 745
Hematocrit 746
Differential Count 747
Red Blood Cell Morphology 748
Complete Blood Count Normal Values 751
■ **Erythrocyte Sedimentation Rate (ESR)** **752**
■ **Automated Hematology Analyzers** **753**
■ **Coagulation Tests** **754**

CHAPTER 27 **Microbiology** **766**

- Microbiology Abbreviation Review 769
- Classification of Microorganisms 769
- Divisions of Microbiology 769
- Binomial Nomenclature System for Bacteria 769
- Characteristics of Bacteria 770
  - Basic Bacterial Cell Structure 770
  - Morphology of Bacteria 770
  - Classification by Staining Reaction 771
- Specimen Collection and Safe Handling Requirements 772
  - General Specimen Collection Guidelines 772
  - Specific Specimen Collection Requirements 773
  - Sources of Contamination 775
- Identification of Bacteria 775
  - The Culture 775
  - Growth Media 776
  - *Streptococcus* Identification 778
  - Rapid Strep Tests 779
- Sensitivity Testing 779
- Special Microscopic Techniques 780
  - The Wet Mount 780
- Virology 781
  - Identification of Viruses 781
- Parasitology 782
  - Identification of Parasites 783
- Mycology 783
  - Identification of Fungi 785
- Quality Control 785
- Lab Requisition and Test Report Forms 785

CHAPTER 28 **Clinical Chemistry and CLIA-Waived Testing** **796**

- Chemistry Abbreviation Review 799
- Clinical Chemistry Tests 799
  - Quality Control 799
- Specimen Requirements 799
  - Serum 799
  - Plasma 800
  - Whole Blood 801
  - Arterial Blood 801
- Appearance of Serum and Plasma 801
- Profiles and Panels 801
  - Hepatic (Liver) Profile 802
  - Renal Profile 803
  - Lipid Profile 803
  - Cardiac Biomarkers 804
  - Thyroid Panel 804

■ **Glucose Testing** 804
Fasting Blood Glucose Level 805
Two-Hour Postprandial Blood Glucose Level 805
Oral Glucose Tolerance Test (OGTT) 805
Glycosylated Hemoglobin ($HbA1_c$) 806
■ **Additional Chemistry Tests** 807
■ **Serology and Immunology Tests** 807
Rapid Tests 808
Common Serology Tests 809
■ **Blood Typing** 810
ABO Blood Typing 811
Rh Blood Typing 811
■ **Drug Testing** 811
Chain of Custody 812
■ **Chemistry Tests Normal Values** 812
■ **Lab Requisition and Test Report Forms** 812

CHAPTER 29 **Diagnostic Imaging** 823

■ **Radiology Overview** 826
■ **Legal Considerations for Diagnostic Imaging** 826
■ **Radiographic Equipment** 826
Digital Radiography 827
■ **The Medical Assistant's Role in Radiographic Procedures** 828
Positioning the Patient 828
■ **Common Types of Radiographs (X-rays) Performed in the Office** 828
■ **Processing and Displaying Radiographic Films** 830
■ **Storing and Disposing of Radiographic Films** 830
■ **Safety Precautions** 831
Personnel Safety Precautions 831
Patient Safety Precautions 832
■ **Scheduling Radiological Procedures outside the Office** 832
Patient Preparation Instructions 833
Explaining the Procedure 833
■ **Radiological Procedures Commonly Performed outside the Office** 834
■ **Other Diagnostic Imaging Procedures** 836
Computed Tomography (CT) Scan 836
Magnetic Resonance Imaging (MRI) 836
Ultrasound/Sonography 837
■ **Molecular Imaging and Nuclear Medicine** 838
■ **Radiation Therapy** 839

CHAPTER 30 **Fundamentals of Pharmacology** 843

■ **Pharmacology** 846
■ **Drug Origins** 846
Drug Sources 846
■ **Medicinal Uses of Drugs** 847
■ **Drug Classifications** 848

■ **Pharmacodynamics** 853
Dose Response 854
Drug Actions 855
Drug Effects 856
■ **Pharmacokinetics** 856
Variables That Affect a Drug's Blood Plasma Level 857
Factors That Affect Drug Actions 857
■ **Drug Names** 857
■ **Medication Tasks** 858
■ **Regulations and Legal Classifications of Drugs** 858
Controlled Substances 859
■ **The Medication Order or Prescription Writing** 861
Prescription Abbreviations 862
Rules for Creating Prescriptions for Controlled Substances 863
Tamper-Resistant Prescription Pads 863
■ **Drug Resources** 864
The Physicians' Desk Reference 864
U.S. Pharmacopeia/National Formulary 865
Drug Product Package Inserts 865
Drug Resources on the Internet and E-versions of Drug References 865
■ **Safe Drug Administration** 865
Seven Rights of Drug Administration 865
Safety and Continuity during Medication Administration 866
■ **Routes of Medication Administration** 867
Enteral Routes 867
Parenteral Routes 870

CHAPTER 31 **Dosage Calculations** **879**

■ **Medication Order** 882
■ **Medication Math Fundamentals** 882
The Apothecary System 882
The Metric System 882
Household Measurements 885
■ **Calculating Drug Dosages for Administration** 886
Rounding Equations 887
Proportional Method 887
Formula Method 887
Calculating Pediatric Dosages 888
■ **Calculating Insulin Dosages** 889
Types of Insulin 890
■ **Reading Medication Labels** 890
Warning Labels 892

CHAPTER 32 **Administration of Parenteral Medications** **896**

■ **Administration of Parenteral Medications** 899
Parenteral Equipment and Supplies 899
Preparing Medications 903
General Guidelines for Parenteral Medications 908

- **Routes of Administration** 910
  - Intradermal Injections 910
  - Subcutaneous Injections 912
  - Intramuscular Injections 912
- **Parenteral Complications** 915
- **Immunizations** 915
  - Contraindications and Precautions in Vaccine Administrations 915
- **Basics of Intravenous (IV) Therapy** 917
  - Equipment and Supplies Employed in Intravenous Therapy 917
  - Documentation of IV Therapy 919
  - Risks, Complications, and Adverse Reactions of IV Therapy 919
  - Discontinuation of Intravenous Infusion Therapy 920
- **Intra-Articular Injections** 921

CHAPTER 33 Responding to Medical Office Emergencies 941

- **Preparing Personnel for Emergencies** 944
  - The Medical Assistant's Role in Office Emergencies 944
  - Assessment and Screening in the Ambulatory Health Care Setting 944
- **Identification and Response to Emergencies** 944
  - Acute Abdominal Emergencies 945
  - Anaphylaxis 947
  - Breathing Emergencies 948
  - Cardiac Arrest 949
  - Cerebrovascular Accident (CVA) 951
  - Bleeding/Pressure Points 953
  - Burns 954
  - Diabetic Ketoacidosis and Insulin Shock 957
  - Poisoning 958
  - Seizures 958
  - Shock 959
  - Syncope 961
  - Vertigo 961
  - Thermal Emergencies 961
  - Wounds 962
  - Musculoskeletal Injuries 963
  - Animal Bite 966
  - Insect Bites and Stings 966
  - Concussion and Other Head and Neck Injuries 966
  - Mentally or Emotionally Distressed Patients 967

Appendix A Medical Abbreviations 977

Appendix B ISMP's List of *Error-Prone Abbreviations, Symbols*, and *Dose Designations* 981

Appendix C Top 50 Drugs (based on number of prescriptions) 983

Glossary 986

Index 1006

List of Procedures

PROCEDURE 1-1	Locate a State's Legal Scope of Practice for Medical Assistants	21
PROCEDURE 1-2	Apply the Patients' Bill of Rights as it Relates to Choice of Treatment, Consent for Treatment, and Refusal of Treatment	22
PROCEDURE 3-1	Create and Organize a Patient's Medical Record	68
PROCEDURE 4-1	Documenting the Administration of a Medication	93
PROCEDURE 4-2	Documenting a Phone Call from a Patient	95
PROCEDURE 5-1	Conduct a Patient Screening	115
PROCEDURE 6-1	Effectively Communicate with Patients from Different Cultures	143
PROCEDURE 6-2	Effectively Communicate with Sight Impaired or Visually Impaired Patients	145
PROCEDURE 6-3	Effectively Communicate with Hearing Impaired or Deaf Patients When an Interpreter Is Present	147
PROCEDURE 6-4	Effectively Communicate with a Hearing Impaired or Deaf Patient Who Speech Reads	148
PROCEDURE 7-1	Coach Patients Regarding Office Policies, Health Maintenance, Disease Management, and Disease Prevention	169
PROCEDURE 7-2	Develop a Current List of Community Resources Related to Patients' Health Care Needs	171
PROCEDURE 7-3	Facilitate Referrals to Community Resources in the Role of a Patient Navigator	172
PROCEDURE 8-1	Perform Medically Aseptic Handwashing	202
PROCEDURE 8-2	Perform an Alcohol-Based Hand Rub	203
PROCEDURE 8-3	Remove Contaminated Gloves	204
PROCEDURE 8-4	Select, Apply, Remove, and Dispose of Appropriate PPE Following Universal or Standard Precautions	205
PROCEDURE 9-1	Sanitization and Lubrication of Instruments	236
PROCEDURE 9-2	Chemical Disinfection of Instruments*	237
PROCEDURE 9-3	Wrapping Items for Sterilization in an Autoclave	239
PROCEDURE 9-4	Operate an Autoclave	241

PROCEDURE 9-5	Apply Skin Closures	242
PROCEDURE 9-6	Suture or Staple Removal	244
PROCEDURE 10-1	Perform a Surgical Handwash and Apply Surgical Gloves	270
PROCEDURE 10-2	Prepare the Patient's Skin for the Surgical Procedure Using a One-Step Scrub	273
PROCEDURE 10-3	Disinfect a Surgical Tray and Place a Sterile Barrier on the Tray	274
PROCEDURE 10-4	Open Sterile Items and Place Them on the Sterile Field	275
PROCEDURE 10-5	Set Up a Complete Sterile Tray and Pour a Sterile Solution	278
PROCEDURE 10-6	Apply Surgical Attire	281
PROCEDURE 10-7	Remove an Old Dressing, Irrigate the Wound, and Apply a New Dressing	284
PROCEDURE 11-1	Obtain the Height and Weight of an Adult Patient	309
PROCEDURE 11-2	Obtain Oral, Aural, Axillary, and Temporal Body Temperatures	311
PROCEDURE 11-3	Obtain a Radial Pulse Rate and Respiration Rate	315
PROCEDURE 11-4	Obtain an Apical Pulse Rate	317
PROCEDURE 11-5	Obtain a BP Measurement Using the Palpatory Method	318
PROCEDURE 12-1	Prepare the Examination Room	338
PROCEDURE 12-2	Position and Drape the Patient	340
PROCEDURE 12-3	Assist with the General Physical Examination	343
PROCEDURE 13-1	Snellen Chart Visual Acuity Testing	366
PROCEDURE 13-2	Screen Near Visual Acuity	368
PROCEDURE 13-3	Ishihara Test for Color Vision	369
PROCEDURE 13-4	Eye Instillation	370
PROCEDURE 13-5	Eye Irrigation	371
PROCEDURE 13-6	Hearing Acuity Testing	373
PROCEDURE 13-7	Ear Instillation	373
PROCEDURE 13-8	Ear Irrigation	375
PROCEDURE 14-1	Perform a Standard 12-Lead Electrocardiogram with a Multichannel Unit	406
PROCEDURE 14-2	Apply the Holter Monitor	408
PROCEDURE 15-1	Perform a Spirometry Test	434
PROCEDURE 15-2	Performing Peak Flow Testing	435
PROCEDURE 15-3	Perform Pulse Oximetry	437
PROCEDURE 15-4	Obtain a Sputum Specimen and Prepare a Smear	438
PROCEDURE 15-5	Administer a Nebulizer Treatment	439
PROCEDURE 16-1	Instruct the Patient on How to Collect a Fecal Specimen	458
PROCEDURE 16-2	Perform a Fecal Occult Blood Test	460
PROCEDURE 16-3	Assist with a Flexible Sigmoidoscopy	462
PROCEDURE 17-1	Instruct the Patient in Breast Self-Examination	498
PROCEDURE 17-2	Assist with a GYN Exam and Pap Test	500
PROCEDURE 17-3	Assist with the Prenatal Exam	503
PROCEDURE 19-1	Perform Allergy Testing	543
PROCEDURE 20-1	Develop a 2,000-Calorie Meal Plan Utilizing Basic Principles of Nutrition	566
PROCEDURE 20-2	Instruct a Patient According to the Patient's Special Dietary Needs	567
PROCEDURE 21-1	Obtain the Height/Length and Weight of an Infant	590
PROCEDURE 21-2	Obtain the Temperature of an Infant or Young Child	591
PROCEDURE 21-3	Perform a PKU on a Newborn	594
PROCEDURE 21-4	Perform a Pediatric Injection	596

PROCEDURE 22-1	Splint an Arm	625
PROCEDURE 22-2	Instruct a Patient to Use a Cane	626
PROCEDURE 22-3	Instruct a Patient to Use Axillary Crutches	628
PROCEDURE 22-4	Instruct a Patient to Use a Walker	629
PROCEDURE 22-5	Assist a Patient from the Wheelchair to the Exam Table and Back to the Wheelchair	631
PROCEDURE 22-6	Administer Heat Therapy Treatments	632
PROCEDURE 22-7	Administer Cold Therapy Treatments	635
PROCEDURE 23-1	Run a Control	661
PROCEDURE 23-2	Review and Report Laboratory Results	662
PROCEDURE 23-3	Specimen Collection for Offsite Testing	663
PROCEDURE 23-4	Use the Microscope	666
PROCEDURE 24-1	Perform Venipuncture (Syringe Method)	691
PROCEDURE 24-2	Perform Venipuncture (Vacuum Tube Method)	694
PROCEDURE 24-3	Perform Venipuncture (Butterfly Method)	697
PROCEDURE 24-4	Perform a Capillary Puncture	700
PROCEDURE 25-1	Instruct a Patient on a Clean-Catch Midstream Urine Collection	725
PROCEDURE 25-2	Perform a Physical and Chemical Urinalysis and Prepare a Microscope Slide for the Provider	728
PROCEDURE 25-3	Utilizing a Urine Transport System for Culture and Sensitivity	730
PROCEDURE 25-4	Urinary Catheterization	732
PROCEDURE 26-1	Perform a Capillary Puncture and Microhematocrit Test	755
PROCEDURE 26-2	Perform a Hemoglobin Using the Hemocue System	758
PROCEDURE 26-3	Perform an Erythrocyte Sedimentation Rate	759
PROCEDURE 26-4	Performing a Prothrombin Time (PT) and INR	761
PROCEDURE 27-1	Collect a Throat Specimen and Perform a Rapid Strep Test	787
PROCEDURE 27-2	Collect a Wound Specimen	789
PROCEDURE 27-3	Prepare a Wet Mount	791
PROCEDURE 27-4	Instruct a Patient on Fecal Specimen Collection for Ova and Parasite Testing	791
PROCEDURE 28-1	Measure Blood Glucose Using a Handheld Monitor	817
PROCEDURE 28-2	Perform a Urine Pregnancy Test	819
PROCEDURE 28-3	Perform a CLIA-Waived Mono Test	820
PROCEDURE 30-1	Write a Prescription	873
PROCEDURE 30-2	Administer an Oral Medication	874
PROCEDURE 31-1	Calculate a Medication Dosage for Administration	893
PROCEDURE 32-1	Withdraw Medication from a Vial	922
PROCEDURE 32-2	Withdraw Medication from an Ampule	924
PROCEDURE 32-3	Reconstitute a Powdered-Base Medication with a Diluent	926
PROCEDURE 32-4	Mix Two Medications into One Syringe	928
PROCEDURE 32-5	Load a Cartridge or Injector Device	930
PROCEDURE 32-6	Administer an Intradermal Injection	932
PROCEDURE 32-7	Administer a Subcutaneous Injection	934
PROCEDURE 32-8	Administer an Intramuscular Injection	936
PROCEDURE 33-1	Performing Basic First Aid in the Medical Office Setting	968

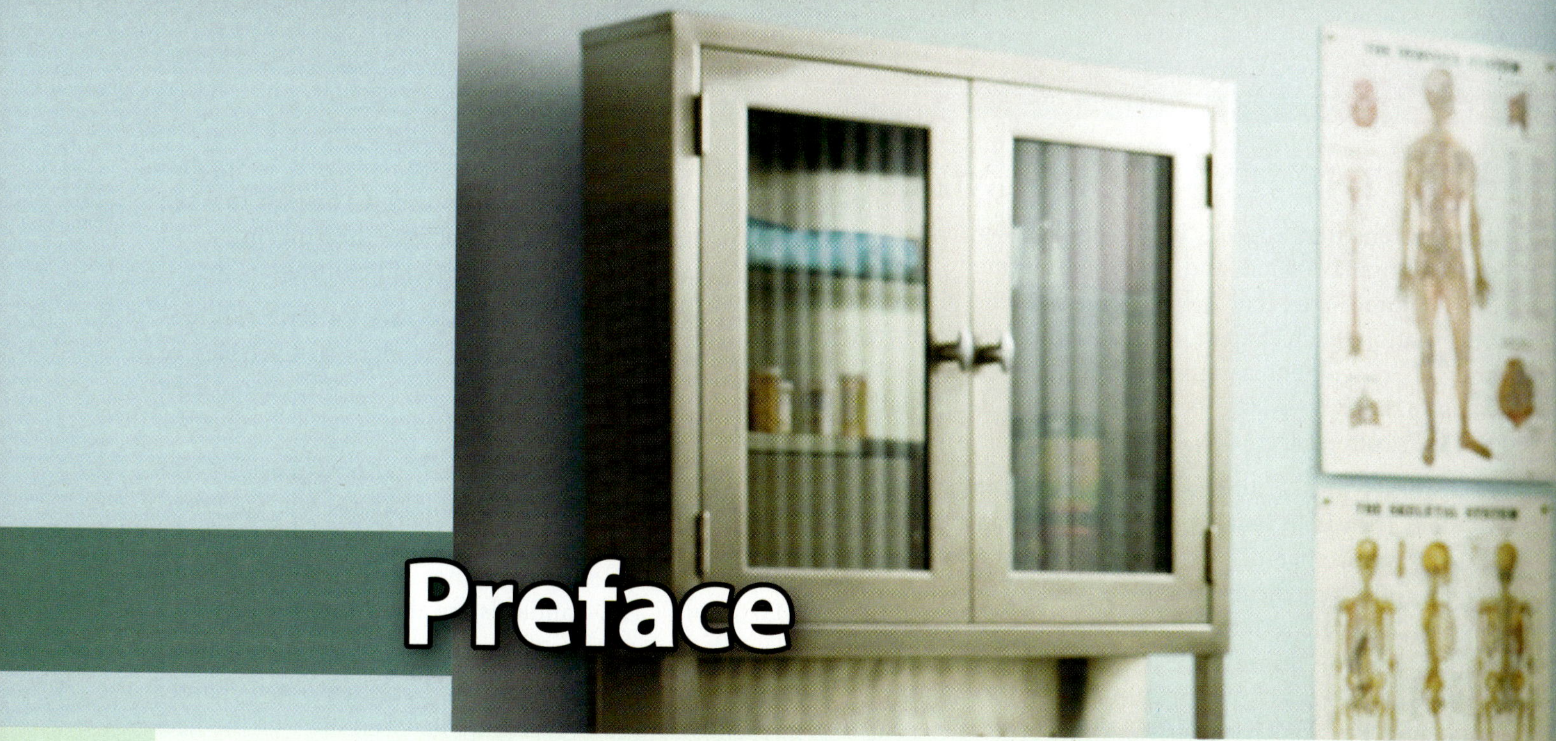

Preface

Welcome to *Clinical Medical Assisting: A Professional, Field Smart Approach to the Workplace, Second Edition*! The field of medical assisting is continually evolving. Today's medical assistant is being called upon to perform more complex tasks and to accept greater loads of responsibility than ever before. This is especially true in the clinical arena. With the implementation of the Affordable Care Act, ambulatory health care centers are relying on medical assistants working in a clinical capacity to possess strong technical skills, patient screening skills, health coaching skills, and wonderful communication skills. Medical assistants must understand that being a good clinician requires more than just being technically proficient—it requires the medical assistant to think on a higher level and to have superb problem-solving skills.

Today's office supervisors are looking for individuals who possess strong professional skills and can internalize the theoretical concepts learned in the classroom and apply them to the workplace. Because we are now living in the digital age, medical assistants must have a good grasp of the latest electronic health record (EHR) functionalities and have a clear understanding of how privacy laws affect health care members working on the clinical team.

This book is designed to empower medical assisting students with the knowledge that is necessary to meet and exceed the expectations of today's health care facilities. This book will help to prepare medical assisting students for the next generation of health care by providing them with educational resources that will not only be valuable in the health care market today, but for many years to come.

MOTIVATION FOR THE CONTENT THAT APPEARS IN THE BOOK

The core material for the book incorporates theoretical and technical information from the clinical standards set forth by the Commission on Accreditation of Allied Health Education Programs (CAAHEP) and The Accrediting Bureau of Health Education Schools (ABHES). The remainder of the book's content is the result of feedback received from educators and office supervisors across the country regarding both the latest trends in ambulatory medicine and common deficiencies among today's medical assistants.

Common areas of concern among supervisors and educators include a lack of professionalism or "soft" skills and weak documentation and screening skills among today's medical assistants. As a result of their important feedback, individual chapters have been designed to specifically address these areas of concern.

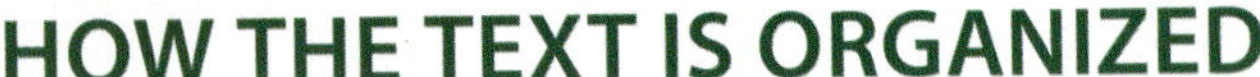

HOW THE TEXT IS ORGANIZED

The content that appears in the book is written in a contemporary format and incorporates many tables and feature boxes that help to organize and simplify information. Each chapter integrates important clinical and general content designed to correlate with institutions that are CAAHEP or ABHES accredited. Chapters are grouped according to subject matter:

Chapters 1 and 2, Journey to Professionalism and Clinical Trends in Health Care These chapters focus on the importance of professionalism and credentialing for today's medical assistant, especially those working in a clinical capacity. These chapters help students understand the importance of a professional mindset when working as a clinical medical assistant. Chapter 1, lists eight keys or characteristics which are necessary to be successful in health care. These keys are woven throughout each chapter to remind students of the importance of soft skills. Chapter 2, sets the foundation for accountable care. As the country moves to "pay for performance," clinical roles are changing. Providers now are reimbursed based on patient outcomes. Medical assistants must understand their role in a team-based care environment and how to assist patients in meeting their health care goals.

Chapters 3 and 4, The Complete Medical Record and the Fundamentals of Documentation These chapters focus on the importance of medical records and teach the student how charts are organized. These chapters also discuss laws that affect medical records and provide tips on how to apply legal principles when using information contained within a chart. Chapter 3 includes an entire section on EHR technology and teaches students about the latest functionalities available from software vendors. Meaningful use and the medical assistant's role in computerized order entry is covered in this chapter. Chapter 4 is devoted to medical documentation. The Dos and Don'ts of medical documentation are addressed, as well as tables with lists of what should be included in each type of documentation. There are a multitude of documentation samples in this chapter.

Chapter 5, Patient Screenings Today, medical assistants working in ambulatory medicine have more responsibility in conducting patient screenings. Effective communication is a very important element in the screening process. Students learn the elements of oral communications using a sender-receiver process and effective and noneffective questioning techniques. Parts of the comprehensive history are described and the role of the medical assistant in obtaining this information is also addressed.

Chapter 6, Assisting Patients with Special Needs This chapter instructs students on how to work with pediatric, geriatric, visually or hearing impaired patients, and patients from different cultures.

Chapter 7, Health Coaching and Patient Navigation This chapter introduces readers to the roles of patient navigator and health coach and discusses how medical assistants are a good fit for both of these roles.

Chapter 8, Principles of Infection Control and Medical Asepsis The steps of the infection cycle are introduced in this chapter as well as ways to interrupt the chain of infection. Guidelines for compliance with OSHA and CDC standards are also addressed.

Chapter 9, Sterilization Procedures, Instrument Identification and Surgical Supplies This chapter presents common instruments used in the medical office and methods used to sanitize, disinfect and sterilize instruments and other medical devices. Students learn common supplies used during a surgical procedure and how to remove sutures and staples.

Chapter 10, Assisting with Minor Office Surgeries and Wound Care Procedures This chapter prepares students to work in a surgical environment. Preparation of the surgical suite, patient skin prep and instructing patients on how to manage their surgical wounds is the central theme of this chapter.

Chapter 11, Vital Signs and Measurements This chapter presents steps for performing vital signs and mensuration procedures. Normal values and indicators for shifts in these values are presented to assist students in determining patient priority during the screening process.

Chapters 12–19, Assisting with Examinations and Procedures These chapters include information that is essential to know when assisting with various types of examinations and procedures in both general practice settings and specialty practices. A very brief overview of anatomical structures and disease processes associated with each system are included in each chapter to assist with health coaching. Each system chapter includes a screening table which lists common questions associated with particular body systems as well as tables which lists diagnostic testing, medications and abbreviations associated with each specialty.

Chapter 20, Diet and Nutrition This chapter presents basic information on the importance of nutrition in overall health. Major nutrients, vitamins, minerals, and the five food groups are core topics within the chapter. Special dietary needs for patients with diabetes, cardiovascular disease, hypertension, and cancer are featured contents in the chapter as well as information about lactose sensitivity, gluten free diets, and food allergies.

Chapter 21, Evaluation and Care of the Pediatric Patient This chapter covers common procedures that occur in pediatric offices as well as immunization updates.

Chapter 22, Orthopedics, Rehabilitation, and Physical Therapy This chapter presents important information to know when working in an orthopedic practice. The application of heat and cold packs and other modalities are also addressed in the chapter.

Chapters 23–28, Medical Laboratory Concepts These chapters focus on the various types of testing that are performed in the physician's office laboratory. Also covered are moderately and highly complex tests that are commonly performed in hospital and reference laboratories. Students will learn how to perform all of the major tests that are performed in waived labs, as well as phlebotomy. Specialty chapters include hematology, urinalysis, clinical chemistry, and microbiology. These chapters incorporate many tables to help simplify information.

Chapter 29, Diagnostic Imaging This chapter focuses on the many diagnostic and radiological exams that are performed in hospitals and other diagnostic centers. Students will learn the purpose of such testing and common prep for each procedure.

Chapters 30–32 Pharmacology These chapters focus on the uses of drugs and how the body metabolizes medications. Dosage calculation formulas, drug classifications, prescription writing, and procedures for administering medications are all covered in these chapters.

Chapter 33, Emergency Care This chapter covers common emergencies that occur in the medical office. The student will learn how to screen for emergencies and how to respond to specific types of emergencies.

CHAPTER ORGANIZATION

Each chapter includes the following components:

- **Essential Terms** are bolded terms that are essential for comprehending the material contained within the chapter.
- The **Chapter Outline** delineates how the material is organized within each chapter.
- **Developmental Objectives** are objectives to focus on when reading each chapter.
- **Solve the Case scenarios** are case studies that appear at the beginning and end of each chapter. The opening "Solve the Case" introduces students to a featured patient. Students are quizzed to see what they know about a specific condition prior to reading the chapter. The final "Solve the Case" is a wrap-up of the patient's appointment with instructions from the provider for discharging the patient. Soft skills are threaded throughout these two features.
- **Professionalism Mentor** is a mentoring feature that weaves the "keys to professionalism," presented in Chapter 1, throughout each mentor feature.
- **Illustrated Procedures** give step-by-step instructions that correlate with the chapter contents. Procedures list the rationales for important steps and many procedures incorporate pictures or illustrations for easy referencing.
- The **Chapter Summary** provides bulleted information of key points presented in each chapter.
- The **Certification Review** quiz consists of ten multiple choice questions written in certification exam style that correspond to the material covered in the chapter.

FEATURE BOXES

This book is loaded with feature boxes that help to simplify and reinforce chapter content. These feature boxes have a variety of themes and help to break up heavy text.

- **Field Smarts:** This feature provides quick facts relevant to book content. Informative facts, time-saving tips, and organizational tips are examples of information found in these boxes.
- **Health Coach:** This feature provides excellent data and tips that can be used during patient educational sessions.
- **EHR Application:** This feature educates on various functionalities of the EHR that can be utilized to help organize and expedite many of the clinical tasks that medical assistants perform.
- **Critical Thinking Challenge:** This feature helps the student think about and deal with issues he or she may face on the job.

NEW TO THIS EDITION

The central theme of this edition focuses on the latest trends in health care and the medical assistant's evolving role in affordable care organizations, such as patient-centered medical homes and patient navigation roles. Medical assistants have more responsibilities in these types of roles and must be able to think and act at a higher level.

Chapter 1, "Journey to Professionalism" sets the stage for the mindset of a clinician. It introduces readers to eight essential keys or character traits that are necessary to possess in order to be successful in health care. These keys are interwoven throughout the text and include the following:

- Key #1: Professional Communications
- Key #2: Performing as a Team Member (Collaboration)
- Key #3: Engagement
- Key #4: Accountability
- Key #5: Respect
- Key #6: Problem-solving
- Key #7: Mindfulness
- Key #8: Adaptability

Each chapter includes a "Professionalism Mentor" box written by a nurse manager of clinical development for Ohio Health Physician's Group. She oversees the training for medical assistants in over 200 physician office practices. Her feature pulls in the keys introduced in Chapter 1 and how they correlate with chapter material. Her factual perspective helps with student "buy in" on why these character traits are essential to succeeding in the industry.

Each of the systems chapters have been expanded to help students think and perform at a higher level. Each systems chapter includes the following:

- **System Snapshot:** This segment includes anatomical information necessary to educate patients about particular conditions.
- **Meet the Specialists:** This segment introduces readers to the different specialists for each system.
- **Abbreviation Review:** This segment of the chapter includes tables of common medical abbreviations for each system chapter.
- **In-Office and Telephone Screening Tips:** This part of the chapter teaches readers typical screening questions that are used when screening patients in the office or over the phone for each specialty area as well as how to set up the room and patient for exams and procedures.
- **Common Diseases:** This segment features a few of the more common diseases for each specialty area (for patient education purposes).
- **Over-the-Life Span:** This feature talks about what happens to organs in each system over the life span.
- **Featured Procedures:** This section introduces students to common procedures they will perform out in the field and the theory behind each procedure. It also includes common outside procedures and the medical assistant's role in educating patients about these procedures.
- **Common Treatments and Medications:** This segment discusses common medications prescribed in each type of practice and common treatments associated with different conditions.
- **Common Lab Tests:** These are common labs which are used for each system.

In addition to the above revisions and expansions, three new chapters have been added to the second edition: Clinical Trends in Health Care, Health Coaching and Patient Navigation, and Other Specialty Procedures.

STUDENT SUPPLEMENTS

Workbook

(ISBN 978-1-3051-1138-7)

Explore the text content through Vocabulary Review, Chapter Review, Certification Practice, and Application Activities for each chapter. The Workbook has been fully revised to align with the content in the second edition. Use the Competency Checklist section to evaluate performance of the text procedures and map to current, specific ABHES and CAAHEP curriculum standards. The Competency Checklists have been completely reformatted to match the text procedures exactly and provide instruction to download the specific material needed to complete the procedure. Procedure Forms can be downloaded from the Student Companion Website.

Student Companion Website

(www.cengagebrain.com)

This student website is designed to provide students with the resources they will need to complete the Competency Checklists. Procedure Forms are provided for the relevant checklists. The forms can be completed electronically and saved, or printed and completed manually.

Critical Thinking Challenge 3.0

(ISBN 978-1-1339-3330-4 or 978-1-1339-3324-3)

The Critical Thinking Challenge 3.0 software simulates a three-month practicum in a medical clinic. You will be confronted with a series of situations in which you must use your critical thinking skills to choose the most appropriate action in response to the situation. Your decisions will be evaluated in three categories: how your decisions affect the practice, the patient, and your career. The 3.0 version includes 12 all-new video-based scenarios with more branching options. After successfully completing the program, print out a Certification of Completion.

Learning Lab

(ISBN 978-1-1336-0956-8 or 978-1-1336-0953-7)

Learning Lab maps to learning objectives and includes interactive activities and case scenarios to build students' critical thinking skills and help retain the more difficult concepts. This simulated, immersive environment engages users with its real-life approach. Each Learning Lab has a preassessment quiz, three to five learning activities, and postassessment quiz. The postassessment scores can be posted to the instructor grade book in any learning management system.

MindTap to Accompany Clinical Medical Assisting: A Professional, Field Smart Approach to the Workplace, Second Edition

MindTap is a fully online, interactive learning experience built upon authoritative Cengage Learning content. By combining readings, multimedia, activities, and assessments into a singular learning path, MindTap elevates learning by providing real-world application to better engage students. Instructors customize the learning path by selecting Cengage Learning resources and adding their own content via apps that integrate into the MindTap framework seamlessly with many learning management systems.

The guided learning path demonstrates the importance of the medical assistant through engagement activities and interactive exercises. Learners can apply their understanding of the material through interactive activities taken from Critical Thinking Challenge 3.0 and the Medical Assisting Learning Lab, in addition to certification style quizzing and case studies. These simulations elevate the study of medical assisting by challenging students to apply concepts to practice.

To learn more, visit www.cengage.com/mintdtap

INSTRUCTOR SUPPLEMENTS

Instructor Companion Site

(ISBN 978-1-3051-1087-8)

(Access at www.cengage.com/login)

Spend less time planning and more time teaching with Cengage Learning's Instructor Resources. Log on to the Instructor Companion Site to gain access to the Instructor's Manual, Cognero Test Bank, and PowerPoint slides. Access at www.cengage.com/login with your Cengage instructor account. If you are a first-time user, click Create a New Faculty Account and follow the prompts.

Instructor's Manual

The Instructor's Manual provides mapping to ABHES and CAAHEP curriculum, lesson outlines, suggestions for classroom activities, and answer keys for the text and Workbook.

Online Cognero Test Bank

An electronic test bank makes and generates tests and quizzes in an instant. With a variety of question types, including multiple choice and matching exercises, creating challenging exams will be no barrier in your classroom. This test bank includes a rich bank of over 1,300 questions that test students on retention and application of what they have learned in the course. Answers are provided for all questions so instructors can focus on teaching, not grading. Each question also contains a reference to the text page number and ABHES and CAAHEP curriculum standard.

Instructor PowerPoint Slides

A comprehensive offering of more than 800 instructor support slides created in Microsoft® PowerPoint outlines concepts and objectives to assist instructors with lectures.

About the Authors

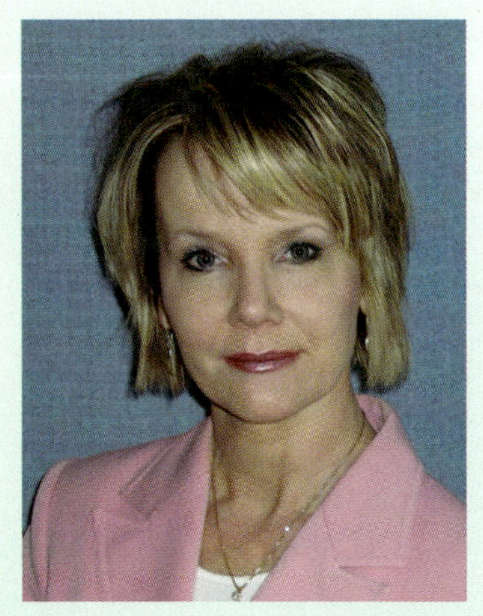

MICHELLE E. HELLER, CMA (AAMA)

Currently a faculty member at the Columbus State Community College, Michelle Heller has worked in health care and health care education for the past 35 years. She has received a number of "Outstanding Teacher" awards from institutions in which she had taught, and from the Ohio Council of Private Career Schools and Colleges. She has authored several books and is invited to give presentations at various forums. Heller served as director of education as well as director of the Medical Assisting Program for the Ohio Institute of Health Careers.

Acknowledgments

The amount of time invested into a project such as this requires huge sacrifices, not only from members of the author's team but also from their family members. This edition has been particularly challenging because of the loss of my coauthor, Lyn Veach, during the early stages of development, and due to some major health challenges my husband, Kevin, had to endure throughout the revision. He is doing much better now, after receiving a kidney transplant. We are so thankful to the donor and donor's family for this precious gift of life. Kev, I am so proud of you for persevering and not giving up! A big thanks to Erin, Aaron, Megan, Justin, Kevin, and Betsy, as well as other family members and friends for their love and support throughout the entire process both professionally and personally. We also welcomed our first grandbaby Gabriella Rose during the revision process. Gabriella, Grandma can't wait to start spoiling you.

I would also like to acknowledge members of my publishing family. I thank Stephen Smith, product team manager, for his support and encouragement during this project and for not giving up on me. But for Virginia Ferrari (special contributor) and Lauren Whalen (senior content developer), there wouldn't have been a second edition. Your contributions and support haven been immeasurable, and I don't know how I will ever adequately thank the two of you. A special thanks to my other contributors, Davene Yankle, Dr. Blake Busey, Dr. MaryEllen Tancred, Barbara Dahl, Colleen Wolf, and Sandy Reuble: Thank you for your hard work on this revision. Because of this extraordinary team effort, this book has turned out to be a product we can all be proud of.

CONTRIBUTORS

The authors and publisher would like to acknowledge the following educators and professionals for contributing to the content of this book:

Virginia Ferrari, MHA, BA, CEHRS
Contributing author for Chapters 1, 3, 6, 7, 11, 17, 19, 29, and 33

Blake Busey, D.O., Medical Director, PCMH Champion at Soldier and Family Medical Clinic, Fort Bliss, TX
Technical Reviewer and Advisor

Barbara Dahl, CMA (AAMA), CPC
Contributing author for Chapters 10, 28, 29, and 31

Sandy Reuble
Contributing author for Chapters 16, 18, 20, and 22

MaryEllen Tancred, Ph.D., MLS (ASCP)^{CM} SH^{CM}
Assistant Professor, Columbus State Community College
Contributing material to Chapters 23-28

Colleen Wolf, PA, UC Health-North, Fort Collins, Colorado
Contributing author for Chapters 12 and 13

Davene Yankle, MS, RN, CCRN, Manager of Clinical Development, OhioHealth Physician Group
Creation of all Professionalism Mentor features and Technical Reviewer

The authors and publisher would also like to acknowledge the following facilities and professionals for helping facilitate and execute the photo shoot which provided so many new photos for this book:

Stock Studios Photography
Saratoga Springs, NY
With special thanks to Tom Stock.

Columbus State Community College
Columbus, OH
With thanks to Connie Grossman, Fauna Stout, and Sabrina Becker (Photoshoot assistant)

REVIEWERS

The following educators provided feedback and thoughtful comments throughout the development process, which helped shape the final product.

Don Lamb, C.S.T., B.T.
Columbus State Community College
Columbus, OH.

Cheryl Baxter, RN MS, Certified Nurse Practitioner
Nation Wide Children's Hospital
Columbus, OH.

Janet Abuita
Ross College
Grand Blanc, MI

Jennifer Chandler
Living Arts College
Advance, NC

Abby Chelstowski
Ross College
Sylvania, OH

Stacy Clark
Ross Medical Education Center
Port Huron, MI

Lisa Cyprowski, RN, BSN
Pittsburgh Technical Institute
Oakdale, PA

Amanda Davis-Smith, AS, NCMA, AHI
Sanford-Brown College
Tinley Park, IL

Rebecca Gibson Lee, MSTE, CMA (AAMA), CPT (ASPT)
The University of Akron
Akron, OH

Elizabeth Hoffman, MA Ed, CMA (AAMA). CPT (ASPT)
Henry Ford College
Dearborn, MI

Mary Jo Jobbitt
Ross Medical Education Center
Port Huron, MI

Amanda Kennedy, LVN
American Commercial College
Wichita Falls, TX

Stacy Kuhn
Ross College
Sylvania, OH

Jessica Le, CMA, AHI
Ross Medical Education Center
Fort Wayne, IN

Lovie Little
Baker College
Southfield, MI

Wilsetta McClain, RMA, PhD
Baker College of Auburn Hills
Auburn Hills, MI

Nancy Measell, BS, AAS, CMA (AAMA)
Ivy Tech Community College
South Bend, IN

Linda Mollino, MSN, RN
Oregon Coast Community College
Newport, OR

Patricia Ricard
Ross College
Sylvania, OH

Kathleen Richards
Herzing University Online
North Huntington, PA

Keegan Richards
Ross College
Muskegon, MI

Lori H. Starnes, AAS, CMA (AAMA)
South Piedmont Community College
Monroe, NC

Kim VanDerMaas
Ross Medical Education Center
Port Huron, MI

Lauree Vasher
Ross Medical Education Center
Ann Arbor, MI

Barbara Westrick, AAS, CPC, CMA
Ross Education
Ann Arbor, MI

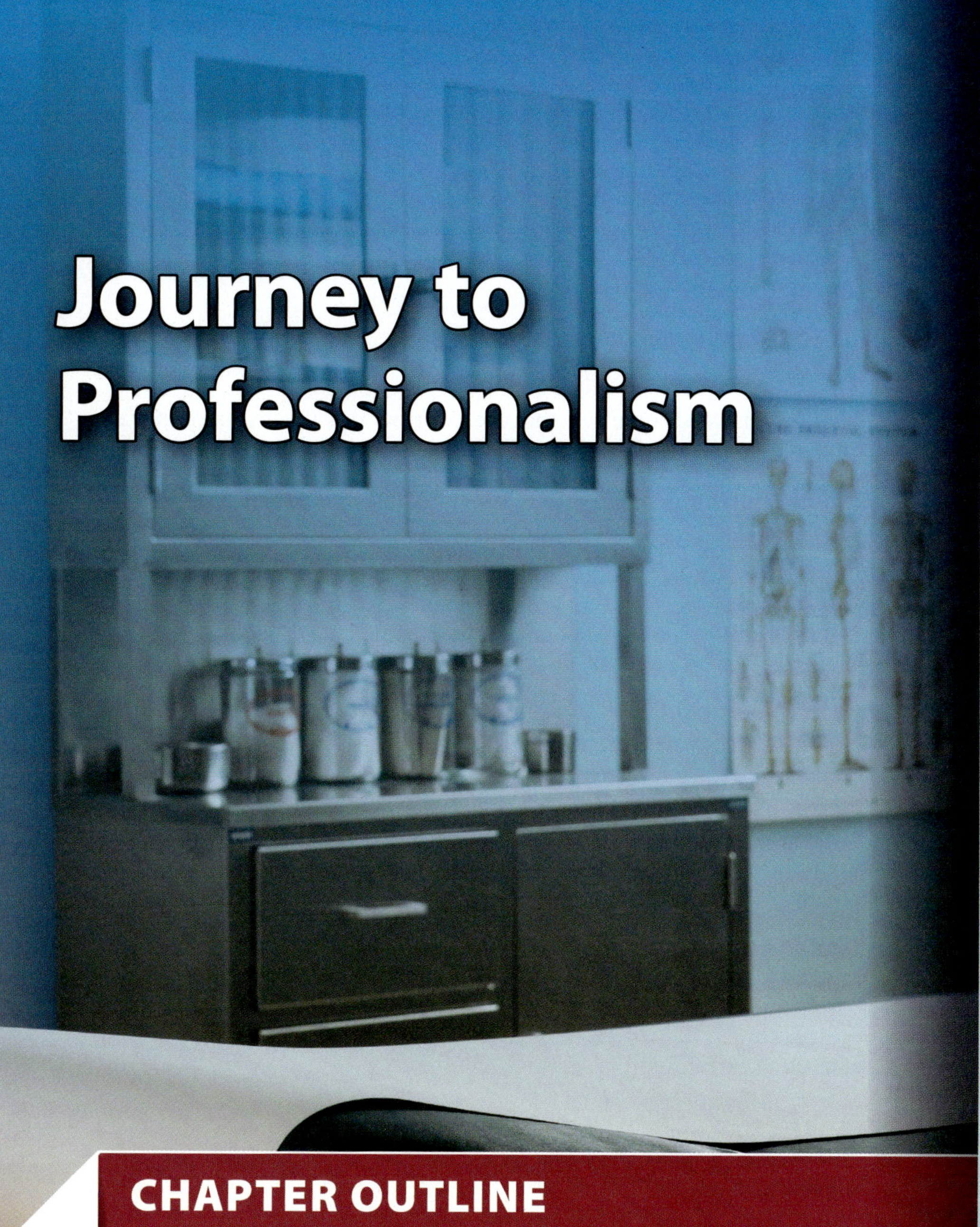

1

Journey to Professionalism

CHAPTER OUTLINE

Professionalism and the Clinical Medical Assistant

- A High Degree of Professionalism
- Scope of Practice and Standard of Care
- Patients' Bill of Rights
- Ethics and Morals

Developing Your Professional Persona

The Keys to Your Professionalism Journey

- Key #1: Professional Communication
- Key #2: Performing as a Team Member (Collaboration)
- Key #3: Engagement
- Key #4: Accountability
- Key #5: Respect
- Key #6: Problem-solving
- Key #7: Mindfulness
- Key #8: Adaptability

Time Management Principles

Developing Professionalism Skills

ESSENTIAL TERMS

accountability
Accrediting Bureau of Health Education Schools (ABHES)
adaptability
aggressive
American Association of Medical Assistants (AAMA)
American Medical Technologists (AMT)
appearance
assertive
attitude
certification
Certified Medical Assistant (AAMA) [CMA (AAMA)]
clinician
collaboration
Commission on Accreditation of Allied Health Education Programs (CAAHEP)
communication
compassion
confidentiality
courtesy
credentialing
dependability
dignity
diplomacy
dynamics
empathy
engagement
ethics
honesty
initiative
integrity
licensing
mindfulness
morals
National Healthcareer Association (NHA)
nonverbal
organizational ethics

continues

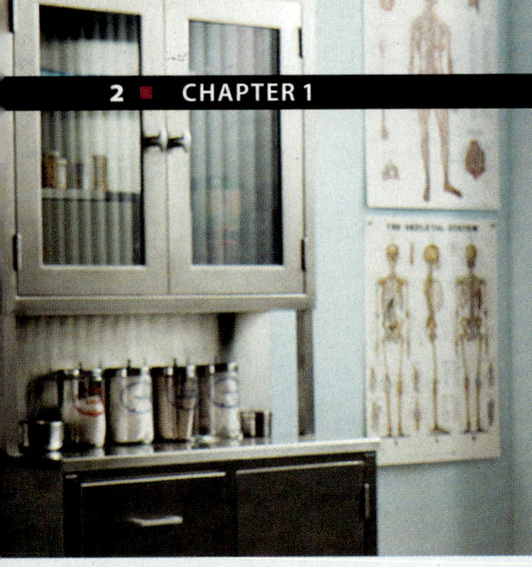

passive
Patients' Bill of Rights
problem-solving
professionalism
Registered Medical Assistant (RMA)
registration
respect
responsibility
scope of practice
service
standard of care
tact
verbal

DEVELOPMENTAL OBJECTIVES

After completing this chapter, you should be able to:

1. Correctly spell and define the essential terms.
2. Explain why a medical assistant working in a clinical capacity is held to a high degree of professionalism.
3. List six character qualities that are essential in a professional medical assistant.
4. Locate and define the scope of practice for the medical assistant within your state.
5. Differentiate between the scope of practice and standards of care for medical assistants.
6. Summarize the Patients' Bill of Rights.
7. Apply the Patients' Bill of Rights as it relates to (a) choice of treatment, (b) consent for treatment, and (c) refusal of treatment.
8. Demonstrate sensitivity to patient rights.
9. Display compliance with Code of Ethics of the profession.
10. Differentiate between personal and professional ethics.
11. Identify the effect of personal morals on professional performance.
12. Recognize the impact personal ethics and morals have on the delivery of health care.
13. Demonstrate empathy.
14. Display professionalism through written and verbal communications.
15. Relate assertive, aggressive, and passive behaviors to professional communication.
16. List five external actions that must be taken in order to expand technical knowledge, communicate more effectively, and demonstrate a caring attitude toward the patient.
17. List two different types of communications and describe ways in which overall communication skills can be improved.
18. List nine types of nonverbal communication and cite examples.
19. Explain the importance of service when working as a medical assistant.
20. List four organizations that credential medical assistants.
21. List three other credentials besides the CMA (AAMA) and RMA (AMT) that medical assistants may be able to obtain with some additional coursework or field experience.

INTRODUCTION

Throughout our working lives, most of us will have many different jobs, each requiring a different level or set of skills. No matter the industry—from customer service to an office job to construction and the trades—all of these jobs have one thing in common: in order to succeed and move ahead, you need to demonstrate **professionalism**. Professionalism does not mean wearing a suit or carrying a briefcase; rather, it means conducting oneself with **responsibility** (a duty or obligation), integrity, accountability, and excellence. According to the U.S. Department of Labor, professionalism means communicating effectively and appropriately and always finding a way to be productive.

The process that will assist you in developing professional skills can be compared to a journey. Your journey to become a professional medical assistant will require you to assess internal and external factors that affect your professional behavior. You must perform an internal inventory of your own character traits and make appropriate adjustments before gaining the respect of patients and other professionals in the industry. To **respect** others means to treat them with a positive feeling and appreciation, and to treat others the way you would want them to treat you. External actions must be taken in order to gain professional knowledge, communicate more effectively, and better serve your patients (Figure 1-1).

The professional journey will require you to conduct some deep soul-searching along the way and will compel you to fine-tune areas both within your mind and within your heart. The journey will stimulate you to take actions that will enhance your persona, resulting in positive communication with patients and colleagues. This will assist you in enhancing personal relationships as well.

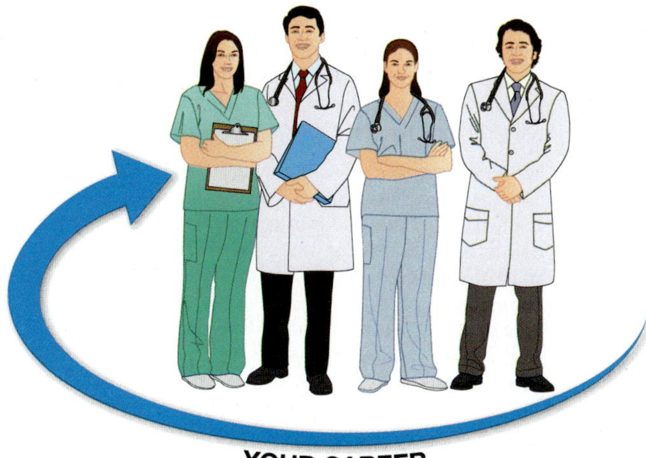

Figure 1-1 ■ You will be working with many other medical professionals throughout your career. It is critical that you gain their respect.

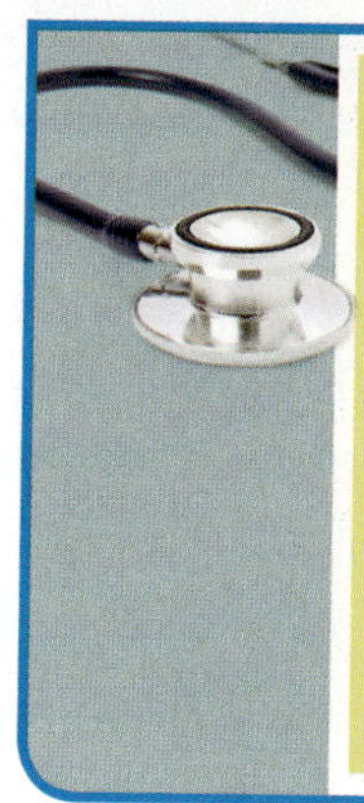

Field Smarts

Employers want workers to be responsible, ethical, and team oriented, and to possess strong communication, interpersonal, and problem-solving skills. Wrap these skills up all together and you've got professionalism.

Source: U.S. Department of Labor.

Professionalism develops over time and requires commitment to serve by placing patients and their families first. It requires you to make a conscious decision to be kinder than you sometimes are and to deny yourself in order to help others. Professionalism requires that you not judge people, but accept them as they are instead of dwelling on the negative, to go to work when you don't feel like going, and to perform duties that you don't feel like doing. It requires you to think on a higher level, become a problem-solver, and to react in all situations with poise and **dignity**, showing respect and assurance.

This chapter will present you with *Key* professionalism components that will help to unlock your professional characteristics.

PROFESSIONALISM AND THE CLINICAL MEDICAL ASSISTANT

Professionalism, both individual and organizational, is an essential element in the compact between the medical profession and society that is based on trust and putting the needs of patients above all other considerations. Health care professionals are bound to a code of ethics. Even though each health care profession has its own set of ethical standards, many health care programs include professionalism courses within their training programs. At the time of graduation, or during a special pinning ceremony, some students or graduates of health care programs recite the ethical creed for the professions in which they have trained and take a vow to implement those standards into their daily professional lives.

The field of medical assisting is no different than any other health care profession. The **American Association of Medical Assistants (AAMA)**, **American Medical Technologists (AMT)**, **National Healthcareer Association (NHA)**, and other medical assisting certifying organizations have

1-1 Solve the Case

Mr. Spadoni, a patient of Dr. Endo, is on a pain management regimen. Mr. Spadoni calls the office on a Thursday requesting a refill that the pharmacy has told him is too early to fill, even though he has only one day of medication left. Using key professionalism characteristics solve the case. You will score service points with the patient and provider by investigating the issue and offering a solution.

1. **What steps would you take to identify the problem?**
2. **After investigating the issue, what solutions can you offer?**
3. **How should these options be communicated to the patient as well as Dr. Endo?**

In this chapter you are going to learn about the characteristics that are essential to possess when working in health care.

4. **With your current level of knowledge, state the professional characteristics that you feel are essential to portray when working with all the parties involved in this scenario?**

established their own code of ethics (Figure 1-2a), standards of practice (Figure 1-2b), and creeds (Figure 1-2c) to which medical assistants must abide.

CODE OF ETHICS
of the American Association of Medical Assistants

The Medical Assisting Code of the Ethics of the AAMA sets forth principles of ethical and moral conduct as they relate to the medical profession and the particular practice of medical assisting.

Members of AAMA dedicated to the conscientious pursuit of their profession, and thus desiring to merit the high regard of the entire medical profession and the respect of the general public which they do serve, do pledge themselves to strive always to:

1. Render service with full respect for the dignity of humanity.
2. Respect confidential information obtained through employment unless legally authorized or required by responsible performance of duty to divulge such information.
3. Uphold the honor and high principles of the profession and accept its disciplines.
4. Seek to continually improve the knowledge and skills of medical assistants for the benefit of patients and professional colleagues.
5. Participate in additional service activities aimed toward improving the health and well being of the community.

Figure 1-2a ■ AAMA Code of Ethics.

AMT STANDARDS OF PRACTICE

The American Medical Technologists is dedicated to encouraging, establishing, and maintaining the highest standards, traditions, and principles of the disciplines which constitute the allied health professions of the certification agency and Registry.

Members of the Registry and all individuals certified by AMT recognize their professional and ethical responsibilities, not only to their patients, but also to society, to other health care professionals, and to themselves.

The AMT Board of Directors has adopted the following Standards of Practice which define the essence of competent, honorable and ethical behavior of an AMT-certified allied health care professional. Reported violations of these Standards will be referred to the Judiciary Committee and may result in revocation of the individual's certification or other disciplinary sanctions.

I. While engaged in the Arts and Sciences that constitute the practice of their profession, AMT professionals shall be dedicated to the provision of competent and compassionate service and shall always meet or exceed the applicable standard of care.
II. The AMT professional shall place the welfare of the patient above all else.
III. When performing clinical duties and procedures, the AMT professional shall act within the lawful limits of any applicable scope of practice, and when so required shall act under and in accordance with appropriate supervision by an attending physician, dentist, or other licensed practitioner.

Figure 1-2b ■ AMT Standards of Practice.

IV. The AMT professional shall respect the rights of patients and of fellow health care providers, shall comply with all applicable laws and regulations governing the privacy and confidentiality of protected healthcare information, and shall safeguard patient confidences unless legally authorized or compelled to divulge protected healthcare information to an authorized individual, law enforcement officer, or other legal or governmental entity.

V. AMT professionals shall strive to increase their technical knowledge, shall continue to learn, and shall apply scientific advances in their fields of professional specialization.

VI. The AMT professional shall respect the law and pledges to avoid dishonest, unethical, or illegal practices, breaches of fiduciary duty, or abuses of the position of trust into which the professional has been placed as a certified healthcare professional.

VII. AMT professionals understand that they shall not make or offer a diagnosis or dispense medical advice unless they are duly licensed practitioners or unless specifically authorized to do so by an attending licensed practitioner acting in accordance with applicable law.

VIII. The AMT professional shall observe and value the judgment of the attending physician, dentist, or other attending licensed practitioner, provided that doing so does not clearly constitute a violation of law or pose an immediate threat to the welfare of the patient.

IX. AMT professionals recognize that they are responsible for any personal wrongdoing, and that they have an obligation to report to the proper authorities any knowledge of professional abuse or unlawful behavior by any party involved in the patient's diagnosis, care and treatment.

X. The AMT professional pledges to uphold personal honor and integrity and to cooperate in protecting and advancing, by every lawful means, the interest of the American Medical Technologists and its Members.

Figure 1-2b ■ *(Continued)*

MEDICAL ASSISTING CREED

The Medical Assisting Creed of the AAMA sets forth medical assisting statements of belief:

I believe in the principles and purposes of the profession of medical assisting.
I endeavor to be more effective.
I aspire to render greater service.
I protect the confidence entrusted to me.
I am dedicated to the care and well being of all people.
I am loyal to my employer.
I am true to the ethics of my profession.
I am strengthened by compassion, courage, and faith.

Figure 1-2c ■ AAMA Creed.

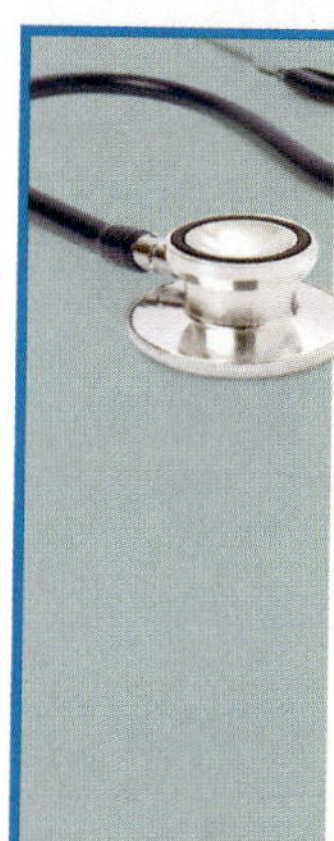

Field Smarts

Read over the AAMA code of ethics and creed (Figures 1-2a and 1-2c) and determine what kinds of adjustments you will need to make in order to comply with the standards. Start implementing these standards within your daily life now so that by the time you graduate, you will have a good grasp of how to develop a professional presence as a medical assistant.

A High Degree of Professionalism

So you may be asking yourself: Why is a clinical text focusing on professionalism training? After all, isn't clinical training just about learning how to perform related technical skills? The answer is no. Before you can become a good **clinician** (used in this context to mean someone working in a clinical capacity), you must possess a professional demeanor. While all health care professionals are held to a professional presence, patients have more intimate contact with health care professionals working in a clinical capacity and therefore may hold those workers to a higher standard. There are several contributing factors that lead to this type of thinking.

The Visibility Factor

The first factor is visibility. The clinical medical assistant is often more visible than the medical assistant working in an administrative capacity. Often much of the patient contact with the administrative medical assistant is on the telephone or at the reception and check-out desk. In contrast, the clinical medical assistant is in full view of the patient when performing clinical duties.

The Proximity Factor

The second factor is the amount of distance that usually exists between the medical assistant and the patient. The administrative medical assistant normally sits at few to several feet away from the patient. The clinical medical assistant, however, works much closer to the patient. On many occasions, a clinical medical assistant is face-to-face with the patient, making it easier for the patient to make observations with regard to the medical assistant's appearance and other professional

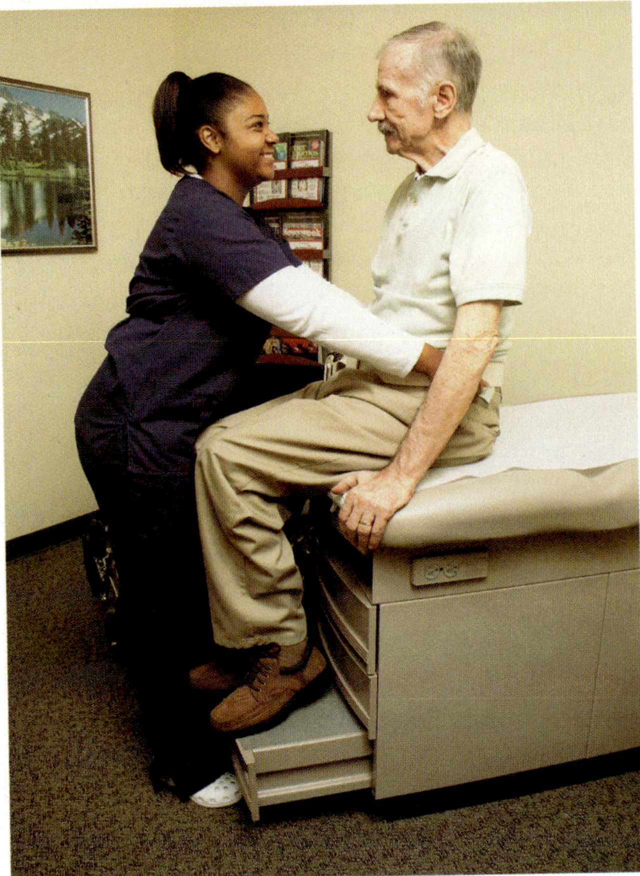

Figure 1-3 ■ Notice the close proximity of the medical assistant to the patient when assisting the patient onto the table from a wheelchair.

characteristics. Figure 1-3 shows the proximity of the medical assistant to the patient when assisting the patient onto an examination table.

The Time Factor

The third factor is the amount of face-to-face time the clinical medical assistant spends with the patient in comparison to the administrative medical assistant. The administrative medical assistant spends anywhere from seconds to a few minutes of physical time with each patient. The clinical medical assistant may spend anywhere from a few minutes to a few hours with the patient, depending on the procedures being performed. This allows more time for the patient to make observations regarding the clinical medical assistant's attitude, appearance, and work ethic.

The Nature of the Work

The fourth factor is the nature of the work being performed. The clinical medical assistant works with the patient on a physical level, which involves a certain amount of professional contact. The clinical medical assistant sees parts of the patient's body that the patient is private about and converses with the patient about sensitive health care matters. The patient needs to fully trust that the medical assistant is not going to share private comments that are made behind closed doors or discuss specific observations made about the patient's body.

The administrative medical assistant usually performs tasks related to scheduling, check-in/check-out, patient billing, and insurance processing. This information is also considered confidential, and should be treated with the highest level of confidentiality and sensitivity.

Errors

Errors may also have a bearing on the patient's expectations. Certain administrative errors (e.g., billing or insurance claims) may be easier to correct and have less consequence than a clinical error. A clinical error is generally not as easily corrected and could result in patient harm or even death to the patient. Your clinical actions will be held to a high degree of scrutiny.

Scope of Practice and Standard of Care

A medical assistant must always perform delegated clinical and administrative duties within his or her **scope of practice**, working under a physician's direct supervision, and consistent with his or her education, training, and experience. There is no uniform, national definition of a medical assistant's scope of practice, and duties will vary according to state law. A medical assistant's duties shall not constitute the practice of medicine and may not supersede what is permitted by law. However, the tasks performed by the medical assistant may be limited by the provider he or she works for. The governing body for doctors and their medical assistants is usually the State Medical Board or the State Board of Medical Examiners. Medical assistants must adhere to the rules, regulations, and requirements mandated by the state in which they work, as well as those imposed by their credentialing body or certification association. To find out more about the scope of practice that applies to the state where you will be working, go to the AAMA website (http://aama-ntl.org) and search under "State Scope of Practice Laws" (see Procedure 1-1).

Standard of care is defined as the diagnostic and treatment process that is reasonable and prudent that a clinician should follow for a certain type of patient, illness, or clinical circumstance. Medical assistants should always perform within the standard of care set forth by the profession and state laws.

Patients' Bill of Rights

Facilities and providers will often post a **Patients' Bill of Rights** developed by the organization as a way to communicate the legal rights patients have while under the care of a provider or facility. President Obama announced on June 22, 2010, new interim final regulations for the Patients' Bill of Rights from a government standpoint. The regulations proposed include a set of protections that apply to health coverage starting on or after September 23, 2010, six months after the enactment of the Affordable Care Act (ACA). The Centers for Medicare & Medicaid Services (CMS) says the Patients' Bill of Rights will help individuals with preexisting conditions gain coverage and keep it, protect all Americans' choice of doctors, and end lifetime limits on the care consumers may receive. These protections as outlined create an important foundation of patients' rights in the private health insurance market that puts Americans in charge of their own health. In Procedure 1-2 you will apply the Patients' Bill of Rights as it relates to choice of treatment, consent for treatment, and refusal of treatment while demonstrating sensitivity to patient's rights. To demonstrate sensitivity, be **courteous** (polite) and treat the patient with dignity and acceptance.

Ethics and Morals

Ethics is one of those intangible elements of life we deal with on a daily basis. Being aware of what is and is not ethical is essential for a successful career as a medical assistant. An ethical dilemma is where two moral principles are in conflict, such as when there is no clear-cut right or wrong on any matter. It might also be true when the right behavior leads to the wrong outcome.

There are three types of categorizing principles: law, ethics, and morals. There are often no clear-cut lines separating the three. For example, that which is legal might not be ethical in certain situations. What seems morally correct might not be legal. Sometimes, these are distinctions without differences; more often, they are joined seamlessly by contours that are not immediately recognizable. Whatever the case, a medical assistant must be able to distinguish among the three.

Organizational ethics represent the values by which an organization conducts its business. Organizations frequently include a values statement as part of their mission and vision statements.

The Effect of Personal Morals on Professional Ethics

The terms *morals* and *ethics* are often used interchangeably. The definition of *morals* references *ethics.* **Morals** can be defined as cultural and religious-based distinctions of right and wrong. Ethics transcends culture, religion, and time, representing the innate knowledge of right and wrong. What does all this mean to you, the medical assistant? Ethical considerations are intended to enhance your professional performance. Whatever your personal perspective might be regarding ethical matters, you must adapt your personal views to be in complete alignment with the ethical standards of your profession and the organization in which you are employed.

DEVELOPING YOUR PROFESSIONAL PERSONA

Developing professional characteristics is not something that just happens overnight. The integration of traits associated with professionalism actually begins early in life and progresses throughout one's lifetime.

If you watch a young child with younger siblings and playmates, you can recognize that the child often mimics what has been learned from parents. If the child's parents continually lash out and belittle the child, there is a good chance that the child will repeat the same behavior with siblings and playmates (Figure 1-4). If the child's parents are disrespectful toward other people, such as individuals in authority positions or in certain ethnic groups, the child most likely will mimic the same behavior patterns and prejudices in adulthood.

On the contrary, if a child is raised in a home where family members are respectful toward one another and talk in a positive manner when referring to people from other cultures, that child will be less likely to

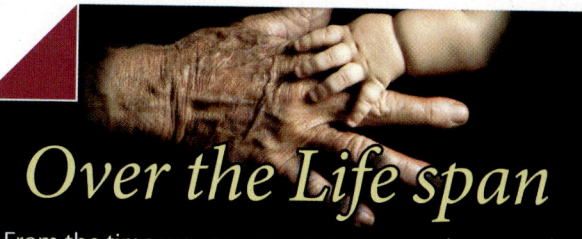

Over the Life span

From the time we are very young, we are instructed to "mind our manners," "address our elders with respect," and "have a good work ethic." These are the characteristics that help define the person we become. Some people are privileged enough to hear those instructions as well as to witness them first-hand through generations and the example of parents, relatives, and other mentors. Use these mentoring opportunities to learn and grow from the experience of caring for patients that span many generations.

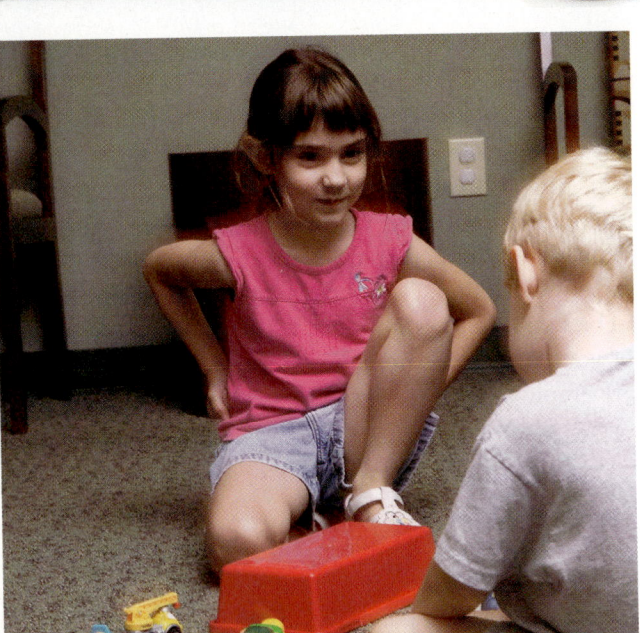

Figure 1-4 ■ Children often mimic their parents. Notice how the older child is scolding the younger child.

feel prejudice toward persons from other ethnic backgrounds and will be more likely to treat all individuals with dignity and respect.

Religion or faith may have an impact on professional skills. Many religious principles are similar to the ethical principles set forth by health care certifying organizations. For those who have been active in their areas of faith, professional standards may already be more familiar and come naturally.

Friends and peers can also influence your professional persona, for better or worse. If you surround yourself with individuals who are continually negative and lack motivation, there is a greater tendency to be negative yourself; however, if you surround yourself with friends and family members who are positive and have great initiative, chances are you will possess similar traits.

THE KEYS TO YOUR PROFESSIONALISM JOURNEY

The introduction of this chapter compared the development of professional qualities to a journey. The internal journey may be the most difficult part of the journey because it requires you to examine personal qualities that are deep within you and to perform the necessary adjustments before you can acquire professional character qualities. This chapter will define the "keys" to your journey that represent important character traits necessary in the development of professionalism. Figure 1-5 is an illustration of the keys that you must possess in order to complete this part of the journey.

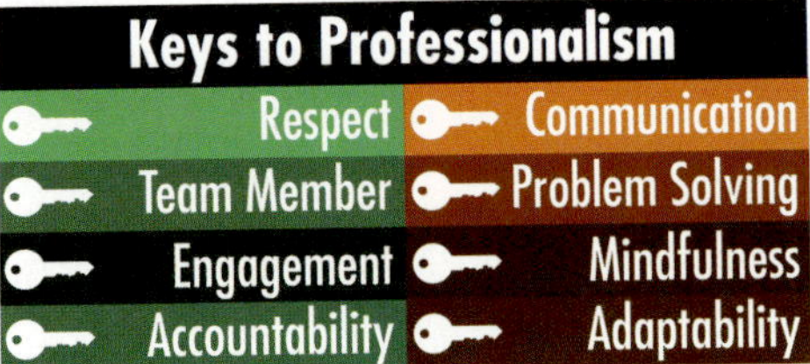

Figure 1-5 ■ The "keys" to your professionalism journey.

Key #1: Professional Communication

Professional communication is the foundation of every action taken in the health care setting. **Communication** takes many forms, including the exchange of thoughts, messages, or information, using speech, signals, writing, or behavior. Both clinical and administrative duties require a constant exchange of **verbal** (written or oral) and **nonverbal** information.

Types of nonverbal communication include:

- *Perception*. Being aware of one's own feelings and the feelings of others.
- *Body language*. Involves unconscious use of posture, gestures, and other forms of nonverbal communication (e.g., professional appearance and expression of confidence and skills).
- *Facial expression*. You wear your expression like a billboard, so you want to convey relaxed and pleasant facial expressions. The most common example of a positive, happy facial expression is a smile.
- *Eye contact*. This tells the person that you are interested in giving and receiving messages of mutual concern and importance. Warning! With electronic health records now dominating the charting process, make a conscience effort to maintain eye contact and personal touch with patients. On the other hand, you must also be sensitive, because in certain cultures making continuous eye contact with a person during a conversation can be interpreted as rude.

- *Gestures.* Body movements (hand and body gestures) that enhance what is being said.
- *Distance.* Comfort zones vary for different people and cultures. You must be respectful and ask if you are not sure of a patient's accepted practice. It would be appropriate to ask "Would you like to take my arm while I escort you to the exam room?"
- *Silence.* Silence is often frustrating for the person to whom it is directed. You must set the tone in the relationship, demonstrate leadership, and show confidence. Always greet the patient by name, listen carefully, and master the art of the open-ended question to avoid awkward situations.
- *Therapeutic touch.* A handshake and a hug are meaningful body movements that convey feelings of warmth and affection. Know when it is appropriate or not appropriate to use which type of touch, and be certain of the acceptable boundaries expressed by the person or by office protocol. Be sensitive to the person's reaction when touching is involved.
- *Active listening.* Participation in a conversation with another by means of repeating words and phrases or giving approving or disapproving nods. This signals that you are hearing and following what is being said. In order to be perceived as empathetic, you must engage in active listening.

Effective Communication

Attributes of an effective communicator include the ability to identify and adapt to the communication styles of others. You need to watch and listen carefully to patients, recognize their style, and then carefully adjust your communication. By listening carefully with empathy, you will establish a rapport with your patients and create a respectful, trusting, and honest relationship. Identify the most appropriate form of communication (verbal, nonverbal, visual, body language), and information technologies to enhance relationships. Conversations should be held in a suitable location, time, and place. Listen in a calm, open, nonjudgmental, and nonthreatening way, using open questions.

You must be able to convey (to impart an idea or message) in an articulate way to many different people and receive vital information in the same manner and demonstrate an appropriate behavior that reflects professional communication skills. This includes distinguishing between assertive, aggressive, and passive behaviors and the ability to apply the appropriate professional behavior applicable to the situation. **Assertive** behavior is being able to articulate and express your ideas, needs, and feelings in a way that is honest and direct. Assertive behavior is described as standing up to express your feelings, rights, and thoughts honestly and directly in a way that respects the feelings of other people. Assertive behavior is the most effective communication in most situations. On the other hand, **aggressive** behavior means to stand up for your rights, but in a way that violates the rights of others. The **passive** behavior characteristic is to typically avoid situations. Passive-aggressive behavior is described as the tendency to express anger or frustration in a silent way rather than expressing it directly.

The medical assistant must possess strong verbal and written communication skills. As a medical assistant, you will be in constant communication with other health care professionals, insurance representatives, and patients from all walks of life. Learning medical terminology is only part of the training that is necessary when developing professional language skills. Students must also learn proper English in addition to medical terminology. Pronounce words correctly so that the receiver can properly interpret what is being stated. Elimination of slang terms and profanity is a must when working in a professional environment. Good communicators are able to converse about many different subjects. Thus, it is important for the medical assistant to keep up with current events by reading and viewing news articles (paper or electronic). A medical assistant should be well informed about many different topics so that he is able to appropriately respond to comments made during casual conversations. While a casual brief conversation may help the patient feel more at ease, conversation topics to avoid include religion, politics, and those of a sexual nature that are not related to the patient's medical history or condition.

Written communication is just as important as verbal communication. A large percentage of the way you will communicate both inside and outside of the office is through written or electronic communication. Documenting in patient's charts (paper or electronic), sending faxes, and composing email messages are just a few of the types of written communication that you will perform. Proper spelling and grammar is essential when documenting in the patient's chart or sending out correspondence.

Key #2: Performing as a Team Member (Collaboration)

A vital component of professionalism is the ability to perform as a team member, demonstrate stewardship of resources, and a commitment to service. **Collaboration** is defined as the action of working with someone to accomplish a task or project, or to produce or create something. Today more than ever, medical assistants are considered essential members of the Patient-Centered Medical Home (PCMH) team. According to a survey by the Healthcare Intelligence Network, medical assistants ranked as one of the top five professionals necessary to the PCMH team (AAMA).

The term **service** means to extend help to others. Figure 1-9 illustrates a medical assistant consoling a patient who is fearful about some tests that need to be performed. The field of medical assisting is a service profession; serve your employer and patients to the best of your ability. Serving others often involves listening with your ears, eyes, and heart. It is extending a hug when someone is hurting and going the extra mile to institute modesty for your patient. It is allowing the alcohol to dry before inserting the needle and making the telephone call before the patient has to call you. The benefits and rewards of serving others is knowing that you have made a difference in the lives of your patients. To serve is a privilege!

Principles of Health Care Team Dynamics

As with most professions, medical assistants must work in harmony with each other to achieve a common goal for optimal outcomes. According to an article by Mitchell, Parker, Giles, and Boyle (2013), more than 70% of medical errors can be attributed to dysfunctional team dynamics. Strategies to improve the functionality of health care team dynamics include leadership, reinforcement of shared values (being patient-centered), and developing a shared group identity. Medical assistants must be able to identify the roles and credentials of health care team members, and work in harmony.

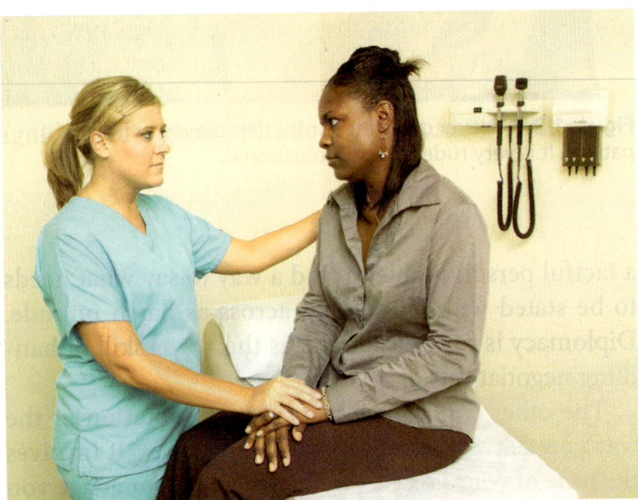

Figure 1-9 ■ The medical assistant should be prepared to console patients who are fearful or hurting.

Everyone must feel they are an essential part of the team and valued for his or her contributions. Part of understanding professionalism is knowing how each of our actions impacts the actions and work of others. The dynamics and expectations of professional team members must demonstrate functional trust, mutual respect, open communication, and cooperation for optimal patient outcomes. **Dynamics** are the unconscious, psychological forces that influence the direction of a team's behavior and performance.

Key #3: Engagement

The concept of engagement encompasses enthusiasm, excellence, work ethic, initiative, and education/credentialing. **Engagement** is the emotional commitment an employee has to the organization and its goals. This emotional commitment means engaged employees care about their work and their company. Demonstrate this commitment by showing up for work on time, with enthusiasm, and the initiative to perform to the best of your ability. Exhibit work ethic and strive for excellence.

The term **initiative** means to take the lead or to work independently. Employers rely on their employees to be proactive and, when an order has been placed, start a procedure or process on their own and see it through to fruition. A good medical assistant will use observation and listening skills to expedite this process.

It is hard to take initiative until you understand your role within an organization. Instead of just standing or sitting at your station waiting for the provider to finish up with the patient, look for things that you can do while you are waiting, such as straightening up the reception room, filing some charts, and scanning documents. On the other hand, the medical assistant must be mindful of boundaries. In eagerness to please your employer, you must never cross the line of your specific role. You must always act within your scope of practice. For instance, it is considered acceptable to anticipate that a provider is going to need a urine specimen when a patient complains of urinary symptoms, but it is not acceptable to perform any testing on that urine until you have received a direct order from that provider to do so.

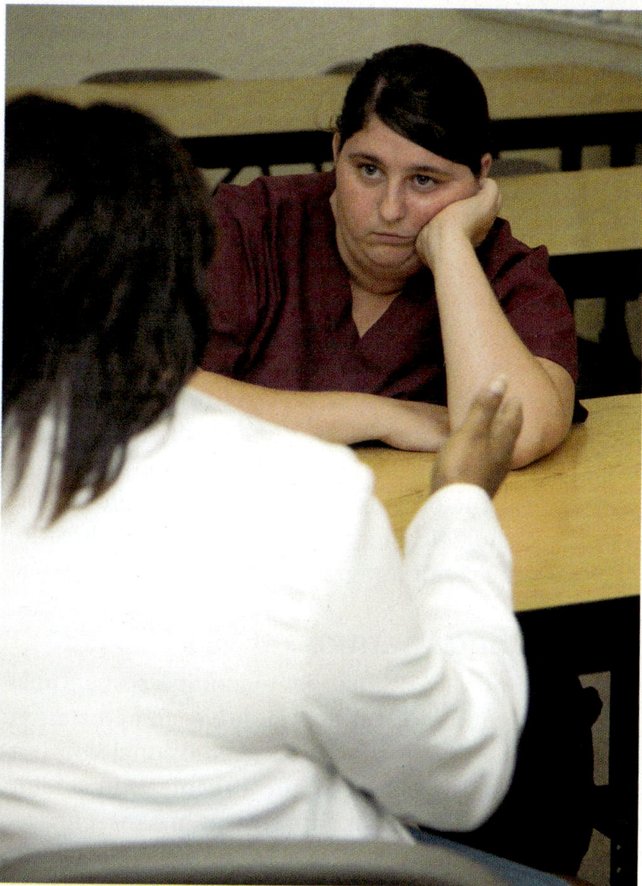

Figure 1-7 ■ Constructive criticism from your instructor may be a bit painful at the time you are receiving it, but it can help you from making errors in the future.

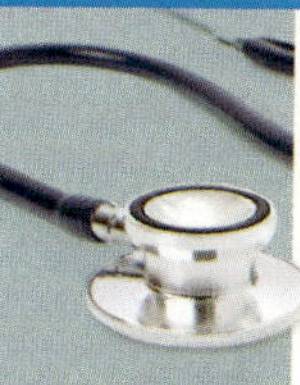

Field Smarts

Never confront another employee in the heat of frustration. Give yourself time to cool down and think about what you are going to say and how you are going to say it. Location is just as important when confronting another employee. Avoid making the situation worse by embarrassing your coworker, or yourself. Find a location where you can ensure privacy. Handle the situation the way that you would want it to be handled if you were on the receiving end. Figure 1-8 shows a picture of one employee confronting another employee in front of a patient. This type of behavior is unacceptable in a professional environment.

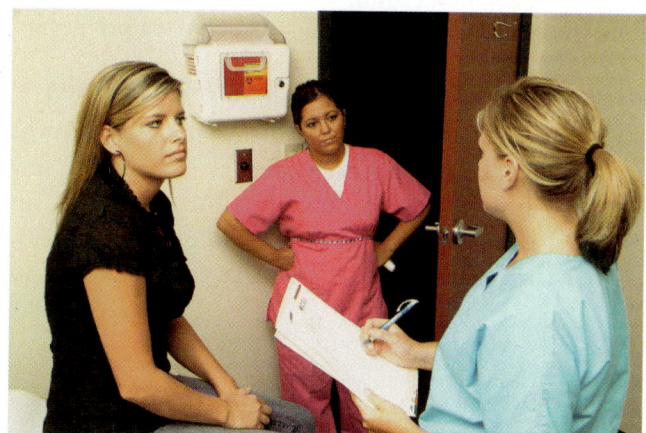

Figure 1-8 ■ Never confront another employee in front of a patient. It is very rude and unprofessional.

beneath you. Work hard to stay away from cliques and people who criticize others.

Actions That Reflect a Positive Attitude The following is a list of actions that reflect a positive attitude to those around you:

- Extend greetings toward coworkers, supervisors, and patients.
- Smile often.
- Accept constructive criticism from those in supervisory or authoritative positions.
- Be flexible in your thinking when things don't necessarily go as planned.

Tact

Tact or tactfulness (sometimes referred to as **diplomacy**) is a character trait that is essential to demonstrate in your professional communication. You may have heard a friend call someone tacky or tactless. A person who possesses tact is sensitive to what is appropriate when dealing with other individuals, including the ability to act or speak without being offensive. During conflict, a tactful person is able to find a way to say what needs to be stated without coming across as harsh or rude. Diplomacy is further defined as the art or skill of handling negotiations or relations.

The other component of tact is presentation or the way you deliver the message to the receiver. It involves the tone of your voice as well as the body language you use. It is deciding when and where you will share the information and who will be present when the message is delivered.

Key #2: Performing as a Team Member (Collaboration)

A vital component of professionalism is the ability to perform as a team member, demonstrate stewardship of resources, and a commitment to service. **Collaboration** is defined as the action of working with someone to accomplish a task or project, or to produce or create something. Today more than ever, medical assistants are considered essential members of the Patient-Centered Medical Home (PCMH) team. According to a survey by the Healthcare Intelligence Network, medical assistants ranked as one of the top five professionals necessary to the PCMH team (AAMA).

The term **service** means to extend help to others. Figure 1-9 illustrates a medical assistant consoling a patient who is fearful about some tests that need to be performed. The field of medical assisting is a service profession; serve your employer and patients to the best of your ability. Serving others often involves listening with your ears, eyes, and heart. It is extending a hug when someone is hurting and going the extra mile to institute modesty for your patient. It is allowing the alcohol to dry before inserting the needle and making the telephone call before the patient has to call you. The benefits and rewards of serving others is knowing that you have made a difference in the lives of your patients. To serve is a privilege!

Principles of Health Care Team Dynamics

As with most professions, medical assistants must work in harmony with each other to achieve a common goal for optimal outcomes. According to an article by Mitchell, Parker, Giles, and Boyle (2013), more than 70% of medical errors can be attributed to dysfunctional team dynamics. Strategies to improve the functionality of health care team dynamics include leadership, reinforcement of shared values (being patient-centered), and developing a shared group identity. Medical assistants must be able to identify the roles and credentials of health care team members, and work in harmony.

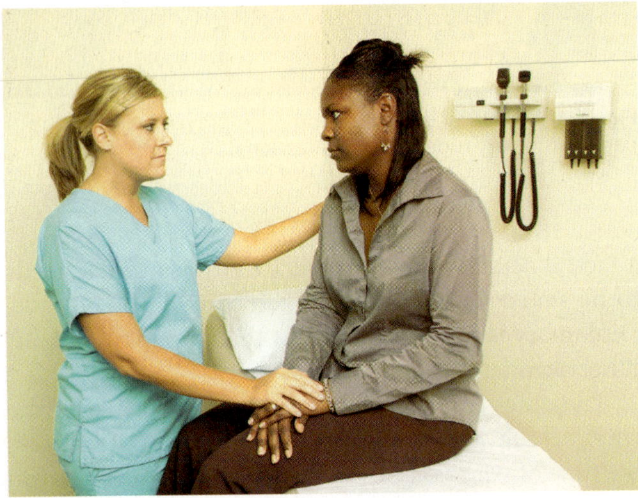

Figure 1-9 ■ The medical assistant should be prepared to console patients who are fearful or hurting.

Everyone must feel they are an essential part of the team and valued for his or her contributions. Part of understanding professionalism is knowing how each of our actions impacts the actions and work of others. The dynamics and expectations of professional team members must demonstrate functional trust, mutual respect, open communication, and cooperation for optimal patient outcomes. **Dynamics** are the unconscious, psychological forces that influence the direction of a team's behavior and performance.

Key #3: Engagement

The concept of engagement encompasses enthusiasm, excellence, work ethic, initiative, and education/credentialing. **Engagement** is the emotional commitment an employee has to the organization and its goals. This emotional commitment means engaged employees care about their work and their company. Demonstrate this commitment by showing up for work on time, with enthusiasm, and the initiative to perform to the best of your ability. Exhibit work ethic and strive for excellence.

The term **initiative** means to take the lead or to work independently. Employers rely on their employees to be proactive and, when an order has been placed, start a procedure or process on their own and see it through to fruition. A good medical assistant will use observation and listening skills to expedite this process.

It is hard to take initiative until you understand your role within an organization. Instead of just standing or sitting at your station waiting for the provider to finish up with the patient, look for things that you can do while you are waiting, such as straightening up the reception room, filing some charts, and scanning documents. On the other hand, the medical assistant must be mindful of boundaries. In eagerness to please your employer, you must never cross the line of your specific role. You must always act within your scope of practice. For instance, it is considered acceptable to anticipate that a provider is going to need a urine specimen when a patient complains of urinary symptoms, but it is not acceptable to perform any testing on that urine until you have received a direct order from that provider to do so.

- *Gestures.* Body movements (hand and body gestures) that enhance what is being said.
- *Distance.* Comfort zones vary for different people and cultures. You must be respectful and ask if you are not sure of a patient's accepted practice. It would be appropriate to ask "Would you like to take my arm while I escort you to the exam room?"
- *Silence.* Silence is often frustrating for the person to whom it is directed. You must set the tone in the relationship, demonstrate leadership, and show confidence. Always greet the patient by name, listen carefully, and master the art of the open-ended question to avoid awkward situations.
- *Therapeutic touch.* A handshake and a hug are meaningful body movements that convey feelings of warmth and affection. Know when it is appropriate or not appropriate to use which type of touch, and be certain of the acceptable boundaries expressed by the person or by office protocol. Be sensitive to the person's reaction when touching is involved.
- *Active listening.* Participation in a conversation with another by means of repeating words and phrases or giving approving or disapproving nods. This signals that you are hearing and following what is being said. In order to be perceived as empathetic, you must engage in active listening.

Effective Communication

Attributes of an effective communicator include the ability to identify and adapt to the communication styles of others. You need to watch and listen carefully to patients, recognize their style, and then carefully adjust your communication. By listening carefully with empathy, you will establish a rapport with your patients and create a respectful, trusting, and honest relationship. Identify the most appropriate form of communication (verbal, nonverbal, visual, body language), and information technologies to enhance relationships. Conversations should be held in a suitable location, time, and place. Listen in a calm, open, nonjudgmental, and nonthreatening way, using open questions.

You must be able to convey (to impart an idea or message) in an articulate way to many different people and receive vital information in the same manner and demonstrate an appropriate behavior that reflects professional communication skills. This includes distinguishing between assertive, aggressive, and passive behaviors and the ability to apply the appropriate professional behavior applicable to the situation. **Assertive** behavior is being able to articulate and express your ideas, needs, and feelings in a way that is honest and direct. Assertive behavior is described as standing up to express your feelings, rights, and thoughts honestly and directly in a way that respects the feelings of other people. Assertive behavior is the most effective communication in most situations. On the other hand, **aggressive** behavior means to stand up for your rights, but in a way that violates the rights of others. The **passive** behavior characteristic is to typically avoid situations. Passive-aggressive behavior is described as the tendency to express anger or frustration in a silent way rather than expressing it directly.

The medical assistant must possess strong verbal and written communication skills. As a medical assistant, you will be in constant communication with other health care professionals, insurance representatives, and patients from all walks of life. Learning medical terminology is only part of the training that is necessary when developing professional language skills. Students must also learn proper English in addition to medical terminology. Pronounce words correctly so that the receiver can properly interpret what is being stated. Elimination of slang terms and profanity is a must when working in a professional environment. Good communicators are able to converse about many different subjects. Thus, it is important for the medical assistant to keep up with current events by reading and viewing news articles (paper or electronic). A medical assistant should be well informed about many different topics so that he is able to appropriately respond to comments made during casual conversations. While a casual brief conversation may help the patient feel more at ease, conversation topics to avoid include religion, politics, and those of a sexual nature that are not related to the patient's medical history or condition.

Written communication is just as important as verbal communication. A large percentage of the way you will communicate both inside and outside of the office is through written or electronic communication. Documenting in patient's charts (paper or electronic), sending faxes, and composing email messages are just a few of the types of written communication that you will perform. Proper spelling and grammar is essential when documenting in the patient's chart or sending out correspondence.

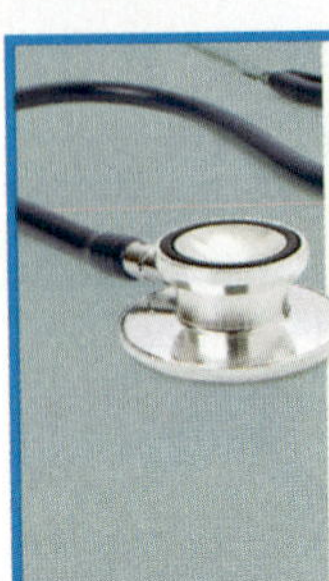

Field Smarts

When documenting in a patient's chart, never use a word that you do not know how to spell. If you do not know a synonym to use in its place, leave space in the chart and look up the word after you meet with the patient. Not only is the chart a legal document that can be used in a court of law, the opinion of your coworkers and supervisors may diminish as a result of misspellings or poor documentation.

Confidentiality

Patients must feel that you will uphold the confidentiality of his or her medical record. The word **confidentiality** means to keep something secret or private. Patient information is considered confidential and must not be shared with anyone without the patient's written authorization. Other privacy issues include comments made to you from a supervisor or other employee that are meant to stay private. A tactful person does not share private information of any kind, and this includes sharing information from your working environment on social media forums.

Attitude

A part of excelling at professional communication is to have a good attitude and tactfulness. **Attitude** refers to the way you feel about someone or something. Attitudes help to mold your personality. Quite often, attitudes are learned. Some popular phrases that demonstrate the magnitude of a good attitude are "Attitude = Altitude" (Figure 1-6) and "Attitude Is Everything." Having a good attitude can help you to flourish both in your professional and personal lives. Your attitude can be a magnet that draws people toward you or a repellant that drives people away.

Attitudes are infectious, which illustrates why employers work hard to find employees with good attitudes. Employers realize that it only takes one staff member with a poor attitude to sour the whole team. On the contrary, staff members who possess positive attitudes will most often influence other staff members to be positive and to work in harmony with one another.

One significant factor that influences our attitude is our emotions. Emotions can trigger our attitudes, especially repeated emotions. Take the woman who feels that all men are "jerks," because she has been hurt by two bad marriages that ended in divorce. The repeated emotions of heartbreak and distrust have caused her to feel that all men are not to be trusted, thus creating a poor attitude toward men in general.

To fix a problem, you must first admit that there is a problem. If an employer or instructor expresses concern with regard to your attitude (Figure 1-7), instead of becoming defensive about it, look inward and recognize that you may have a problem. A helpful practice that may assist in improving your attitude is to log in a notebook or diary the instances in which your attitude diminished. Explore possible triggers that cause your attitude to decline. Do you have a coworker, friend, or peer who causes your attitude to deteriorate? If so, separate yourself from that individual or discuss ways to improve the situation so that your attitude is not affected when you are around that individual.

Look for the good in people instead of focusing on the bad. Realize that everyone is unique and that just because they do not share your same interests or opinions does not mean they are inferior to or

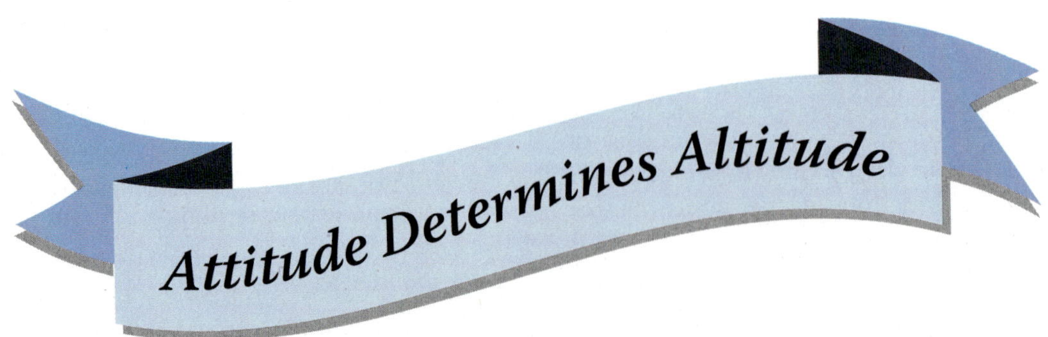

Figure 1-6 ■ A good attitude is essential to climb the ladder of success as a medical assistant.

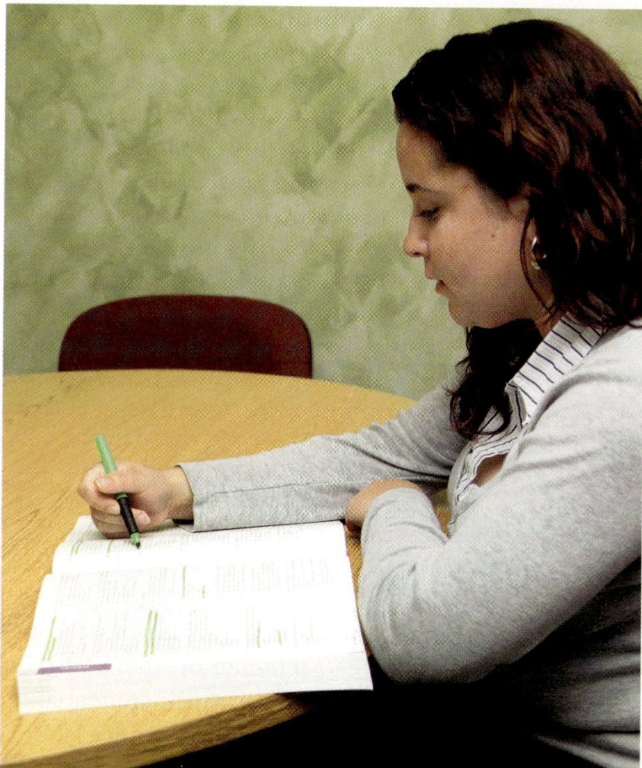

Figure 1-10 ■ Medical assisting students must empower themselves with education so that they can be the best they can be.

Education

Another attribute of engagement is to empower yourself with education (Figure 1-10). Your employer will expect you possess the job-related technical skills as well as the soft skills required to perform your job. The more you know, the better you can serve your employer and patients. You must work hard to learn all you can during the educational process. Listen and adhere to the advice of your instructors. Academic and technical skills are very important, but so are the life experiences that your instructor shares. An instructor has already gone down the road before you, navigating through the rough spots, smoothing out imperfections, and advising you of the many bends and curves that lie ahead. Welcome constructive comments from your supervisors and other seasoned professionals. Their expertise can supply you with wonderful insight and save you a great deal of heartache and energy along the way. Being part of the health care team means you will be a lifelong learner and your education does not stop at the time of graduation. You will never know all you need to know even if you work as a medical assistant for 20 years. Health care is always changing and a professional is always learning.

Get involved in professional societies and attend continuing education workshops, seminars, and conventions. Read professional journals and watch educational programming that can supply you with the latest health information so that you are better able to educate your patients.

Professional Credentials

Becoming credentialed as a medical assistant demonstrates to your patients and supervisors that you are qualified to be working in the capacity in which you have been entrusted. **Credentialing** validates that you have been successful in attaining the educational components that are necessary for the duties that you perform.

There are several terms that are used to validate one's knowledge of a particular profession. The terms that are used most often are *licensed, registered*, and *certified*.

Licensing refers to a legal document that permits or authorizes a person to perform a specific task or tasks. You must be licensed to practice medicine. Examples of professionals who must be licensed to practice medicine include physicians, physician assistants, dentists, and nurse practitioners. Currently, no state offers licensing opportunities for medical assistants. **Certification** is a term that signifies that one has fulfilled the necessary requirements of a specific organization to perform specific tasks. This is usually accomplished through some kind of testing. **Registration** is a term that means to enroll one's name in a register, based on successful completion of a specific program and/or ability to pass an examination designed specifically for that particular specialty.

The earlier part of the chapter discussed certifying organizations for medical assistants. The two major organizations that credential medical assistants are the AAMA and the AMT. The AAMA offers the **Certified Medical Assistant** credential. The initials of the credential are CMA (AAMA). The emblem for the AAMA can be found in Figure 1-11a, and the CMA (AAMA) pin can be found in Figure 1-11b. To sit for the CMA (AAMA) exam, you must be a graduate of an institution that is accredited by the **Accrediting Bureau of Health Education Schools (ABHES)** or the **Commission on Accreditation of Allied Health Education Programs (CAAHEP)**.

The AMT offers the **Registered Medical Assistant (RMA)** credential. Figure 1-12a represents the AMT logo and Figure 1-12b represents the logo that is found on the RMA pin. To sit for an RMA exam you must provide documentation to prove one of the following: you are a graduate from an institution accredited by one of the accrediting bodies listed above; you received formal training from the military; or you have worked in the industry for a minimum of five years.

AMERICAN ASSOCIATION OF MEDICAL ASSISTANTS®

Figure 1-11a ■ AAMA logo. Reprinted with permission of the American Association of Medical Assistants.

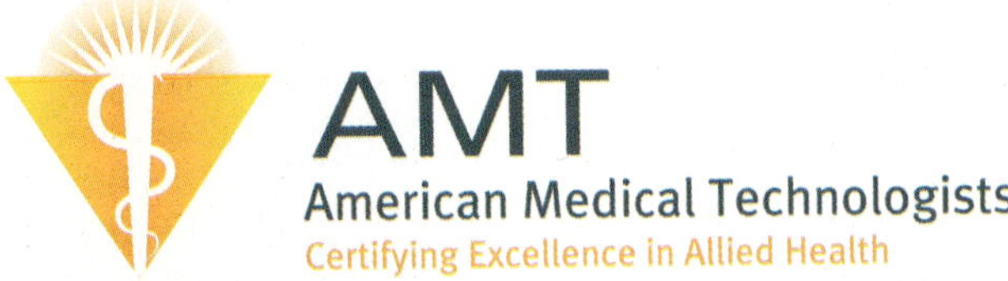

Figure 1-12a ■ AMT logo. Courtesy of the American Medical Technologists.

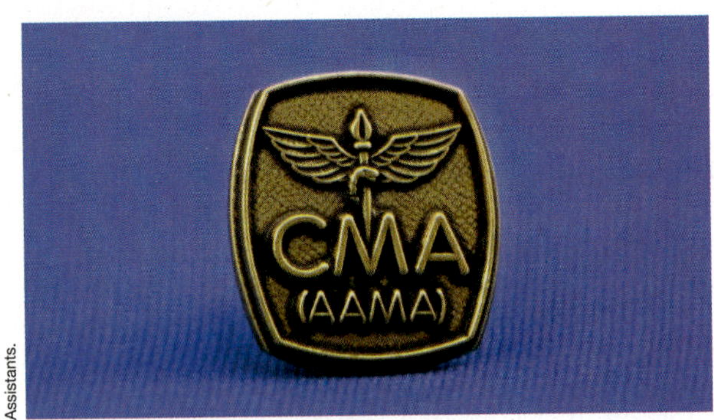

Certifying Board of the American Association of Medical Assistants.

Figure 1-11b ■ CMA (AAMA) pin.

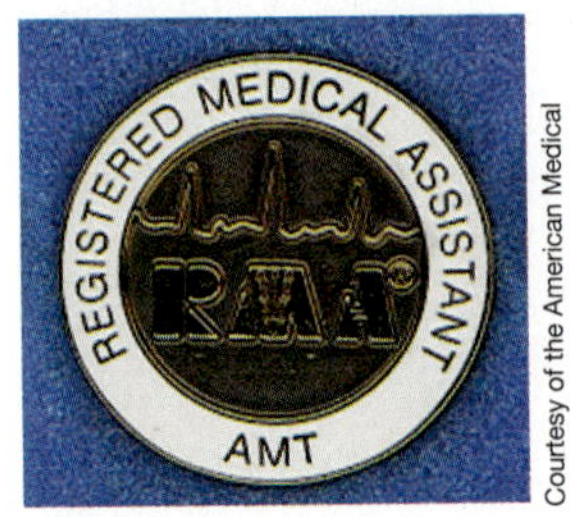

Courtesy of the American Medical Technologists.

Figure 1-12b ■ RMA (AMT) pin.

There are other certifying bodies for medical assistants as well. Refer to Table 1-1 to learn more about other certifying organizations and different credentialing opportunities for medical assistants. Table 1-1 also contains the contact information of the organizations that offer the credentialing.

Medical assistants can also take various clinical specialty exams based on the accreditation status of their school. Different specialty areas in which credentialing is available include phlebotomy, physician office laboratory, and ECGs. Some medical assistants may also be interested in taking classes for a special type of X-ray

Table 1-1 Credentialing/Certification Opportunities for Medical Assistants

Name of Organization	Address of Organization	Testing Requirements	How Often Testing Is Administered and Location of Testing Centers	Credentialing/Certification Opportunities Available (Will Vary According to Each Institution's Accreditation and Training Requirements)
American Association of Medical Assistants (AAMA)	20 N. Wacker Dr., Ste. 1575 Chicago, IL 60606 (800) 228-2262 www.aama-ntl.org	Must have graduated from a CAAHEP- or ABHES-accredited institution	The dates and times tests are given will vary with sites administering the exams. Tests are given at Prometric Testing Centers. Contact the AAMA for a listing of approved sites.	CMA (AAMA)-Certified Medical Assistant through the AAMA
American Medical Technologists (AMT)	10700 West Higgins Road, Suite 150 Rosemont, IL 60018 (847) 823-5169 www .americanmedtech .org	Must have graduated from a CAAHEP- or ABHES-accredited institution or have had related military training or a minimum of five years of field experience	The times tests are given will vary with sites administering the exams. Tests are given at Pearson VUE locations throughout the country and other sites approved by the AMT.	RMA—Registered Medical Assistant MLT—Medical Laboratory Technician CMLA—Certified Medical Laboratory Assistant RPT—Registered Phlebotomy Technician CMAS—Certified Medical Administrative Specialist MT—Medical Technologist
National Center for Competency Testing (NCCT)	7007 College Blvd., Suite 385 Overland Park, KS 66211 (800) 875-4404 www.ncctinc.com/	Programs that are accredited through a national or regional organization	Will vary with each testing center or institution; several testing centers and institutions are located throughout the nation.	NCMA—National Certified Medical Assistant NCPT—National Certified Phlebotomy Technician NCET—National Certified ECG Technician NCMOA—National Certified Medical Office Assistant NCICS—National Certified Insurance and Coding Specialist NCPCT—National Patient Care Technician

Table 1-1 Credentialing/Certification Opportunities for Medical Assistants *(continued)*

Name of Organization	Address of Organization	Testing Requirements	How Often Testing Is Administered and Location of Testing Centers	Credentialing/Certification Opportunities Available (Will Vary According to Each Institution's Accreditation and Training Requirements)
American Registry of Medical Assistants (ARMA)	61 Union Street, Suite 5 Westfield, MA 01085 (413) 562-7336 www.arma-cert.org	Most programs accredited through national or regional bodies; candidates who have worked in the field for a minimum of five years or who have related military training	No testing is required. Requirement for annual renewal is the accumulation of a minimum of 12 Continuing Educational Activities (CEUs)	RMA—Registered Medical Assistant
National Healthcareer Association (NHA)	11161 Overbrook Road Leawood, KS 66211 (800) 499-9092 Email address: info@nhanow.com Website: http://nhanow.com	Must have a high school diploma or equivalency and successfully completed an NHA-approved training program or worked in the field of certification for a minimum of one year	NHA exams are given at different locations throughout the country. Dates will vary. Call the NHA for location and date information.	CPT—Certified Phlebotomy Technician CET—Certified ECG Technician CCMA—Certified Clinical Medical Assistant CBCS—Certified Billing & Coding Specialist CPCT/A—Certified Patient Care Technician/Assistant CMAA—Certified Medical Administrative Assistant
American Society for Clinical Pathology (ASCP)	33 West Monroe Street, Suite 1600 Chicago, IL 60603 (312) 541-4999 Email: info@ascp.org Website: http://ascp.org/	High school graduate or equivalent and successful completion of RN, LPN, or other acceptable accredited allied health professional/occupational education, which includes 100 successful venipunctures, 25 successful skin punctures, and orientation in a full-service laboratory	Test is given at Pearson VUE locations throughout the country; dates and times will vary.	PBT—Phlebotomy Technician MLT—Medical Laboratory Technician
American Society of Phlebotomy Technicians (ASPT)	P.O. Box 1831 Hickory, NC 28603 (828) 294-0078 Email: office@aspt.org Website: www.aspt.org	Will vary with each type of certification; must be a member of the ASPT to participate in all exams	Testing is given at different locations throughout the country and different dates; contact the ASPT for details.	ECG Technician Phlebotomy Technician Medical Assistant

licensing. X-ray licensing will vary from state to state. A limited radiography certificate generally allows the medical assistant to take limited X-rays in ambulatory care centers.

Arrange a meeting with the institution's medical assisting program director or other instructors within the program to determine which credentials you qualify for based on the school's accreditation status and the academia presented within the program.

Key #4: Accountability

As a medical professional, you must demonstrate accountability. Key characteristics of **accountability** include honesty, self-confidence, integrity, and dependability (taking responsibility for one's own actions). The term **dependability** means to be reliable or trustworthy. It starts with an internal mind-set and works its way outward in the form of an action. The word **integrity**

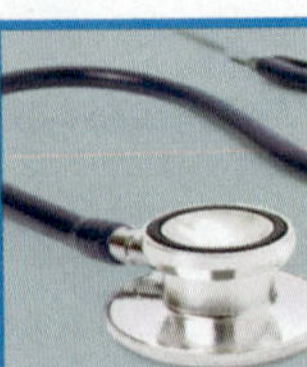

Field Smarts

You will be competing for positions with members of your own class and from competing schools. These candidates will each be working toward or possess their own set of credentials. It is not only important that you gain credentials, but it is also equally important that you have a basic knowledge of the various credentials available, so that you can explain and sell your own credential(s) at the time of your interview. Prospective employers may be confused about the various types of credentials that come across their desk and may ask you to explain why your credential is equal to or better than another candidate's credential. Many of the larger health care systems prefer to hire only credentialed medical assistants or require a newly hired medical assistant to commit to becoming certified within one year of employment.

means to possess sound character. **Honesty** (truthfulness and sincerity) and honor are qualities of a person who possesses integrity. Medical assistants should demonstrate integrity at all times. Never give anyone a reason to doubt your integrity. Lying or taking things that do not belong to you will provoke office staff members to question your integrity. Making false excuses for missing work will result in a loss of respect from coworkers and supervisors. Examples of actions that reflect accountability include the following:

- Showing up for work on time.
- Being honest; admit to any mistakes you make, especially those dependent on the safety of your patient.
- Giving ample notice to your supervisor when you are unable to go to work.
- Returning from breaks and lunch hours on time.
- Following through with assigned tasks in a timely fashion.
- Working past your scheduled time off, when necessary.
- Demonstrating self-confidence.
- Going the extra mile to help your coworkers.
- Taking responsibility for your actions.

To demonstrate the importance of accountability, consider this: When a potential employer calls a school to check a reference for a student, he rarely begins the conversation by asking about the student's grade point average. The first question typically asked is, "How was the student's attendance?" Remember, you are affecting the recommendation from your instructors whether you are present or not.

If you have notoriously poor attendance, realize that you are not going to change overnight. Start off the beginning of your training program by being more dependable. If necessary, arrange for backup childcare and transportation before problems arise. Strive for perfect attendance as a personal goal. Statistics confirm that employers will select candidates with perfect or good attendance over candidates who possess fair or poor attendance, even if those candidates were academically outstanding.

Key #5: Respect

Another key to professionalism is respect. With respect come the attributes of loyalty, trust (honesty), and compassion. Think about trust in terms of the magnitude of trust placed in you as a medical assistant by the patient, provider, and colleagues. The term **compassion** means to show concern and **empathy**. Empathy is having the ability to put yourself in another person's shoes. In the minds of your patients, compassion is paramount.

If you were to suddenly become disabled, you would want your health care provider to do everything possible to make certain that all paperwork was properly completed so that you could receive your weekly benefits. Think about that when a patient "inconveniences" you by asking you to complete paperwork or asks you to make a phone call on his

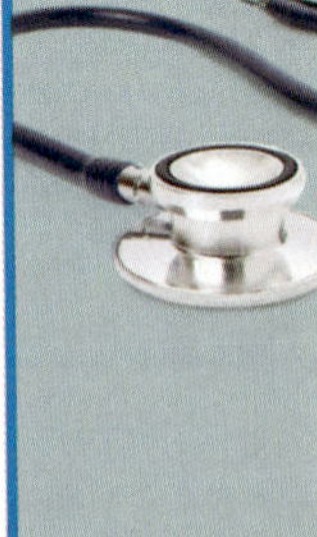

Field Smarts

Avoid putting yourself in a situation where someone can question your integrity. Bending the truth, taking a coworker's lunch or drink, or falsifying information are all ways that your integrity may be challenged. Be completely honest about the hours you record on your time sheet. Never lie to cover up an error. It may be costly to both you and the patient.

> **CRITICAL THINKING CHALLENGE**
>
> You are about a third of the way into your training program. Your instructor has repeatedly stated that a reference is not a gift, but rather something that you have to earn. Your attendance has not been very good up to this point. You are now really starting to see the value of a good reference.
>
> 1. **Is there anything that you can do to salvage your reputation with your instructor at this point in the program?**
> 2. **Do you think that your instructor should bend the truth with potential employers regarding your early attendance problems as long as you correct your attendance for the remainder of the program? Why or why not?**

> **CRITICAL THINKING CHALLENGE**
>
> You are a medical assistant who works for a mid-size family practice. While you are cleaning the examination room, your coworker, Sarah, enters the doorway and asks to speak with you for a moment. Sarah tells you that she believes that another coworker, Kim, lied about being ill today and that the only reason Kim didn't come in is because she is lazy and doesn't want to help on "scanning catch-up day." Sarah ends the conversation by telling you that she doesn't mean to gossip but that she really feels that Kim is a poor worker and that she is tired of picking up the slack for her. You personally have always found Kim to be quite helpful and honest.
>
> 1. **Do you think that it is right for Sarah to voice her concerns about Kim to another coworker?**
> 2. **What is an appropriate way to respond to Sarah's accusations?**
> 3. **Do you feel that you should share this information with Kim when she returns? Explain your response.**

behalf. A compassionate person, even though he is busy, makes every effort to complete the request in a timely manner.

Compassion shouldn't stop with the patient; it should permeate to your coworkers as well. When you observe that a coworker is running behind schedule, ask if there is anything that you can do to help. Someday, he may return the favor.

Key #6: Problem-solving

Today more than ever, two key qualities employers are looking for in employees are problem-solving skills and critical thinking capabilities. Throughout your studies you have been prompted with "critical thinking" activities or challenges. Critical thinking is defined as the disciplined, intellectual process of applying skillful reasoning as a guide to belief or action (Paul, Ennis, & Norris). **Problem-solving** is the process of working through the details of a problem to reach a solution. Today's patient-centered care model uses a conceptual framework that incorporates the patient's needs, caring for the whole person as an individual, and not as the disease or diagnosis. Think about the distinction between critical thinking and problem-solving. While it may be easy to identify a "problem," coming up with solutions to solve problems is a trait deemed valuable by employers.

Key #7: Mindfulness

You may be asking yourself, what is "**mindfulness**"? In simple terms, it means to be aware, alert, and attentive. A key way to display mindfulness is to act using your "intelligence." Think about the attention to detail required to professionally perform your duties as a medical assistant. To be detail-oriented, you will be expected to use your decision-making skills. In addition, you wear your "mindfulness" on your sleeve with your appearance. Do you appear "professional," not only in appearance but in behavior? Remember, you only get one chance to make a first impression.

The patient's initial impression about you as a professional is based on your appearance. You may be very good at phlebotomy, but if the patient looks down and sees that your nails are unkempt, you may never get the opportunity to prove your technical capabilities.

Figure 1-13 shows professional athletes in uniforms that match and demonstrate a professional appearance. The medical assistant can have a similar look and use the motto: "Look professional, feel professional, be professional!" (Figure 1-14).

Professional **appearance** is about much more than the uniform. It is about the amount of sleep you

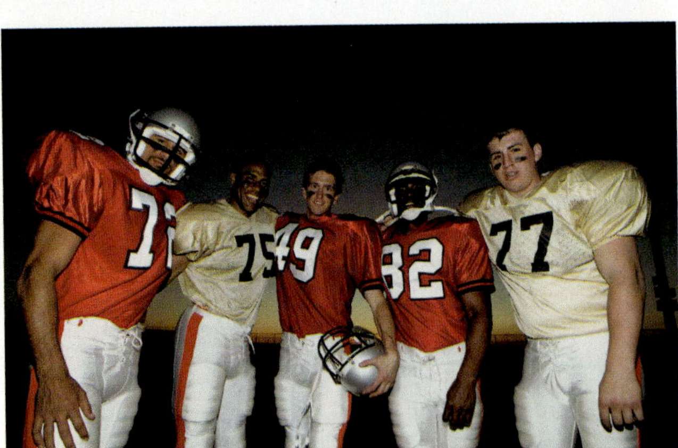

Figure 1-13 ■ These athletes take pride in the way that they look.

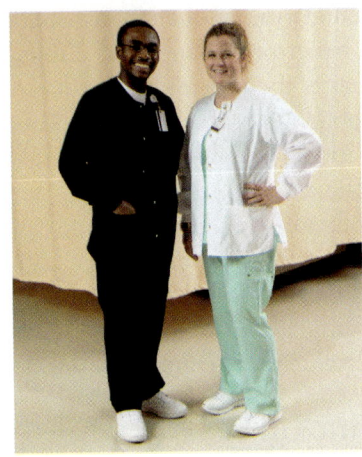

Figure 1-14 ■ Medical assistants should also take pride in the way that they look.

obtain, the food you consume, and the way that you carry yourself. It is about walking into the patient's room and earning their immediate trust and respect because your uniform is clean, neat, and pressed. Your shoes are clean, your hair is neat, and you look rested. Your smile puts the patient at immediate ease and your straight posture and confident voice exude professionalism.

Even though there can be some variance from facility to facility, Table 1-2 depicts typical standards in the industry for appearance.

Key #8: Adaptability

The final "key" to your professionalism journey is adaptability. **Adaptability** can be defined as an effective change in response to an altered situation. Employers will expect that you demonstrate highly effective organizational skills, are flexible in your assignments, and be open-minded to change. This means that you must prioritize your work and plan accordingly. Consider the rapid changes in technology and health care, diversity and society. Employers seek those who are open to new ideas, flexible enough to work through challenges, and cope when things do not go as planned. People who are not adaptable tend to get stressed when faced with change. To demonstrate adaptability, remain poised, calm, and ready to make the required changes necessary to improve patient care.

Table 1-2 Elements of a Professional Appearance

Items	Acceptable	Unacceptable
Personal hygiene	Shower or bathe prior to shift. Use deodorant whether or not you think you need it. Brush teeth, floss, and use mouth rinse. Use breath mints throughout the day to help keep breath fresh.	Body odors. Halitosis. Wearing fragrances such as perfumes or aftershave lotion. Having the aroma of alcohol or cigarettes coming from your body or clothes.
Uniform	Wear scrubs or other styles of uniforms that are in alignment with the rules of the facility in which you are employed. Keep uniforms clean, neat, and free of wrinkles.	Wearing uniforms that are not in alignment with the facility standards. Wearing unprofessional clothing underneath your uniform such as T-shirts with logos or sweatshirts underneath scrub tops. Wearing uniforms that have stains or that are wrinkled.
Shoes/hosiery	Keep shoes and hosiery clean. There are many new styles and colors of professional duty shoes. Adhere to the standards of the facility in which you work.	Wearing dirty shoes or open-toed shoes. Not abiding by facility standards.
Jewelry	Use very simple jewelry or no jewelry. Limit jewelry to one simple ring or wedding set per hand. Use of a watch with a second hand is encouraged.	Wearing facial, tongue, or multiple ear piercings. Wearing earrings that are very large such as large hoops or earrings that dangle. Wearing necklaces, bracelets, and anklets.

Table 1-2 Elements of a Professional Appearance *(continued)*

Items	Acceptable	Unacceptable
Tattoos	Whenever possible, cover tattoos with clothing or a special makeup that helps to conceal them.	Leaving tattoos exposed.
Makeup	Use of light foundations, light blush, and light shades of lipstick is considered professional.	Wearing makeup that is very dark against your natural pigment. Wearing dark shades of lip color or eye makeup.
Hair color and hair styles	Maintain a hair color that is one of the more natural hair colors. Tie back hair when longer than shoulder length. Keep beards well-groomed.	Wearing unnatural hair colors or streaks within the hair, such as pink and purple. Wearing hair longer than shoulder length without tying it back.
Nail care	Keep nails well-manicured and short enough that they do not extend above the fingertip.	Nails that extend beyond the fingertip. Dirty nails, darker shades of nail polish, or nails with chipped polish. Artificial nails or overlays, which can be a breeding ground for microorganisms.
Identification badge and professional pins	Wear with your uniform.	Not wearing an identification badge.
Posture	Stand straight, with shoulders back and chin up.	Slouching with shoulders rolled forward and head bent downward.

Employees with organizational skills are more productive on the job. When you are organized your work will be of better quality, and you will make a positive impression on your provider, patients, and supervisor. Being organized, yet flexible, demonstrates that you are responsible and serious about your job.

TIME MANAGEMENT PRINCIPLES

Time management is a key component of your organizational skills. Are you a procrastinator or do you manage time effectively? Time management means the ability to make appropriate choices about how

CRITICAL THINKING CHALLENGE

Time Management

One way to evaluate time management is to create a list or chart for balancing time. First write down how many hours are in a day and subtract how many hours you should be sleeping. Next, write down and subtract how many hours you are required to be at work/school. The balance of hours in the day can be assigned to free time or other activities in the appropriate categories. Apply this information to creating the list or chart as described. Divide activities into three categories: necessities, school/work, and free time. Using one week (7 days/24 hours per day) for a total of 168 hours for the week, list the type and number of hours spent on each activity for each category. Examples include:

- Necessities: Sleep, eating, bathroom/showering, grooming/dressing, and so on.
- School/work: Commute, employment (or school), homework (if applicable), and so on
- Free time: Reading, shopping, fitness, spirituality, relationships with family/friends, Internet, movies, reading, and so on

1. After completing the chart, divide the total hours in each category by 168 to get a percentage.
2. Does the percentage and balance of activities seem reasonable to you? Why or why not?
3. Did you realize how much time you spend on each activity? List any unexpected outcomes.
4. Describe ways you can improve your work/life balance by improving time management skills.

Present your findings to your instructor for class discussion.

to use time, both professional and personal. Being able to manage time effectively and prioritize responsibilities are highly desirable traits sought by employers. For some people, time management brings relief, satisfaction, and challenge. Others may experience stress, anxiety, and exhaustion. Everyone has experienced the feeling that we have too much to do and not enough time. Being able to manage time efficiently will reduce stress and improve daily life.

DEVELOPING PROFESSIONALISM SKILLS

Because professionalism is such a key component to your success as a medical assistant, not only will the textbook reference the professionalism "keys," but you will also have a "professionalism mentor." Your mentor will give you tips and real-world examples to consider, incorporating "soft" skills with the technical components of professionalism.

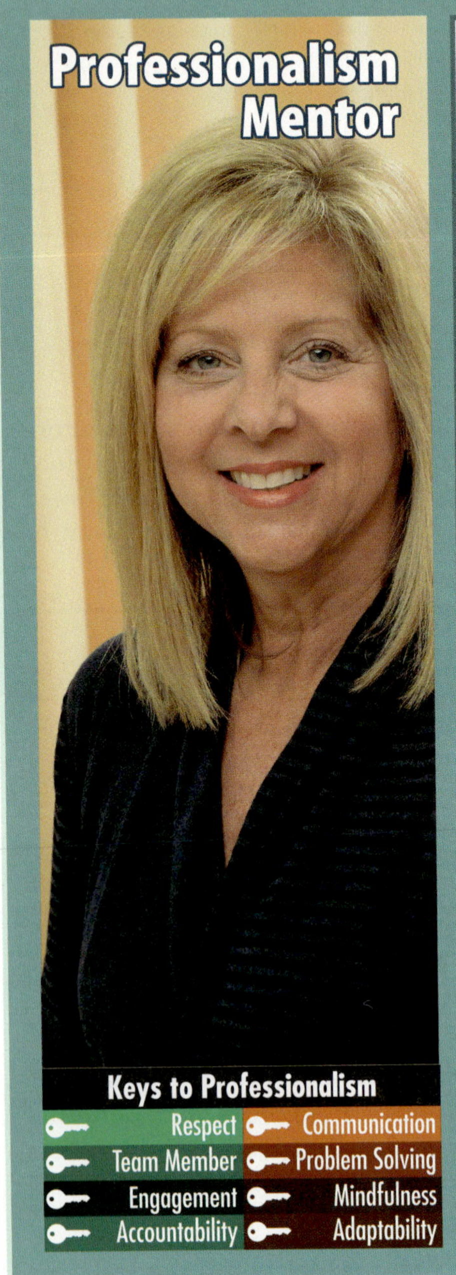

Hello! Allow me to introduce myself to you. My name is Davene Yankle, and I am the nurse manager of Clinical Development for the Ohio Health Physicians Group. I manage a team of clinical nurse educators responsible for training and development of our clinical staff in over 200 physician practices. Our largest percentage of clinicians are medical assistants. As our organization continues to grow, the need for medical assistants is growing as well. However, we often have a hard time finding medical assistants (MAs) with the right interpersonal skills to fit our needs.

In today's health care environment, your personal development is as important as your professional development. As you read each chapter of this book, I want you to also consider those "personality" skills that you will need along with the professional skills this book will teach you. As a 30+ year health care provider myself, I know from experience that in order to be successful, both sets of skills are equally important.

In addition to training and education, I also place new medical assistant students in practices for externships. Practice managers consider the externship program something similar to what you might do when considering the purchase of a new car: you take a new car for a test drive. Practice managers allow a student to come into their practice and watch to see how they interact and communicate with the providers, staff, and most importantly the patient. You may be surprised to learn that your people skills will impact your career prospects more than how well you complete a skill such as taking a blood pressure. I'm fairly certain that after taking a dozen or more blood pressures, you will become proficient at it, but will you be kind and courteous after rooming a dozen or more patients on a busy and stressful day? Over the long run, most employers are seeking medical assistants who have more to offer than just technical skills alone.

So what skills do you need to develop? As your professionalism mentor, I will emphasize the "soft" skills you will need to master along with the technical skills you will be learning as we journey through these chapters together. Always remember that both sets of skills are required in order to be the best medical assistant you can be! ■

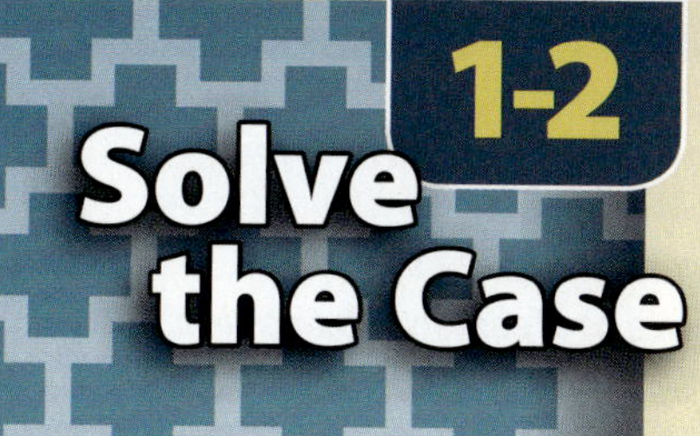

As previously discussed, Mr. Spadoni called the office requesting a refill that the pharmacy has told him is too early to fill, even though he has only one day of medication left. After researching Mr. Spadoni's request, you discover that Dr. Endo had written a new prescription for two tablets of 100 mg tramadol ER daily two weeks ago. This new prescription written by Dr. Endo had increased the dosage of the original prescription from one tablet daily to two in order to meet the needs of post-op pain management. The pharmacy has stated that Mr. Spadoni's insurance will only cover one tablet per day. Using your problem-solving skills, research and provide options and solutions to the issue.

1. **What steps would you take to identify the problem?**
2. **After investigating the issue, what solutions can you offer? Given Mr. Spadoni's insurance coverage, are there any payment options that will allow him to receive the new daily dose of tramadol prescribed by Dr. Endo?**
3. **How should these options be communicated to the patient as well as Dr. Endo?**
4. **Which professionalism keys did you use to "solve the case"?**

PROCEDURE 1-1

Locate a State's Legal Scope of Practice for Medical Assistants

Objective:

To locate a state's legal scope of practice for medical assistants.

Equipment/Supplies:

- Computer with Internet access
- Paper and pen
- Computer with word processing or spreadsheet capabilities

PROCEDURAL STEPS	DETAILS AND/OR RATIONALE
1. Using a computer, access the Internet to locate the legal scope of practice for your state, as noted in Step 2.	
2. Access the AAMA website (www.aama-ntl.org). Search under "State Scope of Practice Laws." Locate the state where you are located (e.g., Ohio).	Medical assistants can only perform duties within their scope of practice. Laws vary from state to state.
3. Using the information obtained in Step 2, click on the Scope of Practice link for your state. Review the information and then access the additional links (if available), for example, Frequently Asked Questions and Laws and Regulations.	Understanding and working within your state's "Scope of Practice" for medical assistants will keep you in legal compliance with your certification and employment.

continues

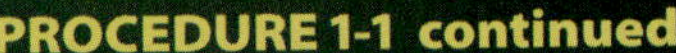

PROCEDURE 1-1 continued

PROCEDURAL STEPS	DETAILS AND/OR RATIONALE
4. Using paper and pen (or computer with a word processing program) prepare a written summary of the scope of practice, what you learned from the website, and how you would apply it to your medical assisting duties. Cite your sources.	Using the information learned, consider how you would ***demonstrate professional behavior*** as a medical assistant.

PROCEDURE 1-2

Apply the Patients' Bill of Rights as it Relates to Choice of Treatment, Consent for Treatment, and Refusal of Treatment

Objective:

To explain both the practice's expectations for patients as well as what legal and ethical rights the patient can expect and to apply the Patients' Bill of Rights as it relates to choice of treatment, consent for treatment, and refusal of treatment.

Equipment/Supplies:

- Quiet room free from distraction
- Printed policy
- Patient education materials
- Patient chart or computer with EHR access
- Paper and pen

PROCEDURAL STEPS	DETAILS AND/OR RATIONALE
1. Identify the patient.	
2. Invite the patient into a room free of distractions and demonstrate sensitivity to the patient's privacy by closing the door to maintain and protect the patient's privacy and integrity of the medical record.	Provide an environment in which the patient can engage in an active discussion.
3. ***Displaying professionalism through verbal communication***, introduce yourself, identify your role in the practice, and tell the patient what to expect from the conversation, using language the patient can understand and making the patient feel at ease. Display tact, diplomacy, and respect for the patient. Be courteous and treat the patient with dignity.	Example: "Good morning, I'm Janet, the medical assistant for Dr. Jones. I would like to give you an explanation of our office policies for new patients. It will help familiarize you with the way our office runs and what you can expect."
4. Explain both the practice's expectations for patients as well as what legal and ethical rights the patient can expect.	Doing this offers the patient a better understanding of what kinds of questions you are prepared to answer. Be sure to demonstrate and include the following points:

continues

PROCEDURE 1-2 continued

PROCEDURAL STEPS	DETAILS AND/OR RATIONALE
	■ Patients should be and should expect to be treated professionally with respect and courtesy at all times and, most important, when they are feeling most vulnerable, such as when receiving unpleasant news. Courtesy is described as showing respect for others and having polished manners. ■ Patients should have a clear understanding of what they can expect regarding how their privacy will be protected and how their personal information will be used. ■ Patients have a right to participate actively in the decisions made in providing their health care and procedures and to undergo only those procedures for which they provide informed consent. ■ Patients should be advised of what means of communications will be used to contact them regarding medical information, how insurance billing will be handled, any safety procedures they are expected to observe while in the office, and what they can expect from the practice's employees in general.
5. Apply the Patients' Bill of Rights as it relates to choice of treatment, consent for treatment, and refusal of treatment.	
6. Provide preprinted information and policies, preferably in the patient's native language (or with verification through a translator followed by documentation of the patient's response to explanations).	Visual reinforcement with printed policies helps the patient understand better and remember key points.
7. ***Demonstrating empathy,*** provide the patient with an opportunity to ask questions. Individualize the conversation and discussion based on the patient's needs and reason for visit. Analyze communications, providing appropriate responses and feedback.	*Relate the appropriate behaviors to professional communication (assertive, aggressive, and passive).*
8. Refer questions to appropriate others for further explanation or clarification.	Confirms that the patient has all the correct and needed information.
9. Document time, date, patient response, and any materials provided in the patient record.	A record provides documentation of the conversation for later reference.

DOCUMENTATION EXAMPLES:

12/1/XX 9:30 am	Office policies discussed with Ms. Hernandez including treatment, compliance, HIPAA, NPP, communication preference, late cancel, no-show appointment, and the assignment of benefits and patient account collections. Discussed policy regarding smoking as patient is a known smoker, especially since compressed oxygen cylinders are used and maintained in office. Stressed importance of compliance with all office policies and procedures, Patient acknowledges and agrees. Signatures obtained as required. Copy of printed practice policies provided to patient. T. Gutierrez, RMA(AMT)--

CHAPTER SUMMARY

- While all health care professionals are held to a high degree of professionalism, patients have more, and more intimate, contact with health care professionals working in a clinical capacity. This may be due to several factors: visibility, proximity, time, and the nature of the work.
- A medical assistant must always perform delegated clinical and administrative duties within his or her scope of practice, working under a physician's direct supervision, and consistent with his or her education, training, and experience. There is no uniform, national definition of a medical assistant's scope of practice and duties will vary according to state law. A medical assistant's duties shall not constitute the practice of medicine. Standard of care is defined as the diagnostic and treatment process that is reasonable and prudent that a clinician should follow for a certain type of patient, illness, or clinical circumstance.
- The Patients' Bill of Rights is a way to communicate the legal rights patients have while under the care of a provider or facility. Federal law of a Patients' Bill of Rights under the Affordable Care Act (ACA) will help individuals with preexisting conditions obtain insurance coverage and ends the lifetime limit on the care consumers may receive.
- The terms *morals* and *ethics* are often used interchangeably. The definition of *morals* references *ethics*. Morals can be defined as cultural and religious-based distinctions of right and wrong. Ethics transcends culture, religion, and time, representing the innate knowledge of right and wrong.
- Developing your professional persona involves making the transition from student to professional and will require a great deal of commitment on your part. It will require you to perform an honest assessment of your character traits and to make the necessary adjustments. The person you are today shouldn't be the same person that walks across the stage during the graduation ceremony. Family members, peers, and instructors should notice differences in your demeanor and the way that you conduct yourself as you progress throughout the training process. Work hard throughout the program to earn the references that are essential in obtaining the job of your dreams.
- Professional communication is the foundation of every action taken in the health care setting and includes verbal and nonverbal communications.
- A vital component of professionalism is the ability to perform as a team member. As with most professions, medical assistants must work in harmony with each other to achieve a common goal for optimal outcomes.
- To empower yourself with education is a great start toward becoming a professional and one form of the key attribute engagement, but you will need to continue your education once you finish your training by attending seminars, workshops, and conventions through one of the professional societies for medical assistants. Certification and/or credentialing solidifies your position in the professionalism arena. Demonstrate enthusiasm and work ethic to achieve excellence.
- Being accountable includes honesty, self-confidence, integrity, and dependability. The term *dependability* means to be reliable or trustworthy. It starts with an internal mind-set and works its way outward in the form of an action. Dependability is one of the most important keys to possess as a professional.

- Another key to professionalism is respect. With respect come the attributes of loyalty, trust (honesty), and compassion. The trust placed in you as a medical assistant by the patient, provider, and colleagues is monumental.
- Today more than ever, two key qualities employers are looking for in employees are problem-solving skills and critical thinking capabilities. Critical thinking is defined as the disciplined, intellectual process of applying skillful reasoning as a guide to belief or action (Paul, Eniss, & Norris). Problem-solving is the process of working through the details of a problem to reach a solution.
- Mindfulness means to be aware, alert, and attentive. A key way to display mindfulness is to act using your "intelligence." Think about the attention to detail required to perform your duties as a medical assistant. In addition, to be detail oriented, you will be expected to use your decision-making skills.
- Adaptability can be defined as an effective change in response to an altered situation. Consider the rapid changes in technology and health care, diversity and society. Employers will expect that you demonstrate highly effective organizational skills, are flexible in your assignments, and be open-minded to change. This means that you must prioritize your work and plan accordingly.
- Time management means the ability to make appropriate choices about how to use time, both professional and personal. Being able to manage time effectively and prioritize responsibilities are highly desirable traits sought by employers.

CERTIFICATION REVIEW QUESTIONS

1. The ability to place yourself in someone else's "shoes" or situation is known as:
   a. sympathy.
   b. empathy.
   c. imitation.
   d. projection.
2. All of the following are keys to unlocking the door to professionalism except:
   a. attitude.
   b. education.
   c. appearance.
   d. talent.
3. Which of the following does not contribute to a professional work environment?
   a. Gossip
   b. Initiative
   c. Helpfulness
   d. Integrity
4. While serving your externship, you observe Sandy—one of the employees at the externship site—slip an ampule of Demerol into her lab jacket. She doesn't record it into the narcotics log, and she has no idea that you saw her take it. The next day the office supervisor calls a meeting and tells everyone that the narcotics count was off last night and that they are missing some ampules of Demerol. What of the following is the best course of action?
   a. Tell Sandy that you saw her take the Demerol.
   b. Tell one of the other staff members that you witnessed Sandy take the Demerol.
   c. Tell the supervisor that you witnessed Sandy take the Demerol.
   d. Say nothing at all.

5. Each of the following organizations credentials medical assistants except the:
   a. AAMA.
   b. ASCP.
   c. NCCT.
   d. AMT.

6. Working under a provider's direct supervision and consistent with his or her education, training, and experience is referred to as:
   a. standard of care.
   b. scope of practice.
   c. certification connections.
   d. Both a and b.

7. According to the Centers for Medicare & Medicaid Services (CMS), the ______________________ will help children (and eventually all Americans) with preexisting conditions gain coverage and keep it, protect all Americans' choice of doctors, and end lifetime limits on the care consumers may receive.
   a. Accountable Care Organization
   b. Patient-Centered Medical Home
   c. Social Security Administration
   d. Patients' Bill of Rights

8. ______________________ can be defined as cultural and religious-based distinctions of right and wrong.
   a. Ethics
   b. Morals
   c. Perception
   d. All of the above

9. Which of the following is not considered nonverbal communication?
   a. Perception
   b. Brochures
   c. Distance
   d. Therapeutic touch

10. Which of the following is not an attribute of a team player?
   a. Getting to work on time
   b. Trying to solve problems
   c. Following safety and company rules
   d. Using company materials and equipment for personal use

STUDY RESOURCES

Resources to Test and Reinforce Your Knowledge:	
Certification Review Questions	Take this end-of-chapter quiz
Workbook	• Complete the activities for Chapter 1 • Perform the procedures for Chapter 1 using the Competency Checklists
Resources to Promote Critical Thinking:	
***Solve the Case* Activities**	• Consider these case studies and discuss your conclusions
Learning Lab	• Module 1: Health Care Roles and Responsibilities
MindTap	• Complete Chapter 1 readings and activities

REFERENCES

American Association of Medical Assistants (n.d.). State Scope of Practice Laws. Retrieved on September 29, 2014 from http://www.aama-ntl.org/employers/state-scope-of-practice-laws.

American Hospital Association Patient Bill of Rights. Retrieved from www.patienttalk.info/AHA-Patient_Bill_of_Rights.htm

American Medical Technologists (n.d.). AMT Standards of Practice. Retrieved on September 29, 2014 from http://www.americanmedtech.org/Portals/0/PDF/Certification/2013%20standards%20of%20practice.pdf

Blesi, Michelle (2017). *Medical assisting administrative and clinical competencies* (8th ed.). Clifton Park, NY: Cengage Learning.

Brennan, Michael D. (May 2014). Professionalism: Good for patients and health care organizations. *Mayo Clinic Proceedings 89*(5): 644–652.

Centers for Medicare & Medicaid Services (n.d.). *Patient's Bill of Rights.* Retrieved on July 12, 2014, from http://www.cms.gov/CCIIO/Programs-and-Initiatives/Health-Insurance-Market-Reforms/Patients-Bill-of-Rights.html.

McCarty, Michael N., Esq. (June 2012). The lawful scope of practice of medical assistants—2012 update. Retrieved on September 29, 2014 from http://www.americanmedtech.org/Portals/0/PDF/News/ScopeOfPracticeArticle_June%202012.pdf

Mitchell, R., Parker, V., Giles, M., & Boyle, B. (2013). The ABC of health care team dynamics: Understanding complex affective, behavioral, and cognitive dynamics in interprofessional teams. *Health Care Management Review* Epub July 15. Retrieved on October 8, 2014, from http://www.ncbi.nlm.nih.gov/pubmed/24304597.

Morals vs. ethics (n.d.). Retrieved on September 29, 2014, from http://www.ethicsdefined.org/what-is-ethics/morals-vs-ethics/.

Norris, S. P. & Ennis, R. H. (1989). *Evaluating critical thinking.* Pacific Grove, CA: Pacific Grove, CA: Midwest Publications, Critical Thinking Press. Retrieved on October 10, 2014, from http://www.criticalthinking.org/pages/critical-thinking-to-think-like-a-nurse/834.

Paul, R.W. (1990). *Critical thinking: What every person needs to survive in a rapidly changing world.* Rohnert Park, CA: Rohnert Park, CA: Center for Critical Thinking and Moral Critique. Retrieved on October 10, 2014, from http://www.criticalthinking.org/pages/critical-thinking-to-think-like-a-nurse/834.

Team Technology (est. 1994). Definition of team dynamics. Retrieved on September 29, 2014, from http://www.teamtechnology.co.uk/team/dynamics/definition/

The Medical Board of California (n.d.). Medical Assistants. Is your medical assistant practicing beyond his or her scope of training? Retrieved on September 29, 2014, from http://www.mbc.ca.gov

U.S. Department of Labor (n.d.). Skills to pay the bills. Professionalism. Retrieved on September 29, 2014, from http://www.dol.gov/odep/topics/youth/softskills/Professionalism.pdf

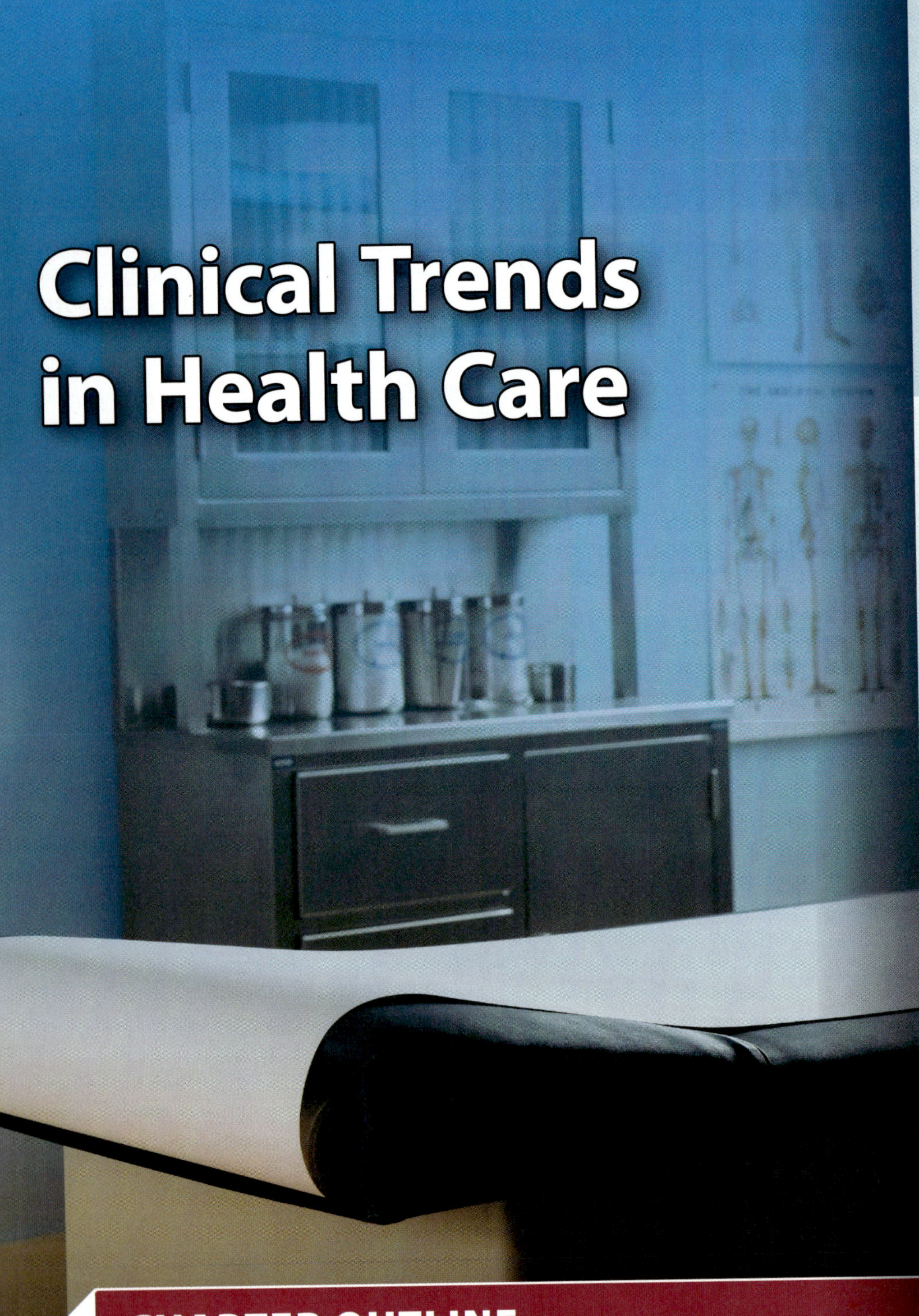

2

Clinical Trends in Health Care

ESSENTIAL TERMS

accountable care organization
health information technology (HIT)
fee for service
National Committee for Quality Assurance (NCQA)
patient-centered
patient-centered medical home (PCMH)
pay for coordination
pay for performance organization
Triple Aim Initiative

CHAPTER OUTLINE

Patient Protection and Affordable Care Act
- Reforming Health Care
- Pay for Performance Organizations
- Patient-Centered Approach
- Pay for Coordination Organizations

The Role of Information Technology in Newer Health Care Delivery Models

The Medical Assistant's Role in New Delivery Models

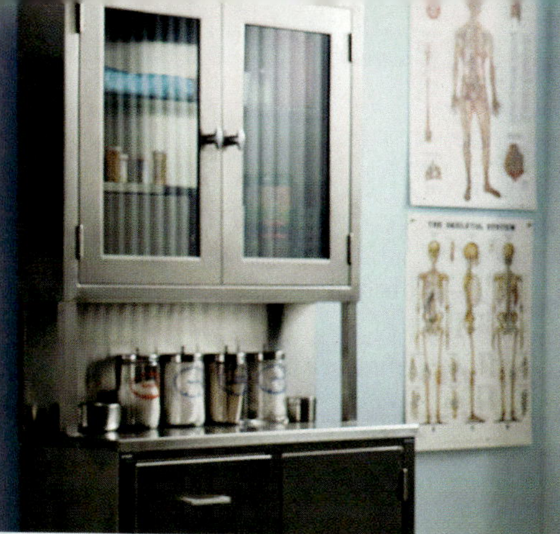

DEVELOPMENTAL OBJECTIVES

After completing this chapter you should be able to:

1. Correctly spell and define the essential terms.
2. Explain the Patient Protection and Affordable Care Act (ACA) and describe how this act impacts the health care team.
3. Describe a patient-centric approach to health care.
4. Discuss the differences between fee for service delivery systems and pay for performance organizations.
5. Define patient-centered medical home (PCMH) and describe the relationship between an accountable care organization (ACO) and a patient-centered medical home.
6. List the six PCMH standards and describe each one.
7. Explain the role of health information technology in the newer health care delivery models.
8. Discuss the medical assistant's role in the newer health care models and describe how the role impacts the patient, employer, and nation.

INTRODUCTION

One of the most common delivery models used for reimbursing providers in the United States is the **fee for service** model. In this model, the provider is reimbursed according to the type and amount of services provided with no emphasis on patient outcomes. Unfortunately, this model emphasizes quantity of services rather than quality. However, this trend is slowly fading as newer payment models reward providers for value and efficiency rather than for services provided.

Some health care professionals may question the relevancy of this topic in a clinical textbook; however, these changes impact everyone on the health care team and the way health care is delivered. Clinical team members must gain a new mind-set that medicine is no longer just about taking vital signs and performing procedures. Every clinician on the health care team will play an integral role in disease prevention, health maintenance, and patient satisfaction.

This chapter will explore these newer health care delivery models and the changing role of the medical assistant as these trends prevail.

PATIENT PROTECTION AND AFFORDABLE CARE ACT

The Patient Protection and Affordable Care Act (PPACA), also known as "Obama Care," was signed into law on March 23, 2010. The most noted portion of the law is Title I, Quality Affordable Health Care for All Americans; however, there are two major provisions in the act that directly impact health care providers. This text will focus on Title III of the act, "Improving Quality and Efficacy of Health Care" and Title IV of the act, "Prevention of Chronic Disease and Improving Health."

Reforming Health Care

Whether or not you agree with recent health care reforms, one thing is very clear: America's ranking for health care efficiency is among the lowest in the world. According to a recent Bloomberg study on health care efficiency, America ranked number 46 out of the 48 countries studied. The study revealed that the United States spends an average of $8,608 per capita on health care, while Hong Kong, the country that placed number

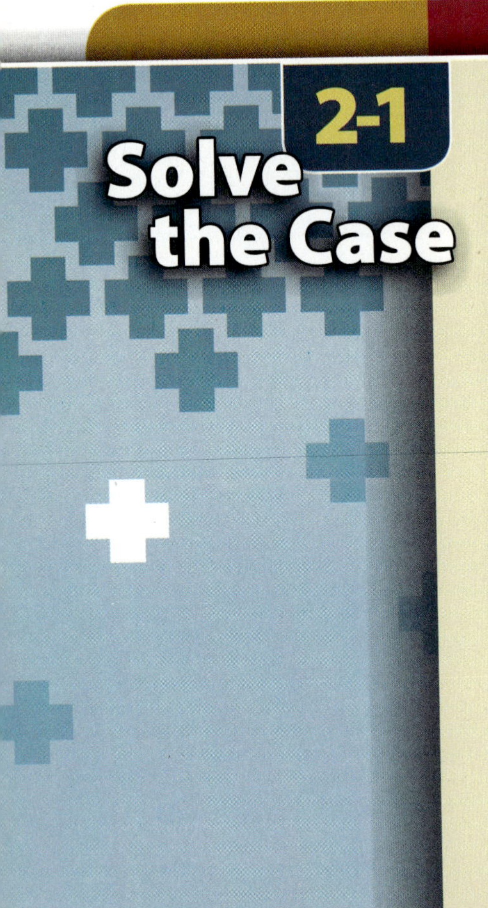

Danielle Anderson is a 42-year-old single mother of three who struggles with hypertension and obesity. Her children range in age from 12 to 16. She has a job with the state working at the Bureau of Motor Vehicles but barely makes enough money to keep her household going. Danielle receives very little in child support because her ex-husband is incarcerated. This is her first visit to a patient-centered medical home. While interviewing the patient, you find out that she smokes 1.5 packs of cigarettes per day and consumes high levels of carbohydrates, caffeine, and fats. She rarely consumes fruits or vegetables and states that the family eats all of their meals in the car or in front of the television. Danielle doesn't monitor her blood pressure because she doesn't have a home monitoring device. She also doesn't take her blood pressure medication as prescribed because she doesn't have time to go to the pharmacy and pick it up. She states that she has no time to exercise and rarely gets more than six hours of sleep per night. She tries to diet but always ends up gaining back the weight she loses.

1. **Using just your current level of knowledge, list the lifestyle choices that are affecting Danielle's current health status.**
2. **What conditions or diseases might be in Danielle's future if she doesn't change her lifestyle quickly?**
3. **What factors may be contributing to Danielle's lifestyle choices? How does Danielle's lifestyle impact her children? How do these lifestyle choices impact future health care costs?**

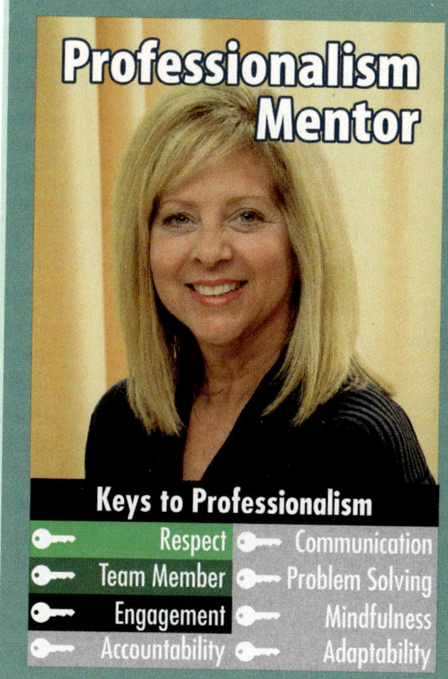

Did you know that many Americans believe that health care professionals demonstrate the highest level of honest and ethical behavior? That's quite an honor and it's also a big responsibility to continue to uphold this perception. I am always amazed at the medical assistant who can, in the midst of a busy practice, focus on specific patients and make them feel like they are the center of attention. Most health care facilities are pressured to maintain or lower costs, while increasing their patient outcomes and satisfaction levels. This is a difficult balance, and the medical assistant plays a key role. Patients will rely on you for information, to be their advocates and above all, for physical and emotional comfort. The medical assistant who possesses the skills to communicate clearly with patients, and advocate for them more effectively will most likely help to decrease unnecessary hospital readmissions, as well as improve patient satisfaction. That's the good news for your patient and a key to success in your profession! ■

one in the study, spends an average of $1,409 per capita on health care. Unfortunately, even though the United States outspends the majority of other countries, it also ranks very poorly in patient outcomes. This downtrend is expected to worsen as the population ages and chronic health problems rise.

How do we change a system that is clearly broken? We, and our culture, have to start by being a part of the solution rather than a part of the problem. There are many wastes in health care. Some of the wastes stem from high-ticket diagnostics, which are not always necessary or duplication of tests that have already been performed. Patients often seek the services of a specialist for procedures or conditions that could easily be managed by a primary care provider. The utilization of hospital emergency rooms for conditions that can be handled in an urgent care center or doctor's office also cause health care costs to rise.

While all of the items listed above contribute to the soaring costs of health care, one factor not mentioned above is the real culprit: chronic disease. According to Ursula Bauer of the Centers for Disease Control and Prevention, chronic health problems such as cardiovascular disease, diabetes, obesity, cancer, and kidney disease account for more than 75% of the nation's $2.7 trillion in annual spending for medical care. Four health risk behaviors—lack of exercise or physical activity, poor nutrition, tobacco use, and drinking too much alcohol—contribute to chronic diseases.

Title IV of the PPACA, "Prevention of Chronic Disease and Improving Health," challenges members of the health care team to improve health spending in this area by helping patients prevent or delay the onset of chronic disease and to guide patients who already have a chronic disease to better manage their disease.

Pay for Performance Organizations

Paying providers for performance is one of the federal government's solutions toward fixing health care costs. In this model, providers are rewarded for such things as better glucose control in their diabetic population, lower blood pressures in their hypertensive patients, and an increase in preventative screenings and procedures in all patient populations. This model uses a team approach, which may include a variety of players including the provider (team leader), nurse case managers, social workers, pharmacists, and of course medical assistants. **Pay for performance organizations** are reimbursed through care processes and measurable goals related to outcomes, as well as overall patient satisfaction.

Accountable Care Organizations

An accountable care organization is an example of a pay for performance organization. According to the Centers for Medicare & Medicaid Services (CMS), **accountable care organizations (ACOs)**, which are sometimes referred to as medical communities, are groups of doctors, hospitals, and other health care providers who come together voluntarily to give coordinated high-quality care to their Medicare patients. The goal of coordinated care is to ensure that patients, especially the chronically ill, get the right care at the right time while avoiding unnecessary duplication of services and preventing medical errors.

Accountable care organizations that are able to deliver quality care while reducing health care costs usually obtain higher reimbursement from governmental insurance organizations. Private payers are also experimenting with this newer model of health care. While many argue that this model isn't perfect due to the burden it puts on the provider and the extra costs to the practice, it does emphasize quality over quantity, which is a step in the right direction.

Patient-Centered Approach

Of course, patients need to be a part of the solution as well. We now know that lifestyle choices contribute extensively to chronic disease, thus patients need to be integral partners in matters of their own health and need guidance in setting goals that promote health. The medical team needs to work collaboratively with one another and institute a **patient-centered** approach to health.

The Institute of Medicine (IOM) defines patient-centered as "Providing care that is respectful of and responsive to individual patient preferences, needs and values, and ensuring that patient values guide all clinical decisions." Figure 2-1 illustrates a patient-centric environment.

A patient-centric approach focuses on the whole person, not just the condition, and measures quality of life as well as quality of health. Patients are provided tools and tracking mechanisms to meet health goals and productive feedback when they fall short.

Pay for Coordination Organizations

Pay for coordination is a type of health care delivery model that is often used in medical home environments and involves payment for specified care coordination services. In this environment, the provider, usually a primary care physician, or the team registered nurse (RN) leads a team of professionals to oversee and coordinate the patient's overall health. This is particularly important in patients with chronic illness. In a fee for service system, chronically ill patients often see multiple specialists with no one really coordinating patient care. In a pay for coordination model, the team coordinator oversees the patient's treatment, creates a care plan, and distributes parts of that care to other members of the team including physician assistants, nurse practitioners, medical assistants, dieticians, social workers, and others. When the patient's condition is beyond the scope of the primary care provider, the patient is sent to a specialist in the medical home community. Team members collaborate with one another through team huddles (Figure 2-2) and electronic exchanges. The following section discusses the patient-centered medical home in detail.

Patient-Centered Medical Homes

The **patient-centered medical home (PCMH)** was defined by the American Academy of Family Physicians, the American College of Physicians, the American Academy of Pediatrics, and the American Osteopathic Association in the 2007 Joint Principles for the Patient-Centered Medical Home. The PCMH model is designed to facilitate partnerships between patients and their physicians and may be part of an accountable care organization.

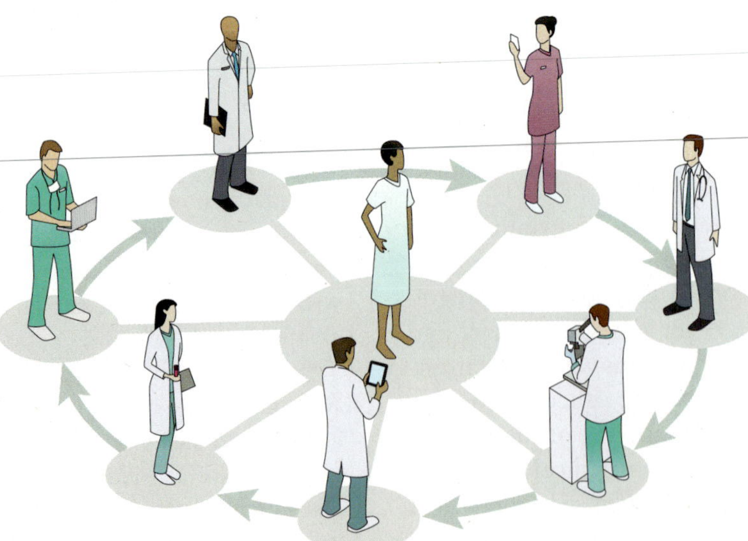

Figure 2-1 ■ In a patient-centric environment, the patient is at the center of health care.

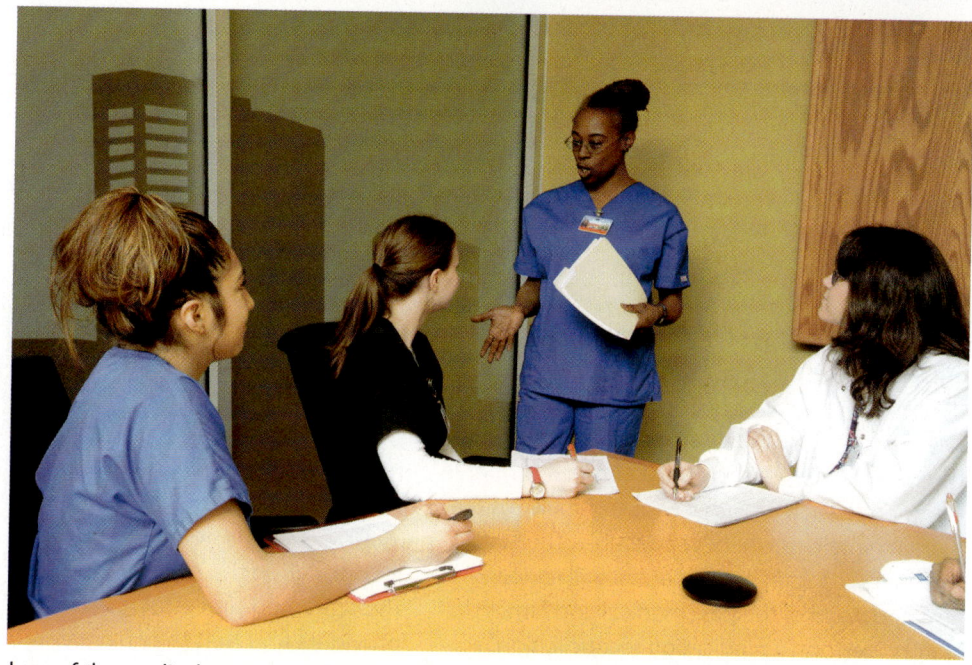

Figure 2-2 ■ Members of the medical team meet for their morning team huddle.

In addition, this model helps to ensure that the patient receives continuity of care, the facility has the ability to mine their data to track patient outcomes, the facility works toward continuous quality improvement, and the care provided is patient centric. The Agency for Healthcare Research and Quality (AHRQ) defines a medical home not simply as a place but as a model of the organization of primary care that delivers the core functions of primary health care.

PCMHs are often accredited through the **National Committee for Quality Assurance (NCQA)**, a nonprofit organization that strives to improve the quality of health care. The NCQA accredits a wide range of health care organizations including health plans, disease management programs, and physician organizations. In order to be accredited through the NCQA, the PCMH must meet a variety of standards. Table 2-1 provides a summary of the NCQA PCMH 2014 Standards and Requirements.

There are three levels of NCQA PCMH Recognition (Figure 2-3). Level 1: 35–59 points; Level 2: 60–84 points; and Level 3: 85–100 points. All three levels must

Table 2-1 Summary of NCQA PCMH 2014 Standards

Standard	Summary of Requirements
PCMH 1: **Patient-Centered Access**	The practice provides 24/7 access to team-based care for both routine and urgent needs of patients/families/caregivers.
PCMH 2: **Team-Based Care**	The practice provides continuity of care using team-based approaches that are culturally and linguistically appropriate.
PCMH 3: **Population Health Management**	The practice provides evidence-based decision support and proactive care reminders based on complete patient information, health assessment, and clinical data.
PCMH 4: **Care Management and Support**	The practice systematically identifies individual patients and plans, and manages and coordinates care based on need.
PCMH 5: **Care Coordination and Care Transitions**	The practice systematically tracks tests and coordinates care across specialty care, facility-based care, and community organizations.
PCMH 6: **Performance Measurement and Quality Improvement**	The practice uses performance data to identify opportunities for improvement and acts to improve clinical quality, efficiency, and patient experience.

Source: National Committee for Quality Assurance.

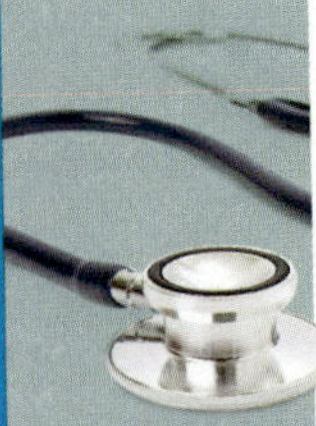

Field Smarts

Dr. Blake Busey set up his clinic's PCMH and received level 3 certification (level 1 being the lowest and level 3 being the highest). Dr. Busey describes the workflow at his clinic as having a morning team huddle to review specific topics: patients that are scheduled and were prescreened the days prior, all labs and orders are ready prior to the patient visit, emergency department visits and hospital admissions, and any important news pertaining to the daily business. At the huddle, a clinical staff member is assigned to each provider, with continuity of the team maintained whenever possible. The staff member who screens the patient will review and update all of the past medical and family history, perform a medication reconciliation, and provide the provider with any changes to the patient's health plan since their last visit. The provider then reviews the encounter and determines what additional studies, procedures, and/or follow-up may be necessary. Dr. Busey's clinic provides a written medication reconciliation and summary of the encounter with an updated care plan to the patient at the end of the visit, and then the patient is handed back to the clinical staff member who screened them for any additional services or education necessary. In addition, Dr. Busey's facility is required to track consults, high-end radiology orders, and specific HEDIS, and ORYX measures. They have also integrated behavioral health consultants (IBHC) for any counseling or classes and have a "transitions of care" coordinator who ensures that inpatient to outpatient transition goes smoothly, which has dropped their readmissions and emergency department visits from those who were hospitalized.

Dr. Busey considers medication reconciliation the most important aspect of the screening process. This is because many providers find that they have to redo the medication reconciliation initially completed by the staff. As a result, it is vital that this process should be practiced during the medical assistant's training program. As the medical team learns from its mistakes and successes, standard operating procedures are updated to continuously improve the patient experience, quality of care, cost effectiveness, and staff satisfaction.

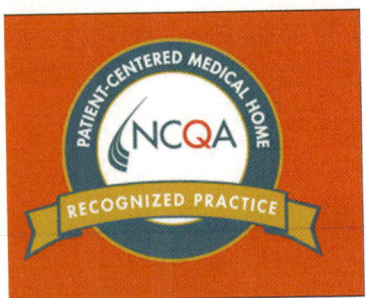

Figure 2-3 ■ PCHM-recognized practice.
Patient Centered Medical Home (PCMH 2014) Standards Training material is reproduced with permission from the National Committee for Quality Assurance (NCQA)

meet all six must-pass elements. Each level reflects the degree to which the practice meets the standards and provides the practice a range of capabilities and sophistication to successfully meet the requirements.

The pace of clinicians and sites adopting the PCMH model has been increasing at a rapid rate. Over 8,678 physicians achieved PCMH recognition through NCQA by November 2014. However, there are four other organizations that accredit PCMH models so the numbers are actually much higher.

Implementing the PCMH model is expected to improve quality of care, reduce costs, and enhance patient experience with their health care provider. External factors to the PCMH will also influence outcomes (see Table 2-2).

Figure 2-4 demonstrates the conceptual framework for the effectiveness of the PCMH. These factors, in

Table 2-2 External Factors to the PCMH

Factors	Examples
Patient	Health risk, motivation, behaviors, socioeconomic status
System-wide	Adoption of health IT, payment policies affecting provider reimbursement, workforce development, community resources, organizational context of the primary care setting, nature and cooperativeness of other providers in the medical neighborhood

Source: U.S. Department of Health and Human Services, Agency for Healthcare Research and Quality.

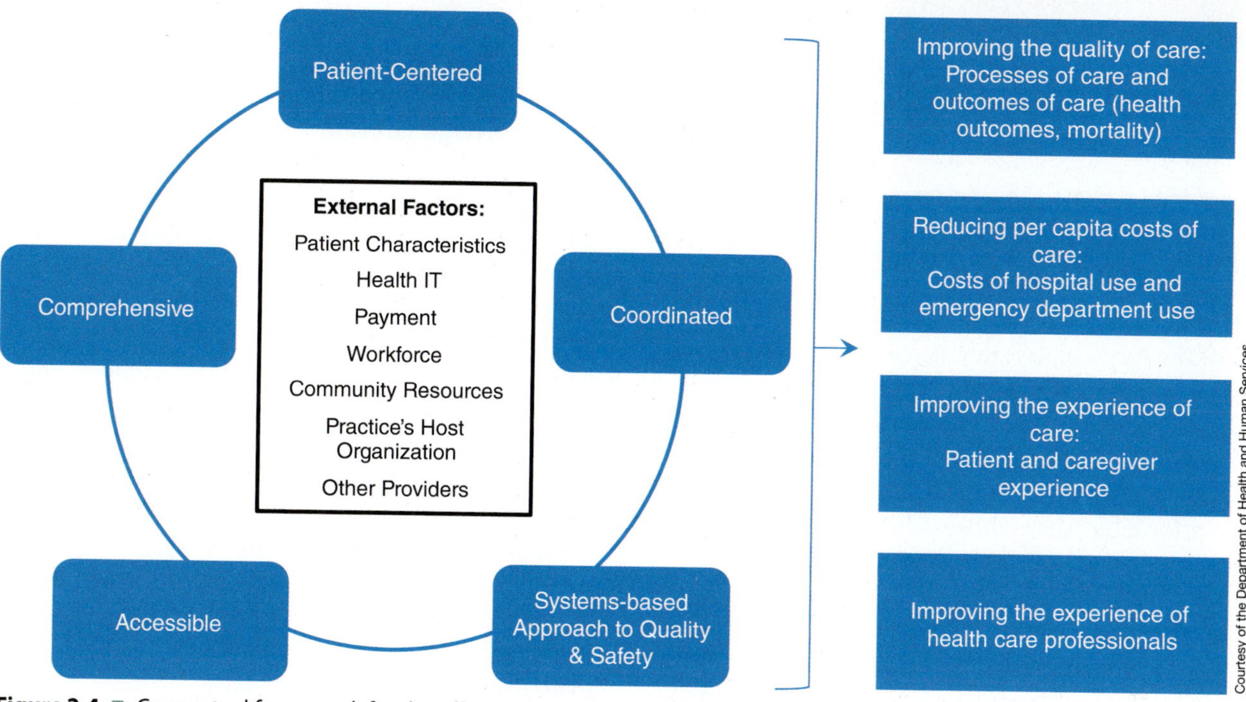

Figure 2-4 ■ Conceptual framework for the effectiveness of the medical home.

addition to the PCMH model, will collectively determine whether an intervention improves outcomes, the degree to which the improvements can be measured, and the applicability of the findings to other settings and populations.

THE ROLE OF INFORMATION TECHNOLOGY IN NEWER HEALTH CARE DELIVERY MODELS

In order for these newer delivery models to be effective, the practice must be actively engaged in **health information technology (HIT)**, which involves the exchange of health information in an electronic environment. The implementation of electronic health records (EHR) is an essential component of HIT. EHRs are the patient's medical records in digital format. Refer to Chapter 3 to learn more about electronic medical records.

The Institute for Healthcare Improvement (IHI) has initiated a movement referred to as the **Triple Aim Initiative** (Figure 2-5). IHI believes that new HIT designs must be developed to simultaneously pursue three dimensions:

- Improving the patient experience of care (including quality and satisfaction)

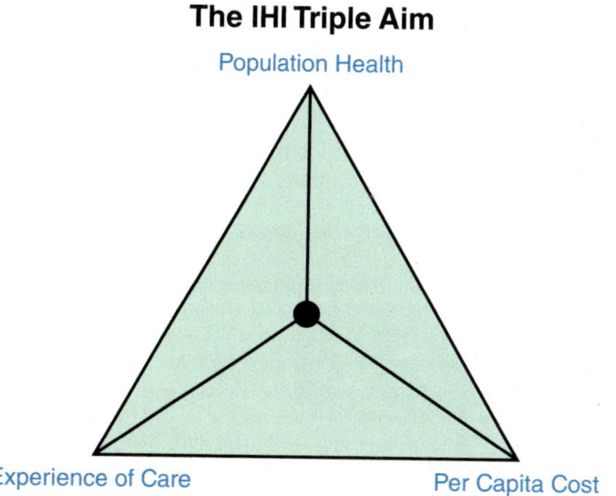

Figure 2-5 ■ Triple Aim Initiative. The IHI Triple Aim Framework was developed by the Institute for Healthcare Improvement in Cambridge, Massachusetts (www.ihi.org).

- Improving the health populations; and
- Reducing the per capita cost of health care.

IHI also believes to do this effectively, it is important to capture the range of determinants within the community, empower the patient and their families, and expand the impact and role of not only the primary care provider, but other services within the health care community. Doing so enables the patient to control his or her health care decision-making and outcomes throughout their life span. There has been recent discussion that a possible fourth measure should be added: a measure that addresses staff satisfaction and physician burnout. With the ever-increasing new standards, reporting requirements, and regulations, many in the health care field often feel overwhelmed.

THE MEDICAL ASSISTANT'S ROLE IN NEW DELIVERY MODELS

The role of the medical assistant is continuously evolving. As health care organizations search for ways to be more efficient with staffing budgets, the profession of medical assisting is gaining momentum. Some of the appeal is due to the fact that medical assisting salaries are more affordable than those of nurses and other health care specialists; however, the versatility of medical assistants is also intriguing.

How do these new delivery models impact the role of the medical assistant? Because the medical assistant is part of an integral team whose reimbursement is contingent on patient outcomes and experience, accountability is greater.

The medical assistant helps to implement care plans by doing the following:

- Carefully screening patients and sharing findings with the provider
- Entering orders into the electronic health record
- Helping patients stay up to date with preventive testing and health maintenance procedures through education and good coaching techniques
- Setting up outside procedures for the patient rather than having the patient set up the procedure
- Tracking the patient to make certain he or she follows through with outside testing
- Keeping a watchful eye on diagnostic reports and ascertaining the provider reviews the reports in a timely manner.
- Making the reports accessible to patients in the patient's health care portal and providing any home care or follow-up instructions
- Developing and maintaining a current list of community resources related to patients' health care needs and directing patients to these resources when applicable

Customer service is essential for fostering patient relationships. Patients must feel valued and know that their health and wellness is important to everyone on the team. Patients take a more active role in their own health care when they feel connected to the team members promoting health.

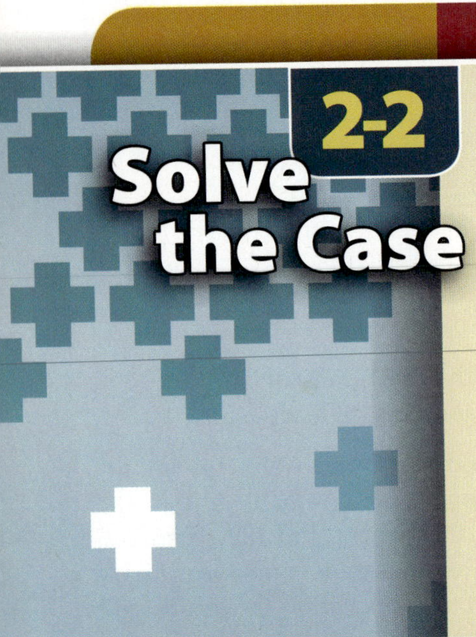

Danielle has just finished her visit with Dr. Dorado. He is very concerned about Danielle's current health problems. Today's assessment includes the following: obesity, hypertension, and bronchitis. Danielle had several tests performed today, including the following: a chest X-ray, electrocardiogram, complete blood count, comprehensive metabolic panel, and lipid panel. The doctor suspects the patient has hyperlipidemia (high cholesterol) and the start of coronary artery disease.

1. **What types of educational materials would benefit Danielle?**
2. **What other types of providers may be good to connect Danielle with based on her personal situation at home and her diet?**
3. **Is there anything you can do to help Danielle get her blood pressure medication on time and assist Danielle in monitoring her blood pressure at home?**

CHAPTER SUMMARY

- Health care reform is necessary due to the country's surging health care debt and poor outcomes.
- A patient-centric approach is an essential key in obtaining better outcomes. This approach focuses on the whole person, not just the condition.
- In a fee for service delivery model, providers are reimbursed according to services performed.
- In a pay for performance approach, the provider is reimbursed through care processes and measurable goals related to outcomes and overall patient satisfaction.
- An accountable care organization is a type of pay for performance organization. In a pay for coordination delivery model, providers are paid for specified care coordination services. This delivery model is often used in medical home environments.
- A patient-centered medical home may be part of a medical community and is designed to foster partnerships between the patients and their physicians.
- The National Committee for Quality Assurance (NCQA) is one of four agencies that accredits the PCMH.
- Health information technology (HIT) involves the exchange of health information between providers, payers, and consumers in a secure electronic environment. Electronic health records are an essential component of HIT.
- The Institute for Healthcare Improvement (IHI) has initiated a movement referred to as the "Triple Aim Initiative." The initiative hopes to do the following: improve the patient experience of care, improve the health populations, and reduce the per capita cost of health care.
- The medical assistant helps to implement care plans by carefully screening patients and sharing information with the provider, helping patients stay up to date with preventive testing and health maintenance, setting up outside appointments for the patient, tracking patients to make certain they followed through with care plan, keeping a watchful eye for diagnostic reports, making reports accessible to patients, and developing and maintaining a list of community resources for patients when applicable.

CERTIFICATION REVIEW QUESTIONS

1. What is one of the most common patient delivery models currently used for reimbursing providers?
   a. Pay for performance
   b. Pay for coordination
   c. Pay for service
   d. Fee for service

2. Which patient populations would benefit most from being a patient in an accountable care organization?
   a. Patients with diabetes
   b. Patients with hypertension
   c. Patients that are generally young and healthy
   d. Both a and b

3. Which of the following titles in the Patient Protection and Affordable Care Act addresses affordable health care for all Americans?
   a. Title I
   b. Title II
   c. Title III
   d. Title IV

4. These organizations are reimbursed through care processes and measurable goals related to outcomes, as well as overall patient satisfaction.
   a. Fee for service organizations
   b. Preferred provider organizations
   c. Pay for performance organizations
   d. None of the above.

5. Which of the following is not the medical assistant's responsibility regarding care plans?
   a. Carefully screening patients and sharing findings with the provider
   b. Creating the care plan
   c. Tracking patients to see if they followed through with the care plan
   d. Keeping a watchful eye on diagnostic reports and making certain the provider reviews the report in a timely manner.

6. Which PCMH standard focuses on 24/7 access to patients and their families?
   a. PCMH 1
   b. PCMH 2
   c. PCMH 3
   d. PCMH 4
7. The health care movement that focuses on improving the patient experience of care, improving health populations, and reducing the per capita cost of health care is referred to as:
   a. Patient Centered Medical Improvement Act
   b. Accountable Care Initiative
   c. Coordinated Care Initiative
   d. Triple Aim Initiative
8. Which NCQA PCMH recognition is the highest?
   a. Level 1
   b. Level II
   c. Level III
   d. Level IV
9. In the "Straight from the Field" box, Dr. Busey stated which of the following is one of the most important aspects of the screening process?
   a. Medication reconciliation
   b. Gathering the patient's history
   c. Stating the patient's chief complaint
   d. Listing the patient's dietary habits
10. In the newer health care models, every clinician including the medical assistant plays a significant role in which of the following?
   a. Disease prevention
   b. Health maintenance
   c. Patient satisfaction
   d. All of the above

STUDY RESOURCES

Resources to Test and Reinforce Your Knowledge:	
Certification Review Questions	Take this end-of-chapter quiz
Workbook	• Complete the activities for Chapter 2
Resources to Promote Critical Thinking:	
***Solve the Case* Activities**	• Consider these case studies and discuss your conclusions
MindTap	• Complete Chapter 2 readings and activities

REFERENCES

Chronic Diseases and Health Promotion. (May 9, 2014). Retrieved from http://www.cdc.gov/chronicdisease/overview/

Committee on Quality of Health Care in America. (March 2001). Crossing the quality chasm: A new health system for the 21st century. *Institute of Medicine*, 1–8.

Features and Announcements. (n.d.). Retrieved on December 23, 2014, from http://www.ncqa.org/

NCQA Patient-Centered Medical Home Brochure. (n.d.). A new model of care delivery. Reform update: New payment models could motivate providers to cut wasteful services. (n.d.). Retrieved from http://www.modernhealthcare.com/article/20140514/NEWS/305149963

Stinson, S. (n.d.). The cost of chronic disease. Retrieved from http://www.foxbusiness.com/personal-finance/2013/08/09/cost-chronic-disease/

Top Questions about ACOs & Accountable Care. (n.d.). Retrieved on December 23, 2014, from http://www.accountablecarefacts.org/topten/what-is-an-accountable-care-organization-aco-1

3

The Complete Medical Record and Electronic Charting

CHAPTER OUTLINE

The Medical Record
- Electronic Medical Records

Important Uses of the Medical Record

Medical Records Formats
- Source-oriented Medical Record (SOMR)
- Problem-oriented Medical Record (POMR)
- Combining Formats

Creating a Paper Chart
- Maintaining the Medical Record

Contents of the Medical Record
- Administrative Information in a Medical Record
- Clinical Information in a Medical Record

EHR Responsibilities for the Medical Assistant
- Checking Electronic Tasks
- Checking Clinical Today or Equivalent in Another EHR

Laws That Affect the Medical Record
- HITECH Act
- The Health Insurance Portability and Accountability Act of 1996 (HIPAA)
- Meaningful Use

Sharing Protected Information with other Health Care Professionals
- Fees Associated with Copying of Medical Records
- Retention of Medical Records
- Disposal of Medical Records
- Confidentiality
- Electronic Access Audit/Activity Log

ESSENTIAL TERMS

accountability
addendum
advance directive
American Recovery and Reinvestment Act (ARRA)
assessment
business associate agreement
Certification Commission for Healthcare Information Technology (CCHIT®)
Computer Physician Order Entry (CPOE)
electronic health record (EHR)
electronic medical record (EMR)
engagement
flow sheet
health information technology (HIT)
Health Information Technology for Economic and Clinical Health (HITECH) Act
Health Insurance Portability and Accountability Act of 1996 (HIPAA)
HIPAA Privacy Rule
HIPAA Security Rule
individually identifiable health information (IIHI)
notice of privacy practices (NPP)
objective impressions
meaningful use
mindfulness
minimum necessary
personal health record (PHR)
plan
practice management
problem list
problem-oriented medical record (POMR)
professional communications
progress notes
protected health information (PHI)

continues

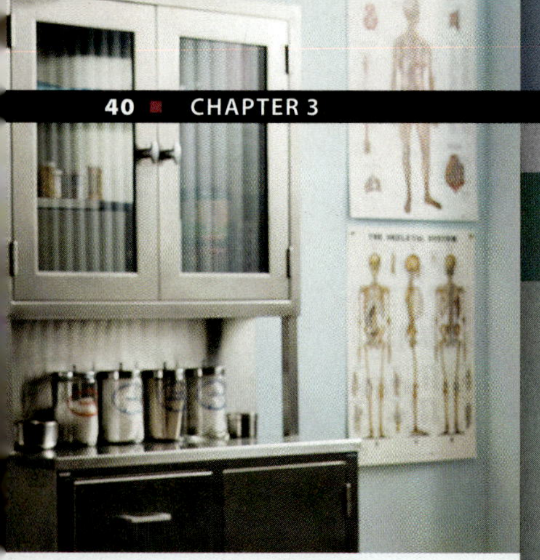

reverse chronological order
Rx Norm
scrub
shingling
source-oriented medical record (SOMR)
subjective impressions
subjective, objective, assessment, plan (SOAP)

DEVELOPMENTAL OBJECTIVES

After completing this chapter, you should be able to:

1. Correctly spell and define the essential terms.
2. Differentiate between electronic medical records (EMR) and a practice management system (PM).
3. List common functionalities of the EHR and the benefits of this system.
4. List three different types of medical records and describe each one.
5. List the two major types of formats that are used for documenting in the patient's record.
6. Identify methods of organizing the patient's medical record based on the problem-oriented medical record (POMR) and the source-oriented medical record (SOMR), and list the pros and cons for using each system.
7. Describe each letter of the SOAP format and list appropriate information to include under each section.
8. Create and organize a patient's medical record.
9. List important reasons for keeping neat, structured medical records.
10. Describe administrative and clinical components of the medical record.
11. Define types of information contained in the patient's medical record.
12. Utilize electronic medical records (EMR) and a practice management (PM) system.
13. Document on a growth chart and analyze healthcare results as reported in graphs.
14. Compose professional correspondence utilizing electronic technology.
15. Identify and describe laws relating to the exchange of information.
16. Define HIPAA and give examples of ways that the office can become HIPAA compliant.
17. Describe elements of meaningful use and reports that are generated.
18. Determine which sections of the medical record are owned by the health care provider and which sections belong to the patient.
19. Describe how long medical records have to be retained and how to properly dispose of them.
20. Discuss applications of electronic technology in professional communication including confidentiality, electronic access, and the audit/activity log.

INTRODUCTION

The medical record is the most important record kept in a medical office. A couple of different formats can be used to set up the medical record and to record entries within the patient's chart. The medical record is divided into several sections, all of which contain different forms.

It is important to have knowledge and understanding of paper medical records; however, electronic health records (EHRs) are now dominant in ambulatory medicine. Therefore, the medical assistant must become familiar with the functions, benefits, and restrictions related to EHRs. You often hear the acronym and terms EMR and EHR used interchangeably, but there is a distinction between the two. **Electronic medical records (EMRs)** are patient records in a digital format. **Electronic health records (EHRs)** refer to the interoperability of electronic medical records, or the ability to share medical records with other health care facilities. An EHR also integrates the administrative functions (known as **practice management**) and the clinical functions, typically referred to as EMR. In this textbook we use the term EMR to refer to only clinical duties, PM for administrative duties, and EHR for the combined PM/EMR electronic application that is interoperable.

There are laws that protect the private information contained in a patient's chart (HIPAA) and dictate how that information may be shared, with whom it may be shared, and how long a patient's information should be stored once the relationship between the provider and the patient is terminated.

After studying the information in this chapter, you will become familiar with various documenting formats used in medical establishments and gain an understanding of laws that are in place to protect patient information. EHRs and their functions are described in depth, providing you with essential information that will assist you when working in paperless offices.

THE MEDICAL RECORD

The medical record is an analysis of a patient's health status. It contains a medical history, current findings, considerations, test results, and treatment information related to conditions or diseases that ail the patient. Notes in the medical record are usually entered by the provider and other members of the health care team, including the medical assistant.

There are two major types of medical records that may be found in a medical practice: paper and electronic, or a combination (hybrid) of the two. Paper records are medical records that are stored in file folders. Paperless records are electronic records or records stored in digital format and are often referred to as electronic medical records (EMRs) or electronic health records (EHRs).

Another type of medical record, the **personal health record (PHR)**, is a copy of the patient's own medical record that may be in paper or digital format. There are websites catering to the needs of patients that include instructions for creating a PHR. Some medical offices create a PHR for patients as a perk for joining the practice, or have a PHR integrated into the practice's EHR.

The maintenance of the medical record is often assigned to administrative staff members; however, clinical staff members also have responsibilities in records

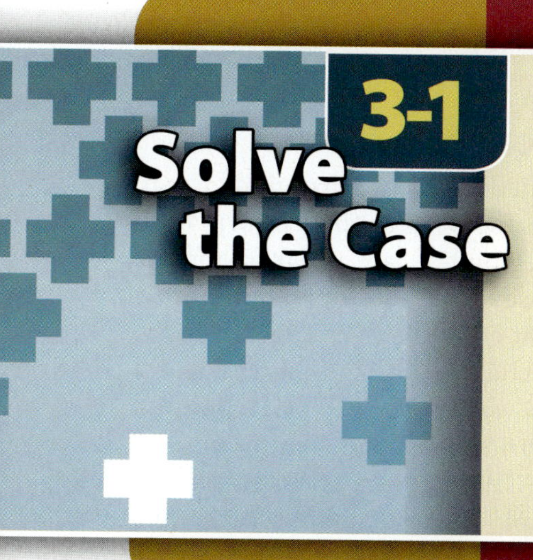

Emil Abello comes to the practice today to obtain copies of his medical record as he is planning to relocate and needs a new primary care provider (PCP) and an orthopedic specialist. Your practice is in the process of converting from paper charts to electronic medical records. Emil wants to be sure he has copies of all his X-ray, MRI, and CT studies included along with his medical history and lab reports.

1. **Using your current level of knowledge, what steps do you need to take to get Emil a copy of his medical records?**
2. **Would you need to obtain approval to release the record? Why or why not, and from who?**

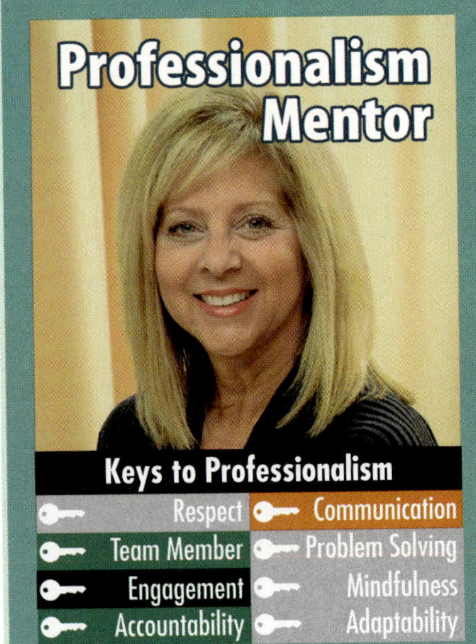

Imagine trying to read a book with missing words or pages. That would be hard to do and not very easy to understand. Documentation in the patient medical record is like telling a story, and incomplete documentation in the patient medical record is like having a book with missing pages. Every office visit is a new chapter and the provider depends on the medical assistant to maintain accurate records of each patient experience. Dependability, especially when it comes to maintaining a complete medical record, is an important key to success in the medical profession. Demonstrate your excellent work ethic by taking the time to tell the patient story correctly. As a medical assistant, maintaining the complete medical record is part of the patient care you provide. Be accountable and don't let your patient's medical record be like the book with missing pages. ■

maintenance. Duties are somewhat different for maintaining paper or electronic records. That is because in electronic records, orders and results are typically generated and received electronically, and documentation can be printed directly from the electronic chart as opposed to having to file paper documentation. Reports not received electronically will need to be scanned into the patient's electronic chart. The clinical team is usually responsible for ensuring that all outstanding lab and imaging results are entered into the paper chart or recorded in the electronic chart. They are also responsible for updating patient history and other data on a regular basis. Clinical staff members may have additional responsibilities such as removing information/data from the paper chart in order to copy the data, send it to other health facilities, and then return any removed data to its original location in the paper chart.

Any time the patient has an encounter with the medical assistant, whether it is over the phone, electronically, or in person, it must be documented in the patient's record. Electronic messaging is automatically recorded in the patient's chart, and a "digital footprint" exists of each and every time you access an electronic chart noting the user, date, and time.

With the latest rules of the **Health Insurance Portability and Accountability Act of 1996 (HIPAA)** and the widespread adoptions of EHRs, it is more important than ever for clinical staff members to have a clear understanding of their roles in entering and retrieving data from patient files and the federal guidelines that dictate how patient information can be shared. Generally you must only release the minimum necessary per HIPAA's rule.

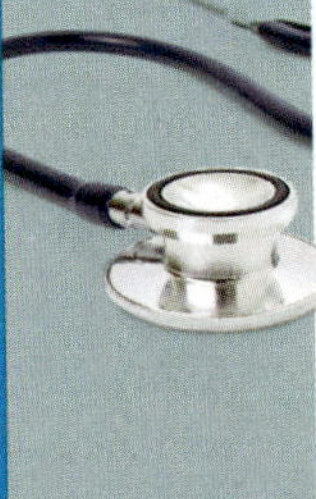

Field Smarts

HIPAA's **minimum necessary** rule:

- Indicates that you must provide only protected health information (PHI) in the minimum necessary amount to accomplish the purpose for which use or disclosure is sought
- Does not apply when patients provide a valid, signed authorization for release of PHI
- Requires that you de-identify information: PHI with all HIPAA identifiers removed

Electronic Medical Records

An EMR is a patient's medical record in digital format. It provides users with secure real-time information about the patient at the point of care and from remote locations. To get a sense of the interoperability of an EHR, consider a patient entering an emergency room (ER) complaining of chest pain. The patient had a physical the previous week with his PCP. Because the patient had some prior chest pain symptoms earlier in the week, the PCP ordered a stress test, heart ultrasound, and multiple lab tests, all of which were performed at an outside facility, but within the health care network.

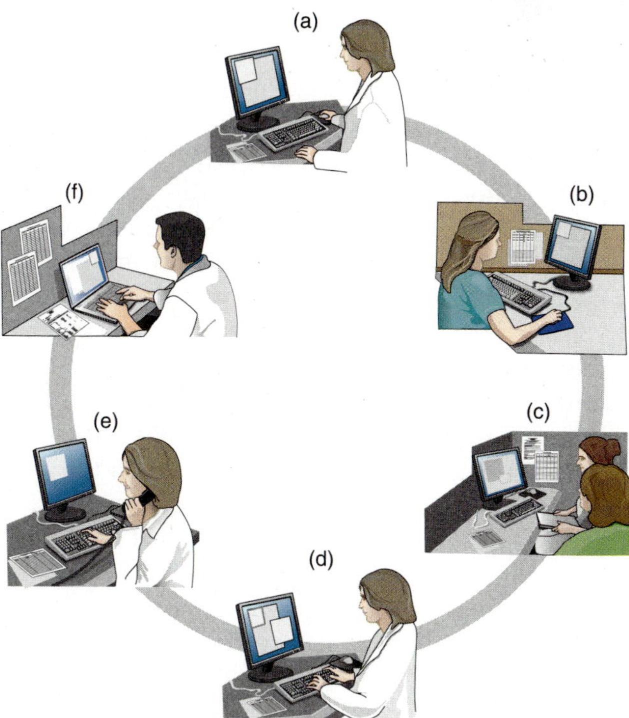

Figure 3-1 ■ A computer network provides health care workers with the necessary information with just a click of a button.

Figure 3-1 illustrates what occurs within an electronic health network. The connection is initiated when the PCP sends an electronic task to the medical assistant asking her to order the tests for the patient (Figure 3-1a). The medical assistant sends electronic orders to the facility where the tests are to be performed (Figure 3-1b). The testing facility receives the orders and sends the results back electronically to the PCP (Figure 3-1c), where they are reviewed and uploaded into the patient's EHR (Figure 3-1d). The ER provider can view the same information that the PCP has in the patient's electronic record, the findings from the physical, all diagnostic and lab reports, and a copy of the patient's clinical summary. If additional information is needed, the ER provider calls the PCP for some insight on the patient's condition, and the PCP sends the information (Figure 3-1e). In a matter of minutes, the ER provider has vital information that is necessary for determining necessary testing, making a diagnosis, and treating the patient (Figure 3-1f).

Features of EHRs

The electronic record has many features designed to improve patient care and staff efficiency. The type of software that a medical practice selects will depend on many factors including the type of practice, the number of providers within the practice, the goals of the practice, and the individual preferences of the clinicians and staff.

Though specific functions will vary depending on the particular program used, general EHR functions include:

- Creating customized progress notes and building notes efficiently through standardized templates and copy/paste features
- Enabling the provider and staff members to electronically transmit or fax progress notes, prescriptions, and orders directly from the point of care
- Allowing team members to schedule appointments from the point of care
- Automatically filing and displaying lab results in a variety of different formats
- Graphing lab values, pediatric growth patterns, and vital signs
- Displaying several parts of the chart at one time
- Allowing multiple users access to different parts of the chart at the same time
- Providing electronic tasking features to help keep staff members organized and greatly improving time management
- Providing full remote access of patient records for those authorized to view them
- Interfacing with the clinic's practice management program, making billing more efficient
- Providing reporting and benchmarking capabilities that allow users to compare patient outcomes or to track other statistical data

EHRs have enhanced the organization and structure of the traditional paper medical record. As more facilities adopt EHRs, the more elaborate these programs will become, providing more options than what are currently available.

Pitfalls of EHRs

EHRs have many benefits, but there are also a few pitfalls such as:

- Cost of the software
- Training time and costs to the facility
- Problems that occur when the system goes down
- Increased risk of unauthorized persons obtaining identifiable health information about the patient; privacy and security concerns
- Loss of "personal touch," meaning that you should not get lost in technology and focus on the computer in front of you. Remember to maintain eye contact and engage in a dialog with the patient.

Creating and Maintaining an EHR

The medical assistant may have the responsibility of maintaining an EHR. The amount of responsibility will be determined by office protocol. In general, the medical assistant may be responsible for any of the following when dealing with EHRs: creating the patient's electronic chart, updating basic demographic information, completing an electronic history, updating legal information, documenting subjective findings within progress notes, documenting vital signs and other procedures into the appropriate sections of the chart, creating electronic lab requisitions and prescriptions based on the provider's order, creating letters from templates stored within the EHR, downloading lab and diagnostic testing results from outside facilities, documenting within specialized patient logs (such as immunization and educational), and scanning paper items into an electronic format.

Attention to detail is important when performing these tasks. The medical record—whether in paper or electronic format—is a legal document that can be used in a court of law. The law also follows the rule of "if it isn't documented, it wasn't done." See Procedure 3-1 on how to create and maintain a medical record.

Amending Information in an EHR

When documenting information within an EHR, the user may need to change (edit) or add items. During your initial charting, information can be updated and changed. Once the information is saved, you will need to "edit" or "amend" the document. There is no "delete" or "undo" function in an EHR. To correct an error, the user must access the record and information that needs to be amended and select the appropriate amendment option. This may vary depending on the specific EHR software. Any changes that are made to the progress note or other electronic entry following submission are tracked and stored for future reference.

An **addendum** is text that is added to a progress note or other electronic entry after it has been signed or saved to the chart. The addendum appears at the end of the original progress note or other electronic entry and helps track any updates made to the record. Additionally, the "Addended By" label displays with the operator's name and the date and time of the addendum (Figure 3-2). This tracks changes made to the record and the person responsible for the change.

Certification of EHRs

In September of 2005, the U.S. Department of Health and Human Services (HHS) awarded a contract to the **Certification Commission for Healthcare Information Technology (CCHIT®)** to develop and evaluate the certification criteria and inspection process for EHRs. CCHIT is the oldest and best known of the six EHR-certifying agencies recognized by the Office of the National Coordinator (ONC). In order for a **health information technology (HIT)** vendor—a company that develops software for health care organizations—to get their product certified, the software must meet the basic criteria for functionality, interoperability, and security. Authorized by the Office of the National Coordinator, ONC-Authorized Testing and Certification Bodies (ONC-ATCBs) test and certify that certain types of EHR technology are compliant with the standards, implementation specifications, and certification criteria adopted by the HHS. An EHR that is certified means that, among other things, it supports meaningful use, which is discussed later in the chapter. CCHIT® announced its first ambulatory certified products in 2006. The CCHIT® certified its first inpatient EHR products in 2007. In November 2014, CCHIT® ceased testing and certification of EHRs. The reason given by CCHIT® was that it had become difficult to plan new services due to the slowing of the pace of ONC 2014 Edition certification, delays to subsequent meaningful use implementation, and the unreliable timing of future federal health IT requirements. For a listing of certification vendors and certified products, visit the HealthIT.gov website (www.HealthIT.gov) and search "Certified Health IT Product List."

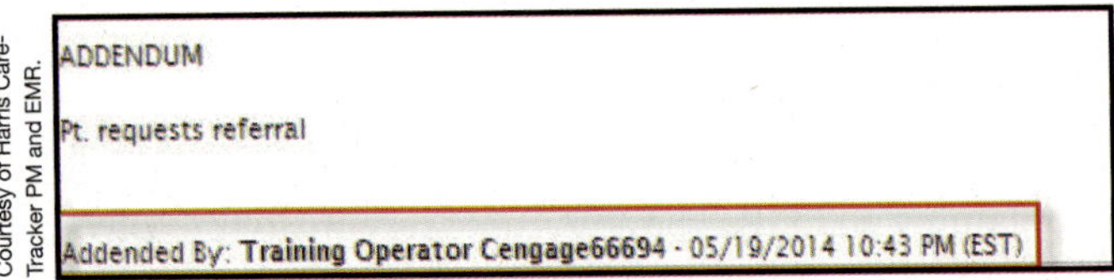

Figure 3-2 ■ Electronic addendum.

The Push for EHR

In 2004, President Bush put forth an executive order pushing for most Americans to have EHRs by 2014. The Centers for Medicare and Medicaid Services (CMS) developed a variety of incentives for health care providers to adopt EHRs, such as increases in Medicare and Medicaid reimbursements to those practices using EHRs and supplying qualifying offices with federal grants to purchase EHR software.

The American Recovery and Reinvestment Act of 2009 dedicated $19 billion to the cause of accelerating the adoption of progressive health information technologies such as EHRs. Incentive payments were made under initiatives through Medicare and Medicaid. Medicare incentives in the amount of $44,000 per provider are paid out over a five-year period to providers in ambulatory medical facilities that use EHRs. Bonus incentive payments are also paid to providers that demonstrate they are meaningful users of a certified EHR.

Medicaid-eligible providers receive cash incentives of up to $63,750 for purchasing and using qualified EHRs.

In addition, $21,250 is offered to every Medicaid-eligible provider to assist in the procurement and implementation of a qualified EHR system. The last year a Medicaid provider may initiate and register is 2016 in order to be eligible for these incentives. Once a Medicaid-eligible provider has adopted an EHR system, Medicaid provides an additional incentive payment of $8,500 to every provider for complying with meaningful use requirements.

IMPORTANT USES OF THE MEDICAL RECORD

The most important purpose of a medical record is to provide the provider with precise health data to assist in formulating an accurate diagnosis, plan an appropriate treatment, and track a patient's progress. The record also assists the provider in formulating disease prevention measures and overall health maintenance goals for the patient.

Other functions of the medical record are:

1. To provide a means of communication: It is a communication tool that is used between providers, health care teams and patients (Figure 3-3) to improve the continuity of care and contains instructions for other health care employees to perform various diagnostic procedures or to administer particular treatments.
2. To be used for financial purposes: Progress notes are used by a medical practice to determine the complexity of the office visit, the diagnostic procedures performed, and any treatment rendered. The insurance company may also use progress notes from the chart to establish medical necessity for specified diagnostic procedures or treatments. The PM side of an EHR captures each patient encounter with CPT® and ICD codes, then **scrubs** [verifies procedure(s) are supported with appropriate diagnoses and meet the approval of the insurance carrier] the claim(s).
3. To serve as a legal document: The chart is a legal document that can protect the provider against frivolous lawsuits. On the other hand, it can be used as an incriminating piece of evidence by a plaintiff to prove negligence in a medical malpractice suit.
4. To be used as an educational tool: The chart may be used by medical students, residents, and health care providers as case studies.
5. To provide statistical data for research purposes: Patients may elect to participate in a clinical trial sponsored by a drug company or a company that manufactures medical devices. The medical record can be used to provide these companies with pertinent data regarding the overall effectiveness of their products and safety performance.

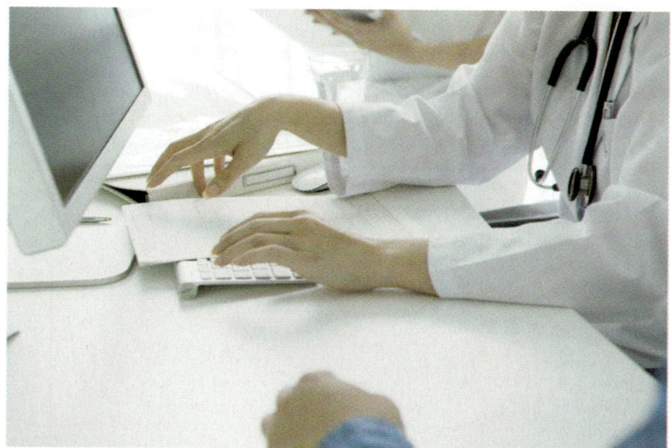

Figure 3-3 ■ The patient's medical chart provides valuable information so that both providers and medical assistants know how to proceed with the patient.

MEDICAL RECORDS FORMATS

There are two different documentation formats that are used for paper medical records, the source-oriented medical record (SOMR) and the problem-oriented medical record (POMR).

Source-Oriented Medical Record (SOMR)

The more traditional format used for recording data in the medical record is the **source-oriented medical record (SOMR)**. Charts in which the SOMR format is used are divided into specific sections including: History and Physical, Progress Notes (notes that track the patient's progress), Nursing/Medical Assisting Notes, Laboratory, and Diagnostic Testing. The "source" or individual providing the data enters the information within the appropriate section of the chart. There is no systematic cross-referencing of data from one section to the next. **Progress notes** are usually recorded in a narrative format, making it necessary to read the entire progress note before determining what is wrong with the patient. All reports and notes are kept in a **reverse chronological order**, meaning the most recent note is on top.

Problem-Oriented Medical Record (POMR)

The **problem-oriented medical record (POMR)**, also known as the POR, was developed by Lawrence L. Weed in the early 1970s. The POMR system incorporates structure and organization within the medical chart, stimulating better communication between those reading and those entering data within the chart. The POMR is developed using four categorizations or stages:

1. Develop a database: The database should include patient history and current medications, physical findings, and baseline readings for diagnostic and laboratory testing.
2. Assemble a detailed **problem list:** The problem list should record specific problems identified from the patient history form and should list new problems as they arise. Each problem is numbered and should include the name of the condition or diagnosis. Each time the patient is seen for a particular problem, the progress note will reference the number listed on the problem list. If the problem is resolved, the date that the problem is resolved is entered onto the problem list. See Figure 3-4A for an example of a detailed problem list in paper format. Figure 3-4B represents the problem list in an electronic format.
3. Formulate a plan of action for each problem: The plan for each problem may be found as a separate listing within the chart or may be included in the problem list. This section should include plans for testing, treatment, and education.
4. Provide ongoing progress notes for each problem on the problem list.

SOAP Notes

The POMR system uses the **subjective, objective, assessment, plan (SOAP)** note format for each progress note. Table 3-1 lists each section of a SOAP note, the type of information included in each section, and states which personnel is responsible for entering information within each section. Figure 3-5 illustrates an example of a complete SOAP note.

DOUGLASVILLE MEDICINE ASSOCIATES
5076 BRAND BLVD
DOUGLASVILLE, NY 01234
(123) 456-7890

MASTER PROBLEM LIST

Patient's Name: Green, Kelly **DOB:** 05-16-1955 **Chart #** 129876

Date	Problem/ Diagnosis/RO	Problem Number	Plan Abbreviations:	Practitioner	Date of Resolve	Recurrence Date
02/14/XX	L. Otitis Media	1	DP: None	Legg	2/26/XX	
			RX: Amoxicillin, 500 mg			
			CE: Ear Infection Fact Sheet			
07/15/XX	VTI	2	DP: Complete VA and C&S	Legg	7/25/XX	
			RX: TMP-SMX			
			CE: VTI Fact Sheet			
09/22/XX	Hypertension	3	DP: None Presently	Legg		
			RX: Atenolol, 25 mg & Life style changes			
			CE: BP Fact Sheet			
			DP:			
			RX:			
			CE:			

Legend:
DP: Diagnostic Plan
RX: Therapeutic Plan
CE: Client education
FUP: Follow-Up Plan

Figure 3-4A ■ A detailed problem list (in paper format) makes it easy for anyone using the chart to track patient problems and treatments without reading the entire chart.

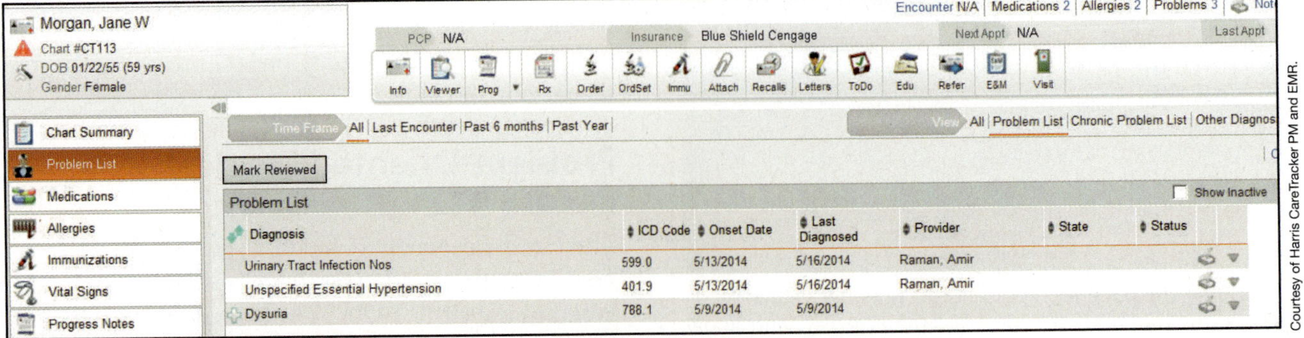

Figure 3-4B ■ A detailed problem list in an electronic format.

Courtesy of Harris CareTracker PM and EMR.

Table 3-1 SOAP Notes Defined

Section Name	Description	Examples of What is Included in Each Section	Personnel Who Typically Documents within Each Section
Subjective impressions (S)	Information provided by the patient	Patient's chief complaint or reason for visit in the patient's own words	Medical assistant, nurse
Objective impressions (O)	Information provided by the health care professional; includes a list of measurable reproducible data	Provider's physical findings, patient's vital signs, height and weight, laboratory results, or other diagnostic data	Provider, nurse, medical assistant, other health care personnel who perform diagnostic testing
Assessment (A)	Interpretation of the subjective and objective findings	Diagnosis	Provider
Plan (P)	Provider's plan for diagnosing and treating the patient	Names of lab and diagnostic tests to be performed, forms of treatment, and educational plans	Provider

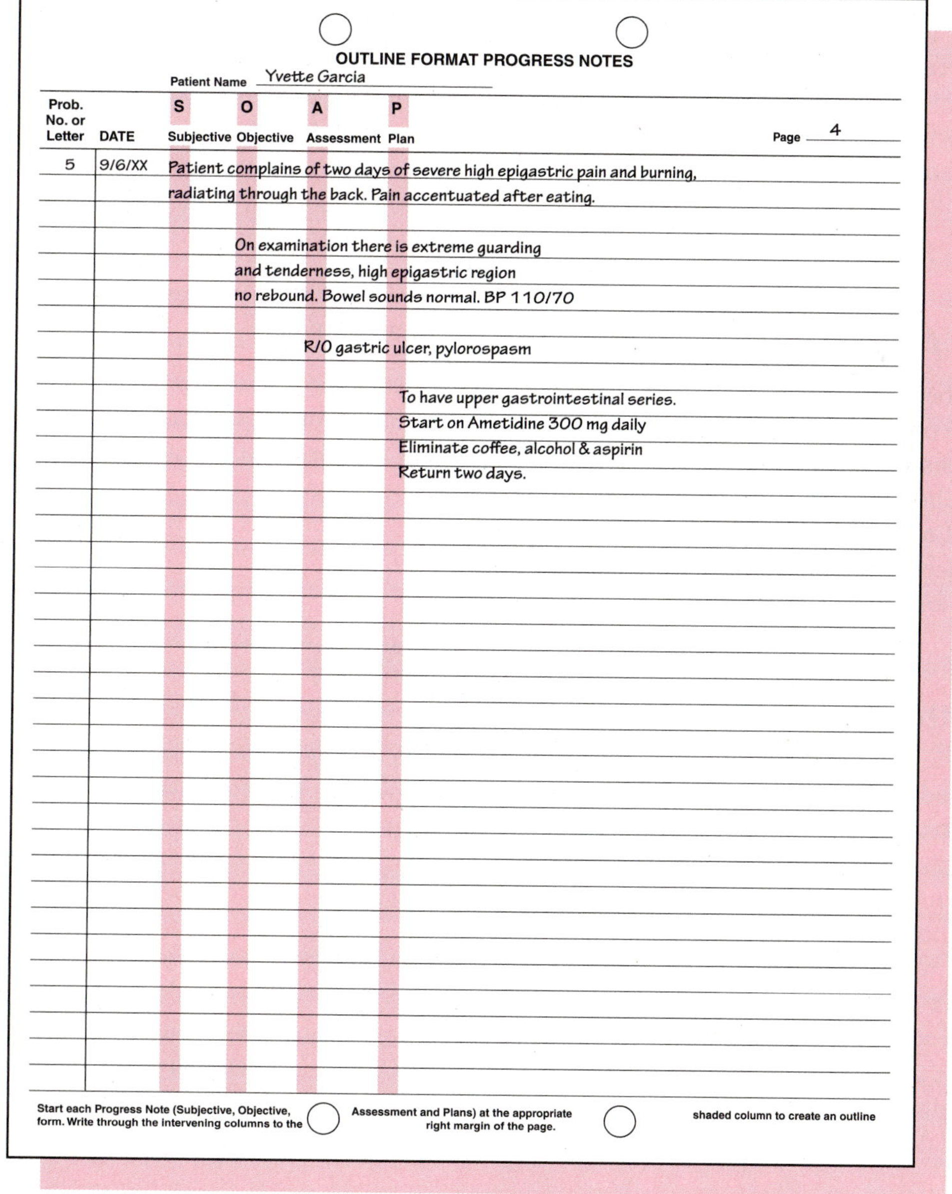

OUTLINE FORMAT PROGRESS NOTES

Patient Name Yvette Garcia

Page 4

Prob. No. or Letter	DATE	S Subjective O Objective A Assessment P Plan
5	9/6/XX	Patient complains of two days of severe high epigastric pain and burning, radiating through the back. Pain accentuated after eating.
		On examination there is extreme guarding and tenderness, high epigastric region no rebound. Bowel sounds normal. BP 110/70
		R/O gastric ulcer, pylorospasm
		To have upper gastrointestinal series. Start on Ametidine 300 mg daily Eliminate coffee, alcohol & aspirin Return two days.

Start each Progress Note (Subjective, Objective, Assessment and Plans) at the appropriate shaded column to create an outline form. Write through the intervening columns to the right margin of the page.

Figure 3-5 ■ An example of a POMR progress note page.

There are a number of advantages of using the POMR including:

1. It makes exploration of the chart much more efficient.
2. It decreases ambiguity of prior problems and treatment goals.
3. It encourages uniformity amongst those using the chart.
4. It simplifies record keeping.

Combining Formats

Some offices may combine particular aspects of the SOMR and POMR formats. The record may be set up using the SOMR format, but the provider may use the SOAP approach when entering information on the progress note and may include an abbreviated problem list on the front *inside* cover of the paper chart. Regardless of which system is used, the medical assistant will need to learn how paper charts are set up within each office and the proper method for documenting information in the medical record. Being familiar with the setup of paper charts will help you understand electronic charts as well because many of the features used in these formats are also used in electronic charts.

CREATING A PAPER CHART

Steps for creating the medical record will vary depending on whether the office is using a paper or paperless system. The paper chart is usually created by administrative staff members, but maintained by both clinical and administrative staff members (see Procedure 3-1). The clinical staff may need to file items within the patient's chart, insert new forms, and make minor repairs to the chart.

Maintaining the Medical Record

Once a paper patient record is created it must be properly maintained. The chart is regularly inspected and any physical tears mended. Loose labels should be firmly reattached. Misplaced reports should be reviewed to determine if they have been released for filing and then placed in the appropriate section of the record. When forms such as progress notes and flow sheets are over 75% complete, new forms should be placed nearby so that they are easily assessable when needed.

Part of maintaining a chart is making certain that all information is updated. The record should be checked regularly to make certain that all labs are up to date and that the patient is current on health maintenance screenings. Once the provider and medical assistant are finished using the chart, it should be released for filing.

CONTENTS OF THE MEDICAL RECORD

Sections contained within the medical record will vary from one office to the next for both paper and electronic records.

Factors that influence which sections will be incorporated into the medical record include:

- Provider's personal preference
- Type of practice
- Costs
- Regulatory requirements

Many of the forms found in a paper medical chart can be purchased through a supplier and can be printed with the name, address, and phone number of the practice located at the top of each form. Generally, charts are divided into two major sections:

- Administrative information
- Clinical information

The paper chart's front cover should include the patient's name or identification number, and color-coded stickers that identify the last year the patient was seen (Figure 3-6). It may also include stickers that alert staff members when a patient is allergic to a particular drug.

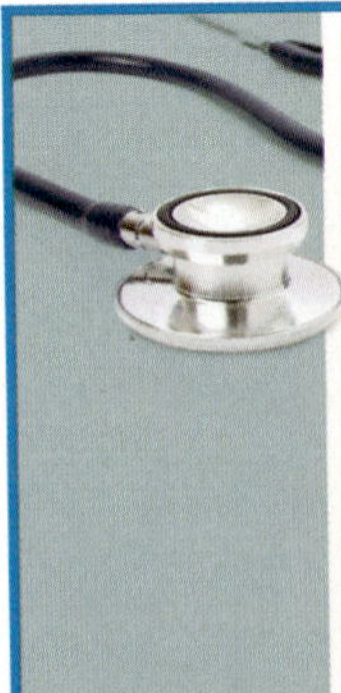

Field Smarts

Documenting within the patient's record is a key task performed by medical assistants. All patient encounters are to be documented within the patient's chart. Documentation should be accurate and thorough, yet concise. Medical assisting students should practice all types of documentation throughout their training period (see Chapter 4 for documentation guidelines).

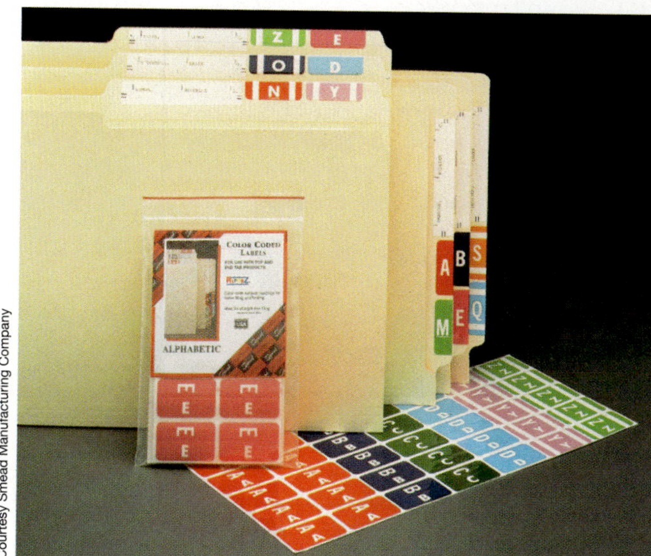

Courtesy Smead Manufacturing Company

Figure 3-6 ■ Paper charts.

Administrative Information in a Medical Record

Administrative information is most often used by administrative staff members and occasionally members of the clinical team. Administrative sections within the medical record may include the following:

- Demographics: A patient registration form that includes personal information about the patient including address, phone number, insurance information, etc.
- Insurance: Copy of the insurance card, referrals, and precertification (authorization) requests
- Correspondence: Letters from insurance companies, attorneys, etc.
- Legal: Copy of the patient's privacy statement, living will, and advance directives
- (EHR) Claims: Visit capture, claims scrubbing, electronic submission of claims and remittances
- (EHR) Billing: Ages patient accounts receivable

Information within each section is usually placed in reverse chronological order, or the most recent date on top.

Clinical Information in a Medical Record

The majority of information found in a patient's chart is considered to be clinical data. Clinical data is information that providers use to help diagnose, prescribe, and treat patients. Clinical information should also be placed in reverse chronological order in the paper chart. Other clinical documentation includes advanced features such as working on the progress note, manually entering results, recording messages in the patient's chart, creating patient recall letters, and generating immunization reports. The following is a description of each section of clinical data found in a patient's chart.

Medical History

The medical history form is normally completed during the patient's initial visit and updated during subsequent visits. This form may be completed by the patient, provider, or medical assistant. It is a tool used for assessment purposes. It gives the provider subjective information about the patient and patient's family and provides a database that can be used to build upon. See Chapter 5 for more information regarding the medical history section.

Updating Medications, Immunizations, Drug Allergies, and Preventive Screenings

Additional documentation in a patient's medical record includes updating medications, immunizations, drug allergies, and preventive screenings. In the paper chart, this information is generally noted on the progress note for the encounter in question.

EHR Application

Some EHR software programs have a medical history component that can be completed rather easily. The user simply identifies each disease or condition that is applicable by clicking on the "Yes" response and clicking on the "No" response for conditions that are nonapplicable. A new template of questions may appear, allowing the user to expand on "Yes" responses. The majority of software programs allow users an opportunity to personalize the medical history to coincide with their particular specialty. Patients may also participate in completing the electronic history by using a kiosk in the examination room or by completing the requested health information online, prior to the first appointment. If there is no medical history component built within the EHR software, the medical assistant may need to scan the history form within the patient's electronic file. Figure 3-7 illustrates an example of an electronic history form.

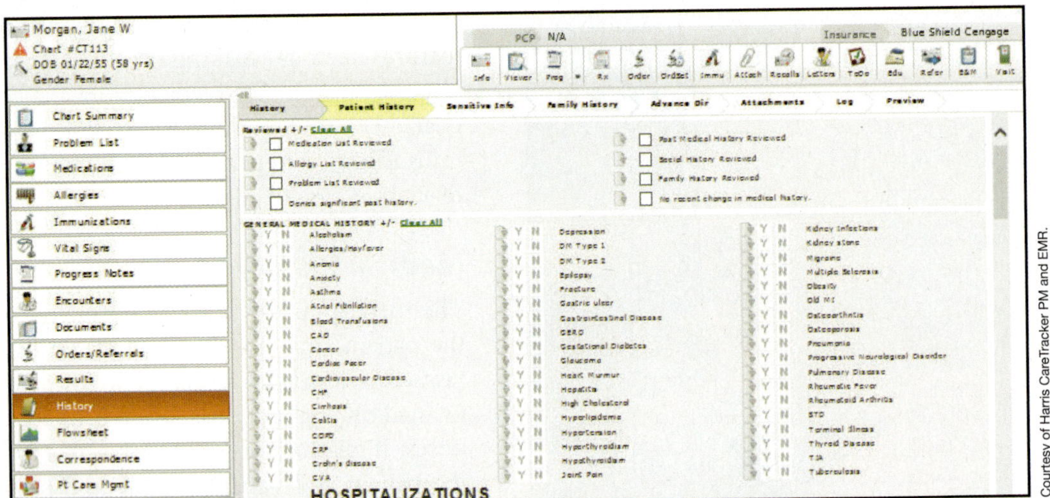

Courtesy of Harris CareTracker PM and EMR.

Figure 3-7 ■ An example of an electronic patient history form.

Physical Exam

The physical examination is a key component of the diagnostic approach for each patient and provides an overview of the patient's general condition. The physical exam involves a head-to-toe evaluation of the patient, organized by body system. It is an important tool for discovering any new problems and monitoring previously identified problems. A physical exam is usually performed during the patient's initial office visit and every one to three years thereafter. The frequency of physical exams depends on the following:

- The patient's overall health status and age
- Insurance protocol
- The type of physical (annual, sports, work, or presurgical)

The patient's insurance company or payer, and recent regulations set forth by the Affordable Care Act (ACA) and Medicare, usually set specific guidelines for the time span between physicals. When a patient requests a physical, the office staff should check to determine that the timing or reason for the physical falls within the payer's parameters. If the parameters do not meet insurance guidelines, the patient should be warned by a member of the health care team beforehand of the exact financial responsibility.

It is also customary for patients to have a physical prior to a surgical procedure. The patient may be examined by the surgeon or the primary care provider. A copy of the history form should be faxed or electronically transmitted to the hospital where the surgery is to be performed.

Specialty forms may be used for physical exams or the physical exam findings may be documented on a standard progress note.

Progress Notes

Progress notes are the heart of the patient record. They serve as a chronological listing of the patient's overall health status. Data pertaining to the findings from the visit are entered on a progress note, usually in the SOAP format. The progress note form may also be used for recording telephone encounters, procedures, treatments, and other interactions that take place with the patient. The header on the progress note should include the patient's name, birth date, and any allergy alerts. Before entering any information on the progress note, ensure that you have the correct chart by asking the patient for two identifiers such as his or her full name and birth date.

Medication Records

Some offices using paper charts have a separate section for medication entries; other offices have team members document medication treatments directly onto the progress note. Medication reconciliation is a key component of the patient record. Prescribed drugs may be logged in a separate section from those administered or dispensed. The medical assistant should avoid using abbreviations when documenting medications or use only standard abbreviations that are not listed on the "Do Not Use" abbreviation list. The list can be viewed by accessing the Joint Commission website (www.joint-commission.org) and searching for the Official "Do Not Use" List. The Institute for Safe Medical Practices

EHR Application

Features of an EHR, such as Harris CareTracker, include the patient's *Chart Summary*, and *Medications* applications that allow you to manually update the patient's medication list. New prescriptions can also be added. It is important to ensure that all active medications are recorded to screen for interactions when prescribing new medications. Additional features of the Harris CareTracker EHR include:

- The *Immunizations* module allows you to enter previous immunizations as well as new immunizations that you administer in your office.
- The *Allergies* application helps add new and existing allergies to a patient's medical record. It is important to ensure that all active allergies are recorded for accurate drug–allergy contraindication checks when prescribing medications and ordering immunizations.
- The *Patient Care Management* application is used as a proactive reminder tool to improve the care management process (Figure 3-8). The patient is evaluated and moved to specific health maintenance and disease management registries based on measures that are activated within the practice. The application helps manage the recurring preventive care items pertinent to a patient, flags overdue items, enables you to manually move the patient to a high-risk registry, and more. The care recommendations in the *Health Maintenance* and *Disease Management* registries are based on CDC and National Committee for Quality Assurance/Healthcare Effectiveness Data and Information Set (NCQA/HEDIS) guidelines.

EHR Application

Entering information within the progress note is quite simple. The user may use standardized templates for entering patient data or may copy and paste information from prior visits and make the appropriate adjustments. The user can integrate information from other sections of the chart directly onto the progress note—such as lab findings, history information, and the patient's medication history—by simply clicking on the appropriate tabs. EHR reduces documentation time significantly and can save the practice thousands of dollars in the long run. Figure 3-9 illustrates a progress note in which information from other parts of the chart have been integrated within the progress note.

(ISMP) publishes a more extensive list of abbreviations, symbols, and dose designations that are prone to error. You can access the most current information available by logging on to the ISMP website (www.ismp.org) and searching for "List of Error-Prone Abbreviations, Symbols, and Dose Designations." Medical assistants should always check the individual policies of the office in which they work.

Vital Signs

Monitoring a patient's vital signs can help detect health changes. Vital signs include height, weight, heartbeat, respiration rate, pulse oximetry, temperature, body mass index (BMI), blood pressure, and pain level. Health care providers will watch, measure, and monitor vital signs to check a patient's level of physical

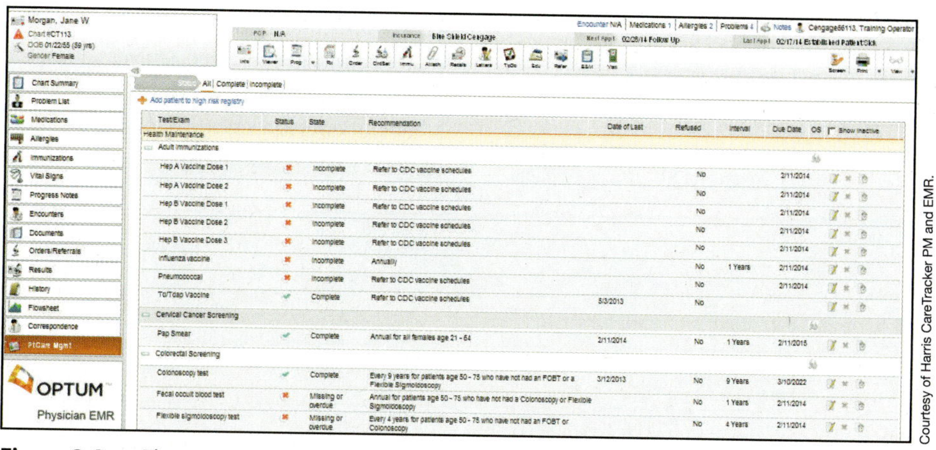

Courtesy of Harris CareTracker PM and EMR.

Figure 3-8 ■ Electronic Patient Care Management application.

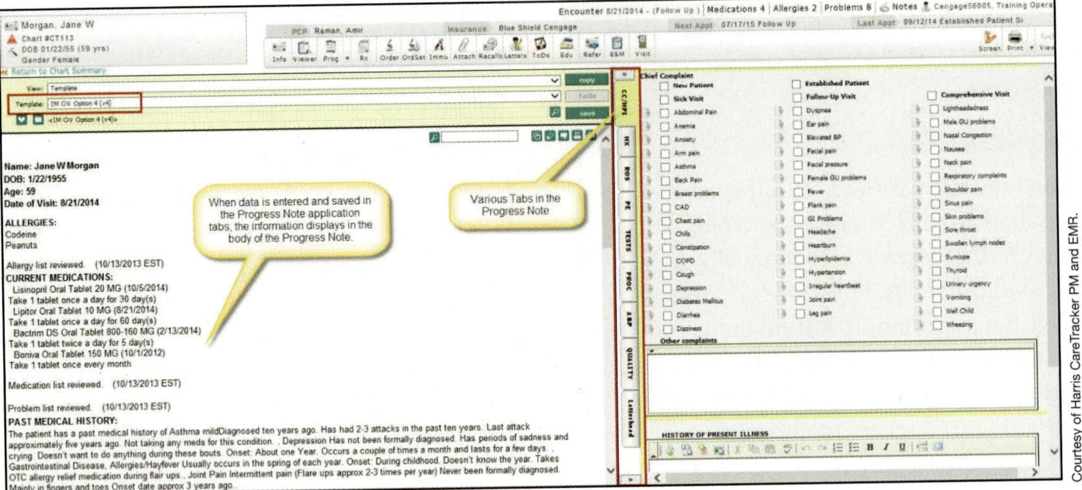

Courtesy of Harris CareTracker PM and EMR.

Figure 3-9 ■ An example of electronic progress note tabs.

functioning. In a paper chart, vital signs are typically recorded on the progress note for the encounter with the patient.

Phone Reports

Any time a patient calls to change an appointment, give a progress report, obtain test results, or request a

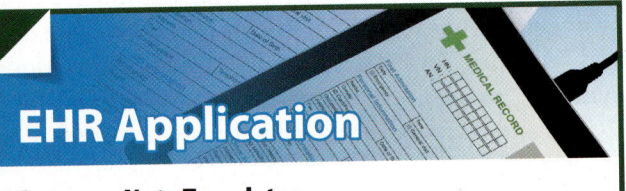

Progress Note Templates

There are predefined specialty and condition specific templates available in most EHRs (Figure 3-10) such as pediatric, internal medicine, and dictation. Use of templates simplifies the process of documenting a patient encounter at the point of care. Each template offers a specific layout and custom options. These options allow providers to select the template that best suits their documenting needs. Staff members can also pull in sections of a prior note and insert documents and images into templates if necessary. Standard templates can be broken down by specialty and template styles.

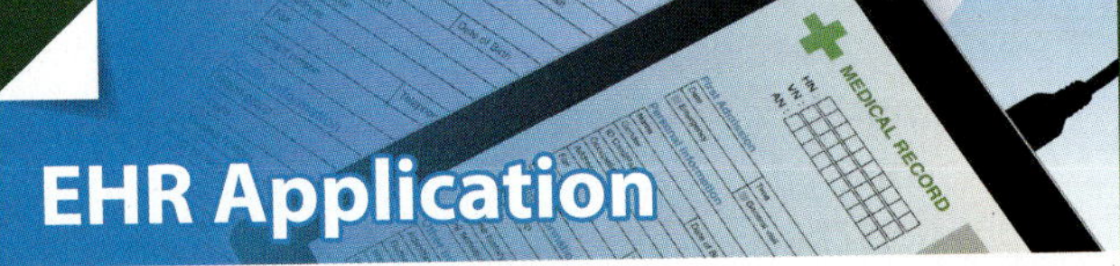

The *Rx* application allows you to create prescriptions for both controlled (scheduled) and noncontrolled drugs. The prescription software can store thousands of common drug names with their usual dosages. The user brings up the patient's electronic chart, clicks on the prescription tab, and selects the name and dosage of the ordered drug (Figure 3-11). The number of refills to be given is selected, as well as the name of the provider ordering the prescription. There is normally an option for printing, faxing, or electronically transmitting the order. All prescriptions created through the *Rx Writer* application are recorded in the *Medications* application with the name, Rx Norm code, dosage, and other pertinent data. **Rx Norm** is a standardized nomenclature for clinical drugs and drug delivery devices produced by the National Library of Medicine (NLM). The Rx Norm code supports interoperability between EHR systems. The software may have individual patient logs for immunizations, narcotics, and other drugs administered within the office. Universal or global logs may also be stored within the EHR to track drugs administered to all patients for reporting purposes.

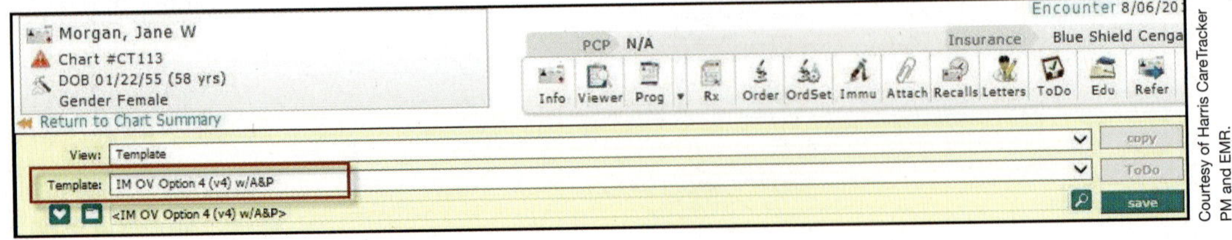

Courtesy of Harris CareTracker PM and EMR.

Figure 3-10 ■ Progress note templates.

Courtesy of Harris CareTracker PM and EMR.

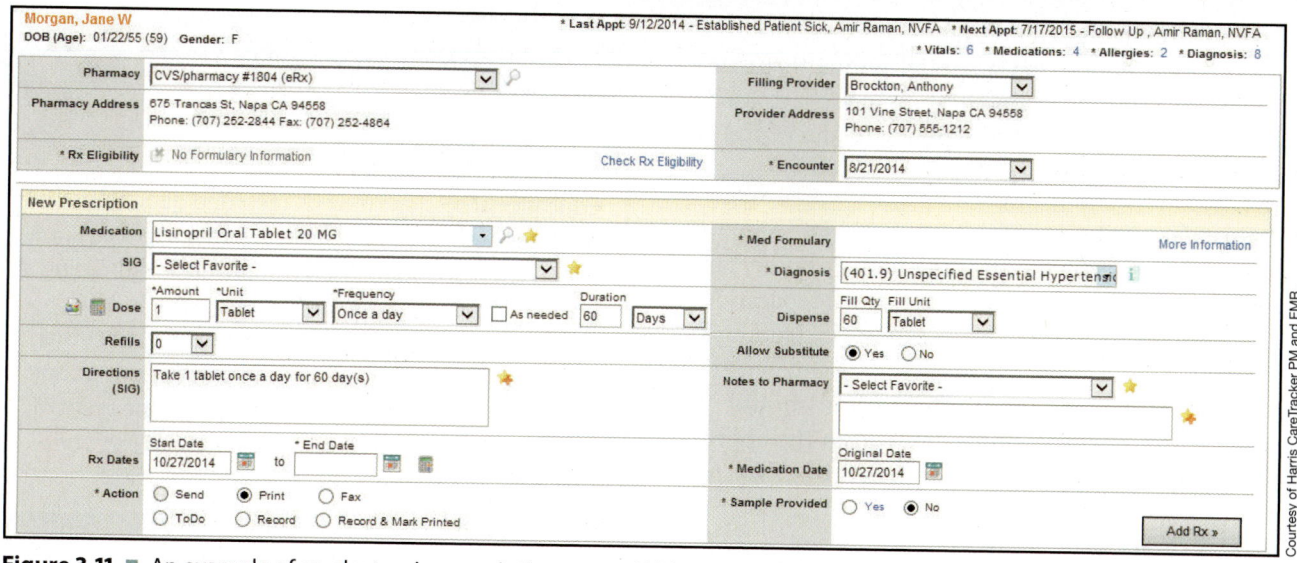

Figure 3-11 ■ An example of an electronic prescription screen. With just a few clicks, an entire prescription can be created.

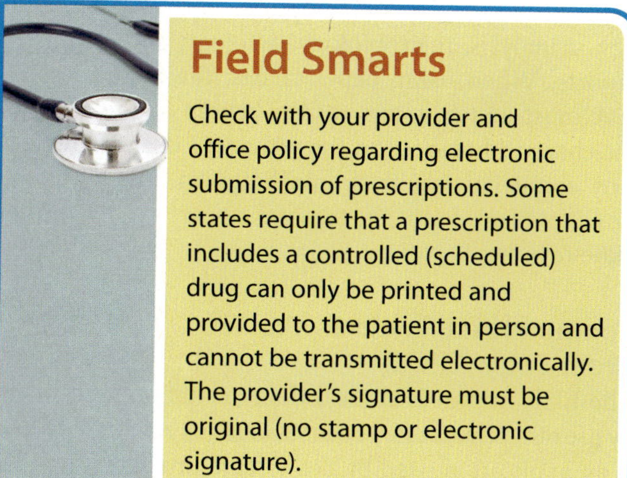

Field Smarts

Check with your provider and office policy regarding electronic submission of prescriptions. Some states require that a prescription that includes a controlled (scheduled) drug can only be printed and provided to the patient in person and cannot be transmitted electronically. The provider's signature must be original (no stamp or electronic signature).

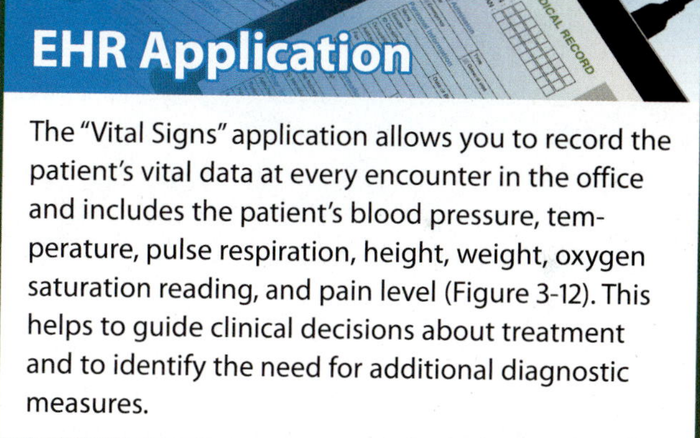

EHR Application

The "Vital Signs" application allows you to record the patient's vital data at every encounter in the office and includes the patient's blood pressure, temperature, pulse respiration, height, weight, oxygen saturation reading, and pain level (Figure 3-12). This helps to guide clinical decisions about treatment and to identify the need for additional diagnostic measures.

Courtesy of Harris CareTracker PM and EMR.

Figure 3-12 ■ Electronic vital signs.

prescription refill, the call should be recorded either on the progress note or on a special phone form and placed within a special section of the paper chart. Medical assistants should check the policy of the office in which they work for specific details.

Education Sessions

At times, it is necessary to give the patient home care instructions including postoperative, test preparation, disease management, and medication instructions. The patient should be given both verbal and written instructions with repeat back. The session should be documented on a progress note and within the appropriate logs.

Laboratory Documents

In the paper chart, all lab forms should be placed in reverse chronological order and placed in the lab section of the chart. Some offices use the **shingling** method for filing lab reports when reports are not on a standard size piece of paper. Lab reports are attached to a special shingling form that coincides with the lab reporting form. The forms may be color coded

> **EHR Application**
>
> Many EHRs have special telephone message templates that make it easy to record information. The user clicks on the telephone icon or message tab and completes the requested information by clicking on a few more tabs (Figure 3-13). A message is sent to the "Task" box of the provider instructing the provider to pull up the message. The provider may then send a message back to the medical assistant with instructions to perform a specific action.

> **EHR Application**
>
> Educational sessions may be recorded directly into the progress note or can be tracked within a special application (correspondence, education, etc.) when using electronic records. Some software programs have educational data stored directly within the electronic software. The software allows the user to print a copy of the educational data for the patient at the point of care, or to send the material to the patient electronically through a patient portal (PHR) application.

to match one another. Only like or similar reporting forms are placed on the same shingling form (e.g., all urinalysis reports and all CBC reports).

Common laboratory reports include hematology, urinalysis, microbiology, cytology, and chemistry reports. When using paper charts, the medical assistant must attach a copy of the report to the front of the chart and place it on the provider's desk for review. Any abnormal results should be given directly to the provider or placed at the top of the chart pile for immediate review.

Computerized Physician/Provider Order Entry (CPOE)

The EHR improves clinical documentation and orders by use of **Computer Physician Order Entry (CPOE)**. CPOE is an application used by health care providers to enter patient care information. Using CPOE for medication and orders will allow results to be automatically checked for potential errors or problems. CPOE entails the provider's use of computer assistance to directly enter medication orders from a computer or mobile device. The order is also documented or captured in a digital, structured,

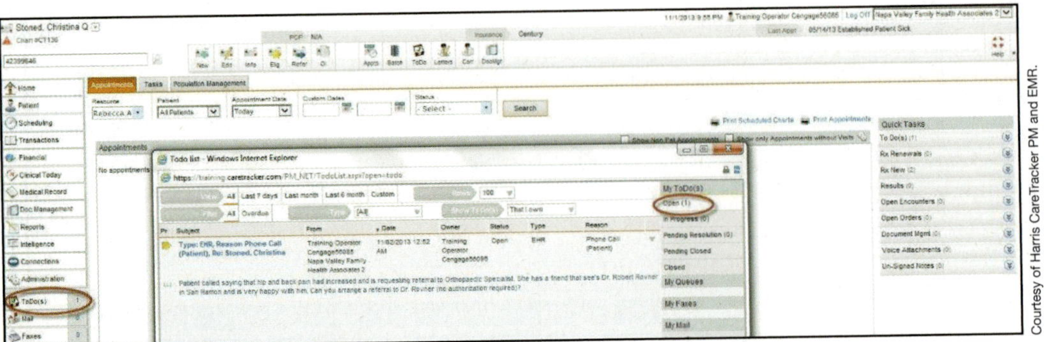

Courtesy of Harris CareTracker PM and EMR.

Figure 3-13 ■ Electronic "Tasks" tab.

and computable format for use in improving safety and organization. EHRs with the CPOE feature also provide support tools that result in improved care and patient outcomes. Use of CPOE supports Measure 1 of 13, Stage 1 of Meaningful Use.

Credentialed medical assistants are now allowed to enter medication, laboratory, and radiology orders into a CPOE, a process that was previously limited to licensed medical professionals. Providers can now delegate credentialed medical assistants to input orders electronically, thus improving workflow and efficiencies. This transfer of duties can help providers meet Meaningful Use criteria (both Stages 1 and 2).

EHR Application

Many programs feature an orders management section that allows users to order lab testing (Figures 3-14A and 3-14B). Once a test is ordered, it is stored in the patient's electronic record.

Orders placed electronically are received electronically if the lab is integrated with the practice EHR (Figure 3-15) and provides a link to the order. Alternatively, designated personnel may access the lab information by downloading it from the appropriate website and transferring it into the patient's electronic record. An electronic message is sent to the "Task" box of the ordering provider. Abnormal labs are flagged (in Figure 3-15 abnormal results appear in bold red) for immediate review. Once reports are reviewed, providers can commit the result to the electronic chart by clicking on "Sign." In addition, providers will often send a message to the medical assistant's "Task" box with instructions for handling each lab, such as notifying the patient. The medical assistant will perform the task and make an entry within the electronic chart stating that the task has been completed. There are many customizable options for displaying lab reports depending on the software used including displaying by test category, by individual test, alphabetically, and even in a graphing format. Medication levels that affect various lab results may also be displayed in a cell beside the corresponding lab result, making decisions about medication changes much easier. The medical assistant should monitor results on a continuous basis, ascertaining that results are received, reviewed, and handled in an efficient manner.

Diagnostic Reports

In the paper chart, copies of the patient's nonlab-related procedures should be placed in the diagnostic reports section of the chart. Procedures such as imaging reports, ECGs, and heart catheterizations are examples of diagnostic procedures. When using paper charts, the medical assistant must attach a copy of the report to the front of the chart and either place it on the provider's desk or hand it directly to the provider when results are abnormal.

In the EHR, reports may be received electronically in to the patient's chart (Figure 3-16), or a hard copy must be scanned into the chart.

Consultation Reports

The days of one provider treating all that ails the patient are all but gone. Providers frequently send patients to specialists for further examination. The specialist will send thank-you letters to the referring provider and will provide a report of particular findings and plans for the referral patient. When using paper charts, the medical assistant must attach a copy of the consultation report to the front of the chart before giving it to the provider. In the EHR, referrals and letters are generated and stored electronically.

Nursing Home Reports, Therapeutic Service Reports, and Hospital Reports

Other reports that may be placed under the Consultation, Miscellaneous, or Correspondence tabs include reports from nursing homes, providers of therapeutic services, and hospitals.

Nursing Home Reports

Nursing home documents are frequently faxed from nursing homes and extended care facilities. This is especially true in family practice and geriatric offices. It is very important that these documents be given to the provider prior to being filed or scanned in the patient's chart. If the office is using paper charts, the correspondence is attached to the front of the chart prior to giving it to the provider. With EHR, the information is either uploaded or scanned into the patient's electronic chart either after being reviewed by the provider or attached to an electronic message prompting the provider to review and sign.

Therapeutic Reports

Therapeutic reports may also be faxed or sent electronically from various facilities and may include reports from medical personnel, such as a physical

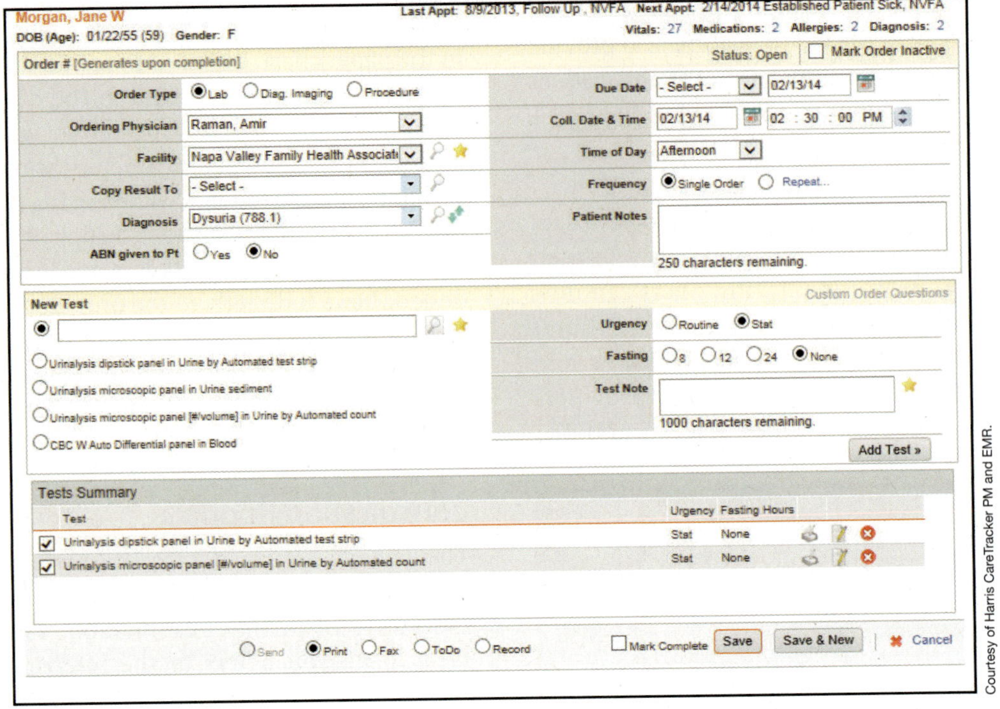

Morgan, Jane W
DOB (Age): 01/22/55 (59) Gender: F
Last Appt: 8/9/2013, Follow Up , NVFA Next Appt: 2/14/2014 Established Patient Sick, NVFA
Vitals: 27 Medications: 2 Allergies: 2 Diagnosis: 2

Order # [Generates upon completion] Status: Open Mark Order Inactive

Order Type	◉ Lab ○ Diag. Imaging ○ Procedure	Due Date	- Select - 02/13/14
Ordering Physician	Raman, Amir	Coll. Date & Time	02/13/14 02 : 30 : 00 PM
Facility	Napa Valley Family Health Associat	Time of Day	Afternoon
Copy Result To	- Select -	Frequency	◉ Single Order ○ Repeat...
Diagnosis	Dysuria (788.1)	Patient Notes	250 characters remaining.
ABN given to Pt	○ Yes ◉ No		

New Test — Custom Order Questions

○ Urinalysis dipstick panel in Urine by Automated test strip
○ Urinalysis microscopic panel in Urine sediment
○ Urinalysis microscopic panel [#/volume] in Urine by Automated count
○ CBC W Auto Differential panel in Blood

Urgency: ○ Routine ◉ Stat
Fasting: ○ 8 ○ 12 ○ 24 ◉ None
Test Note: 1000 characters remaining.
Add Test »

Tests Summary

Test	Urgency	Fasting Hours
☑ Urinalysis dipstick panel in Urine by Automated test strip	Stat	None
☑ Urinalysis microscopic panel [#/volume] in Urine by Automated count	Stat	None

○ Send ◉ Print ○ Fax ○ ToDo ○ Record ☐ Mark Complete Save Save & New Cancel

Courtesy of Harris CareTracker PM and EMR.

Figure 3-14A ■ Electronic lab order.

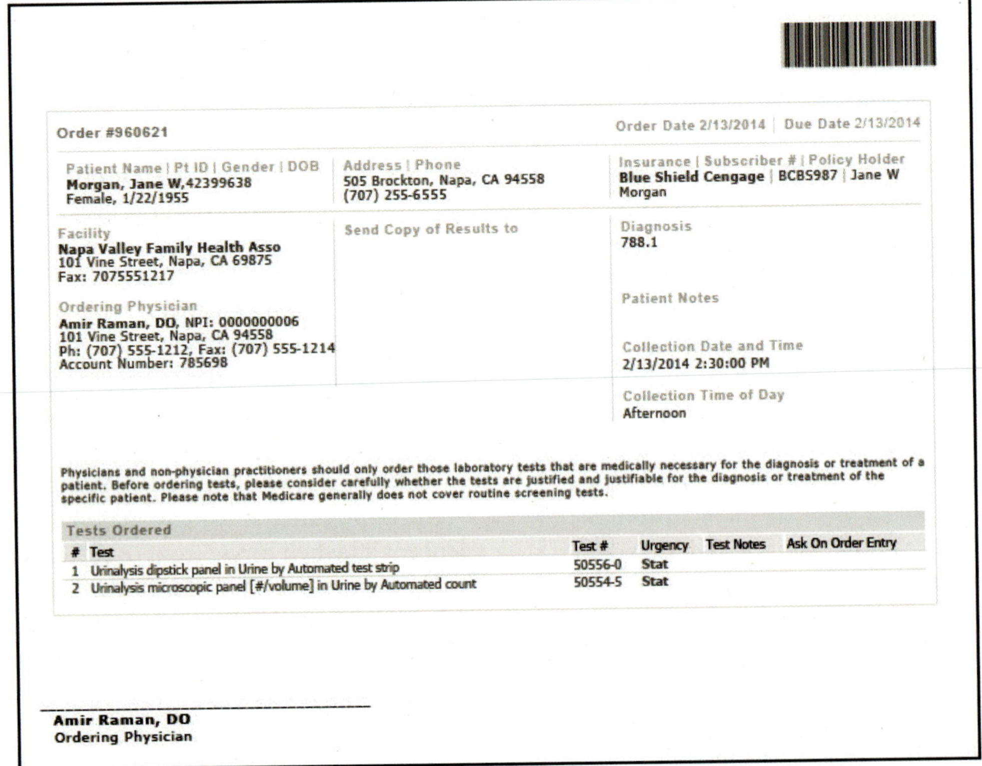

Order #960621 Order Date 2/13/2014 | Due Date 2/13/2014

Patient Name | Pt ID | Gender | DOB
Morgan, Jane W,42399638
Female, 1/22/1955

Address | Phone
505 Brockton, Napa, CA 94558
(707) 255-6555

Insurance | Subscriber # | Policy Holder
Blue Shield Cengage | BCBS987 | Jane W Morgan

Facility
Napa Valley Family Health Asso
101 Vine Street, Napa, CA 69875
Fax: 7075551217

Send Copy of Results to

Diagnosis
788.1

Ordering Physician
Amir Raman, DO, NPI: 0000000006
101 Vine Street, Napa, CA 94558
Ph: (707) 555-1212, Fax: (707) 555-1214
Account Number: 785698

Patient Notes

Collection Date and Time
2/13/2014 2:30:00 PM

Collection Time of Day
Afternoon

Physicians and non-physician practitioners should only order those laboratory tests that are medically necessary for the diagnosis or treatment of a patient. Before ordering tests, please consider carefully whether the tests are justified and justifiable for the diagnosis or treatment of the specific patient. Please note that Medicare generally does not cover routine screening tests.

Tests Ordered

#	Test	Test #	Urgency	Test Notes	Ask On Order Entry
1	Urinalysis dipstick panel in Urine by Automated test strip	50556-0	Stat		
2	Urinalysis microscopic panel [#/volume] in Urine by Automated count	50554-5	Stat		

Amir Raman, DO
Ordering Physician

Courtesy of Harris CareTracker PM and EMR.

Figure 3-14B ■ Electronic lab order completed with bar scan.

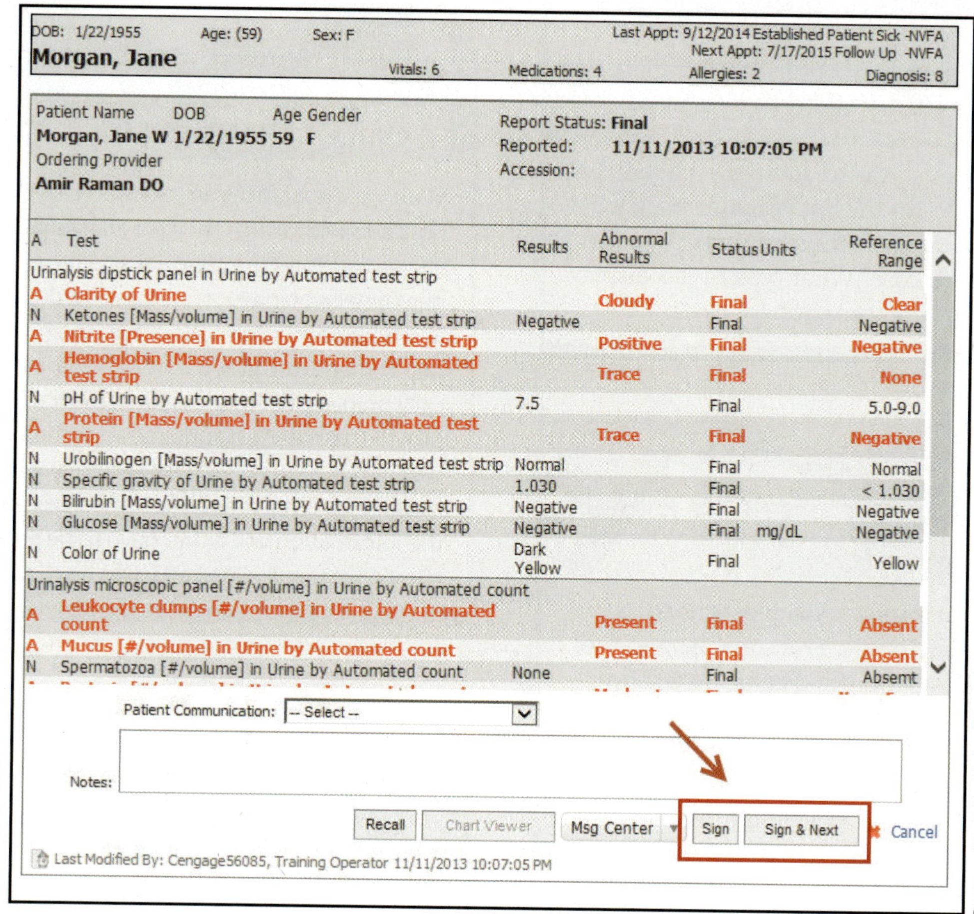

DOB: 1/22/1955 Age: (59) Sex: F
Morgan, Jane
Last Appt: 9/12/2014 Established Patient Sick -NVFA
Next Appt: 7/17/2015 Follow Up -NVFA
Vitals: 6 Medications: 4 Allergies: 2 Diagnosis: 8

Patient Name DOB Age Gender
Morgan, Jane W 1/22/1955 59 F
Ordering Provider
Amir Raman DO

Report Status: **Final**
Reported: **11/11/2013 10:07:05 PM**
Accession:

A	Test	Results	Abnormal Results	Status	Units	Reference Range
	Urinalysis dipstick panel in Urine by Automated test strip					
A	Clarity of Urine		Cloudy	Final		Clear
N	Ketones [Mass/volume] in Urine by Automated test strip	Negative		Final		Negative
A	Nitrite [Presence] in Urine by Automated test strip		Positive	Final		Negative
A	Hemoglobin [Mass/volume] in Urine by Automated test strip		Trace	Final		None
N	pH of Urine by Automated test strip	7.5		Final		5.0-9.0
A	Protein [Mass/volume] in Urine by Automated test strip		Trace	Final		Negative
N	Urobilinogen [Mass/volume] in Urine by Automated test strip	Normal		Final		Normal
N	Specific gravity of Urine by Automated test strip	1.030		Final		< 1.030
N	Bilirubin [Mass/volume] in Urine by Automated test strip	Negative		Final		Negative
N	Glucose [Mass/volume] in Urine by Automated test strip	Negative		Final	mg/dL	Negative
N	Color of Urine	Dark Yellow		Final		Yellow
	Urinalysis microscopic panel [#/volume] in Urine by Automated count					
A	Leukocyte clumps [#/volume] in Urine by Automated count		Present	Final		Absent
A	Mucus [#/volume] in Urine by Automated count		Present	Final		Absent
N	Spermatozoa [#/volume] in Urine by Automated count	None		Final		Absemt

Patient Communication: -- Select --
Notes:
Recall | Chart Viewer | Msg Center | Sign | Sign & Next | Cancel
Last Modified By: Cengage56085, Training Operator 11/11/2013 10:07:05 PM

Courtesy of Harris CareTracker PM and EMR.

Figure 3-15 ■ Electronic lab results.

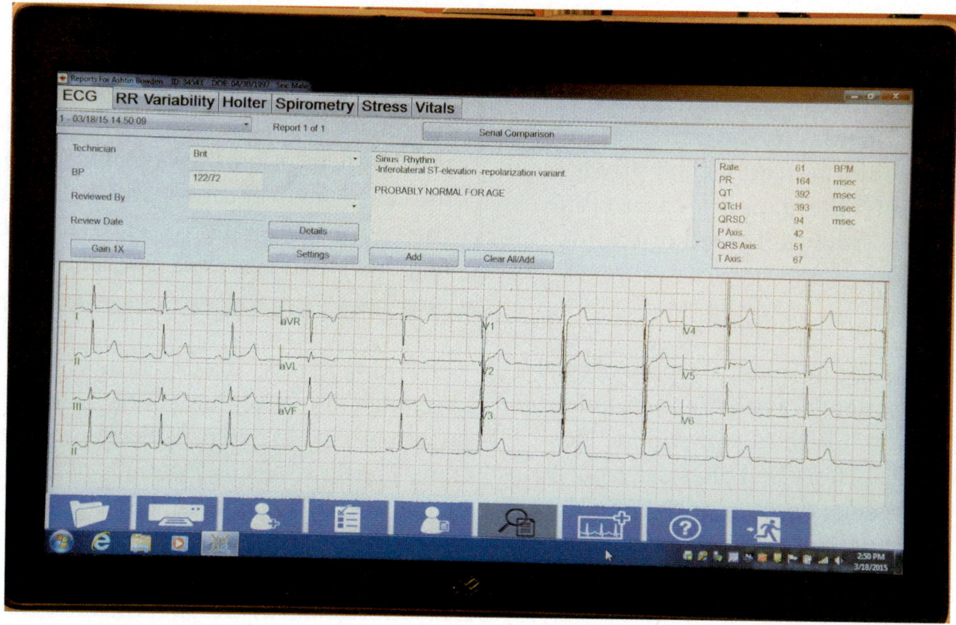

Figure 3-16 ■ Electronic ECG.

CRITICAL THINKING CHALLENGE

The provider wants you to show the patient his blood sugar results for the last year and track what medications appear to be most responsive to lowering his blood glucose. What type of lab display would be best for this scenario?

EHR Application

The procedure for inserting diagnostic reports will vary depending on the EHR software and the electronic capabilities of the diagnostic testing center. If there is a direct link between the two, the reports are handled similarly to the way that lab tests are handled; otherwise the results are scanned directly into the EHR. In-house digital diagnostic equipment may link directly to the EHR software. Once the test is performed, the medical assistant is able upload the results electronically into the patient's electronic record for the provider to review and "sign" (commit to the electronic chart).

or occupational therapist, who provide rehabilitative or therapeutic treatments for the patient. Once again, these reports should be read by the provider before they are filed into the patient's chart. With EHR, the information is either uploaded or scanned into the patient's EHR.

Hospital Reports

Any time a patient visits the hospital, a report of that visit will be sent to the patient's primary care provider (PCP) and other pertinent health care providers. Hospital reports may include history and physical reports, operative reports, emergency room reports, and discharge summaries. Most patients will be instructed to follow up with their PCP once they leave the hospital.

Flow Sheets

Flow sheets are logs found in the patient's chart that assist the provider in monitoring specific repetitive information, at one glance. These may also be referred to as "health care screenings." Types of flow sheets include PT/INR results, glucose or HgbA1c results, blood pressure readings, and more. The flow sheet is especially useful for patients who are diabetic, on Coumadin therapy, or hypertensive. Any time a patient has a test or procedure performed that is listed on the flow sheet, it should be documented onto the flow sheet as well as the lab form. Flow sheets may also be used to track routine health screenings such as mammograms, pap smears, and PSA levels. Figure 3-18A shows an example of an electronic flow sheet and Figure 3-18B represents a flow sheet in a paper chart.

EHR Application

Many medical offices are electronically linked to hospitals with which they are affiliated. This type of affiliation allows the provider and other health care personnel who have special pass codes to explore and download information from the hospital's various department websites or the information is automatically uploaded in to the patient's electronic chart. The provider can track diagnostic and laboratory tests as well as the status of patients who have been hospitalized. If a hospital opts to fax reports to the provider, the information will either have to be scanned into the chart or manually entered using a special template.

EHR Application

Electronic exchange of information makes it much easier for providers to communicate with one another. When using EHR, referral letters, thank-you letters, and consultation reports can be sent electronically between the primary care provider and specialist. A clinical summary (Figure 3-17) that displays the patient's problem list, medication list, allergy list, and family history is usually sent to the consultant at the time the referral is made. Once reports are received, they are uploaded and saved in the consultation or correspondence section of the chart. An electronic task is sent to the provider referring them to the patient's chart and report.

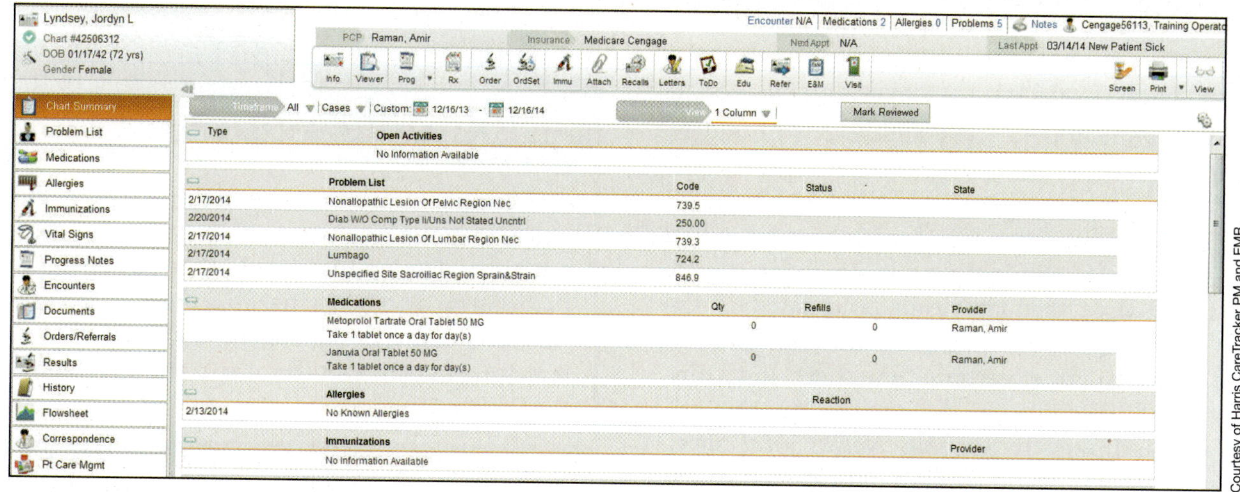

Courtesy of Harris CareTracker PM and EMR.

Figure 3-17 ■ Electronic Chart Summary.

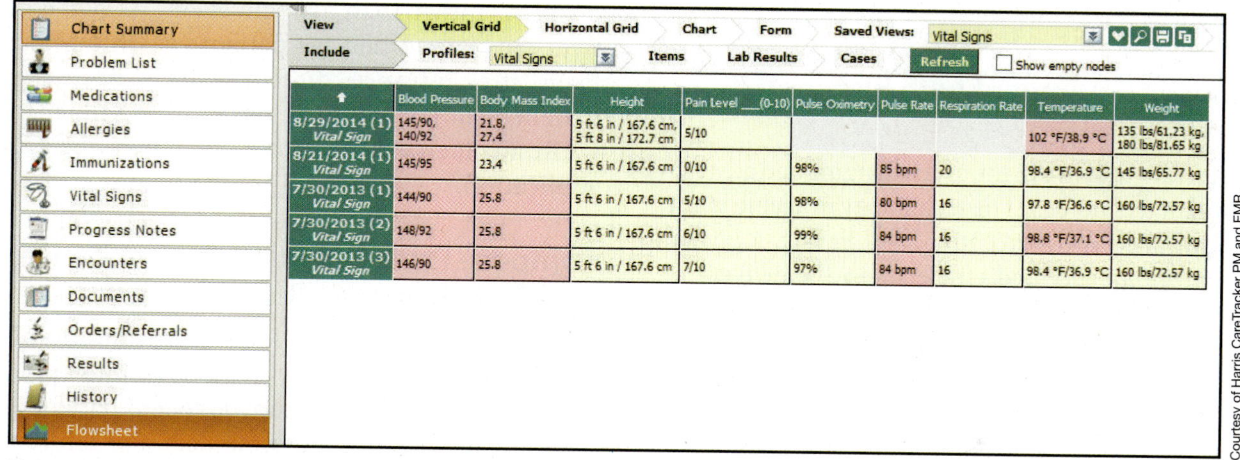

Courtesy of Harris CareTracker PM and EMR.

Figure 3-18A ■ Electronic vital signs flow sheet.

DOUGLASVILLE MEDICINE ASSOCIATES
5076 BRAND BLVD
DOUGLASVILLE, NY 01234
(123) 456-7890

HgbA1c FLOW SHEET

Patient's Name: Cindy McDonald **Patient's Birth Date: 03/17/1967**

Patient's ID # 45687 **Provider's Name: Dr. Laura Samoni**

Date of Test	Result	Current Med	Current Dosage	Recommended Change in Dose (If any)	Provider Making the Change
10/10/XX	6.8	*Avandia* *Triglide*	*8 mg* *160 mg*	*None* *None*	
03/16/XX	8.2	*Avandia* *Triglide*	*4 mg* *160 mg*	*8 mg* *None*	*Dr. Samoni*
09/19/XX	7.0	*Avandia* *Triglide*	*4 mg* *160 mg*	*None* *None*	
03/20/XX	6.6	*Avandia* *Triglide*	*4 mg* *160 mg*	*None* *None*	
08/29/XX	6.8	*Avandia* *Triglide*	*4 mg* *160 mg*	*None* *None*	

Figure 3-18B ■ A flow sheet in a paper chart.

Flow Sheets (Analyze Healthcare Results as Reported in Graphs)

The *Flow Sheet* application provides electronic management of clinical data entry and review of patient progress over time using different flow sheet templates. A flow sheet template is a profile with selected items. Data in a patient medical record can be pulled into a flow sheet, eliminating the need for double entry. Every time that lab result is updated in the patient's lab file, the test name, result, and date will also be added to the electronic flow sheet. It accommodates multidisciplinary documentation requirements and is linked to *Progress Notes, Vital Signs*, and the *Results* applications. The application displays patient information that includes lab results, medications, vitals, and other medical data in a table or graph view (Figure 3-19).

Diagnostic Equipment with Bluetooth® Capabilities

We are fortunate to live in the ever-changing and advancing world of technology. The technology available in the health care field is no exception, and in fact, a pivotal change in the quality and efficiency in the delivery of health care. Bluetooth® Smart technology is a wireless communication system that replaces the need for cable connecting many types of devices such as mobile phones, headsets, heart monitors, and other medical equipment. Refer to Figure 3-16, which represents some of the latest electronic technology available.

Living Will (Advance Directives)

Advance directives are the legal documents, such as the living will, durable power of attorney, and health care proxy that allow people to convey their decisions about end-of-life care ahead of time. Advance directives provide a way for patients to communicate their wishes to family, friends, and health care professionals and to avoid confusion later on, should they become unable to do so. Ideally, the process of discussing and writing advance directives should be ongoing, rather than a single event. Advance directives can be modified as a patient's situation changes. Even after advance directives have been signed, patients can change their mind at any time. In the EHR, advance directives are entered in the *History* application.

EHR Application

EHR flow sheets work well not only because of their ability to group results but also because they can automatically alert the provider when a patient is past due for a particular health screening. The user just clicks on the designated button and a message comes up that informs the user of any screenings the patient is behind on.

Compose Professional Correspondence Utilizing Electronic Technology

In an EHR the *Letter* application provides the ability to use letter templates to create letters for patients. You can include the company logo and patient information, such as progress note data and lab reports, in the letter. You can utilize the editor that is similar to other desktop editors like MS Word® to format and edit each letter. After creating the letter, you can save, print, or attach the letter to a message, mail, or fax. The *Correspondence* application displays any correspondence your practice has had with the patient in context and with another provider regarding the patient. This includes items such as messages, emails, phone calls, letters pertaining to the patient, and patient education material given to the patient. This helps keep track of all communications associated with the patient in a central location.

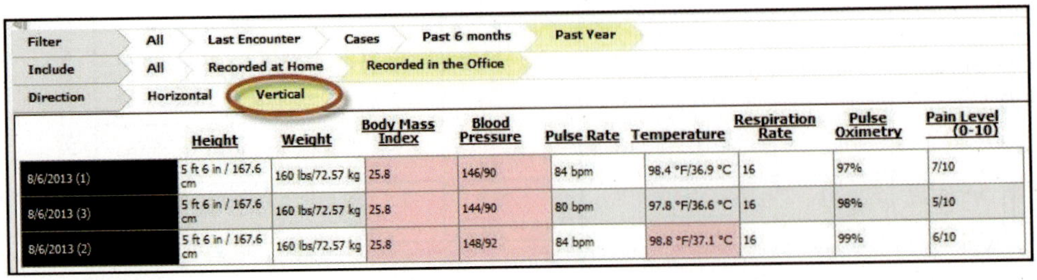

Filter: All | Last Encounter | Cases | Past 6 months | Past Year
Include: All | Recorded at Home | Recorded in the Office
Direction: Horizontal | Vertical

	Height	Weight	Body Mass Index	Blood Pressure	Pulse Rate	Temperature	Respiration Rate	Pulse Oximetry	Pain Level (0-10)
8/6/2013 (1)	5 ft 6 in / 167.6 cm	160 lbs/72.57 kg	25.8	146/90	84 bpm	98.4 °F/36.9 °C	16	97%	7/10
8/6/2013 (3)	5 ft 6 in / 167.6 cm	160 lbs/72.57 kg	25.8	144/90	80 bpm	97.8 °F/36.6 °C	16	98%	5/10
8/6/2013 (2)	5 ft 6 in / 167.6 cm	160 lbs/72.57 kg	25.8	148/92	84 bpm	98.8 °F/37.1 °C	16	99%	6/10

Courtesy of Harris CareTracker PM and EMR.

Figure 3-19 ■ Flow Sheets example.

EHR RESPONSIBILITIES FOR THE MEDICAL ASSISTANT

Your responsibilities as an electronic health record specialist will consist of a wide variety of duties. You will be responsible for documenting patient's health information, medical history, symptoms, examination and test results, treatments, and other information. Duties will vary according to the size of the facility and the type of practice (specialist or general). Typical responsibilities include:

- Assembling patient's health information to ensure information is complete and accurate
- Entering data, such as demographics, history and extent of disease, diagnostic procedures and treatment into computer
- Statistical and data analysis for quality improvement measures
- Assisting with special studies and research for public health agencies
- Compiling medical care and census data for statistical reports on diseases treated, surgery performed, and use of hospital beds for clinical audits
- Managing data backup and retention of records as well as maintaining a variety of health record indexes, storage, and retrieval systems
- Working National Database Registries as a registrar and contacting discharged patients, their families, and providers to maintain registry with follow-up information, such as quality of life and length of survival of cancer patients
- Working with department managers to review policies and develop new workflows for EHR, coordinating training resources, and providing ongoing end-user training
- Assisting with the daily operations of the office; duties such as answering the phone, inputting notes from the patient's charts, scheduling appointments, and general reception area duties

(*Source*: CEHRS™ Exam)

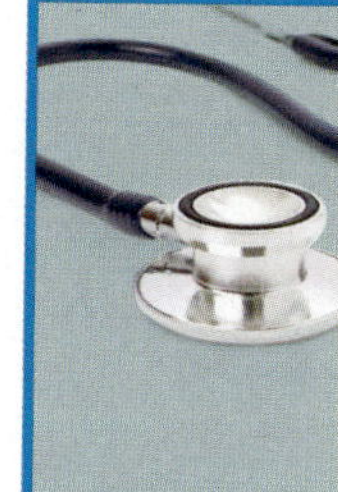

Field Smarts

Viewing the electronic "Tasks" list helps you to efficiently manage routine tasks occurring throughout the practice and provide improved patient services. To leave at your regularly scheduled time each day, it is vital that you work on tasks between patients. Tasks usually require two to three steps (reviewing the task, alerting the provider, and following up with the patient when applicable). Keep yourself and your provider on course to manage outstanding tasks.

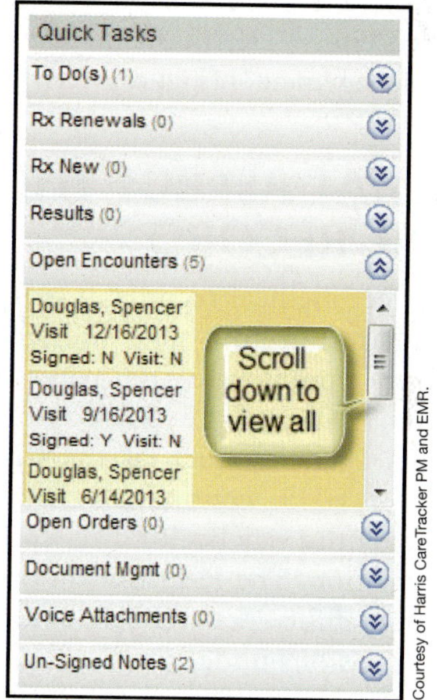

Figure 3-20 ■ Electronic "Tasks" application provides an integrated view of all open and active tasks that require attention.

Checking Electronic Tasks

Throughout the day, medical assistants must effectively manage time and keep current with tasks. As referred to earlier in the chapter, you may view tasks in a "Task" Tab/Module (refer to Figure 3-13), or a "Quick Tasks" Pane (Figure 3-20). The "Tasks" menu displays an up-to-date number of any outstanding activities, such as lab results pending review, incomplete encounters, and documents pending review. The "Tasks" application provides an integrated view of all open and active tasks that require attention.

Checking Clinical Today or Equivalent in Another EHR

The clinical medical assistant will complete most of his or her activities in a "Clinical Today" or equivalent module in an EHR. In addition to the "Tasks" tab, there is usually an "Appointments" tab (which displays patient appointments within the date range entered)

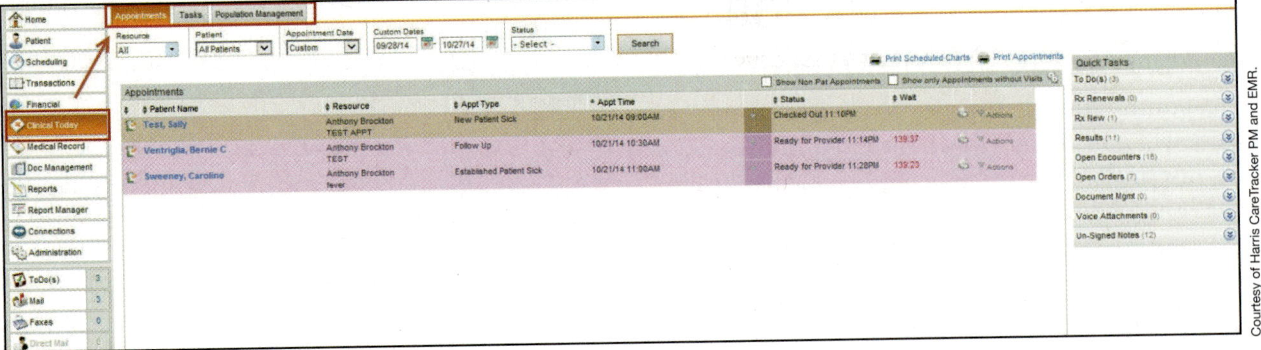

Courtesy of Harris CareTracker PM and EMR.

Figure 3-21A ■ Appointments in "Clinical Today".

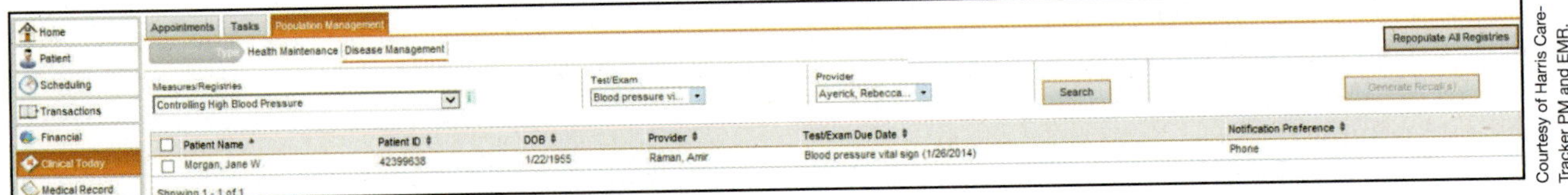

Courtesy of Harris CareTracker PM and EMR.

Figure 3-21B ■ Population Management tab in "Clinical Today" module.

(Figure 3-21A), and a "Population Management" tab (which displays either "Health Maintenance" measures or "Disease Management") (Figure 3-21B).

LAWS THAT AFFECT THE MEDICAL RECORD

Many laws affect medical records. It is important to become familiar with both state and federal guidelines to ensure compliance and avoid noncompliance penalties related to the violation of such laws. Governmental agencies, such as the CMS and the Department of HHS, continuously make changes that may impact the way health care workers handle patient information. The Health Insurance Portability and Accountability Act (HIPAA) and subsequent privacy rule revisions under the Health Information Technology for Economic and Clinical Health Act (HITECH) changed how covered entities approach a patient's right to access and amend protected health information (PHI). Generally, all consumers now have the ability to view, copy, and amend information collected and maintained about them.

HITECH Act

The **Health Information Technology for Economic and Clinical Health (HITECH) Act** was signed into law on February 17, 2009, to promote the adoption and meaningful use of health information technology. HITECH was enacted as part of the **American Recovery and Reinvestment Act (ARRA)**, also known as the "stimulus bill." HITECH provides the Department of Health and Human Services (HHS) with the authority to establish programs to improve health care quality through the promotion of Health Information Technology (HIT). Components of HITECH are promoted through incentives paid to providers for complying with the act. In future years, providers will face penalties through payment reductions for noncompliance of the bill. HITECH created additional provisions that:

- Give consumers the right to request electronic access to their health information (with a few exceptions noted)
- Expand the accounting of disclosure requirements to include treatment, payment, and operations
- Require the federal government to provide covered entities with greater guidance on the HIPAA minimum necessary requirements

The Health Insurance Portability and Accountability Act of 1996 (HIPAA)

In 1996, Congress passed the Health Insurance Portability and Accountability Act, also known as HIPAA. HIPAA as written was to ensure that an employee leaving his or her job could take at least some insurance coverage with him or her. At the same time, Congress addressed the growing concern about the erosion of patient privacy (Freudenheim, 1991).

There are two reasons the question of confidentiality of records is so important: First, sometimes there is a legitimate public interest in having records released, perhaps even over the patient's objection. The second purpose is to protect the individual's interest in making an informed, independent decision regarding his or her care and not being forced to accept a predetermined course of action.

HIPAA is divided into the Privacy Rule (Title I) and the Security Rule (Title II). To assure the accountability of those who have access to the patient's private health information (known as **protected health information (PHI)** or **individually identifiable health information (IIHI)**, Congress requires the imposition of civil and criminal penalties for any person or entity that uses PHI improperly. Patients should receive a **Notice of Privacy Practices (NPP)** of how their personal medical information may be used. This will be expanded upon below.

The **HIPAA Privacy Rule** provides federal protections for personal health information held by covered entities and gives patients an array of rights with respect to that information. At the same time, the Privacy Rule is balanced so that it permits the disclosure of personal health information needed for patient care and other important purposes (Summary of the HIPAA Privacy Rule, Department of Health & Human Services, 2014).

The **HIPAA Security Rule** establishes national standards to protect individuals' electronic personal health information that is created, received, used, or maintained by a covered entity. The Security Rule requires appropriate administrative, physical, and technical safeguards to ensure the confidentiality, integrity, and security of electronic protected health information (Department of Health & Human Services, 2014).

Confidentiality issues are serious. Unauthorized access to medical information can affect the patient's employment status, family life, and personal relationships. Accessing patient records without cause may result in termination from employment. Many health care facilities have software that can track where employees have accessed patient records and identify who is adding or changing information in the medical record. This is referred to as an "audit trail" and is a vital component toward maintaining patient confidentiality. Because of the sensitivity and confidentiality issues related to patient information, it is crucial for all providers and staff to avoid situations in which personal integrity can be challenged. Table 3-2 represents good privacy practices and practices to avoid pertaining to HIPAA.

With the rules and regulations constantly evolving, it is wise to visit the CMS and HHS websites to view the most current rules.

Meaningful Use

Meaningful use is the set of standards defined by CMS incentive programs that governs the use of EHRs and allows eligible providers and hospitals to earn incentive payments by meeting specific criteria. For EHR software to be certified, it must meet meaningful use. Stage 1 and Stage 2 requirements are listed in Appendix A.

Table 3-2 Good Privacy Practices and Practices to Avoid

Good Privacy Practices	Practices to Avoid
Only access a patient's file when it is absolutely necessary.	Never access a patient's file because a friend or relative wants to find out information about the patient.
When sending information about a patient to a covered entity, only send the minimal amount of information that is necessary to handle the request.	Never send more information than what is necessary.
Turn computer monitors away from patients, or keep them out of the patient's sight, or utilize screen protectors.	Do not allow computer monitors to display patient files in areas where the patients are in viewing range. (If using electronic records in the patient exam rooms, be certain all information from the previous patient has been cleared before bringing in a new patient.)
Use sign-in sheets that require minimal information to acknowledge the patient's arrival and the time of arrival or have patients sign in via computer.	Sign-in sheets should not ask patient to list any changes since the last visit, such as changes in insurance or other demographic information.
Talk to the patient in private regarding billing or health-related information.	Do not discuss private information about or with a patient in an area where others can hear what you are discussing.
Allow the patient access to the patient's medical record and the ability to review and request changes within 30 days of request.	Do not forbid the patient access to the patient's medical record. Remember the patient is the owner of the information stored in the chart.
Only discuss parts of the patient's record or health status with those individuals who have the authority to receive the information.	Do not discuss parts of the patient's record with anyone other than the patient or those listed in the privacy statement. Do not discuss PHI with members of the health care team, unless it is absolutely necessary in order for them to carry out the duties of their job.
In the event of an emergency, provide the minimal amount of information that is necessary to handle that emergency.	Do not communicate more information than is absolutely necessary to handle an emergency. Keep voices low to ensure privacy.
Respect the patient's right to privacy away from the office.	Do not tell friends or family members that a particular patient was in for an appointment. Even if you do not disclose the reason for the visit, it is a violation of HIPAA rules.

CRITICAL THINKING CHALLENGE

Mr. Walker calls the office and states that he heard a message on his answering machine that his wife needed to call the office. He states that his wife is out of town and asks you to give the information to him.

1. Are you allowed to release the information to the husband?
2. Where in the chart can you find out if you can release the information?
3. If after checking the documentation in the chart you find that you can release the information to the husband, how much information should you release?

Figures 3-22A and 3-22B illustate the Meaningful Use Dashboard in an EHR. Figure 3-22A shows the Core Requirements and Figure 3-22B represents the Menu Item Tab. These standards ensure that providers are using their EHR software to its fullest potential, promoting accuracy, access, patient empowerment, and better coordination of care. These incentives specify three components of meaningful use:

- The use of a certified EHR in a meaningful manner
- The use of certified EHR technology for electronic exchange of health information to improve quality of health care
- The use of certified EHR technology to submit clinical quality and other measures

Benefits of meaningful use include complete and accurate medical records, better access to information, and patient empowerment. One of the major goals of meaningful use is to make medical records interoperable so that immediate access can be given to any provider who works with the patient. There are three stages associated with meaningful use.

Stage 1: Data Capture and Sharing Stage

In August 2014 CMS released its final rule for Stage 1 requirements. This stage focuses on the following:

- Electronic capturing of health information in a coded format
- Using electronically captured health information to track key clinical conditions and communicate information for care coordination purposes
- Implementing clinical decision support tools to facilitate disease and medication management
- Reporting information for quality improvement and public health information

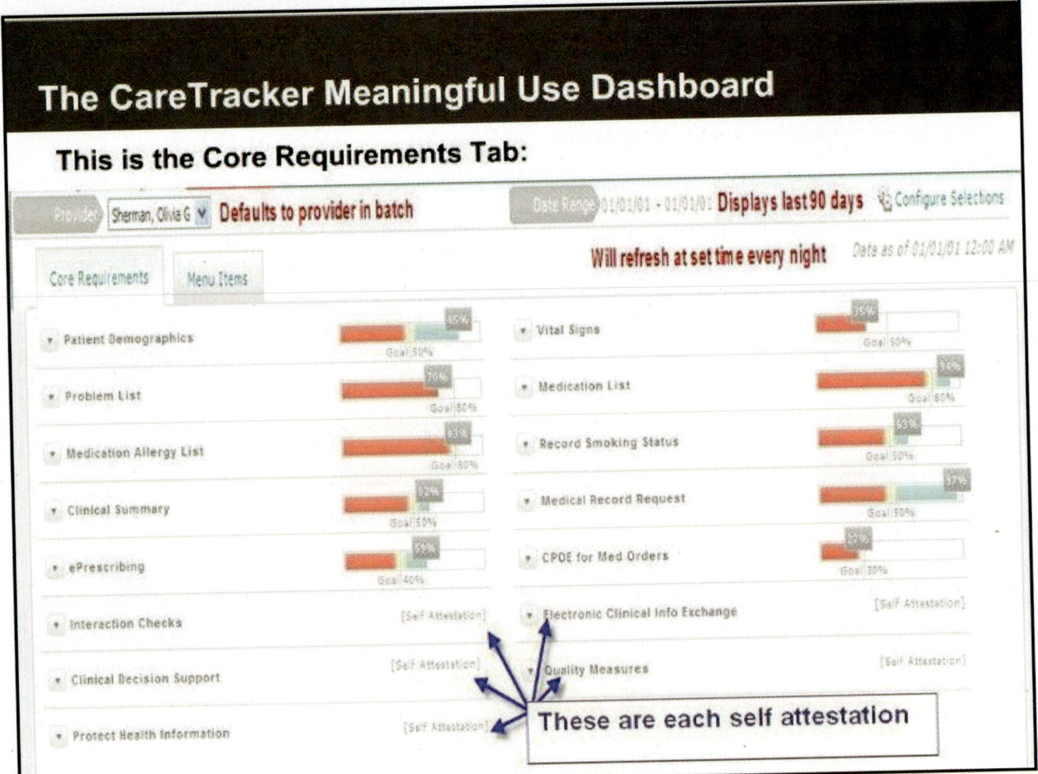

Figure 3-22A ■ Example of Stage 1 Meaningful Use Core Requirements.

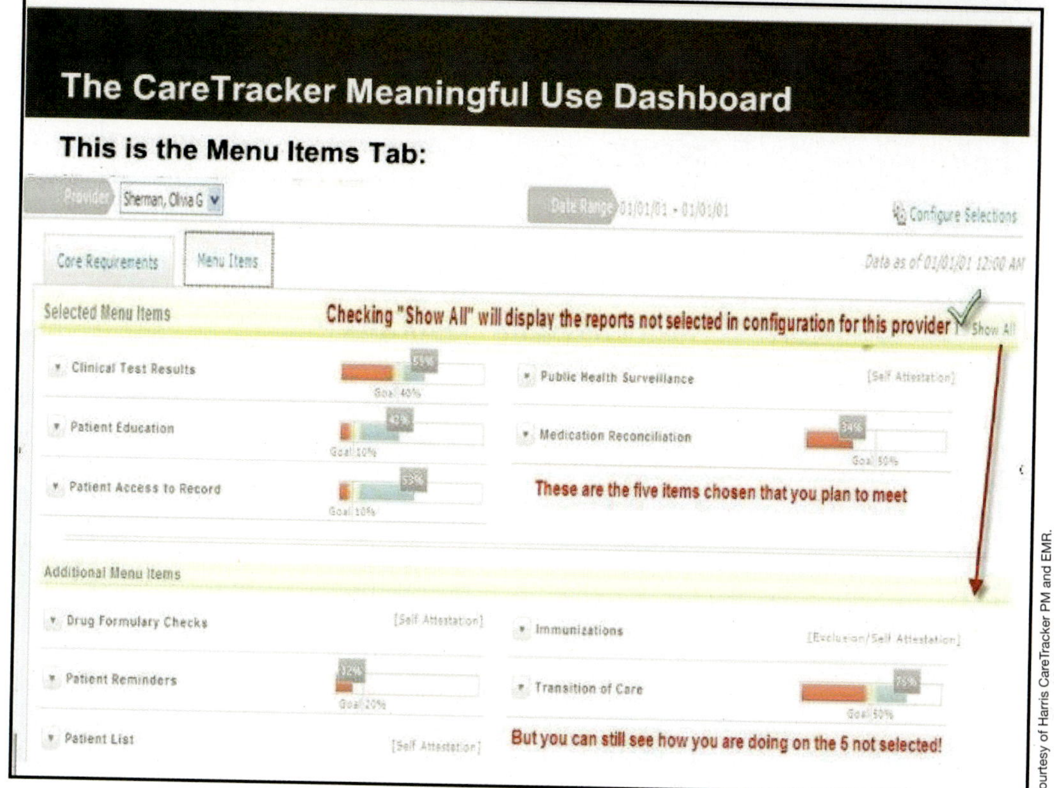

Figure 3-22B ■ Example of Stage 1 Meaningful Use Menu Items.

Courtesy of Harris CareTracker PM and EMR.

There are two sets of objectives that must be met to prove attestation for this stage: core and menu. All of the core objectives are required; however, eligible providers may choose which menu set objectives to follow. Eligible professionals (EPs) must be credentialed with Medicare and may be a doctor of medicine or osteopathy, doctor of dental surgery or medicine, doctor of podiatric medicine, doctor of optometry, or a chiropractor. Medicaid EPs include physicians, dentists, certified nurse-midwives, nurse practitioners, and physician assistants. Providers in the health care setting can only apply for attestation with either Medicare or Medicaid but not both.

Meaningful Use Criteria for Eligible Professionals

Meaningful use criteria require providers to meet 13 core objectives, 5 menu objectives from a list of 9, for a total of 18 objectives. EPs are required to report the following clinical quality measures (CQMs) using a certified EHR during each year of participation in order to receive an incentive: health outcomes, clinical processes, patient safety, efficient use of health care resources, care coordination, patient engagements, population and public health, and adherence to clinical guidelines. Figure 3-23 is an example of Quality Measures in an electronic progress note.

Refer to Appendix A for tables that illustrate what is included in the eligible professional meaningful use core and menu set objectives (Stage 1 [2013 definition] last updated July 2014). Visit the CMS website (www.cms.gov) and search "meaningful use" to obtain the most current information available.

Stage 2: Advance Clinical Processes

This stage focuses on expanding on Stage 1 criteria to encourage the use of HIT for continuous quality improvement at the point of care and the exchange of health information in the most structured format possible. Criteria for Stage 2 include:

- More rigorous health information exchange (HIE)
- Increased requirements for e-prescribing and incorporating lab results
- Electronic transmission of patient care summaries across multiple settings
- More patient-controlled data

The final rule for Stage 2 was released in October 2012. Compliance with Stage 2 has been extended until 2016 as proposed by CMS. In Stage 2, eligible providers must meet 17 core objectives and 3 of 6 menu objectives. In Appendix A you will find figures that illustrate the objectives for Stage 2 meaningful use.

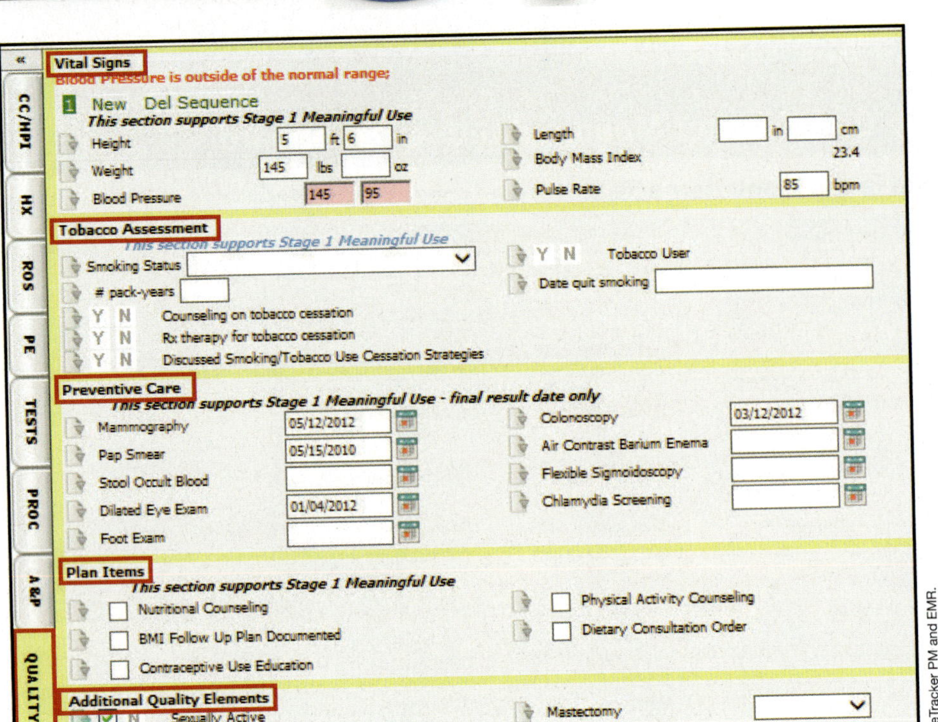

Courtesy of Harris CareTracker PM and EMR.

Figure 3-23 ■ Electronic Quality Measures tab.

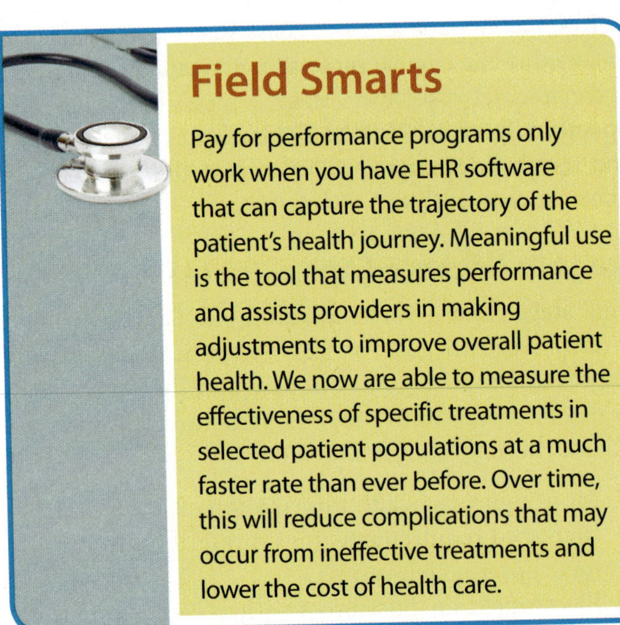

Field Smarts

Pay for performance programs only work when you have EHR software that can capture the trajectory of the patient's health journey. Meaningful use is the tool that measures performance and assists providers in making adjustments to improve overall patient health. We now are able to measure the effectiveness of specific treatments in selected patient populations at a much faster rate than ever before. Over time, this will reduce complications that may occur from ineffective treatments and lower the cost of health care.

Stage 3: Improved Outcomes

This stage focuses on the following:

- Promoting improvements in quality, safety, and efficiency
- Clinical decision support for national high-priority conditions
- Patient access to self-management tools
- Access to comprehensive patient data through patient-centered HIE
- Improving population health

Stage 3 is expected to be implemented in 2017.

SHARING PROTECTED INFORMATION WITH OTHER HEALTH CARE PROFESSIONALS

Rules relating to the ownership, retention, and disposal of medical records can vary by state.

In general, medical records are the property of the practice or treating provider or hospital. The practice or provider owns the physical part of the record, but the patient is the owner of the information stored within the chart. Patients are entitled access to their medical records and may request copies of it.

Fees Associated with Copying of Medical Records

"Reasonable fees" for copying a patient's medical records will usually be dictated by state statutes. In most cases, the practice can charge fees for retrieving, copying, and mailing the medical record. Check each state's policies for specific details.

Retention of Medical Records

Federal and state guidelines for retention of medical records will vary depending upon the type of record. In general, adult records should be retained for 7 to 10 years and records of minors should be retained several years past the age of majority. Check the state and federal laws that apply to the practice. It is prudent to follow the guidelines of the agencies that have the most stringent standards.

If a practice decides to cease operations or providers within the practice plan to change locations, the practice should notify patients to determine how their records should be handled. Each patient should be consulted to determine if records should be transferred to another location of the patient's choice, or if they should be moved with the transferring provider. If neither occurs, the patient should be alerted to where the records are being stored in case the information is needed by the patient at a later date.

Disposal of Medical Records

Occasionally, the medical record itself or parts of the medical record need to be discarded. Privacy laws state that PHI disposal must occur by shredding the documents; therefore, a shredder should always be used when disposing of information from a patient's medical record. Many businesses hire a shredding company to perform their shredding. In that case, the medical facility must select a reliable vendor that has thorough knowledge of HIPAA guidelines and should have the company sign a **business associate agreement** that states that the records are not to be used for any other purpose but for shredding and that the company is to provide a certificate of destruction once the task has been performed.

Confidentiality

Throughout this chapter we have discussed the need for and rules regarding confidentiality of the medical record and the various laws (HIPAA Privacy Rule and HIPAA Security Rule) and the HITECH Act that govern electronic transmission of records. A major goal of the Privacy Rule as outlined by the Department of HHS is to assure that individuals' health information is properly protected while allowing the flow of health information needed to provide and promote high-quality health care and to protect the public's health and well-being. The rule strikes a balance that permits important uses of information, while protecting the privacy of people who seek care and healing. Given that the health care marketplace is diverse, the rule is designed to be flexible and comprehensive to cover the variety of uses and disclosures that need to be addressed.

The HIPAA Security Rule establishes national standards to protect individuals' electronic personal health information that is created, received, used, or maintained by a covered entity. The Security Rule requires appropriate administrative, physical, and technical safeguards to ensure the confidentiality, integrity, and security of electronic protected health information.

Electronic Access Audit/Activity Log

The *Operator Audit Log* maintains an audit trail of all actions performed in an EHR by each operator (Figure 3-24). This log is helpful to monitor each operator's usage. The audit log can be customized by operator, activity type, and date range. Regardless of the filters you set, the operator log always includes the date, time, operator's log-in identification (ID), operator's name, the name of the patient whose record was accessed, the group in which the action was taken, and a comment (the action performed). The *Operators Log* (a different report) tracks the number of operators who log in to the EHR each day. The log can be viewed for the current month or for a specific time period.

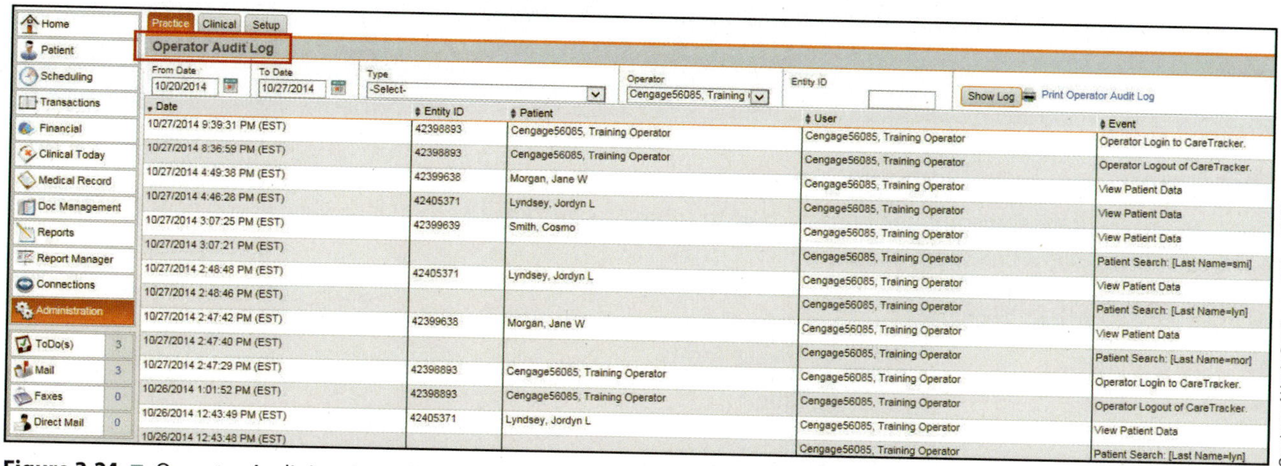

Home
Patient
Scheduling
Transactions
Financial
Clinical Today
Medical Record
Doc Management
Reports
Report Manager
Connections
Administration
ToDo(s) 3
Mail 3
Faxes 0
Direct Mail 0

Practice | Clinical | Setup

Operator Audit Log

From Date 10/20/2014 | To Date 10/27/2014 | Type -Select- | Operator Cengage56085, Training | Entity ID | Show Log | Print Operator Audit Log

Date	Entity ID	Patient	User	Event
10/27/2014 9:39:31 PM (EST)	42398893	Cengage56085, Training Operator	Cengage56085, Training Operator	Operator Login to CareTracker.
10/27/2014 8:36:59 PM (EST)	42398893	Cengage56085, Training Operator	Cengage56085, Training Operator	Operator Logout of CareTracker.
10/27/2014 4:49:38 PM (EST)	42399638	Morgan, Jane W	Cengage56085, Training Operator	View Patient Data
10/27/2014 4:46:28 PM (EST)	42405371	Lyndsey, Jordyn L	Cengage56085, Training Operator	View Patient Data
10/27/2014 3:07:25 PM (EST)	42399639	Smith, Cosmo	Cengage56085, Training Operator	View Patient Data
10/27/2014 3:07:21 PM (EST)			Cengage56085, Training Operator	Patient Search: [Last Name=smi]
10/27/2014 2:48:48 PM (EST)	42405371	Lyndsey, Jordyn L	Cengage56085, Training Operator	View Patient Data
10/27/2014 2:48:46 PM (EST)			Cengage56085, Training Operator	Patient Search: [Last Name=lyn]
10/27/2014 2:47:42 PM (EST)	42399638	Morgan, Jane W	Cengage56085, Training Operator	View Patient Data
10/27/2014 2:47:40 PM (EST)			Cengage56085, Training Operator	Patient Search: [Last Name=mor]
10/27/2014 2:47:29 PM (EST)	42398893	Cengage56085, Training Operator	Cengage56085, Training Operator	Operator Login to CareTracker.
10/26/2014 1:01:52 PM (EST)	42398893	Cengage56085, Training Operator	Cengage56085, Training Operator	Operator Logout of CareTracker.
10/26/2014 12:43:49 PM (EST)	42405371	Lyndsey, Jordyn L	Cengage56085, Training Operator	View Patient Data
10/26/2014 12:43:48 PM (EST)			Cengage56085, Training Operator	Patient Search: [Last Name=lyn]

Courtesy of Harris CareTracker PM and EMR.

Figure 3-24 ■ Operator Audit Log in an EMR.

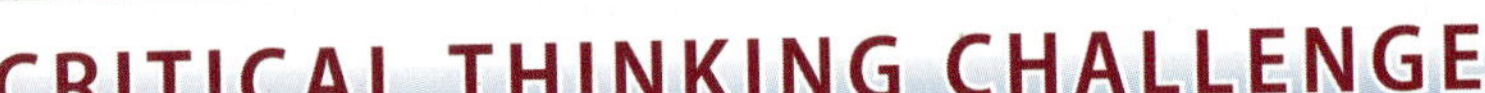

CRITICAL THINKING CHALLENGE

As a medical assisting student, you perform your externship in an office that uses EHR. You were able to see the wonderful advantages of EHR and are hopeful that you will get a position in an office that uses EHR. Unfortunately, the office that hires you still uses paper records. The provider has stated several times that he is hesitant to use EHR because of the software cost.

Research the topic and write a proposal using a SWOT (Strengths, Weaknesses, Opportunities, and Threats) format to the provider stating why the office should convert from paper records to EHR. To help you prepare, complete the following:

1. On a separate sheet of paper, list at least 10 functions of EHR.
2. List at least five advantages for using EHR.
3. Using an Internet search engine, look up three different EHR software vendors and price their software. Compare and contrast your findings.

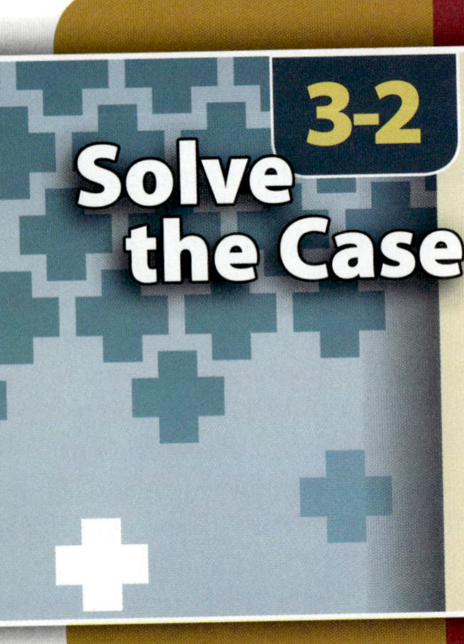

Emil Abello comes to the practice today to obtain copies of his medical record as he is planning to relocate and needs a new primary care provider (PCP) and an orthopedic specialist. Your practice is in the process of converting from paper charts to electronic medical records. Emil wants to be sure he has copies of all his X-ray, MRI, and CT studies included along with his medical history and lab reports. Having completed your studies in Chapter 3, answer the following questions:

1. **What, if any, documents would Emil need to complete?**
2. **Where would you locate the documents Emil is requesting?**
3. **Can you charge Emil for providing the copies?**
4. **Is any approval required prior to releasing the records? If so, who? If not, why not.**

PROCEDURE 3-1
Create and Organize a Patient's Medical Record

Objective:

To prepare an accurate and complete patient chart to submit to the provider for final review (if you have access to an EHR, create a patient's medical record)

Equipment/Supplies:

- Chart or folder
- Patient records
- Privacy forms
- Tabs

continues

PROCEDURE 3-1 continued

PROCEDURAL STEPS	DETAILS AND/OR RATIONALE
1. Prepare chart or folder for patient (electronic or paper). Verify accurate spelling of name. Include demographics, insurance information, privacy forms, and emergency contact information.	In an EHR, this step is what actually creates the chart and assigns a number that will link the patient to other applications within the EHR.
2. Retrieve and compile available reports and information. Verify that all records are for the correct patient before including in the record.	Misfiled and misidentified records are very difficult to locate later.
3. Sort and organize records by type: operative notes, progress notes from various providers, laboratory reports, radiology, medication flow sheets, immunization records, and so on.	Organize and tab appropriate sections of the chart. Look for gaps in records where additional information might need to be requested or clarified. Follow the same organizational format for all patients to help avoid omitting important information.
4. Verify accuracy and completeness and submit to provider for final review.	Provides an opportunity for any desired information to be requested.

CHAPTER SUMMARY

- The medical record is an important tool in maintaining patient health. Understanding the sections of the medical record and knowing what information pertains to each section will save time for everyone who uses the chart. An organized medical record promotes good communications from one staff member to the next and better care for the patient.
- Meaningful use is the set of standards defined by CMS incentive programs that governs the use of EHRs and allows eligible providers and hospitals to earn incentive payments by meeting specific criteria. There are three stages of meaningful use. Credentialed medical assistants entering orders into a CPOE will count toward meaningful use reimbursement.
- Electronic health records (EHRs) have for the most part replaced paper records. The advantages of using EHRs include better communication, organization, electronic networking with outside facilities, and increased efficiency.
- The most important purpose of a medical record is to provide the provider with precise health data to assist in formulating an accurate diagnosis, plan an appropriate treatment, and track a patient's progress. The record also assists the provider in formulating disease prevention measures and overall health maintenance goals for the patient.
- There are two different documentation formats that are used for paper medical records: the source-oriented medical record (SOMR) and the problem-oriented medical record (POMR).
- The paper chart is usually created by administrative staff members, but maintained by both clinical and administrative staff members (see Procedure 3-1). The clinical staff may need to file items within the patient's chart, insert new forms, and make minor repairs to the chart.
- The majority of information found in a patient's chart is considered to be clinical data. Clinical data is information that providers use to help diagnose, prescribe, and treat patients.
- Your responsibilities as an electronic health record specialist will consist of a wide variety of duties. You will be responsible for documenting patient's health information, medical history, symptoms, examination and test results, treatments, and other information.

- Many laws affect medical records. It is important to become familiar with both state and federal guidelines to ensure compliance and avoid noncompliance penalties related to the violation of such laws.
- Federal and state laws dictate how the medical community uses PHI, what rights patients have to medical information, security measures designed to protect patient information and the length of time records should be kept.
- Rules relating to the ownership, retention, and disposal of medical records can vary by state.
- In general, medical records are the property of the practice or treating provider or hospital. The practice or provider owns the physical part of the record, but the patient is the owner of the information stored within the chart. Patients are entitled access to their medical records and may request copies of it.

CERTIFICATION REVIEW QUESTIONS

1. Important uses of the medical record include all of the following except:
   a. means of communication.
   b. statistical data.
   c. payment data.
   d. information to pharmaceutical companies.
2. Which format has no systematic cross-referencing of information?
   a. POMR
   b. Organizational
   c. SOAP
   d. SOMR
3. In the POMR format, the category that includes patient history, provider findings, and baseline results is the:
   a. problem list.
   b. database.
   c. plan.
   d. progress notes.
4. Which is one of the organizations that has been approved to certify products from HIT vendors?
   a. CCHIT
   b. CMS
   c. OSHA
   d. HHS
5. HIPAA's minimum necessary rule:
   a. indicates that you must provide only Protected Health Information (PHI) in the minimum necessary amount to accomplish the purpose for which use or disclosure is sought.
   b. does not apply when patients provide a valid, signed authorization for release of PHI.
   c. requires that you de-identify information (PHI with all HIPAA identifiers removed).
   d. All of the above
6. Which of the following would be considered a subjective finding?
   a. Vital signs
   b. Physical exam findings
   c. Diagnostic test results
   d. Patient's chief complaint
7. Nonlaboratory test results should be filed in which section of the paper medical record?
   a. Demographic section
   b. Diagnostic reports
   c. Progress notes
   d. Lab reports
8. HIPAA helps protect:
   a. PHI.
   b. IHI.
   c. PMI.
   d. PPE.
9. In order to give personal health information to a relative, the patient must:
   a. state the name of the individual on the privacy statement.
   b. have written consent from the patient to share information.
   c. Both a and b
   d. None of the above
10. ______________ provides the Department of Health and Human Services (HHS) with the authority to establish programs to improve health care quality through the promotion of Health Information Technology (HIT).
    a. CCHIT
    b. HIPAA
    c. HITECH
    d. ONC

STUDY RESOURCES

Resources to Test and Reinforce Your Knowledge:	
Certification Review Questions	Take this end-of-chapter quiz
Workbook	• Complete the activities for Chapter 3 • Perform the procedure for Chapter 3 using the Competency Checklist
Resources to Promote Critical Thinking:	
***Solve the Case* Activities**	• Consider these case studies and discuss your conclusions
MindTap	• Complete Chapter 3 readings and activities

REFERENCES

American Medical Association (n.d.). HIPAA Violations and Enforcement. Retrieved October 27, 2014, from http://www.ama-assn.org/ama/pub/physician-resources/solutions-managing-your-practice/coding-billing-insurance/hipaahealth-insurance-portability-accountability-act/hipaa-violations-enforcement.page?

Blesi, Michelle. (2017). *Medical assisting administrative & clinical competencies* (8th ed.). Clifton Park, NY: Cengage Learning.

Bluetooth® (n.d.). What is Bluetooth technology. Retrieved October 27, 2014, from http://www.bluetooth.com/Pages/what-is-bluetooth-technology.aspx

Centers for Medicare & Medicaid Services (May 2104). Eligible Professional Meaningful use Core Measures. Measure 1 of 13. Stage 1 (2014 Definition). Last updated: May 2014. CPOE for Medication Orders. Retrieved October 31, 2014, from http://www.cms.gov/Regulations-and-Guidance/Legislation/EHRIncentivePrograms/downloads/1_CPOE_for_Medication_Orders.pdf

Centers for Medicare & Medicaid Services (n.d.). 2014 Definition Stage 1 of Meaningful Use. Retrieved October 27, 2014, from http://cms.gov/Regulations-and-Guidance/Legislation/EHRIncentivePrograms/Meaningful_Use.html

Centers for Medicare & Medicaid Services (n.d.). Stage 2. Retrieved on October 27, 2014, from http://cms.gov/Regulations-and-Guidance/Legislation/EHRIncentivePrograms/Stage_2.html

Cunningham, Patricia (January 2011). AHIMA. "Patient Access and Amendment to Health Records (Updated)." Retrieved October 27, 2014, from http://library.ahima.org/xpedio/groups/public/documents/ahima/bok1_048587.hcsp?dDocName=bok1_048587

Ferrari, V. and Heller, M. (2015). *The paperless medical office: Using Harris CareTracker*. NY: Clifton Park, NY: Cengage Learning.

Freudenheim, M. (1991). "Guarding Medical Confidentiality." *New York Times*, January 1, p.1.

HealthIT.gov (n.d.). EHR Incentives & Certification. Retrieved October 27, 2014, from http://www.healthit.gov/providers-professionals/how-attain-meaningful-use

HealthIT.gov (n.d.). Certified Health IT Products List. The Office of the National Coordinator for Health Information Technology. Retrieved November 1, 2014, from http://oncchpl.force.com/ehrcert/ehrproductsearch

Institute for Safe Medication Practices (2013). ISMP's list of error-prone abbreviations, symbols, and dose designations. Retrieved December 6, 2014, from http://www.ismp.org/Tools/errorproneabbreviations.pdf

The Joint Commission (June 2014). Facts about the Official "Do Not Use" List. Retrieved December 6, 2014, from http://www.jointcommission.org/assets/1/18/Do_Not_Use_List.pdf

U.S. Department of Health & Human Services (n.d.). Civil Rights. Retrieved October 27, 2014, from http://www.hhs.gov/ocr/civilrights/index.html

U.S. Department of Health & Human Services (n.d.). Health Information Privacy: The Security Rule. Retrieved October 27, 2014, from http://www.hhs.gov/ocr/privacy/hipaa/administrative/securityrule/

U.S. Department of Health & Human Services (n.d.). Summary of the HIPAA Privacy Rule. Retrieved October 27, 2014, from http://www.hhs.gov/ocr/privacy/hipaa/understanding/summary/privacysummary.pdf

4

Fundamentals of Documentation

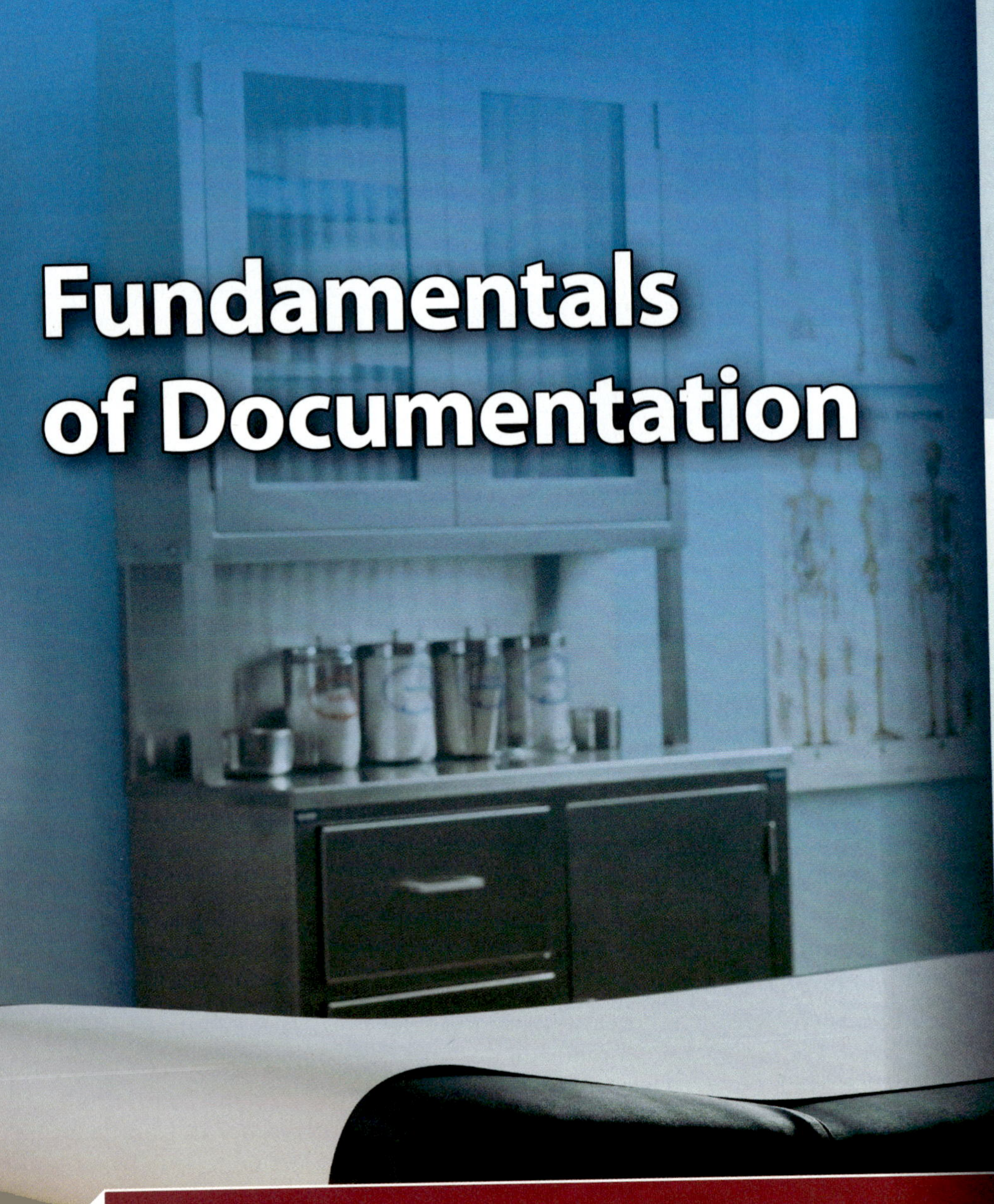

ESSENTIAL TERMS

addendum
chief complaint
consumer-mediated exchange
directed exchange
"Do Not Use" abbreviations list
informed consent
Institute for Safe Medication Practices (ISMP)
Joint Commission (JC)
participating provider
progress note

CHAPTER OUTLINE

Guidelines for Documenting in the Patient's Chart

- Documenting for Legal Success
- General Guidelines for Documenting in the Patient's Medical Record
- The Use of Medical Abbreviations in Chart Entries
- Documenting Chief Complaints and Progress Notes
- Documenting Laboratory Procedures
- Documenting In-Office Procedures
- Documenting Medications
- Documenting Prescriptions
- Documenting Patient Education Sessions
- Documenting Telephone Calls
- Identifying Critical Information for Scheduling Outside Procedures

Making Corrections or Addendums to Chart Notes

Compose Professional Correspondence Using Electronic Technology

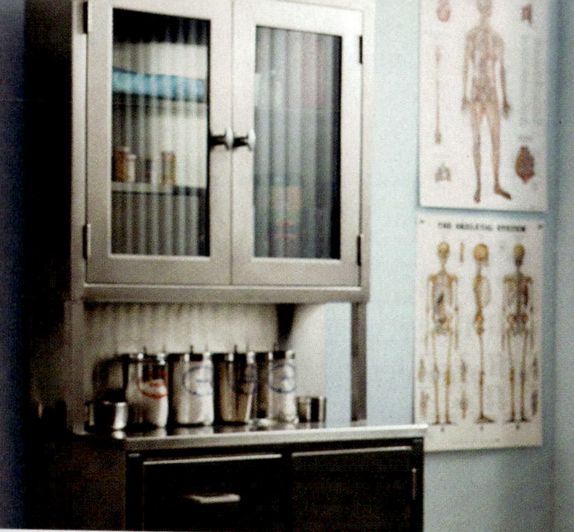

DEVELOPMENTAL OBJECTIVES

After completing this chapter, you should be able to:

1. Correctly spell and define the essential terms.
2. Follow documentation guidelines that will aid in the provider's defense should the record be subpoenaed in a court of law.
3. List 11 "Documentation Dos" and five "Documentation Don'ts" when documenting in the medical record.
4. Define and use medical abbreviations when appropriate and acceptable.
5. Identify critical information required for documenting laboratory procedures, in-office procedures, medication procedures, prescription orders, patient education sessions, patient telephone calls, and when scheduling patient procedures.
6. Compare and contrast the general differences between documentation in a paper chart and documentation in an electronic health record.
7. List the steps that should be taken when making a correction or an addendum to both a paper and paperless record.
8. Discuss application of electronic technology in professional communication.
9. Document the administration of a medication.
10. Appropriately document a patient telephone screening.

INTRODUCTION

A large percentage of the communication between health care professionals today is through written or typed communications. A provider discovers the reason for the patient's office visit by reading the documentation recorded in the patient's chief complaint. If a patient calls the office requesting a prescription refill, it is more than likely communicated to the provider through an electronic task in the electronic health record (EHR) or through a written message.

Other types of professional communication also transpire through written or typed messages and may include faxes, emails, and electronic messaging in the patient's health portal.

How well medical assistants communicate can set the stage for how far they progress in the industry. What type of impression will supervisors get if they continually find spelling errors within the medical assistant's documentation or are unable to decipher what the medical assistant has written in paper charts due to poor handwriting or incomplete documentation? Even though the majority of offices have gone to EHR, spelling and grammar errors may still occur.

Moreover, poor documentation within the patient's chart may cause the office to become more vulnerable when lawsuits arise. Employers just cannot take those kinds of risks.

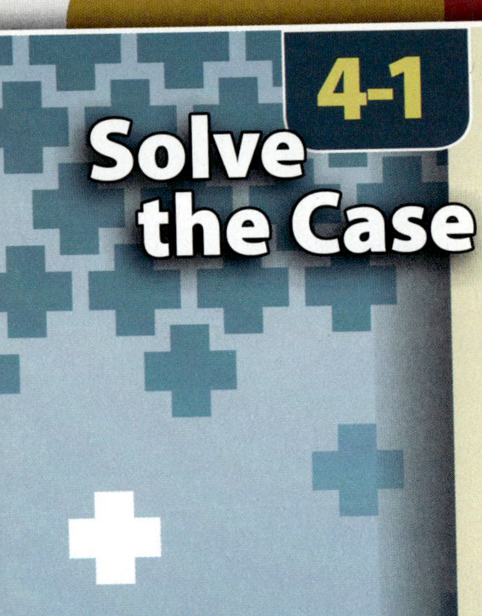

John Wilcox is a 36-year-old male complaining of intermittent headaches over the past three weeks (approximately five to six headaches ranging from 5 to 10 on the pain scale). The headaches are often accompanied with severe nausea, vomiting, and diarrhea and often start in the middle of the night. As a matter of fact, Mr. Wilcox is experiencing a severe headache right now. The pain rating is a "10" and he has been vomiting all morning. Mr. Wilcox has no previous history of headaches prior to the ones he has been experiencing over the past three weeks. He is begging to see the Dr. Timmons right away because he can't stand the pain. You know the doctor is running about a half hour behind.

1. **What can you do to make Mr. Wilcox feel more comfortable while waiting for the doctor?**
2. **Given the circumstances, is there anything you can do to decrease the wait for Mr. Wilcox?**

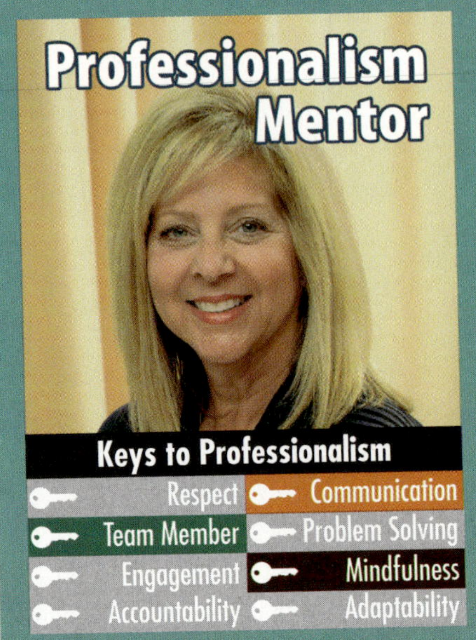

Have you ever heard the saying "if it isn't documented, it wasn't done"? That is the mantra taught in every documentation class, especially in health care, where the medical record is used in a court of law. I have heard from many medical assistants who say that documentation is their least favorite thing to do because they feel it takes them away from doing patient care. Sometimes we have to remind our medical assistants to document in "real time" meaning as soon as they perform patient care in order for it to be most accurate. Providers will often read over your notes so attention to detail is an important key to success when documenting. Take the initiative to follow through with all your assignments, and then take credit for what you do by documenting it! ■

GUIDELINES FOR DOCUMENTING IN THE PATIENT'S CHART

The medical record conveys a story about the patient. It houses the patient's history, progress notes, and lab data so that anyone caring for the patient will have a foundation to build upon. It also assists administrative staff members in knowing what services need to be billed and to which parties. In professional liability cases, the medical record may become evidence aiding judges and jury members in determining the guilt or innocence of those involved.

Documentation within the patient's chart is the essential tool that providers and health care workers use to communicate with one another regarding the patient's overall health status. There are several state and federal guidelines in place that protect documentation stored within the chart such as the Privacy Act. There are also federal guidelines in place designed to help reduce the risk of injury to the patient due to undecipherable documentation. Medical assistants must become familiar with these guidelines to avoid infractions to the office and harm to the patient.

Chapter 3 introduced laws that govern the medical record and listed components of the medical record. This chapter specifically addresses general documentation guidelines, both within and outside the chart.

Documenting for Legal Success

Chart notes within the medical record can be a dynamic defense against frivolous lawsuits or can be the trigger for a disastrous defeat (Figure 4-1). Accurate and thorough documentation is essential when documenting in the medical record. Electronic templates are designed to reduce missing documentation.

The chart is a legal document that is used in *all professional liability cases* and much of the jury members' opinions will be formed by what is written or typed in the chart. Poor documentation may equate to poor medical care in the eyes of jurors.

Procrastination is a pitfall to avoid when referring to the task of documentation because as time passes the accuracy of documentation decreases. The medical assistant should document findings either during or immediately following each patient encounter to promote comprehensive and accurate documentation. Documenting procedures hours after they occur may cause the medical assistant to forget important facts related to the patient encounter or medical procedures. It could even cause the medical assistant to forget the encounter or procedure altogether.

Refer to Figure 4-2 for a common adage that is used in many medical programs and in medical facilities all over the country.

Lack of documentation has been the deciding factor in many professional liability cases that were lost.

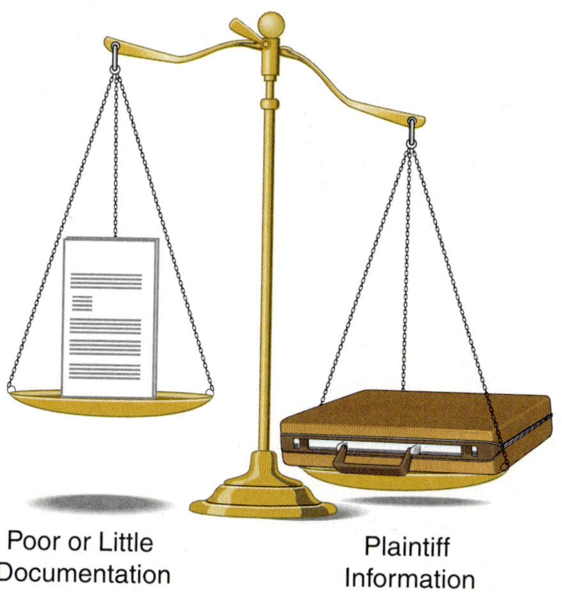

A Win for the Plaintiff

Thorough and Complete Documentation

Plaintiff Information

A Win for the Practice

Figure 4-1 ■ Notice that the practice's chance of winning a medical professional liability case is much greater when records are thorough and documentation is complete.

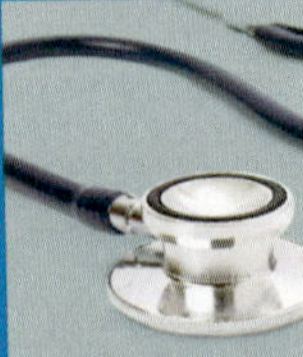

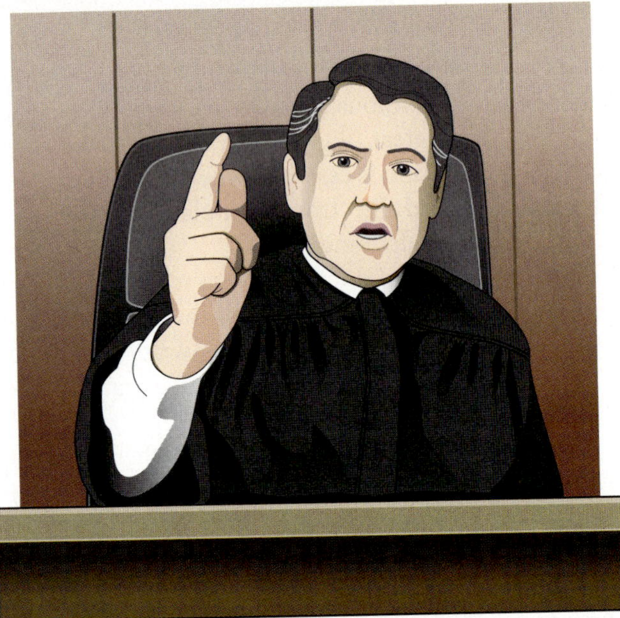

"IF YOU DIDN'T DOCUMENT IT, YOU DIDN'T DO IT!"

Figure 4-2 ■ The judge's comments emphasize the importance of documentation in the patient's chart.

Field Smarts

The latest "National Patient Safety Goals" are a set of required standards for all institutions accredited by the Joint Commission (JC). One of the goals mandates the use of two patient identifiers when identifying patients for medication administration or lab testing. First, you should compare the name on the chart with the patient. In addition, use at least one other identifier such as the patient's birth date or the last four digits of the patient's social security number to ascertain that you have the correct chart. Following these guidelines will help prevent needless errors that could harm the patient and lead the practice into litigation.

Any time the medical assistant has an encounter with the patient, even if it the encounter appears to be minor or trivial, it should be documented in the medical record.

Statements such as, "It doesn't appear that the patient changed her bandage since the last appointment," could appear insensitive and judgmental in the eyes of a juror. A better way to address this type of scenario would be to state, "The patient's dressing was soiled with dirt and dried blood and was torn in several places." This type of statement presents straight facts without appearing subjective and may indicate negligence on the part of the patient in the event that a lawsuit does transpire.

General Guidelines for Documenting in the Patient's Medical Record

Now that you understand some of the legalities associated with medical documentation, the following section will address basic foundational guidelines that must be adhered to when documenting in the patient's chart.

The following is a list of "Documentation Dos":

1. Do Make Certain That You Use the Correct Chart: Always use two identifiers before recording in the patient's chart. Recording information in the wrong chart may set the patient up to receive the wrong treatment or wrong procedure. It also creates havoc for the billing office.
2. Do Document All Patient Encounters: Document each office visit, all procedures, each telephone call, and all appointment-related changes such as broken, cancelled, or rescheduled appointments. Multiple appointment changes, especially cancellations, illustrates that the patient was neglectful in his or her duty to follow up with the provider.
3. Do Chart Thoroughly: As stated previously, professional liability cases are frequently lost due to incomplete or missing documentation. Thorough documentation aids in the communication process among all those using the chart, which equates to better care for the patient.
4. Do Document Accurately: Make certain that each entry is accurate. Inaccurate documentation may generate many problems from inaccurate diagnosis to wrongful treatment and incorrect billing.
5. Do Use Correct Spelling: Proper spelling is imperative when documenting in the patient's chart. Spelling errors in a chart entry makes the medical assistant who made the entry appear deficient and also creates an overall negative impression of the office to outsiders reading the chart notes. *You can't always rely on spell check to pick up on spelling errors in the EHR.* Refer to the student companion website for a list of common misspelled everyday words and for a list of common misspelled medical words.
6. Do Document the Date and Time of Each Entry: Documenting the date and time can be very important when referring to times of medication administ ration or when a procedure or treatment is administered. It can also be very important for worker's compensation and personal injury cases. *Electronic health*

record entries automatically record the date; however, you may need to provide times for specific entries.

7. Do Chart Legibly: *This should resolve itself as the country moves entirely to electronic health records.*
8. Do Identify Your Chart Entries by Documenting an Approved Documentation Identifier: This is only necessary when documenting in paper charts. The medical assistant should sign her name by recording her first initial, last name, and credential. Always check the protocol of the office. *It is not necessary to sign entries when using electronic health records. This is because audit logs identify each individual making entries in the chart.*
9. Do Document Informed Consent or Refusal to Follow Directions: **Informed consent** is a legal doctrine that requires practitioners to provide patients with a complete set of facts prior to surgical procedures or medical experiments. Information must include the nature of the treatment, possible benefits, possible risks, and possible alternative treatments. The provider is usually responsible for presenting this information and will ask the patient to sign a consent form at the conclusion of the explanation. The medical assistant may be responsible for preparing the form prior to the explanation of the procedure or treatment. The encounter is usually documented on the progress note as well. Refer to Figure 4-3 for a copy of a procedure consent form. When a patient refuses treatment or to follow office instructions such as waiting the allotted time following an allergy injection, it should be documented in the chart with the patient's signature beside it. Some offices have the patient sign a "Refusal of Medical Advice" form (Figure 4-4).

CONSENT TO
OPERATION, ADMINISTRATION OF ANESTHETICS AND
RENDERING OF OTHER MEDICAL SERVICES

1. I hereby authorize and direct Dr. James Soldano, my physician, and whomever he/she designates as his/her assistants (associates and/or resident physicians), to perform upon (state name of patient or myself) Megan Donaldson the following procedures: Tubal Ligation

   If any unforeseen condition arises in the course of this operation for the physician's judgment to perform procedures in addition to or different from those now contemplated, I further request and authorize him/her to do whatever he/she deems advisable and necessary in these circumstances. Such additional services may include, but are not limited to, the administration and maintenance of anesthesia and the performance of services involving pathology and radiology.

2. The following information has been explained to me to the degree that I wish to have it discussed:
   - The nature and character of the proposed treatment or procedure;
   - The anticipated results;
   - Possible recognized alternative methods of treatment, including non-treatment;
   - Recognized serious possible risks, complications, and anticipated benefits involved in proposed and alternative treatments, including non-treatment.

   My questions have been answered to my satisfaction. I acknowledge that no guarantee, warrantee, or assurance has been made as to the results or cure that may be obtained.

3. Federal Regulations (21 CFR Part 821) require manufacturers to track certain medical devices, and assist the U.S. Food and Drug Administration (FDA) with notification to individuals in the event that a certain medical device presents serious health risks. I authorize and agree to the release of my contact information to the manufacturer: Not Applicable for this tracking purpose only. I understand that the manufacturer may notify me, if necessary, of important safety information about my medical device, and may release my information to the FDA if ordered to do so. I understand that this consent is valid for the life of the medical device.

Any sections below that do not apply to the proposed treatment may be crossed out. The patient must initial any section crossed out.

4. I consent to the administration of blood and blood products if deemed medically necessary. I understand that all blood and blood products involve the risk of allergic reaction, fever, hives, and in rare circumstances infectious diseases such as hepatitis and HIV/AIDS. I understand that precautions are taken by the blood bank in screening donors and in matching blood for transfusion to minimize those risks.
5. I hereby consent to the disposal or use for research purposes any tissues, parts, or products of conception, which may be removed.
6. I authorize and agree to the presence of observers during my surgical procedure. These observers may include persons other than the medical staff that are considered appropriate by my health care provider during my care and treatment. The purpose of these individuals observing would be for instruction and medical study.

I certify that I have read this form and understand its contents.

PATIENT NAME & ID #
Megan Donaldson
ID # 459098C

Signature of Patient or Legally Responsible Party
Megan Donaldson

Relationship to patient, if not signed by patient

Signature of Witness
Blake Peterson, RMA

Printed Name of Witness Blake Peterson, RMA

Date 05/28/XX Time 1:15 a.m. (p.m.)

MRD: HOSP1
DISTRIBUTION: 1-WHITE – CHART 2-CANARY – PATIENT COPY

Figure 4-3 ■ An example of a patient consent form.

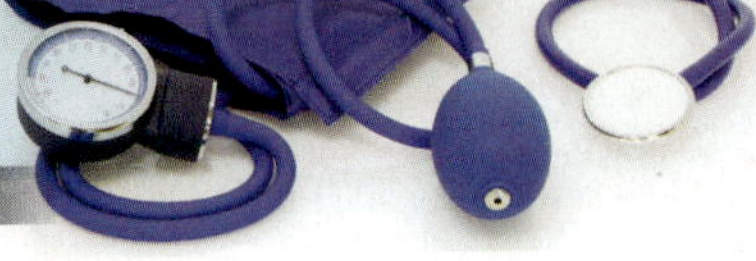

DOUGLASVILLE MEDICINE ASSOCIATES
5076 BRAND BLVD
DOUGLASVILLE, NY 01234
(123) 456-7890

REFUSAL OF MEDICAL ADVICE FORM

I Debbie Johnson do hereby refuse the following medical test, treatment, procedure, or **advice** as recommended by Dr. Karl Valentine at Douglasville Medicine Associates.

Proposed Advice: Waiting 30 Minutes Following an Injection.

I have been fully instructed regarding the possible consequences of not following the advice listed above. Complications may include but are not limited to:

Developing an allergic reaction to the medication and going into anaphylaxis which could lead to death.

I am fully aware of my condition and understand the possible consequences that exist by refusing to follow medical advice.

I certify that I have read this form and completely understand its contents.

Name of Patient or Person Acting on Behalf of the Patient: **Debbie Johnson**

Signature of Patient or Person Acting on Behalf of the Patient: Debbie Johnson

Relationship to Patient: **Self**

Signature of Witness: Roger Wong, CMA (AAMA) Today's Date: 05/19/XX

****

Refusal to Sign:

Patient or representative of patient has received a full explanation in regards to the possible consequences in not following the advice listed above but refuses to sign the form.

Signature of Witness: ____________________ Today's Date: __________

Figure 4-4 ■ An example of a refusal to follow medical advice form.

10. Do Only Use Standard Abbreviations: Because abbreviations can easily be misinterpreted, many medical facilities are reducing the number of abbreviations that they allow workers to use or are eliminating them altogether. Refer to the Documentation Don'ts to learn more about the Joint Commission's list of "Do Not Use" abbreviations.

11. Do Document on Every Line: When using paper records, leave no open lines that can be altered at a different time and draw a line to the end of the margin when the last line extends only partially across the page. *When recording in the electronic health record, each entry is separate and cannot be altered by other individuals. To amend an entry an addendum is created.*

Just as there is a list of "Documentation Dos," there is also a list of "Documentation Don'ts":

1. Don't Procrastinate: Never rely on your memory. Information is much clearer during or immediately following a patient encounter.
2. Don't Diagnose: List the symptoms only. If the patient states that she feels she may have a urinary tract infection or migraine, use the patient's exact wording placed in quotation marks.
3. Don't Document for Someone Else and Don't Allow Others to Document for You: Allowing others to document for you may set you up for an array of problems. The other person may intentionally or inadvertently leave out important facts. If you administer an injection, you should follow the injection from preparation to documentation. There should be no breaks in the chain. When you document the injection, you are taking ownership of the injection from start to finish.
4. Don't Alter Records: Altering records may appear that you have something to hide. Any alteration or addendum is visible in the EHR; however, when using paper charts, never scribble over or use correction fluid to correct an error and never rewrite a progress note. Lawyers who suspect wrongdoing may hire handwriting specialists to review patient records they feel may have been tampered with or recreated. If you need to make a correction, follow the directions under the section entitled, "Making Corrections or Addendums to Chart Notes" found toward the end of this chapter.
5. Don't use abbreviations on the Joint Commission's "Do Not Use" list.

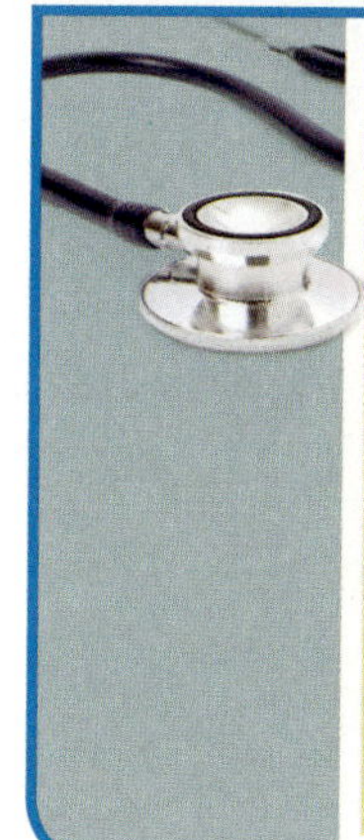

Field Smarts

Chart auditors will check to see if health care workers making entries in the charts are using abbreviations that appear on the Joint Commission's "Do Not Use" abbreviations list. This is much easier now that records are in digital format. Continued use of these abbreviations may result in infractions against the practice.

The Use of Medical Abbreviations in Chart Entries

To assist with time management and reduce the length of chart entries, standard medical abbreviations may be used when entering information within the medical record. The use of medical abbreviations, particularly medication abbreviations and symbols, has been heavily scrutinized over the past few years due to the number of errors related to their use.

The **Joint Commission (JC)**, a national organization that focuses on improving the quality and safety of services provided by health care organizations, published a "Do Not Use" abbreviations list as part of their 2004 National Patient Safety Goals. The **"Do Not Use" abbreviations list** is a list of abbreviations that are commonly misinterpreted and should no longer be used when documenting any orders within the patient's medical record, or when sending orders to other health care facilities. Always check the Joint Commission's website to see if the list has been updated. There have been no abbreviations added or deleted to the list since the original list was published in 2004; however, changes may occur at any time.

The **Institute for Safe Medication Practices (ISMP)** is a governmental organization that specifically seeks ways to promote medication safety. The ISMP has also compiled a list referred to as the "List of Error-Prone Abbreviations, Symbols, and Dose Designations." This list includes all of the JC's "Do Not Use" abbreviations and several other dangerous abbreviations.

Refer to Appendix A for a list of approved medical abbreviations and symbols that may be used in chart entries and Appendix B for the ISMP "List of Error-Prone Abbreviations, Symbols, and Dose Designations" that should not be used when recording entries within the chart.

Documenting Chief Complaints and Progress Notes

The **chief complaint** is the reason that the patient is being seen. It is a listing of the patient's symptoms and should be written using the patient's own words whenever possible. The chief complaint should be short, concise, and flow well. Often the chief complaint is as simple as "productive cough for 3 days." The history of present illness (HPI) follows the chief complaint and is where the facts regarding the complaint are developed.

A **progress note** is a follow-up note from a previous visit. This information elaborates on the patient's progress between visits.

Refer to Chapter 5 for items that should be included when documenting a patient screening.

Documenting Laboratory Procedures

Often times, the medical assistant will be asked to obtain patient specimens and send them to an in-house laboratory or an outside reference facility; however, the medical assistant may also be responsible for performing the testing. The medical assistant must be thorough in the documentation by listing the type of specimen collected (blood, urine, stool, sputum, etc.), from where it was collected (antecubital vein in left arm, right hand, throat, etc.), and whether or not the test was performed in the office or sent to an outside laboratory. If testing was performed by the medical assistant, the entry should also include the results of the test.

Items Listed When Documenting Laboratory Procedures

Table 4-1 lists items that should be recorded when documenting laboratory procedures. The medical assistant should document the procedure in both the patient's chart and onto a lab log when using paper records. The purpose of the log is to track outstanding labs.

EHR Application

Recording lab procedures in the electronic health record is much different than in the paper record. Instead of documenting the procedure on a progress note, the entry is created when you create the order for the test (Figure 4-5). All of the necessary documentation appears in the order including patient notes giving specifics about the procedure. The medical assistant does not have to sign her name anywhere in the order's window because it appears in the EHR tracking log (Figure 4-6).

Table 4-1 Items Listed When Documenting Lab Procedures

Information to be Documented	Description or Facts
1. The date and the time of collection or testing	This is very important because specimens must be tested within the proper time frame to guarantee that the results are accurate.
2. What type of specimen was collected and from what location when applicable. If procedure is a blood draw, list the following information:	Type of specimen: stool, sputum, blood, urine. Location from where the specimen was collected: throat, wound, L. hand, and so on (List if patient was fasting if applicable and for how long). The method used to collect the blood, such as vacuum, syringe, or butterfly method. Location of blood draw, such as antecubital vein in left arm, right hand, and so on. Color and number of tubes drawn (e.g., two lavender top tubes and one red top tube).
3. The name(s) of the test(s) to be performed	Make certain that you list all the tests to be performed. Providers often order multiple tests, for example, CBC, Complete UA, Metabolic Panel, and so on.
4. The name of provider ordering the testing	You must show an order for any test that is performed.
5. The results of the tests when applicable	If the testing was performed in-house, document the results in both the patient's chart (with reference ranges) and the lab log.
6. Where specimens were sent when applicable	This is important because it illustrates that the specimen was sent out and to which lab it was sent should problems occur.
7. Any reference numbers assigned to the test such as an acquisition number	Many labs will assign a number to the specimen for tracking purposes.
8. Any complications that occurred during or following the procedure	Examples of complications that may occur include: fainting, vein collapsed, patient experienced prolonged bleeding following the blood draw, and so on. This information can assist those who take care of the patient during future visits to take steps to prevent such complications.
9. Documentation identifier	First name or initial and last name, followed by your credential [e.g., Megan Speck, CMA (AAMA)].
10. Record information in the outstanding lab log	The lab log helps to keep track of who had lab procedures and where they were sent. This also assists with tracking.

DOCUMENTATION EXAMPLE #1: DOCUMENTING LAB PROCEDURES

05-16-XX 1115	Blood draw (Syringe Method), L. arm (antecubital vein) for a CBC, PT and INR per Dr. Chow. 1 lavender and 1 light blue top tube sent to Quest Labs. Acquisition #2357A. Pt. tolerated procedure well. No complications. Sam Brown, CMA (AAMA)------------------------

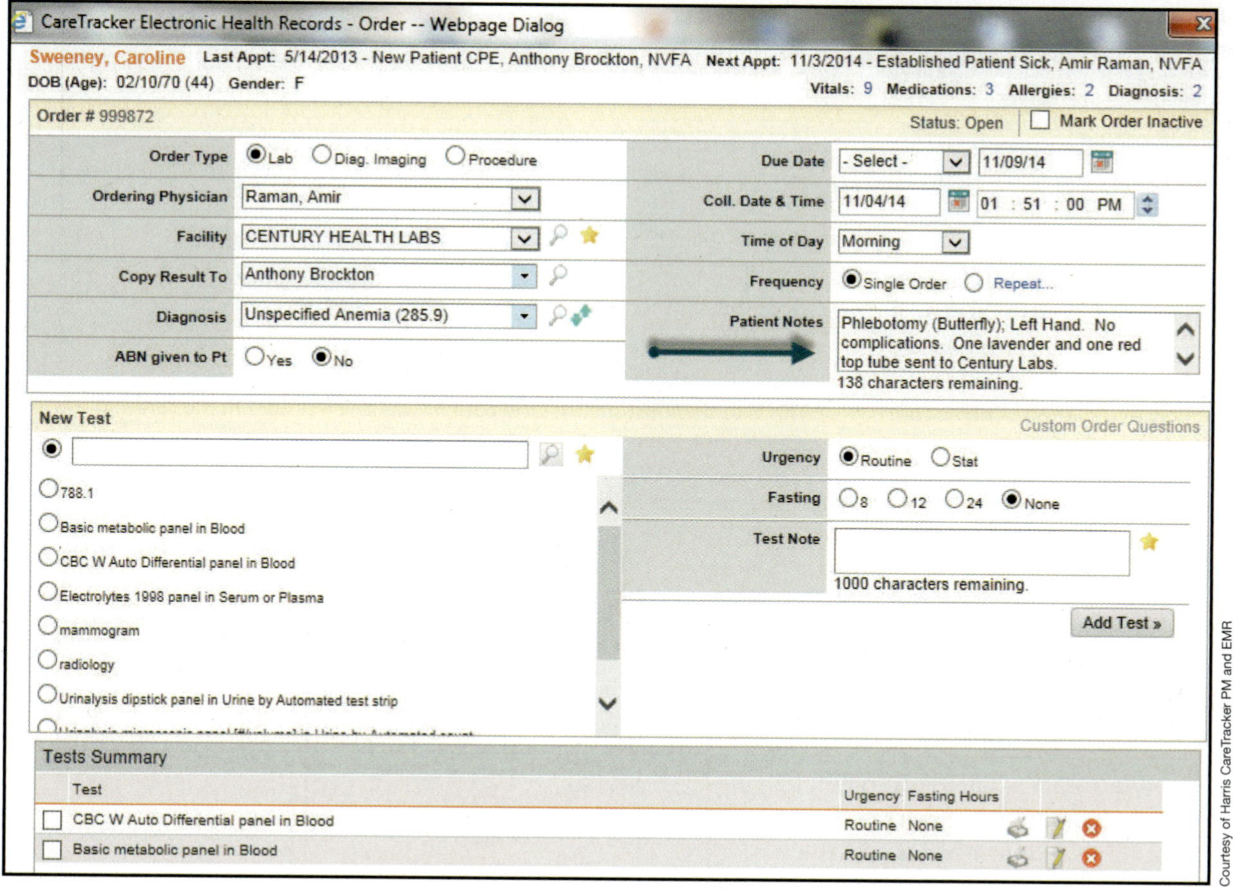

Courtesy of Harris CareTracker PM and EMR

Figure 4-5 ■ In the EHR, you don't have to create a separate note for the procedure. Patient notes can be entered directly within the order.

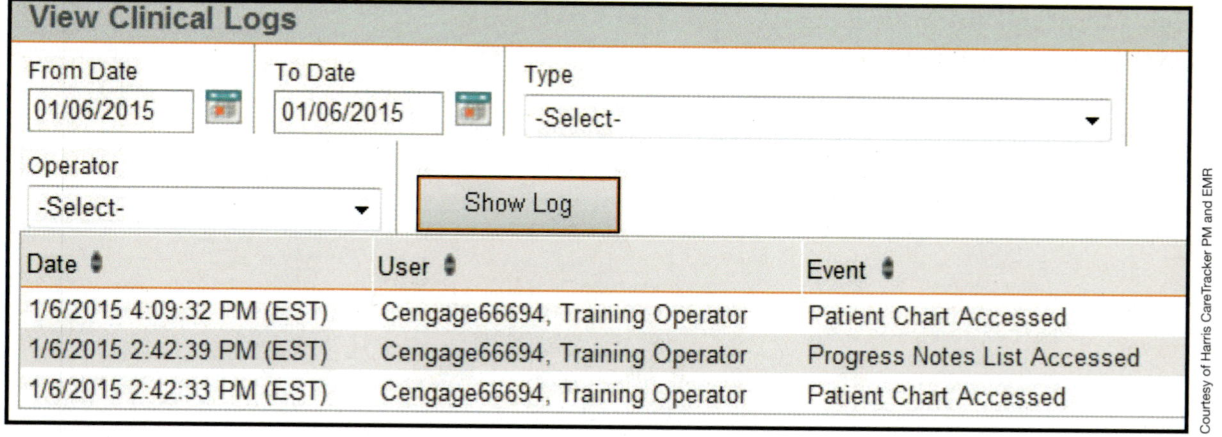

Courtesy of Harris CareTracker PM and EMR

Figure 4-6 ■ Any time the medical assistant accesses the patient's electronic health record or documents in the medical record it is tracked in the audit log; therefore, the medical assistant does not need to sign entries.

Documenting In-Office Procedures

Medical assistants routinely perform other types of diagnostic tests and procedures in addition to laboratory tests. These procedures may include vital signs, ECGs, pulmonary function tests, and results for pulse oximetry testing. The medical assistant should document the name of the procedure, where it was performed (if applicable), the results (if applicable), and who ordered the testing.

Items Listed When Documenting In-Office Procedures

Table 4-2 lists specific items that should be listed when documenting procedures that are performed in the office.

Table 4-2 Items Listed When Documenting In-Office Procedures

Information to be Documented	Description or Facts
1. Date and time of the procedure	
2. Name of the procedure	May use standard abbreviations such as ECG, UA/C&S, and PFT testing.
3. Name of the provider ordering the procedure	You must always show an order for all procedures performed in the office. This is for legal and reimbursement purposes.
4. Location when applicable	Applied splint to right arm, 6 Steri-Strips applied to left leg.
5. Special steps that were taken to perform the procedure	What solution was used to clean the wound, what ointment was applied to wound, and other steps.
6. Complications either during or following the procedure	Patients may have problems with certain procedures. Recording those problems will help other health care workers for future procedures.
7. Any educational information or home care instructions given to the patient	This is to demonstrate that the patient was given proper home care instructions.
8. Documentation identifier	First name or initial and last name, followed by your credential.

EHR Application

A lab log is not necessary when using an EHR because the order's module is connected to a tasks module in most EHRs. Figure 4-7 illustrates the *Open Orders* tab in the medical assistant's quick task pane in Harris CareTracker and Figure 4-8 illustrates what the Open Orders tab looks like when opened. Once the results for each order are uploaded, downloaded, or manually entered in the patient's EHR, the open order no longer appears in the task bar.

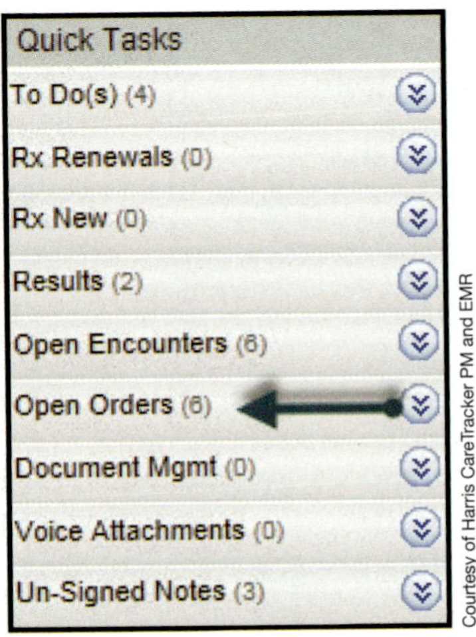

Figure 4-7 ■ The EHR tracks every outstanding lab order, thus a separate tracking log is not necessary when entering orders electronically.

Open Orders — Show Inactive

Order #	Due Date	Patient	Type	Test Description	Provider	Enc Date	Status
973761	05/09/14	Morgan, Jane W	Lab	Urinalysis dipstick panel in Urine by Automated test strip (S)	Raman, Amir	05/09/14	Open
973793	05/09/14	Morgan, Jane W	Diag Imag	Patient information entered into a reminder system with a target due date for the next mammogram (RAD) (S)	Raman, Amir	05/09/14	Open
973794	05/09/14	Thompson, Adam	Lab	CBC W Auto Differential panel in Blood (S); Electrolytes 1998 panel in Serum or Plasma	Brockton, Anthony	05/09/14	Open
973981	05/09/14	Morgan, Jane W	Lab	Urinalysis microscopic panel [#/volume] in Urine by Automated count	Raman, Amir	05/09/14	Open
974223	05/21/14	Hernandez, Julia	Lab	Basic metabolic panel in Blood	Ayerick, Rebecca	05/21/14	Open
989589	08/29/14	Patient, Claire	Lab	Urinalysis dipstick panel in Urine by Automated test strip (S); CBC W Auto Differential panel in Blood (S)	Raman, Amir	08/29/14	Open
999875	11/02/14	Sweeney, Caroline	Proc	12-Lead Electrocardiogram Performed	Raman, Amir	11/03/14	Open

Courtesy of Harris CareTracker PM and EMR

Figure 4-8 ■ An example of the open orders screen when opened. Once results are uploaded or entered and reviewed by the provider, the order is removed from the screen.

Documenting Medications

The medical assistant is often responsible for administering and dispensing medications and calling in prescriptions. Anytime the medical assistant performs a medication procedure or calls in a prescription, it must be documented in the patient's chart (see Procedure 4-1). Chapters 30, 31, and 32 address procedures for these tasks. This chapter will concentrate on the documentation of these procedures.

DOCUMENTATION EXAMPLE #2: CHARTING ROUTINE IN-OFFICE PROCEDURES

03-02-XX 1445	12-Lead ECG per Dr. Walker. Pt. was unable to lie in a supine position due to a neck injury thus was placed in a semi-fowler's position. No complications during or following the procedure. Milli Thomas, SMA--

DOCUMENTATION EXAMPLE #3: CHARTING IN-OFFICE PROCEDURES

07-12-XX 1330	Steri-Strip application × 4 to the pt's lower L. leg per Dr. Green. Irrigated wound with 60 mL of sterile H_2O and dried with sterile gauze prior to the procedure. Applied "Tincture of Benzoin" to improve the adhesiveness of the strips. Good approximation of wound. Covered with sterile dressing and discussed home care instructions with pt. Pt. appeared to comprehend the instructions. Gave pt. written instructions as well. Pt. to return in 6 days for a F/U appointment. Taylor Steager, CMA (AAMA)--

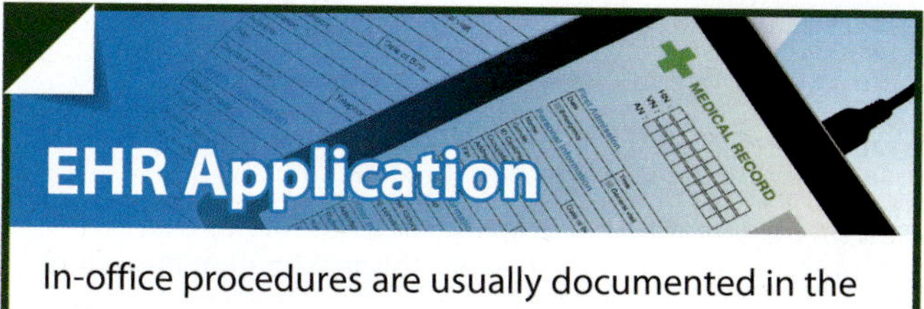

In-office procedures are usually documented in the order's management screen of the EHR as well. Refer to Figure 4-9 for a documentation sample of an ECG in the order's management section of a patient's chart in Harris CareTracker.

Items Documented When Recording a Medication Entry

Table 4-3 lists important components that should be included when documenting medications. The medical assistant should make certain that this information is placed in the appropriate log when applicable.

Documenting Prescriptions

Medical assistants may have the task of calling in, writing, or creating prescriptions in the EHR per the

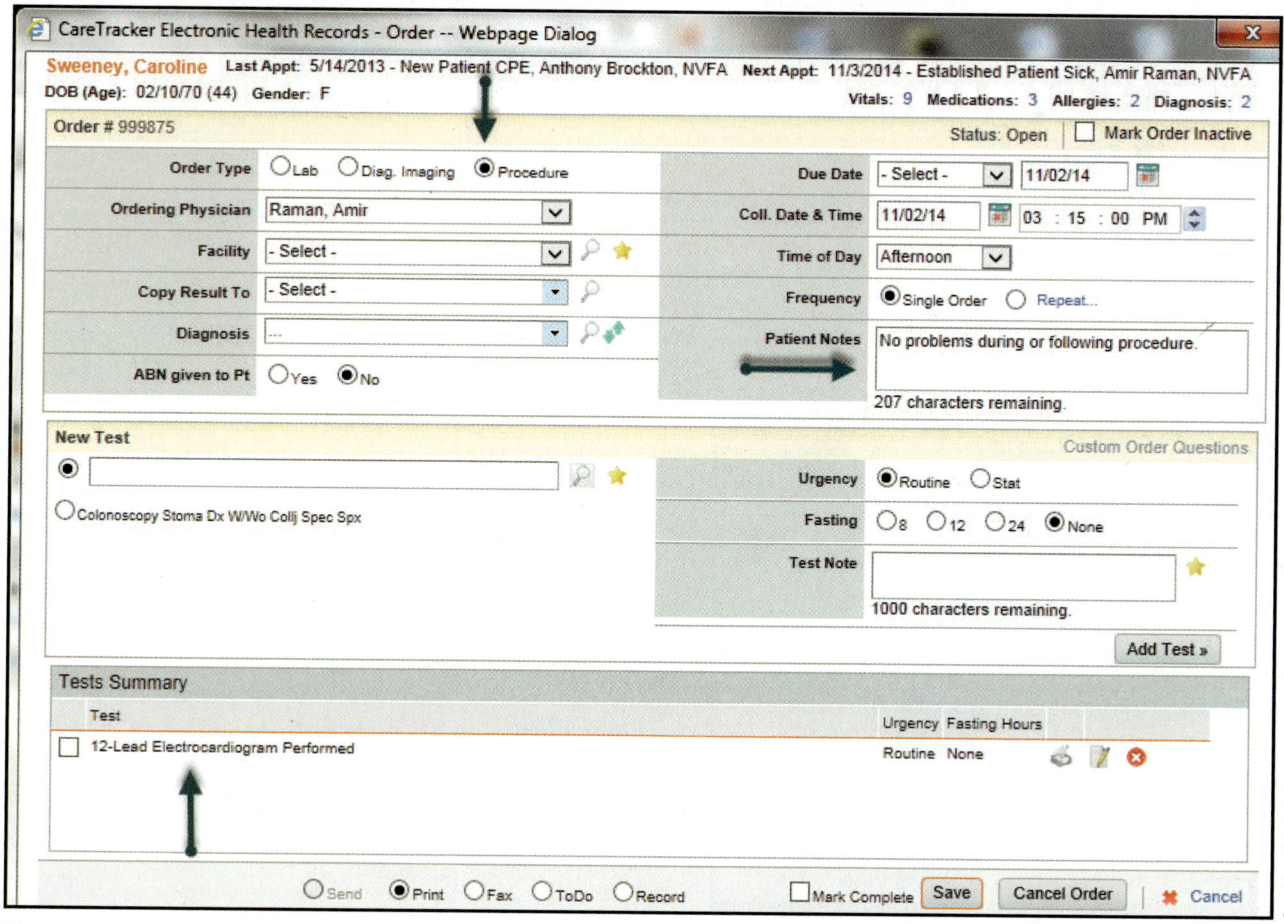

CareTracker Electronic Health Records - Order -- Webpage Dialog

Sweeney, Caroline Last Appt: 5/14/2013 - New Patient CPE, Anthony Brockton, NVFA Next Appt: 11/3/2014 - Established Patient Sick, Amir Raman, NVFA
DOB (Age): 02/10/70 (44) Gender: F Vitals: 9 Medications: 3 Allergies: 2 Diagnosis: 2

Order # 999875 Status: Open Mark Order Inactive

Order Type: Lab / Diag. Imaging / ● Procedure — Due Date: - Select - 11/02/14
Ordering Physician: Raman, Amir — Coll. Date & Time: 11/02/14 03 : 15 : 00 PM
Facility: - Select - — Time of Day: Afternoon
Copy Result To: - Select - — Frequency: ● Single Order / Repeat...
Diagnosis: --- — Patient Notes: No problems during or following procedure. 207 characters remaining.
ABN given to Pt: Yes / ● No

New Test — Custom Order Questions
Colonoscopy Stoma Dx W/Wo Colj Spec Spx
Urgency: ● Routine / Stat
Fasting: 8 / 12 / 24 / ● None
Test Note: 1000 characters remaining.
Add Test »

Tests Summary

Test	Urgency	Fasting Hours
12-Lead Electrocardiogram Performed	Routine	None

Send / ● Print / Fax / ToDo / Record — Mark Complete — Save — Cancel Order — Cancel

Courtesy of Harris CareTracker PM and EMR

Figure 4-9 ■ Other diagnostic tests such as ECGs and imaging studies are created very similar to lab orders. Notice the box for Patient Notes. This greatly simplifies the documentation process.

Table 4-3 Items Listed When Documenting a Medication Entry

Information to be Documented	Description or Facts
1. Date and time of administration	Timing is critical so that the patient receives the appropriate amount of medication within the proper time frame.
2. Name of medication	Write out the entire name to avoid confusion or misunderstandings. For example, if you write "Depo shot," it could be read as Depo-Provera, Depo-Medrol, or Depo-Testosterone.
3. Strength of medication (dose given)	When the physician orders a particular strength of medication, it should be documented the way it was ordered. For example, the physician orders 100 mg of Toradol. It comes stocked as 100 mg per 1 mL of medication, so you give the patient 1 mL of medication. You should record it as Toradol, 100 mg, not Toradol, l mL. Immunizations are usually recorded in milliliters (mL), such as 0.5 mL of adult tetanus toxoid. Allergy medications are usually recorded in mL, such as 0.1 mL of allergy serum.
4. Route of administration	Was medication given intramuscularly (IM), subcutaneously (Sub-Q), intradermally (ID), intravenously (IV), or by mouth (PO)?
5. Site of administration	Where was the medication given? Right deltoid, L. ventrogluteal, etc.
6. Name of physician who ordered the medication	You need to show that you had an order to give the medication. If this information is not listed, it will appear as though *you* ordered the medication.
7. Manufacturer's name, lot number, and expiration date (when applicable)	Some practices will want this information documented in the patient's chart, however the majority of practices will have the MA put this information into a log.
8. Any problems encountered	The medical assistant should document any local or systemic reactions, list the patient's specific symptoms or signs, and document actions taken to counteract or ease the symptoms.
9. Consent form confirmation	If the patient was to sign a consent form, confirm that it was signed. This is common with vaccinations, experimental drugs, and drugs not covered by insurance.
10. Any educational material distributed	Educational material may include a vaccination information statement (VIS), side effects to watch for after receiving certain medications, etc. Make certain that you list the VIS date when applicable. Figure 4-10 illustrates where the dates can be found on the VIS.
11. Documentation identifier	First name or initial and last name, followed by your credential.

DOCUMENTATION EXAMPLE #4: DOCUMENTING MEDICATIONS

06-26-XX 0900	Adult Hepatitis B Vaccine, 0.5 mL, IM, L Deltoid per Dr. Miller. Neg complications during or following procedure. Consent form signed. Gave pt. Hep B VIS (10-25-XX) Catrina McDonald, RMA (AMT)--

EHR Application

When documenting immunizations or other medications administered in the office, you usually just need to click a few buttons and the order and administration information is stored in the patient's EHR. Refer to Figure 4-11 for an illustration of the immunization screen in Harris CareTracker. You will not need to use a medication log when using an EHR because an electronic log can be generated at any time.

provider's order. All prescriptions should be documented in the patient's chart. Whether or not the medical assistant is able to create prescriptions will largely depend on the type of prescription, the policy of the office, and state statutes. When assigned this task, the medical assistant must be diligent in maintaining patient safety and take precautions to minimize documentation errors. Even though medical assistants may create prescriptions, the provider must sign all prescriptions either manually or electronically.

This chapter focuses on documenting prescription information in the chart. To learn more about writing prescriptions, see Chapter 30.

3 Some people should not get hepatitis A vaccine or should wait.

- Anyone who has ever had a severe (life threatening) allergic reaction to a previous dose of hepatitis A vaccine should not get another dose.
- Anyone who has a severe (life threatening) allergy to any vaccine component should not get the vaccine.
- **Tell your doctor if you have any severe allergies**, including a severe allergy to latex. All hepatitis A vaccines contain alum, and some hepatitis A vaccines contain 2-phenoxyethanol.
- Anyone who is moderately or severely ill at the time the shot is scheduled should probably wait until they recover. Ask your doctor. People with a mild illness can usually get the vaccine.
- Tell your doctor if you are pregnant. Because hepatitis A vaccine is inactivated (killed), the risk to a pregnant woman or her unborn baby is believed to be very low. But your doctor can weigh any theoretical risk from the vaccine against the need for protection.

4 What are the risks from hepatitis A vaccine?

A vaccine, like any medicine, could possibly cause serious problems, such as severe allergic reactions. The risk of hepatitis A vaccine causing serious harm, or death, is extremely small.

Getting hepatitis A vaccine is much safer than getting the disease.

Mild problems

- soreness where the shot was given *(about 1 out of 2 adults, and up to 1 out of 6 children)*
- headache *(about 1 out of 6 adults and 1 out of 25 children)*
- loss of appetite *(about 1 out of 12 children)*
- tiredness *(about 1 out of 14 adults)*

If these problems occur, they usually last 1 or 2 days.

Severe problems

- serious allergic reaction, within a few minutes to a few hours after the shot *(very rare)*.

5 What if there is a serious reaction?

What should I look for?

- Look for anything that concerns you, such as signs of a severe allergic reaction, very high fever, or behavior changes.

  Signs of a severe allergic reaction can include hives, swelling of the face and throat, difficulty breathing, a fast heartbeat, dizziness, and weakness. These would start a few minutes to a few hours after the vaccination.

What should I do?

- If you think it is a severe allergic reaction or other emergency that can't wait, call 9-1-1 or get the person to the nearest hospital. Otherwise, call your doctor.
- Afterward, the reaction should be reported to the Vaccine Adverse Event Reporting System (VAERS). Your doctor might file this report, or you can do it yourself through the VAERS web site at **www.vaers.hhs.gov**, or by calling **1-800-822-7967**.

VAERS is only for reporting reactions. They do not give medical advice.

6 The National Vaccine Injury Compensation Program

The National Vaccine Injury Compensation Program (VICP) is a federal program that was created to compensate people who may have been injured by certain vaccines.

Persons who believe they may have been injured by a vaccine can learn about the program and about filing a claim by calling **1-800-338-2382** or visiting the VICP website at **www.hrsa.gov/vaccinecompensation**.

7 How can I learn more?

- Ask your doctor.
- Call your local or state health department.
- Contact the Centers for Disease Control and Prevention (CDC):
  - Call **1-800-232-4636** (**1-800-CDC-INFO**) or
  - Visit CDC's website at **www.cdc.gov/vaccines**

Vaccine Information Statement (Interim)
Hepatitis A Vaccine

→ 10/25/2011

42 U.S.C. § 300aa-26

Office Use Only

Figure 4-10 ■ The date of the VIS must appear in your documentation of all immunizations.

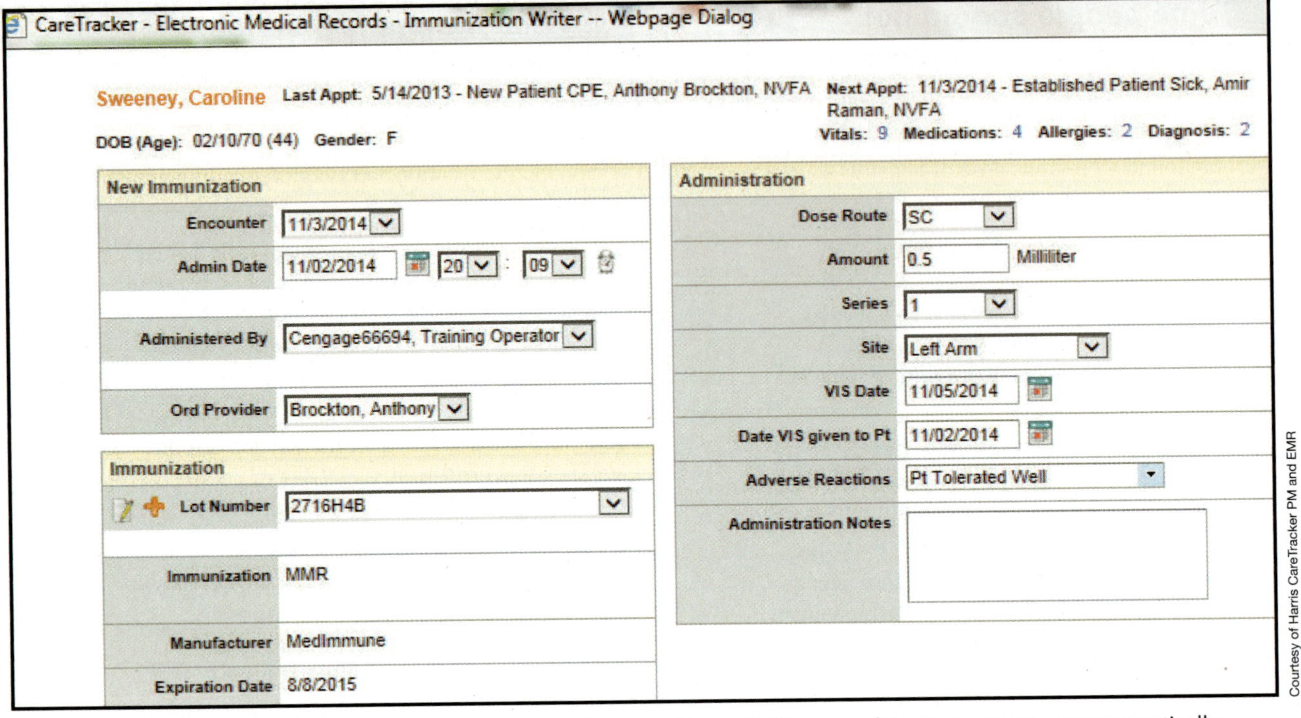

Courtesy of Harris CareTracker PM and EMR

Figure 4-11 ■ When the lot number of the immunization is entered in the EHR, many of the items necessary automatically populate in the window. The VIS Date window is where you will enter the date from the back of the VIS form.

Items Listed When Documenting a Prescription Order in the Patient's Chart

Table 4-4 lists items that should be listed when documenting prescription orders.

Documenting Patient Education Sessions

Today we live in a society where patient education is essential. Education is particularly important in

Table 4-4 Items Listed When Documenting a Prescription Order

Information to be Documented	Description or Facts
1. The date and the time that you called in the prescription or gave the patient a copy of the written prescription	This is important when the patient calls to see what time the prescription was called in to the pharmacy.
2. If calling in the prescription to a pharmacy, the pharmacy's name, location, phone number, and pharmacist's name	This will help to alleviate any misunderstandings as to which pharmacy was used and to whom you spoke.
3. Name of medication	Write out the entire name of the drug. Many drugs sound alike and using abbreviations could increase the risk of error.
4. Strength of medication	The strength should be clearly written so that the patient is not under or overmedicated.
5. Amount to be dispensed	The amount to be dispensed is the amount of medication that the patient is to receive, such as the number of pills or number of mL. You may write the numeral for the amount to be dispensed but it should also be spelled out to minimize confusion and to decrease the ability for someone to change the number.
6. Special instructions	This part of the prescription lists how the medication is to be taken and how much is to be taken per dose.
7. Number of refills	List the number of refills designated by the physician.
8. Who ordered the prescription	The medical assistant must show an order when documenting any medication orders.
9. Documentation identifier	First name or initial and last name, followed by your credential.

DOCUMENTATION EXAMPLE #5: DOCUMENTING A PRESCRIPTION ORDER

09-12-XX 1015	Called in Rx to ABC Pharmacy (South High Location), 292-6778. Spoke w/ pharmacist Julie Moore. TOPROL-XL 25mg; Take 1 tab daily, #90 (Ninety), no refills per Dr. Stevenson. Ray Biggs, CMA (AAMA)------------------------------

DOCUMENTATION EXAMPLE #6: DOCUMENTING A PRESCRIPTION ORDER

05-12-XX 1300	Written Rx: Ery-Tab, 250 mg, #40 (forty), Take 1 tab q.i.d. per Dr. Dorado. Tom Lehamn, RMA (AMT)

EHR Application

When you create prescriptions in the patient's EHR, there is no need to document the information anywhere else in the chart. The information is saved in the patient's EHR when you create the prescription. Refer to Figure 4-12 for an illustration of a prescription screen in Harris CareTracker and refer to Figure 4-13 to illustrate how the prescription automatically populates in the patient's EHR after creating the prescription.

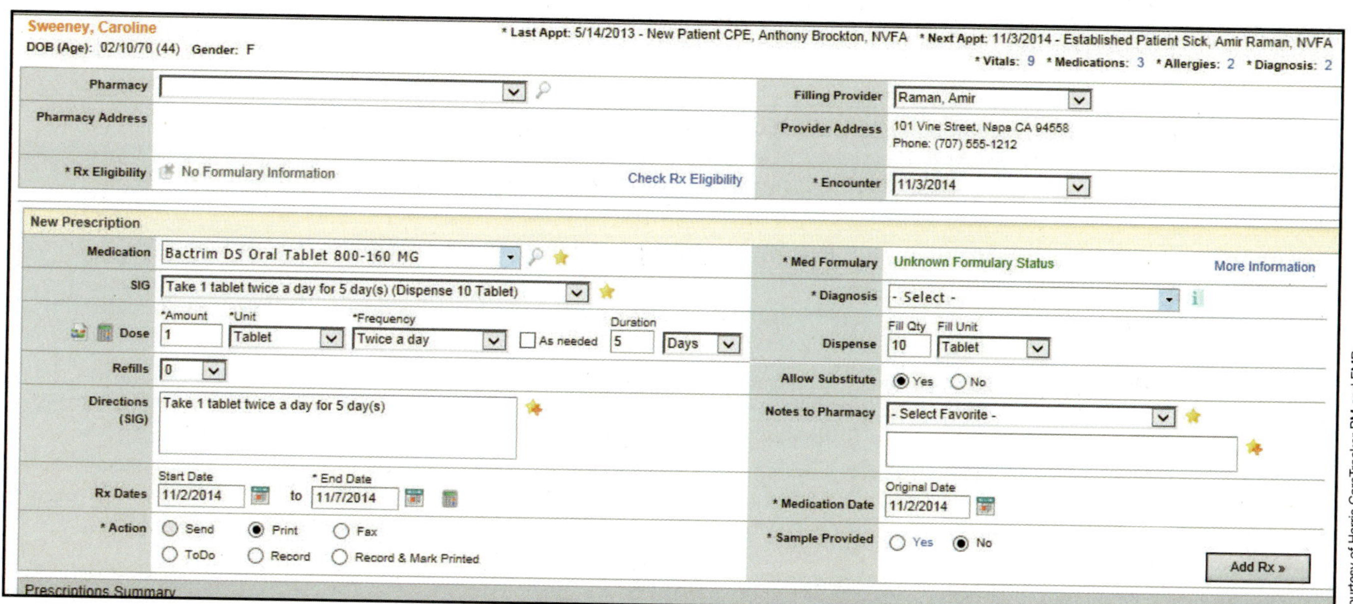
Sweeney, Caroline
DOB (Age): 02/10/70 (44) Gender: F
* Last Appt: 5/14/2013 - New Patient CPE, Anthony Brockton, NVFA * Next Appt: 11/3/2014 - Established Patient Sick, Amir Raman, NVFA
* Vitals: 9 * Medications: 3 * Allergies: 2 * Diagnosis: 2

Pharmacy: | Filling Provider: Raman, Amir
Pharmacy Address: | Provider Address: 101 Vine Street, Napa CA 94558 Phone: (707) 555-1212
* Rx Eligibility: No Formulary Information — Check Rx Eligibility | * Encounter: 11/3/2014

New Prescription
Medication: Bactrim DS Oral Tablet 800-160 MG | * Med Formulary: Unknown Formulary Status — More Information
SIG: Take 1 tablet twice a day for 5 day(s) (Dispense 10 Tablet) | * Diagnosis: - Select -
Dose: *Amount 1 *Unit Tablet *Frequency Twice a day ☐ As needed Duration 5 Days | Dispense: Fill Qty 10 Fill Unit Tablet
Refills: 0 | Allow Substitute: ◉ Yes ○ No
Directions (SIG): Take 1 tablet twice a day for 5 day(s) | Notes to Pharmacy: - Select Favorite -
Rx Dates: Start Date 11/2/2014 to * End Date 11/7/2014 | * Medication Date: Original Date 11/2/2014
* Action: ○ Send ◉ Print ○ Fax ○ ToDo ○ Record ○ Record & Mark Printed | * Sample Provided: ○ Yes ◉ No
Add Rx »
Prescriptions Summary

Courtesy of Harris CareTracker PM and EMR

Figure 4-12 ■ An example of a prescription order screen in the electronic health record.

Medications

	Medication	Original	Renewal	Order #	Fill Provider	Qty	Re	Status	Diag
☐	Bactrim DS Oral Tablet 800-160 MG	11/02/14							
	Take 1 tablet twice a day for 5 day(s)		11/02/14	11872177	Raman, Amir	10	0	Rx Printed	
☐	Sertraline HCl Oral Tablet 50 MG	03/15/14							
	Take 1 tablet once a day for days		03/15/14	11872176	Brockton, Anthony	30	0	Med Entered (Manual)	

Courtesy of Harris CareTracker PM and EMR

Figure 4-13 ■ Notice how the prescription information automatically populates in the patient's medication pane after creating the prescription.

pay-for-performance organizations. Patients who typically benefit from education include patients with chronic disease, presurgical patients, postsurgical patients, and patients who need to follow special preparation instructions for diagnostic procedures. Because of the emphasis on prevention, medical assistants may also educate patients on the importance of keeping up with specific screenings.

Table 4-5 lists important components that should be included in each patient education entry.

EHR Application

Most EHRs are stocked with a full set of instructional materials for all kinds of conditions, procedures, and medications. When you click on the educational sheet, it automatically loads the information in the patient's EHR. Depending on the software, you may need to develop a progress note regarding the session and the patient's understanding. Figure 4-14 illustrates a patient education screen in Harris CareTracker.

Documenting Telephone Calls

Clinical staff members are often called upon to screen patient symptoms over the phone (see Procedure 4-2). Because medical statutes vary from state to state always check your state's medical practice act before conducting telephone screenings. Screening patient calls is an important task and medical assistants should have specialized training before attempting to perform telephone screenings. Medical assistants should never attempt to screen calls without the aid of an approved office protocol manual or telephone screening manual. Refer to Table 4-6 for a complete listing of the items that should be included in the documentation of a telephone screening.

Table 4-5 Items Listed When Documenting Patient Education Sessions

Information to be Documented	Description or Facts
1. The date and time of the education session	
2. The topic and purpose of the education session	For instance, smoking cessation, diabetes education, and medication management.
3. Who ordered the education session	This could be especially important if there is any kind of charge associated with the session.
4. Who was present for the education session	Family members quite often assist with home care. Documenting who was present for the session illustrates that someone besides the patient also received the training.
5. Patient's comprehension and any reactions to the session	It is important to establish that those members in attendance understood the educational components that were delivered. This is usually accomplished by having the patient and family members in attendance repeat back the instructions.
6. Any educational materials that were distributed to the patient	Giving the patient educational materials helps the patient to remember the instructions when they get home.
7. Any verbal information that was given to the patient that wasn't listed in the brochures	If special instructions were given, such as encouraging the patient to call with any questions or to follow up in a certain time span, these should be noted in the chart.
8. Documentation identifier	First name or initial and last name, followed by your credential.

DOCUMENTATION EXAMPLE #7: DOCUMENTING PATIENT EDUCATION SESSIONS

03-12-XX 1530	Breast health education session per Dr. Gutile. Demonstrated how to perform a breast self-exam and the signs to look for when performing a breast exam. Pt. appeared to comprehend the information and performed a successful breast exam on the breast model. Gave pt. breast health brochures and set up pt's first baseline mammogram at Blackwell Radiology on 03-17-XX at 1400. Pt instructed to call with any questions. Molly Brown, CMA (AAMA)--

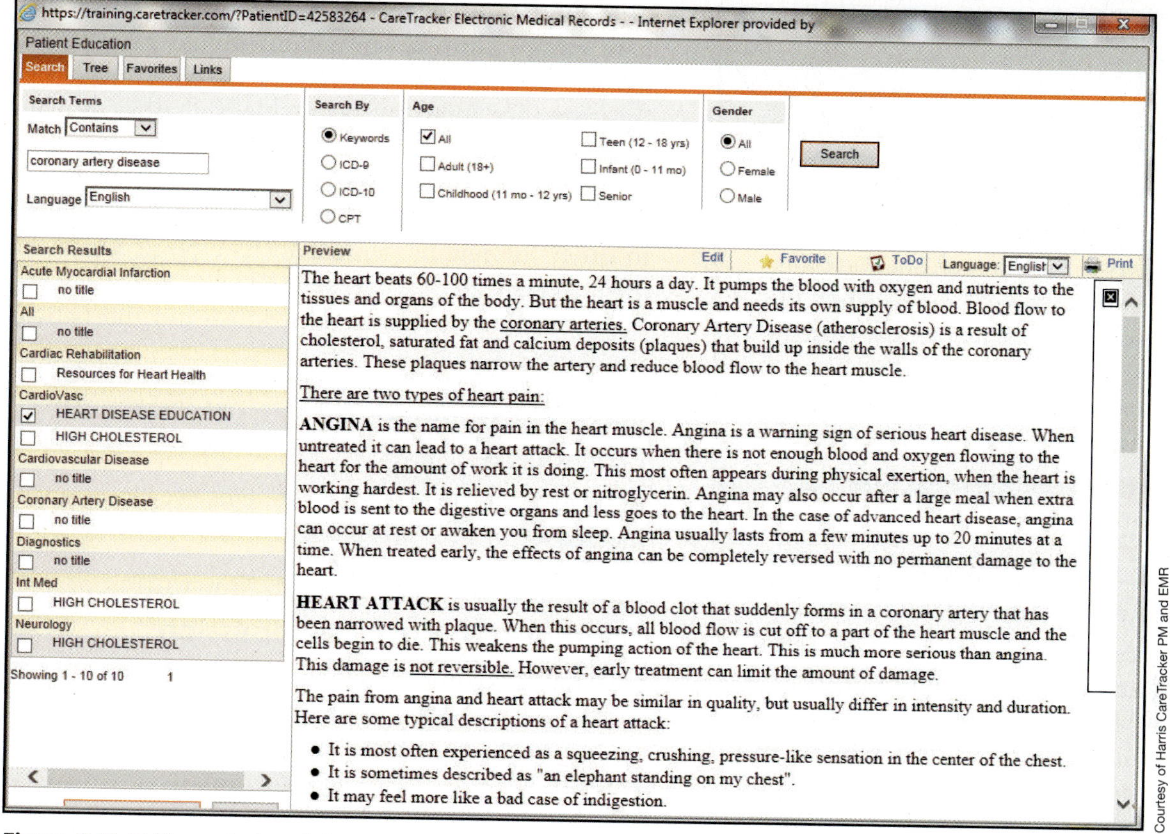
https://training.caretracker.com/?PatientID=42583264 - CareTracker Electronic Medical Records - - Internet Explorer provided by

Patient Education

Search | Tree | Favorites | Links

Search Terms

Match Contains

coronary artery disease

Language English

Search By: Keywords, ICD-9, ICD-10, CPT

Age: All, Adult (18+), Childhood (11 mo - 12 yrs), Teen (12 - 18 yrs), Infant (0 - 11 mo), Senior

Gender: All, Female, Male

Search

Search Results

Acute Myocardial Infarction
no title
All
no title
Cardiac Rehabilitation
Resources for Heart Health
CardioVasc
HEART DISEASE EDUCATION
HIGH CHOLESTEROL
Cardiovascular Disease
no title
Coronary Artery Disease
no title
Diagnostics
no title
Int Med
HIGH CHOLESTEROL
Neurology
HIGH CHOLESTEROL

Showing 1 - 10 of 10 1

Preview | Edit | Favorite | ToDo | Language: English | Print

The heart beats 60-100 times a minute, 24 hours a day. It pumps the blood with oxygen and nutrients to the tissues and organs of the body. But the heart is a muscle and needs its own supply of blood. Blood flow to the heart is supplied by the coronary arteries. Coronary Artery Disease (atherosclerosis) is a result of cholesterol, saturated fat and calcium deposits (plaques) that build up inside the walls of the coronary arteries. These plaques narrow the artery and reduce blood flow to the heart muscle.

There are two types of heart pain:

ANGINA is the name for pain in the heart muscle. Angina is a warning sign of serious heart disease. When untreated it can lead to a heart attack. It occurs when there is not enough blood and oxygen flowing to the heart for the amount of work it is doing. This most often appears during physical exertion, when the heart is working hardest. It is relieved by rest or nitroglycerin. Angina may also occur after a large meal when extra blood is sent to the digestive organs and less goes to the heart. In the case of advanced heart disease, angina can occur at rest or awaken you from sleep. Angina usually lasts from a few minutes up to 20 minutes at a time. When treated early, the effects of angina can be completely reversed with no permanent damage to the heart.

HEART ATTACK is usually the result of a blood clot that suddenly forms in a coronary artery that has been narrowed with plaque. When this occurs, all blood flow is cut off to a part of the heart muscle and the cells begin to die. This weakens the pumping action of the heart. This is much more serious than angina. This damage is not reversible. However, early treatment can limit the amount of damage.

The pain from angina and heart attack may be similar in quality, but usually differ in intensity and duration. Here are some typical descriptions of a heart attack:

- It is most often experienced as a squeezing, crushing, pressure-like sensation in the center of the chest.
- It is sometimes described as "an elephant standing on my chest".
- It may feel more like a bad case of indigestion.

Figure 4-14 ■ The majority of electronic health records have educational materials that can be printed or emailed to the patient. Any time you print or email information to the patient, it automatically is recorded in the patient's EHR.

Table 4-6 Items Listed When Documenting a Patient Telephone Screening

Information to be Documented	Description or Facts
1. The date and time of the telephone call	Establish the date and time of the call in case the "timing of the call" becomes an issue in a legal dispute.
2. General complaint	A description of why the patient is calling. If talking to someone other than the patient, list the name of the person with whom you spoke (spoke with Emily's mother, Mrs. Booker).
3. The responses to the screening questions listed in the protocol or telephone screening manual	Once the patient has stated the general complaint and duration of the symptoms, proceed directly to the protocol or telephone screening manual and ask the patient the corresponding questions that best match the patient's complaint. Document the patient's responses to each question. (If it is determined that the patient is in the middle of a life-threatening emergency, do not proceed any further, but rather give the instructions listed in the action column of the screening manual.)
4. Instructions given to the patient and list where the instructions came from	This is to illustrate that you followed a specific protocol approved by the provider.
5. The patient's comprehension of the instructions and the patient's intentions in following the instructions	This applies if the patient was given instructions to follow at home.
6. Documentation identifier	First name or initial and last name, followed by your credential.

DOCUMENTATION EXAMPLE #8: DOCUMENTING A TELEPHONE SCREENING

11-07-XX 1530	TC: Pt. c/o a continuous headache (10) × 2 days. "Pain starts in the front of my head and radiates to the back of my head."⊕Nausea & Vomiting (3 episodes in last 2 hours).⊕Light sensitivity,⊖fever,⊖trauma,⊖neck pain,⊖sinus symptoms. No history of migraines. OTC: Tylenol Extra Strength 1000 mg every 4–6 hours. "Little relief." Scheduled pt. for SDA per page 24 of screening manual. Pt. scheduled for 1630 appointment today with Dr. Song. Mary Brown, CMA (AAMA)--

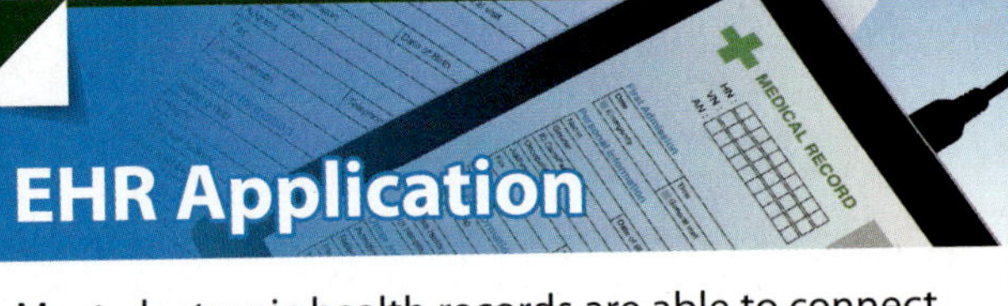

Most electronic health records are able to connect phone messages to the provider's task module. The provider is able to see the message once he clicks on the task. Refer to Figure 4-15 for an example of "To Do" messages created by the medical assistant to the provider in Harris CareTracker. Once the message is created it can be found in the correspondence box in the patient's electronic health record.

Identifying Critical Information for Scheduling Outside Procedures

There will be occasions when the patient will need to be scheduled at an outside facility to have particular procedures performed such as lab tests, X-rays, and certain diagnostic testing. The clinical medical assistant may be responsible for scheduling these procedures and must check the patient's insurance plan to determine if the patient should be sent to a **participating provider** (a facility that contracts with the insurance company to provide laboratory or diagnostic services) before scheduling the procedure. The medical assistant will also need to determine if the procedure needs to be precertified by the payer in order for reimbursement to take place. Once the medical assistant has checked the insurance coverage, the procedure should be scheduled and the patient should be notified.

Items Documented for Outside Procedures

Refer to Table 4-7 to learn what items need to be documented for outside procedures.

Items Recorded in the Chart When Scheduling a Hospital Admission

Hospital admissions should be recorded in the patient's record. Refer to Table 4-8 for a list of items that should be recorded in the chart when scheduling a hospital admission.

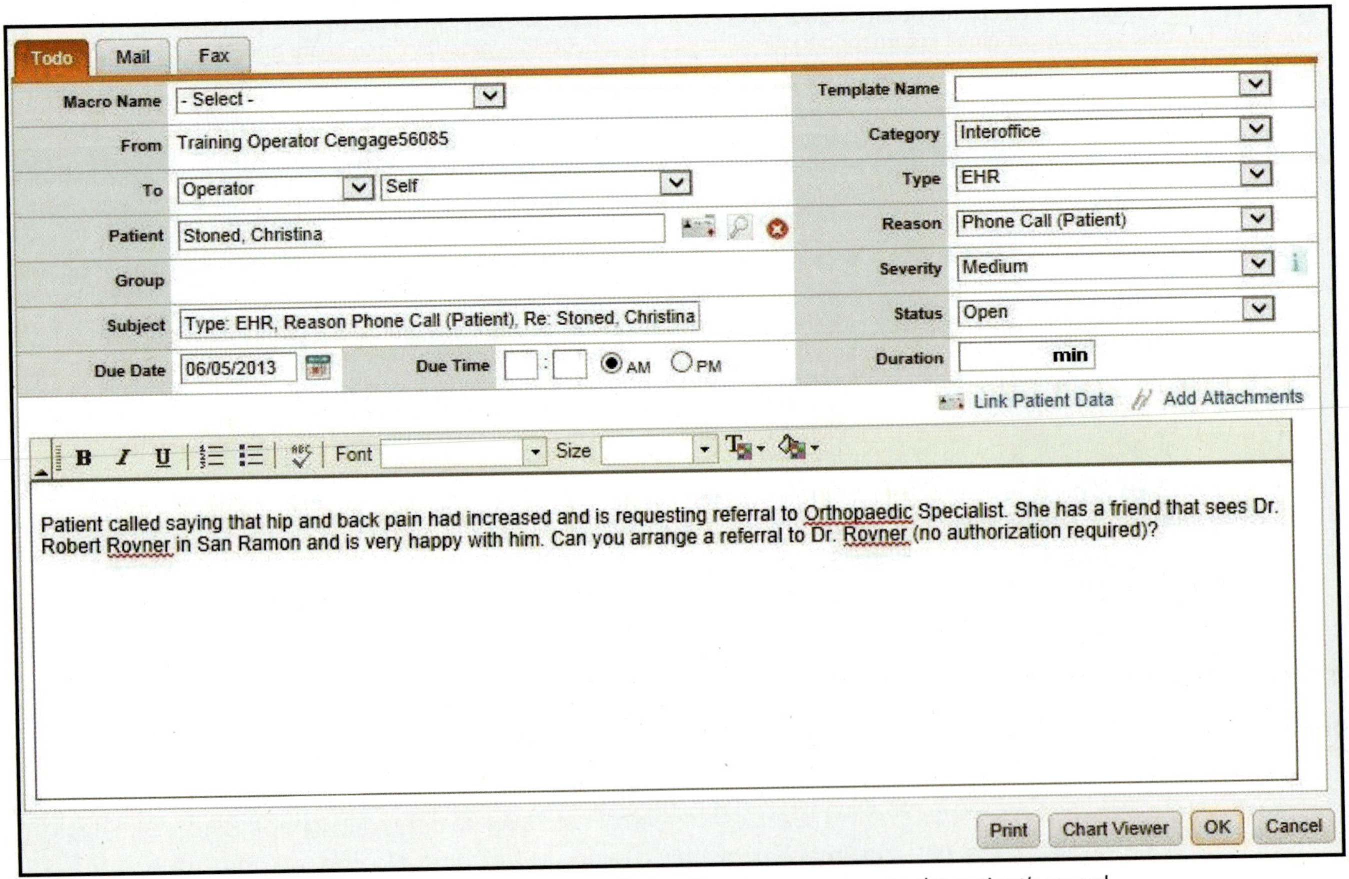

Todo | Mail | Fax

Macro Name	- Select -	Template Name	
From	Training Operator Cengage56085	Category	Interoffice
To	Operator / Self	Type	EHR
Patient	Stoned, Christina	Reason	Phone Call (Patient)
Group		Severity	Medium
Subject	Type: EHR, Reason Phone Call (Patient), Re: Stoned, Christina	Status	Open
Due Date	06/05/2013 Due Time : AM PM	Duration	min

Link Patient Data Add Attachments

B I U Font Size

Patient called saying that hip and back pain had increased and is requesting referral to Orthopaedic Specialist. She has a friend that sees Dr. Robert Rovner in San Ramon and is very happy with him. Can you arrange a referral to Dr. Rovner (no authorization required)?

Print | Chart Viewer | OK | Cancel

Figure 4-15 ■ The ToDo screen in an electronic health records ties all patient messages to the patient's record.

Table 4-7 Items Listed When Documenting an Outside Procedure

Information to be Documented	Description or Facts
1. The date and time that the procedure was set up	
2. Name of procedure(s) or test(s) to be performed and diagnosis when applicable. (CPT and ICD codes are often necessary when setting up these procedures.)	Examples: MRI of the brain and spinal cord, chest X-ray PA and lateral, tubal ligation.
3. Name and location of facility performing the procedure and location within the facility where patient is to report	This is important because many health facilities have more than one location. It is also to give the patient information where they should report once they arrive at the center.
4. Name of person at facility who scheduled the procedure	This is important in case there are any problems.
5. Date and time of procedure	The date and time that the procedure is to be performed.
6. Name of provider ordering procedures	You must always show an order for any diagnostic or lab procedures in order for the insurance company to cover the procedures.
7. Any special instructions for the patient	Does the patient need to fast before the testing, follow special preparations prior to the testing, or arrive early to fill out the appropriate paperwork?
8. Confirmation to the patient	You will need to confirm that you have shared this information with the patient once the procedure is scheduled.
9. Documentation identifier	First name or initial and last name, followed by your credential.

DOCUMENTATION EXAMPLE #9: DOCUMENTING AN OUTSIDE PROCEDURE

05-22-XX 0900	Scheduled pt. for a uterine ultrasound at Washington Hospital on Tuesday 05-23-XX at 0800. Spoke with Judy Allen in the ultrasound lab. "Pt. should arrive 30 minutes early to complete the appropriate paperwork and should drink 4–6 glasses of water before arriving and bring a water bottle just in case the bladder is not completely full." Called and confirmed this info with pt. Jessica Holtsberry, CMA (AAMA)--

Table 4-8 Items Listed When Documenting a Hospital Admission

Information to be Documented	Description or Facts
1. Name of the hospital and location when applicable	Some hospitals have multiple locations.
2. Date of admission	The date the patient should be admitted.
3. Reason for admission	The diagnosis or condition that created the need for the patient to be hospitalized.
4. Provider ordering the admission	What provider ordered the hospitalization?
5. Person to whom you spoke to set up the admission	This is in case there are any problems.
6. Any special instructions given to the hospital	This generally includes orders for diagnostic testing, medication orders, special diet requests, and so on.
7. Any special instructions given to you by the hospital	Time for the patient to arrive and room number if applicable.
8. Documentation identifier	First name or initial and last name, followed by your credential.

DOCUMENTATION EXAMPLE #10: DOCUMENTING A HOSPITAL ADMISSION

10-12-XX 1445	Spoke w/ Terry Pike in Admissions at Riverside Hospital (East). Scheduled pt. for direct admission regarding an acute flare up of colitis per Dr. Scottler. "Pt. is to go straight to the admission's department upon arrival." Pt. given written orders from Dr. Scottler to take to the hospital. Bianca Walker, RMA (AMT)--

MAKING CORRECTIONS OR ADDENDUMS TO CHART NOTES

On occasion, it may be necessary to make a correction or an addendum to a previous chart entry. An **addendum** is an addition or supplement to a previous chart note. Health care workers should never paint correction fluid over an error, scratch over the error with a pen or marker, or rewrite the record. Applying those kinds of corrections could make it appear that the person making the correction is trying to hide something.

When making a correction in a paper chart, do the following:

1. Draw a single line through the error.
2. Write in the correction.
3. Write CORR above the correction.
4. Initial and date the correction.

The procedure for correcting or amending electronic entries will vary according to the program being used. A nice advantage of using electronic records is that until you finalize the note you can make all of the corrections you want, but once you click on the tab to complete the note, the information will be permanently stored within the system's software. You can usually make addendums by clicking on the Addendum or Changes button within the patient's individual file. The addendum function may allow you to add information but not change the contents of the original note. Some programs will allow you to make changes to the original note but stores all of the original notes so that they can be tracked for future reference.

COMPOSE PROFESSIONAL CORRESPONDENCE USING ELECTRONIC TECHNOLOGY

The majority of health care facilities are now digital; however, the depth of digitization will vary from one facility to another. As a result of these technological advances, much of the way we communicate with individuals inside and outside of the medical office will be through electronic exchanges.

According to the federal government, electronic health information exchanges allow health care providers and patients to appropriately access and securely share medical information electronically—improving the speed, quality, safety, and cost of patient care. This type of exchange helps to meet the Meaningful Use Stage 2 requirements in regards to the use of Health Information Exchange (HIE). The types of HIE are described below.

Directed exchange is used by providers to easily and securely send patient information—such as laboratory orders and results, patient referrals, or discharge summaries—directly to another health care professional, according to the healthit.gov website. The medical assistant may be responsible for sending patient information to outside health care providers through this type of exchange.

Consumer-mediated exchange is a means that is often used to communicate with patients. The patient's health portal is an example of a consumer-mediated exchange. This is the safest way to communicate with patients. The patient portal may be compared to an online banking portal in which the patient can view different parts of their medical record. Through this exchange the patient may have access to clinical summaries, chart notes, and diagnostic testing results. Electronic messaging can also be conducted through patient portals. Medical office team members control what the patient can see through the portal.

Before sending electronic exchanges, or entering information into the patient portal, the medical assistant should review the following:

- Be sure that you are using a very secure HIE that meets all HIPAA standards when sharing protected health information.
- Make certain the provider has authorized content for the patient to review before making available in the patient's portal.
- Be sure that all exchanges are professional and do not contain any spelling or grammatical errors.

When sending e-mails through a secure exchange:

- Always include the subject in the subject line box.
- Include a salutation and a closing when sending exchanges to patients or other providers.
- Insert numbers or bullets when making a point.
- Avoid using all capital letters in electronic messages, as this could be interpreted as shouting at the individual with whom you are corresponding (such as "DID YOU RECEIVE SAMPLE #541432 YET?").
- Avoid using common jargon or abbreviations in professional electronic exchanges.
- Avoid using emoticons in professional exchanges.
- Make certain that your subject line matches the content in your message.

- Make certain that you attach your attachments when applicable.
- You should only use the high-priority symbol (!) when you truly have a high-priority message.

In general, medical assistants should never use the Internet for personal endeavors while at work. This includes shopping online, checking or sending personal email, or going to inappropriate websites.

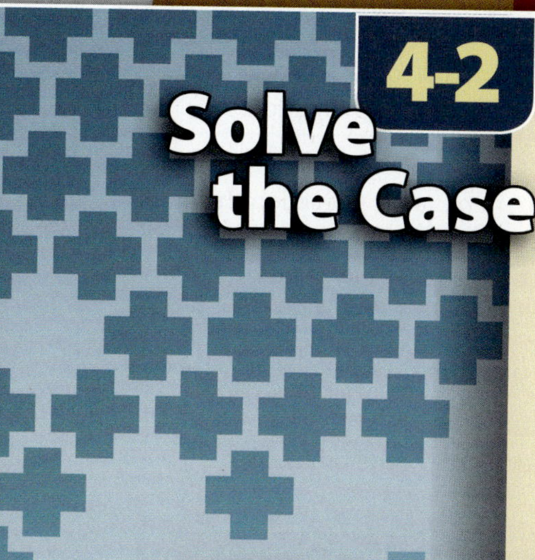

Dr. Timmons finished his exam and asks you to combine Demerol 100 mg and Phenergan 50 mg into a single syringe and to administer it IM to Mr. Wilcox. (*Note*: Some states allow medical assistants to administer controlled substances; however, several states do not. Always check your state's standards!). Dr. Timmons asks you to give the patient a handout on "Different Types of Headaches" and also asks you to set up a CT of the head and neck. Using the information you learned in this chapter, document three different entries on a progress note or lined paper illustrating the performance of these tasks. Entries should include: Medication administration information, patient education information, and setting up a CT of the head and neck (outside procedure). Insert fictional data to complete your entries such as the location of the injection, how the patient tolerated the injection, who was present for patient education, and where you sent the patient for the CT scan.

PROCEDURE 4-1

Documenting the Administration of a Medication

Objective:

To document a medication you just administered.

Equipment/Supplies:

- Patient's chart/EHR
- Black Pen (if applicable)
- Medication Information

PROCEDURAL STEPS	DETAILS AND/OR RATIONALE
1. Assemble required information for medication entries such as medication labels and provider orders.	Having these items saves time.
2. Record the date and time of administration.	This is for legal purposes.

continues

PROCEDURE 4-1 continued

PROCEDURAL STEPS	DETAILS AND/OR RATIONALE
3. Record the full name of the medication.	Many medications are similar. Recording full name eliminates any confusion.
4. Record the strength of the medication.	Medications come in different strengths.
5. Record the route of administration.	Drugs are intended to give a specific route. Make certain that you are specific in your documentation.
6. Record the site of administration.	This is especially important when patients have multiple injections. If a patient has a local reaction the provider needs to know which medication was given and where it was given to properly identify which medication caused the reaction.
7. Record the name of physician that ordered the medication.	You must always show an order for medications.
8. Record any problems during or following administration and actions taken.	This is to make the provider aware of the problem and for legal purposes.
9. Record any consent forms signed.	This is necessary when administering immunizations, experimental medications, and medications not covered by insurance.
10. Record educational material distributed.	This is to illustrate the patient was given home care instructions.
11. Record information in the medication log (if applicable).	
12. Record documentation identifier.	First name or initial and last name, followed by your credential.
13. Document accurately in the patient's chart and make certain there are no spelling errors. Only use standard medical abbreviations that do not appear on the Joint Commission's "Do Not Use List."	

DOCUMENTATION EXAMPLE

12-10-XX 1335	Allergy serum, 0.3 mL, Sub-Q, R. arm per Dr. Kim. Observed a small wheal the size of a dime at the injection site during the post exam. ⊖erythema or rash at injection site. ⊕warm to the touch. ⊖dyspnea. Informed Dr. Kim of reaction. Dispensed one 50 mg caplet of Benadryl, PO per Dr. Kim. Pt's husband will drive her home. Dr. Kim would like allergy dose reduced to 0.1 mL the next visit. Pt. to call with any problems. A Muhammad, CMA (AAMA)--

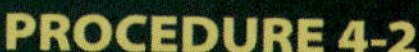

PROCEDURE 4-2

Documenting a Phone Call from a Patient

Objective:

To document a call from the patient.

Equipment/Supplies:

- Patient's chart/EHR
- Black Pen (if applicable)
- Telephone Screening or Triage Manual

PROCEDURAL STEPS	DETAILS AND/OR RATIONALE
1. Assemble patient's chart, black pen (if applicable), and telephone screening manual.	
2. Document the date and time of the telephone call.	Important for legal purposes.
3. Document the general complaint and to whom you are speaking, if not the patient. (Check privacy statement to see if you have permission to discuss patient information with caller.) If not, you will need to speak directly with patient.	You need to show the nature of the call and who you spoke with if not the patient. You need to verify that you can speak with the caller if the caller is someone other than the patient or you will violate HIPAA policies.
4. Open screening manual and document responses to the screening questions listed in the protocol or telephone screening manual	This will illustrate that you followed the protocol in the screening manual.
5. ***Incorporate critical thinking skills when performing patient assessment.***	It is important that you use good critical thinking skills when screening patients over the phone. When the screening manual doesn't match the patient's symptoms, it is important to that you provide the patient with the best directions possible.
6. Document instructions given to the patient and list where the instructions came from.	This illustrates what the patient was told and where you obtained the instructions.
7. Document the patient's comprehension of the instructions and the patient's intentions in following the instructions.	This is for legal purposes.
8. Record documentation identifier.	First name or initial and last name, followed by your credential.
9. Document accurately in the medical record. There should be no spelling errors and you should only use standard medical abbreviations that are not on the Joint Commission's "Do Not Use List."	

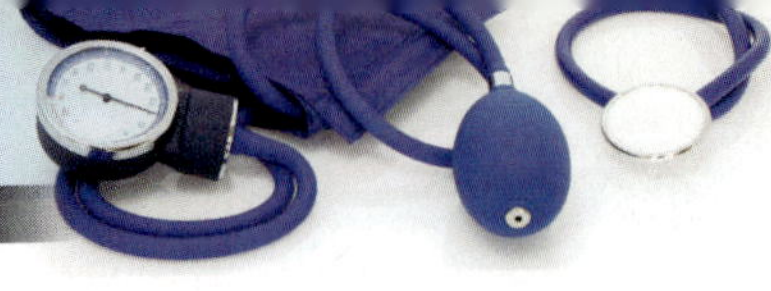

DOCUMENTATION EXAMPLE

Todo | Mail | Fax

Macro Name:
From: Training Operator Cengage66694
To: Operator | Cengage66694, Training Operato
Patient: Smith, Cosima
Group:
Subject: Type: EHR, Reason Phone Call (Patient), Re: Smith, Cosima
Due Date: 4/19/2015 Due Time: : AM PM

Template Name:
Category: Interoffice
Type: - Select -
Reason: - Select -
Severity: Critical
Status: Open
Duration: min

Link Patient Data Add Attachments

B I U Font Size A- A-

TC: Pt called complaining of "chest pain" for the past 30 minutes. Pain starts in the center of chest and radiates to the left side of chest. Pain level (5/10) No radiation of pain to other parts of the body. +SOB, Negative N/V. Instructed patient to hang up and call 911 per screening manual, page 26 so that she can be evaluated by the EMS. Patient stated she would.

Print | Chart Viewer | OK | Cancel

CHAPTER SUMMARY

- Documentation within the patient's chart is the essential tool that providers and health care workers use to communicate with one another.
- There are several state and federal guidelines that protect patient information in the chart.
- The chart is a legal document used in all professional liability cases.
- Lack of documentation has been the deciding factor in many professional liability cases that were lost. Any time the medical assistant has an encounter with the patient, even if the encounter appears to be minor or trivial, it should be documented in the medical record.
- Objectivity is important when documenting for legal success. The medical assistant should avoid comments that could appear subjective or trite.
- Documentation Dos include the following: Do use the right chart, Do document all encounters, Do chart thoroughly, Do document accurately, Do use correct spelling, Do document the date and time of each entry, Do chart legibly, Do use an approved documentation identifier, Do document informed consent of refusal to follow directions, Do use only standard and approved abbreviations, and Do document on every line.
- Documentation Don'ts include the following: Don't procrastinate, Don't diagnose, Don't document for someone else, and Don't alter records.
- Avoid using abbreviations on the Joint Commission's "Do Not Use List" or the ISMP's "Error-Prone Abbreviation List."
- A chief complaint is the reason the patient is being seen and a progress note is a follow-up from a previous visit.

- Types of documentation performed by the clinical medical assistant include the following: Chief complaints, progress notes, laboratory procedures, in-office procedures, medication administration, prescriptions, patient education sessions, telephone calls from patients, outside procedures, and hospital admissions.
- Documentation in the EHR is much different than in paper charts because of templates within the EHR and the ability for items to populate to other areas in the EHR.
- If you make an error in the patient's paper chart, draw a single line through it, write in the correction, write CORR above the error, and initial and date the error. Once a note is saved in the electronic health record it cannot be changed. An amendment will need to be made.
- Send patient emails only through secure servers such as the patient portal in the EHR. Watch spelling and grammar when sending emails; include a subject line in the subject line box; include a salutation and closing; use bullets when you want to make specific points; and avoid using all capital letters, jargon, or emoticons when sending emails. Attach your attachments before writing the message and use the high-priority symbol only when it truly is a high-priority email.

CERTIFICATION REVIEW QUESTIONS

1. Which of the following would not be considered a "Documentation Do"?
   a. Do document accurately.
   b. Do include the date and time for each entry.
   c. Do document subjectively.
   d. Do use only standard abbreviations that have been approved by the practice.

2. Which of the following items should be included when documenting an in-house procedure?
   a. The name of the procedure.
   b. The location where the procedure was performed.
   c. The storage cabinet from where you obtained supplies to perform the procedure.
   d. Both a and b.

3. Which of the following practices would be harmful to the provider if the record went to court?
   a. Documentation that was illegible and incomplete.
   b. An error that had been scratched out and rewritten.
   c. A chart containing abbreviations that were on the "Do Not Use" abbreviations list.
   d. All of the above.

4. Which of the following should be included when documenting a laboratory entry in the patient's chart?
   a. The name of the lab test.
   b. Where the specimens were sent.
   c. Any problems experienced during or following the procedure.
   d. All of the above.

5. What items should not appear in a professional email?
   a. The name of the person to whom you are sending the email.
   b. Emoticons.
   c. Common email jargon used in personal emails such as "lol".
   d. Both b and c.

6. Which of the following should not be done when correcting an error in the chart?
   a. Drawing a single line through the error.
   b. Recording the date that you make the correction.
   c. Starting a new progress note and rewriting the entry so that the entry doesn't look messy.
   d. Placing your initials next to the error.

7. What is the name of the organization that provides a list of "Do Not Use" abbreviations?
   a. HIPAA.
   b. CCHIT.
   c. Joint Commission.
   d. FDA.
8. The medical assistant is able to create what types of prescriptions?
   a. Nonscheduled.
   b. Scheduled and nonscheduled.
   c. The medical assistant cannot write any prescriptions.
   d. The types vary from office to office and state to state.
9. What information does not need to be documented for a patient education session?
   a. The topic and purpose of the session.
   b. Who was present for the session.
   c. Patient's comprehension of the session.
   d. All of the above responses are correct.
10. How should the medical assistant handle telephone screenings?
    a. A medical assistant should never perform telephone screenings because it is against the law.
    b. A medical assistant should provide instructions to patients on what has worked for her in the past.
    c. A medical assistant should schedule appointments for anyone who calls the office.
    d. A medical assistant should follow an approved screening manual if given the responsibility of screening patient calls.

STUDY RESOURCES

Resources to Test and Reinforce Your Knowledge:	
Certification Review Questions	Take this end-of-chapter quiz
Workbook	• Complete the activities for Chapter 4 • Perform the procedures for Chapter 4 using the Competency Checklists
Resources to Promote Critical Thinking:	
***Solve the Case* Activities**	• Consider these case studies and discuss your conclusions
MindTap	• Complete Chapter 4 readings and activities

REFERENCES

Consumer-Mediated Information Exchange. (2011). 968–976. Retrieved January 5, 2015, from http://www.gahin.org/sites/default/files/pictures/GA%20Consumer%20Mediated%20Information%20Exchange%2012_06_11_FINAL.pdf

HealthIT.gov. (n.d.). Retrieved January 5, 2015, from http://www.healthit.gov/providers-professionals/health-information-exchange/what-hie

The Joint Commission. (n.d.). Retrieved January 5, 2015, from http://www.jointcommission.org/facts_about_the_official_/

The Joint Commission. (n.d.). Retrieved January 5, 2015, from http://www.jointcommission.org/standards_information/npsgs.aspx

Practices, I. F. (n.d.). *ISMP's List of Error-Prone Abbreviations, Symbols, and Dose Designations*. Retrieved January 5, 2015, from http://www.ismp.org/Tools/errorproneabbreviations.pdf

Today's Hospitalist. Charting 101: Making sure your documentation is on time and legible. (n.d.). Retrieved January 5, 2015, from http://www.todayshospitalist.com/index.php?b=articles_read&cnt=528

5

Conducting a Patient Screening

ESSENTIAL TERMS

active listening
body language
comprehensive medical history
family medical history
genogram
gesture
history of present illness (HPI)
past history (PH)
past health history (PHH)
personal medical history
social history
subjective information
symptoms
therapeutic communication
usual childhood diseases (UCHD or UCD)

CHAPTER OUTLINE

The Communication Cycle

Therapeutic Communication
- The Use of Nonverbal Communication or Body Language

Incorporating Effective Interviewing Techniques
- Effective Questioning Techniques
- Ineffective Questioning Techniques
- Effective Listening Techniques

The Screening Process
- Greeting Stage
- Performance of Height, Weight, and Vital Signs
- Medication Reconciliation
- Drug Allergies
- Obtaining the Chief Complaint and History of Present Illness

The Role of the Medical Assistant in History Collection

Tools Used to Collect Medical History Information

The Comprehensive Medical History
- Personal Medical History
- Family Medical History
- Social History
- Depression Screening
- Preventive Care Section
- Concluding the Interview

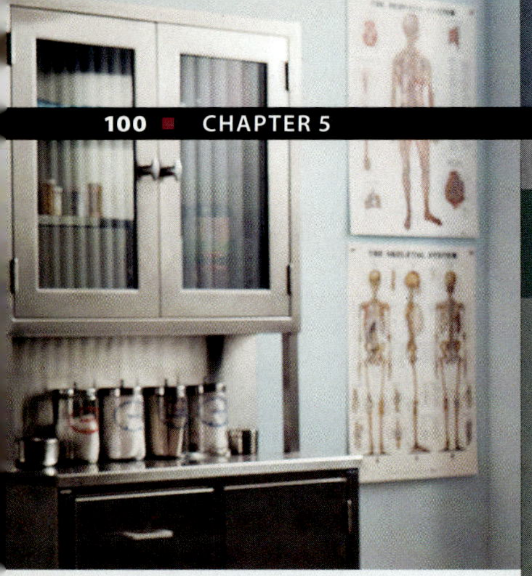

DEVELOPMENTAL OBJECTIVES

After completing this chapter, you should be able to:

1. Correctly spell and define the essential terms.
2. Recognize the element of oral communication using a sender-receiver process.
3. Recognize barriers to communication and techniques for overcoming barriers.
4. Explain how therapeutic communication improves the interviewing process.
5. Identify different forms of nonverbal communication and respond appropriately.
6. Identify and describe three types of questioning techniques and list examples for each technique.
7. List and describe eight different types of ineffective questioning techniques and explain why they are ineffective.
8. List various senses that are used during listening and why active listening is so important during the interview process.
9. Identify and describe four different listening techniques and list examples of each technique.
10. List two methods that are used to collect patient data.
11. List and describe three parts of the medical history.
12. List five questions that should be posed when a patient answers "Yes" to a disease or condition during a health history.
13. Develop a family history using the genogram method.
14. Describe why the reproductive health section and social part of the history may be more sensitive than other parts of the history.
15. Perform patient screening using established protocols.
16. Use feedback techniques to obtain patient information including reflection, restatement, and clarification and demonstrate principles of self-boundaries.

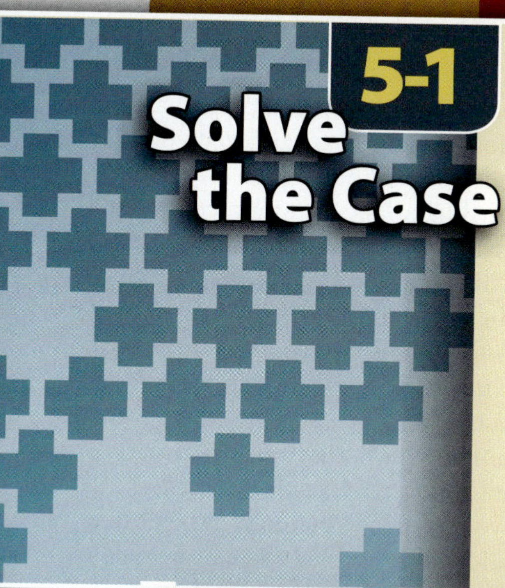

You are conducting a patient screening on 80-year-old Dillon Anderson. His daughter remains in the room during the interview. You notice that the patient is barely answering any questions; instead the daughter is answering all of the questions. Mr. Anderson appears very frail, unkempt, and has some bruises on his forearms, which may be related to blood thinners he is taking. He appears to have had a black eye; however, the bruising is very faded at this point. Mr. Anderson appears frustrated that his daughter continues to stay in the room. All of a sudden, the daughter gets a cell phone call and runs out to the lobby.

1. **How can the daughter staying in the room during the patient history hamper the communication process?**
2. **What questions might you ask the patient while the daughter is away?**
3. **How can you gently steer the daughter back out to the reception area when she returns?**

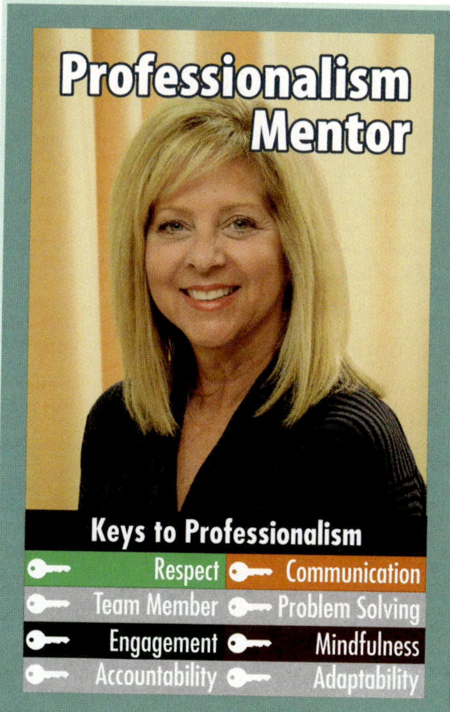

Are you a good listener? An important characteristic to possess when conducting a patient interview is "attention to detail." This is especially true when listening to a patient describe why they are being seen. Active listening demonstrates respect toward your patient. Consider the following scenario that I happened to witness firsthand at a very busy practice: A relatively new medical assistant was taking a patient history. Before the patient was situated, the medical assistant began the interview. With eyes on the computer and not really ever lifting her head up to look at the patient, the interview felt cold and the medical assistant seemed uncaring. The patient was having a hard time articulating what her chief complaint was. I wanted the medical assistant to stop typing and make eye contact with the patient. The simple act of giving your full attention can make the biggest difference when communicating because it makes the patient feel valued. This medical assistant did not show respect for her patient and in turn missed the opportunity to really connect with her. Over time, this connection helps to build trust that leads to a positive experience for both you and your patient. ■

INTRODUCTION

Conducting patient screenings is one of the most common tasks that medical assistants perform. Patient screenings usually consists of taking the patient's vital signs and measurements, updating the patient's medication and allergy history, obtaining the chief complaint, and conducting a medical history.

The medical history is one of the most vital documents found in the patient's chart. It gives providers an instant replay of diseases and conditions that the patient has encountered from the time of birth to the time when the history is developed. Figure 5-1 illustrates a medical assistant performing a history on the patient.

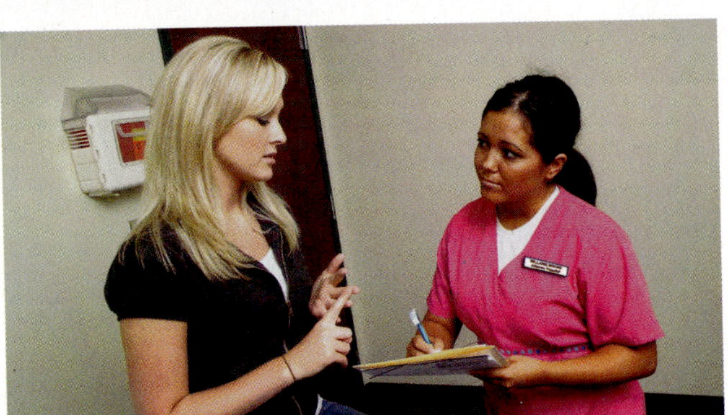

Figure 5-1 ■ An important task of the medical assistant is to take the patient's history.

The patient's personal, family, and social history are explored for possible clues in determining what ails the patient. The history also assists the provider in predicting future ailments and provides an opportunity for intervention that will either prevent or delay these possible conditions from occurring.

THE COMMUNICATION CYCLE

To be a successful communicator you must understand how the communication cycle works (Figure 5-2). In every communication encounter there is a *sender* or source. The sender is the person that conveys the message. *Encoding* is transferring the message in a manner that can be fully understood by the receiver during the decoding process. A good communicator will try to anticipate barriers that may impede communication and make the appropriate adjustments. Barriers may include items such as language deficiencies, distractions from family members, and behavioral, physical, or mental challenges in specific patients. *Channel* is the mode in which the message is delivered. In the office, the message is usually delivered face to face, but as we evolve with technology, the mode may be through videoconferencing or other forms of technology. It is important to select channels that best suit the receiver. *Decoding* information is just as important as encoding. It involves active listening and waiting to process the information until you have all the facts. During the decoding process you must free yourself from stereotyping or passing judgment on someone because of their race, religion, gender, sexual orientation, or socioeconomic status. The patient must trust that you are going to keep information private and that you have only their best interest at heart during the screening process. The *receiver* during any communication exchange is the one for whom the message is intended. The medical assistant will play both the sender and receiver throughout the screening process. *Noise* includes barriers that were listed earlier. The interviewer must take every measure to prevent all forms of noise during the encounter. For example, if you have a patient with a limited proficiency in English, you will arrange for an interpreter to be present during the interview; if you have a pediatric patient, you will adjust your communication style so that you can better connect with the child. *Feedback* is the verbal and nonverbal reactions provided by your audience, which is usually the patient but may be a parent, spouse, or another person acting on the patient's behalf. This is the segment of the interview in which you can assess the patient's comprehension of the questions at hand and an opportunity to make adjustments if necessary. The application of critical thinking is very important during this part of the interview.

THERAPEUTIC COMMUNICATION

Beyond the basic communication cycle, the medical assistant must understand how to communicate in a therapeutic manner. **Therapeutic communication** may be best described as an exchange of information between the health care worker and patient that leads to the advancement of the patient's physical and emotional well-being. In order to communicate at a therapeutic level, the medical assistant must learn how to create an environment that promotes active cooperation on the part of the patient during the interview

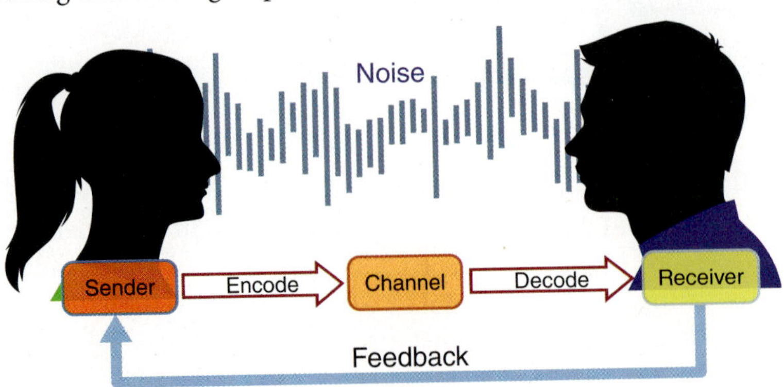

Figure 5-2 ■ What occurs during the communication cycle.

process. The medical assistant should display a trustful and compassionate demeanor and convey to the patient that all information collected during the interview will remain confidential.

Medical assistants must choose their words wisely and make certain that their body language is congruent with what is being stated verbally.

The Use of Nonverbal Communication or Body Language

Body language is nonverbal communication that includes unconscious body movements, gestures, and facial expressions; it often accompanies verbal messages. The use of body language is important during the patient interview. Body language can change the meaning of what is conveyed verbally. Studies suggest that less than 10% of what is perceived during a communication encounter is actually spoken while over 90% is the direct result of body language and tone of voice.

Body posture should be direct, open, and relaxed while still maintaining a professional posture. Medical assistants should avoid facial expressions or body language that make it appear that they are bored or preoccupied. Eye contact should be frequent, though excessive eye contact may be interpreted as staring, causing the patient to feel uncomfortable. This is especially true in certain cultures.

Touching may be used in instances where the medical assistant wants to convey concern or compassion (Figure 5-3), but may seem insincere if overly used or used in an inappropriate manner.

The medical assistant must also pay attention to the patient's body language and assess if it aligns with the patient's verbal communication. If not, the medical assistant must redirect her questions to obtain an accurate assessment.

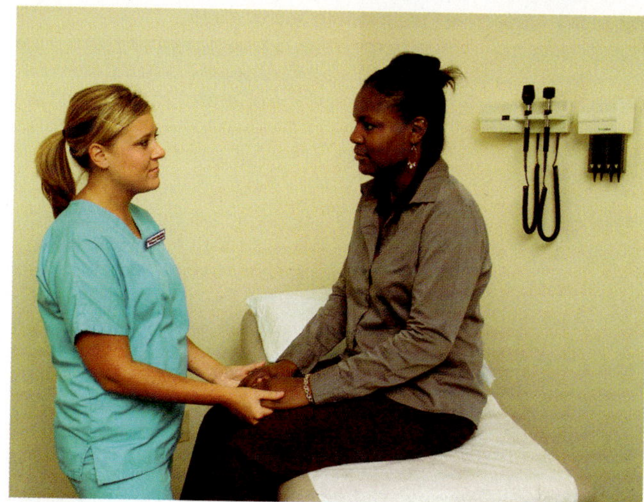

Figure 5-3 ■ The medical assistant is conveying that she cares about the patient through a gentle touch.

INCORPORATING EFFECTIVE INTERVIEWING TECHNIQUES

Becoming an effective interviewer is a skill that needs to be developed over a period of time. Medical assisting students should practice patient screenings several times throughout the training process so that by the time they graduate, they are comfortable with the process.

Effective Questioning Techniques

Effective questioning is necessary to facilitate a good exchange between the patient and medical assistant. The medical assistant should display interest and concern regarding what troubles the patient. For instance, one might respond to a patient by saying, "Mrs. Jones, it sounds as though you have gone through a rough time this past month." Interest in what the patient is saying can be demonstrated both verbally and nonverbally. Reinforce your concern by gently patting the patient on the shoulder or arm.

A **gesture** is a sign, signal, or cue that is used to communicate in combination with or apart from words. Gestures help to enhance the message that is being sent and are often incorporated during the questioning phase of the patient interview.

There are three types of questioning techniques that can be incorporated during the interview to help facilitate patient responses. Table 5-1 identifies those techniques and lists examples.

Ineffective Questioning Techniques

Just as good communication techniques encourage patient input, poor communication techniques impede the communication process. Table 5-2 lists examples of ineffective interviewing techniques.

Effective Listening Techniques

Listening is a difficult skill to master. It requires the medical assistant to enter the interview process with a clear mind. You cannot be an effective listener if your mind is wandering during the interview.

A good listener is an active listener. **Active listening** involves more than just your sense of hearing; it encompasses other senses as well. Observe the patient's facial expressions and body language as they respond to certain questions. Does the patient's body language match what is being stated verbally?

Table 5-1 Effective Questioning Techniques

Technique	About the Technique	Examples
Asking open-ended questions	Ask this type of question when you are opening up the interview. Open-ended questions often begin with what, when, how, where, and who, and often elicit a more comprehensive response.	"What brings you to the office today, Mr. Jones?"
Asking close-ended questions	You should avoid asking close-ended questions unless it is necessary to expand on a response that was given after asking an open-ended question. This type of question can frequently be answered with a *yes* or *no* response or a single-word answer. You should be careful not to overuse these questions because they restrict the patient's response and may make the patient feel as though you are controlling and uninterested in what the patient has to say.	*Effective*: "How many episodes of vomiting have you had over the past two days?" or "On a scale from 0 to 10, how would you rate your pain?" *Ineffective*: "Would you say that your rash is better than the last time you were here?"
Periods of silence	Periods of silence can also be effective during the questioning phase of the interview. It demonstrates that you are still waiting on a response while allowing the patient time to think about the question.	*Medical assistant*: "Out of all your symptoms, which symptom is bothering you the most today?" *Patient*: "I don't know, they all give me grief." *Medical assistant*: (silent) *Patient*: "Oh gee, probably my foot pain."

Table 5-2 Ineffective Interview Techniques

Technique	About the Technique	Examples
Asking leading questions	This may indicate a desired response rather than the patient's real feelings.	"Megan, please tell me that you are not sexually active, are you?"
Demanding an explanation	This may appear to threaten or challenge the patient to justify a response for certain actions.	"Why didn't you come in sooner for this condition?"
Agreeing or disagreeing with the patient	It is not your job to side with or against a statement made or a feeling expressed by the patient.	"I am in total agreement with you, Mrs. Jones," or "I don't think that you should go on vacation when you are eight months pregnant."
Interrupting the patient	You should allow patients to complete their train of thought. Interrupting minimizes the value of the patient's input and may suppress important information.	*Medical assistant*: "Has anyone in your family ever been diagnosed with cardiovascular disease?" *Patient*: "Well, my sister's husband ..." *Medical assistant*: "No, we only want to know about blood relatives."
Using medical terminology	Patients often do not understand medical terms. The patient may not ask for interpretation because of being fearful that the medical assistant will think he is unintelligent or uneducated. Use terms that can be easily understood by the patient.	"Have you noticed any edema in your ankles, Mr. Lacy?"
Diagnosing the patient	You must be careful to never offer an opinion regarding what may be wrong with the patient. Medical assistants do not have a license to practice medicine.	"I bet you just have a case of the stomach flu, Mrs. Wilson. It's been going around."
Advising the patient	You must be careful to never advise patients on what procedures to have or what medications to take.	"I use calamine lotion when I have poison ivy."
Offering false reassurance	When patients are uneasy or anxious about a condition or procedure, you may want to ease the patient's anxiety by offering reassurance. However, you must never promise that everything is going to be just fine or that you are certain there will be no problems when a certain procedure is performed. Statements like these can set up the office for legal problems if problems are incurred.	"Mrs. Bean, I know everything is going to be just fine. There is no need to worry."

Table 5-3 Effective Listening Techniques

Listening Techniques	Description	Example
Clarification	*Clarification* means to clear confusion or uncertainty. This is a process that is used when the patient uses a phrase or term that needs further interpretation or the patient sends mixed signals either verbally or nonverbally.	*Patient*: "I have a weird feeling when I go to the bathroom." *Medical assistant*: "What do you mean by 'weird feeling'?"
Restatement	*Restatement* means to state again or to state in a new form. This is repeating or rephrasing the main idea of the sentence and validating what the patient just stated. It also lets the patient know that you are listening to what they are trying to convey.	*Patient*: "I am so tired and weak and just do not feel like doing anything." *Medical assistant*: "So, you are so weak you don't feel like doing anything, even working in your beautiful garden?"
Reflection	*Reflection* means to ponder or think. Reflecting gives the patient an opportunity to expound on something that is bothering him and stimulates the patient to revisit his original thought.	*Patient*: "I just want to give up the fight. I am sick of taking all these pills every day." *Medical assistant*: "Mr. Baker, do you really want to give up?" *Patient*: "No, I don't want to give up, but I am sick of taking all of these expensive, horrible pills every day." *Medical assistant*: "You sound upset, Mr. Baker. What is upsetting you the most: the expense of the medication or taking the pills?"
Summarizing	This listening response is usually incorporated at the conclusion of the interview. It recaps the patient's concerns. This listening component helps to separate what is relevant from what is irrelevant.	*Medical assistant*: "Okay, Mrs. Jones, so your main concerns today are your inability to lose weight and your high blood pressure readings. Is that correct?"

Active listening sometimes requires the medical assistant to respond to a patient's response with an additional question to fully understand the patient's original response. Refer to Table 5-3 for effective listening responses.

THE SCREENING PROCESS

Before performing any patient screenings, you must know the protocols of the office. Information you will need to know includes the following:

- What parts of the screening are your responsibility?
- What conditions warrant specific procedures (e.g., collect a urine sample for all patients with urinary symptoms, perform a throat swab and rapid strep on all patients with sore throat, set up all patients with urogenital symptoms for STI cultures, etc.)?
- What are the boundaries of a medical assistant in the state and the particular office in which you are employed? Are you allowed to share results with the patient such as vital signs, blood sugars, and rapid strep results before the provider reviews the results?

It is vital to create an atmosphere that helps place the patient at ease. Begin by selecting a room that is private and free of distractions. Check the room's appearance. Make certain that it is clean, neat, and free of odors. The thermostat for the room should be set at a temperature that is comfortable for the patient. There should be comfortable seating for both the patient and the patient's family members when applicable. The medical assistant should perform questioning so that she is at the same level as the patient. Seating is arranged so that the medical assistant's stool or chair is directly across from the patient's chair about a distance of 4 to 6 feet. Some health care professionals question the patient on the exam table; however, this can be quite uncomfortable for the patient. If the patient is to have a special procedure, trays should be placed out of the view of the patient. Trays that are left in the open may trigger the patient to become anxious and less focused on questioning.

Greeting Stage

The greeting may take place in the reception room or in the examination room if someone other than person performing the intake takes the patient back

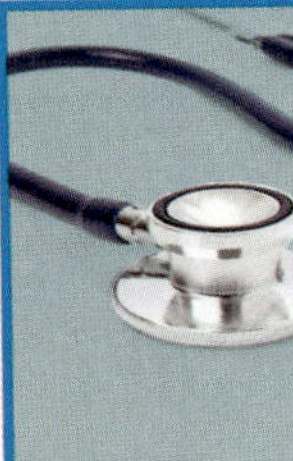

Field Smarts

If a patient has a language barrier, an interpreter that speaks the patient's native language will need to be available to assist with communication. Some patients may use family members who are bilingual to aid with communication; however, this may not be a good idea. The family member may not possess the language skills that are essential for "effective communication." Also the patient may not feel as free to speak if a family member is in the room. Watch for signs that could suggest the patient's discomfort with the person performing the interpreting. Share your findings with the provider.

to the exam room. Address adult patients by using their title (Mr., Mrs., Dr., and so on) followed by their last name. Children should be addressed by their first name. The medical assistant should ask the patient how they prefer to be addressed for the remainder of the interview and for future visits. Take a little extra time to document this information in the chart so that anyone working with the patient in the future will be cognizant of the patient's preference. Acknowledge family members or friends that may also be present. Once you have properly identified the patient, you should identify yourself and state your title.

Performance of Height, Weight, and Vital Signs

The patient's height, weight, body mass index (BMI), and vital signs are usually performed and recorded in the patient's chart at the beginning of the visit; however, this will vary from office to office. Vital signs include the patient's temperature, pulse, respiration, and blood pressure. Some offices also include oxygen saturation level and pain rating in this part of the screening. Refer to Chapter 11 to learn more about vital signs and height and weight procedures.

Medication Reconciliation

At the time the appointment is scheduled, patients should be directed to bring a current list of medications with them to the appointment. During the appointment, patients should be asked about prescribed medications, over-the-counter medications, and supplement information such as vitamin intake and herbal remedies. After documenting the name of the medication, the dose, amount, and how often the medication is taken should be recorded (i.e., lisinopril 20 mg tab/bid). All EHR programs have a medication section that contains the names of thousands of medications. The user just clicks on a dropdown list and selects the appropriate information. Lots of drugs have similar spellings so make certain you click on the correct drug.

Drug Allergies

Patients can develop a drug allergy at any time, so it is important to inquire about drug allergies on a regular basis. When recording in a paper chart, the allergy is usually recorded in red so that it will stand out; however, when recording in the EHR, the user will select the type of alert that should appear for the allergy such as a soft or hard alert. A hard alert in most programs is an alert box that automatically opens up when you access the chart. Soft alerts are usually an icon in a tool bar that you click on and are often used for allergies like peanuts or other foods that aren't as essential to know when prescribing medications.

Obtaining the Chief Complaint and History of Present Illness

The chief complaint or reason that prompted the patient to seek medical attention is referred to as **subjective information** because it is information that is supplied by the patient. **Symptoms** are a list of signals or signs experienced by the patient that indicate a specific disease or condition and may include pain, fever, itching, and a host of other physical or mental ailments.

Table 5-4 provides tips for expanding on common signs or symptoms that may come up during the screening.

Table 5-4 Tips for Expanding on Common Signs and Symptoms

Symptom	Tips
Location	Always provide the exact location of the symptoms such as the left ear, right-sided lower abdominal pain, right fourth finger, etc.
Amounts or size	When documenting size, use comparison terms such as the following, "the clots are comparable to the size of a quarter." When documenting amounts, you may use a comparison such as the following: "The patient states that her vaginal bleeding is so heavy that she is going through 1 Ultra Tampon per hour" or "The patient is using two boxes of tissues per day."
Color	Be specific about color, especially when describing the color of drainage: "The patient states that her sputum is a mixture of white mucus with tinge of yellow from time to time."
Pain	Always have the patient rate her pain on a scale from 0 to 10 (Figure 5-4); however, some offices use a 1 to 10 scale. For children or patients with limited proficiency in English, you may use the OUCHER! pain rating scale as shown in Figure 5-5. Have the patient point to the face that describes her pain.
Related symptoms	These are symptoms that are specific to particular body systems.

Along with the chief complaint the medical assistant may also be responsible for conducting a *brief* **history of present illness (HPI)**, which is a series of questions that are related to the patient's complaint. Developing a brief HPI will assist the medical assistant in knowing how to properly prepare the patient and set up the room for the examination. The provider, however, will need to thoroughly develop the HPI for diagnostic and reimbursement purposes.

Each of the system chapters in this text include a system screening table, which lists questions to be asked when a particular system is involved along with disrobing information, possible procedures, or treatments that may be ordered and telephone screening tips.

Refer to Table 5-5 for a summary of items that should be documented during an in-office screening.

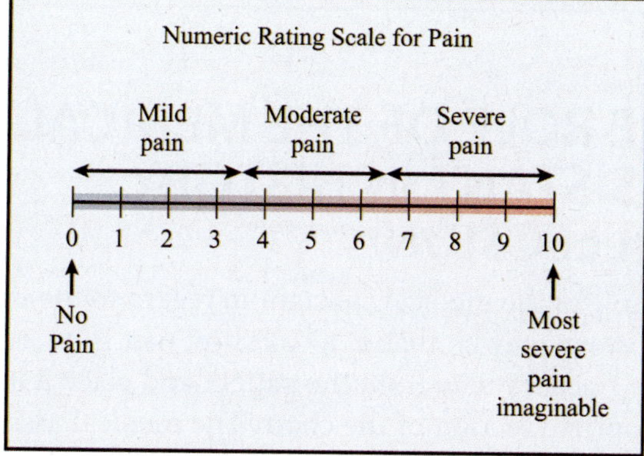

Figure 5-4 ■ The Visual Analog Scale for pain assessment.

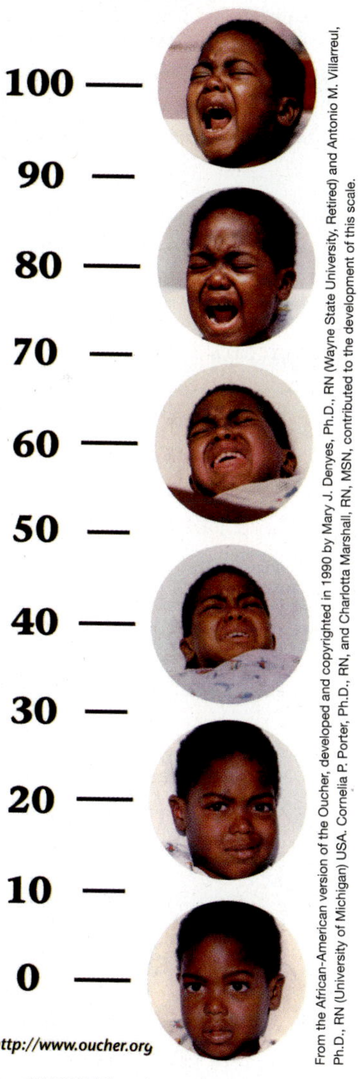

Figure 5-5 ■ The OUCHER! pain scale.

Table 5-5 Items That Should Be Documented When Conducting an In-Office Screening

What Should Be Documented	Description
1. The date and time of the visit	These items automatically populate in the EHR. If using paper charts, the date should be recorded using the 2/2/4 format, two-digit day, two-digit month and four-digit year, i.e., 05/18/2020. Military time is commonly used in the medical industry, especially in hospitals, because of its preciseness. Refer to Figure 5-6 for a military 24-hour conversion clock. Always check the policy of the office in which you are working.
2. Vital signs	This is the temperature, pulse, respiration, blood pressure, and BMI. Some offices also record oxygen saturation and pain rating as part of the vital signs. In the EHR, BMI is automatically populated after entering the height and weight.
3. Medication information	Medications should include all prescribed, over-the-counter (OTC), and nutritional supplements along with the dosage, the amount, the route (if other than by mouth), and how often the patient takes the medication. The database in most EHR programs include thousands of medications along with usual dosages. The medical assistant just clicks on the appropriate medication and dose and the medication information populates into the progress note.
4. Allergy status	For medication allergies, the medical assistant will usually include the name of the medication and what happens when the patient takes the medication. In the EHR, this may consists of a dropdown list with several different symptoms that occur when the patient takes the medication, e.g., anaphylaxis, breaks out in hives, etc. The medical assistant just clicks on all that apply. The medical assistant may also include other allergy information such as latex, food, and seasonal allergies.
5. The chief complaint or reason for the visit	This is a description of what is wrong with the patient, using the patient's own words whenever possible. Medical terms should not be used in this part of the note.
6. History of present illness (HPI) [Usually recorded by provider]	The HPI includes the following: *location* (where the symptoms occur), *quality* (description of the symptoms such as colors and type of pain), *severity* of symptoms (if pain is involved, rate on a 0–10 scale), *duration* (how long the symptoms have been present), *timing* (when symptoms occur, morning, during sleep, and so on), *context* (are the symptoms related to an event such as an accident, following an illness, and so on), *modifying factors* (what makes symptoms better or worse), *associated symptoms or signs* (other findings that the patient presents with, related or not related to the chief complaint).
7. Identification of person making the entry	Not necessary in the EHR because this information is automatically tracked. When using paper charts, place first initial, last name, and credential as your identifier.

WRITTEN DOCUMENTATION SAMPLE FOR AN IN-OFFICE SCREENING

02/20/XXXX 1300	Ht: 67" Wt: 136 # BMI: 21.3 T: 98.6 P: 72 R: 16 BP: 110/68 Prescribed Medications: Levoxyl (one 125 mg tab daily); Supplements: Vitafusion Women's Multivitamin (One gummy/day). Medication Allergies: NKDA ------------------------- CC: Pt c/o chest pain x 1 hour. Pain is located in the center of the chest and radiates slightly to the left shoulder and arm. Pain is continuous and is a "10" on 0-10 pain scale. The patient states that the pain feels like a squeezing sensation. Associated symptoms include, shortness of breath and nausea and vomiting. Pt took two 325 mg aspirin 30 minutes ago, (no relief). A. Pugh, CMA (AAMA) --

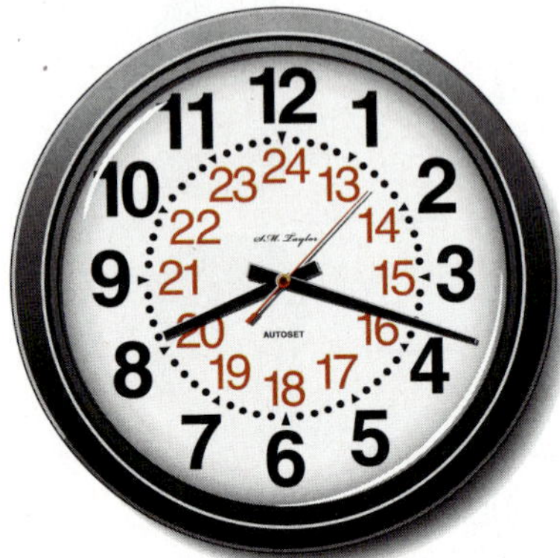

Figure 5-6 ■ This clock is an illustration of a 24-hour clock for practices that use military time.

THE ROLE OF THE MEDICAL ASSISTANT IN HISTORY COLLECTION

The role of the medical assistant in regard to the medical history may be that of a collector, that is, to collect related history data from the patient and place it in the appropriate section of the chart. The medical assistant may also act as an interviewer, to complete the history form for the patient, or to review the form once it has been completed by the patient, making certain that all questions have been answered and all "Yes" responses have been developed. This is accomplished by asking a series of questions that are specifically related to the disease or disorder that is marked.

TOOLS USED TO COLLECT MEDICAL HISTORY INFORMATION

There are two types of tools that are used to collect data for the patient history. The first is the standard paper medical questionnaire (Figure 5-7), which requires the person completing the form to write in the correct responses. This form may be initially completed by the patient and then further developed by the medical assistant or provider. The second tool used to collect patient data is the computer. The electronic history is a major component found in many EHR programs. The electronic medical history (Figure 5-8) may be completed by the patient prior to the appointment if the patient has access to a computer, or it may be completed in the examination room using an electronic kiosk with

CONFIDENTIAL HEALTH HISTORY

Name:______ Date:______
Birthdate:______ Age:______ Date of last physical examination:______
Occupation:______
Reason for visit today:______

MEDICATIONS List all medications you are currently taking	**ALLERGIES** List all allergies

SYMPTOMS Check (✓) symptoms you currently have or have had in the past year.

GENERAL
☐ Chills
☐ Depression
☐ Dizziness
☐ Fainting
☐ Fever
☐ Forgetfulness
☐ Headache
☐ Loss of sleep
☐ Loss of weight
☐ Nervousness
☐ Numbness
☐ Sweats

MUSCLE/JOINT/BONE
Pain, weakness, numbness in:
☐ Arms ☐ Hips
☐ Back ☐ Legs
☐ Feet ☐ Neck
☐ Hands ☐ Shoulders

GENITO-URINARY
☐ Blood in urine
☐ Frequent urination
☐ Lack of bladder control
☐ Painful urination

GASTROINTESTINAL
☐ Appetite poor
☐ Bloating
☐ Bowel changes
☐ Constipation
☐ Diarrhea
☐ Excessive hunger
☐ Excessive thirst
☐ Gas
☐ Hemorrhoids
☐ Indigestion
☐ Nausea
☐ Rectal bleeding
☐ Stomach pain
☐ Vomiting
☐ Vomiting blood

CARDIOVASCULAR
☐ Chest pain
☐ High blood pressure
☐ Irregular heart beat
☐ Low blood pressure
☐ Poor circulation
☐ Rapid heart beat
☐ Swelling of ankles
☐ Varicose veins

EYE, EAR, NOSE, THROAT
☐ Bleeding gums
☐ Blurred vision
☐ Crossed eyes
☐ Difficulty swallowing
☐ Double vision
☐ Earache
☐ Ear discharge
☐ Hay fever
☐ Hoarseness
☐ Loss of hearing
☐ Nosebleeds
☐ Persistent cough
☐ Ringing in ears
☐ Sinus problems
☐ Vision - Flashes
☐ Vision - Halos

SKIN
☐ Bruise easily
☐ Hives
☐ Itching
☐ Change in moles
☐ Rash
☐ Scars
☐ Sores that won't heal

MEN only
☐ Breast lump
☐ Erection difficulties
☐ Lump in testicles
☐ Penis discharge
☐ Sore on penis
☐ Other

WOMEN only
☐ Abnormal Pap Smear
☐ Bleeding between periods
☐ Breast lump
☐ Extreme menstrual pain
☐ Hot flashes
☐ Nipple discharge
☐ Painful intercourse
☐ Vaginal discharge
☐ Other
Date of last menstrual period______
Date of last Pap Smear______
Have you had a mammogram?______
Are you pregnant?______
Number of children______

MEDICAL HISTORY Check (✓) the medical conditions you have or have had in the past.

☐ AIDS
☐ Alcoholism
☐ Anemia
☐ Anorexia
☐ Appendicitis
☐ Arthritis
☐ Asthma
☐ Bleeding Disorders
☐ Breast Lump
☐ Bronchitis
☐ Bulimia
☐ Cancer
☐ Cataracts
☐ Chemical Dependency
☐ Chicken Pox
☐ Diabetes
☐ Emphysema
☐ Epilepsy
☐ Gall Bladder Disease
☐ Glaucoma
☐ Goiter
☐ Gonorrhea
☐ Gout
☐ Heart Disease
☐ Hepatitis
☐ Hernia
☐ Herpes
☐ High Cholesterol
☐ HIV Positive
☐ Kidney Disease
☐ Liver Disease
☐ Measles
☐ Migraine Headaches
☐ Miscarriage
☐ Mononucleosis
☐ Multiple Sclerosis
☐ Mumps
☐ Pacemaker
☐ Pneumonia
☐ Polio
☐ Prostate Problem
☐ Psychiatric Care
☐ Rheumatic Fever
☐ Scarlet Fever
☐ Stroke
☐ Suicide Attempt
☐ Thyroid Problems
☐ Tonsillitis
☐ Tuberculosis
☐ Typhoid Fever
☐ Ulcers
☐ Vaginal Infections
☐ Venereal Disease

CONFIDENTIAL HEALTH HISTORY

Figure 5-7 ■ An example of a paper medical history form.

HOSPITALIZATIONS

Year	Hospital	Reason for Hospitalization and Outcome

Have you ever had a blood transfusion? ☐ Yes ☐ No
If yes, please give approximate dates: ______

OCCUPATIONAL CONCERNS Check (✓) if your work exposes you to the following:	HEALTH HABITS Check (✓) which substances you use and indicate how much you use per day/week.	PREGNANCY HISTORY Year of Birth	Sex of Birth	Complications if any
☐ Stress	☐ Caffeine			
☐ Hazardous Substances	☐ Tobacco			
☐ Heavy Lifting	☐ Drugs			
☐ Other	☐ Alcohol			

SERIOUS ILLNESS/INJURIES	DATE	OUTCOME

FAMILY HISTORY Fill in health information about your family.

Relation	Age	State of Health	Age at Death	Cause of Death	Check (✓) if your blood relatives had any of the following Disease	Relationship to you
Father					☐ Arthritis, Gout	
Mother					☐ Asthma, Hay Fever	
Brothers					☐ Cancer	
					☐ Chemical Dependency	
					☐ Diabetes	
					☐ Heart Disease, Strokes	
Sisters					☐ High Blood Pressure	
					☐ Kidney Disease	
					☐ Tuberculosis	
					☐ Other	

I certify that the above information is correct to the best of my knowledge. I will not hold my doctor or any members of his/her staff responsible for any errors or ommisions that I may have made in the completion of this form.

______ Signature ______ Date

______ Reviewed By ______ Date

Figure 5-7 ■ *(Continued)*

patient portal access. The medical assistant or provider will review the electronic history with the patient and make certain that all information is accurate.

Many electronic medical histories allow the person completing the information to select various diseases and conditions from a dropdown list. When the user clicks on a "Yes" response, another set of questions may populate on the screen that expounds further on that particular condition or disease.

Electronic histories can be developed in a quicker time frame than the standard paper history, and are easier to read.

History formats may also vary according to the specialty of the practice. Some specialties will emphasize questions that parallel with their particular specialty.

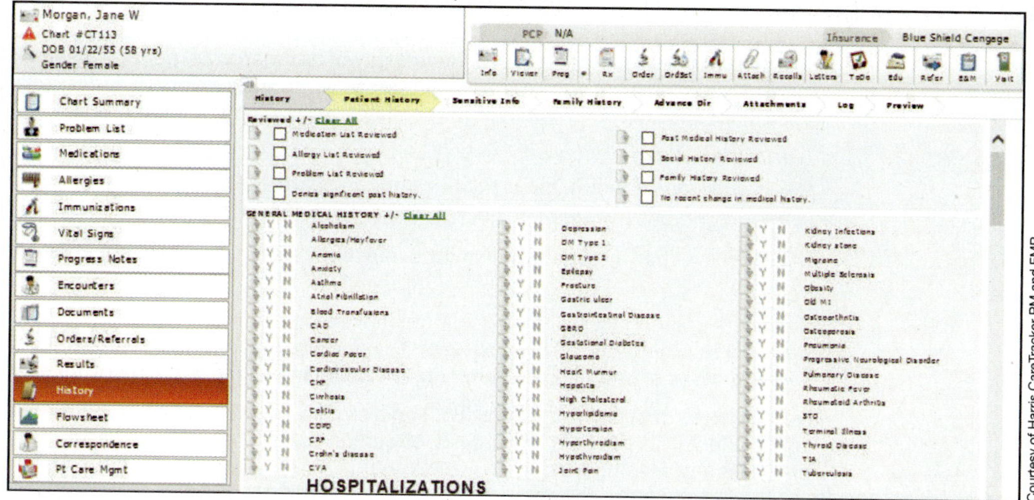

Courtesy of Harris CareTracker PM and EMR

Figure 5-8 ■ An electronic medical history screen from Harris CareTracker.

THE COMPREHENSIVE MEDICAL HISTORY

The **comprehensive** (or complete) **medical history** is a head-to-toe look at the patient and is divided into three major sections:

1. Personal medical history
2. Family medical history or family history (FH)
3. Social history (SH)

A depression screening and preventive care information may be integrated within the history; however, there may be a specific place in the chart other than within the history where this information is stored.

Personal Medical History

The patient's **personal medical history** includes the patient's previous health concerns, current health concerns, and a current medication list. Previous health concerns include the patient's **past history (PH)** also known as **past health history (PHH)**. This part of the history includes **usual childhood diseases (UCHD or UCD)**, previous major illnesses, previous injuries, previous surgical procedures, and immunization information. Current health concerns include a review of systems (ROS) or systems review (SR) and the patient's chief complaint (CC). The ROS is a list of symptoms that coincide with different body systems that the patient is currently experiencing or has experienced in the past year. This part of the history is completed by the provider. When asked to elaborate on the patient's past medical history, use Table 5-6 to elaborate on "Yes" responses.

OB-GYN History

The OB-GYN section of a personal history requests information regarding a female's reproductive health. This section contains sensitive information. The medical assistant must make every effort to help the patient feel at ease during this section of questioning. Refer to Table 5-7 for specifics on the information to be gathered.

Table 5-6 Questions That Should Be Asked When a Patient Responds with a "Yes" to a Particular Symptom, Disease, or Condition

Question	Definition or Information About the Question
Exact name of symptom, disease, or condition	Many questionnaires are categorized to include only general information such as, "Have you ever experienced heart problems?" If the patient indicates "Yes", list the name of the disorder.
When first diagnosed or duration of illness or condition	How long ago was the patient diagnosed with the particular illness or condition?
Course of treatment	What type of treatment did the patient receive to remedy the condition or illness (medication, surgery, diet, and so on)? If the patient had a surgical procedure, list the name and date of the procedure and the name of the provider who performed the procedure.
Current status of the illness or condition	Does the patient still suffer from this condition or illness?
Date of resolve (if applicable)	List time frame or date of resolve when applicable.

Table 5-7 Female Reproductive Health

GYN information	*Last menstrual period (LMP)* (record the first day of last menstrual period), *menarche* (age of first menstrual cycle), *menopause* (age when periods completely stopped), *history of abnormal pap smears* (list specifics such as classification, dates, and treatment information)
Birth control and barriers	*Type of birth control* *Risk stratification*: monogamous relationship (one partner), multiple partners, and so on *Barriers*: Condoms (sometimes, always, never)
History of sexually transmitted infections or disease	Have you ever had a sexually transmitted infection? List type and date of onset.
OB-History	*Gravida* (# of pregnancies), *term* (# of pregnancies that went full term), *pre-term* (# of pregnancies that occurred prior to week 37) *abortions* (# of pregnancies terminated), *miscarriages* (# of pregnancies terminated involuntarily), *live children* (# of children still living)
Breast history	Do you perform breast self-exams (BSE) on a regular basis? Date of last mammogram if applicable. Any history of cancer, cysts, or benign tumors? Any discharge, dimpling, or lumps in breast? Breast feeding history.

Male Reproductive Health Information

Males may have a specific category as well; however, it usually is not nearly as lengthy as the female reproductive health section. This section also includes sensitive information. Refer to Table 5-8 for information that may be found in this category.

Surgical Histories and Hospitalizations

The surgical histories and hospitalization information is part of the personal medical history section. Refer to Table 5-9 for specifics.

Family Medical History

The **family medical history** provides detailed information about the present and past health of the patient's family members. The family history can provide insight to possible risks of future diseases or conditions for the patient. Medical histories should include a minimum of two to three generations whenever possible. The family history should contain the age and health status of living family members and list the age at which nonliving members died and their cause of death. Family members should include siblings, parents, grandparents (both paternal and maternal), aunts, uncles, and children. Some history forms also include information regarding the spouse's health status. Another type of medical history is referred to as a **genogram**. It resembles a family tree. Squares represent male family members and circles represent female members. Refer to Figure 5-9 for an example of a genogram.

Table 5-8 Male Reproductive Health Information

Testicular information	How often do you perform regular testicular self-examinations (TSE)? Have you ever been diagnosed with testicular cancer?
Prostate information	When was your last prostate exam? When was your last PSA test? Have you ever been diagnosed with prostate cancer?
Barriers	*Risk stratification*: monogamous relationship (one partner), multiple partners, etc. *Barriers*: Condoms (sometimes, always, never)
History of sexually transmitted infections or disease	Have you ever had a sexually transmitted infection? List type and date of onset.

Table 5-9 Information Necessary When Developing Surgical Histories and Hospitalizations

Listing	Definition	Example of Documentation on the History Form
Surgical history	List type of surgery, date of procedure, name of surgeon, where the surgery was performed, and any complications.	*Surgical Procedures*: Appendectomy, 03-07-15, Dr. Carl Valentine, Grant General, no complications
Hospitalizations	List dates of hospitalizations, name of hospital, reasons for and length of hospitalization, and any complications.	*Hospitalizations*: 07-15-16: Riverside Hospital × 6 days for double pneumonia, no complications

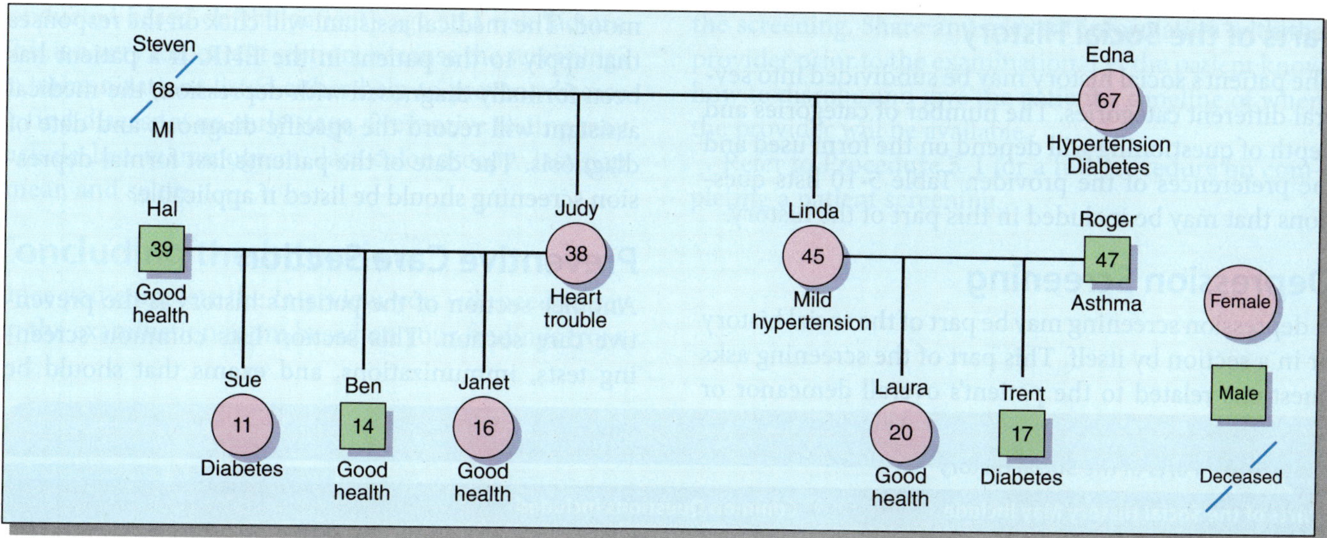

Figure 5-9 ■ An example of a completed genogram.

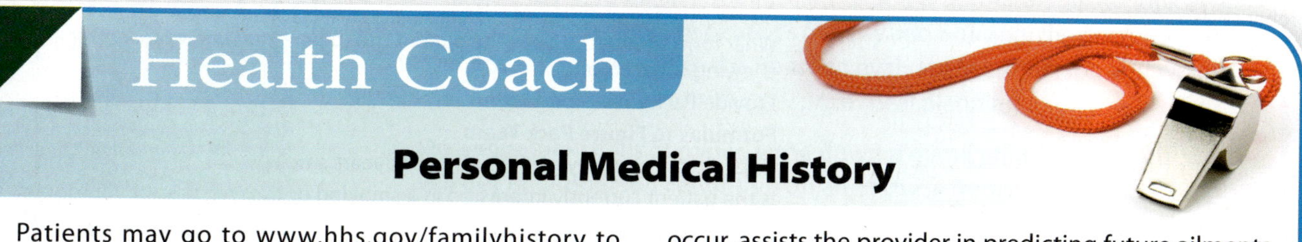

Health Coach

Personal Medical History

Patients may go to www.hhs.gov/familyhistory to download a tool called, "My Family Health Portrait." Entering personal and family health data into this electronic template creates a personalized medical history form that can be used throughout the patient's life span. The form, which can be updated when changes occur, assists the provider in predicting future ailments and provides an opportunity for intervention that will either prevent or delay these possible conditions from occurring. Patients should print a copy of the history and take it with them when visiting new providers or whenever changes occur in their medical history.

Information that should be obtained when gathering health data about each family member should include the following:

1. The family member's current age or age at the time of death
2. All diseases or disorders for each family member
3. If family member is deceased, the cause of death

Example:

Family Member	Health Status or Deceased	Current Age or Age at the Time of Death	Diseases or Disorders (Cause of Death)
Father	Fair	66	Hypertension and type 2 diabetes
Mother	Fair	64	Hypertension and MVP
Maternal grandmother	Deceased	77	Cause of death: Heart attack
			Other diseases: Hypertension and breast cancer

Social History

The **social history** refers to lifestyle questions. Lifestyles can have a large impact on the prevention or launching of certain diseases or conditions. Patients frequently feel anxious during this part of the interview due to the sensitivity of the questioning.

PROCEDURE 5-1 continued

PROCEDURAL STEPS	DETAILS AND/OR RATIONALE
2. Once the patient has been escorted to the examination room, identify yourself, list your title, and identify the patient using two different identifiers. Ask the patient if she has a certain preference for the way she wants to be addressed throughout the remainder of the interview and future visits.	It is important for medical assistants to identify themselves and to list their title so that the patient knows that they have authority to perform this task.
3. Obtain a height and weight and vital signs on the patient.	These measurements help the provider properly assess the patient.
4. Update the patient's medication list. Include the name of the medication, the strength, the route if other than oral, and how often the patient takes the medication.	The patient's medication list is continuously evolving. You must have an updated list to avoid medication interactions.
5. Update the patient's allergy history.	The patient can develop an allergy at any time.
6. Obtain the patient's chief complaint and a brief history of present illness if office protocol.	The chief complaint describes the reason for today's visit. (The provider is usually responsible for the HPI but may want the medical assistant to obtain a brief HPI.)
7. Explain the rationale for gathering the history and inform the patient that everything that is shared during the interview will remain confidential, ***demonstrating empathy***.	Explaining the purpose of the history will help the patient to understand why the information is necessary. Letting the patient know that information will remain confidential will help the patient feel more at ease when discussing the more sensitive information.
8. If the patient completed the form prior to the visit, review all information and check for possible omissions or incomplete responses, ***incorporating critical thinking skills when performing patient assessment***. If the medical assistant is completing the entire form, address all questions on the form, ***demonstrating active listening***.	Patients may have omitted important information or possibly misunderstood certain questions. Reviewing the form and expanding on applicable responses will help save time for the provider later on.
9. Properly develop all "Yes" responses in the past medical history section. List the exact name of the disease or condition, duration or onset of the disease, treatment, current status, and date of resolve if applicable.	Properly developing the "Yes" responses will save the provider a great deal of time.
10. Properly expand on all "Yes" responses listed in the family and social history sections.	Properly expanding on all "Yes" responses will save the provider time.
11. Make certain that all hospitalizations and surgeries are listed on the medical history form.	This gives the provider a look at some of the more serious conditions the patient has encountered and helps the provider to anticipate future events.
12. Answer depression screening questions that can be completed by someone other than the provider.	The provider may want to complete the entire depression screening. Know the office protocol.
13. Update the patient's preventive care information.	Updating this information will aid in identifying outstanding immunizations or preventive screenings so that measures can be taken to get the patient updated on these procedures.

continues

conducted based on the patient's age and risk factors. This is a very important section, because the screenings or immunizations listed either help to prevent disease or find disease at an early stage. Preventive testing may include last mammogram, last colonoscopy, last pap smear, and so on.

Concluding the Interview

Once you complete the interview, you will need to set up the examination room based on your findings from the screening. Share any relevant information with the provider prior to the examination. Let the patient know how to disrobe and give the patient a timeline of when the provider will be available.

Refer to Procedure 5-1 for a full procedure on completing a patient screening.

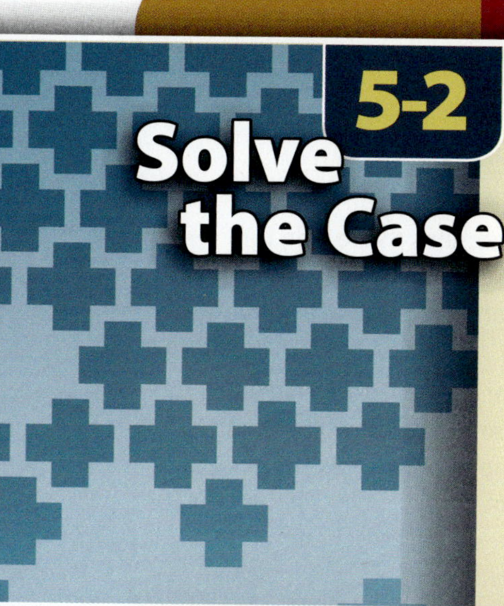

The doctor concludes her exam. She wants you to get Mr. Anderson caught up on all of the outstanding items in the preventive screening section which includes his shingles vaccine, flu shot, and tetanus shot. He also needs a PSA test and she would like you to schedule an appointment with the dermatologist to look at a suspicious mole. Because of the patient's fragility and bruising, the doctor would like to get a social worker out to the house to evaluate Mr. Anderson and would like to get a dietician to assist Mr. Anderson in meal planning.

1. **On a separate sheet of paper, write down a game plan for how you will get Mr. Anderson caught up on all of these items.**
2. **How can you keep the patient and the daughter from becoming suspicious about having a social worker come out to the house?**
3. **Are there any other services that Mr. Anderson may benefit from?**

PROCEDURE 5-1

Conduct a Patient Screening

Objective:

To accurately complete a patient screening while promoting good therapeutic communications.

Equipment/Supplies:

- Patient history form/EHR
- Writing instruments if applicable

PROCEDURAL STEPS	DETAILS AND/OR RATIONALE
1. Wash hands and prepare the interview area. The interview area should be private, comfortable, and free of distractions.	Properly preparing the room will make the patient feel more comfortable and more receptive to answering the questions.

continues

PROCEDURE 5-1 continued

PROCEDURAL STEPS	DETAILS AND/OR RATIONALE
2. Once the patient has been escorted to the examination room, identify yourself, list your title, and identify the patient using two different identifiers. Ask the patient if she has a certain preference for the way she wants to be addressed throughout the remainder of the interview and future visits.	It is important for medical assistants to identify themselves and to list their title so that the patient knows that they have authority to perform this task.
3. Obtain a height and weight and vital signs on the patient.	These measurements help the provider properly assess the patient.
4. Update the patient's medication list. Include the name of the medication, the strength, the route if other than oral, and how often the patient takes the medication.	The patient's medication list is continuously evolving. You must have an updated list to avoid medication interactions.
5. Update the patient's allergy history.	The patient can develop an allergy at any time.
6. Obtain the patient's chief complaint and a brief history of present illness if office protocol.	The chief complaint describes the reason for today's visit. (The provider is usually responsible for the HPI but may want the medical assistant to obtain a brief HPI.)
7. Explain the rationale for gathering the history and inform the patient that everything that is shared during the interview will remain confidential, ***demonstrating empathy***.	Explaining the purpose of the history will help the patient to understand why the information is necessary. Letting the patient know that information will remain confidential will help the patient feel more at ease when discussing the more sensitive information.
8. If the patient completed the form prior to the visit, review all information and check for possible omissions or incomplete responses, ***incorporating critical thinking skills when performing patient assessment***. If the medical assistant is completing the entire form, address all questions on the form, ***demonstrating active listening***.	Patients may have omitted important information or possibly misunderstood certain questions. Reviewing the form and expanding on applicable responses will help save time for the provider later on.
9. Properly develop all "Yes" responses in the past medical history section. List the exact name of the disease or condition, duration or onset of the disease, treatment, current status, and date of resolve if applicable.	Properly developing the "Yes" responses will save the provider a great deal of time.
10. Properly expand on all "Yes" responses listed in the family and social history sections.	Properly expanding on all "Yes" responses will save the provider time.
11. Make certain that all hospitalizations and surgeries are listed on the medical history form.	This gives the provider a look at some of the more serious conditions the patient has encountered and helps the provider to anticipate future events.
12. Answer depression screening questions that can be completed by someone other than the provider.	The provider may want to complete the entire depression screening. Know the office protocol.
13. Update the patient's preventive care information.	Updating this information will aid in identifying outstanding immunizations or preventive screenings so that measures can be taken to get the patient updated on these procedures.

continues

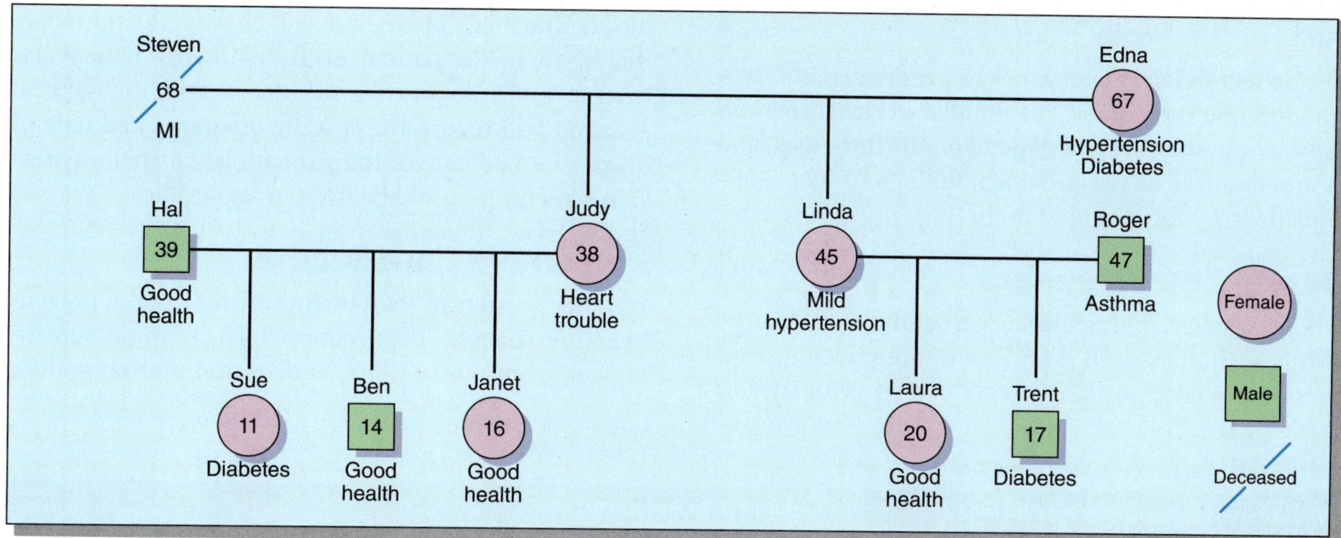

Figure 5-9 ■ An example of a completed genogram.

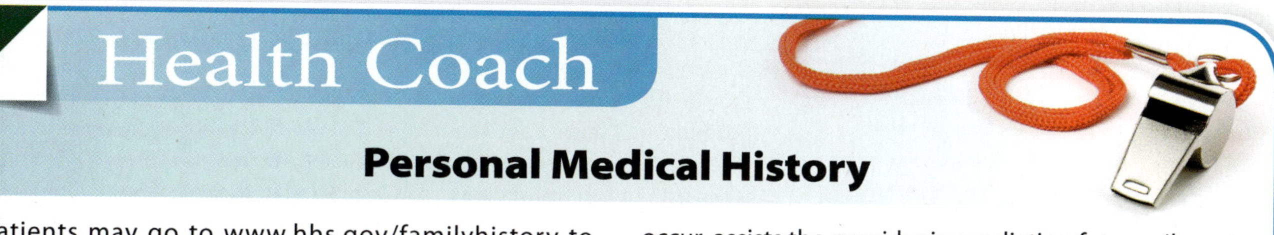

Health Coach

Personal Medical History

Patients may go to www.hhs.gov/familyhistory to download a tool called, "My Family Health Portrait." Entering personal and family health data into this electronic template creates a personalized medical history form that can be used throughout the patient's life span. The form, which can be updated when changes occur, assists the provider in predicting future ailments and provides an opportunity for intervention that will either prevent or delay these possible conditions from occurring. Patients should print a copy of the history and take it with them when visiting new providers or whenever changes occur in their medical history.

Information that should be obtained when gathering health data about each family member should include the following:

1. The family member's current age or age at the time of death
2. All diseases or disorders for each family member
3. If family member is deceased, the cause of death

Example:

Family Member	Health Status or Deceased	Current Age or Age at the Time of Death	Diseases or Disorders (Cause of Death)
Father	Fair	66	Hypertension and type 2 diabetes
Mother	Fair	64	Hypertension and MVP
Maternal grandmother	Deceased	77	Cause of death: Heart attack
			Other diseases: Hypertension and breast cancer

Social History

The **social history** refers to lifestyle questions. Lifestyles can have a large impact on the prevention or launching of certain diseases or conditions. Patients frequently feel anxious during this part of the interview due to the sensitivity of the questioning.

Parts of the Social History

The patient's social history may be subdivided into several different categories. The number of categories and depth of questioning will depend on the form used and the preferences of the provider. Table 5-10 lists questions that may be included in this part of the history.

Depression Screening

A depression screening may be part of the social history or in a section by itself. This part of the screening asks questions related to the patient's overall demeanor or mood. The medical assistant will click on the responses that apply to the patient in the EHR. If a patient has been formally diagnosed with depression, the medical assistant will record the specific diagnosis and date of diagnosis. The date of the patient's last formal depression screening should be listed if applicable.

Preventive Care Section

Another section of the patient's history is the preventive care section. This section lists common screening tests, immunizations, and exams that should be

Table 5-10 Parts of the Social History

Parts of the Social History May Include	Common Questions Included
Alcohol use	List what type of alcohol the patient consumes (beer, wine, hard liquors) How much alcohol is consumed weekly and how often does the patient drink alcohol (daily, only on weekends, and so on)?
Tobacco assessment	Age of onset What form of tobacco does the patient use (pipe, cigars, cigarettes, e-cigarettes, chewing tobacco, and so on)? Provide Pack Year Information **Formulas to Figure Pack Years** Cigarettes: # cigs/day ÷ 20 × number of years smoked Is the patient currently interested in a smoking or tobacco cessation program?
Caffeine intake	List the types of beverages that the patient drinks that contain caffeine. How many of those beverages does the patient consume on average per day (i.e. four 12 ounce cups of coffee/day)?
Seatbelts	This is usually just a "Yes" or "No" response Record if the patient uses a seatbelt. If not, list reason for not wearing seatbelt.
Sun protection	List what protection the patient uses when in the sun (sunblock and number, sun glasses, sun hat, and so on)
Tattoos	This is usually just a "Yes" or "No" response Inquire if procedures were performed in a sterile environment
Body piercings	This is usually just a "Yes" or "No" response Inquire if procedures were performed using sterile technique
Physical or domestic abuse	Describe the abuse; What type of violence occurred? How often does the violence occur? Have injuries ever provoked a hospital visit? Has the individual performing the violence ever been formally charged? Has patient ever gone to a shelter?
Sexual orientation refers to the patient's physical and/or emotional attraction to the same and/or opposite gender.	Describe the patient's sexual orientation: heterosexual or straight, gay, lesbian, or bisexual.
Gender identity should not be confused with sexual orientation. Refers to the patient's psychological identification as a man or woman which may or may not correspond with the sex listed on the birth certificate.	*Transgender*: Umbrella term used to describe one whose gender (identity or expression) is different from the sex assigned at birth. May or may not have gone through gender transition surgery. *Gender transition*: in the process of transitioning to the gender with which the patient identifies
Patient's native language	Insert the patient's native language: English, German, Spanish, and so on.
Patient's occupation	List current occupation and any occupations in the past that have a high risk of environmental illness such as firefighters, coal miners, construction workers, and so on.
Exercise	State forms of exercise and regularity of exercise

PROCEDURE 5-1 continued

PROCEDURAL STEPS	DETAILS AND/OR RATIONALE
14. Use feedback techniques to obtain patient information including reflection, restatement, and clarification. Make adjustments if necessary.	Using feedback techniques will help you assess if the patient truly understands the questions and you truly understand the intended responses.
15. ***Demonstrate empathy, active listening, and professional nonverbal communication throughout the screening.***	Demonstrating empathy, active listening, and using professional nonverbal communication demonstrates that you care about the patient and the messages you are sending back to your patient.
16. Monitor the patient's nonverbal communication throughout the screening.	Monitoring nonverbal communication helps in assessing the patient's comprehension and feelings about questions that come up during the interview.
17. Once the form is completed, summarize the information with the patient.	Summarizing the information will help to confirm that the information is factual.
18. Ask the patient if she would like any additional information added to the history form.	This gives the patient an opportunity to address anything that was not listed on the form and validates that what the patient states is important.
19. Thank the patient for his or her assistance during the interview process.	This demonstrates appreciation toward the patient.
20. Instruct the patient how to disrobe prior to the exam. Give patient a timeline when the provider will be in and properly exit the room.	Giving the patient appropriate disrobing directions will save time for the provider later on.
21. Report relevant information concisely and accurately to the provider.	Reporting relevant information to the provider will help the provider in his overall assessment of the patient.
22. ***Demonstrate the principles of self-boundaries*** by staying within the boundaries of medical assisting throughout the screening.	The medical assistant must be aware of self-boundaries so that she doesn't go beyond her scope of practice.

CHAPTER SUMMARY

- A communication encounter consists of a sender that sends the message, encoding the message (which is transferring the message in a manner that can be understood by the receiver), deciding the channel of communication to be used, and a decoding of the message by the receiver. Noise is a barrier that can hamper the communication process. Feedback is the verbal and nonverbal reactions provided by your audience.
- Therapeutic communication is an exchange of information between the health care worker and patient that leads to the advancement of the patient's physical and emotional well-being.
- Body language includes gestures, postures, and facial expressions by which a person manifests various physical, mental, or emotional states and communicates nonverbally with others.

- Effective questioning techniques include asking open-ended questions, asking close-ended questions when applicable, and periods of silence in order to give the patient ample time to formulate an accurate response.
- Ineffective interview techniques include asking leading questions, demanding an explanation, agreeing or disagreeing with the patient, interrupting the patient, using medical terminology, diagnosing the patient, advising the patient, and offering false reassurance.
- Active listening involves more than just your sense of hearing; it encompasses other senses as well.
- Effective listening techniques include clarification, restatement, reflection, and summarizing.
- Before conducting a patient screening, you need to know what parts of the screening you are responsible for, what conditions warrant specific procedures, and your boundaries as a medical assistant.
- Stages of a patient screening usually include the greeting, height and weight measurement, vital signs measurement, medication reconciliation, drug allergy history, obtaining the chief complaint and HPI if applicable, performing a patient history, and updating the patient's preventive screening section of the chart.
- The comprehensive history usually is divided into three major sections: the personal medical history, family medical history, and social history.

CERTIFICATION REVIEW QUESTIONS

1. Transferring the message in a manner that can be fully understood by the receiver is associated with which of the following?
   a. Encoding
   b. Decoding
   c. Feedback
   d. Channel
2. The type of questioning technique that is usually used at the beginning of the interview is referred to as:
   a. open-ended questions.
   b. close-ended questions.
   c. silence.
   d. asking leading questions.
3. Which of the following would be considered an ineffective interviewing technique?
   a. Asking leading questions
   b. Demanding an explanation
   c. Strongly agreeing or disagreeing with the patient
   d. All of the above
4. What is the name of the listening technique that stimulates the patient to ponder on their last response?
   a. Clarification
   b. Restating
   c. Reflecting
   d. Summarizing
5. What type of family history is also considered a family tree?
   a. Famogram
   b. Genogram
   c. Genofam
   d. None of the above
6. What information would be included in the patient's personal medical history?
   a. Past medical history
   b. Review of systems
   c. Current medication listing
   d. All of the above
7. Which of the following is not part of the patient screening?
   a. Performing a physical exam on the patient
   b. Obtaining the chief complaint
   c. Obtaining the patient's vital signs
   d. Updating the patient's preventive testing section
8. Effective listening techniques include:
   a. asking leading questions.
   b. demanding answers.
   c. clarifying the patient's answers.
   d. None of the above
9. What part of the history would include the patient's surgical history?
   a. Personal history
   b. Family history
   c. Social history
   d. Depression screening
10. What part of the screening would include whether or not the patient wears a seatbelt?
    a. Personal history
    b. Family history
    c. Social history
    d. None of the above

STUDY RESOURCES

Resources to Test and Reinforce Your Knowledge:	
Certification Review Questions	Take this end-of-chapter quiz
Workbook	• Complete the activities for Chapter 5 • Perform the procedure for Chapter 5 using the Competency Checklist
Resources to Promote Critical Thinking:	
***Solve the Case* Activities**	• Consider these case studies and discuss your conclusions
Learning Lab	• Module 20: Patient Intake
MindTap	• Complete Chapter 5 readings and activities

REFERENCES

GLAAD Media Reference Guide - Transgender Issues. (2011, September 09). Retrieved August 18, 2015, from http://www.glaad.org/reference/transgender

My Family Health Portrait, A tool from the Surgeon General | NIH MedlinePlus the Magazine. (n.d.). Retrieved from http://www.nlm.nih.gov/medlineplus/magazine/issues/winter10/articles/winter10pg4.html

My Family Health Portrait Tool. (n.d.). Retrieved from http://www.hhs.gov/familyhistory/portrait/index.html

Theories of Communication and the Communication Cycle. (n.d.). Retrieved August 18, 2015, from http://yourbusiness.azcentral.com/theories-communication-communication-cycle-11318.html

Therapeutic Communication and Behavioral Management. (n.d.). Retrieved August 18, 2015, from http://www.ncchc.org/cnp-therapeutic-communication

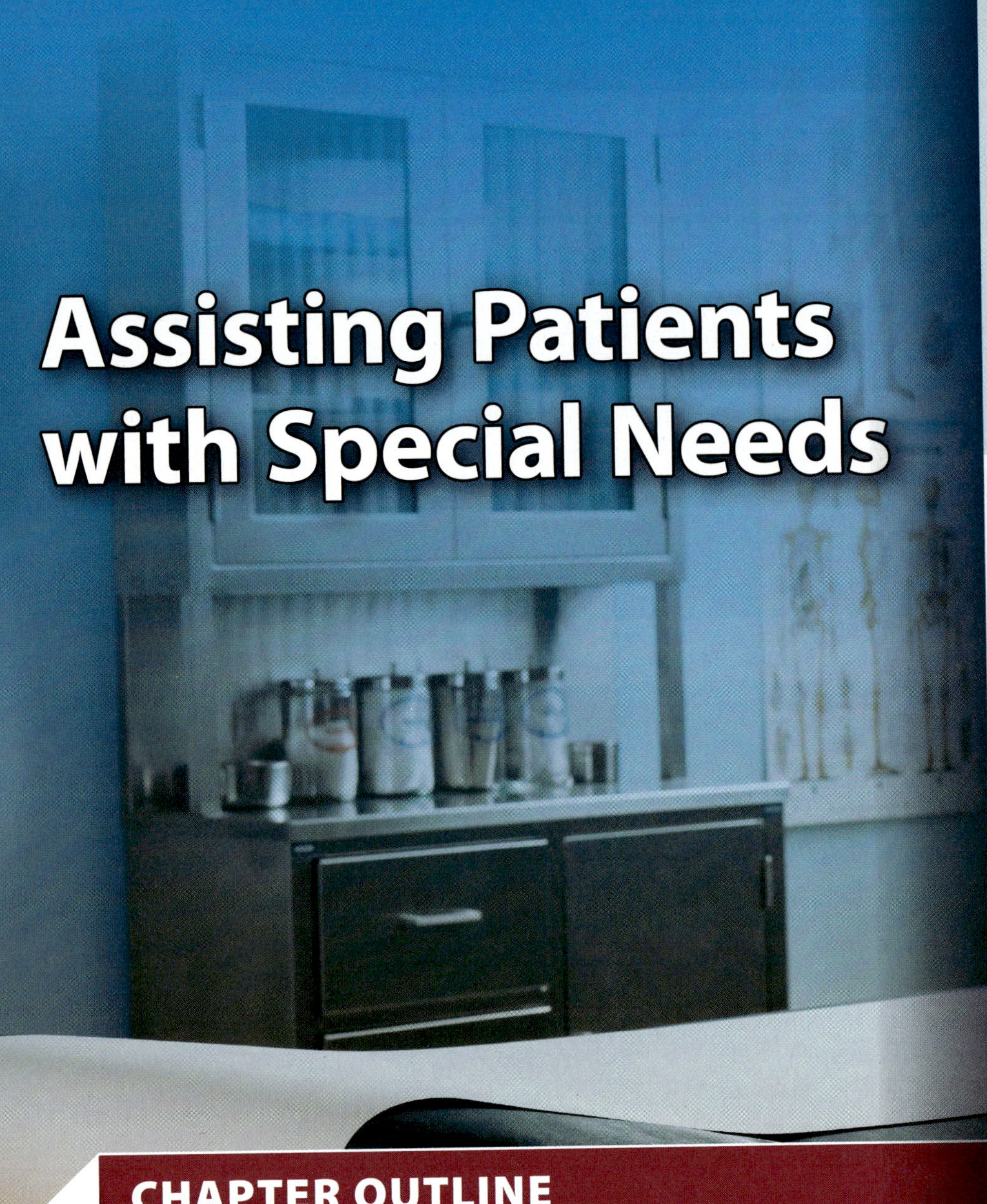

6

Assisting Patients with Special Needs

CHAPTER OUTLINE

Legal Issues and the Special Needs Patient

- Laws for the Hearing Impaired Patient
- Laws Assisting the Visually Impaired Patient
- Accessible Design Standards for Persons with Physical Disabilities
- Laws for Non-English-Speaking Patients

Working with Patients with Special Needs

- Diversity in Health Care
- Barriers to Communication and Techniques to Overcome
- Working with Visually Impaired Patients
- Working with Hearing Impaired and Deaf Patients
- Working with Older (Geriatric) Adults
- Working with Pediatric Patients
- Working with Physically Disabled Patients
- Working with Patients Who Have Intellectual Disabilities

ESSENTIAL TERMS

activities of daily living (ADLs)
ADA Standards for Accessible Design
Alzheimer's disease
American Sign Language (ASL)
Americans with Disabilities Act (ADA)
Americans with Disabilities Act Amendments Act (ADAAA)
auxiliary services
Civil Rights Act
conceptually accurate signed English (CASE)
cultural diversity
dementia
diversity
elder abuse
exploitation
frail senior
guide dogs
limited English proficiency (LEP)
mental health
mental illness
mental impairment
mentally challenged
neglect
physical disability
postlingual
prelingual
senior abuse
sighted guide assistance
signed English
signed exact English (SEE)
telecommunications device for the deaf (TDD)
Telecommunications Relay Services (TRS)
teletypewriter (TTY)

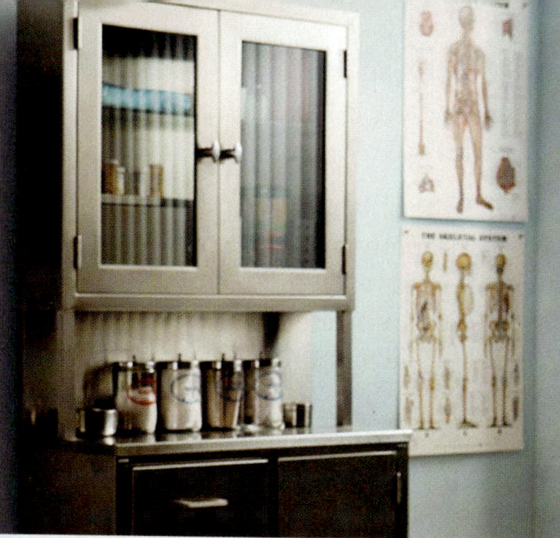

DEVELOPMENTAL OBJECTIVES

After completing this chapter, you should be able to:

1. Correctly spell and define the essential terms.
2. Identify and comply with federal, state, and local health laws and regulations as they relate to health care settings.
3. Explain the purpose of the Americans with Disabilities Act (ADA) and Amendments Act (ADAAA) and list what groups are included under this provision.
4. List ways that the office can become compliant with ADA guidelines to assist visually impaired patients.
5. Give four examples of auxiliary services and aids that can be used to assist the hearing impaired patients.
6. List six examples of "accessible design" features that can accommodate patients who have disabilities.
7. Describe obligations of the medical office in providing an interpreter for the non-English-speaking patient.
8. Explain the term *diversity* and discuss examples of cultural, social, and ethnic diversity, and ways to demonstrate respect for individual diversity including gender, race, religion, age, economic status, and appearance.
9. Recognize communication barriers and identify techniques to overcome barriers.
10. Describe why the use of certain gestures is discouraged.
11. Explain the procedure for providing sighted guide assistance and briefly describe the procedures for accessing elevators, stairways, and doorways.
12. List tips for working with older adults and pediatric patients.
13. List tips for working with physically disabled patients.
14. List tips for working with patients who have an intellectual disability.
15. Analyze the effect of hereditary, cultural, and environmental influences on behavior, and demonstrate sensitivity to patient rights.

INTRODUCTION

A health care worker must have excellent communication skills. The majority of responsibilities for the clinical medical assistant involve direct patient care. Because a clinical medical assistant spends a great deal of time with patients, effective communication with all types of patients is vital.

Before a medical assistant can be a good technician, she must be a good communicator. If the assistant lacks the ability to properly communicate, it can impede the ability to perform well technically.

Illness or injury can strike anyone at any time, regardless of age, religion, ethnic background, or disability. The medical assistant must learn how to work with all types of individuals in spite of language or cultural differences and how to properly accommodate individuals with disabilities.

Learning how to effectively communicate with individuals having special needs is a lifelong process that begins during medical assistant training. This chapter will set the foundation for working with patients who have special needs, and their families. You will build on the foundation throughout your professional career by attending continuing education courses, and through your own learning experiences. Just as your technical skills improve with time and practice, so will your communication skills.

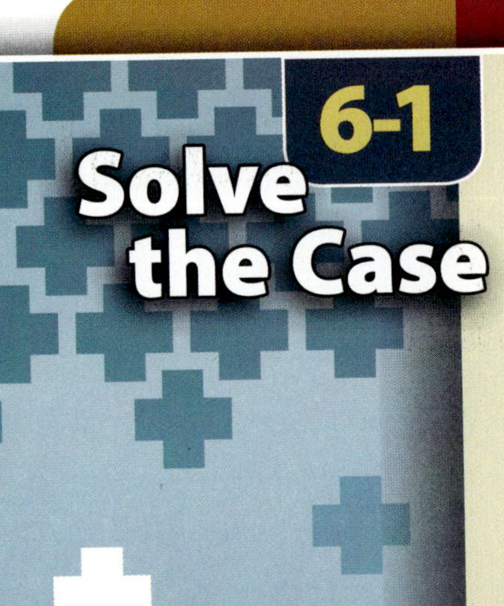

Mrs. Adams, a visually impaired patient, has an appointment to see Dr. Brockton today for symptoms of a urinary tract infection. She is accompanied by her guide dog. You are ready to take her back to the exam room.

1. **How should you approach Mrs. Adams in the reception area?**
2. **Your office has a policy that no pets are allowed in the facility. Will you permit Mrs. Adams to allow the dog to lead her back to the blood drawing area? Why or why not?**
3. **What should you do if you see people in the reception area trying to pet and talk to the dog?**
4. **Will Mrs. Adams need sighted guide assistance?**

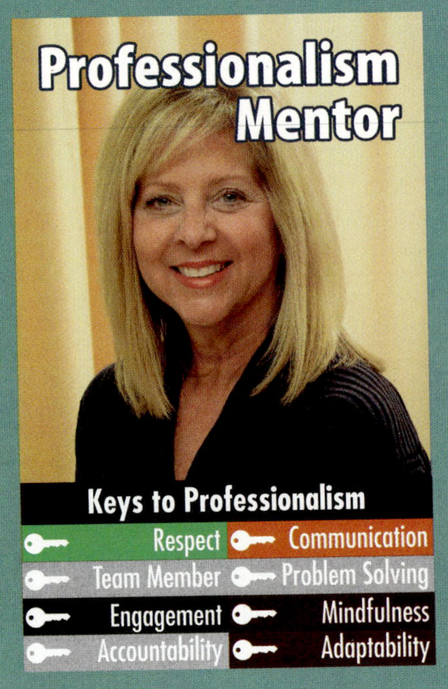

Assisting the patient with special needs is probably one of the toughest yet most rewarding services a medical assistant can provide. I recently had the opportunity to visit one of our pediatric clinics and witnessed firsthand the compassion of the staff caring for a young boy with Down's syndrome. He was by nature a sweet boy but was visibly afraid when it came time for his yearly vaccinations. The medical assistant in the office was fairly new but she greeted the little boy and his mother with a big smile. His mother seemed on the edge herself, probably worried about the staff and how they would react to her son. The medical assistant spoke softly to the mother and told her, everything would be "okay." Her voice and demeanor exhibited patience and empathy, two important keys to success when caring for a child with special needs having a somewhat painful procedure. I cannot in all honesty say it was an easy task giving that little boy his injection, but the medical assistant did her best to provide the care that mother and child needed that day. As they left the clinic, the medical assistant handed the little boy his "sticker" and gave him a big hug and in return he smiled at her. That was a good day! ■

LEGAL ISSUES AND THE SPECIAL NEEDS PATIENT

In addition to being able to effectively communicate with special needs patients, the medical assistant must have a good grasp of laws that assist some of the special needs patients who frequent the medical office. Failure to adhere to these laws can set the office up for possible litigation. Accessibility of doctors' offices, clinics, and other health care providers is essential in providing medical care to people with disabilities. Accessibility is not only legally required, but it is also important medically so that minor problems can be detected and treated before turning into major and possibly life-threatening problems.

The **Americans with Disabilities Act (ADA)** of 1990 is referred to as civil rights legislation designed to prohibit discrimination against individuals based on disability. The Act defined "disability" as "a physical or mental impairment that substantially limits a major life activity" (42 U.S.C. sec. 12112, 1990). On September 25, 2008, President Bush signed the **Americans with Disabilities Act Amendments Act (ADAAA)** (the "Act"). The Act became effective January 1, 2009. The Act emphasizes that the definition of disability should be construed in favor of broad coverage of individuals to the maximum extent permitted by the terms of the ADA and generally shall not require extensive analysis. The Act made important changes to the definition of the term *disability* by rejecting the holdings in several Supreme Court decisions and portions of EEOC's ADA regulations. The effect of these changes is to make it easier for an individual seeking protection under the ADA to establish that he or she has a disability within the meaning of the ADA (EEOC, n.d.). According to the U.S. Department of Labor, "The purpose of the ADA or Americans with Disabilities Act is to extend to people with disabilities, including disabled veterans, civil rights similar to those now available on the basis of race, color, sex, national origin, and religion through the **Civil Rights Act** of 1964. It prohibits discrimination on the basis of disability in: private sector employment, services rendered by state and local governments, places of public accommodation, transportation, and telecommunication services." To learn more about the ADAAA, log on to the EEOC website (www.eeoc.gov) and search the topic ADAAA.

Laws for the Hearing Impaired Patient

Businesses, including medical offices, are required by law to ensure effective communication with individuals who have hearing, vision, or speech impairments by furnishing appropriate **auxiliary services** and aids whenever necessary (Title III of the Americans with Disabilities Act, section 36.303). Table 6-1 lists some examples of auxiliary aids and services provided under the ADA.

Because each patient's ability to communicate is different, the office will need to determine what services, materials, or devices are necessary to effectively communicate with each individual hearing impaired or deaf patient. In many instances, this is determined at the time the appointment is scheduled by either the patient or caregiver of the patient.

To effectively communicate when scheduling appointments, some medical offices have a device referred to as a **teletypewriter (TTY)** or **telecommunications device for the deaf (TDD)**. These devices allow users to type messages between each other. When the office does not have a TTY/TDD, the deaf caller may use **Telecommunications Relay Services (TRS)**. There are also new technologies that give consumers a wider variety of choices such as voice carryover; hearing carryover; captioned telephone service; and Internet-based communication through text relay services (Internet Protocol or IP Relay), video relay services (VRS), and captioned telephone services. It is your responsibility as a medical assistant to be aware of the laws and device/services offered to assist hearing and speech impaired patients.

Table 6-1 Auxiliary Aids and Services That Aid in Communication

Aids That Require the Services of Other People	Aids That Require Special Equipment	Aids That Require a Computer or Television
Qualified Interpreters Interpreters for the deaf who are specially trained to interpret what is being stated during a medical office or hospital visit	**Assisted Listening Headsets and/or Devices** Devices that help to amplify sound, such as hearing aids, head sets, and so on	**Computer-Aided Transcription Services** Turns verbal audio-taped information into a written transcript
Notetaker A specially trained individual who takes written notes for deaf patients during meetings, office visits, and school and college courses	**Telecommunication Devices for Deaf Persons (TDDs)** A device that allows a deaf person to type information over the phone lines to another person with a TDD	**Closed and Open Caption** Captions that display dialog being stated on a TV screen. May be used during a video presentation or video conference.

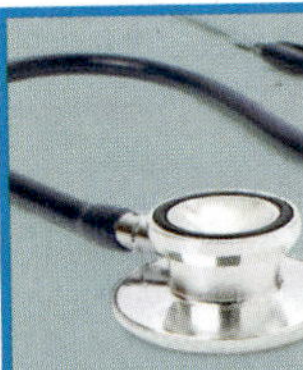

CRITICAL THINKING CHALLENGE

A deaf patient schedules an appointment using a relay operator. You ask the operator to ask the patient if she will need the office to schedule an interpreter for the visit. The operator states that the patient doesn't feel an interpreter will be necessary because her friend is going to come with her and she just finished a sign language class at the community college.

1. List at least three reasons why using the friend in this scenario is not a good decision.
2. What would be an appropriate response for you to give to the patient?

Field Smarts

Don't make assumptions about a patient's visual acuity or the functional effects associated with his or her vision loss. The same patient may have perfectly adequate travel vision during the day but may find mobility to be much more difficult at night under low lighting conditions. Respond to your patient's needs on an individual basis. As a general matter, be guided by his or her request for assistance. The simple question: "How can I be of assistance to you, Mr. Jessup?" is one of the most powerful ADA compliance tools (AFB).

Wireless carriers provide a variety of features for hearing impaired or deaf customers including text messaging, instant messaging, email, and vibrating ringers and alerts. Numerous smartphone apps have been developed that can be a powerful communication tool.

Laws Assisting the Visually Impaired Patient

The federal ADA law requires that visually impaired patients have a right to receive health care information in "alternative formats," the most common formats being Braille, large print, audio recording, email, and electronic or digital documents. In addition, admission of service animals must be permitted for patients with disabilities who would require them. A guide dog should always be under the control of the patient. New building codes require office entrance ways, exit signs, bathrooms, and elevator controls to have Braille plates for identification purposes (Figure 6-1). For more information about laws that assist the visually impaired, explore the American Foundation for the Blind (AFB) website at www.afb.org.

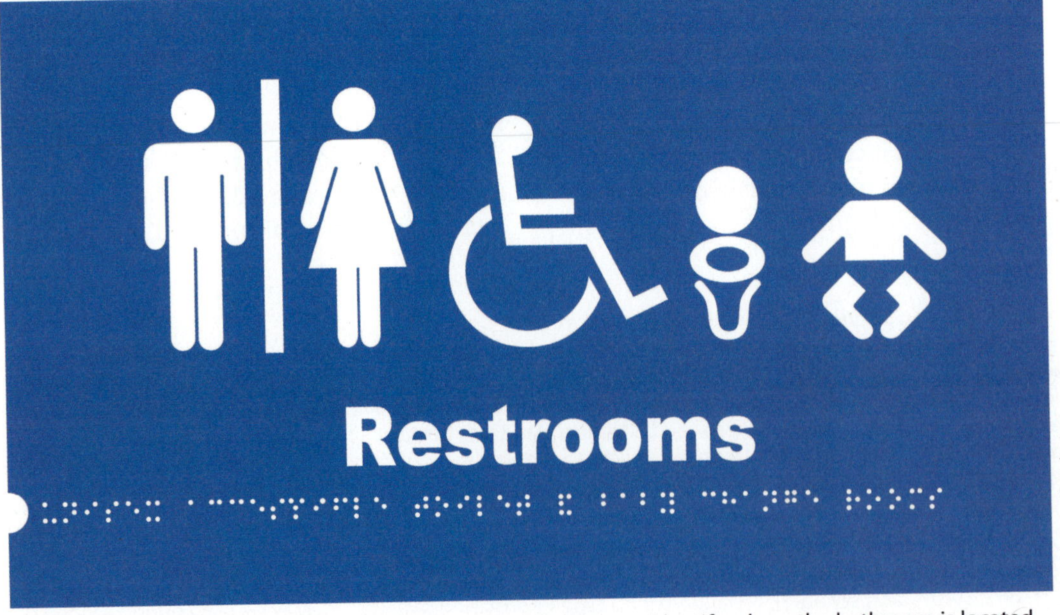

Figure 6-1 ■ A Braille plate allows a visually impaired patient to identify where the bathroom is located.

Accessible Design Standards for Persons with Physical Disabilities

Since 1992, the ADA has required all new public and commercial facilities to comply with the **ADA Standards for Accessible Design**. Revised regulations were published on September 15, 2010, called the 2010 ADA Standards of Accessible Design (2010 Standards), which became effective March 15, 2012. These standards mandate construction companies to design buildings that are accessible to all persons, including those who have dexterity and limited mobility problems. Other groups addressed in this standard include individuals with visual and hearing impairments. Examples of ADA standards for handicap and wheelchair accessibility features include the following:

- Parking: Detectable warnings on curb ramps
- Adequate number of handicapped parking spaces
- Wheelchair ramps to buildings with elevated entrances
- Wider elevators, doorways, and hallways (maneuvering clearances)
- Specifications for knee and toe space
- Exterior doors: Automation recommended
- Lower service counters
- Plumbing elements and access: Handicapped bathrooms designed to accommodate patients who are in wheelchairs.

While many of these guidelines do not directly affect the communication process, failure to comply with the guidelines can directly affect the patient's mental state before, during, and following the appointment. It can also lead to legal difficulties for the office. Because of this the clinical medical assistant should routinely scan hallways and patient rooms to make certain that there are no barriers that would impede physically handicapped patients from getting through or potentially cause patients to injure themselves. The U.S. Department of Justice, Civil Rights Division, and the U.S. Department of Health and Human Services created a document titled "Americans with Disabilities Act: Access to Medical Care for Individuals with Mobility Disabilities" that provides not only the specific requirements, but also offers visual aids for how the medical office and equipment should be configured and how to assist patients. For more information view or download the document from the ADA website (www.ada.gov). Additional information is also available from the U.S. Access Board (www.access-board.gov).

Laws for Non-English-Speaking Patients

Another act that must be considered for special needs patients is Title VI of the Civil Rights Act. This act requires entities receiving federal assistance from the Department of Health and Human Services (HHS)—including providers who participate in Medicare or Medicaid programs—to provide interpreters for non-English-speaking patients and patients with **limited English proficiency (LEP)**.

An individual is considered LEP when English is not the primary language or the patient is not literate. Providers must demonstrate that they have taken the appropriate steps to provide those patients with limited English-speaking or reading abilities the services that are necessary to ensure effective communication.

Methods Used to Assist Patients with LEP

The medical office has an obligation to provide written and oral language assistance to all patients with LEP. Methods that can be used for assistance include the following:

- Hiring competent bilingual staff members and interpreter services
- Providing patients verbal offers and written notices in their preferred language, informing them of their right to receive language assistance services
- Making available easily understood patient-related materials in the patient's native language (including consent forms, privacy statements, and a listing of services that are provided by the medical office)
- Posting signage in the languages commonly encountered and/or presented in the service area.

Brochures should be designed to accommodate the non-English-speaking populations that reside in the community. They should state that interpreting services are available to the patient at no additional charge.

In order for providers to be in compliance with agencies that provide certification and accreditation, such as The Joint Commission (JC) and the National Committee for Quality Assurance (NCQA),

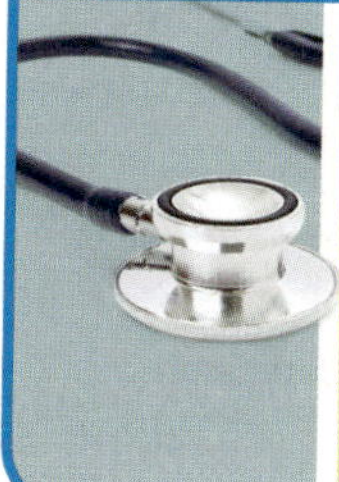

Field Smarts

Being bilingual or multilingual will give you added value to employers in offices that have great diversity within their patient population.

the provider must establish that the interpreters used are qualified, meaning that they have been specially trained for the assignment. Qualified medical interpreters should be fluent in both the patient's language and English and have gone through special training for medical assignments, demonstrating mastery of the skill through competency testing. The American Translators Association (ATA) provides a testing exam for Certified Translators, which helps to ensure that the translator is proficient. For more information, log on to the ATA website (www.atanet.org) and search "ATA Certification."

Most interpreting companies provide interpretation for multiple cultural groups. These companies usually provide training and testing for their interpreters and require the interpreters to be bonded. The company will provide HIPAA training and require each interpreter to sign a confidentiality statement, simplifying the amount of work that the office has to perform. The office can schedule an in-office interpreter or may choose to use a special interpreter telephone service line that can provide immediate translators 24 hours a day, seven days per week. Telephone interpreting is usually more economical and can be accessed quickly.

To learn more about assisting patients with LEP, go to the website www.usdoj.gov and search "LEP." You can also visit the website www.LEP.gov for more information.

WORKING WITH PATIENTS WITH SPECIAL NEEDS

The remainder of this chapter focuses on various types of special needs patients and the challenges a medical assistant may face when caring for them. The medical assistant must find ways to effectively communicate with special needs patients in order to provide the best possible care. Families of special needs patients are especially helpful in interpreting their family member's needs. Include them whenever possible to make communication as effective as possible.

Diversity in Health Care

Diversity means something different to each and every person. **Diversity** encompasses and includes different types of people (such as people of different races or cultures) into a group. The term **cultural diversity** incorporates several variables including ethnicity, race, and religious beliefs. *Culture* includes a person's customs and beliefs, social forms, and traits of racial, religious, or varying social groups. *Diversity* is a term that identifies the unique differences in various cultures.

The United States is one of the most culturally diverse countries in the world. Data from the 2010 U.S. Census states that almost 40 percent of the U.S. population is from racially, ethnically, or culturally diverse groups and that rate is predicted to continue growing.

As diversity numbers continually increase, it is vitally important for medical assistants to learn about different cultures and gain a better understanding of the customs and practices for the cultural groups that they serve.

Barriers to Communication and Techniques to Overcome

Cultural variances will impact the communication process with patients and can at times provide challenges to the medical assistant. Examples of cultural variances are the following:

- Not all patients are familiar with or accepting of "Western medicine" and may in fact believe in holistic, homeopathic, folk remedies, rituals, and ceremonies.
- Personality traits vary. In certain cultures people are outgoing and in others the tendency may be to be quiet and reserved.
- Nonverbal signals may have different meanings.
- Eye contact is an important tool in body language and conveying a message; however, certain cultures find eye contact disrespectful or aggressive.
- Therapeutic touch is generally accepted in Western medicine; however, there are patients or employees who may be offended by touching or whose religious beliefs, culture, or ethnic origin does not allow this. When touching someone to offer comfort or praise, it would be best to do so in the presence of other professionals to protect against possible misunderstandings (Figure 6-2).

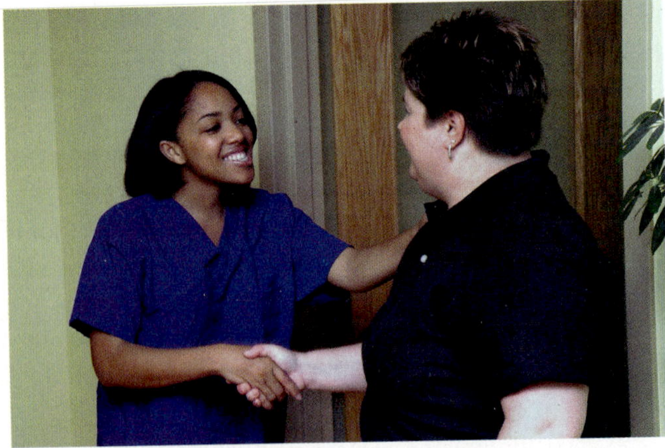

Figure 6-2 ■ Therapeutic touch is generally accepted in Western medicine; however, there are patients or employees who may be offended by touching or whose religious beliefs, culture, or ethnic origin do not allow this.

Table 6-2 Common Communication Barriers

Barrier	Example	Techniques to Overcome
Physical disabilities	Hearing or vision impairment	Adjust volume of speech; offer Braille or large print materials
Psychological attitudes and prejudice	Personal opinions formed (e.g., alternative lifestyles, certain ethnic or religious groups)	Avoid touching or eye contact if there is a cultural or religious barrier; family member present with patient in exam room
Cultural diversity, language	Non-English-speaking; limited English proficiency	Use qualified interpreter services for patient and family members; printed material available in multiple languages
Age	Children or elderly patients	Use terminology and tone appropriate to each patient; schedule appointments convenient to the age group
Outside influences	Noise	Move to a quiet room/area; focus on communication versus distraction

You will encounter barriers to the communication process. A barrier is defined as anything that gets in the way of clear communication. Table 6-2 outlines common barriers, examples, and techniques to overcome.

Ways to demonstrate good intercultural communication skills:

- Withhold judgment
- Show respect
- Empathize
- Tolerate ambiguity
- Recognize your own cultural biases
- Emphasize common ground
- Send clear messages
- Learn when to be direct

Hereditary, Cultural, and Environmental Influences on Behavior

Today, researchers generally agree that heredity and environment have an interactive influence on intelligence and behavior. Environmental factors are thought to be the primary cause of cultural differences.

Easing the Culturally Diverse Patient

Good medical assistants work hard to make every patient feel at ease. The following information lists a step-by-step approach that can be taken to help culturally diverse patients and their families feel more comfortable during the office visit.

1. Begin the visit by introducing yourself and stating your title.
2. If you are a different gender than the patient, ask the patient if she would prefer someone of her gender to conduct the interview (Figure 6-3).
3. Ask the patient for assistance with the correct pronunciation of her name.

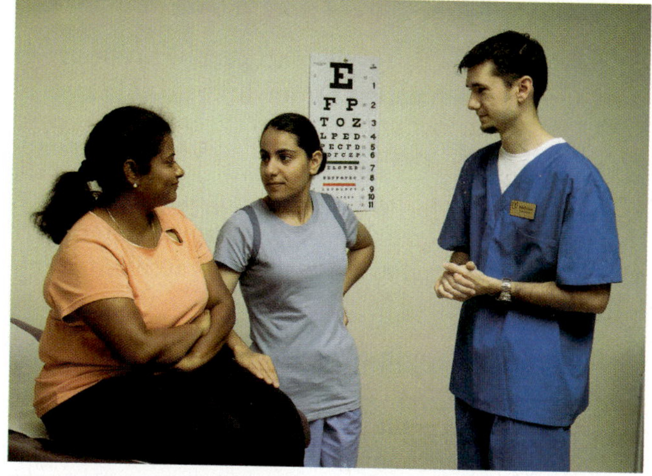

Figure 6-3 ■ Always ask patients of the opposite gender if they would prefer a medical assistant of the same gender.

4. Ask the patient to introduce any family members or friends who are present.
5. Be conversational by starting with a question about the patient's family or career. This demonstrates a caring attitude toward the patient and family members.
6. Before starting the formal patient intake questioning, ask the patient and family members to state their goals for the visit.
7. If an interpreter is not present and the patient has limited English proficiency, give the patient written materials that explain his or her rights to have a qualified interpreter present during the interview process. If the patient is going to use a family member to perform the interpreting, ensure that the family member understands the importance of the task. Using nonadult children as interpreters is usually discouraged.
8. Instruct the patient and patient's family members to stop you at any time if they need something more clearly stated.

9. Observe the patient for cues on how she feels regarding eye contact, gestures, and proxemics (the amount of distance that one needs in order to feel comfortable when sitting or standing next to another person). This will help you get a feel for what is and is not comfortable to the patient. Do not ask the patient to do anything that would make her feel uncomfortable unless absolutely necessary.
10. Do not judge or criticize the patient about her cultural or religious beliefs.
11. Be sensitive to the patient's cultural beliefs with regard to disrobing. Use extra drapes and keep the patient covered completely except during times when it is absolutely necessary to remove articles of clothing.
12. Explain all procedures before you perform them.

In Procedure 6-1 you will practice how to effectively communicate with patients from different cultures.

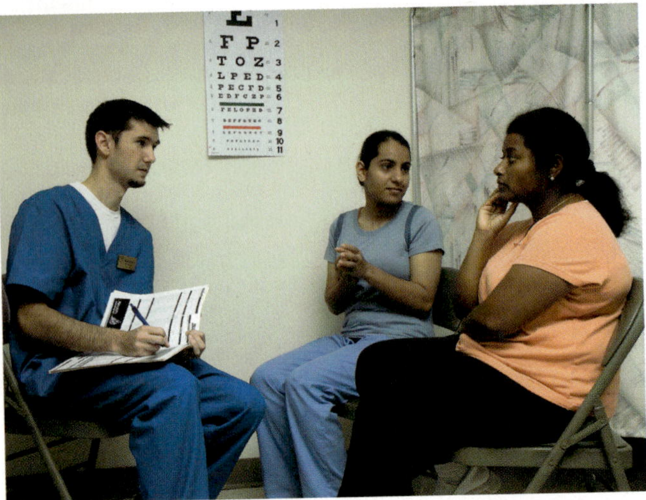

Figure 6-4 ■ A room should be set up properly when working with an interpreter and a patient with limited English proficiency.

Working with Interpreters

When the patient has limited English proficiency, the services of a qualified or professional interpreter should be used whenever possible, because of the following reasons:

- Qualified and professional interpreters have specialized training in medical interpreting to handle the types of communication that are common during medical encounters.
- Although family members may be bilingual, they may not possess the language skills that are necessary to properly translate medical information.
- The patient may withhold information if a family member is performing the interpreting to avoid revealing sensitive personal information.
- The patient's family member may be hesitant to translate certain findings from the provider to the patient because she may not want to worry the patient.

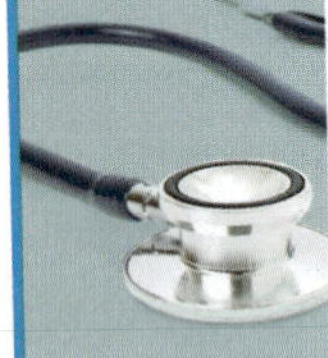

Field Smarts

If an interpreter is present, place the interpreter's chair next to the patient's chair and angle the chairs so that they just slightly face each other. Place your chair across from the patient's chair centered between both the patient and the interpreter (Figure 6-4). Talk clearly and avoid using slang or medical jargon. Speak in simple phrases and avoid long sentences. Always speak in the first person as though you are speaking directly to the patient. Avoid saying phrases like, "Ask the patient" or "Tell her…." The conversation should be directed toward the patient, but you should make certain that the interpreter can understand what is being said as well.

Timing is critical when working with a translator. The translator must listen to the question, process it, and translate the question from English into the language of the patient. The patient will then respond to the question, and the translator once again will need to translate the patient's response into English. Make certain that the translator is finished before proceeding with the next question.

You should be looking for nonverbal cues from the patient and make certain that they match with what the interpreter is relaying. Always ask the patient to repeat any instructions to ensure a complete understanding of the instructions. Figure 6-4 illustrates a room that has been properly set up when working with an interpreter.

Table 6-3 Interpretation of Body Language and Gestures by Different Cultures

Eye contact	Considered respectful in Western civilization; however, patients from other cultures may not return eye contact as a way of demonstrating respect, and yet others may consider direct eye contact to be aggressive or disrespectful in particular situations.
Touching	Therapeutic touch is generally accepted in Western medicine; however, there are patients or employees who may be offended by touching or whose religious beliefs, culture, or ethnic origin does not allow this. When touching someone to offer comfort or praise, it would be best to do so in the presence of other professionals to protect against possible misunderstandings (see Figure 6-2).
Gestures	Gestures are body movements that enhance what is being said. Using hand and body gestures to accentuate a point can help the receiver understand your meaning. To emphasize the subject matter in a conversation, gestures help to convey the message. Gestures not only reinforce what is being said, they also reveal a person's attitude. Gestures may be perceived as either warm or cold. Warm gestures might include leaning toward people, directly facing them, maintaining eye contact while smiling, touching, and gesturing expressively. Conversely, cold gestures could be keeping your hands on your hips, slumping, avoiding eye contact, not smiling, and displaying nervous gestures, such as drumming your fingers and fiddling with jewelry, hair, or objects.
Proxemics (the use of space)	Westerners usually require more space when conversing with another individual than persons from other countries. Distances (comfort zones) vary for different people and cultures. You must be respectful and ask if you are not sure of a patient's accepted practice. It would be appropriate to ask, "Would you like to take my arm while I escort you to the exam room?"

Body Language and the Communication Process

Body language is an integral part of the communication process. Even when working with persons from the same or similar cultures, gestures or body language can change the entire meaning of what is stated. Table 6-3 provides general information regarding communication facts and beliefs and how the use of body language and gestures might be perceived by patients from other cultures.

Commonalities among Different Cultures and Avoiding Stereotypes

It is important to note commonalities in various cultures in order to improve communication, which ultimately means better service and care for the patient. A better understanding of what is considered "offensive" or what is considered "acceptable" for the different populations served will help to keep the communication door open. Offending the patient by making gestures or saying things that are not considered appropriate can jeopardize the relationship, which may cause both emotional and physical stress to the patient.

Just as there are unique differences in various cultures, there are also individual differences and preferences within each person that may be influenced by gender, education, religion, subcultures, age, reason for migration, and socioeconomic status.

It is important that medical assistants examine their personal views on cultural issues and replace negative thoughts with positive thinking. Neither past experiences with individuals from other cultures nor family prejudices can be allowed to influence the service that a patient receives.

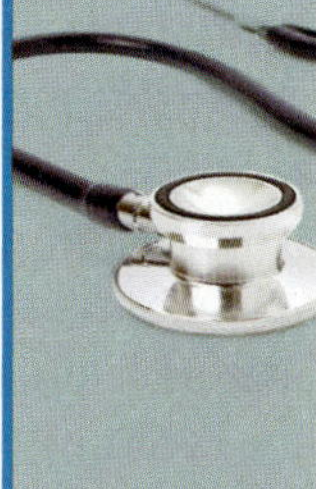

Field Smarts

If your patient backs away from you or moves toward you, do not be offended and do not reposition your chair. This could well be a sign that the patient is uncomfortable with the spacing of the chairs. Allow patients to position the chairs in a manner that is comfortable for them.

CRITICAL THINKING CHALLENGE

During the chief complaint segment of an in-office screening, a Middle-Eastern female patient complains of lower abdominal pain. She also has some vaginal symptoms. You instruct the patient to remove her clothes from the waist down. The patient and her husband appear quite distressed by the instructions and refuse to comply.

1. How should you respond to the couple's distress?
2. What types of reinforcement techniques can you use to help the patient and husband comply with the instructions?

Working with Visually Impaired Patients

Attitude is important when working with visually impaired patients. The medical assistant's views regarding the patient's abilities, needs, and interests can have a great effect on the patient, family members of the patient, and coworkers. Never assume that patients will be unable to perform a specific function just because they are visually impaired. Visually impaired patients have learned how to maneuver in spite of their disability and hence, are capable individuals. A large percentage of visually impaired people live independently.

Some individuals make the mistake of speaking loudly or shouting at visually impaired people. Visually impaired patients may not be able to see, but they are not deaf, and this is insulting to the patient. Avoid "talking down" to visually impaired patients; that is, do not make them feel as though they have a comprehension problem or a learning disability just because they are visually impaired. Continually communicate with visually impaired patients so that they know what is going on, but communicate at the patients' level of understanding. Consider this situation: A medical assistant, without identifying herself, enters the exam room of a patient who is visually impaired and noisily places an object on the counter. The patient wonders "What is it happening?" Solution: The medical assistant should identify herself and her purpose for entering the room: "Good afternoon, I'm Carla Smith, Dr. Brockton's medical assistant. I've placed a procedure tray on the counter as requested by Dr. Brockton. Can I get you anything before Dr. Brockton arrives?"

Most visually impaired patients have learned to be independent. Never assume they want your help. Always ask if they need sighted guide assistance before trying to assist them. The following list presents tips that are helpful to know when assisting visually impaired patients:

- Use verbal cues. Always let the patient know when you have entered an area by introducing yourself and stating your title. Alert the patient when you are going to leave an area as well.
- Out of respect for the patient, you should look directly at the patient as you speak, and position yourself at the same level as the patient. Visually impaired people have a very good sense of proxemics.
- Shake hands only if the patient extends the hand.
- Introduce new people as they enter the area and let the patient know where people are positioned in reference to the patient. Using positions of the clock may be helpful in this situation (for instance, "Mrs. Jones, Carrie is on your left side at about the 9:00 position").
- Alert the patient before you touch any part of the body so that the patient is not startled (e.g., "Mr. Tedrow, I am getting ready to clean your right arm with alcohol.").
- Continue using "sighted words" such as look, see, or read, as well as phrases such as "I'll see you later." Visually impaired patients have the same language as the sighted. Avoiding these words will make both parties uncomfortable.
- Never move a visually impaired patient's personal belongings without the patient's knowledge and consent.
- Keep the area safe. Make certain that there is nothing in the path of the patient to trip over or run into.

Providing Sighted Guide Assistance

There will be times when the patient may benefit from some extra help in maneuvering around the office. This is especially true if the patient is not a regular patient and is unfamiliar with the office surroundings. The patient may use a white cane or have a guide dog. With a guide dog, the patient may not need extra assistance, but always ask if you may be of any assistance. If a guide dog is not present, the patient may be more accepting of assistance. The following list gives some suggestions for providing **sighted guide assistance**:

- Ask the patients if they would like to have sighted guide assistance. Do not be offended if they refuse. They may feel strongly about their independence or have experienced a negative encounter in the past with someone who did not know how to properly lead.
- Stand next to the patient and gently touch the patient's elbow, forearm, or back of the hand with your hand. This will signal the patient to take your arm.
- Keep your arm relaxed and down by your side, allowing the patient to grasp your arm rather than you grasping the patient's arm. The patient will usually embrace your arm just above the elbow.
- Walk about a half step in front of the patient toward the inside of the patient so that the patient can feel your body movements (Figure 6-5).
- Walk at a comfortable pace and avoid dragging the patient.

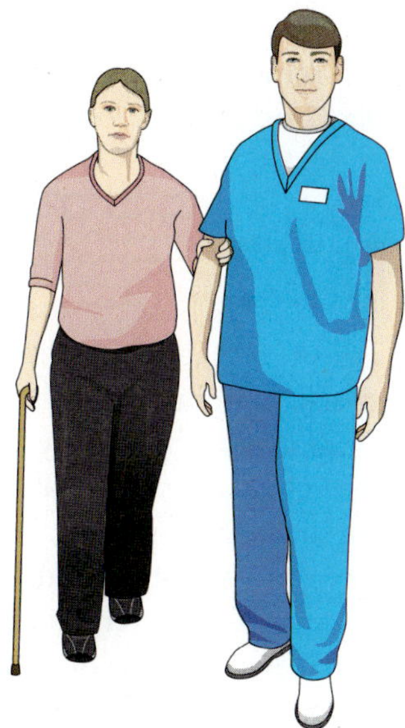

Figure 6-5 ■ Notice how the medical assistant walks about a half step in front of the visually impaired patient toward the inside of the patient so that the patient can feel the medical assistant's body movements.

- When moving through a narrow area, warn the patient and move your arm diagonally across your back. The patient should straighten her arm and walk directly behind you. This will permit you and the patient to move single file through the narrow area.
- Warn the patient when there are obstacles ahead or when you are going to make a turn, pass through a doorway, or go up or down steps.

See Procedure 6-2 for more information.

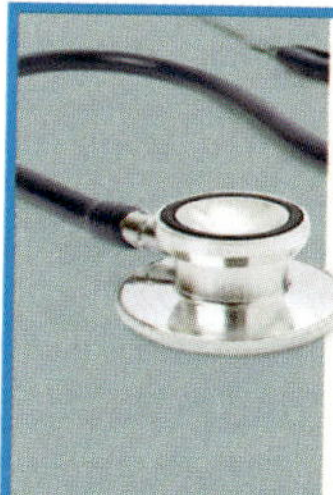

Field Smarts

Navigating Stairs: Pause and alert the patient when you are at the top or bottom of a stairway. Inform the patient of the number of steps and whether you are going up or down the stairs. Have the patient grasp the railing with his free hand as he holds on to your arm with the other hand. Pause when you get to the edge of the first step so the patient can touch the edge of the step with his foot. Both you and the patient should walk in rhythm with one another and you should always be one step ahead of the patient (Figure 6-6). Pause and alert the patient when you have reached the last step.

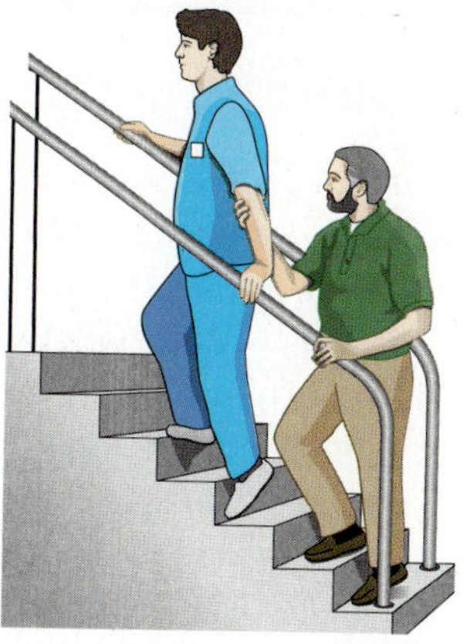

Figure 6-6 ■ An example of the proper way to lead a visually impaired person when ascending stairs.

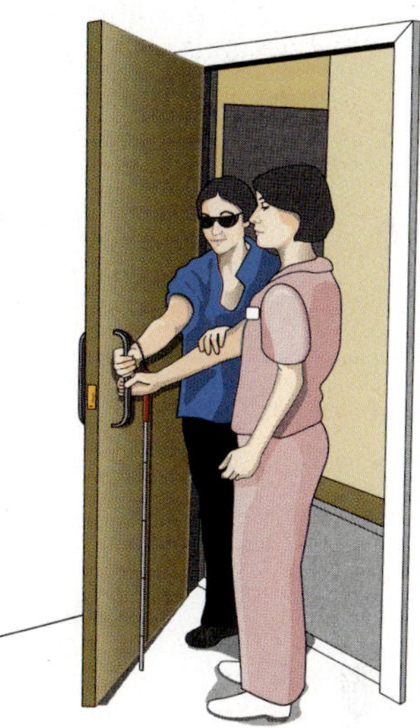

Figure 6-7 ■ An example of the proper way to lead a visually impaired person through a doorway.

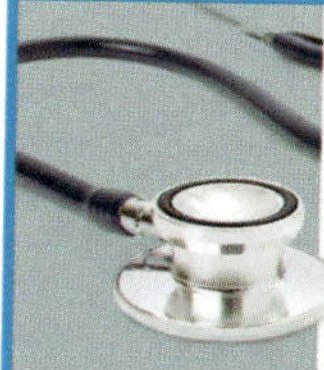

Field Smarts

Navigating Doorways: Let the patient know that you are at a doorway and describe whether it is a push or pull door and on what side the door opens. Position the patient so that she is on the hinged side of the door. Open the door with your guiding arm so that the patient senses where the handle is located. Have the patient place her free hand against the door, sliding it over to replace your hand on the handle (Figure 6-7). Release your hand from the handle and guide the patient through the doorway.

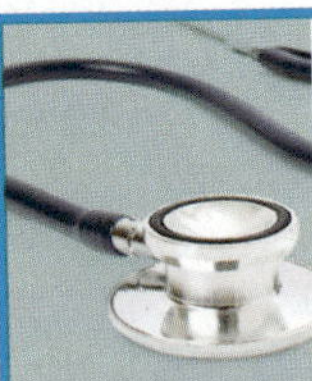

Field Smarts

Seating a Visually Impaired Patient: Before seating a visually impaired patient, explain the details of the seating. Describe whether the seating is a couch or chair, the height of the seating, and whether the seating has arms. When approaching the seating from the front, walk the patient up to the front of the chair, allowing her knees to just slightly touch the front side of the seat. Place the patient's hand on the handle of the chair and allow the patient to take over. When approaching the chair from the rear, walk the patient in a forward motion toward the back of the chair, placing the patient's hand on the back of the seat (Figure 6-8). Release the patient's hand and allow her to seat herself.

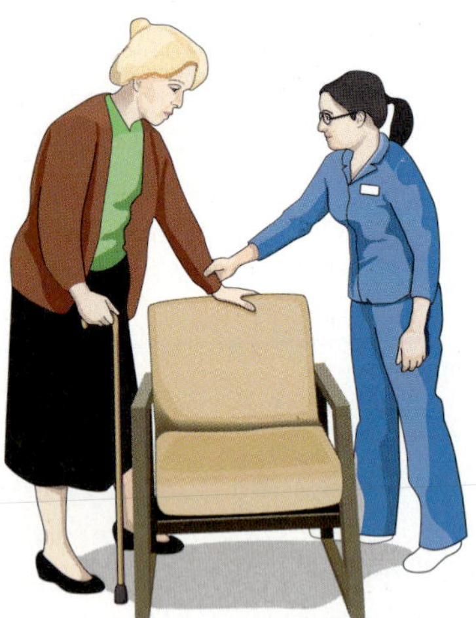

Figure 6-8 ■ An example of the proper way to seat a visually impaired patient.

Working with Guide Dogs

Many people have dogs and are intrigued when they see a guide dog. **Guide dogs** have been specially trained to guide visually impaired patients. Whenever a guide dog has a harness on, it means that the dog is "working." Both the blind person and the dog are a team. Do not try to feed, speak to, or pet the dog when the harness is on to prevent the dog from becoming distracted. Once the harness has been removed, the dog is like any other dog and can eat, play, and sleep.

Working with Hearing Impaired and Deaf Patients

Many people struggle with hearing loss but may be embarrassed to admit it. Hearing impairments can range from slight to moderate impairments and in some cases the patient may be totally deaf. Patients with mild-to-moderate hearing loss may be referred to as hearing impaired or hard of hearing. The term *hearing impaired,* however, may not be considered culturally acceptable to some deaf patients for a number of reasons. The National Association of the Deaf (NAD) expands on why it may be offensive: "Deaf and hard of hearing people are by no means 'silent' at all and use sign language, lip-reading, vocalizations, and so on to communicate" (n.d.). Accommodation factors for each patient will be based on the type and degree of hearing loss as well as the individual preference of the patient. The following list provides some tips that can be useful when working with patients with slight to moderate hearing impairments:

- Encourage patients to use their assistive hearing devices during the visit.
- Place the patient in a quiet room. Select rooms that are well-insulated with fabrics and carpeting. This will assist in reducing background noise.
- Sit directly across from and at the same level as the patient so that the patient can see your lip movement.
- Speak clearly and in a normal tone. Avoid shouting at the patient.
- Use gestures to enhance what is being stated.
- There may be times when you need to speak to the patient when she is not in full view of you. When this is necessary, gently tap the patient on the shoulder or use another means to let her know you are going to speak.
- Ask the patient to repeat any instructions given so that you can ascertain that the patient understood the information, without being condescending or insulting.
- Always give the patient written instructions and include family members in the discussion when appropriate.

The beginning of the chapter discussed the office's responsibility in providing an interpreter for hearing impaired patients as well as auxiliary services and aids available. The medical assistant may be responsible for

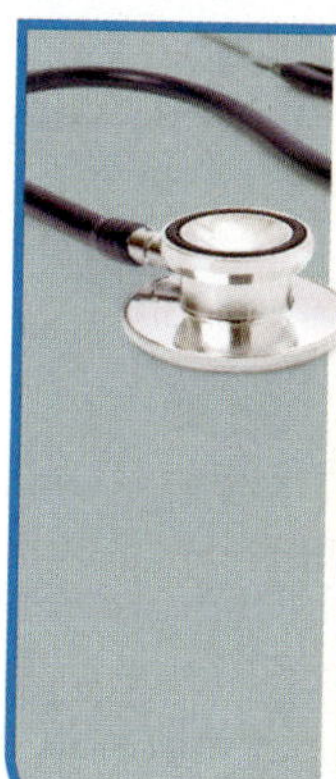

Field Smarts

Reflect on the use of "labels" when referring to culturally diverse or special needs patients and how it may be interpreted. Words and labels can have a profound impact on people. The one commonality we all have is that we all want to be treated with respect.

contacting an interpreting service to arrange for an interpreter to be present on the day of the appointment or to arrange a teleconference or video conference through an interpreting service during the time of the visit.

Communication styles will vary among deaf patients based on several factors including the age of onset of the deafness—**prelingual** (before the patient started talking) versus **postlingual** (after the patient started talking)—the educational background of the patient, current age of the patient, gender of the patient, and the patient's interest level. Some deaf patients are able to use and comprehend sign language, read lips, and read written materials, while others will only be able to communicate through the services of an interpreter.

Just as there are different spoken languages from region to region, there are also different kinds of sign languages. The most common sign language used in the United States and parts of Canada is **American Sign Language (ASL)**. ASL is a distinct language for the deaf and is considered the native language of the deaf. It is not English translated into different gestures and finger movements, which is why some deaf patients have difficulty when reading written material. Other types of sign languages common in the United States include the following:

- **Signed Exact English (SEE)**: This form of signing codes English words into a visual form.
- **Signed English**: Similar to SEE but often borrows vocabulary terms from ASL. This language is more similar to ASL than SEE.
- **Conceptually Accurate Signed English (CASE)**: Formerly pidgin signed English (PSE), this system uses ASL conceptual signs but in English word order.

The medical assistant should ask patients which form of sign language they feel most comfortable with and arrange for the right interpreter. Most interpreters are able to adapt to the patient's specific language needs.

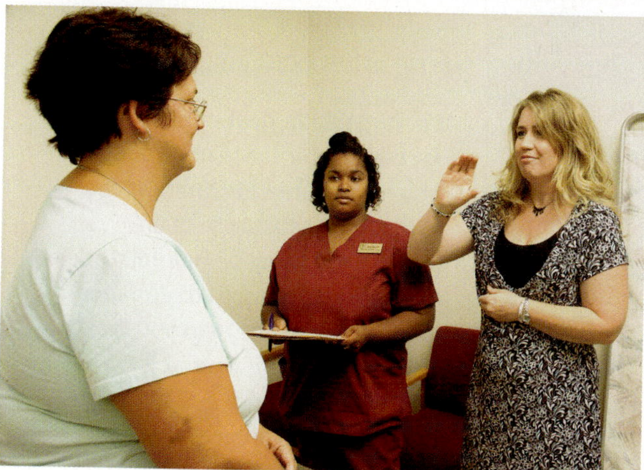

Figure 6-9 ■ The proper way to set up a room when using an interpreter for a deaf patient. Notice that the patient can see both the medical assistant and the interpreter. This allows the deaf patient to observe both the parties simultaneously.

The following list provides some tips that can be useful when working with an interpreter (see Procedure 6-3):

- Set the room up in a triangular pattern. The provider and medical assistant should be beside the interpreter and the patient should be centered across from members of the medical team and interpreter (Figure 6-9).
- Look and speak directly to the patient, not the interpreter, while communicating. For example, say to the patient, "What brings you to the office today?" but don't say to the interpreter, "Ask the patient the purpose of today's office visit."
- Give patients time to think about their response and make certain that they are completely finished with their response before asking a new question.

Working with Patients Who Speech Read

Patients who speech read usually have some hearing, although it may be limited. Speech reading (also known as reading lips) is hard to master and even the best speech readers can only interpret about 30 percent of the words formed with the lips during a verbal encounter. Because of this, speech readers use other cues to assist them, including tongue movement, cheek positioning, throat positioning, and facial gestures. They will also look for other body gestures to assist them in the communication process. The following list provides other helpful tips when working with speech-reading patients (see Procedure 6-4):

- Choose a room that is quiet, well lit, and glare free.
- Position yourself directly across from the patient at the same level as the patient. When possible, lighting should be angled toward your face.

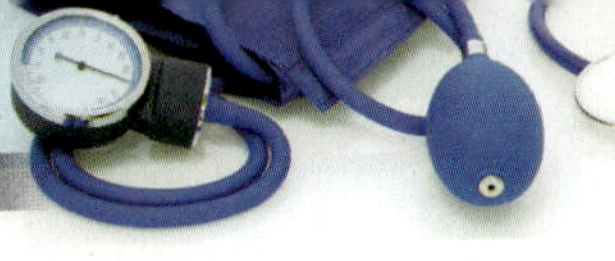

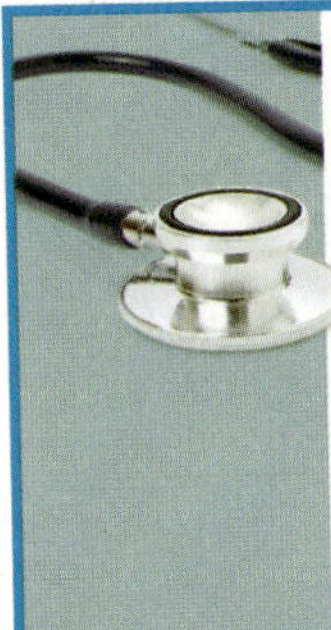

Field Smarts

Working with a deaf patient does not have to be awkward. Many deaf patients are able to communicate without the assistance of an interpreter. It may be helpful to take sign language classes to enhance your skills. This will help you feel more confident in your ability to communicate when a deaf patient comes into the office.

- Do not turn away from the patient when speaking, which can occur as you write or reach for something.
- Do not chew gum.
- When the patient does not understand a statement that you have made, try rephrasing it instead of repeating it.
- Use gestures and hand cues to assist in the communication process.
- Do not yell and do not slow down or overenunciate your words. Speech readers read speech at a normal speaking rate.
- Make certain that the patient understands what is stated by having the patient repeat the information to you.

Assistance Dogs

Assistant animals are individually trained to perform tasks for people with disabilities: "Guide dogs" for guiding visually impaired persons, "signal dogs" for alerting people who are deaf, and "service dogs" for alerting people who have seizures, and so on. Just as some visually impaired patients have guide dogs, some deaf patients have "hearing guide dogs," also known as "signal dogs." These dogs are trained to alert teammates of special sounds and will physically lead them to the sound. Knocks on the door, doorbell rings, telephone rings, and the sounds of a honking car are just a few of the sounds the dog is trained to respond to. Deaf people that typically use hearing guide dogs are those who became deaf later in life. Signal dogs generally wear bright orange leashes when they are working and should not be distracted.

Working with Older (Geriatric) Adults

The average life expectancy in 2015 in the United States is somewhere around the age of 79. According to the U.S. Census, an estimated 43 million Americans today are above the age of 65 and that number is expected to almost double to 83.7 million by the year 2050. Currently, 50 percent of the patients who are seen seeking health care services are senior adults.

Examination and Screening of the Geriatric Patient

When initially screening the geriatric patient, some special considerations might need to be addressed. Physical limitations need to be considered along with communication. As with the pediatric patient, communication may involve caregivers in addition to the patient.

Age can be deceiving. Just because a person is over a certain age does not mean that the individual will have a hearing or visual impairment or will be in failing health. Seniors want to be respected and included in health care decisions. They do not want to be patronized or treated as though they are children. They expect quality health care and want to know that the professionals caring for them are knowledgeable, respectful, and considerate.

Now more than ever, those working in health care must have an understanding of how to better serve their senior patients.

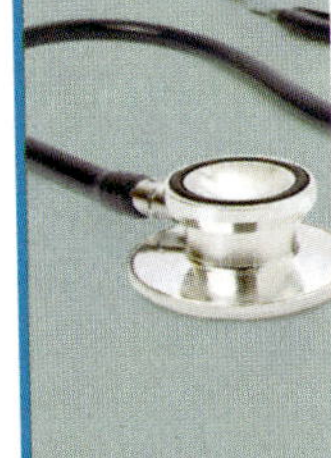

Field Smarts

Allow the older adult ample time for new paperwork or any reading of health information. Make sure there is adequate lighting. You may need to place the patient in a quiet exam room or education room rather than the reception area. It may be difficult for the older adult to perform any task while trying to ignore other sensory distractions (see Figure 6-10).

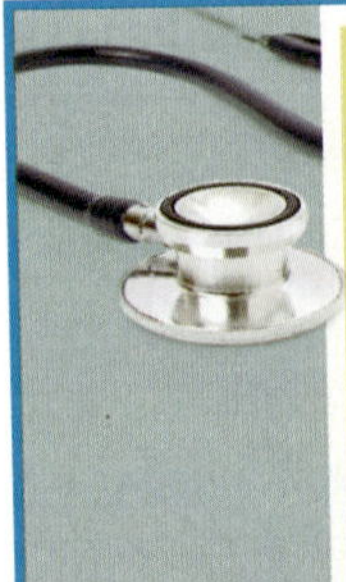

Field Smarts

It is important to remember that aging is not synonymous with disease or illness. With advancements in new treatment methods for chronic as well as acute illnesses, people are living longer and having a better quality of life.

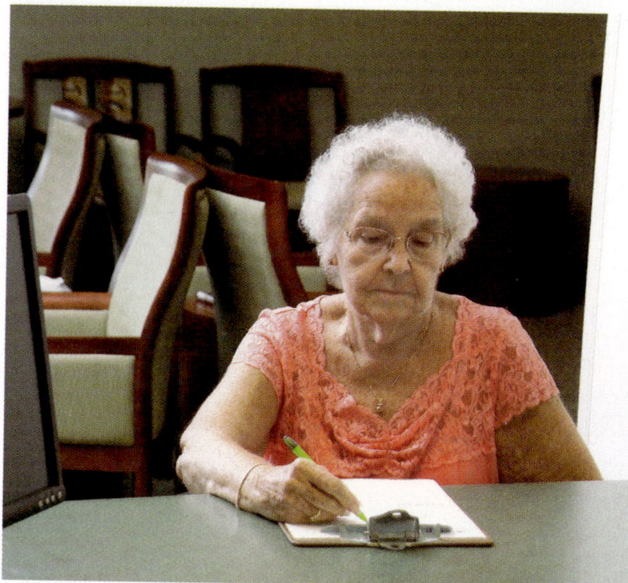

Figure 6-10 ■ The patient is much more at ease in quiet surroundings where she can concentrate.

What Seniors Are Thinking

This chapter focuses on cultural and communication issues that affect the senior patient. Although cognitive functioning and development may diminish to varying degrees in older adults, some limited areas of cognition and sense appear to heighten with age. Aesthetic senses and appreciation of nature tend to increase as we age. Creativity may be rediscovered and wisdom certainly surfaces and becomes apparent. As health care workers interact with the senior patient, these changes in life, either positive or negative, must be considered and incorporated into the screening, assessment, and provision of care.

Regardless of the patient's health status, some philosophies or thought patterns are relatively common among persons over the age of 65. Again, not all seniors will feel the same, but as a culture, there may be some similarities. Knowing these commonalities will help the medical assistant use communication techniques that are pleasing to the patient and avoid communication anomalies that may cause stress. The following list depicts some of those views:

- Most seniors prefer to be addressed as Mr. or Mrs. ________________, but always ask patients how they would like to be addressed for future encounters.
- Professional appearance of the medical staff is important to many seniors. They will quite often perform a head-to-toe appearance inventory, checking hair, uniform, nails, and shoes for cleanliness. They are often distressed by body piercings and tattoos in "unusual" places and may even request that someone else draw their blood or give their injection in such cases.
- Professional behavior is paramount in the eyes of most seniors. They may become quite disturbed when they observe the medical assistant talking and joking with coworkers instead of appearing busy with work. They appreciate compliments and nice gestures; however, it is unprofessional to call a patient hon, honey, sweetie, pops, or by any other name that is not his or her given name. Seniors usually detest being spoken down to or being patronized.
- Most seniors have a playful side and enjoy a bit of humor from time to time, but remember there is a time and place for everything.

Physical Aspects of Working with Senior Patients

As the body ages, the muscles and skin become much more sensitive. The medical assistant must be careful when assisting senior patients onto tables or into chairs. Assisting a senior patient onto an examination table can be quite traumatic for both the patient and medical assistant (Figure 6-11). The patient may say things like

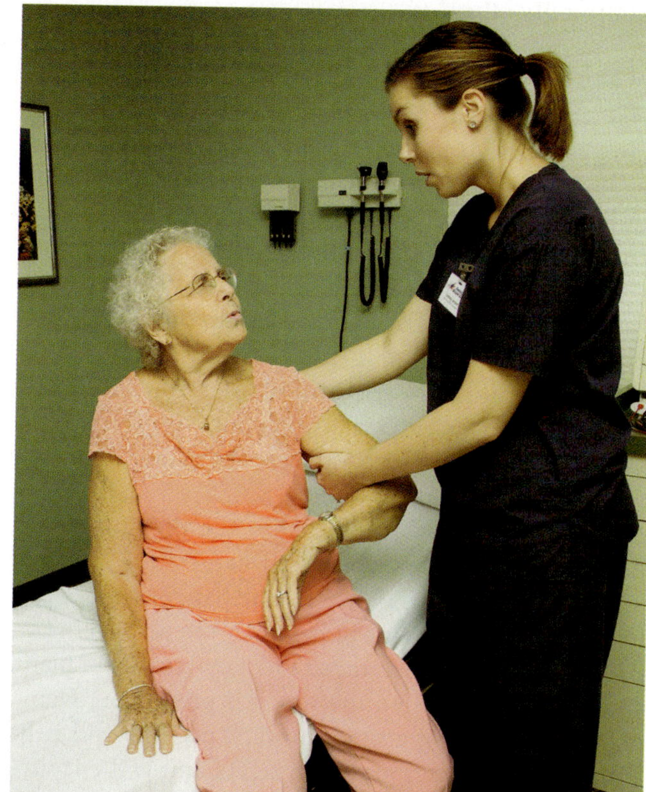

Figure 6-11 ■ Minute amounts of pressure can be uncomfortable or painful to senior patients.

"You are so rough" or "You are not very gentle." The patient's skin is sensitive and even though you don't feel like you are exerting a great deal of pressure, you may be exerting more force than you realize. Ask the patient to tell you if you do anything to make him or her feel uncomfortable or cause pain. Check your thermostats on a regular basis and make certain that they are at a comfortable setting for the patient. Give the patient a drape or a blanket that can be placed over the lap until the provider examines the patient. It is appropriate to consider whether or not a senior patient should be left alone in the exam room seated on the exam table. Use your best professional judgment. Always treat patients the way that you would want others to treat your own family members.

The **frail senior** patient is defined as one who cannot complete three or more **activities of daily living (ADLs)** independently. These include bathing, eating, dressing, walking, and using the restroom. As the number of senior patients increase, the care of the frail patient needs to be considered. Often caregivers and family members are now involved in the office visits. This may include the spouse or adult children. Observe the relationships shown in Figure 6-12. Home health nurses might be incorporated and nursing homes may be transporting patients for medical appointments. Caring for the frail senior patient is a community effort.

The Mental Outlook of Senior Patients

Many seniors may suffer from loneliness and depression, especially seniors who are widows or widowers. Their loneliness may be due to a lack of interaction and communication with family members and friends. To these seniors, going to the doctor may be more of a social event than a health assessment. Seniors often view the office staff as extended family and unknowingly monopolize staff members' time. The medical assistant should be respectful and listen whenever time permits. The health care worker may gently pat the patient on the shoulder or squeeze the patient's hand to demonstrate a caring attitude.

Medical assistants should alert the provider when they observe signs of dementia, depression, or signs of neglect. Often it is easier for the patient to open up to the medical assistant rather than the provider. The patient should be encouraged to follow treatment plans and to take medication the way it is prescribed. Demonstrating a caring attitude toward patients will help patients feel better about themselves and will encourage compliance on their part.

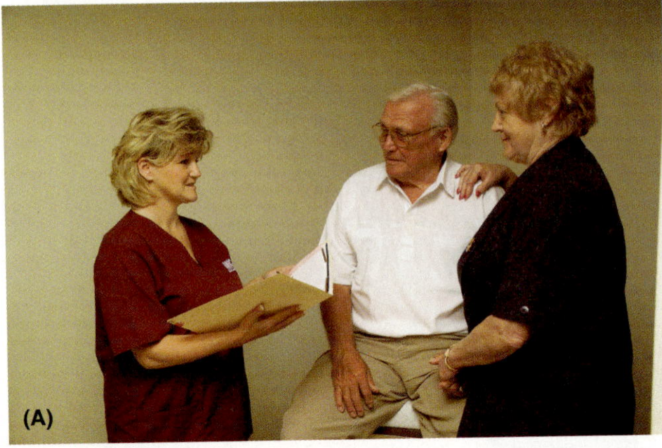

(A)

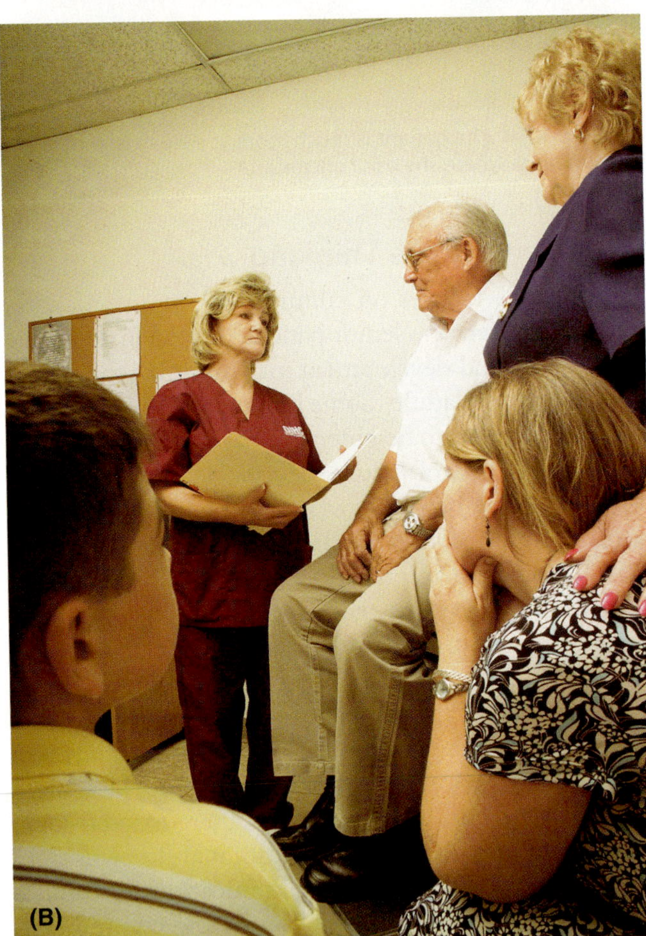

(B)

Figure 6-12 ■ (a) The medical assistant speaks with the patient and his spouse. (b) Often other family members such as adult children are involved in a senior's care.

Tips for Improving Care for Senior Patients

Caring for seniors may present some challenges, but overall it is quite rewarding. The best thing to do for senior patients is to show them that they are valued not just as patients but as individuals. The following is a list of tips that can improve communications with senior patients:

- Address them using their last name (e.g., Mrs. Adams). Ask them what they prefer to be called for the remainder of the visit and for future encounters.
- If the patient is hearing impaired, give the patient time to adjust the hearing aid and sit on the side of the patient in which the patient's ear has the best hearing.
- Take a few moments to learn about the patient's personal life before the interview begins. If you know about a recent event that occurred between the last visit and the current visit, such as a wedding or a birthday, inquire about it.
- Offer assistance with the removal and putting on of clothing.
- Ask the patient about the temperature of the room. If you can't adjust the thermostat, give the patient a warm blanket or sheet to cover up with.
- Warm up anything that will touch the patient's skin, such as your stethoscope, speculums, or other items.
- Give patients an opportunity to participate in their health care by saying things like, "Do you have a preference as to which arm I use?"
- Follow through when you say that you are going to do something for the patient.
- When distributing reading materials, make certain that the patient has plenty of light to assist with vision.
- End the encounter with a little therapeutic touching. Many seniors appreciate the gesture and affection. Try rubbing the patient's shoulder, patting the patient's hand, or extending a little hug at the end of the visit.
- Offer to assist the patient to the reception room or car if the patient is struggling.

Caring for Patients with Dementia

Dementia is a deterioration of intellectual functioning that affects the patient's memory and ability to concentrate. The patient's ability to react and judge becomes severely impaired, and the patient may suffer from personality changes as a result of the disease. Dementia usually progresses with time, and may force the caregiver to place the patient into an extended care facility.

Alzheimer's and Dementia

A frightening diagnosis for patients and their families is when they are told they have Alzheimer's disease. Although this is the most common form of dementia, there is no known cure to date. In the past, it was believed that only younger adults with recall difficulties had this dreaded disease. The older patients were only senile. This is no longer the acceptable description.

Alzheimer's disease occurs when certain areas of the brain that control thinking, communication, and behavior deteriorate. Some of the deterioration may be caused by a decrease of the neurotransmitter acetylcholine. Correct levels of this neurotransmitter are needed for the nerve cells in the brain to work properly and a decrease creates difficulty with memory, decision making, and daily living. As the disease progresses, the level of independence diminishes, requiring increased care by family members and facilities specializing in the treatment of Alzheimer's patients.

It is estimated that 5.2 million Americans of all ages have Alzheimer's disease in 2014. One in nine people aged 65 and older have Alzheimer's disease based on the 2010 census. Estimates from the Aging, Demographics, and Memory Study (ADAMS) indicate that 13.9 percent of people aged 71 and older in the United States have dementia. Tips for working with dementia patients include the following:

- Be empathetic toward both the patient and the caregiver. Caregivers often become ill themselves from the physical and emotional strain of caring for the patient. After addressing the patient's needs, address the needs of the caregiver preferably in an area away from the patient.

EHR Application

Many EHR programs have a patient education section that stores patient handouts. These fact sheets may be printed off for the patient at the point of care or may be sent electronically via a patient portal to the patient. Many older adults have computers and access to the Internet. Most EHRs have a field for entering the patient's email address within the software to better communicate with patients. Patient portals are often the preferred method of electronic communications due to HIPAA privacy concerns with email. You will be able to send patient handouts, lab test results, appointment reminders, and even some holiday messages—all with a click of a button.

- Simplify instructions. Patients with dementia often experience difficulties with the smallest of tasks. Keeping the instructions simple will help to prevent the patient from becoming anxious. Break down procedures into step-by-step directions. For example, "Mr. Jones, I need to weigh you today so the first thing that I need you to do is to remove your shoes.... Great.... Now I need you to follow me to the scale.... Okay Mr. Jones, I need you to step up onto the scale."
- Ask the patient's caregiver for assistance when the communication process appears to be in a state of decline.
- Avoid laughing at comments that appear nonsensical or irrational. Remember that the patient's condition is a significant stress already and laughter may provoke the patient to become angry or feel hurt or unimportant.
- Above all, practice patience! Because dementia patients take more time, ask your coworkers to watch your rooms ahead of time so that you can give the patient and caregiver your full attention.

In advanced cases of dementia, the patient may drift in and out of various time periods or may even think that they are somewhere other than the provider's office. They may not recognize you even though you have been caring for them for several years or they may think that you are someone else such as a friend or a relative. Try to gently correct the patient, but if the patient appears to become more agitated as a result of the correction, you may want to look to the caregiver for cues. Some of the most recent research states that in some cases, it is better to go along with the patient, rather than to force the patient into reality.

CRITICAL THINKING CHALLENGE

An 83-year-old male patient with dementia appears confused by instructions that you give him for urine collection. His caregiver, his daughter, also tries to explain the procedure, but the patient just doesn't understand. The daughter volunteers to help her father, but he quickly refuses the daughter's assistance.

1. **What are some things that you can do to help the patient with the instructions?**
2. **What might be an alternative if the patient refuses or just never comprehends the instructions?**

Public Health Statutes: Abuse, Neglect, and Exploitation

As our society continues to increase in age, many challenges develop that need to be addressed. Many senior patients are often alone and unable to care for themselves. Others receive care from family and friends, often creating additional stress on the caregiver.

As more senior patients want to stay in a home environment, more families are called upon to provide the needed care. This can prove to be a rewarding experience for all involved. It draws generations together again, and grandparents are becoming part of the nuclear family. Conversely, it also presents some challenges for families: financially, physically, emotionally, and psychologically. New skills must be learned by family members as many seniors need assistance with medical treatments. Relationships need to be developed that may not have existed in the past. For example, helping a parent bathe and use the restroom requires a different level of interaction than in the past. Roles are often reversed. Family members must also have time and support to provide care for themselves in order to maintain their own individual quality of life. It is also important to help the patient retain independence to the highest degree possible. All of this can be fulfilling, yet exhausting.

As a medical assistant, you may come in contact with forms of abuse, neglect, and exploitation. The Centers for Disease Control and Prevention (CDC) defines **elder abuse** as any abuse and neglect of persons aged 60 and older by a caregiver or another person in a relationship involving an expectation of trust. At times, this relationship fails, either at home or in a facility. This may create a dangerous or abusive situation, referred to as **senior abuse**. Refer to Table 6-4 to help identify signs of abuse.

Physical abuse is defined as the use of physical force that may result in bodily injury, physical pain, or impairment. Physical punishments of any kind are examples of physical abuse. Forms of abuse can include physical abuse, sexual abuse, psychological or emotional abuse, neglect, abandonment, and financial abuse or exploitation (CDC, 2014). **Neglect** is further defined as the failure or refusal of a caregiver or other responsible person to provide for an elder's basic physical, emotional, or social needs, or failure to protect them from harm. Examples include not providing adequate nutrition, hygiene, clothing, shelter, or access to necessary health care; or failure

Table 6-4 Signs of Senior Abuse

Type of Abuse	Definition	Signs and Symptoms
Physical abuse (Figure 6-13)	Hitting, pushing, scratching, slapping, kicking, burning, pinching, restraining, force feeding, drugging	Bruising, black eyes, welts, rope marks, cuts, fractures, open wounds, dislocations, broken glasses, unprescribed medications found in the blood after testing, change in behavior
Sexual abuse	Nonconsensual touching, rape, sodomy, sexual photography	Bruises at genitals or breasts, venereal disease, genital infections, vaginal bleeding, anal bleeding, torn or bloody underwear
Emotional abuse	Verbal assaults, threats, intimidation, humiliation, insults, isolating socially	Agitated, withdrawn, and rocking behavior
Neglect (Figure 6-14), or patient not given his prescription medications	Refusing duties or responsibilities to the patient Not providing food, water, clothing, payments for care, hygiene	Malnutrition, dehydration, unsanitary conditions, lice, fleas, dirty clothing, fecal smell
Abandonment	Deserting the patient	Patient left alone at home or in a facility
Exploitation	Forging checks, stealing possessions, coercion into signing papers	Forged signatures on medical statements and checks, valuables missing, funds withdrawn from financial institution
Self-neglect	The patient behaves in a manner that threatens the patient's health and safety	Malnutrition, dehydration, not taking medications as prescribed, lack of clothing, fecal smell, lack of medical aids, such as glasses, and dentures.

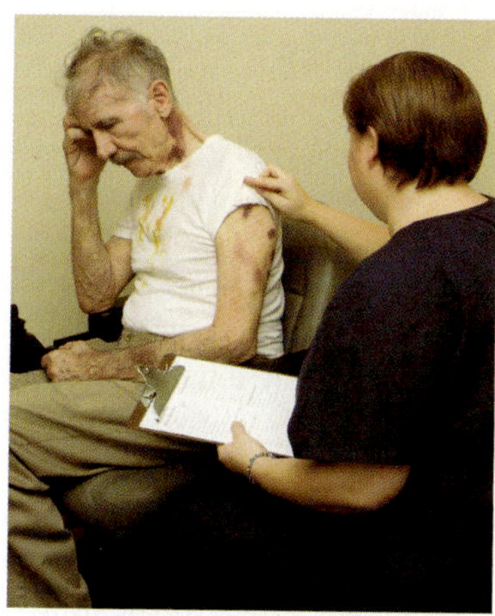

Figure 6-13 ■ The medical assistant notices bruises on the patient's arm.

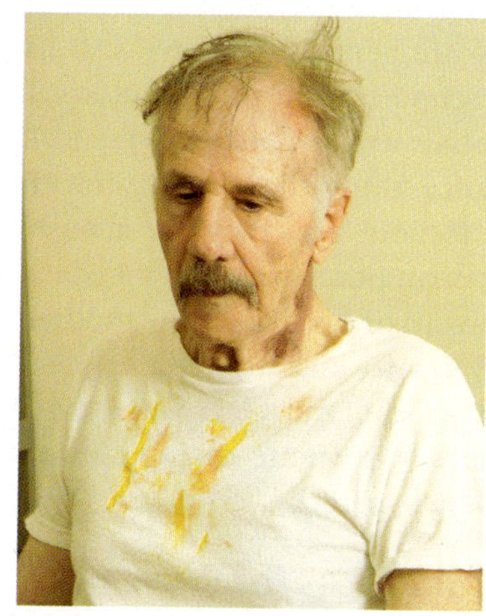

Figure 6-14 ■ The patient appears to be disheveled with dirty hair and stained clothing, which may be signs of neglect.

CRITICAL THINKING CHALLENGE

While you are helping a senior male patient get ready for the provider's exam, he tells you that he has not been feeling very well because he hasn't been eating very much lately. He says his medications are so expensive that there is no money left for food. He can't drive anymore, so he can't even visit his local food pantry.

1. What assistance can you offer this patient?
2. What other options may be available to him?

to prevent exposure to unsafe activities and environments. Financial abuse or **exploitation** is defined as the unauthorized or improper use of the resources of an elder for monetary or personal benefit, profit, or gain. Examples include forgery, misuse, or theft of money or possessions; use of coercion or deception to surrender finances or property; or improper use of guardianship or power of attorney (CDC, 2014).

Working with Pediatric Patients

Working with pediatric patients can be entertaining, but may also present unique challenges (Figure 6-15). Pediatric offices are usually fast-paced, which means that the office sees a high volume of patients in a short amount of time.

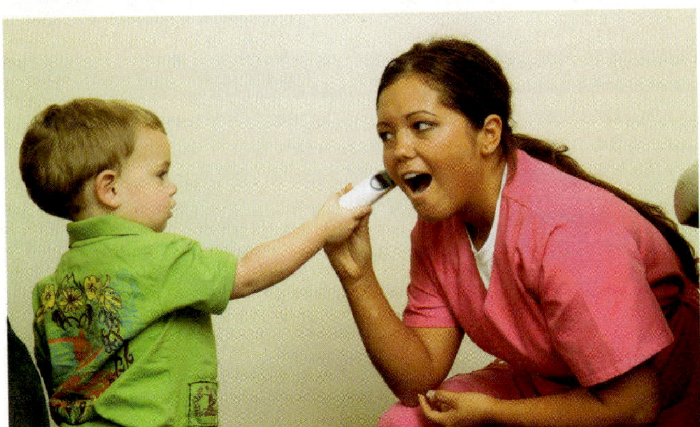

Figure 6-15 ■ The medical assistant works to gain the child's acceptance by stooping down to his level and using lots of expressions.

Children are usually fun to observe and to carry on a conversation with but generally they have no concept of a schedule. Therefore, the medical assistant must learn how to gain the child's cooperation early during the visit to avoid running behind schedule.

Infants are usually easy to prepare for examinations because they are generally passive and used to being handled. Preschoolers and young children, on the other hand, are not always as cooperative and may demonstrate resistance along the way. By the time children reach the preschool age, they are accustomed to the usual events of an office visit and may be anxious. The child may scream or hold on to the mother's leg, and in rare cases, even slap, kick, or bite the medical assistant. The medical assistant must learn effective communication techniques to promote cooperation with pediatric patients and their parents.

General Guidelines for Working with Younger Children

This chapter provides communication guidelines for working with pediatric patients. Medical assistants working in pediatric offices must be patient and should genuinely enjoy working with children. Children are quite intuitive and can discern when adults do not care for them. They may be fearful and become frightened by nonthreatening procedures such as being weighed or having their blood pressure measured. Children may also be playful and want to play with the equipment that is being used such as the stethoscope. They may prefer to dance and sing when their vision is tested instead of reading the symbols on the eye chart. The following list provides tips on how to effectively communicate with young children:

- Involve the child in the discussion.
- Use terms that the child understands.

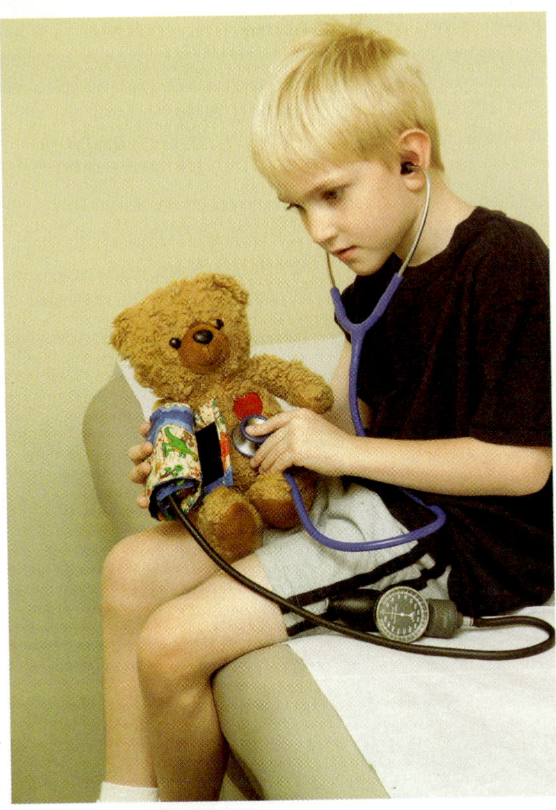

Figure 6-16 ■ Allowing a child to investigate the equipment before you use it is a good way to gain cooperation from the child.

- Start the discussion out by asking the child about nonhealth-related items such as school, pets, or siblings. This will help the child to gain trust in you.
- Gently and in a nonthreatening manner, explain to the child what you are going to do and why you are going to do it. Ask the child to assist you whenever possible. Use phrases such as the following: "Adam, I am going to take your blood pressure to make certain that your heart is working okay. Before I do, can you point to where the heart is located on this little bear? Would you like to listen to the bear's heart before we get started?" (Figure 6-16).
- End every visit with some kind of prize such as stickers, a cartoon adhesive bandage, or other items that promote a positive attitude.

Performing Invasive Procedures on a Young Child

The following is a list of tips for performing invasive procedures on pediatric patients:

- Never lie to a child. Be honest and upfront. Explain what you are going to do, such as "Hello Johnny! I need to give you some medicine in your leg today so you will start feeling better."

- To minimize the child's anxiety, keep the needle out of the child's view.
- Children may feel more secure holding on to their mom or dad or sitting on their parent's lap during invasive procedures; however, do not involve parents who appear to be apprehensive.
- Provide something for the child to squeeze during the procedure such as a little stuffed animal or large sponge ball. It is best if the toy is something that he can take with him so that he doesn't have to give it up at the end of the procedure. Make certain the toy is safe for the child's age range.
- Work quickly. The longer the procedure takes, the more traumatic it is for the child.
- Praise the child and offer a prize for good behavior, such as, "Johnny, you did so good today that I am going to let you choose something special from the toy chest."

Performing Noninvasive Tests on a Young Child

Start out by explaining the procedure to the child. Make certain that the child has a good grasp of the procedure by doing some practice testing first. Once you are certain that the child understands the procedure, you may begin the testing.

Working with Physically Disabled Patients

A **physical disability** refers to an impairment that restricts or prevents normal functioning of a particular limb or group of limbs. The condition may be temporary or it may be permanent. The medical assistant may need to make special accommodations for these types of patients.

If the disability involves the upper extremities, the medical assistant may need to offer the patient assistance with writing, disrobing, and dressing. If the disability involves the lower limbs, the patient may be using some type of assisted device such as a cane, walker, or crutches. If the disability involves both lower limbs, the patient may need the assistance of a wheelchair.

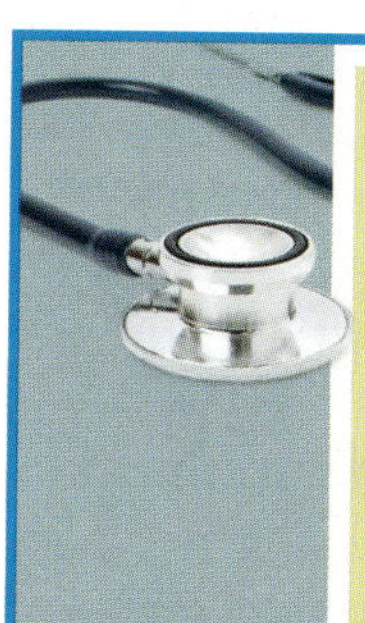

Field Smarts

Some offices use distraction techniques while performing invasive procedures. You may give the child a noisemaker to blow until the procedure is over. Or the child can count as loud as she can from 1 to 10.

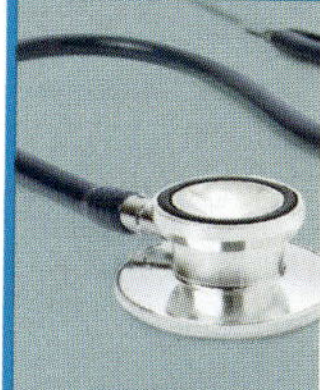

Field Smarts

Before performing visual acuity testing on a young child, start by having the child stand close to the chart. Ask the child to identify the shapes, or explain which way the legs are positioned on the "Big E Chart." This will establish that the patient can identify the objects correctly and will stimulate more involvement from the child once the testing begins.

Hygiene Issues and the Physically Disabled Patient

Physical disabilities that involve casting may impair the patient's ability to properly shower or bathe. If the patient's hand or arm is fractured, not only can she not submerge her cast in water, but she does not have the mechanical ability to properly wash herself, especially if the affected limb involves her dominant hand. If the lower limbs are involved, it may be difficult for the patient to get into a tub or to go the store to buy soap products for cleansing purposes.

The patient may feel embarrassed when she comes to the office and even apologize at the beginning of the appointment for her "poor hygiene." The medical assistant must never make the patient feel uncomfortable by making faces or comments that are derogatory toward the patient. Nor should the medical assistant make derogatory comments about a patient's hygiene to other coworkers. Those working in health care should be kind and compassionate and put themselves in the place of their patients.

General Guidelines for Working with Physically Disabled Patients

It is important to know that not everyone with a physical disability will need assistance. Many disabled patients, especially those with permanent disabilities, are independent and are perfectly capable of getting around. Others, however, will welcome assistance. Some basic rules for working with physically disabled patients are the following:

- Prepare the room ahead of time. Gather supplies or equipment that will assist in the patient's overall comfort.
- Always offer assistance, but do not insist on providing assistance.
- Question the patient about home needs. Some patients may not know that there are special devices that can assist them with daily tasks such as bathing, eating, and opening cabinet doors.
- Always reflect a caring attitude.

Assisting Patients in Wheelchairs

The following are guidelines for working with patients in wheelchairs:

- Prepare the examination room for the wheelchair and clear anything in the path between the reception room and examination room that could impair the patient's ability to maneuver the wheelchair around it.
- Always offer to wheel the patient from the reception room to the examination room. This also provides the patient or caregiver rest from operating the wheelchair.
- Be careful not to run the wheelchair into walls or doors.
- When the patient is unable to walk, check with the provider to see if the patient can remain in the wheelchair for the examination. Many procedures can be performed directly from the wheelchair.
- When necessary, offer the patient assistance with clothing removal and re-dressing.
- Offer to wheel the chair out to the patient's vehicle. This will assist the caregiver and demonstrate a caring attitude to the patient and patient's family.

Working with Patients Who Have Intellectual Disabilities

The Substance Abuse and Mental Health Services Administration (SAMHSA), a division of the HHS, defines **mental health** as "how people look at themselves, their lives, and the other people in their lives; evaluate their challenges and problems; and explore choices." **Mental illness** is a disorder that disrupts the person's ability to think, feel, and relate to others. Examples of mental illness include the following:

- Major depression
- Bipolar disease
- Certain anxiety disorders (panic disorders, obsessive compulsive disorder, and posttraumatic stress disorders)
- Schizophrenia

Most mental illnesses are believed to be organic in nature caused by neurochemical imbalances. These conditions are usually treated with psychotherapy and psychiatric medications. Some experts believe that lifestyle changes in combination with social and environmental support can also assist those suffering from various types of mental illness.

The term **mental impairment** refers to a condition or illness that impairs the mind's ability to process information in a "normal" fashion. Impairment may be brought on by a mental illness, brain damage, or dementia.

The National Institute of Mental Health (NIMH) estimates that one in four adults suffer from a diagnosable mental disorder in a given year. The degree or type of impairment will determine the amount of extra intervention that is necessary to assist these patients.

Guidelines for Working with Patients with Mental Disorders or Impairments

The first step toward working with patients who suffer from mental disorders or impairments is to drop any preconceived notions that are negative. People who suffer from mental impairment come from all walks of life and quite often are very aware. As stated earlier, many of these disorders are due to an imbalance of various neurochemicals. Like any other disease, sometimes the patient responds well to treatment; however, in other cases, the provider may have to experiment with various psychotropic medications combined with various forms of psychotherapy before discovering the right treatment. Other tips for working with mentally impaired patients include the following:

- Demonstrate compassion and empathy toward the patient.
- Understand that each condition has its own array of symptoms, emotional struggles, and communication challenges.
- Avoid talking down to the patient.
- Be respectful and treat the patient with the same level of dignity as other patients.
- Direct your questions toward the patient whenever possible.
- Never laugh or snicker at a comment that appears to be nonsensical or irrational.

Guidelines for Working with Patients Who Are Mentally Challenged

Some patients with mental impairments may also be **mentally challenged**. When a patient is diagnosed as being mentally challenged, it means that the brain functions at a subnormal intellectual level. Patients who are mentally retarded are sometimes referred to as mentally challenged or mentally deficient. The causes of mental retardation include congenital defects, brain injuries, and disease. Patients with such impairments may find it difficult to think in a clear, organized manner and may struggle with instructions that are abstract or that constitute multiple directions. Guidelines for working with mentally challenged patients include the following:

- Question caregivers to learn more about the patient's level of understanding. Caregivers understand the patient and will be able to interpret various cues that might normally go unnoticed.
- Use language that can be easily understood by the patient.
- Give simple instructions that only involve one direction at a time.
- Realize that directions may need to be given several times.
- Do not become agitated if the patient refuses to follow instructions. Instead, give the patient a break before trying the procedure again.

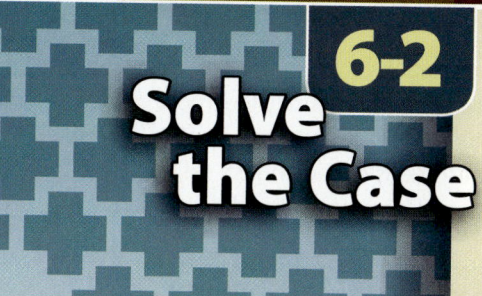

Dr. Brockton has now completed his exam of Mrs. Adams. Dr. Brockton has ordered a "Urinalysis dipstick panel in urine by automated test strip" and "Urinalysis microscopic panel [#volume] in urine by automated count," has written a prescription for "Bactrim DS Oral Tablet 800-160MG," and requested a follow-up visit in one week with Mrs. Adams. Since Mrs. Adams is visually impaired, what instructions and steps should you follow to complete the orders as requested by Dr. Brockton?

PROCEDURE 6-1

Effectively Communicate with Patients from Different Cultures

Objective:

To use effective communication techniques when working with patients from other cultures.

Equipment/Supplies:

- Patient's chart/EHR
- Pen

PROCEDURAL STEPS	DETAILS AND/OR RATIONALE
1. Prepare the interview area. The interview area should be private, comfortable, and free of distractions. The furniture should be set up to accommodate the patient and anyone who may be with the patient, including an interpreter. The medical assistant's chair should be set up at least 4 to 12 feet directly across from the patient and interpreter if present.	Properly preparing the room will make the patient feel more comfortable and more receptive to answering the questions.

continues

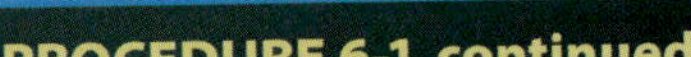

PROCEDURE 6-1 continued

PROCEDURAL STEPS	DETAILS AND/OR RATIONALE
2. Identify yourself, list your title, and identify the patient. If you are uncertain how to properly pronounce the patient's name, ask the patient for the proper pronunciation. Write the phonetic spelling somewhere in the chart.	Foreign names are quite often difficult for English speakers to pronounce. Asking the patient for clarification communicates respect toward the patient.
3. If you are not the same gender as the patient, ask the patient if she would prefer to have a medical assistant of the same gender, ***demonstrating respect for individual diversity***.	This will help the patient and possibly the patient's spouse to feel more comfortable. Patients from certain cultures are especially concerned about this.
4. Ask the patient to introduce any family members who are present.	An introduction assists in building trust with family members and acknowledges their role in the patient's health care.
5. Ask the patient a little bit about her family or career.	This type of conversation can help the family feel more at ease and gives the medical assistant an opportunity to check the patient's English skills or the English skills of the family member who will be performing the interpreting.
6. If the patient has limited English proficiency and a professional interpreter is not present, give the patient written materials that explain the patient's right to a professional interpreter in his or her native language.	Patients may not know that interpreting is available or may be fearful about using an interpreter. They may not want to hurt a loved one's feelings or may be fearful about admitting that they do not want the family member present.
7. If the patient states that a family member will be performing the interpreting, explain to the family member the importance of accurate interpreting. If an interpreter is required, contact the agency (or qualified interpreter). Wait until the interpreter is available before proceeding with questioning.	Making the suggestion to have a professional interpreter tactfully allows the patient to avoid using a family member as the interpreter.
8. Ask the patient to explain the goals for today's visit.	Setting goals sets the tone for the visit. It provides an agenda and allows the patient to express personal goals as well.
9. Speak clearly and avoid using any slang or medical jargon. Talk directly to the patient even if an interpreter is present. Avoid using many gestures as some common gestures may be considered offensive in some cultures.	Using medical terms or slang could cause the interpreter to become confused. Use common everyday words whenever possible.
10. Have the patient repeat any instructions to ensure that the patient understands the information.	Comprehension promotes compliance on the patient's part.

continues

PROCEDURE 6-1 continued

PROCEDURAL STEPS	DETAILS AND/OR RATIONALE
11. Direct and demonstrate which clothes need to be removed and explain why. Provide the patient with items such as gowns, sheets, or drapes to help ensure modesty.	Modesty is very important to most patients, but in particular to people from specific cultures. The more you can assist in protecting the patient's modesty, the more cooperative the patient will be.
12. Thank the patient and family members for their cooperation and let them know that the provider will be in shortly.	If the provider is running behind, let the patient know. Keep the patient informed if there are further delays and provide an expected wait time, if possible.
13. Document the visit and record and explain any paperwork that was given to the patient, as well as if an interpreter was present.	Documenting that an interpreter was present illustrates that the office did everything possible to promote effective communication.

DOCUMENTATION EXAMPLE:

03-12-XX 1300	Pt. here for immigration physical today. Arabic Translator Amani Barakat was present and translated during the interview process. Pt. has no current physical concerns. See attached medical history form. Theresa Pugh, CMA (AAMA)--

PROCEDURE 6-2

Effectively Communicate with Sight Impaired or Visually Impaired Patients

Objective:

To assist a patient that is visually impaired by using effective communication techniques.

Equipment/Supplies:

- Patient's chart/EHR
- Pen

PROCEDURAL STEPS	DETAILS AND/OR RATIONALE
1. Prepare the patient's room by clearing anything that could cause the patient to trip or fall. Also prepare the walkway from the reception room to the examination room to make certain that it is free of any obstacles.	This is for safety purposes.
2. When you go into the reception room, gently call out the patient's name and tell her that you are ready to assist her back to the room. ***Demonstrating the principles of self-boundaries***, do not shake the patient's hand unless the patient extends her hand first.	You do not want to startle the patient. A gentle hello, followed by the patient's name will let the patient know that you are nearby.

continues

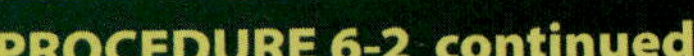

PROCEDURE 6-2 continued

PROCEDURAL STEPS	DETAILS AND/OR RATIONALE
3. Identify yourself and state your title.	This allows the patient to place a name with the voice and tells the patient that you have authority to take them back to the room.
4. If the patient has a guide dog, do not touch or talk to the guide dog while the harness is on. Have the patient and the dog follow you back to the room.	Talking to the dog or touching the dog can distract the dog, making it difficult for the owner to get the dog to perform its duties. ***Incorporate critical thinking skills when performing patient care.***
5. If the patient does not have a guide dog, ask the patient if she would like to have sighted guide assistance.	Sighted guide assistance is a nice gesture to show the patient that you would like to help them. Do not insist on sighted guide assistance.
6. If the patient wants sighted guide assistance, ask the patient which side she prefers to be assisted on.	Some patients feel more comfortable being assisted on one side or the other.
7. Position yourself on the side that the patient indicates and allow the patient to grasp your arm, usually just above the elbow (Figure 6-17).	Allowing the patient to grasp your arm prevents you from dragging the patient.
8. Walk with your arm down to the side about a half step in front of the patient toward the inside of the patient.	This makes it easier to feel your body movements and allows the patient to anticipate the next move.
9. Warn the patient about the surroundings and any obstacles, such as a doorway, an elevator, or a staircase.	This gives the patient time to prepare for the change in elevation or width.
10. Approach seating in a forward motion. Describe the type of seating that the patient will be placed in, such as a low sofa, upright chair, or an armchair.	This allows the patient the ability to assess the seating so that she can judge how far down she will need to bend when sitting down.
11. Walk the patient to the front of the chair, allowing her knees to just gently touch the front of the cushion or seat.	This assists the patient in knowing the height of the chair.
12. Place the patient's hand on the arm of the chair and allow the patient to finish seating herself.	Grasping the arm of the chair will assist with security as the patient sits down.
13. Interview the patient in the way that you would any other patient.	
14. Lay out all gowns and drapes beside the patient. Let her know their exact location before leaving. Ask the patient if she needs any assistance getting dressed.	This helps the patient be more at ease with her new surroundings.

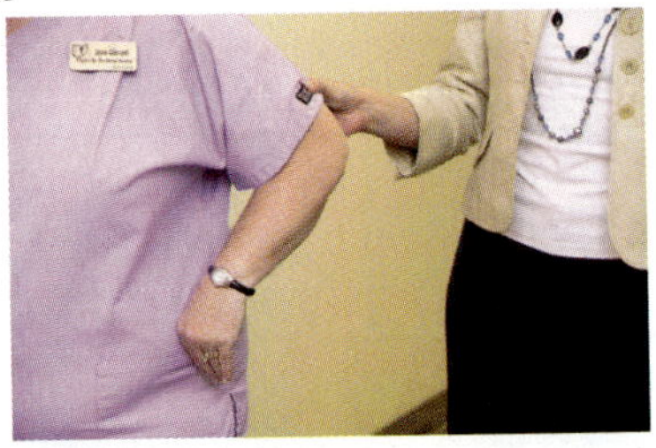

Figure 6-17 ■ When providing sighted guide assistance, allow the patient to grasp your arm.

continues

PROCEDURE 6-2 continued

PROCEDURAL STEPS	DETAILS AND/OR RATIONALE
15. When performing procedures, alert the patient to every step before you perform it, ***showing awareness of the patient's concerns related to the procedure being performed***.	This ensures that she is not startled when you touch her.
16. Notify the patient that you are leaving and tell the patient that the provider will knock before entering.	This lets the patient know that she will be temporarily alone.

PROCEDURE 6-3

Effectively Communicate with Hearing Impaired or Deaf Patients When an Interpreter Is Present

Objective:

To assist a patient who is hearing impaired or deaf by using effective communication techniques.

Equipment/Supplies:

- Patient's chart/EHR
- Pen

PROCEDURAL STEPS	DETAILS AND/OR RATIONALE
1. Set the chairs up in a triangular pattern. The patient's chair should be centered and directly across from both the medical assistant and interpreter.	***Incorporate critical thinking skills when performing patient care***. The triangular pattern will allow the patient to look at both the interpreter and the medical assistant without turning her head.
2. Ask the interpreter to introduce herself.	
3. Look directly at the patient during the communication encounter, not at the interpreter. Keep in mind, however, that the patient will be focusing on the interpreter.	Many deaf patients can also do minimal lip-reading. It also shows the patient that she is your focus, not the interpreter.
4. Talk at a normal rate of speed.	Interpreters and speech readers are trained to interpret at a normal conversation rate.
5. Ask the patient to repeat any instructions.	This ensures effective communication and comprehension on the part of the patient.
6. Give the patient written instructions to take home.	This is a nice reference item that the patient can refer to later.
7. Thank both the patient and interpreter for their participation. If the patient indicates that she really liked this interpreter, make a note of it in the patient's chart.	It is important to use interpreters that patients trust and understand.
8. Document the encounter and state that the interpreter was present.	Documenting that an interpreter was present illustrates that the office did everything possible to promote effective communication.

DOCUMENTATION EXAMPLE:

09-15-XX 1400	Pt. here to discuss lab results from the last visit. Cheryl Taylor, interpreter from Medical Interpreting, Inc., was present for today's visit. Pt. still c/o of joint pain and fatigue. No changes in medications. Michael Allen, CMA (AAMA)---

PROCEDURE 6-4

Effectively Communicate with a Hearing Impaired or Deaf Patient Who Speech Reads

Objective:

To use effective communication techniques for patients who are hearing impaired and who can speech read.

Equipment/Supplies:

- Patient's chart/EHR
- Pen

PROCEDURAL STEPS	DETAILS AND/OR RATIONALE
1. Prepare the interview area. Choose a quiet room that is well lit and glare free. Lighting should point toward your face.	***Incorporate critical thinking skills when performing patient care.*** Choosing a room that is well lit and glare free will assist the patient in viewing your lips and facial cues.
2. Position yourself directly across from the patient at the same level as the patient.	This will provide a good angle for the patient to speech read. Remember that the patient will be viewing your throat, tongue, and cheeks and will also be looking at your expressions.
3. Speak at a normal rate of speed. Do not turn your head away when speaking to the patient.	People who speech read are trained to read speech at a normal talking rate. Speeding up or slowing down or over enunciating your words will distort what is being stated.
4. Use gestures, hand cues, and written materials to assist in the communication process.	These cues and written items will assist with effective communication.
5. When the patient doesn't understand a statement that you have made, try rephrasing it instead of repeating it.	Repeating the same sentence will probably not remedy the problem, so try rephrasing with different words. The patient may be able to read the next phrase more easily than the first phrase.
6. Have the patient communicate back to you any instructions that you have given. This may be through gestures, speaking, or writing.	You need to ascertain that the patient comprehended any instructions that were given.

CHAPTER SUMMARY

- Medical assistants must have a good grasp of laws that assist some of the special needs patients who frequent the medical office. Failure to adhere to these laws can set the office up for possible litigation. Accessibility of doctors' offices, clinics, and other health care providers is essential in providing medical care to people with disabilities.
- The Americans with Disabilities Act (ADA) of 1990 is referred to as civil rights legislation designed to prohibit discrimination against individuals based on disability. The Act (and Amendments Act—ADAAA) defined *disability* as "a physical or mental impairment that substantially limits a major life activity."
- Title VI of the Civil Rights Act requires entities receiving federal assistance from the Department of Health and Human Services (HHS)—including providers who participate in Medicare or Medicaid programs—to provide interpreters for non-English-speaking patients and patients with limited English proficiency (LEP).
- The medical assistant must find ways to effectively communicate with special needs patients in order to provide the patient with the best possible care.
- Diversity is the condition of having or being composed of differing elements, especially the inclusion of different types of people (people of different races or cultures) in a group. The term *cultural diversity* incorporates several variables including ethnicity, race, and religious beliefs.
- Cultural variances will impact the communication process with patients and can provide challenges to the medical assistant.
- You will encounter barriers to the communication process. A barrier is defined as anything that gets in the way of clear communication. Good communication skills and techniques assist in obtaining important information that can be used to properly diagnose and treat the patient.
- Each patient has his or her own array of social, physical, and emotional challenges.
- Medical assistants who learn techniques to accommodate all patients, regardless of their unique set of needs, will earn greater respect from their patients, coworkers, and supervisors.
- It is important to remember that aging is not synonymous with disease or illness. With developments in new treatment methods for chronic as well as acute illnesses, people are living longer and having a better quality of life.
- Other special needs patients include pediatric patients, physically disabled patients, and patients with intellectual disabilities. Being able to adapt to a diverse patient population and their special needs is a key component to your success.

CERTIFICATION REVIEW QUESTIONS

1. Examples of special needs patients include all but which of the following?
   a. Visually impaired patients
   b. Deaf patients
   c. Culturally diverse patients
   d. Patients who work in health care
2. Which of the following acts/laws make it mandatory for offices to provide auxiliary aids or services to ensure "effective communication"?
   a. Title I of the American Disabilities Act
   b. Title III of the American Disabilities Act
   c. HIPAA
   d. The Civil Rights Act
3. When working with patients from other cultures, the medical assistant should:
   a. use lots of gestures to enhance what is being stated.
   b. ask the patient for the correct pronunciation of her name.
   c. insist that the patient remove clothing regardless of the patient's modesty concerns.
   d. ask the patient about her religion to gain a better understanding of her beliefs.

4. Direct eye contact is considered disrespectful among:
   a. Westerners.
   b. Middle Easterners.
   c. Latin Americans.
   d. All of the above
5. Keeping your hands on your hips, slumping, and avoiding eye contact are examples of:
   a. Western culture.
   b. therapeutic touch.
   c. proxemics.
   d. cold gestures.
6. When pediatric patients are to receive an invasive procedure, the medical assistant should do all but which of the following?
   a. Tell them that it probably will not hurt
   b. Be honest and tell them that they may feel some discomfort
   c. Give them something to hold during the procedure like a stuffed animal or ball
   d. Explain the purpose of the procedure
7. Patients with mental impairments should:
   a. be treated with respect and kindness.
   b. be addressed directly during the patient interview.
   c. be assessed to determine their ability to communicate.
   d. All of the above
8. Which of the following is not a prerequisite to be considered a "qualified interpreter" under ADA guidelines?
   a. Must be extremely fluent in the patient's native language and English
   b. Must be properly trained to provide interpretation in a medical facility
   c. Must demonstrate competence in medical interpreting
   d. Must be a U.S. citizen
9. Signal dogs are trained dogs that:
   a. guide visually impaired patients.
   b. alert people who have seizures.
   c. alert people who are deaf.
   d. All of the above
10. The deterioration of intellectual functioning that affects a patient's memory and ability to concentrate is known as:
    a. aging.
    b. dementia.
    c. Alzheimer's disease.
    d. cognitive dysfunction.

STUDY RESOURCES

Resources to Test and Reinforce Your Knowledge:	
Certification Review Questions	Take this end-of-chapter quiz
Workbook	• Complete the activities for Chapter 6 • Perform the procedures for Chapter 6 using the Competency Checklists
Resources to Promote Critical Thinking:	
***Solve the Case* Activities**	• Consider these case studies and discuss your conclusions
MindTap	• Complete Chapter 6 readings and activities

REFERENCES

Alzheimer's Association. (2014). Alzheimer's disease facts and figures. *Alzheimer's & Dementia* 10, Issue 2. Retrieved November 15, 2014, from http://www.alz.org/downloads/facts_figures_2014.pdf

Alzheimer's Foundation of America (n.d.). About Alzheimer's: Statistics. Retrieved November 18, 2014, from http://www.alzfdn.org/AboutAlzheimers/statistics.html

American Foundation for the Blind (May 2006). ADA Checklist: Health Care Facilities and Service Providers. Ensuring Access to Services and Facilities by Patients Who Are Blind, Deaf-Blind, or Visually Impaired. Retrieved November 14, 2014, from http://www.afb.org/info/programs-and-services/public-policy-center/ada-checklist-health-care-facilities-and-service-providers/125

Anonymous (n.d.). The Influence of Heredity and Environment. Retrieved November 14, 2014, from http://www.sparknotes.com/psychology/psych101/intelligence/section3.rhtml

Assistance Dogs (Guide, Signal and Service Dogs) (n.d.). Retrieved November 18, 2014, from http://www.cdss.ca.gov/cdssweb/entres/pdf/ODA/AssistanceDogs.pdf

Blesi, Michelle (2017). *Medical assisting administrative and clinical competencies*, 8th ed. (Clifton Park, NY: Cengage Learning).

Centers for Disease Control and Prevention (2014). Elder Abuse: Definitions. Retrieved August 19, 2014, from http://www.cdc.gov/violenceprevention/elderabuse/definitions.html.

Duckworth, Ken (March 2013). Mental Illness Facts and Numbers. National Alliance on Mental Illness. Retrieved November 15, 2014, from http://www.nami.org/factsheets/mentalillness_factsheet.pdf

Humes, Jones, and Ramirez (March 2011). Overview of Race and Hispanic Origin: 2010. Retrieved November 18, 2014, from http://www.census.gov/prod/cen2010/briefs/c2010br-02.pdf

Limited English Proficiency (LEP) (n.d.). LEP.gov. Retrieved November 14, 2014, from http://www.lep.gov/

Mateo, Julio and Gallardo, Elia (n.d.). Providing health care to limited English proficient (LEP) patients: A manual of promising practices. Retrieved November 14, 2014, from http://www.hhs.gov/ocr/civilrights/resources/specialtopics/lep/providinghealthcare-toleppdf.pdf

National Association of the Deaf (n.d.). Community and Culture-Frequently Asked Questions. Retrieved November 18, 2014, from http://nad.org/issues/american-sign-language/community-and-culture-faq

National Association of the Deaf (n.d.). Telephone and relay services. Retrieved November 14, 2014, from http://nad.org/issues/technology/telephone-and-relay-services

U.S. Department of Justice (July 2010). Access to medical care for individuals with mobility disabilities. Retrieved November 14, 2014, from http://www.ada.gov/medcare_mobility_ta/medcare_ta.htm#part1

U.S. Department of Justice (n.d.). Executive Order 13166: Improving access to services for persons with Limited English Proficiency. Retrieved November 14, 2014, from http://www.justice.gov/crt/about/cor/13166.php

U.S. Equal Employment Opportunity Commission (n.d.). Fact sheet on the EEOC's final regulations implementing the ADAAA. http://www.eeoc.gov/laws/regulations/adaaa_fact_sheet.cfm.

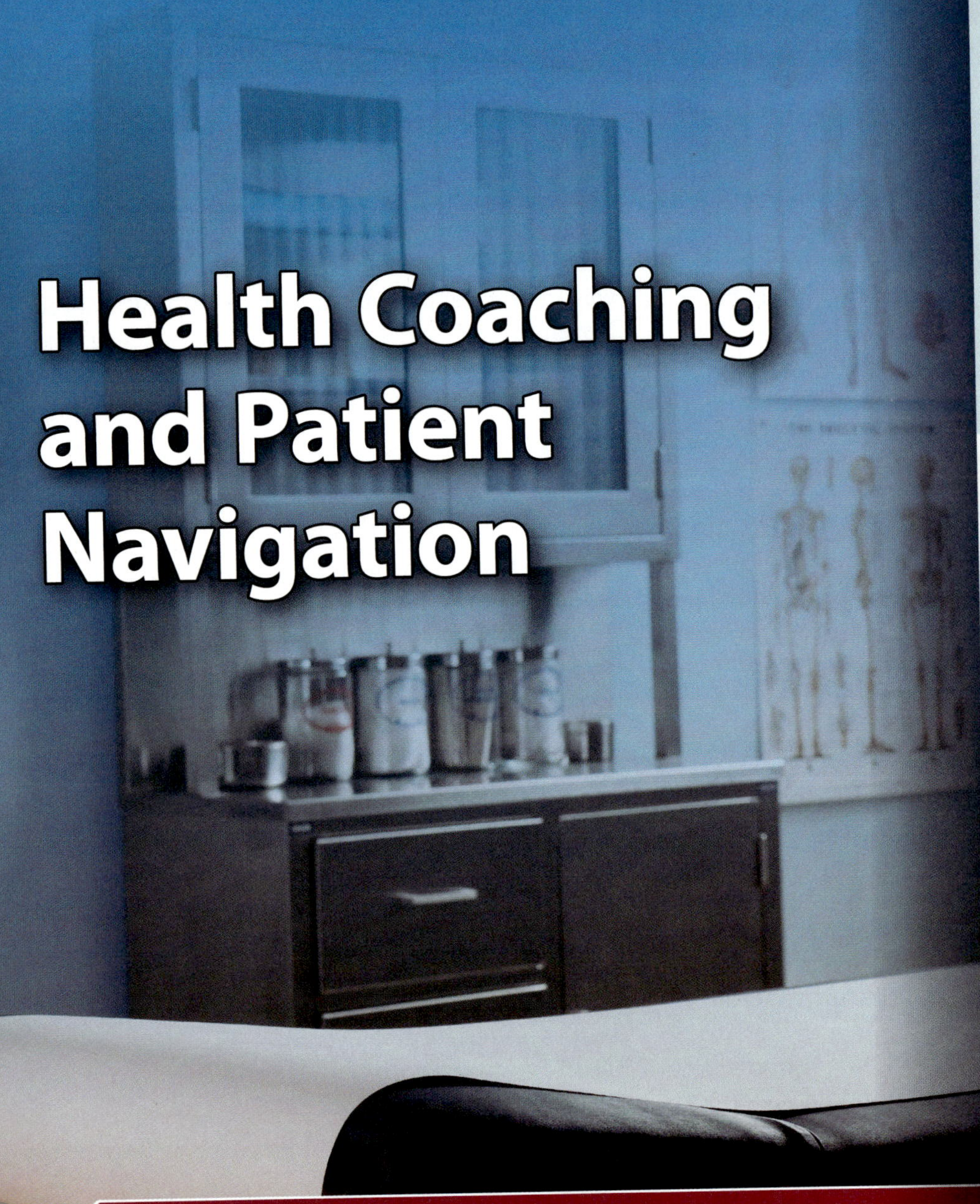

7

Health Coaching and Patient Navigation

ESSENTIAL TERMS

active listening
antidote
case manager
empathy
health coach
patient advocate
patient navigator
population management

CHAPTER OUTLINE

Population Management

What Is Health Coaching?

- Resources
- Demonstrate Respect for Individual Diversity
- Patient Concerns
- Self-Boundaries

Focus of Health Coaching

- Office Policies
- Hygienic Practices
- Health Maintenance and Disease Prevention
- Osteoporosis Screening and Bone Density Scan
- Pre- and Post-Op Care Instructions
- Provide Support for Terminally Ill Patients
- Recognition of Substance Abuse
- Domestic Violence Screening and Detection

The Role of the Patient Navigator or Advocate

- Resource Information
- Transition of Care

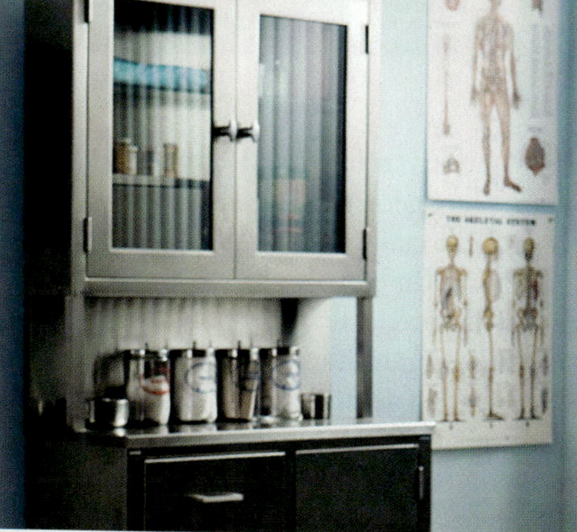

DEVELOPMENTAL OBJECTIVES

After completing this chapter, you should be able to:

1. Correctly spell and define the essential terms.
2. List resources available for health coaching.
3. Demonstrate respect for individual diversity as a health coach/patient navigator.
4. Demonstrate empathy for patient concerns and set self-boundaries as a health coach/patient navigator.
5. Describe office policies and expectations when acting as a health coach/patient navigator.
6. Educate patients and family members on hygienic practices.
7. Educate patients and family members on health maintenance and disease prevention.
8. Provide pre- and post-op care instructions.
9. Identify common stages that terminally ill patients experience.
10. Demonstrate empathy and provide support for terminally ill patients, including providing resources (organizations/support groups) that can assist the patients and their families.
11. Recognize patients who may be substance abusers.
12. Screen and detect patients for domestic violence.
13. Manage appointments in the role of a patient navigator.
14. Facilitate referrals to community resources and follow up on referrals acting as a patient navigator.
15. Intervene on behalf of the patient in the role of a patient navigator.
16. Summarize the components of transition of care of the patient.

INTRODUCTION

In Chapter 2, you learned about the latest trends in health care reimbursement. The pay-for-performance model of health care has rapidly grown with both federal and private payers. As a result, health care establishments are looking for ways to improve patient outcomes. In order to assist patients in taking charge of their own health, offices now utilize the services of health coaches, patient navigators, and case managers. These professionals assist patients in staying current with preventive health screenings and immunizations, transitional care (hospital to home), and disease management.

Medical assistants may be asked to take on the role of health coach and patient navigator in different health care settings, especially, the patient-centered medical home (PCMH) and accountable care organization (ACO) models. These roles may be blended within the usual duties of a medical assistant or separate roles altogether.

This chapter will introduce you to the roles of a patient navigator and health coach and discuss how medical assistants are a good fit for both of these roles.

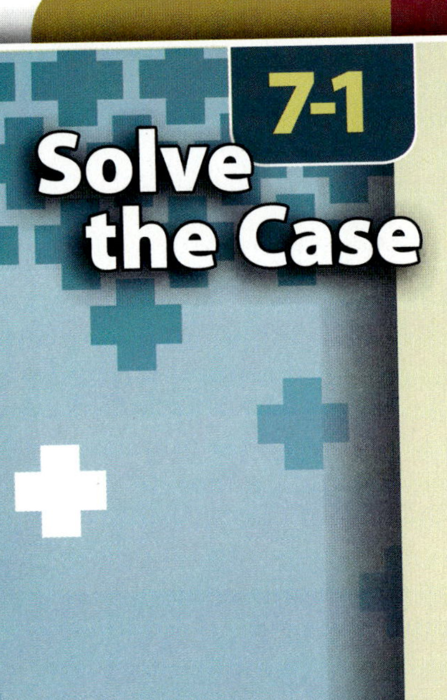

Patient Helene Oslosky has an appointment with staff cardiologist, Dr. Chang, today. Ms. Oslosky is an elderly patient who has limited financial resources and does not drive. The patient has a history of hypertension and hypercholesterolemia. She was recently diagnosed with atrial fibrillation (Afib), a condition that causes the patient's heart to beat out of rhythm. Dr. Chang called her with the results and asked the patient to schedule an appointment to discuss her options. The patient tells you that she is on Medicare but does not have prescription coverage, therefore does not take her blood pressure and cholesterol medication as prescribed. She is anxious about her visit with Dr. Chang today as she does not understand what Afib is and does not know what to expect. Using your current level of knowledge, answer the following questions.

1. **What flags should you share with Dr. Chang right away?**
2. **The patient's recent diagnosis of Afib means that she will probably be placed on yet another medication. Can you think of anything you can do to assist this patient in getting the medications she needs?**
3. **What professionalism keys would be most helpful in coaching Ms. Oslosky?**

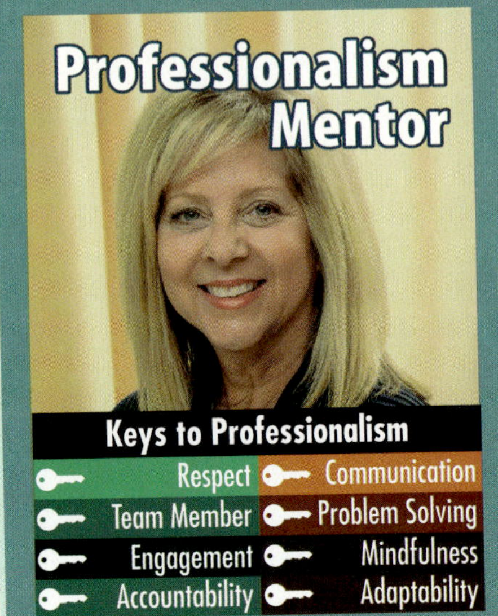

Imagine having a horrible illness and having to deal with it all by yourself. I cannot imagine anything worse! Now imagine that someone who understands the health care world is there to help coach you through your patient care experiences and help you "navigate" your way through the tests and appointments and mountains of paperwork. How would you feel about that person? An important key to being a patient navigator involves building trust with your patients. Patients need to be able to depend on you to guide them in the right direction, and trust that you will do it with empathy because heath care can be a scary experience. Even the strongest person needs a little help now and then. Will you be there to coach your patients and navigate them to safety? ■

POPULATION MANAGEMENT

Population management is identifying and monitoring groups of patients with similar diagnoses. Patient registries within the EHR identify patients in specific populations and their providers. Examples of "groupings by chronic disease" in these patient registries include patients with asthma, diabetes, hypertension, and congestive heart failure. Health organizations must be able to monitor the patient's control of chronic disease. Patients should receive a report card of how they are doing at the completion of each visit. This may include graphing examples of lab results, blood pressure readings, or weight measurements and a summary of kept, broken, or canceled appointments. Each provider and members of the provider's team also receive monthly or quarterly report cards which measure outcomes in specific patient populations. Registries include measurable goals such as blood pressure readings, Hgb A1Cs, the patient's last appointment, emergency room visits, and so on. The goal is to see improvement in these areas. If there is an overall decline in specific populations, the team meets to review what is and isn't working and creates a plan for moving forward. As a member of the health care team, you will need to understand your specific responsibilities for improving outcomes. One of the best ways to improve patient outcomes is through health coaching.

WHAT IS HEALTH COACHING?

A **health coach** is a person who provides individualized evaluation and subsequent management and encouragement to achieve superior patient health outcomes. The number of possible topics to be covered by a health coach is vast, but some common topics include diabetes management, heart health, prevention and management of osteoporosis, and smoking cessation. Health coaching involves the understanding and use of resources available to assist with educating the patient and demonstrating empathy and respect for patient concerns.

The medical assistant should develop a coaching style that he or she is comfortable with, as well as one that can be adapted to the individual needs of the patient. Instructional material may be gathered through different organizations such as the American Diabetes Association or the National Alzheimer's Association. The Internet provides hundreds of resources on popular topics, including downloadable brochures, animations, and interactive websites, but you must be careful to use online resources only from reputable sources. Medical and pharmaceutical representatives often provide great teaching tools in the form of teaching models, DVDs, and wall charts. Medical assistants may also be called upon to develop instructional handouts and brochures for common topics within the practice where they are employed.

To be an effective health coach, you must demonstrate effective verbal and nonverbal communication skills. Verbal communication generally refers to the spoken word. Although verbal communication can be very effective, nonverbal communication is also an essential tool to enhance the learning process. Nonverbal cues include the use of body language, eye contact, and most importantly, active listening. To learn more about verbal techniques that can assist you in effectively communicating with the patient, refer to Chapter 5.

Active listening involves focusing on the information at hand. It is important not to let your mind wander to the next topic. Patient cues must be observed, including the emotional level during the interaction. This will direct the speed and course of the educational session. Active listening usually employs good eye contact. This draws the patient into the conversation, again increasing patient understanding.

It is important to have an understanding of the "whys" and "how's" of patient learning. Employ good communication skills, establish an environment conducive to learning, and provide appropriate coaching and resources to improve the outcome of each individual educational session.

There are times when you will provide coaching or education over the phone. The provider will usually write specific instructions on the progress note or lab form (or message the medical assistant in the electronic health record [EHR]) identifying goals that should be discussed with the patient.

Examples of health coaching topics that may take place over the phone include the following:

- The introduction of a new medication or a change in the way the patient is taking current medication
- Special dietary changes due to an abnormal lab result (such as elevated lipids or glucose)
- Instructions for the patient to see a specialist, dietician, or to have specific testing

Verbal communication skills are even more important when speaking over the phone because facial expressions and body language cannot be seen. Always have the patient repeat information to confirm that she understands. Encourage the patient to obtain a pen and piece of paper at the beginning of the call and to write out the instructions. If the patient has access to the Internet, it may be beneficial to send the patient electronic instructions prior to placing the call via the secure patient portal. The patient is then able to concentrate on listening to the instructions while reading the information.

Throughout this text, "Health Coach" feature boxes have been inserted with examples of how clinical medical assistants may be expected to administer patient education.

Resources

Various resources may be utilized to enhance the educational (coaching) process. For example, you may use models, the Internet, brochures, pharmaceutical companies, pharmacists, etc. Figure 7-1 illustrates some tools that might be incorporated into the coaching session. Combining verbal instructions along with written materials has proven to increase topic retention for the patient. The addition of diagrams will also enhance the learning process. The more senses used in learning, the more information the patient will remember.

The appropriate setting will enhance the success of the health coaching session (see Figure 7-2). The following guidelines will prove most effective:

- Provide a quiet, comfortable environment for the session.
- Make certain the amount of lighting is sufficient to read any literature or view any diagrams.
- Avoid any distractions (loud noises, odors, children, etc.).
- Have comfortable chairs all at the same level so that eye contact can be maintained.
- Have all supplies, brochures, and paperwork prepared and ready prior to the session.
- If possible, have your phone and intercom temporarily quieted. Eliminate anything that creates the feeling that the patient is being rushed or infringing on the time of the health coach.
- Based on the comfort of the patient, the relationship with the patient, and the type of education provided, the chairs should be positioned either with the desk between the medical assistant and the patient (more formal) or with the chairs alone facing each other (more casual and personal). Using a round table when there are multiple family members participating in the session allows everyone to see the presenter and each other.

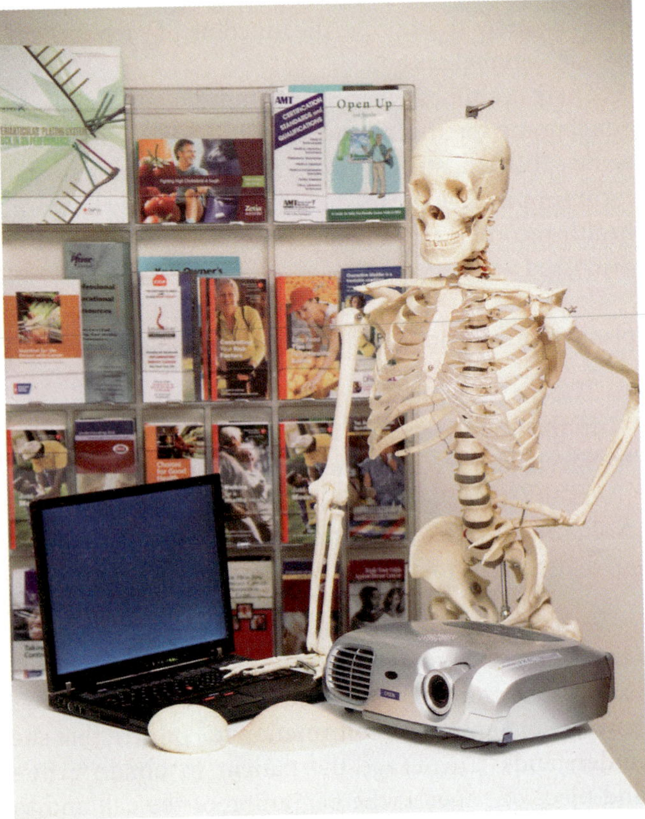

Figure 7-1 ■ Useful supplies needed for a patient education session.

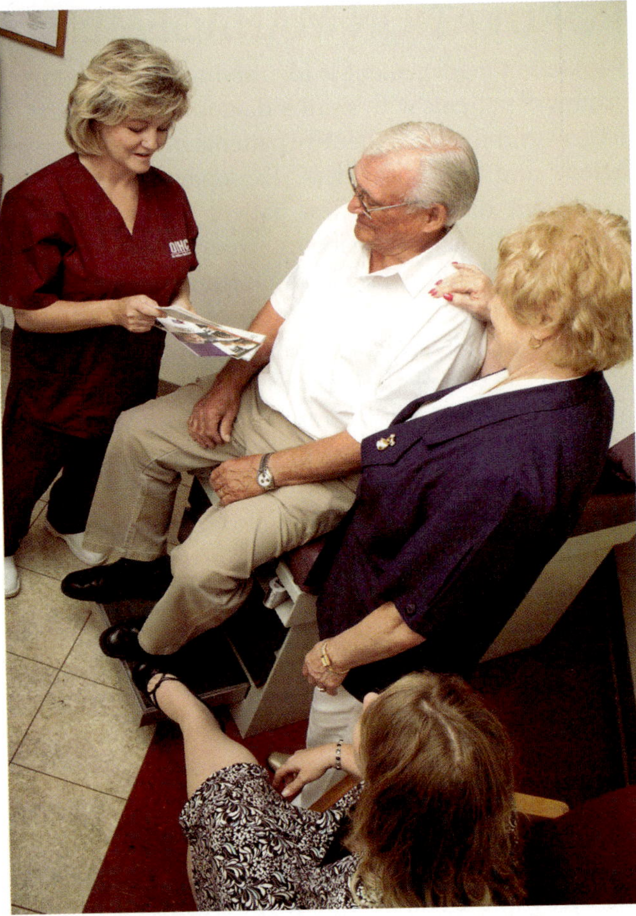

Figure 7-2 ■ It is important to include in the educational sessions family members who can help clarify information when the patient returns home.

CRITICAL THINKING CHALLENGE

You are presenting an important health coaching session to the patient regarding cancer prevention and awareness. The patient's mother and sister both died from ovarian cancer. The patient brought her four-year-old niece to the session. The niece continually interrupts the patient throughout the session.

1. What are some activities that you can introduce to keep the four-year-old busy during the health coaching session? Can you incorporate some assistance from other members of the health care team?

There are also barriers to health coaching that must be considered. These include, but are not limited to the following:

- *Time*. Be certain there is enough time to allow for adequate instruction. Instruction may not be provided during the initial office visit. The medical assistant may need to schedule another visit to allow for ample time.
- *Money*. The patient may not have the financial means to include all of the practices taught. This must be considered when providing the instruction or plan of action. Perhaps a certain drug or procedure is not the most financially feasible. Alternative protocols might need consideration.
- *Interest*. If the patient has no interest in making the changes, instruction will be totally ineffective.
- *Child care*. If a child is interrupting the educational session, the patient may lose interest, focus, or patience. Another time may need to be scheduled for maximum compliance.
- *Transportation*. It may be difficult for the patient to obtain adequate transportation for future health coaching sessions. It may also be a problem to require a patient to stay longer than expected for health coaching following a physical exam. These challenges need to be considered. Instruction over the phone, although not the best setting, might be a better alternative for the individual patient and situation.

Demonstrate Respect for Individual Diversity

We live in a multicultural world that is becoming more diverse each day. As medical professionals, you have a

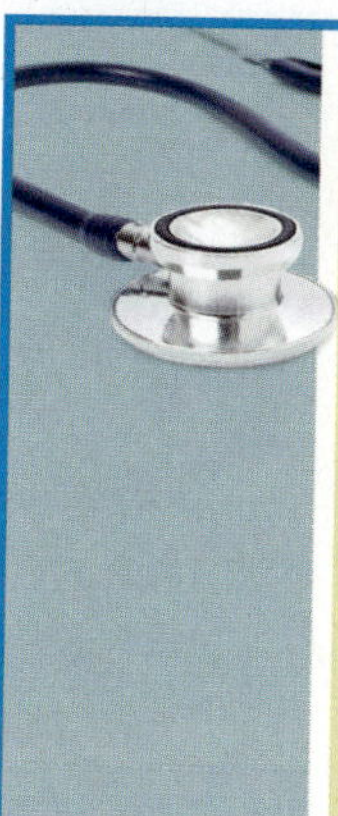

Field Smarts

Be aware of your own biases, such as against obesity, smoking, or body piercing. Remain professional when providing health coaching. Ask yourself, "Is this for me or for the patient?" If a patient is not ready or prepared for discussing or learning the health related content, the time spent may not be effective.

responsibility to care for all people equally. The medical assistant must always demonstrate respect for individual diversity including gender, race, religion, age, socioeconomic status, physical challenges, special needs, appearance, sexual orientation, lifestyle choices, and primary language. (Refer to Chapter 6 for additional information on assisting patients with special needs.)

It is important to set the tone for communication at the start of the session. Begin each session by setting goals together regarding what each party wants to obtain from the session. Be respectful of the patient and acknowledge family members. Many times, family members will be more instrumental in patient compliance than the patient alone. This is especially relevant during dietary training sessions. If the patient's spouse does all the cooking and the session is geared toward lowering the patient's cholesterol, the spouse should be drawn into the session as well as the patient. If the session is related to wound care, the spouse may need to take ownership in caring for the wound due to its location or the patient's inability to comprehend the instructions.

Patient Concerns

When acting as a health coach, inevitably there will be challenges and patient concerns. Patients often do not have a comprehensive understanding of disease processes and home care responsibilities, and the "how and why" to take their medications as prescribed. In addition, many patients avoid seeking medical care out of fear of diagnosis of a life-changing disease or illness. Many patients also experience fear of dying, fear of losing their job, and not being able to support their family. Financial concerns often weigh heavily on the patient as they seek medical care. It is important that you factor in patient concerns when acting as a health coach or patient navigator. The professionalism keys you learned in Chapter 1 will be invaluable.

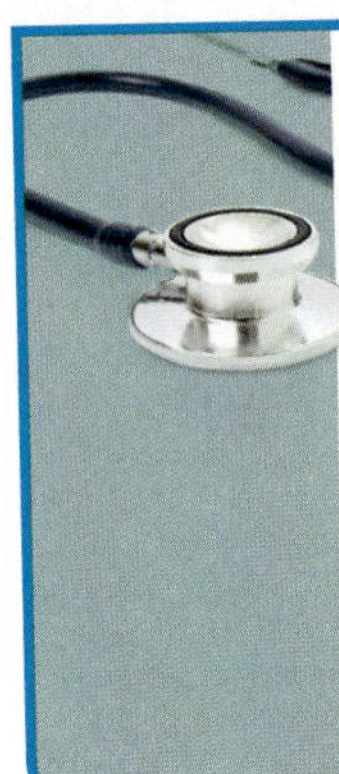

Field Smarts

Motivation has been discussed as a significant part of health coaching. Determine early in the session the level of motivation in the patient. Why does the patient want or need to receive the instruction? This will provide direction for a successful interaction.

Self-Boundaries

To be an effective health coach or patient navigator, you must demonstrate self-awareness and the principles of self-boundaries. Consider how you react when someone invades your "personal space." When someone gets too close, your first reaction may be to take a step back. Doing so sends a message to the other person that he or she is invading your personal space. Consider nonverbal cues given by the patient so that you are aware of and respect his or her boundaries. Other examples of boundary issues include blaming others for problems, telling others how to act or what to think, or allowing the mood of another person to dictate your mood. On a daily basis you will observe patient's mental and emotional states. Using adaptive coping skills as a tool for self-awareness will have a direct impact on both your and your patient's behavior.

FOCUS OF HEALTH COACHING

Health coaching will focus on the dissemination of information such as office policies, as well as teaching patients and their family's basic hygienic practices. In addition, the clinical medical assistant will coach patients on health maintenance and disease prevention topics, and on pre-op and post-op care instructions. As health coach you will also provide support for terminally ill patients, be able to recognize substance abuse and domestic violence, and provide necessary coaching and resources.

Office Policies

In order to effectively manage the medical practice, it is important that patients are fully informed of office policies. In the course of medical treatment, patients tend to feel anxious about all the new and unfamiliar experiences of interviews, tests, examinations, and financial issues they encounter. One way to ease fears and maintain a good relationship with patients is to communicate clearly what is expected from them as well as what patients can expect from the office staff. As a well-informed health coach and patient navigator, you will explain the office policies and patient responsibilities, which include understanding and complying with the financial policy, keeping scheduled appointments, following instructions given by the provider (home care, prescriptions, follow-up, etc.), complying with assessment and plan, and being honest about health issues (see Procedure 7-1).

Office policies should be outlined briefly at the initial patient visit with an offer to answer specific questions and provide more in-depth explanations as needed throughout the patient's subsequent visits. Policies relating to patients are developed and derived from both the legal and ethical responsibilities of the practice to its patients.

In addition to patient responsibilities, the practice will post a Patient's Bill of Rights as a way to communicate the legal rights of the patient while under the care of a practitioner or facility. The Patient Bill of Rights typically should state that patients

- are to be treated professionally with respect and courtesy at all times;
- will have a clear understanding of what they can expect regarding how their privacy will be protected and how their personal information will be used (following HIPAA guidelines and the Notice of Privacy Practices [NPP]);
- have a right to participate actively in the decisions made regarding their health care and procedures, and to undergo only those procedures for which they provide informed consent; and
- should be advised of what means of communications will be used to contact them regarding medical information, how insurance billing will be handled, any safety procedures they are expected to observe while in the office, and what they can expect from the practice's employees in general.

Hygienic Practices

Patients and their families must be coached on hygienic practices such as handwashing techniques, cough etiquette, and using personal protective equipment (PPE) to improve health outcomes. The best way to prevent disease or illness and promote recovery at home is to practice good hygiene at all times. Your responsibility will be to coach the patient and family members and explain the reasoning for good hygiene. For example, you may want to start your coaching by saying "when caring for a loved one …," and then complete the instruction.

Handwashing

Keeping hands clean through improved hand hygiene is one of the most important steps to avoid getting sick and spreading germs to others. Many diseases and conditions are spread by not washing hands with soap and clean, running water. As health coach, you will instruct patients and their families on proper handwashing techniques. Refer to Chapter 8 for handwashing recommendations from the CDC.

Cough Etiquette

To prevent transmission of all types of respiratory infections, infection control measures should be implemented at the first point of contact and incorporated into infection control practices at home and in the health care setting. To contain respiratory secretions, coach the patient (and family members) to do the following:

- Cover their mouth and nose with a tissue when coughing or sneezing, or if tissue is not available to cough or sneeze into their sleeve.
- Dispose of the tissue in the nearest waste receptacle after use.
- Perform hand hygiene (e.g., handwashing with non-antimicrobial soap and water, alcohol-based hand rub, or antiseptic handwash) after having contact with respiratory secretions and contaminated objects/materials.

Donning Personal Protective Equipment (PPE)

Similar to coaching for cough etiquette, you will instruct patients and their families on the use of PPE. PPE can include the use of a mask, gloves, face shields, eye protection, gown, and shoe coverings. This is especially relevant for family members caring for patients with suppressed immune systems. Transplant patients and patients going through chemotherapy are very vulnerable to infection, therefore, infection control practices are essential to keep the patient healthy. Demonstrate excellent hygienic practices and be a role model to patients and their families by displaying good hygienic practices. Refer to Chapter 8 for more information regarding the use of PPE.

Health Maintenance and Disease Prevention

In order to encourage patient compliance, the patient will need to both understand and comply with instructions given during the session. Your role as a health coach is vital in producing positive outcomes. You must demonstrate good hygiene, a positive attitude, and knowledge of the subject matter. Some tips for patient compliance include the following:

- Be a good role model. For example, if you are conducting a session on smoking cessation and you smell like cigarettes, it is going to be difficult to convince the patient to stop smoking.
- Include family members in the session.
- Look for indicators that the patient understands and agrees with the material being presented. This should be assessed several times throughout the session.
- Have the patient repeat back the information at the conclusion of the session.
- Follow up each session with written materials.
- With the provider's permission, give the patient supplies that will help with compliance (e.g., bandaging materials, drug samples).
- One to two days following the session, call the patient to see how things are going and to determine if the patient has any additional questions.
- During follow-up sessions, acknowledge patient compliance, and tactfully question noncompliance.

Diabetic Teaching and Home Care

Diabetes mellitus is a condition in which the body produces no insulin (type 1 diabetes) or insufficient insulin (type 2 diabetes). When insulin is absent or ineffective, cells import inadequate amounts of glucose, a starvation process that causes the liver to release more glucose into the blood in an attempt to feed other tissues. Since this additional glucose still cannot enter the cells, glucose levels in the blood rise. The appropriate treatment for an individual depends on the type of diabetes and its severity. Type 2 diabetes is managed with a combination of exercise, diet, and medication. The first treatment is weight reduction, diabetic diet, and exercise. When these measures fail to control the elevated blood sugars, oral medications are used. If oral medications are still insufficient, insulin therapy, or other newer injectable therapies are considered. Type 1 diabetes requires insulin in addition to exercise and a diabetic diet.

A good health coach will help the patient formulate an action plan to meet goals to treat her diabetes. For example, if the patient states she has tried dieting and exercise, but fails every time, the health coach may ask the patient to make a list of what really stresses her out

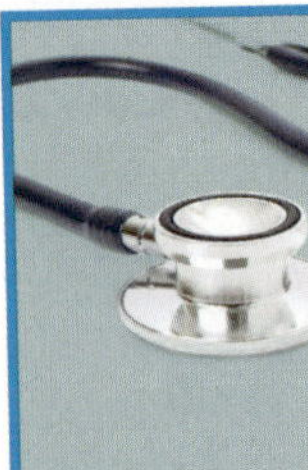

Field Smarts

Some of the newer community patient-centered medical home (PCMH) models have incorporated industrial kitchens into the model where patients and their family members work with dieticians to learn how to make delicious healthy meals in a matter of minutes. The PCMH may partner with food pantries and coalitions to establish that patients have the resources they need to make healthy meals. It is hopeful that this new practice will escalate better nutrition, not just for the patient but for the entire family.

and how she might deal with it. If work or traffic is stressful, causing the patient to get home late for dinner, her meal choices may not be ideal for managing diabetes. She may not "have time" to cook or check her blood glucose levels. By taking the approach of how to deal with the "stressors," the patient may be able to find ways to properly manager her disease. The health coach and patient should work together to create solutions that are both suitable and attainable. Some ideas include having a family member prepare the evening meal one or two times a week that follows a healthy diabetic diet; setting a timer for checking blood glucose levels; not checking personal messages on her smartphone (text or email) prior to 8 A.M., only checking messages one to two times a day, and using that extra time to take walks or exercise. A health coach does not "tell the patient what to do," but works with the patient to set goals and manage her disease.

Home Blood Sugar Monitoring

In addition to diet and exercise, anyone with diabetes would benefit from having a home blood-glucose monitor. The monitor can help the patient be more aware of blood-sugar control. How often to test depends on the patient's individual situation. For some people, testing once each morning for a few days before a visit to the doctor may be sufficient; for others, testing two or more times daily may be needed to adjust medication doses. As health coach, you will need to know if the patient has type 1 or type 2 diabetes, and what instructions the provider has ordered in regards to testing and treatment. With the monitor at the coaching session, assist the patient in reading and following the instructions to test his or her blood sugar (Figures 7-3a, b, and c).

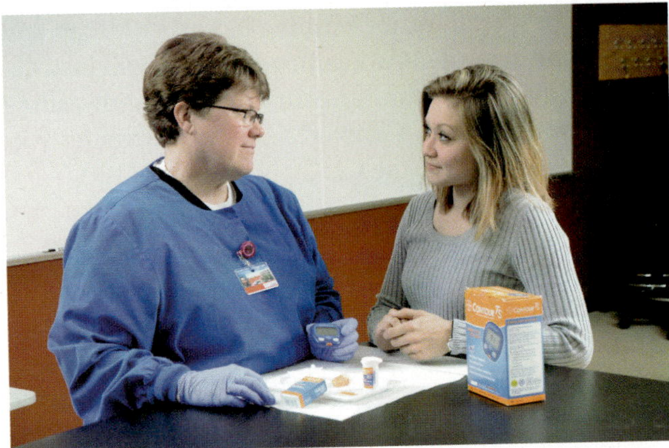

Figure 7-3a ■ The medical assistant sets up the patient's brand new meter and supplies to practice testing.

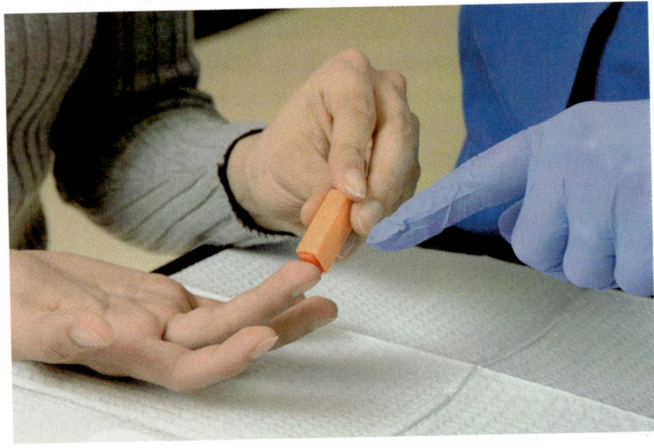

Figure 7-3b ■ The patient performs a finger puncture on herself in front of the medical assistant.

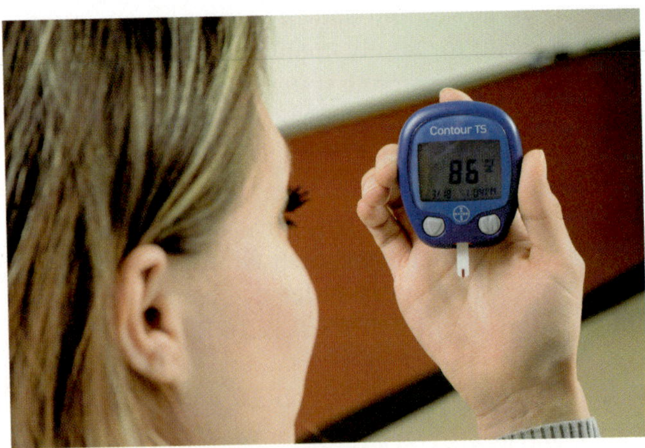

Figure 7-3c ■ The patient reads the LCD display to get the reading. Notice that the patient is not wearing gloves; this is because this is her meter and she will not be wearing gloves at home.

Home Injection Therapies

Patients with insulin-dependent diabetes often need training on how to administer insulin. This training may be incorporated following glucose monitor testing (Figure 7-4). The following Health Coach provides a step-by-step procedure for insulin administration.

Patients may be asked to self-administer other types of injections as well, especially patients with chronic conditions. It is important that patients feel comfortable with the procedure and that they have plenty of time to practice before leaving the office. Provide patients with written materials and other visuals that they can refer to while at home.

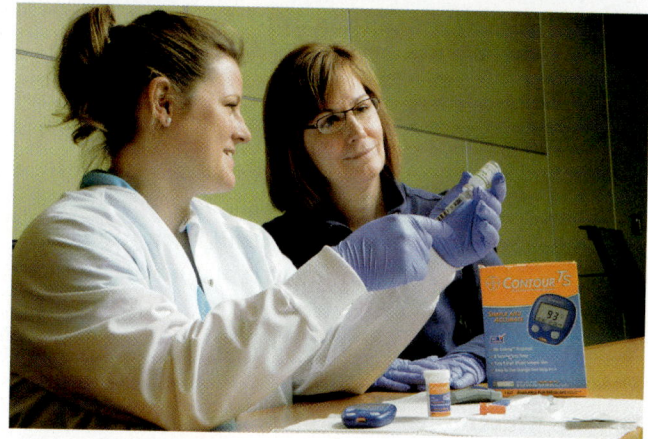

Figure 7-4 ■ The medical assistant is teaching the patient how to draw up her insulin.

Health Coach

Procedure for Administering Insulin

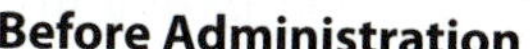

Before Administration

1. Gather supplies (syringe/needle unit, alcohol pad, insulin vials, gauze pad, and adhesive bandage).
2. Roll the insulin vial(s) between your hands to mix. (Do not shake.)
3. Remove plastic cap from the insulin vial(s) and clean with alcohol pad.
4. If using two vials of insulin, always pull up the clear insulin first (short-acting), then the cloudy (intermediate or long-acting).
5. Pull back on the plunger so that the top ring of the rubber stopper is equal to the number of units you are going to remove from the vial.
6. Insert the needle into the vial and push all the way forward on the plunger. (If using two vials, push air into the cloudy vial first and remove the needle right away, then repeat the procedure with the insulin in the clear vial.)
7. Turn the bottle upside down with the syringe/needle unit and pull the plunger down to the volume ordered by your provider.
8. Tap on the syringe to get rid of air bubble and remove needle from insulin bottle. (Move the needle to the cloudy vial and pull the plunger to the required number of total units of insulin needed if applicable.) Place cap on syringe.

During Administration

1. Insulin is administered in the fatty layer of tissue and can be administered anywhere you can find fat on arms, thighs, and abdomen. (Always rotate sites.)
2. Alcohol the injection site starting at the middle and working outward.
3. Remove the needle cap with your dominant hand.
4. With the other hand, grasp a two- to three-inch fold of tissue on either side of the cleansed area between the thumb and index finger.
5. Insert the entire needle at a 90-degree angle or 45-degree angle if you are very thin into the cleansed area.
6. Push in on the plunger until the all the insulin is deposited into the tissue.
7. Swiftly pull the needle out of the skin at the same angle you used upon insertion of the needle. Do not rub the injection site.
8. Apply gentle pressure with gauze pad if bleeding occurs.

Patient Mobility Equipment and Assistive Devices

Patients with physical disabilities may need assistance using mobility devices such as walkers, crutches, wheelchairs, and canes. These tasks are usually taught by a physical or occupational therapist; however, patients may need reminders while visiting their providers. Refer to Chapter 22 for more information on mobility equipment and assistive devices.

High Cholesterol Teaching

Patients with coronary artery disease often need education for reducing cholesterol in their diets. There are different types of cholesterol. The good cholesterol, high-density lipoprotein (HDL), assists with removal of the bad cholesterol (low-density lipoproteins [LDL] and triglycerides). Methods used to lower cholesterol include the following:

- Stay away from foods that are high in trans- and saturated-fats, including fried foods, baked treats, red meats, and dairy products. Instead, eat foods such as whole grains, beans, fish, poultry, and fruits such as apples, grapes, and strawberries.
- Stop smoking.
- Increase exercise.
- Try supplements such as high doses of fish and krill oil.
- Take your cholesterol medication as prescribed.

Cholesterol numbers that patients should strive for include the following:

- Total cholesterol score less than 200
- LDL less than 99
- HDL that is 40 or above.

Although these numbers are important, providers now use HDL and total cholesterol as well as age, sex, race, history of hypertension, blood pressure, and smoking history to assess the patient's 10-year and lifetime risk of atherosclerotic cardiovascular disease. To learn more about cardiovascular disease refer to Chapter 14.

Home Cholesterol Monitoring

Patients who struggle with high cholesterol may be encouraged to perform cholesterol testing in the home. Patients should report their results to the provider so that medication changes can be made if necessary. A common group of drugs that are used to treat hyperlipidemia (increased lipids in the blood) are known as statins. Patients taking these drugs should have liver enzyme studies as well because these drugs can cause liver damage in some patients.

Smoking Risks and Cessation Programs

It is no surprise today that smoking is a contributor to several diseases including lung cancer, throat cancer, emphysema, bronchitis, and cardiovascular disease. Cigarettes, cigars, and pipes are all culprits in these diseases. The jury is still out on vapor cigarettes; however, some studies have shown an increase in the incidence of lung cancer in this population of smokers. Patients should be encouraged to stop all forms of smoking. There are many products available to assist patients with smoking cessation including Zyban, Chantix, Nicorette, and Habitrol. These products may be in the form of inhalers, patches, gum, or lozenges. Patients may also be encouraged to join a support group or pair up with an accountability partner. To learn more about lung health refer to Chapter 15.

Anticoagulation Teaching

Patients who have conditions that predispose them to the formation of blood clots include patients who have been diagnosed with atrial fibrillation, patients who have undergone heart valve replacement, and patients with certain genetic disorders. Patients who have a history of blood clot formation such as those who have had a stroke, heart attack, pulmonary embolism, or deep vein thrombosis (DVT) are also likely to form new clots. As a result, these patients are usually put on anticoagulants to prevent the blood from clotting. Warfarin sodium or Coumadin (trade name) is commonly prescribed for these conditions; however, there are many new drugs on the market that may be used for some of these conditions. Patients should take their anticoagulants exactly as directed and at the same time each day and should receive education regarding foods, medications, and herbal supplements that affect blood clotting. Patients should avoid liver, mango, and herbal products that increase one's risk for bleeding including garlic, ginkgo, ginseng, and fish oil. Vitamin K, as well as certain leafy vegetables, including lettuce, spinach, and turnip greens, stimulates clot formation. Patients on anticoagulation therapy should also avoid ibuprofen, aspirin, naproxen, and aspirin products such as Alka-Seltzer and Pepto-Bismol. Other medications will also affect blood clotting levels, which is why it is so important to have a complete listing of all the patients' medications.

Home Anticoagulation Monitoring

Anticoagulation monitoring can now be performed in the privacy of the patient's home. Patients should be taught how to use the monitor and encouraged to keep a log of their readings to share with the provider. Routine testing performed for patients taking warfarin is a prothrombin time (PT) level and international normalized ratio (INR), which is a formula used to standardize test results from one lab to the next. This formula is built into the home monitoring systems and will automatically populate at the end of testing. A normal PT range can be anywhere from 10 to 14 seconds. INR values are usually therapeutic between 2 and 3 in patients taking warfarin but may be different for some patients. The provider will set the therapeutic range for each patient.

Home Monitoring Equipment

Home monitoring equipment is fairly similar for all of the tests mentioned above including glucose testing, cholesterol testing, and PT/INR testing. The following are steps that should be taken for home monitoring testing.

1. Wash hands and gather supplies.
2. Turn monitor on and follow manufacturer's instructions for readying the unit for testing. (A control may need to be performed prior to testing.)
3. Cleanse fingertip (index, middle, or ring finger) with an alcohol pad.
4. Puncture cleansed fingertip with lancet.
5. Gently squeeze fingertip to bring blood to the surface.
6. Wipe away the first drop of blood with a gauze square.
7. Apply blood to monitor strip following manufacturer's instructions.
8. Perform testing according to manufacturer's instructions.
9. Read result in the LCD display, throw away used supplies and bloody strip, and apply adhesive bandage to the area.
10. Record results in log. Follow provider's instructions in response to any abnormal results.

Oral Medications

Instructing patients on how to take their medications is one of the most frequent topics for health coaching. In order for the medical assistant to be a good coach, she must be familiar with the medication. If needed, do some research on the medication before presenting the session. Know the reason the provider has prescribed the medication (e.g., for treatment of high blood pressure). Additional information that should be acquired includes the following:

- The classification and use of the drug
- The directions for taking the drug
- Common side effects of the drug
- Contraindications for not using the drug
- Economical information (Knowing the economic resources of your patient will help in determining if compliance is even an option. When patients are limited in their funds, talk to the provider and drug company representatives to determine if there are any workable solutions.)

After the coaching session, the medical assistant must ask the patient to repeat back the information and document the session in the patient's chart. Figure 7-5 illustrates a medical assistant providing instruction for a patient about how to keep track of when to take medications using a special medication container.

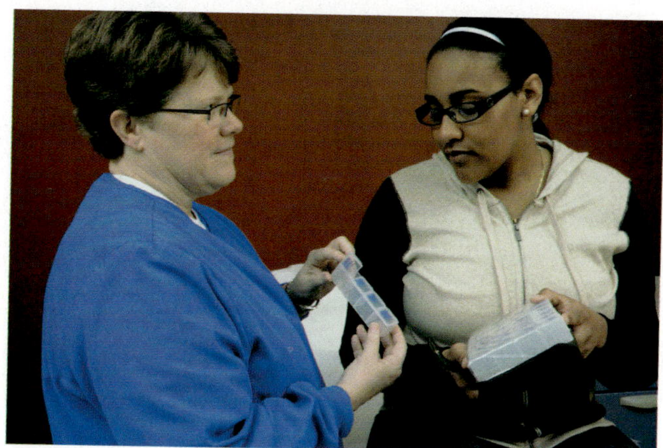

Figure 7-5 ■ The medical assistant provides a pill case for the patient so that she doesn't forget her medications on specific days.

Health Coach

Anticoagulation Therapy

Of important note is that warfarin is currently the only drug used for anticoagulation therapy for which there is an **antidote** (meaning a way to reverse the effect of the drug); however, frequent blood draws are necessary to determine the patient's PT/INR in order to make any necessary adjustments in the dosage. Currently there is no antidote for the newer drugs such as Xarelto, Eliquis, and Pradaxa, which may put the patient at higher risk for serious bleeding complications, although research and development is continuing and that may change in the future.

Blood Pressure Monitoring

Blood pressure measures the amount of force exerted on the arterial walls as the heart ventricles contract and relax. Any blood pressure under 140/90 is considered controlled for most adult patients, but a goal of less than 150/90 is used for patients over 60 years old. Hypertension, if left untreated, may result in coronary artery disease, heart failure, or kidney failure.

Patients with hypertension (high blood pressure) should be encouraged to check blood pressure at home. Many of these monitors are automated and very affordable through the patient's pharmacy. Always ask the patient to bring in their blood pressure unit after purchasing so that you can assist with education. Compare the reading with the patient's unit with one in the office that has been recently calibrated to confirm the patient's unit is in good working order. Patients should be encouraged to check their blood pressures one to two times per day and to take it at the same time each day. Tell the patient to alternate arms and to record which arm was used for each reading. Patients should bring in their blood pressure logs each time they have an office visit.

Osteoporosis Screening and Bone Density Scan

Osteoporosis is a disease that thins and weakens the bones to the point that they become fragile and break easily (Figure 7-6). Women and men with osteoporosis most often break bones in the hip, spine, and wrist, but any bone can be affected. According to the National Institutes of Health, more than 40 million people in the United States either have osteoporosis or are at high risk due to low bone mass. Osteoporosis is most common among older people, especially older women. With healthy lifestyle choices such as proper diet, exercise, and treatment medications, osteoporosis can often be prevented or treated. To detect osteoporosis, a bone mineral density test is performed. The most common and accurate diagnosis is obtained with a dual-energy X-ray absorptiometry (DEXA) scan. As health coach and patient navigator, you will be tasked with providing information about the disease, risk factors, preventive steps, and appropriate testing and diagnosis.

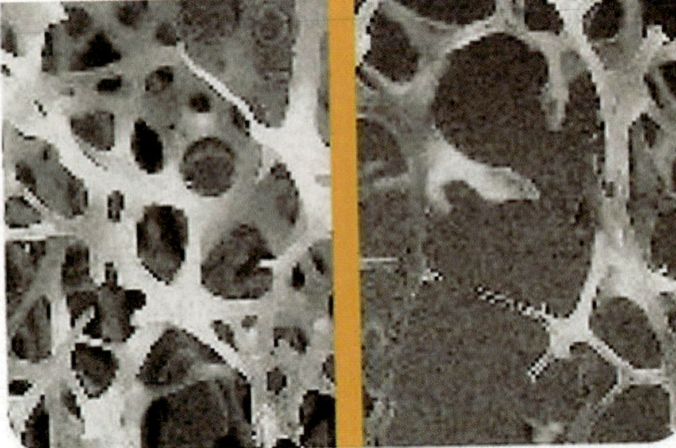

Figure 7-6 ■ Example of normal bone and a bone with osteoporosis. Image courtesy of *The 2004 Surgeon General's Report on Bone Health and Osteoporosis: What It Means to You*. U.S. Department of Health and Human Services, Office of the Surgeon General, 2004.

For more information about osteoporosis and the bone density scan, visit the National Institutes of Health website (www.nihseniorhealth.gov) and search "osteoporosis." View the video "Coping with Osteoporosis" as a useful health coaching/patient navigator tool on the subject of osteoporosis. Chapter 22 includes a health coaching feature on osteoporosis.

Pre- and Post-Op Care Instructions

As a health coach, you will also be responsible for assisting the patient with pre-op and post-op care instructions. Refer to Chapter 10 (Assisting with Minor Surgeries) for more information on this topic.

Provide Support for Terminally Ill Patients

To provide support for terminally ill patients and their families, it is important that you use empathy in your communications. You must also be able to identify the common stages of grief that terminally ill patients experience. Having a ready list of resources will assist you in your role as health coach and patient navigator.

Use Empathy in Communication

Empathy is having the ability to put yourself in another person's shoes. In the minds of your patients, compassion is paramount. This is a way to identify the patient's feelings and respond with understanding. Empathy is used to strengthen rapport with the patient and is crucial in your role as health coach and patient navigator.

Identify Common Stages of Grief

Understanding some fundamentals of psychology is an important element in your job as a medical assistant. Erik Erikson's theory on psychosocial development, Abraham Maslow's hierarchy of needs, and Dr. Elisabeth Kübler-Ross's (author of *On Death and Dying*) five stages of grief are often studied. Being knowledgeable of these studies will assist you in becoming an effective communicator during different stages of development and in understanding patient needs and grief in your role as health coach or patient navigator.

Kübler-Ross's grief model was developed initially as a model for helping dying patients cope with death and bereavement; however, it has been expanded to provide insight and guidance for coming to terms with personal trauma and change and for helping others make emotional adjustments and cope, whatever the cause. Kübler-Ross found that most people went through a process of five stages when dealing with grief, especially over terminal illness and death. The five stages are as follows:

- *Denial*. The person is trying to shut out the reality and magnitude of their situation, often creating a false reality.
- *Anger*. In this stage, patients become difficult to care for because of the misplaced feelings of anger for what has happened to them.
- *Bargaining*. The patient believes that somehow they can undo what has happened by changing their lifestyle or negotiating a compromise to live a little longer.
- *Depression*. The patient is now overcome with the reality that they are going to die but become despondent over their fate, often feeling that there is no point in going on or doing anything.
- *Acceptance*. At this point the patient has come to terms with the inevitable future and plans accordingly in preparation for their impending death.

Recommend Organizations and Support Groups

In your role as health coach and patient navigator, you will often rely on resources such as organizations and support groups that can assist patients and their families when faced with the devastating diagnosis of a terminal illness. Examples of organizations and support groups that can assist patients and family members of patients experiencing terminal illnesses include a local chapter of Hospice, the American Cancer Society, Compassion and Choices, Children's Hospice International, Center to Advance Palliative Care, and your local hospital resources.

Recognition of Substance Abuse

As a medical assistant, health coach, and patient navigator, you will need to know how to recognize the signs of substance abuse. Substance abuse is the excessive use of a drug (alcohol, narcotics, or cocaine) without medical justification. Most addiction starts with experimental use in social situations. It is sometimes difficult to distinguish "moodiness" from signs of drug abuse. The Mayo Clinic has compiled a list of possible indications of substance abuse:

- *Problems at school or work*. Frequently missing school or work, a sudden disinterest in school activities or work, or a drop in grades or work performance
- *Physical health issues*. Lack of energy and motivation
- *Neglected appearance*. Lack of interest in clothing, grooming, or looks
- *Changes in behavior*. Exaggerated efforts to bar family members from entering his or her room or being secretive about where he or she goes with friends; or drastic changes in behavior and relationships with family and friends
- *Spending money*. Sudden requests for money without a reasonable explanation; or your discovery that money is missing or has been stolen, or that items have disappeared from your home

Signs and symptoms of drug use or intoxication may vary, depending on the type of drug. For more information visit the Mayo Clinic website at www.mayoclinic.org and search "drug addiction" or "substance abuse."

Domestic Violence Screening and Detection

The Office of Women's Health (a department of the U.S. Department of Health and Human Services) provides information on the signs of abuse, healthy versus unhealthy relationships, and more. Health care professionals should learn to recognize signs of domestic violence and other forms of abuse (Figure 7-7). Table 7-1 provides a list of possible signs of abuse women may suffer at the hand of their partner. Some are illegal. All of them are wrong. Use the signs outlined in Table 7-1

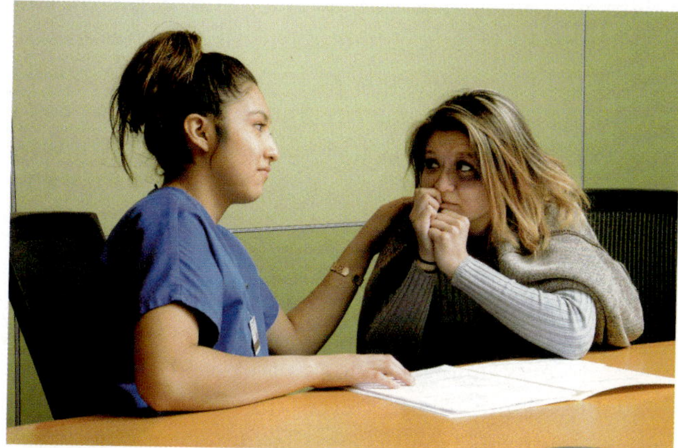

Figure 7-7 ■ The medical assistant consoles the patient as she obtains facts of the patient's injuries.

Table 7-1 Possible Signs of Abuse

You may be abused if your partner:	
Monitors what you're doing all the time	Unfairly accuses you of being unfaithful all the time
Prevents or discourages you from seeing friends or family	Prevents or discourages you from going to work or school
Gets very angry during and after drinking alcohol or using drugs	Controls how you spend your money
Controls your use of needed medicines	Decides things for you that you should be allowed to decide (like what to wear or eat)
Humiliates you in front of others	Destroys your property or things that you care about
Threatens to hurt you, the children, or pets	Hurts you (by hitting, beating, pushing, shoving, punching, slapping, kicking, or biting)
Uses (or threatens to use) a weapon against you	Forces you to have sex against your will
Controls your birth control or insists that you get pregnant	Blames you for his or her violent outbursts
Threatens to harm himself or herself when upset with you	Says things like, "If I can't have you then no one can."

Source: U.S. Department of Health and Human Services (May 2011).

to initiate a discussion, coaching session, or to act as a patient navigator. Abuse can have serious emotional and physical effects.

You may also come in contact with additional forms of abuse, neglect, and exploitation. The nature of privileged communications in the relationship is that a patient has a right to expect his or her communications with his or her provider to be kept confidential. The privilege, however, is not without some exceptions. The provider is required by statutes in most states to report child abuse and elder abuse.

THE ROLE OF THE PATIENT NAVIGATOR OR ADVOCATE

The health care industry is quite complex. In order for patients to access and receive quality health care, a patient navigator can play a unique role in improving health outcomes. The **patient navigator** is the person who is able to assist a patient navigating the health system. A **patient advocate** is an impartial party who listens to the patient's concerns and provides them access to the systems in place that would resolve their conflict. A **case manager** is usually a registered nurse (RN) who can manage and consolidate the information acquired through multiple modalities.

In the role of patient navigator, the medical assistant will use and develop resource information, manage appointments, and provide referrals and follow up to available community resources. In addition, the medical assistant must be prepared to intervene on behalf of the patient regarding a variety of issues including financial matters, insurance information, procedures, and provider orders.

The patient navigator can help with care coordination, insurance resolution, and clinical advocacy. In order to create a less stressful environment for patients and their families, the patient navigator coordinates with patients, their medical team, and social workers.

Resource Information

In addition to patient navigation, additional resources should be made available, including appropriate patient brochures and informational materials. It is important to understand and utilize proper documentation of patient encounters and instruction. A medical assistant should be able to develop, assemble, and maintain appropriate brochures and informational materials.

Appointment Management

The medical assistant as the patient navigator helps set up future patient appointments with his or her provider, specialist(s), and for any procedures or testing ordered. Your responsibility would be to monitor and follow up to see that the patient kept all scheduled appointments and that the patient portal is available and explained to the patient for appointment management ease. In addition, you would make sure the patient has the phone number, address, and directions to any outside facilities he or she is visiting, set up reminder calls, and follow up with the patient after the outside visit, testing, or procedure.

Community Resources

There are times when the patient needs more than just coaching to improve their health and overall well-being. Patients may have physical, health, or financial constraints that limit their ability to comply with treatment plans. In such cases, the medical assistant may need to assist the patient in obtaining resources necessary for improving health and the quality of life.

At times, the patient may benefit from a support group. Support groups are especially useful for patients who have been diagnosed with a disease or condition that will greatly impact the patient's lifestyle or mental outlook. The medical office should have a listing of community resources that can assist patients in times of need.

Medical assistants can find many resources in the phonebook or on the Internet. Providing the patient the resources that are needed will assist in patient compliance and in improving the overall quality of the patient's life.

The patient navigator should keep an up-to-date index of the most frequently called numbers, as well as resources for patients, and emergency preparedness. Table 7-2 is an example of a list of some of the frequently called numbers in a medical office. You will be able to locate these resources through such means as office materials and directories, the Internet, intranet, and telephone book. Use the Internet and health system portals for access to telephone numbers and addresses to research available additional community resources for patient health services. (See Table 7-3 for sample lists. Please note that these are just a sampling of numbers that might be helpful, not a complete list.) This can be a good tool for researching not only local resources but also state and federal resources such as the CDC, Medicare, Department of Motor Vehicles (DMV), the Federal Emergency Management Agency (FEMA) and their website (www.ready.gov), a national public service advertising (PSA) campaign. You may also use such sources as the Yellow Pages (www.yellowpages.com) and MapQuest (www.mapquest.com). Using these search engines can often cut down on your research time and give you options if looking for multiple sites and locations. Keep a copy of the most current telephone book, as well as the current directory for the local emergency clinics, hospitals, providers (in network), and specialists, on hand in the office. In Procedure 7-2 you will develop a current list of community resources related to patients' health care needs.

Table 7-2 Frequently Called Numbers (Partial List)

911	Insurance companies	Answering services
Local hospital(s)	Referrals and authorizations department	Office manager
Ambulance/patient transport systems	Provider specialists	Pager/cell phone for provider
Lab services	Home health services	Quality department; HR department
IT department	Senior services	Office extensions
Pharmacies		

Table 7-3 Community Resources for Patient Health Care Needs (Partial List)

Senior services	Osteoporosis centers	Child protective services
Home health services	Research department	Emergency medical services
Lab services and locations	DMV	Education and training services
Diabetes programs	CDC (including vaccine information, travel advisories, etc.)	Public health department information (Department of Health and Human Services)
Battered women's shelter information	Hospice	Dietician
Adult day care centers	Transportation services	Physical therapy and occupational therapy services
Support group information: • Cancer support groups • Alzheimer support groups	Support group information: (continued): • Alcoholics Anonymous • Smoking cessation	Social service organizations
Mental health centers	Interpreting services	Pharmaceutical company phone and/or website information for free or reduced cost medications

Other factors should be considered when providing resources to a patient. The patient's level of education may dictate the most appropriate tool for the best success. The native language of the speaker will also affect which materials will be beneficial. For example, there are many resources available in multiple languages for non-English-speaking patients who indicate a language preference other than English. Having an employee fluent in the patient's spoken language or using an interpreter service will assist in instruction, allow for questions, and help verify understanding of the material.

Referrals to Community Resources

Having created a list of community resources, you will be responsible for facilitating referrals to community resources in the role of patient navigator (Procedure 7-3). Once you have initiated a referral, it must be fully documented in the patient's medical record (Figure 7-8). As patient navigator, you will follow up with the patient regarding the referral and confirm the patient attended his appointment and find out if any further visits, testing, or procedures are required, ask the patient if he has any questions, and complete any further appointments or referrals on his behalf.

Intervene on Behalf of the Patient

Many times patients are reluctant to seek medical care or face barriers to accessing quality health care. Intervention may be required to assist patients with clinical concerns such as understanding physician or provider order, medications, testing, and procedures. Barriers that are nonmedical may be related to income, health insurance (lack of or high deductible), transportation, cultural differences, and more. As patient navigator, it is your responsibility to intervene on behalf of the patient and find solutions to overcome barriers. Use the community resources available to you as you navigate the often difficult challenges patients may face. Utilize all of your professionalism skills as outlined in Chapter 1. Think of ways to incorporate these key skills in your role as patient navigator.

Transition of Care

Transition of care is the movement of a patient from one setting of care (hospital, ambulatory primary care practice, ambulatory specialty care practice, long-term care, home health, rehabilitation facility) to another. A provider who transitions or refers their patient to another setting of care or provider of care should provide summary care records for each transition of care or referral. Transition of care is Measure 7 of 9 of the Meaningful Use Menu Set Measures. The Joint Commission summarizes that health care organizations can do a better job in contacting the receiving provider to identify what information is required about the patient to ensure a safe transition, and that the need for collaboration was the most common

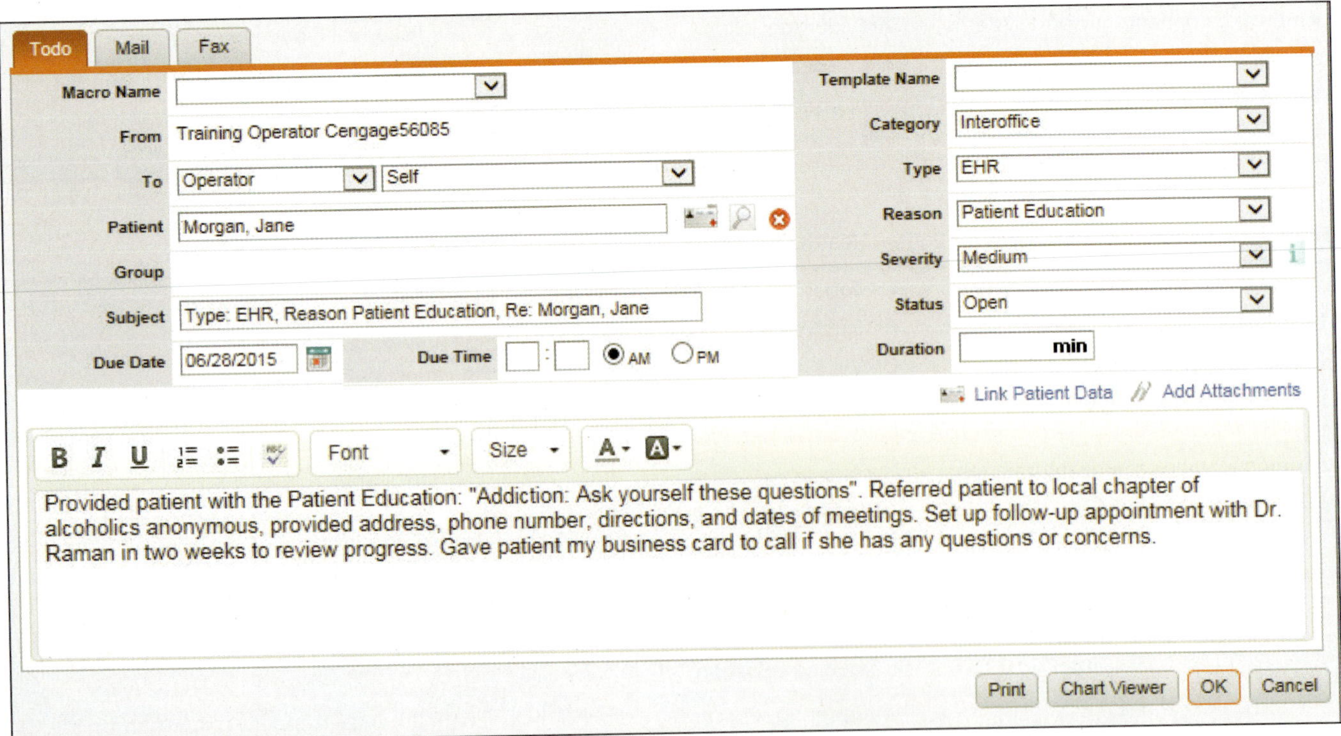
Todo | Mail | Fax

Macro Name:
From: Training Operator Cengage56085
To: Operator | Self
Patient: Morgan, Jane
Group:
Subject: Type: EHR, Reason Patient Education, Re: Morgan, Jane
Due Date: 06/28/2015 Due Time: : AM PM

Template Name:
Category: Interoffice
Type: EHR
Reason: Patient Education
Severity: Medium
Status: Open
Duration: min

Link Patient Data | Add Attachments

B I U Font Size

Provided patient with the Patient Education: "Addiction: Ask yourself these questions". Referred patient to local chapter of alcoholics anonymous, provided address, phone number, directions, and dates of meetings. Set up follow-up appointment with Dr. Raman in two weeks to review progress. Gave patient my business card to call if she has any questions or concerns.

Print | Chart Viewer | OK | Cancel

Figure 7-8 ■ EHR documentation of a patient referral to Alcoholics Anonymous. EHR digitally tracks the operator, date, and time of the documentation.

thread throughout transitions. To ensure safe transitions, planning is essential as is medication management, patient and family action/engagement, and a seamless transfer of information. As patient navigator, you will be implementing and monitoring the transition of care of your patients.

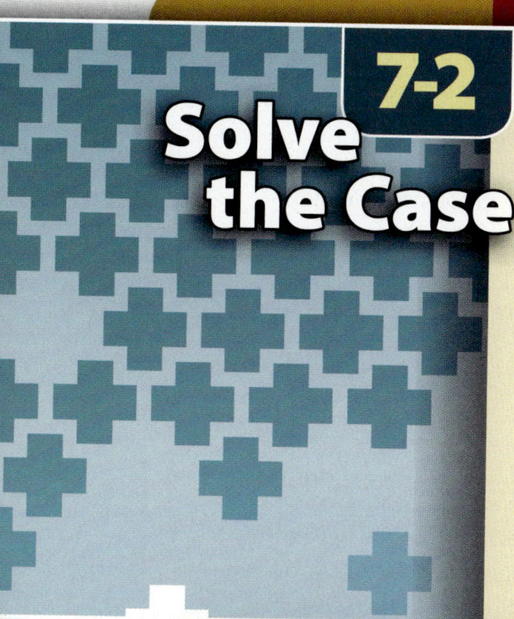

After completing her exam of Ms. Oslosky, Dr. Chang ordered a new prescription medication, Eliquis, to treat her Afib symptoms. While speaking to Ms. Oslosky about the newly prescribed medication, you notice that she appears even more stressed than she was before seeing Dr. Chang. She once again emphasizes that she has no medication coverage. There is no generic substitute for this drug, and it is important in the patient's recovery. Dr. Chang prescribed this medication because it does not require routine blood testing or dietary restrictions that other anticoagulants do.

1. **What should be your first course of action?**
2. **What are some additional actions that you may take or resources you can provide to assist the patient in getting some financial relief?**
3. **What should you do if the patient refuses assistance and states that she doesn't want the drug and that everyone would be much better off if she would die?**

PROCEDURE 7-1

Coach Patients Regarding Office Policies, Health Maintenance, Disease Management, and Disease Prevention

Objective:

To provide a successful health coaching session regarding office policies by collecting the appropriate learning materials, and obtaining the names and numbers of resources that can assist with compliance.

Equipment/Supplies:

- Learning tools (pamphlets, brochures, models, multimedia projector, computer, Internet access)
- Community resource information
- Patient's chart/EHR
- Black pen and paper

PROCEDURAL STEPS	DETAILS AND/OR RATIONALE
1. Read and clarify the order from the provider.	It is important to understand what the provider would like the patient to get out of the session.
2. Collect the learning tools necessary for the session.	
3. Collect numbers or email addresses of community resources, if applicable.	Patients that will need assistance such as in-home help or financial assistance with drugs should be given a list of resources for such services.

continues

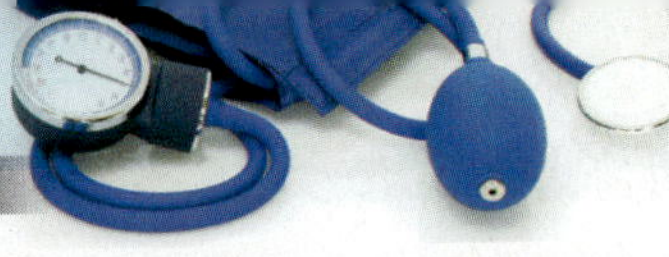

PROCEDURE 7-1 continued

PROCEDURAL STEPS	DETAILS AND/OR RATIONALE
4. Review the information and ask the provider questions if unclear about certain aspects of the material.	You cannot do an adequate job of coaching if you yourself do not understand the material that is being presented.
5. Set up the room so that everyone in the session has a seat and can see each other. Make certain that the room is free from distractions and has plenty of electrical outlets for necessary equipment.	Each individual should be able to see the presenter and each other to assist with communication.
6. Identify the patient using two identifiers. Identify any family members or friends who have accompanied the patient.	Family members will more than likely assist the patient with compliance.
7. Identify yourself and state your title.	
8. Explain the purpose of the session.	
9. Find out the patient's preferred learning style and set goals to determine what the patient and family members want to accomplish from the session. *If educating patients on office policies:* a. Go over policies regarding missed appointments, co-pays, and the privacy policy. b. Have patient sign privacy statement and establish who can have access to their information. c. Go over the patient bill of rights and the patient's responsibilities as a patient. d. Instruct patient how to use the patient portal and set up the patient's account if time permits. *If educating the patient on health maintenance and disease prevention:* a. Review patient's status on preventive testing and immunizations. b. Work on a plan for catching the patient up on these items. c. Discuss other health care goals with patient including BMI and nutrition goals. d. Provide patient with a copy of the goals. *If educating the patient on managing current disease:* a. Go over educational materials detailing the disease. b. Train the patient how to use any monitoring devices and how to properly administer his medications.	Assessing the patient's preferred learning style will assist you in knowing how to proceed with the presentation. Setting goals will help you know what the patient hopes to achieve from the session.
10. Present the information in a clear manner, checking with the patient and family members along the way to make certain that they have a clear understanding of what is being presented.	Having checkpoints throughout the session helps to ensure that the patient comprehends the material.

continues

PROCEDURE 7-1 continued

PROCEDURAL STEPS	DETAILS AND/OR RATIONALE
11. Summarize the information at the end of the session.	
12. Have the patient repeat the information. If a demonstration was incorporated into the session, have the patient demonstrate the procedure back to you.	This illustrates patient comprehension.
13. Praise the patient for acknowledgment of the material.	This helps to validate to the patient that the material has been comprehended.
14. If applicable, give the patient learning pamphlets, information sheets, prescriptions, and supplies, and provide a list of resources that can assist the patient with any special needs (Figure 7-9).	Giving the patient tools to take home will assist in patient compliance.
15. Give the patient your card or a piece of paper with your name and office phone number. Encourage the patient to call you with any questions.	Giving the patient your card lets the patient know that you care and want to be contacted.
16. Dismiss the patient and document the session.	

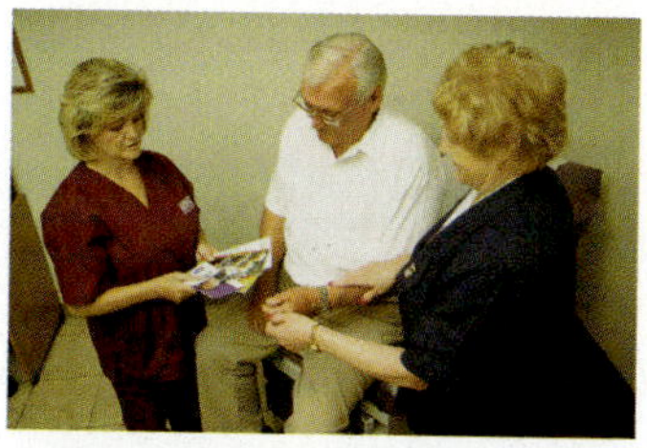

Figure 7-9 ■ The patient should be given pamphlets, brochures, and information sheets that will help with any questions the patient may have once home.

DOCUMENTATION EXAMPLE:

04-15-XX 0930	Educational session on diabetes management per Dr. Fisher. Pt.'s wife present for session. Gave pt. several educational brochures and names and numbers of organizations that may be able to assist pt. with obtaining free test strips and supplies. Also gave the pt. the names and numbers of several dieticians in the area and instructed pt. to set up an appointment with dietician in the next week. Pt. repeated back information, and stated that he would set up an appt with the dietician tomorrow. Encouraged pt. to call back with any questions. Sandy Jancowski, CMA (AAMA) --

PROCEDURE 7-2

Develop a Current List of Community Resources Related to Patients' Health Care Needs

Objective:

Use research tools and techniques to create a list of community resources related to patients' health care needs.

Equipment/Supplies:

- Computer with Internet access
- Telephone
- Telephone directory
- Local hospital directory
- Pen and paper, or computer with word processing program

continues

PROCEDURE 7-2 continued

PROCEDURAL STEPS	DETAILS AND/OR RATIONALE
1. Assemble required items (telephone, telephone directory, hospital directory, pen, paper, computer with Internet access).	
2. Using the telephone directory and Internet, research the community resources available in your area, create a list of available health care resources, and identify the services provided by each.	You might have to use more than one search engine and verify resources for accuracy.
3. Verify the information with a follow-up telephone call to the community resource for most current information to be documented.	Information might be outdated; you want to include the most current information available and update periodically.
4. Create a list in a spreadsheet format (using Microsoft Excel or Word, for instance). In the spreadsheet, identify the community resource(s), services provided, and contact information.	Refer to Table 7-2 as an example.
5. Print the resource document.	

PROCEDURE 7-3
Facilitate Referrals to Community Resources in the Role of a Patient Navigator

Objective:

Use research tools and techniques to facilitate referrals to community resources as a patient navigator.

Equipment/Supplies:

- Computer with Internet access
- Telephone
- Telephone directory
- Local hospital directory
- Pen and paper and patient's chart, or computer with EHR program

PROCEDURAL STEPS	DETAILS AND/OR RATIONALE
1. Assemble required items (telephone, telephone directory, pen, paper, computer with Internet access, patient's chart, or computer with EHR program).	
2. Using the telephone book, Internet, and current list of community resources created in Procedure 7-2 facilitate referral in the role of a patient navigator (coaching the patient during the referral process). ***Demonstrate respect for individual diversity.***	You might have to use more than one search engine and verify resources for accuracy. With patient in the exam room (or on the telephone), offer a variety of community resources that fit the scenario of a patient in an abusive environment needing referral to a women's shelter for domestic abuse.

continues

PROCEDURE 7-3 continued

PROCEDURAL STEPS	DETAILS AND/OR RATIONALE
3. Verify the information with the patient while in the exam room (or on the telephone). Then place a follow-up telephone call to the patient (or caller) following HIPAA guidelines within 48 hours, ***demonstrating empathy and active listening skills.***	Document the contact information (telephone numbers, websites, name of the facility, referral guidelines, etc.) in the patient's chart. Document the request for referral, the type of referral(s) made, and the results of the follow up contact.
4. Print the referral information and document in the patient's chart.	Refer to Table 7-3 as examples of community resources.
5. Give the patient your card or a piece of paper with your name and office phone number. Encourage the patient to call you with any questions.	Giving the patient your card lets the patient know that you care and want to be contacted.
6. Dismiss the patient and document the session.	

DOCUMENTATION EXAMPLE:

07-31-XX 1045	Patient navigator session: Gave pt. several brochures and names and numbers of organizations that may be able to assist pt. regarding abusive environment/domestic violence, counseling services, and social services. Made referral to Hearts to Hands Women Shelter. Arranged transportation to shelter, and an FCC LifeLine Assistance program cell phone. Set up follow up appointment with Dr. Ayerick next week. Pt. repeated back information, and stated that she would call back with any questions to clinic's 24-hour answering service. James Jackson, CMA (AAMA) ----------------------------

CHAPTER SUMMARY

- A health coach is a person who provides individualized evaluation and subsequent management and encouragement to achieve superior patient health outcomes. Health coaching involves the understanding and use of resources available to assist with educating the patient and demonstrating empathy and respect for patient concerns.
- Various resources may be utilized to enhance the educational (coaching) process include use of models, the Internet, brochures, pharmaceutical companies, pharmacists, and more.
- It is important to set the tone for communication at the start of the session. The medical assistant must always demonstrate respect for individual diversity including gender, race, religion, age, socioeconomic status, physical challenges, special needs, appearance, sexual orientation, lifestyle choices, and primary language. Be respectful of the patient and acknowledge family members.
- To be an effective health coach or patient navigator, you must demonstrate self-awareness and the principles of self-boundaries. Consider nonverbal cues given by the patient so that you are aware of and respect his or her boundaries. Using adaptive coping skills as a tool for self-awareness will have a direct impact on both your and your patient's behavior.
- Health coaching focuses on the dissemination of information such as office policies, teaching patients and their family's basic hygienic practices, health maintenance and disease prevention topics, and pre-op and post-op care instructions.

As health coach you will also provide support for terminally ill patients, be able to recognize substance abuse and domestic violence, and provide necessary coaching and resources.

- In the role of patient navigator, the medical assistant will use and develop resource information, manage appointments, and provide referrals and follow up to available community resources. In addition, the medical assistant must be prepared to intervene on behalf of the patient regarding a variety of issues including financial matters, insurance information, procedures, and provider orders.
- The patient navigator can help with care coordination, insurance resolution, and clinical advocacy. In order to create a less stressful environment for patients and their families, the patient navigator coordinates with patients, their medical team, and social workers.
- Transition of care is the movement of a patient from one setting of care (hospital, ambulatory primary care practice, ambulatory specialty care practice, long-term care, home health, rehabilitation facility) to another. To ensure safe transitions, planning is essential as is medication management, patient and family action/engagement, and a seamless transfer of information. As patient navigator, you will be implementing and monitoring the transition of care of your patient(s).

CERTIFICATION REVIEW QUESTIONS

1. A barrier to a successful patient education session would be:
   a. time.
   b. money.
   c. interest.
   d. All of the above

2. Tips for patient compliance include all of the following except:
   a. preventing family members from being in the room during the education session.
   b. looking for indications that the patient understands and agrees with the material being presented.
   c. being a good role model.
   d. giving the patient related supplies.

3. A ____________________ is usually a registered nurse who can manage and consolidate the information acquired through multiple modalities.
   a. patient navigator
   b. health coach
   c. patient advocate
   d. case manager

4. When acting as a health coach, inevitably there will be challenges and patient concerns. Which of the following may be a patient concern you may encounter?
   a. Fear of dying
   b. Fear of diagnosis
   c. Financial concerns
   d. All of the above

5. Which of the following would not be considered a possible indication of substance abuse?
   a. Frugal with money
   b. Neglected appearance
   c. Change in behavior
   d. Frequently missing school or work

6. To be an effective health coach or patient navigator, you must demonstrate self-awareness and the principles of self-boundaries. Which of the following is an example of boundary issues?
   a. When someone gets too close, you take a step forward.
   b. Never blaming others for your problems.
   c. Telling others how to act or what to think.
   d. All of the above

7. Which of the following is not generally one of the possible signs that a patient may be suffering abuse from her partner?
   a. Humiliates patient in front of others.
   b. Destroys patient's property or things that she cares about.
   c. Exhibits no interest in what patient is doing.
   d. Prevents or discourages patient from seeing friends or family.

8. Which of the following examples is not one of the five stages when dealing with grief, especially with a terminally ill patient?
   a. The person is trying to shut out the reality and magnitude of their situation, often creating a false reality.
   b. Patients may become difficult to care for because of the misplaced feelings of anger for what has happened to them.
   c. The patient believes that somehow they cannot undo what has happened by changing their lifestyle.
   d. The patient has come to terms with the inevitable future and plans accordingly in preparation for their impending death.

9. To ensure a safe transition of care, which of the following would be considered an essential component?
   a. Planning
   b. Medication management
   c. Patient and family action/engagement
   d. All of the above

10. The medical assistant as patient navigator helps set up patient appointments. Which of the following would not be considered a role for the medical assistant as patient navigator?
   a. Monitor and follow up to see that the patient kept all scheduled appointments.
   b. Direct the patient to the portal to make his or her own appointments.
   c. Make sure the patient has the phone number, address, and directions to any outside facilities he or she is visiting.
   d. Set up reminder calls, and follow up with patient after the outside visit, testing, or procedure.

STUDY RESOURCES

Resources to Test and Reinforce Your Knowledge:	
Certification Review Questions	Take this end-of-chapter quiz
Workbook	• Complete the activities for Chapter 7 • Perform the procedures for Chapter 7 using the Competency Checklists
Resources to Promote Critical Thinking:	
***Solve the Case* Activities**	• Consider these case studies and discuss your conclusion
Learning Lab	• Module 4: Professional Communications
MindTap	• Complete Chapter 7 readings and activities

REFERENCES

Blesi, M. (2017). *Medical Assisting: Administrative & Clinical Competencies* (8th ed.). Clifton Park, NY: Cengage Learning.

Centers for Disease Control and Prevention (Oct. 2104). Clean Hands Save Lives. Retrieved April 26, 2015, from http://www.cdc.gov/handwashing/when-how-handwashing.html

Centers for Disease Control and Prevention (2014). Elder Abuse: Definitions. http://www.cdc.gov/violenceprevention/elderabuse/definitions.html. Retrieved August 19, 2014.

Centers for Medicare and Medicaid Services (May 2014). Transition of Care Summary. Retrieved April 26, 2015, from http://www.cms.gov/Regulations-and-Guidance/Legislation/EHRIncentivePrograms/downloads/8_Transition_of_Care_Summary.pdf

Ferry Jr., Robert MD (n.d.). Diabetic Home Care and Monitoring. Retrieved April 27, 2015, from http://www.medicinenet.com/diabetic_home_care_and_monitoring/page2.htm

Finn, Leila (June 2013). Integrative Health Coaching. Retrieved April 27, 2015. from http://www.diabetesselfmanagement.com/about-diabetes/diabetes-basics/integrative-health-coaching/

Mayo Clinic (Aug. 2014). Bone Density Test. Retrieved April 26, 2015, from http://www.mayoclinic.org/tests-procedures/bone-density-test/basics/definition/prc-20020254

Mayo Clinic (Dec. 2014). Diseases and Conditions Drug Addiction. Retrieved April 26, 2015, from http://www.mayoclinic.org/diseases-conditions/drug-addiction/basics/symptoms/con-20020970

Merriam-Webster Dictionary (n.d.). Definition of Substance Abuse. Retrieved April 26, 2015, from www.merriam-webster.com/dictionary/substance%20abuse

Minnesota Department of Health (n.d.). Cover Your Cough. Retrieved April 26, 2015, from http://www.health.state.mn.us/divs/idepc/dtopics/infectioncontrol/cover/gen/cycpgeneng.pdf

National Center for Emerging and Zoonotic Infectious Diseases (NCEZID) (Oct. 2008). Hands Together. Retrieved April 26, 2015, from http://www.cdc.gov/CDCTV/HandsTogether/

National Institutes of Health (Nov. 2013). Bone Mineral Density Test. Retrieved April 26, 2015, from http://www.nlm.nih.gov/medlineplus/ency/article/007197.htm

National Institutes of Health: Senior Heath (March 2013). What is Osteoporosis? Retrieved April 26, 2015, from http://nihseniorhealth.gov/osteoporosis/whatisosteoporosis/01.html and http://nihseniorhealth.gov/osteoporosis/whatisosteoporosis/video/osteo5_na_intro.html

The Administration for Children and Families and the Administration on Aging in the U.S. Department of Health and Human Services (1998). The National Elder Abuse Incidence Study. http://www.aoa.gov/AoARoot/AoA_Programs/Elder_Rights/Elder_Abuse/docs/ABuseReport_Full.pdf. Retrieved August 19, 2014.

The Joint Commission (n.d.). Transitions of Care: The Need for Collaboration across Entire Care Continuum. Retrieved April 26, 2015, from http://www.jointcommission.org/assets/1/6/TOC_Hot_Topics.pdf

U.S. Department of Health and Human Services. Office of Women's Health (May 2011). Violence against Women. Retrieved April 26, 2015, from http://www.womenshealth.gov/violence-against-women/am-i-being-abused/

8

Principles of Infection Control

CHAPTER OUTLINE

Medical Abbreviation Review

The Infection Process

The Infection Cycle

- Infectious (Causative) Agents
- Reservoir
- Susceptible Host
- Means of Transmission
- Portal of Entry
- Portal of Exit

Environmental Requirements for Microorganisms

Stages of Infection

- Invasion and Multiplication Stage
- Incubation Stage
- Prodromal Stage
- Acute Stage
- Declining Stage
- Convalescent Stage

The Body's Natural Defenses

- The Process of Inflammation
- The Immune System
- The Immune Response
- Types of Immunity
- Immunizations
- Types of Vaccines

Infection Control

- Medical Asepsis
- Surgical Asepsis

Universal Blood and Body Fluid Precautions

- Standard Precautions
- The Biohazard Label
- Transmission-Based Precautions

Bloodborne Diseases

- HIV/AIDS
- Hepatitis

OSHA Regulations

- Bloodborne Pathogens Standard
- Blood, Body Fluids, and OPIM
- Exposure Determination
- Exposure Control Plan
- Regulated Waste

Exposure to Hazardous Chemicals

- OSHA's Chemical Hygiene Plan

Safeguards in the Educational Environment

ESSENTIAL TERMS

antibody
antigen
asepsis
aseptic technique
biohazard
bloodborne pathogens
body substance isolation (BSI)
cell-mediated immunity
Centers for Disease Control and Prevention (CDC)
disinfection
epidemiology
endospores
exposure control
fomites
humoral immunity
immunoglobulin
immunosuppressed
infectious waste
inflammatory response
medical asepsis
normal flora
Occupational Safety and Health Administration (OSHA)
opportunistic infections
other potentially infectious material (OPIM)
pathogen
personal protective equipment (PPE)
resistance
sanitization
sharps
Standard Precautions
sterilization
surgical asepsis
Transmission-Based Precautions
Universal Precautions
vector
work practice controls

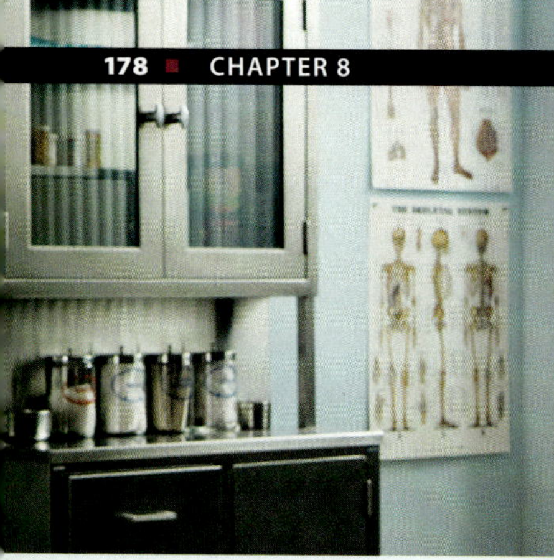

DEVELOPMENTAL OBJECTIVES

After completing this chapter, you should be able to:

1. Correctly spell and define the essential terms.
2. Illustrate and describe the six steps in the infection cycle.
3. Name five types of infectious agents and categorize two diseases within each classification.
4. Clarify six conditions that infectious agents need in order to grow and explain how controlling those conditions can interrupt their life cycle.
5. Match the six stages of infection with their characteristics.
6. Discuss seven of the body's natural barriers to combat invaders and categorize them into either mechanical or chemical.
7. Describe and explain the inflammatory response, differentiating it from infection.
8. Describe the four different types of immunity and cite an example of each.
9. List and describe the four different forms of vaccines available.
10. Compare and contrast medical and surgical asepsis.
11. Demonstrate proper handwashing technique.
12. Define the principles of Standard Precautions.
13. Explain the means of transmission for HIV, its four stages of infection, and the criteria used to diagnose AIDS.
14. List the three most common types of hepatitis and explain how each is transmitted.
15. Summarize the development of OSHA's Bloodborne Pathogen Standard.
16. Participate in bloodborne pathogen training.
17. List six examples of body fluids and other potentially infectious material (OPIM).
18. Select appropriate types of PPE and clarify when each should be worn.
19. Develop a written employee exposure control plan.
20. Design a poster for the proper protocol for disposal of regulated waste.
21. Explain an MSDS/SDS manual and categorize the information it contains.
22. Compile a list of safeguards to be followed in your medical assistant program laboratory.
23. Recognize the implications of not complying with CDC and OSHA regulations.

INTRODUCTION

One of the most important objectives in the ambulatory care setting is to prevent the spread of infectious disease. This chapter will discuss the infection process as well as infection control standards and guidelines developed by the **Centers for Disease Control and Prevention (CDC)** and the **Occupational Safety and Health Administration (OSHA)**. For our own protection and the protection of our patients, coworkers, and the public, we must respect and strictly comply with these guidelines.

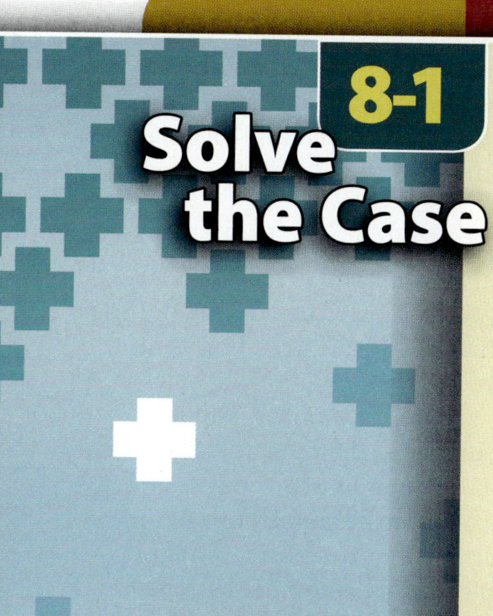

Susan Groves is in the office today to discuss her lab results, which were drawn during her last visit. The physician contacted her by phone to tell her that she was positive for hepatitis C. The purpose of today's visit is to discuss a treatment plan. Susan appears very upset during the screening portion of the exam. She explains that she used illegal drugs in the past, many years ago, but has been clean and sober for the past 12 years. She had surgery last year for a total knee replacement and is positive that is where she contracted the virus. She asks you if you agree with her assessment. She also asks you if she is going to die.

1. **Why is it a possibility that Susan could have obtained the virus from either the illegal drug use or knee replacement surgery?**
2. **Based on your current knowledge, which scenario seems more probable for where Susan obtained the virus and why?**
3. **How would you respond to Susan's queries regarding how she contracted the virus and whether or not she is going to die?**

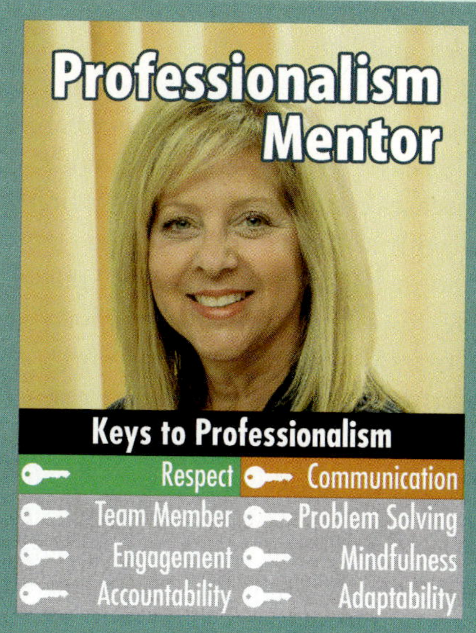

There are a lot of reasons to wash your hands when working in health care. Hopefully you are one of the diligent medical assistants who remembers to foam in and foam out each time you enter an exam room. What would you do if one of your coworkers failed to wash his hands each time he entered and exited an exam room? You know it's the right thing to do and that washing your hands is the best way to prevent the spread of infection. What if it was the provider who failed to wash her hands? Would you feel comfortable telling her not to forget to use good hand hygiene? In your professional journal, put in writing some of the phrases you might use to tactfully remind other providers to wash their hands. Are there any keys or components of keys not listed at the beginning of this mentor box that you feel is necessary in order to be successful in encouraging your co-workers to change their behavior. ■

Table 8-1 Common Abbreviations Associated with Asepsis and Sterilization

Abbreviation	Meaning	Abbreviation	Meaning
AIDS	Acquired immunodeficiency syndrome	OSHA	Occupational Safety and Health Administration
BSI	Body substance isolation	OPIM	Other potentially infectious material
CDC	Centers for Disease Control and Prevention	PPE	Personal protective equipment

MEDICAL ABBREVIATION REVIEW

Medical assistants working in the clinical areas should be familiar with the medical abbreviations associated with asepsis and sterilization as listed in Table 8-1.

THE INFECTION PROCESS

In earlier centuries, infectious diseases were the most common causes of death. Many lives were lost to diseases such as smallpox, tuberculosis, pneumonia, and influenza. **Epidemiology** (the study of infectious diseases), sanitization practices, and the development of vaccines have helped us prevent and control most illnesses.

Microorganisms are present everywhere in our environment—on our bodies, furniture, books, handles, clothing, and even in the food and water supply. Some microorganisms are helpful and necessary for normal life processes of plants, animals, and humans. These microorganisms are called **normal flora**. Microorganisms that cause disease are known as **pathogens** or infectious agents and are able to enter our bodies and multiply, often causing us to become sick.

THE INFECTION CYCLE

For a communicable disease to be infectious from one person to another, a definite series of steps known as the infection cycle must take place (Figure 8-1). An interruption to any of the links in the cycle will stop the infection process.

Medical assistants who are familiar with the steps in the cycle of infection can prevent the spread of many diseases by simply breaking the cycle.

The elements in the infection cycle are as follows:

- Infectious agent
- Reservoir or source
- Portal of Exit
- Means of transmission
- Portal of entry
- Susceptible Host

Infectious (Causative) Agents

In order to design an appropriate treatment plan for a patient with an infectious disease, it is first necessary to identify the pathogen that caused the disease, in other words, the causative agent. Infectious organisms are divided into five different classifications: bacteria, viruses, protozoa, fungi, and parasites.

Bacteria

Bacteria are microscopic, single-celled organisms that do not have a nucleus, yet are capable of carrying out everyday life functions. Bacteria are the most prevalent of all organisms and live everywhere—in soil, water, plants, and in animals, as well as humans. Millions of bacteria live on the surface of the human skin, in mucous membranes of the nose and mouth, and in the gastrointestinal tract. Bacteria can be nonpathogenic or pathogenic in nature. Normal flora, described earlier in the chapter, is an example of nonpathogenic bacteria. Interestingly, normal flora, which is normally harmless and even helpful to us, can become harmful and even deadly if transferred to different parts of our bodies. *Escherichia coli* is a current example. *E. coli* is normally and naturally present in the colon (large intestine) but can be dangerously infective if it enters our mouth through contaminated food, water, or unwashed hands.

Rickettsia is a type of bacteria that is generally transmitted by fleas, ticks, and lice.

Diseases caused by pathogenic bacteria include strep throat, tuberculosis, *E. coli* poisoning, tetanus, bacterial pneumonia, Lyme disease, and bacterial meningitis.

Luckily, most diseases caused by bacterial pathogens can be combatted with antibiotics or our body's own immune systems. Some bacteria are extremely resilient by creating unique resting phases called **endospores**, which can live for years in dry, non-nutrient areas, and then burst to growth and propagation when exposed to moist nutrients. Endospores are very difficult to destroy due to their impermeable coating. This coating surrounds the spore, protecting it from many environmental factors including heat, ultraviolet radiation, chemicals, acids, and drying. The only methods that can eliminate endospores altogether are steam under

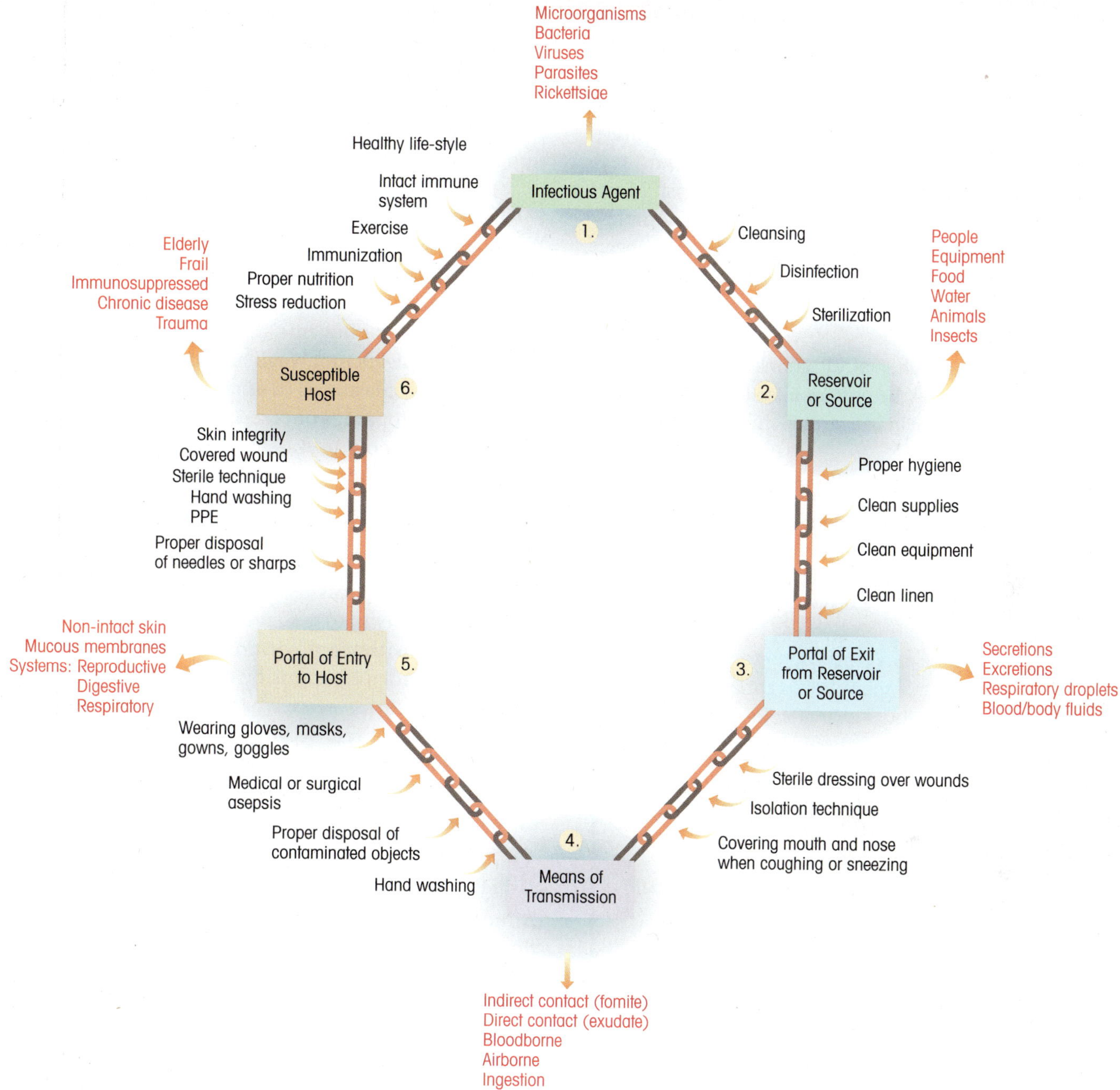

Figure 8-1 ■ The infection cycle.

pressure (autoclaving, which will be discussed under Sterilization Techniques in Chapter 9), certain gases such as ethyl oxide, some chemical sterilization agents, and prolonged exposure to radiation.

Tetanus, anthrax, and botulism are examples of illnesses caused by bacteria that create spores.

Viruses

Viruses are the smallest of all living pathogenic organisms, about a thousand times smaller than bacteria. They are often referred to as *nonliving* because they lack the enzymes necessary for many independent life processes. They need a living host in order to divide and multiply. Because viruses need a living cell within the body in order to reproduce, they are classified as intracellular parasites.

Viruses function by changing bits of genetic material (like DNA and RNA) within the cells they invade. They possess the unusual quality of being able to change certain characteristics of cells and, over time, are capable of adapting to their surroundings. This quality makes it difficult to develop drugs to cure a viral infection since they are constantly changing and treatments that kill the viruses also kill the body cells they are living in.

Viruses can "live" outside of a host body for a brief period of time, from minutes to 24 hours, depending on the surface it is on and the type of virus, but they are incredibly weak until they enter a living host. Most viral diseases are spread by direct contact. Examples of diseases caused by viruses include colds, influenza, HIV, and chicken pox.

Protozoa

Protozoa are the smallest of all animals, and most are microscopic. They may be present in soil, water, and animals. They are parasitic in nature, ingesting bacteria, fungi, and even other protozoa. They can be either pathogenic or nonpathogenic, and are actually environmentally helpful by making and giving off nitrogen that plants can use. They can cause diseases, though, such as malaria, dysentery, trichomoniasis, and toxoplasmosis (transmitted through cat feces).

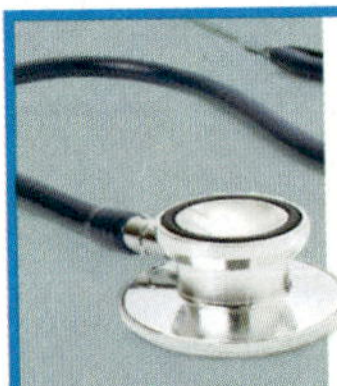

> **Field Smarts**
>
> Normal flora in the body helps to control the growth of yeast in the body. This is because the normal flora and yeast compete for the same nourishment. When patients take antibiotics over a prolonged period of time or take large doses of antibiotics, the antibiotics can kill helpful bacteria as well as the targeted pathogenic bacteria. Without good bacteria, there is room for yeast to multiply, and this may eventually cause what is referred to as a yeast infection. The types of yeast infections most commonly manifested in patients during or following antibiotic therapy include thrush (a yeast infection of the mouth) and vaginal yeast infections. If the antibiotic destroys the good bacteria needed in the digestive system, the patient can experience cramping and diarrhea. Sometimes replacing the intestinal bacteria by eating live active culture yogurts, acidophilus supplements, and other probiotics can be helpful, although used with caution in some conditions. Your physician/clinic will establish protocol for you to follow in educating patients on helpful treatments. Of course, preventing dehydration with diarrhea is always good advice.

Fungi

Fungi, which include yeast and molds, develop as single cells (unicellular) or multiple cells (multicellular). Some fungi are nonpathogenic, such as mushrooms, while others are pathogenic, causing conditions such as ringworm, athlete's foot, vaginal and other yeast infections, and histoplasmosis (a lung infection transmitted through the droppings of certain birds and bats). Yeast infections are most prevalent in patients with weakened immune systems, pregnant women, and people with diabetes. Fungi also create endospores.

Parasites

Parasites are organisms that must live in or on another organism to receive their nutrients. Parasites may be pathogenic or nonpathogenic. Parasitic diseases include infections by tiny protozoa, but also worms (pinworms, tapeworms, and hookworms) and arthropods (lice, bedbugs, and scabies), many of which are not microscopic. Some diseases are caused directly by the parasite, others by the toxins the parasite releases.

Reservoir

Almost anything can serve as a reservoir in the infection cycle. Humans, animals, **vectors** (carriers such as insects or rodents), water, food, surfaces, and equipment can all be reservoirs in the spread of infectious diseases. The following actions can be taken to break the cycle at the reservoir link:

- Wash hands frequently.
- Disinfect work surfaces, equipment, and supplies that are potentially contaminated by the infectious agent.
- Wear gloves and other **personal protective equipment (PPE)** while working with blood and other body fluids.

Portal of Exit

In order for a pathogen to be spread from one person to the next, it must have a portal of exit, meaning it must have a way to leave an infected individual. Often times, the portals of exit and entry are the same. Pathogens can leave the body through fluids or drainage in the respiratory tract, gastrointestinal tract, urinary tract, skin, reproductive tract, and mucous membranes. Patients should be advised to cover their mouth while coughing or sneezing, wash their hands frequently, refrain from direct contact with another when infected, and to keep open wounds properly bandaged.

Means of Transmission

The pathogen must have a method of moving from one individual to another—a mode of transmission. Sometimes, this method will depend on the type of microorganism. There are numerous means of transmission, and they are often redundant and very similar. Some of the more common are listed here:

- Direct contact occurs when an infected person transmits pathogens to another individual through physical contact. This contact can include kissing, sexual contact, or coming into direct contact with drainage or blood from an open wound on an infected individual.
- Indirect contact occurs through ingestion of contaminated foods or drinks, poor handwashing after bathroom use, vectors, and **fomites**, which are contaminated nonliving objects such as water glasses, computer keyboards, telephones, doorknobs, dressings, catheter tubing, needles, and IV tubing.
- Airborne transmission occurs when a pathogen is transmitted through the air. This can be raising dust and air pollutant through air conditioners, vents, or from biological waste deposited in enclosed areas such as attics and basements.
- Droplet transmission occurs when an infected person sneezes or coughs. Tiny droplets containing the pathogen can be carried on air currents and may settle on surfaces.
- Inhalation transmission occurs when a person inhales the pathogen, which may be airborne or droplet.
- Vertical transmission is from mother to child, in utero, through breast milk or during birthing.
- Iatrogenic transmission is due to medical treatments, procedures, injections, and surgeries.

Portal of Entry

When the pathogen is transmitted, it must find a portal of entry in a new host. Pathogens may be inhaled through the respiratory tract, ingested through the gastrointestinal tract, absorbed through an open wound in the skin, or transmitted through sexual contact. The medical assistant and other health care professionals should practice careful aseptic techniques at all times to prevent pathogens from finding a portal of entry. Examples of portal-of-entry prevention are the use of face shields, wound bandages, and gloves.

Susceptible Host

Numerous factors determine whether a person is susceptible to a pathogen once it enters the body. General physical and emotional health and underlying disease conditions are all factors that cause a person to be susceptible to illness. Patients who are **immunosuppressed** (meaning that their immune system has been suppressed or weakened) or who have undergone trauma or surgical procedure are especially at risk. Susceptible patients should be taught ways to avoid exposure and prevent infections. Maintaining a healthy lifestyle with good nutrition, fresh air and exercise, positive emotional health, personal hygiene, and adhering to the recommended immunization schedule can all help lessen the body's susceptibility to disease.

Table 8-2 provides information on some infectious diseases, including the causative agents, means of transmission, and recommended patient care.

ENVIRONMENTAL REQUIREMENTS FOR MICROORGANISMS

Several conditions must exist for microorganisms to survive and prosper, including the following:

- Microorganisms must have certain nutrients to grow. Organic materials within the body and in body fluids provide many types of microorganisms with their nutritional needs.
- Some microorganisms grow best without oxygen and are referred to as anaerobes. Microorganisms that are dependent on oxygen are referred to as aerobes. Some can grow in either environment and are referred to as facultative aerobes.
- Optimal temperatures will vary from one microorganism to the next, but most microorganisms thrive at normal body temperatures (98.6°F or 37°C). However, ranges can fluctuate between 77°F and 104°F (25°C and 40°C).
- Most microorganisms grow best in neutral pH environments (approximately 7.0 on the pH scale), but this will vary depending on the microorganism.
- Most microorganisms grow best in darkness.
- Moisture provides a good environment for microorganisms to grow and multiply, as it facilitates cell metabolism.

Interrupting the optimum growth requirements will interfere with the ability of the pathogens to thrive and is the basis of **sanitization** (cleaning), **disinfection**

Table 8-2 Common Infectious Diseases

Disease	Causative Agent	Means of Transmission	Patient Care
HIV/AIDS	HIV (virus)	Unprotected sex, needle sticks from a contaminated needle, and mother to fetus	Antiviral drugs, supportive care, management of symptoms
Chlamydia	*Chlamydia trachomatis* (bacteria)	Primarily sexual and mother to infant contact	Antibiotics
Chicken pox	Varicella zoster (virus)	Airborne	Supportive care, antiviral drugs
Ebola	Ebola virus	Bloodborne and body fluids, unprotected contact with blood and body fluids and vectors	IV fluids, supportive care, treating other infections as they occur
E. coli infection (gastritis, systemic)	*Escherichia coli* (bacteria)	Foodborne, person-to-person through poor hygiene/ handwashing. Normally found in the lower intestinal tract of animals and humans.	Antibiotics, supportive care, treat dehydration and other symptoms
Enteroviruses(severe respiratory illness)	Hundreds of types, enterovirus EV-D68 specifically	Carried in the intestinal tract, spread by close contact	No vaccine, no antibiotics, self-limiting, supportive care
Gonorrhea (STD)	*Neisseria gonorrhea* (bacteria)	Unprotected sex, direct contact with exudates of mucous membranes	Antibiotics
Hepatitis A (liver inflammation)	HAV (virus)	Contaminated food, water	Supportive care, rest, nutrition
Hepatitis B (liver inflammation)	HBV (virus)	Blood or body fluids	Antiviral medication, interferon, liver transplant
Hepatitis C (liver inflammation)	HCV (virus)	Bloodborne	Medication, liver transplant
Influenza (respiratory illness)	Influenza viruses A, B, C	Inhalation of droplets and transmission through contact with fomites	Supportive care, treatment of symptoms
Legionnaires' disease (respiratory illness)	*Legionella pneumophila* (bacteria)	Airborne from soil or water source	Antibiotics
Lyme disease (systemic infection)	*Borrelia burgdorferi* (bacteria)	Vector (deer ticks)	Antibiotics
Meningococcal (spinal) meningitis (infection of membranes in CNS)	*Neisseria meningitidis* (bacteria)	Airborne inhalation of respiratory droplets, direct contact with patient's respiratory secretions	Antibiotics
Salmonellosis (gastritis, food poisoning)	*Salmonella* (bacteria)	Foodborne, infected animals, turtles, iguanas, some reptiles	Supportive care, treatment of symptoms, antibiotics as needed
Shigellosis (gastritis, food poisoning)	*Shigella* (bacteria)	Person-to-person, contact with infected feces, foodborne, waterborne	Antibiotics as needed, supportive care, treat dehydration
Tetanus (nervous system infection)	*Clostridium tetani* (bacteria)	Puncture wounds or cuts	Supportive care, treatment of symptoms
Tuberculosis (initially respiratory)	*Mycobacterium tuberculosis* (bacteria)	Droplet inhalation	Long-term antibiotic therapy often monitored for compliance

(destroy microorganisms usually through chemical means), and **sterilization** (process that destroys even the toughest of microorganisms usually through steam under pressure) to be discussed in Chapter 9. Maintaining clean, dry surfaces will deny pathogens nutrients and moisture. Plenty of light and fresh air, or creating an anaerobic environment, raising or lowering the pH, and applying heat are all measures that will interfere with the life cycle of pathogens.

STAGES OF INFECTION

When a person becomes infectious, there are several stages that occur. Each stage has its own characteristics although each stage might not always be distinct or obvious. Sometimes the type and duration of treatments will depend on which stage the patient is in.

Invasion and Multiplication Stage

The invasion and multiplication stage is the first stage of the infection process. During this stage, the pathogenic microorganism enters the body and begins to multiply. There may be no identifiable signs or symptoms during this stage.

Incubation Stage

The period of time between exposure to the pathogen and the appearance of the first signs and symptoms of the disease is known as the incubation stage. Some diseases have a short incubation period while in others this stage can last for years.

Prodromal Stage

The prodromal stage is the interval of time between the appearance of first signs and symptoms and the appearance of definitive symptoms such as fever and rash. During this stage, the patient may present with a general complaint of malaise and often isn't aware he is sick.

Acute Stage

The infection process reaches its peak during the acute stage. This is usually when the patient will seek medical assistance. During this stage, symptoms are usually well developed and obvious, which helps with a diagnosis.

Declining Stage

During the declining stage, symptoms begin to subside. The infection is still present; however, the patient begins to return to the previous state of health.

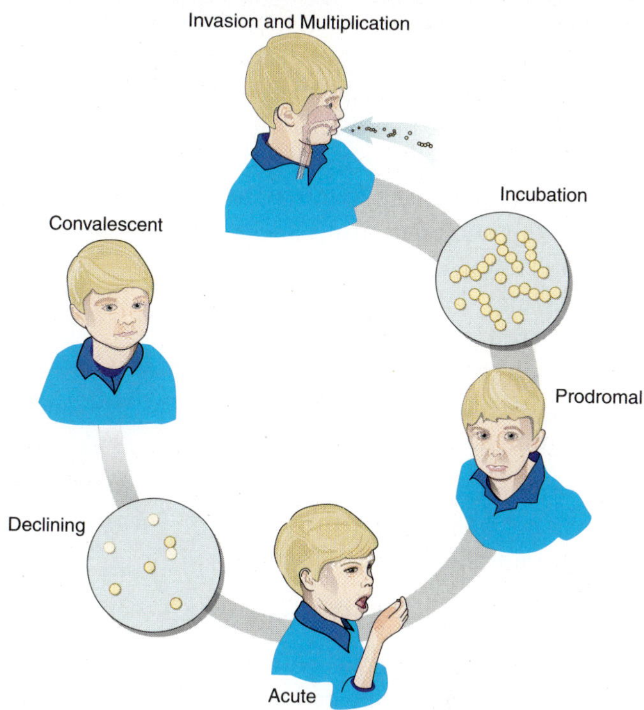

Figure 8-2 ■ The stages of infection.

Convalescent Stage

The convalescent stage is the point at which the patient recovers from the infectious disease and returns to the original state of health.

Refer to Figure 8-2 for a synopsis of the stages of infection.

THE BODY'S NATURAL DEFENSES

Our bodies have many internal and external defenses to protect us against infectious diseases. These defense mechanisms may be nonspecific (to combat all and any threats) or very specific against one particular pathogen. Sometimes these defense mechanisms are able to completely ward off an infection. At other times, the pathogens multiply, gain strength, and overcome our body's defenses.

Physical and chemical nonspecific barriers that assist in preventing infection include the following:

- Intact skin keeps contamination and microorganisms from entering deeper tissue.
- Eyelids, eyelashes, and eyebrows help to keep debris and foreign matter away from the eye.
- Tears wash debris out of the eye and contain an enzyme to protect against pathogens.

- Mucous membranes secrete mucus within the respiratory tract, genital structures, and gastrointestinal (GI) tract that help to trap microorganisms, and white blood cells within the mucus assist in destroying pathogenic microorganisms.
- Cilia are small hairs found in the respiratory tract that trap microorganisms and continually sweep debris toward the outside of the body.
- Coughing and sneezing reflexes help rid the body of microorganisms.
- Acids in the stomach and vagina provide a hostile environment that hinders the growth of microorganisms.

In addition to these barriers, the body's two primary defense mechanisms are the process of inflammation and the immune system.

The Process of Inflammation

The changes that occur within body tissues as a response to an injury or a pathogen invasion are known as inflammation. The **inflammatory response** is the body's attempt to protect itself from microorganisms that enter the body and to heal and replace injured tissue. The terms *inflammation* and *infection* are not synonymous. Inflammation is the body's natural reaction to injury. Infection is caused by a pathogen. A person can have inflammation without infection; however, a person cannot have infection without inflammation. Signs and symptoms of inflammation may be classified as local or systemic. Table 8-3 differentiates local signs of inflammation from systemic signs of inflammation.

Sometimes the process of inflammation is not adequate enough to stop the infection. This is indicated by the formation of pus, the swelling of the lymph nodes, and a systemic feeling of illness. At this point, medical intervention might be needed.

The Immune System

The immune system is a complex system that guards the body against pathogens and abnormal cell growth (which stimulates conditions such as cancer). The immune system works like a small military defense system within our bodies, with each component having a specific function. The immune system works to recognize, suppress, fight, and remove pathogens. The main components of the immune system are the white blood cells, specifically macrophages (that engulf or swallow up pathogens), and lymphocytes known as T-cells and B-cells. Protein particles known as antibodies are produced by the lymphocytes to promote immunity and provide **resistance** to specific pathogens.

The Immune Response

When a pathogen enters the body, it is recognized as a foreign invader and the immune system begins to respond. Two immune responses may occur; cell-mediated immunity and humoral immunity. These mechanisms help us create immunity to certain diseases.

During **cell-mediated immunity**, T-cells, which are white blood cells that mature in the thymus gland or tonsils and are stored in lymph tissue, become activated. These specialized lymphocytes are involved in attacks against cancer cells and infections caused by fungi and viruses. They are also the cells responsible for delayed hypersensitivity reactions associated with organ transplants. This type of immune response is referred to as cell-mediated because the T-cells are directly involved in the attack.

During **humoral immunity**, B-cell lymphocytes that are stored in lymph tissue produce **antibodies** that neutralize rather than destroy the **antigen** (the invading antagonistic organism) directly, like the T-cell does. Antibodies are specially designed by the B-cells so that they can lock directly into the antigen, similar to interlocking jigsaw puzzle pieces (Figure 8-3). The antibody is able to release chemicals that flag the antigen for destruction.

Types of Immunity

Following exposure to an infectious disease, the immune response causes cells within the immune system to store information about the specific antigen (pathogen) into their memory so the next time the same antigen enters the body the immune system

Table 8-3 Local and Systemic Signs of Inflammation

Local signs	*Redness and heat:* blood vessels dilate at the site of injury to bring more white blood cells *Pain and swelling:* dilated blood vessels cause pressure on nerve endings
Systemic signs	*Leukocytosis:* more white blood cells are created to meet the demands of fighting the infection *Increased pulse rate:* to circulate the extra white blood cells *Swollen lymph nodes:* due to the increased activity and lymphocyte production *Fever:* elevation in temperature as an attempt to destroy the pathogens by moving away from their comfort zone of 97°F.

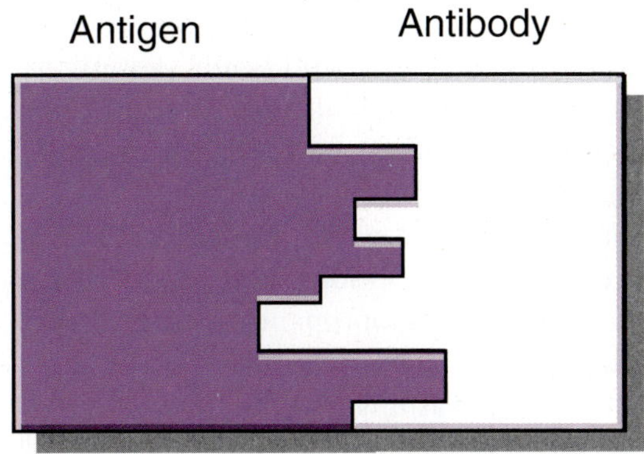

Figure 8-3 ■ Antigens and antibodies attach to each other in a "jigsaw puzzle" fashion.

is able to respond and eradicate that specific antigen before it causes disease.

Immunity, the body's ability to defend itself against pathogens and toxins, can occur in a variety of different ways:

- Natural immunity occurs as a result of being exposed to the pathogen. It can be further broken down into the following:
    - Natural passive immunity is acquired when antibodies are passed from mother to fetus and is usually a temporary immunity until the baby can acquire his own protections.
    - Natural active immunity is developed as a result of direct exposure to the antigen (such as when infection occurs) and the body builds its own protection.
- Artificial immunity occurs as a result of being given (usually through injections) either the antigen or antibodies and can be further broken down into the following:
    - Artificial passive immunity develops when the patient is injected with antibodies (**immunoglobulins**) to fight off infection. These antibodies were not actively created so are temporary, lasting usually about six months.
    - Artificial active immunity occurs when the patient is given small amounts of the antigen (through immunization) to stimulate an antibody reaction so that by the time the body is exposed to the antigen it already has a small arsenal of antibodies ready to attack.

Immunizations

Immunizations can provide immunity against specific infectious diseases. They also help to protect the general population, especially children and the elderly who are most vulnerable to infection. The U.S. Department of Health and Human Services (HHS) strongly recommends that preschoolers under age two be fully vaccinated according to a set schedule and protocol. Refer to Chapter 21 for more specific information and the recommended childhood immunization schedule.

Types of Vaccines

A vaccine is an agent capable of producing immunity to an infectious disease. There are several categories of vaccines:

1. Live Attenuated: These vaccines are a weakened form of a pathogen, altered by the manufacturer using a specific chemical or mechanical process. This type of vaccine stimulates the immune system to produce antibodies against the pathogen without causing the patient to contract the disease itself (although in some cases, the patient may experience mild symptoms). Measles, mumps, rubella (MMR), varicella (chicken pox), influenza nasal spray, shingles, and rotavirus are examples of live attenuated vaccines.
2. Toxoid Vaccines or Antitoxins: These vaccines are inactivated toxins produced by pathogens, which have been extracted from the gamma-globulin portion of the blood from humans and animals who have been vaccinated against a specific disease. By injecting the inactivated toxins produced by some pathogens, the immune system is stimulated to produce antibodies against the specific pathogen. Diphtheria and tetanus are two examples of toxoid vaccines.
3. Killed Vaccine: These vaccines are inactivated (chemically or physically) pathogens. This type of vaccine will stimulate antibody production by the immune system, although a series of vaccines may be required to produce long-term immunity. Polio, hepatitis A, and rabies are examples of killed vaccines.
4. Subunit and Conjugate Vaccines: These vaccines contain a tiny part of the target pathogen to create a response from the immune system. While the piece of the pathogen cannot cause illness, it can generate immunity. Hepatitis B, influenza injection, *Haemophilus influenzae* (Hib), pertussis, pneumococcal, meningococcal, and human papillomavirus (HPV) are examples of subunit/conjugate vaccines.

INFECTION CONTROL

The term **asepsis** means free of germs. **Aseptic technique** is the effort that is employed to reduce the spread of microorganisms. **Medical asepsis** and **surgical asepsis** are two types of infection control that are regularly practiced in the medical office.

Medical Asepsis

Medical asepsis applies to the destruction of microorganisms *after* leaving the body (in other words, removing gloves and washing hands after performing a urine test) to greatly decrease the number of microorganisms and prevent them from being passed from one person to another.

The purpose of medical asepsis is to decrease the risk of spreading infection by blocking or destroying pathogens from hands, instruments, and surfaces. Techniques used to institute medical asepsis include performing handwashing on a regular basis; practicing Standard, Universal, and Transmission-Based Precautions (discussed later in this chapter); and cleaning and disinfecting contaminated surfaces such as countertops, floors, and exam tables. Refer to Figure 8-4 for examples of instituting medical asepsis.

Handwashing and Gloving

Handwashing is the first line of defense in reducing the spread of infection and should be performed by the medical assistant frequently throughout the workday. When soap and water is not available, alcohol-based hand rubs may be used. Antimicrobial soaps are not recommended and have proven to be no more effective at killing pathogens than soap and water. Antimicrobial soaps are even considered harmful since they may lead to the development of resistant bacteria, making it harder to kill these pathogens in the future.

Alcohol-based hand rubs, which are available in several forms, including gels, lotions, and foams should contain at least 60 percent isopropanol or ethanol alcohol (see Figure 8-5).

Since frequent handwashing and the frequent use of alcohol rubs can dry and irritate the skin, causing hands to become rough and inflamed, choosing a product that contains moisturizers is beneficial as well as the frequent application of hand lotion. Refrain from applying oil-based lotions or those containing lanolin just prior to gloving because the oils and lanolin can compromise the protective integrity of latex gloves.

Refer to Procedures 8-1 and 8-2 for step-by-step instructions on handwashing and using alcohol-based hand rubs.

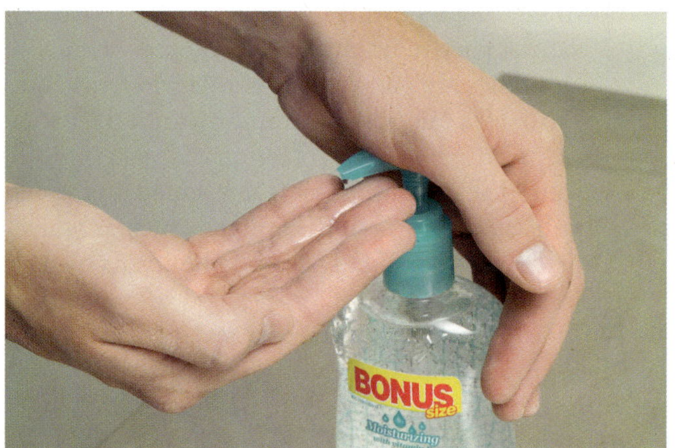

Figure 8-5 ■ Applying alcohol-based hand rub in lieu of handwashing.

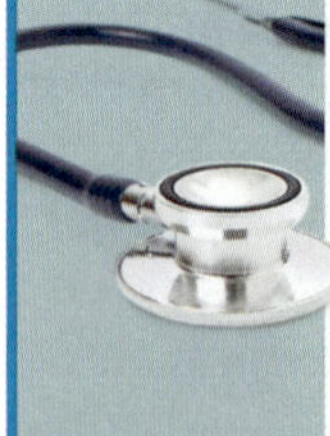

Figure 8-4 ■ Different methods of practicing medical asepsis in the medical office.

Field Smarts

All blood and body fluids should be considered potentially infectious, regardless of the source. A skilled health care professional never becomes careless when handling specimens or contaminated equipment. Trying to judge the likelihood of a particular patient being infected based on their age or lifestyle is dangerous and a poor substitute for good safety practices.

Table 8-4 CDC Recommendations for Hand Hygiene

When to wash hands with detergent or antimicrobial soap	• If hands become soiled with dirt or body fluids • After using the restroom • Before eating or drinking
When to apply an alcohol-based hand rub	• Before applying gloves and after removing them • Before and after each patient contact • If hands are not visibly soiled, after contact with body fluids, non-intact skin, soiled dressings • During patient care, after moving from a contaminated site to a clean site • After using any medical equipment, computer keyboard, or telephone, during the performance of health-care-related job duties
General recommendations	• Keep nails short, less than 1/4 inch long. No acrylic or adorned nails. Maintain healthy cuticles. • Do not add more soap to a dispenser that is low or empty. Cleaning the dispenser before refilling will decrease contamination. • Use disposable paper towels to dry hands • Apply lotions and creams after frequent handwashing to keep hands from drying out • Wash hands and change gloves if moving from a contaminated site to a clean site • Wear a clean pair of gloves for each patient

The CDC recommends wearing gloves (see Table 8-4) whenever there is potential contact with:

- blood;
- body fluids or **other potentially infectious material (OPIM)** that have potential to transmit disease, including any body fluid that is visibly contaminated with blood; cerebrospinal, amniotic, pericardial, pleural, and peritoneal fluids; any unidentifiable body fluid; saliva during dental procedures; semen and vaginal secretions; any unfixed human tissue;
- non-intact skin;
- mucous membranes; and
- contaminated equipment.

All body fluids (except sweat) are treated as potentially infectious. Using gloves as recommended by the CDC standards and removing contaminated gloves properly will prevent infectious materials from coming into contact with your hands. Refer to Procedure 8-3 for step-by-step instructions for safely removing contaminated gloves.

Surgical Asepsis

Surgical asepsis includes procedures and practices used to destroy and eliminate all microorganisms from instruments and other objects before they have an opportunity to enter an individual. It includes measures taken to prevent the transfer of microorganisms to the patient during surgical procedures. Refer to Chapter 9 for more information on surgical asepsis.

UNIVERSAL BLOOD AND BODY FLUID PRECAUTIONS

Universal Precautions are a set of rules that were established in 1987 by the CDC in response to the HIV/AIDS epidemic. Since the implementation of those regulations, there has been a significant decrease in the risk of spreading all infectious diseases, including HIV, hepatitis B virus (HBV), and hepatitis C virus (HCV).

Standard Precautions

In 1996, the CDC added new two-tiered sections (Part III) entitled **Standard Precautions and Transmission-Based Precautions**. Standard Precautions include the previous Universal Precautions, as well as an additional practice called **body substance isolation (BSI)**. BSI takes Universal Precautions to the next level by requiring barriers for *all body substances*, (except for sweat), such as tears, saliva, urine, mucus secretions, and wound drainage. Additional guidelines to Standard Precautions include respiratory hygiene/cough etiquette, safe injection practices, and the use of masks for insertion of catheters or injection of material into spinal or epidural spaces via lumbar puncture procedures. All of these regulations, standards, and guidelines can be confusing, however, their purpose is to prevent the spread of infection. Table 8-5 might help clarify these guidelines.

To reduce the likelihood of transmitting infectious disease, the CDC recommends that *every* patient be considered potentially infectious for *all* bloodborne pathogens. As part of an effective and

Table 8-5 Federal Standards, Guidelines, and Precautions for Blood, Body Fluids, and OPIM

CDC Standards, Guidelines and Precautions (Controls Infections and Educates)	
Universal Precautions	In reaction to HIV and AIDS, relates to blood and body fluids and Other Potentially Infectious Materials (OPIM)
Standard Precautions	Includes Universal Precautions but adds Body Substance Isolation (BSI), which requires barriers to all body substances regardless of potential
Transmission-Based Precautions	Added to Standard Precautions, designed to specifically address the transmission of infection by direct, indirect, and droplet routes
OSHA Standards, Guidelines, and Precautions (Protects the Worker/Employee)	
Bloodborne Pathogen Standards (and Needlestick Safety)	Rules to protect workers from pathogens transmitted through blood and OPIM
Exposure Determination	Determines which workers are at risk (health care professionals and housekeeping, laundry staff)
Exposure Control Plans	Compliance rules for exposure prevention, including vaccinations and employee training, engineering controls, and regulating infectious waste List of all hazards must be available to employees Postexposure evaluation and follow-up procedures Reporting and recordkeeping
Chemical Hygiene Plan	Protection from exposure to hazardous chemicals Safety Data Sheets (SDS)

Table 8-6 Infection Control Standards

Consider *all* blood and body fluids to be contaminated.
Wash hands before and after each patient, and when hands become contaminated with blood or body fluids.
Wear gloves when performing any task, such as venipuncture, finger sticks, heel sticks, and laboratory tests in which there could be contact with a patient's blood, body fluids, mucous membranes, broken skin, wounds, or body tissue.
Change gloves after each patient. *Never* wear the same pair of gloves for more than one patient.
Wash hands before donning gloves and after removing gloves.
When there is a risk of contamination due to splashing or droplets of blood or body fluids, wear protective barriers (such as a gown, mask, goggles/face shield) in addition to gloves (Figure 8-6).
When handling **sharps** (which include needles, sharp instruments, scalpels, glass slides, glass tubes, and pipettes), exercise extreme caution. Place anything sharp into an approved puncture-proof container (Figure 8-7) that displays the **biohazard** symbol (Figure 8-8). These containers should be placed in convenient and easily accessible locations throughout the work area.
Clean all spills (blood and body fluids) immediately with an approved disinfectant or a simple 10% sodium hypochlorite solution, which is used as a household bleach (Figure 8-9).
Immediately report any exposure to contaminated materials (such as splashes into the face or needlesticks) and follow the established postexposure evaluation and follow-up protocol.
Use a barrier mask when performing mouth-to-mouth resuscitation.
Cover any break in your skin.

responsible infection control program, the standards listed in Table 8-6 should be instituted.

The Biohazard Label

The biohazard label alerts everyone to the presence of actual and potential biological hazards. It must be placed on all containers and in all areas where exposure to blood, body fluids, and OPIM is possible. Anything contaminated with blood, body fluids, or OPIM—including gloves, gowns, masks, gauze, and wipes—must be labeled as a biohazard and placed in an appropriate container. Biohazard label requirements include the following:

- The label must be fluorescent orange or red in color.
- The biohazard symbol must appear on the label.
- The label must be secured to all containers.

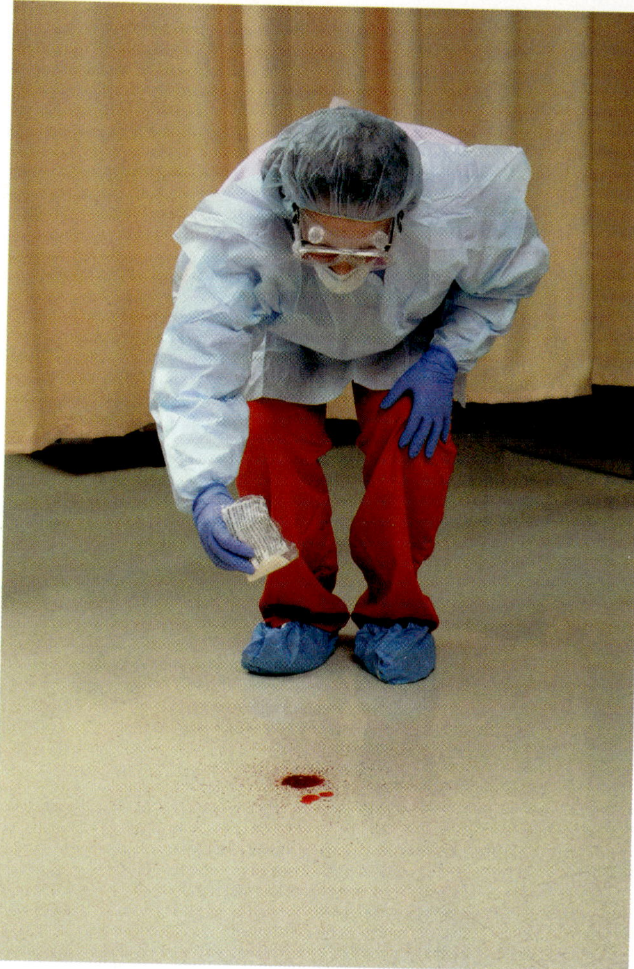

Figure 8-6 ■ A medical assistant wearing full personal protective equipment (PPE).

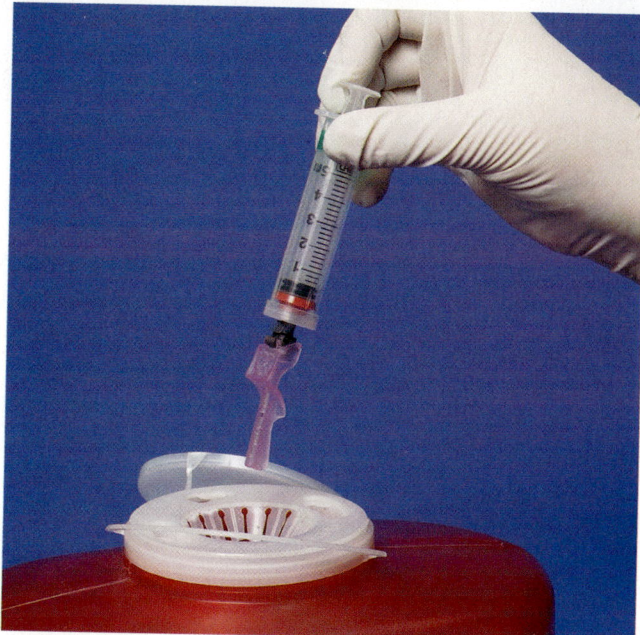

Figure 8-7 ■ Place all used sharps into an approved puncture-proof sharps container.

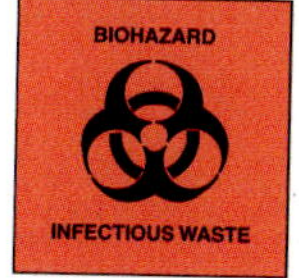

Figure 8-8 ■ A biohazard label.

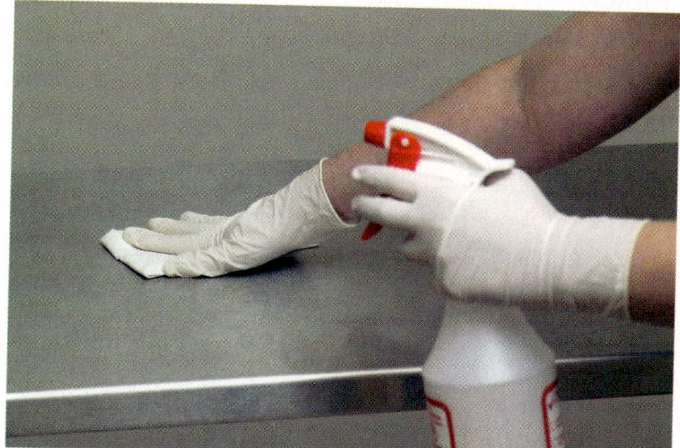

Figure 8-9 ■ Clean all contaminated work surfaces with a solution of 10 percent bleach.

- Red bags or containers may be used in place of the biohazard label.
- Refrigerators used to store blood, blood products, body fluids, and OPIM must clearly display the biohazard label.

Figure 8-10 displays a list of Standard Precaution symbols and an explanation of each one.

Transmission-Based Precautions

Transmission-Based Precautions were designed to decrease the risk of transferring pathogens when dealing with patients with known highly infectious diseases. Examples of Transmission-Based Precautions include the following:

- Indirect Contact/Airborne Precautions: Include the use of respirators and surgical masks as well as placing the patient in a private room with filtered air
- Direct Contact Precautions: Include the use of all PPE and the cleaning and disinfecting of all equipment if used by or for more than one patient
- Droplet Precautions: Include wearing a mask and eye protection or a complete face shield when there is the potential of droplet contamination

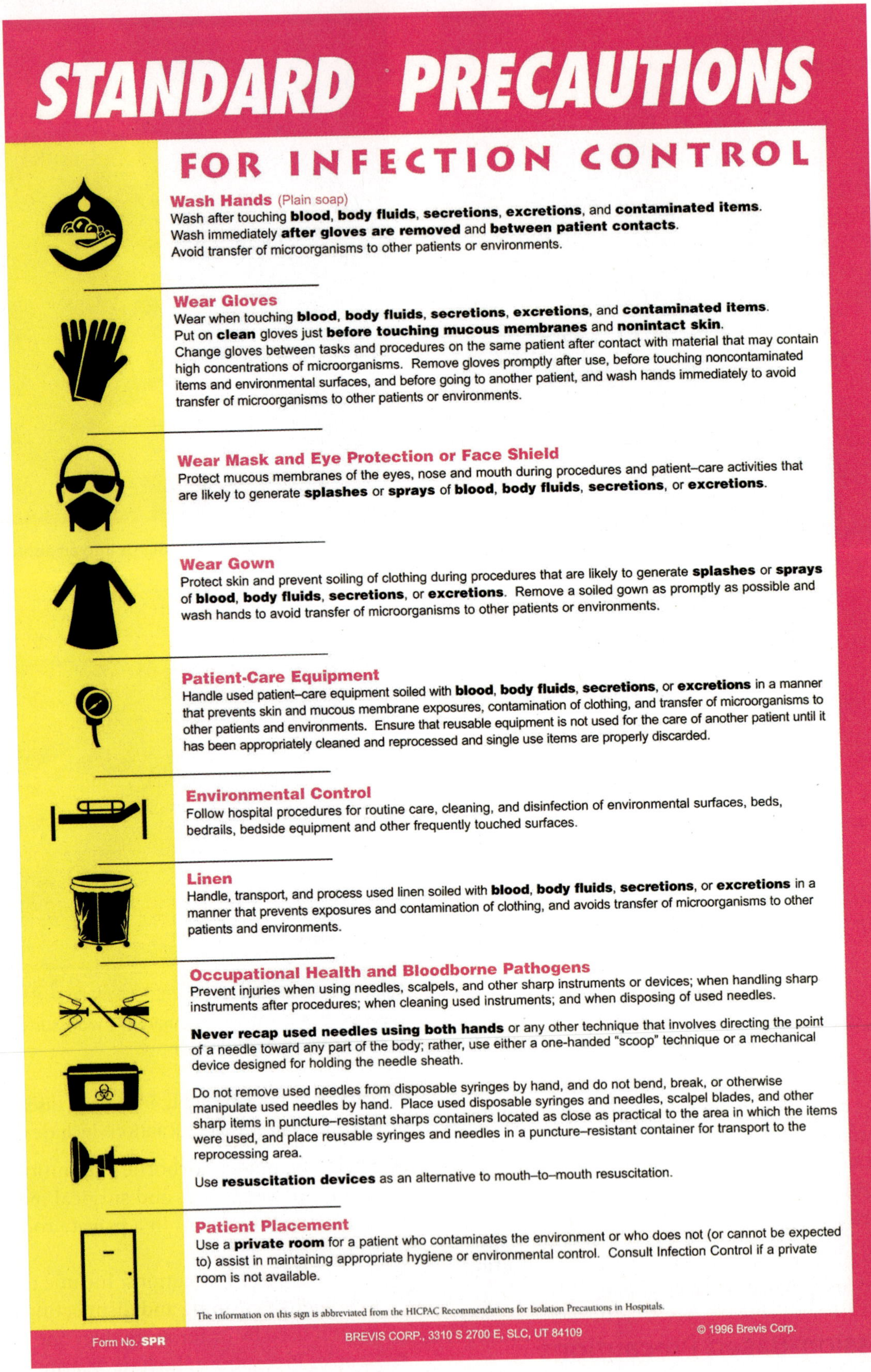

STANDARD PRECAUTIONS

FOR INFECTION CONTROL

Wash Hands (Plain soap)
Wash after touching **blood**, **body fluids**, **secretions**, **excretions**, and **contaminated items**.
Wash immediately **after gloves are removed** and **between patient contacts**.
Avoid transfer of microorganisms to other patients or environments.

Wear Gloves
Wear when touching **blood**, **body fluids**, **secretions**, **excretions**, and **contaminated items**.
Put on **clean** gloves just **before touching mucous membranes** and **nonintact skin**.
Change gloves between tasks and procedures on the same patient after contact with material that may contain high concentrations of microorganisms. Remove gloves promptly after use, before touching noncontaminated items and environmental surfaces, and before going to another patient, and wash hands immediately to avoid transfer of microorganisms to other patients or environments.

Wear Mask and Eye Protection or Face Shield
Protect mucous membranes of the eyes, nose and mouth during procedures and patient–care activities that are likely to generate **splashes** or **sprays** of **blood**, **body fluids**, **secretions**, or **excretions**.

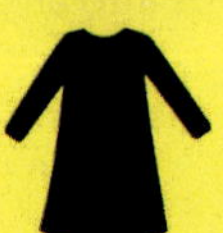

Wear Gown
Protect skin and prevent soiling of clothing during procedures that are likely to generate **splashes** or **sprays** of **blood**, **body fluids**, **secretions**, or **excretions**. Remove a soiled gown as promptly as possible and wash hands to avoid transfer of microorganisms to other patients or environments.

Patient-Care Equipment
Handle used patient–care equipment soiled with **blood**, **body fluids**, **secretions**, or **excretions** in a manner that prevents skin and mucous membrane exposures, contamination of clothing, and transfer of microorganisms to other patients and environments. Ensure that reusable equipment is not used for the care of another patient until it has been appropriately cleaned and reprocessed and single use items are properly discarded.

Environmental Control
Follow hospital procedures for routine care, cleaning, and disinfection of environmental surfaces, beds, bedrails, bedside equipment and other frequently touched surfaces.

Linen
Handle, transport, and process used linen soiled with **blood**, **body fluids**, **secretions**, or **excretions** in a manner that prevents exposures and contamination of clothing, and avoids transfer of microorganisms to other patients and environments.

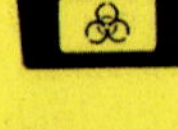

Occupational Health and Bloodborne Pathogens
Prevent injuries when using needles, scalpels, and other sharp instruments or devices; when handling sharp instruments after procedures; when cleaning used instruments; and when disposing of used needles.

Never recap used needles using both hands or any other technique that involves directing the point of a needle toward any part of the body; rather, use either a one-handed "scoop" technique or a mechanical device designed for holding the needle sheath.

Do not remove used needles from disposable syringes by hand, and do not bend, break, or otherwise manipulate used needles by hand. Place used disposable syringes and needles, scalpel blades, and other sharp items in puncture–resistant sharps containers located as close as practical to the area in which the items were used, and place reusable syringes and needles in a puncture–resistant container for transport to the reprocessing area.

Use **resuscitation devices** as an alternative to mouth–to–mouth resuscitation.

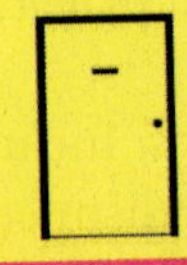

Patient Placement
Use a **private room** for a patient who contaminates the environment or who does not (or cannot be expected to) assist in maintaining appropriate hygiene or environmental control. Consult Infection Control if a private room is not available.

The information on this sign is abbreviated from the HICPAC Recommendations for Isolation Precautions in Hospitals.

Form No. **SPR** BREVIS CORP., 3310 S 2700 E, SLC, UT 84109

Figure 8-10 ■ Standard Precaution symbols.

BLOODBORNE DISEASES

Bloodborne diseases are not easily transmitted but the following situations are examples of how it may happen:

- Accidental puncture with contaminated sharp objects such as needles, scalpels, or broken glass
- Sharing of needles by IV drug users
- Receiving a transfusion of contaminated blood or blood products, although this risk is now rare due to current screening and testing.
- Unprotected sexual contact with an infected person (both homosexual and heterosexual)
- Any break in the skin coming in contact with contaminated blood and body fluids
- Infection passed from the mother to the fetus
- Contaminated tools and needles used for body piercing and tattooing.

HIV/AIDS

HIV is a bloodborne virus that attacks the white blood cells known as T-cells, which protect the body against many types of infections. As the disease progresses, the immune system become more and more compromised since fewer T-cells are available to fight off infections and cancers. Persons infected with HIV are often vulnerable to frequent infections that do not normally bother people with healthy immune systems. These illnesses are called **opportunistic infections** and are referred to as AIDS-defining illnesses because they are typical illnesses that are seen only in patients with progressed HIV or those patients who have progressed to the end stage called AIDS.

Examples of opportunistic infections can be found in Table 8-7.

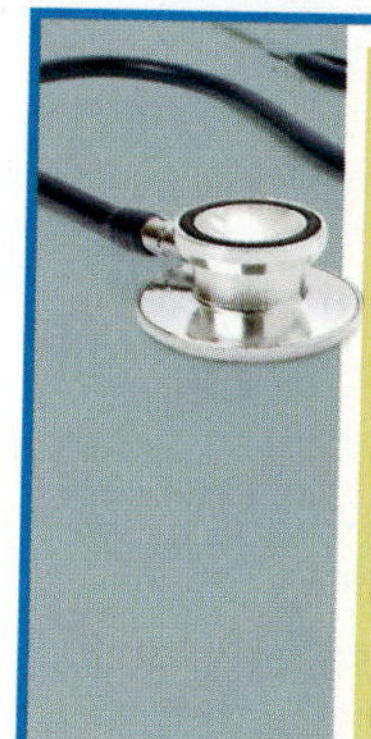

Field Smarts

It is a mistake to refer to an HIV-infected person as having AIDS, since a person can live many healthy years without entering the AIDS stage and not everyone who has an opportunistic infection or an infection that is listed as an AIDS-defining illness has AIDS.

Stages of HIV

There are usually four stages associated with HIV, although some infected individuals may not experience every stage.

Stage 1: Primary HIV Infection Stage

This stage begins within two weeks of exposure, when an individual becomes infected with the virus and may experience flu-like symptoms. There are large amounts of HIV antigens present during this stage and the body starts to manufacture antibodies against the virus. *Seroconversion* refers to the stage when detectable antibodies are present in the serum, causing a positive antibody test and can occur anywhere from two weeks to six months following exposure. HIV antibody testing may present a false-negative during initial testing until seroconversion occurs.

Stage 2: Clinically Asymptomatic Stage

This stage may last for several years, often with no detectable symptoms, other than some enlarged lymph nodes. The level of HIV present in the peripheral blood

Table 8-7 Examples of Opportunistic Infections and Causative Agents

Candida infections (candidiasis) of the trachea, bronchi, lungs, or esophagus
Cytomegalovirus: infections affecting areas of the body other than the liver, spleen, or lymph nodes
Cytomegalovirus retinitis: causing loss of vision
Herpes simplex: chronic ulcers of the mouth of longer than 1 month's duration, bronchitis, pneumonitis, or esophagitis
Mycobacterium avium or *Mycobacterium kansasii*: extrapulmonary infections or disseminated
Mycobacterium tuberculosis: pulmonary or extrapulmonary infections
Pneumocystis carinii pneumonia
AIDS-related cancers:
• Kaposi's sarcoma
• Burkitt's lymphoma
• Primary brain lymphoma
• Immunoblastic lymphoma
• Invasive cervical cancer

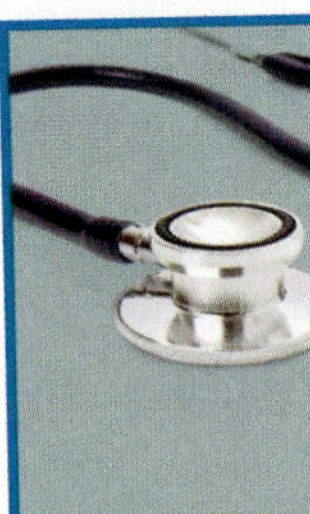

Field Smarts

Confidentiality

The results of all testing must be kept completely confidential. For this reason, many facilities assign patients who are undergoing HIV testing a tracking number that identifies that patient, their specimen, and all correspondence regarding the HIV testing, including the results. A positive HIV test result can adversely affect a patient's lifestyle. Always follow Health Insurance Portability and Accountability Act (HIPAA) guidelines when handling test orders and results.

stream drops during this stage, but HIV antibody testing will still reveal a positive HIV antibody test.

Stage 3: Clinically Symptomatic Stage

Signs of AIDS begin to show, starting slowly and progressing to more severe symptoms including swollen glands, diarrhea, fatigue, mouth ulcers, nail fungus, thrush, and significant weight loss.

Stage 4: Progression of HIV to AIDS

This stage is the fourth and final stage of an HIV infection, when the person becomes very sick. With the latest treatment options, many patients are able to live with HIV for many years. Most patients do not succumb to the disease itself, but rather to opportunistic infections and cancers allowed by their weakened immune state.

The CDC estimates that over one million Americans are now living with HIV, and a quarter of those people are unaware of their HIV infection. While HIV/AIDS is a disease that is at the forefront of the minds of most health care workers, both the HBV and HCV actually pose more of a threat.

Hepatitis

Hepatitis literally means inflammation of the liver. Since the liver is the "blood filter" of the body, it is susceptible to damage by toxic substances such as drugs, alcohol, and poisons as well as by biliary (gall bladder) obstruction. This chapter will discuss the viral causes of hepatitis. There are three viral hepatitis diseases prevalent within the United States: hepatitis A (HAV), B (HBV), and C (HCV) (see Table 8-2).

HAV is contracted through ingesting fecal contamination and is the less severe form; it does not become chronic and the person does not become a carrier. Vaccination is the best way to prevent HAV. HBV is bloodborne and poses the greatest threat to health care workers through needlesticks. A vaccine is available for HBV and is recommended for all health care workers and people working in other high-risk environments. HCV, although not as prevalent as HBV, is another form of bloodborne hepatitis that can be transmitted in the health care setting. Both HBV and HCV infections are almost entirely preventable by strictly observing the Standard Precautions. There is no vaccine against HCV and it tends to become chronic and is more likely to become fatal.

OSHA REGULATIONS

The **Occupational Safety and Health Administration (OSHA)** was created in 1971 by the federal government to establish standards and regulations for all employers to ensure that employees work in a safe and healthy work environment. All workers, everyone employed in any profession within the United States, from teachers to construction workers to waiters to clerks to bus drivers and beyond, are covered by OSHA. However, since OSHA does not have jurisdiction over state or municipal employees or inmates, individual states have their own employee safety laws. Every profession has its own set of safety issues, but health care professional have high risks due to the potentially infectious materials and dangerous chemicals they are exposed to. Two of OSHA's standards protect employees in the health care field: *The Hazard Communication Standard,* which includes rules to notify workers of chemical risks and to protect against exposure to hazardous chemicals in the medical laboratory; and *The Bloodborne Pathogens Standard,* which helps protect against infectious exposures. See Table 8-5 for clarification.

Bloodborne Pathogens Standard

OSHA's Bloodborne Pathogens Standard, published in 1991, was established to protect health care workers from bloodborne diseases. These standards include rules for exposures to blood, body fluids, and OPIM; exposure determination; exposure control plans; exposure prevention (including employee training, vaccinations, and engineering controls); regulating, labeling, and disposal of biohazard waste; postexposure follow-up; housekeeping and laundry procedures; reporting; and recordkeeping.

Blood, Body Fluids, and OPIM

OSHA and the CDC have listed the following as potentially infectious substances from which health care workers should protect themselves:

- Blood and blood components
- Body fluids such as cerebrospinal fluid, synovial fluid, pleural fluid, peritoneal fluid, and pericardial fluid
- Any body fluid visibly contaminated with blood
- Saliva during dental procedures
- Semen and vaginal secretions
- Unfixed human tissues, such as biopsy specimens
- Specimens of unknown origin
- Remember, when a facility is following Standard Precautions, all body fluids are considered potentially infected.

Exposure Determination

Exposure determination requires that employers maintain a list of job classifications in which the employees will be exposed to biohazard substances, such as medical assistants, nurses, doctors, housekeepers, janitors, and laundry workers.

Exposure Control Plan

OSHA requires that a written **exposure control** plan be developed, which would include prevention rules, vaccinations available, postexposure evaluation and follow-up procedures, lists of all hazards to the employees, guidelines for reporting, and recordkeeping procedures. The exposure control should be available to employees and must be kept current.

Compliance Rules for Exposure Prevention

Exposure prevention includes wearing appropriate PPE, implementing engineering controls and work practice controls, properly disposing of regulated waste, and maintaining a clean workspace.

Employers must provide adequate and easily accessible handwashing stations and ensure that all employees wash their hands and any contaminated skin, with soap and water following exposure to blood and OPIM. If mucous membranes have been exposed, they must be flushed immediately with water (Figure 8-11).

PPE should be worn to provide a protective barrier between the employee and blood and OPIM. Figure 8-12 displays examples of PPE.

Some facts about PPE include the following:

- Employers must provide PPE to all employees at no cost and it must be easily accessible. Employers must also clean, launder, and dispose of all PPE.
- Gloves must be readily available throughout the work area and are to be worn when the hands

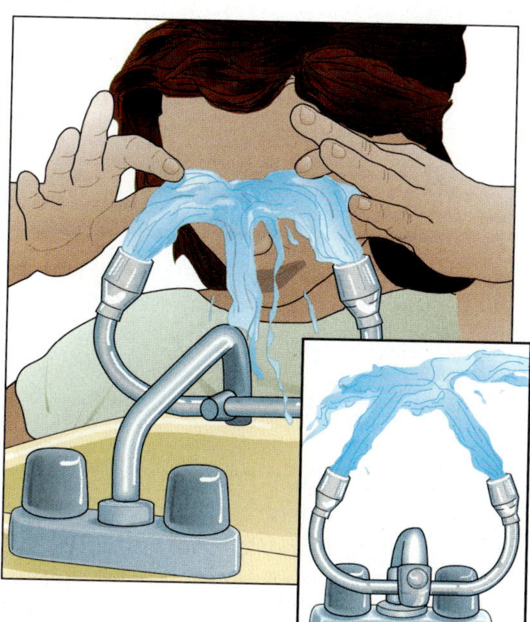

Figure 8-11 ■ An emergency eye-wash station provides a continuous flow of water to flush the eyes.

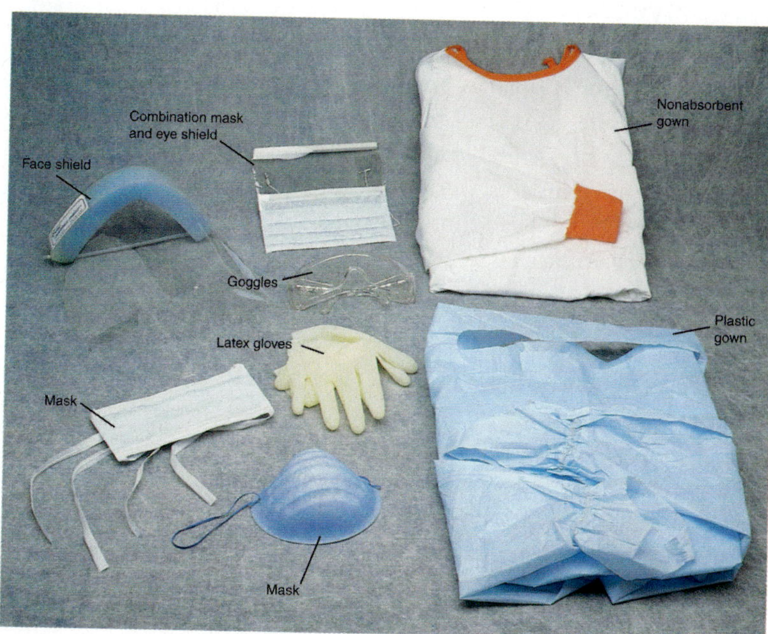

Figure 8-12 ■ Examples of personal protective equipment (PPE).

could possibly come in contact with blood or OPIM, mucous membranes, and broken skin. Gloves must be changed immediately if torn or punctured. Gloves must be provided in the size that best fits the employee. If an employee is allergic to latex, the employer must provide an alternate type of gloves.

- Masks, eye protection, and face shields must be used when there is a possibility of splashing or spraying of blood or OPIM. The eyes, nose, and mouth must be protected. Glasses alone are not considered sufficient protection for the eyes.
- Gowns, aprons, or lab coats must be worn to protect clothing from exposure. All PPE must be safely removed and placed in appropriate containers before leaving the workplace.

Refer to Procedure 8-4 for a procedure on applying and removing PPE.

Vaccinations

Employers must provide all employees at risk for occupational exposure to blood and OPIM with the HBV vaccine free of charge and at a convenient time and place. In the event that an employee refuses the vaccine, she must sign a declination form, which must be kept on file. The employee may decide to be vaccinated at a later date, also at the employer's expense. Other suggested vaccinations include catch-up on appropriate childhood vaccines, varicella, measles, rubella, and annual influenza vaccines.

Employee Training

Employees need to know the risks in their workplace, how to prevent exposure, and what to do if accidently exposed to infectious substances. Safety information should be readily available and training sessions should be offered and updated periodically. A safety officer is an assigned employee who maintains training records and assesses employee safety.

Engineering Controls

Engineering controls are those devices used to separate employees from hazards and **work practice controls** (methods by which a task is performed) are the means used to minimize or eliminate employee exposure. These controls deal with the use of safer equipment and mechanical devices such as safety needles for injections and venipuncture. See Chapter 24 (Blood Collection Techniques) and Chapter 32 (Administration of Parenteral Medications) for more information about safety needles. Puncture-resistant sharps containers also fall under the category of engineering controls (Figure 8-13).

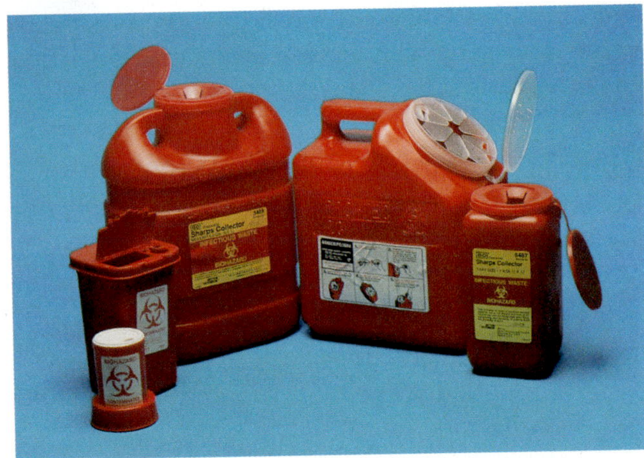

Figure 8-13 ■ Examples of various sharps containers.

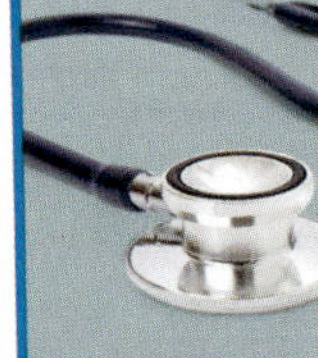

Field Smarts

Hundreds of thousands of U.S. health care workers are accidently stuck with needles each year. Many of these needles are contaminated and pose a risk of transmitting infectious pathogens. Congress asked the CDC to revise the Bloodborne Pathogens Standard to include Needlestick Safety and Prevention. Employers are now required to provide safer needles and medical devices for health care professionals. The workers using the needles are to assist in selecting the preferred safety devices, and a sharps injury log needs to be maintained to record the details of any accidental needlestick injuries. Safety devices include the following:

- Syringes with protective shields that cover the needle
- Needles that retract into the barrel of the syringe after use
- Plastic blood collection tubes
- Self-blunting needles
- Retracting lancets

The following is a list of engineering controls and work practice controls that should be instituted when working in medical establishments:

- Eating, drinking, applying cosmetics, and handling contact lenses are all prohibited in any area where biohazard exposure is likely.
- Food and drinks must never be stored in the refrigerators, on shelves, or in cabinets used for the storage of blood or OPIM.
- Specimens of blood and OPIM must be placed in properly labeled containers identified as a biohazard. These containers must be leakproof for safe handling and transport.
- Broken glass should be cleaned up with dustpans, brushes, tongs, or forceps and the glass must be placed in a sharps container.
- Contaminated needle should never be recapped.
- Needles should be dropped, never pushed, into the sharps container.
- All equipment and work surfaces must be appropriately cleaned and decontaminated after exposure to blood and OPIM.

Regulated Waste

Regulated waste, also known as **infectious waste**, is any medical waste contaminated with blood, body fluids, or OPIM. According to OSHA's **Bloodborne Pathogens** Standard, regulated waste includes: (1) liquid or semiliquid blood or OPIM; (2) any item contaminated with blood or OPIM that, if compressed, would release the blood or OPIM; (3) any item caked with dried blood or OPIM that would flake off if handled; (4) contaminated sharps; and (5) any pathology or microbiology wastes that contain blood or OPIM.

> **CRITICAL THINKING CHALLENGE**
>
> While cleaning the exam room after a minor surgical procedure, you accidentally stick your thumb with sharp scissors that the provider used on the patient. The patient is HIV positive.
>
> 1. What should be your first step in the process following a needlestick incident?
> 2. What prophylactic medications can be given to you?
> 3. How long may it take before you produce a positive antibody test for HIV?

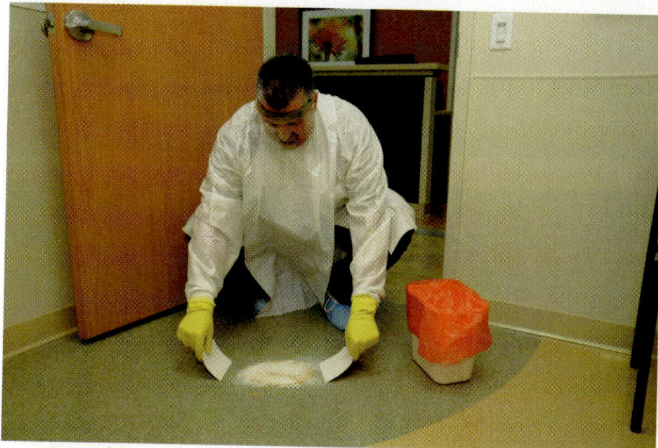

Figure 8-14 ■ The medical assistant properly cleans up a spill, wearing full PPE and using a spill kit.

When cleaning spills that involve biohazard waste, use of a commercially available *spill kit* is recommended (Figure 8-14). Spill kits contain everything needed to properly clean up spilled biohazard material and should be readily available in places where they might be needed. See Table 8-8 for contents of a spill kit. Refer to Figure 8-15 for an example of contents contained in a spill kit. Other guidelines include the following:

- All contaminated sharps must be disposed of immediately in approved sharps containers that are easily accessible. Sharps containers should always remain upright and should not be overfilled. If the outside of the sharps container becomes punctured or broken, it should be placed inside a second container to prevent leakage.
- Approved biohazard containers, such as the one shown in Figure 8-16, must be used to store all nonsharp-regulated waste.
- Contaminated laundry should not be handled more than necessary and must be placed in a clearly labeled bag or container. If the laundry is wet, it must be double-bagged or placed in a second leak proof container.
- Employees must wear eye protection along with other appropriate PPE when handling contaminated laundry.

Refer to Table 8-9 for specific guidelines for the proper disposal of biohazard waste. *Important note:* Table 8-9 follows OSHA guidelines; however, disposal guidelines may vary from one facility to another according to county and state regulations. When following

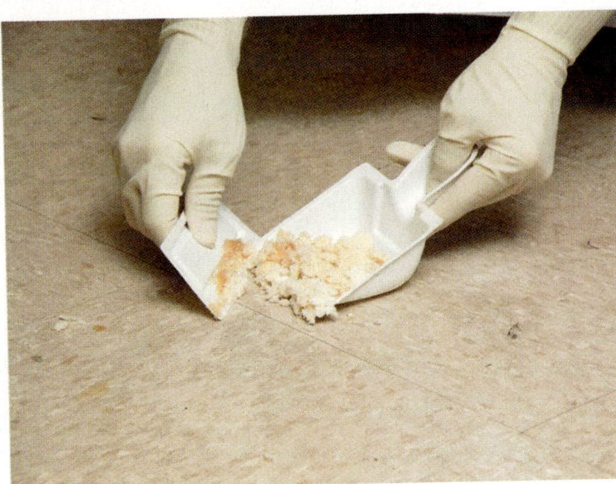

Figure 8-15 ■ A medical assistant cleans up a spill using a scoop from a spill kit.

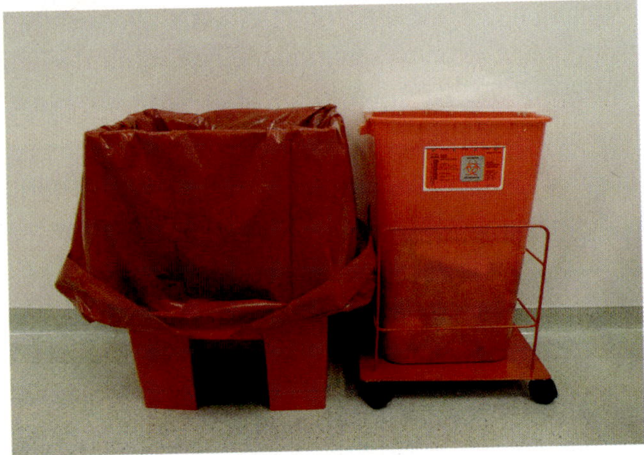

Figure 8-16 ■ The medical assistant disposes of the spill in the biohazardous waste container.

Table 8-8 Contents of a Commercially Available Spill Kit

Plastic water-proof outer bag	Gloves (with options for other PPE)
Absorbent powder (to coagulate and dry any wet biohazard substance)	Instructions compliant with OSHA Standards
Disinfectant wipes	Handheld scoop, scraper, or spatula
Forceps for picking up glass or dangerous sharps	Biohazard bag and closure
Paper towels	Antimicrobial hand wipes

Table 8-9 OSHA Guidelines for Proper Disposal of Biohazard Waste

Class of Waste	Biohazard Container with Red Bag	Sharps Container	Regular Trash
Blood, blood products, blood contaminated materials, microbiology specimens for culture, used nonglass culture plates and culture tubes	X		
Nonglass containers of cerebrospinal, synovial, pleural, peritoneal, pericardial, or amniotic fluid	X		
Fluid-filled containers from patient	X		
Surgical pathology specimens	X		
Needle/syringe units, needles, scalpels, suture needles, other sharps		X	
Glass slides and cover slips, pipettes, tubes of blood, microhematocrit tubes		X	
Used urine containers, diapers, under pads, and empty urinary drainage bags (unless visibly contaminate with blood)			X
OPIM contaminants, stool and other specimen containers	X		
Dressings, bandages, gauze pads, and cotton swabs, unless contaminated with blood or OPIM			X
Used gloves, aprons, masks, and shoe and head covers, unless saturated with blood or OPIM			X
Paper towels used for handwashing, food waste, computer paper, and packaging materials			X
Materials used to clean up nonhazardous spills			X

Note: Always check facility guidelines before disposing of biohazard waste.

Standard Precautions, anything that has any type of a body fluid on it or in it, regardless of the amount, should be placed in the biohazard trash.

Employers must maintain a clean and sanitary work environment and should have a written schedule for cleaning and decontamination. All work surfaces that become contaminated with blood and OPIM must be decontaminated following use, especially at the end of the workday. Gloves must be worn when cleaning any surface that may be contaminated with blood or OPIM. A 10 percent solution of bleach is an effective disinfectant. Paper towels and gloves should be used when cleaning a spill and then placed in an appropriate biohazard container.

Postexposure Evaluation and Follow-Up

Should exposure to blood, body fluids, or OPIM occur, the following steps should be taken:

- The wound or exposed area should be immediately cleansed with soap and water, and if necessary, covered with a sterile bandage.
- If the eyes are contaminated, they should be flushed with tepid water for several minutes.
- If mucous membranes, such as the mouth or eyes, are contaminated, they should be thoroughly rinsed with copious amounts of water.
- After first-aid measures have been instituted, the exposure should be reported to the immediate supervisor.
- An exposure report form must be completed and filed.
- The exposed employee should be tested for HBV and HIV (the employee must give consent to be tested).
- The source or individual whose blood was involved in the exposure must give permission for his or her blood to be tested for HBV and HIV. If permission is granted by the source individual, the employee is permitted to know the results of the tests.
- The exposed employee should be offered gammaglobulin or other preventative medications.
- The exposed employee should be offered counseling both to alert the employee regarding precautions to avoid further transmission to others and for stress management.

Recordkeeping and Reporting

Medical records associated with the exposure incident must be kept separate from the employee's personnel record and must be on file for the *length of employment plus 30 years*. The employer must provide the exposed employee with a written report from the treating provider within 15 days following testing. The employee must be informed of the results of all postexposure tests and evaluations, including any conditions that may require follow-up, treatment, and evaluation. Records are confidential but must be available to OSHA, the employee, and anyone with the employee's written permission.

Employers must provide training for all at-risk employees at the time they assume their duties and annually after that. Anytime an employee's job description or duties change, retraining is required. All training sessions must be documented and placed on file for three years. Employee training programs should include the following:

- Full description and explanation of the Bloodborne Pathogens Standard, symptoms of bloodborne diseases, and means of transmission
- Step-by-step explanation of the exposure control plan
- Engineering and work practice controls
- PPE to be used
- HBV vaccination information
- Postexposure procedures
- Information explaining postexposure evaluation
- Information explaining the biohazard label and color-coding of containers

EXPOSURE TO HAZARDOUS CHEMICALS

Medical assistants not only face the possibility of exposure to biological hazards but may be exposed to hazardous chemicals as well. Many chemicals are used in the laboratory. Exposure can occur through inhalation, injection, or by direct contact to skin. The medical assistant must be aware of these hazards and the guidelines for proper handling, storage, and disposal of hazardous chemicals.

OSHA'S Chemical Hygiene Plan

A written chemical hygiene plan is required by OSHA and must be in place to provide information and training in facilities where chemicals are stored and handled by employees. Compliance is not optional—it is the law.

Some labs are not required to adhere to these standards if the test methods used in the particular lab do not put employees at risk for exposure to hazardous chemicals, such as dipstick procedures or test kits that contain sealed chemicals. Some examples of hazardous chemicals are acetone, formaldehyde, bleach, ethyl alcohol, blood and tissue stains, tissue fixatives, and chemotherapeutic agents.

Standards for a chemical exposure plan include the following:

- Inventory of all hazardous chemicals that lists chemical name, quantity, physical state, hazard class, and manufacturer
- A safety data sheet (SDS) with OSHA's required information must be kept in a manual and readily available to all employees. (Figure 8-17)

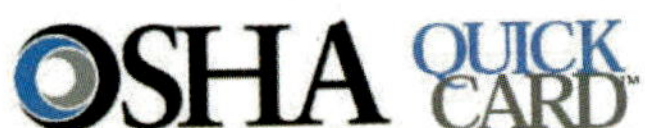

Hazard Communication Safety Data Sheets

The Hazard Communication Standard (HCS) requires chemical manufacturers, distributors, or importers to provide Safety Data Sheets (SDSs) (formerly known as Material Safety Data Sheets or MSDSs) to communicate the hazards of hazardous chemical products. As of June 1, 2015, the HCS will require new SDSs to be in a uniform format, and include the section numbers, the headings, and associated information under the headings below:

Section 1, Identification includes product identifier; manufacturer or distributor name, address, phone number; emergency phone number; recommended use; restrictions on use.

Section 2, Hazard(s) identification includes all hazards regarding the chemical; required label elements.

Section 3, Composition/information on ingredients includes information on chemical ingredients; trade secret claims.

Section 4, First-aid measures includes important symptoms/ effects, acute, delayed; required treatment.

Section 5, Fire-fighting measures lists suitable extinguishing techniques, equipment; chemical hazards from fire.

Section 6, Accidental release measures lists emergency procedures; protective equipment; proper methods of containment and cleanup.

Section 7, Handling and storage lists precautions for safe handling and storage, including incompatibilities.

Section 8, Exposure controls/personal protection lists OSHA's Permissible Exposure Limits (PELs); Threshold Limit Values (TLVs); appropriate engineering controls; personal protective equipment (PPE).

Section 9, Physical and chemical properties lists the chemical's characteristics.

Section 10, Stability and reactivity lists chemical stability and possibility of hazardous reactions.

Section 11, Toxicological information includes routes of exposure; related symptoms, acute and chronic effects; numerical measures of toxicity.

Section 12, Ecological information*

Section 13, Disposal considerations*

Section 14, Transport information*

Section 15, Regulatory information*

Section 16, Other information, includes the date of preparation or last revision.

*Note: Since other Agencies regulate this information, OSHA will not be enforcing Sections 12 through 15(29 CFR 1910.1200(g)(2)).

Employers must ensure that SDSs are readily accessible to employees. See Appendix D of 1910.1200 for a detailed description of SDS contents.

For more information: www.osha.gov

OSHA
U.S. Department of Labor
(800) 321-OSHA (6742)

Courtesy of U.S. Department of Labor, Occupatational Safety & Health Administration

Figure 8-17 ■ OSHA's required information on a Safety Data Sheets.

lists what should be included in a safety data sheet. All SDS must be in alphabetical order within the manual. Information can be obtained from the manufacturer and the information should be reviewed regularly and updated as needed. Figure 8-18 shows an example of a chemical inventory form that should be used to list all chemicals stored on the premises.

- All chemicals are labeled according to OSHA's chemical labeling requirements. The manufacturer of the chemical is required to create and provide the label and labeling information.
- OSHA requires pictograms and hazards information (see Figure 8-19).
- All employees must participate in a training program within 30 days of the start of employment or before handling hazardous chemicals. The program must provide information on location and storage of hazardous chemicals, reading and understanding chemical labels, location of SDS manual, PPE required, and directions on how to clean up a chemical spill.

HAZARDOUS CHEMICALS INVENTORY LIST

Chemical Name	Quantity	Physical State	Hazard Class	Manufacturer	Comments

Figure 8-18 ■ An example of a chemical inventory form.

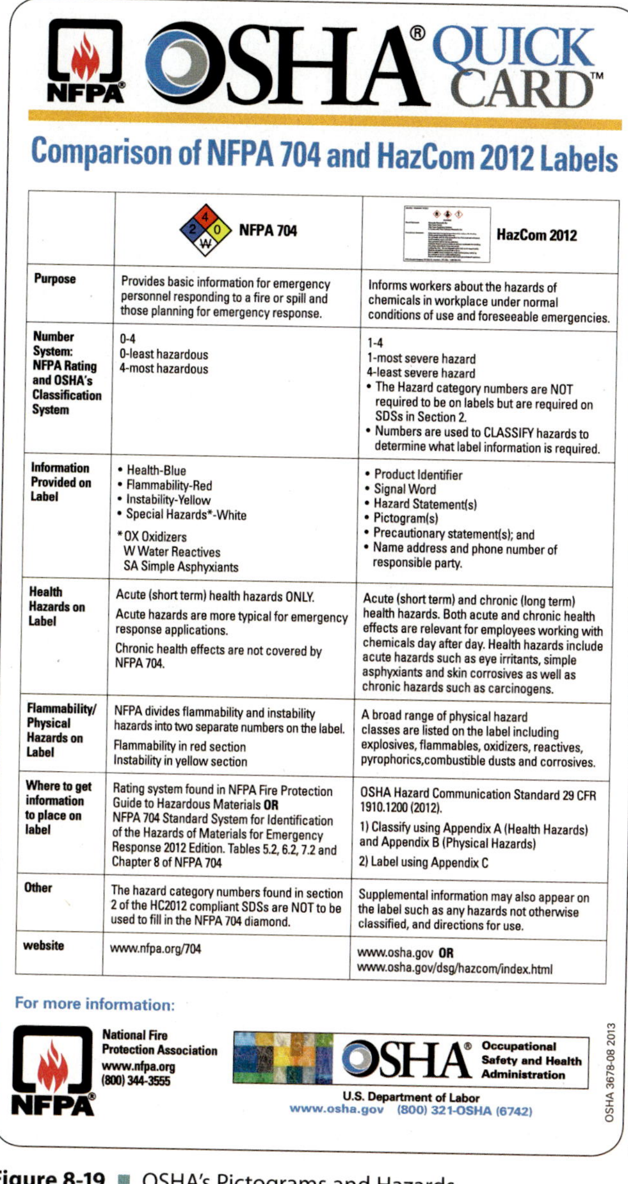

NFPA OSHA® QUICK CARD™

Comparison of NFPA 704 and HazCom 2012 Labels

	NFPA 704	HazCom 2012
Purpose	Provides basic information for emergency personnel responding to a fire or spill and those planning for emergency response.	Informs workers about the hazards of chemicals in workplace under normal conditions of use and foreseeable emergencies.
Number System: NFPA Rating and OSHA's Classification System	0-4 0-least hazardous 4-most hazardous	1-4 1-most severe hazard 4-least severe hazard • The Hazard category numbers are NOT required to be on labels but are required on SDSs in Section 2. • Numbers are used to CLASSIFY hazards to determine what label information is required.
Information Provided on Label	• Health-Blue • Flammability-Red • Instability-Yellow • Special Hazards*-White *OX Oxidizers W Water Reactives SA Simple Asphyxiants	• Product Identifier • Signal Word • Hazard Statement(s) • Pictogram(s) • Precautionary statement(s); and • Name address and phone number of responsible party.
Health Hazards on Label	Acute (short term) health hazards ONLY. Acute hazards are more typical for emergency response applications. Chronic health effects are not covered by NFPA 704.	Acute (short term) and chronic (long term) health hazards. Both acute and chronic health effects are relevant for employees working with chemicals day after day. Health hazards include acute hazards such as eye irritants, simple asphyxiants and skin corrosives as well as chronic hazards such as carcinogens.
Flammability/ Physical Hazards on Label	NFPA divides flammability and instability hazards into two separate numbers on the label. Flammability in red section Instability in yellow section	A broad range of physical hazard classes are listed on the label including explosives, flammables, oxidizers, reactives, pyrophorics,combustible dusts and corrosives.
Where to get information to place on label	Rating system found in NFPA Fire Protection Guide to Hazardous Materials **OR** NFPA 704 Standard System for Identification of the Hazards of Materials for Emergency Response 2012 Edition. Tables 5.2, 6.2, 7.2 and Chapter 8 of NFPA 704	OSHA Hazard Communication Standard 29 CFR 1910.1200 (2012). 1) Classify using Appendix A (Health Hazards) and Appendix B (Physical Hazards) 2) Label using Appendix C
Other	The hazard category numbers found in section 2 of the HC2012 compliant SDSs are NOT to be used to fill in the NFPA 704 diamond.	Supplemental information may also appear on the label such as any hazards not otherwise classified, and directions for use.
website	www.nfpa.org/704	www.osha.gov **OR** www.osha.gov/dsg/hazcom/index.html

For more information:

NFPA National Fire Protection Association www.nfpa.org (800) 344-3555

OSHA® Occupational Safety and Health Administration U.S. Department of Labor www.osha.gov (800) 321-OSHA (6742)

OSHA 3678-08 2013

Courtesy of U.S. Department of Labor, Occupatational Safety & Health Administration

Figure 8-19 ■ OSHA's Pictograms and Hazards.

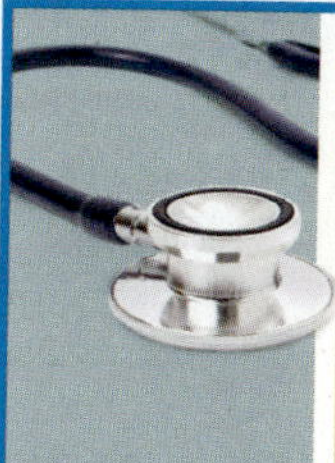

Field Smarts

Safety inspectors may be inspecting the facility for unsafe practices and checking for all required OSHA records. Complete records must be kept documenting current OSHA training and SDS training for all current employees. Assist your practice manager by maintaining your own professional documents and credentials as required by your certification.

SAFEGUARDS IN THE EDUCATIONAL ENVIRONMENT

Students involved in an educational program do not fall under OSHA guidelines (students are not considered to be in the same category as an employee). However, all necessary precautions should be performed in the educational setting to safeguard students against exposure to potentially infectious blood and body fluids as well as hazardous chemicals.

Students should practice Standard Precautions and use PPE when handling biological samples in the classroom and lab. They should also be aware of the use and location of the OSHA and SDS manuals, the location of hazardous chemicals, and the procedure for cleaning up a chemical spill. Commission on Accreditation of Allied Health and Education Programs (CAAHEP) and Accrediting Bureau of Health Education Schools (ABHES) program accreditation standards require that students follow safety precautions.

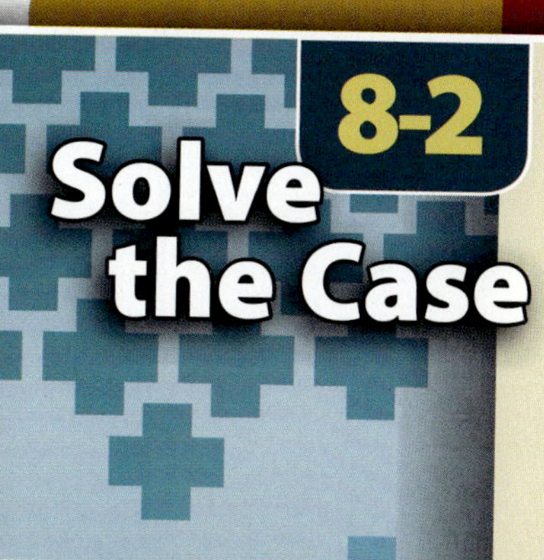

Susan Groves has been taking very good care of herself, physically and mentally, since her diagnosis of HCV infection last year. She has not been feeling very energetic lately and wonders if she might be pregnant.

1. **What might be causing Susan's lack of energy?**
2. **If she is pregnant, would the baby have the virus?**
3. **What changes should she make in her life moving forward from here?**
4. **Is there a vaccination for HCV?**

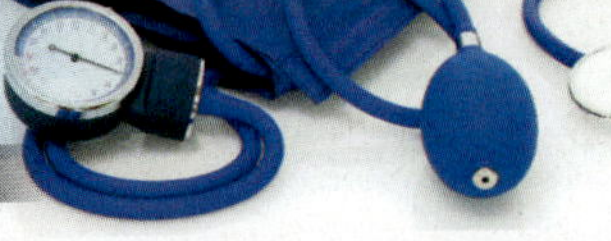

PROCEDURE 8-1

Perform Medically Aseptic Handwashing

Objective:

To clean all surface bacteria off the hands and wrists to prevent the spread of pathogenic microorganisms.

Equipment/Supplies:

- Soap (preferably liquid and not antibacterial)
- Sink with free moving water
- Paper towels
- Orange stick and/or brush for cleaning fingernails

PROCEDURAL STEPS	DETAILS AND/OR RATIONALE
1. Remove all jewelry on hands and wrists.	Microorganisms can hide in crevices in jewelry.
2. Stand at the sink, but do not touch the sink with hands or clothing.	The sink is considered contaminated.
3. Turn on the faucet, and adjust the water temperature (Figure 8-20a).	Water temperature should be warm, not hot.
4. Wet the hands, wrists, and forearms and apply soap; using a circular motion and friction, scrub the backs and palms of hands, wrists, and forearms, interlace fingers and thumbs and rub back and forth to clean surfaces in-between; keep the hands pointing down during the entire washing process (Figures 8-20b and Figure 8-20c).	Friction and running water are best for cleansing; by keeping hands pointed downward and lower than the forearms, contaminants run off the hands and down the drain, instead of back up onto the clean forearm.
5. Clean the nails and cuticles with a cuticle stick or soft brush (Figure 8-20d).	Microorganisms can collect under the nails (especially acrylic and adorned nails) and around the cuticles.
6. Rinse the hands and wrists well with the hands pointed downward and not touching the sink (Figure 8-20e).	Residue soap can irritate the skin; avoid contaminating hands.
7. Repeat if this is the first handwashing of the day or when the hands are contaminated with blood or OPIM. ***Recognize the implications for failure to comply with CDC regulations in the health care setting.***	
8. Blot the hands, wrists, and forearms, dry with a paper towel, and discard the towel. Turn the faucet off with a clean paper towel (Figure 8-20f).	Rubbing the skin with a towel can cause irritation. Touching the faucet will contaminate clean hands.
9. Apply lotion.	Frequent handwashing can irritate and dry the skin. Lotion can help, but do not use lanolin lotions immediately prior to donning gloves.

continues

PROCEDURE 8-1 continued

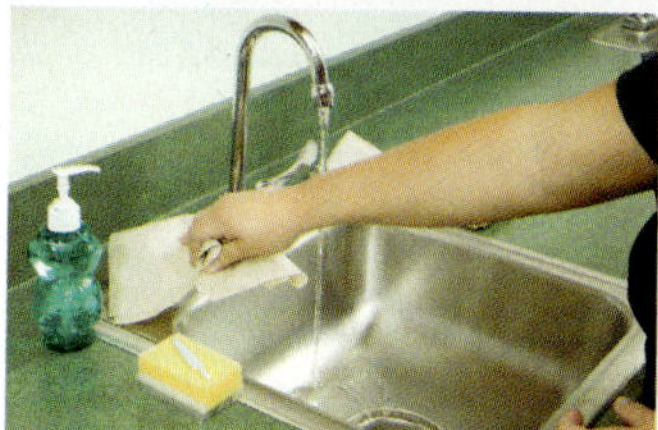
Figure 8-20a ■ Adjust the water temperature.

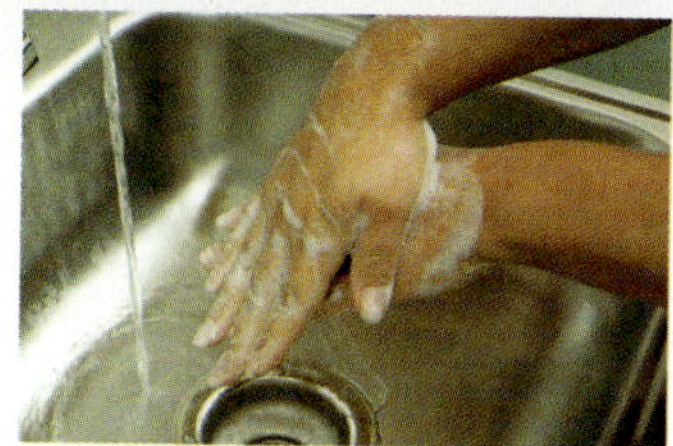
Figure 8-20b ■ Wet hands, apply soap, hands pointed downward and not touching sink.

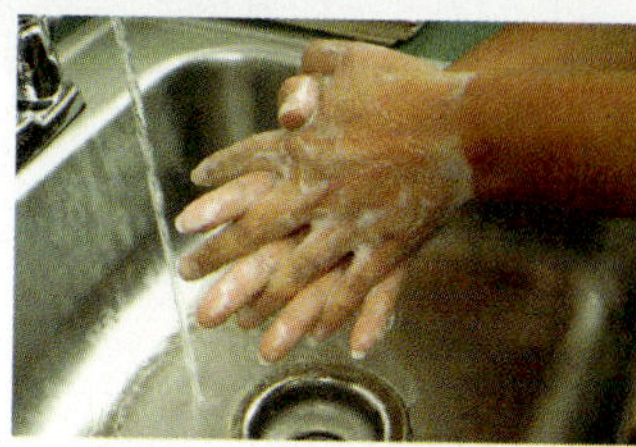
Figure 8-20c ■ Wash all surfaces front and back of hands, between fingers using mild friction.

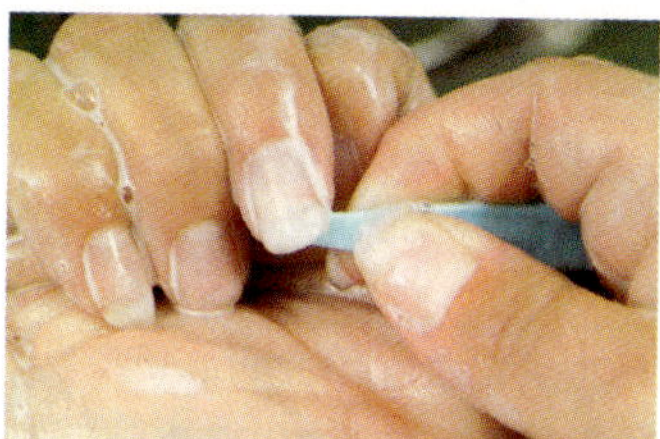
Figure 8-20d ■ Clean fingernails with cuticle stick or nail brush.

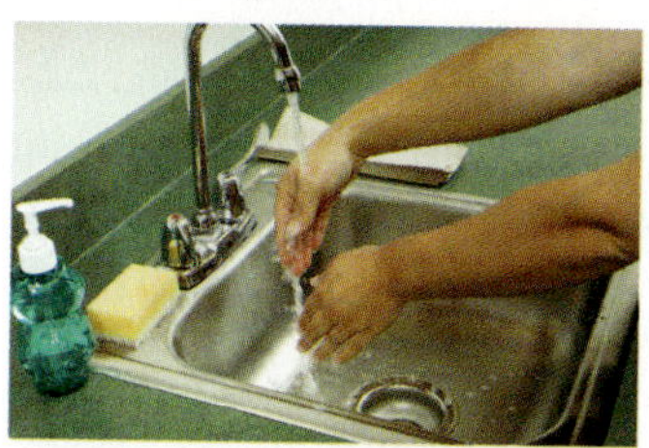
Figure 8-20e ■ With fingers pointing downward, rinse hands without touching the sink.

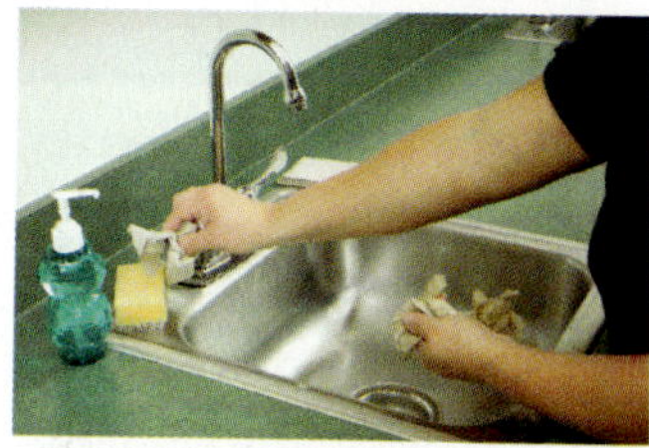
Figure 8-20f ■ Turn off the faucet with a clean paper towel.

PROCEDURE 8-2

Perform an Alcohol-Based Hand Rub

Objective:

To properly perform an alcohol-based hand rub in lieu of handwashing.

Equipment/Supplies:

- Alcohol-based hand sanitizer

PROCEDURAL STEPS	DETAILS AND/OR RATIONALE
1. Inspect the hands for any visible soil or contamination. If present, the hands must be washed first.	An alcohol-based hand sanitizer is not used on visibly contaminated hands.
2. Remove all jewelry on hands and wrists.	Jewelry can harbor microorganisms.
3. Apply the recommended amount of alcohol-based hand sanitizer (Figure 8-21a).	Gels and lotions require a smaller amount than foam, manufacturer's guidelines may vary.
4. Smooth the hand rub over all surfaces of the hand.	All areas must be coated to ensure effective hygiene.
5. Rub the hands together (approximately 15 to 30 seconds) until dry (Figure 8-21b).	Moist hands could attract microorganisms.

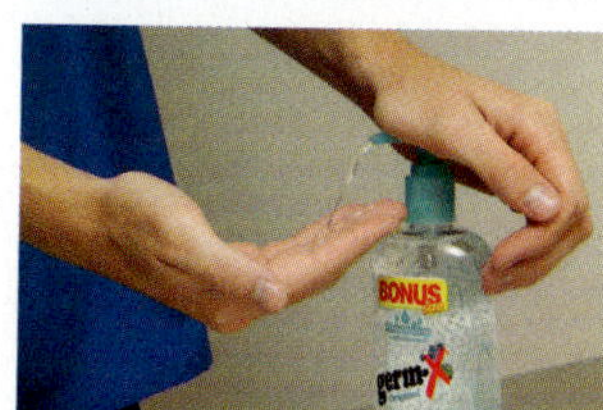

Figure 8-21a ■ After jewelry is removed, apply the alcohol-based gel.

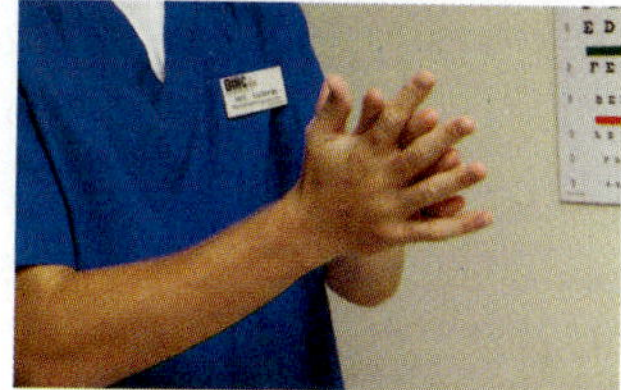
Figure 8-21b ■ Rub the gel into all surfaces of the hands until absorbed.

PROCEDURE 8-3

Remove Contaminated Gloves

Objective:

To properly remove and dispose of contaminated gloves without contaminating hands or other areas.

Equipment/Supplies:

- Biohazard waste container with step-on lid opener

PROCEDURAL STEPS	DETAILS AND/OR RATIONALE
1. With the hands pointed downward and away from the body, grab the palm of the right glove with the left hand (Figure 8-22a).	By keeping the hands pointed downward and away from the body, the risk of exposure to biohazard material is reduced.
2. Turn the right glove inside out, drop it into the left gloved hand, and crumple it into a ball in the left hand (Figures 8-22b, c, d, and e).	Turning the glove inside out places contaminants on the inside and away from the body. Dropping it into the left hand prevents cross contamination between the still gloved left hand and the ungloved right hand.
3. Form a fist with the left hand, containing the right glove, invert the fist, and insert two fingers of the ungloved hand between the wrist and under the cuff of the back of the contaminated left glove (Figure 8-22f).	By inserting ungloved fingers under the back of the cuff, contact with the outside of the contaminated glove is avoided.
4. Turn the left glove inside out over the fist containing the crumpled other glove (Figures 8-22g and h).	Contaminated surfaces of both gloves are reversed and the gloves can be handled without risk of exposure.
5. Dispose of the contaminated gloves by dropping them into a biohazard waste container, preferably controlled with a step-on lid opening pedal (Figure 8-22i). ***Recognize the implications for failure to comply with CDC regulations in health care settings.***	Contaminated gloves should be placed in a red, water-proof biohazard bag. Foot-controlled lid opener pedal prevents having to touch the lid with hands.
6. Wash hands.	Washing the hands after removing gloves cleans away any possible contamination and powder left behind from inside the gloves.

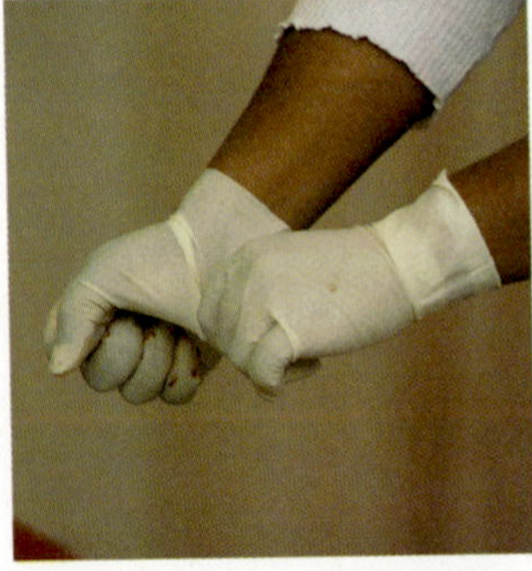

Figure 8-22a ■ Grasp the palm of the contaminated right glove with the left hand.

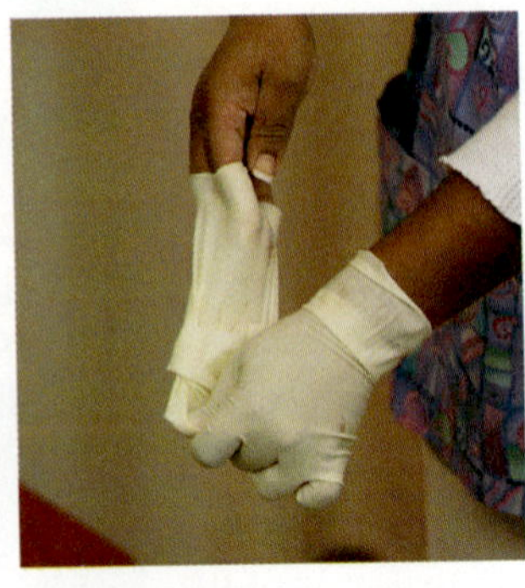

Figure 8-22b ■ Remove the right glove, turning it inside out.

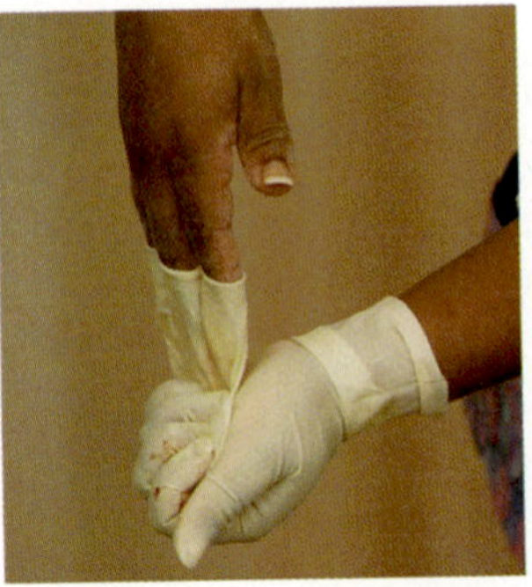

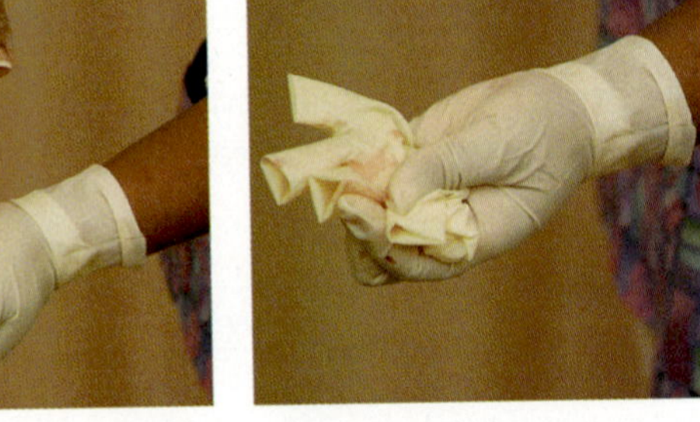

Figure 8-22c and d ■ Remove the right glove, turning it inside out.

continues

PROCEDURE 8-3 continued

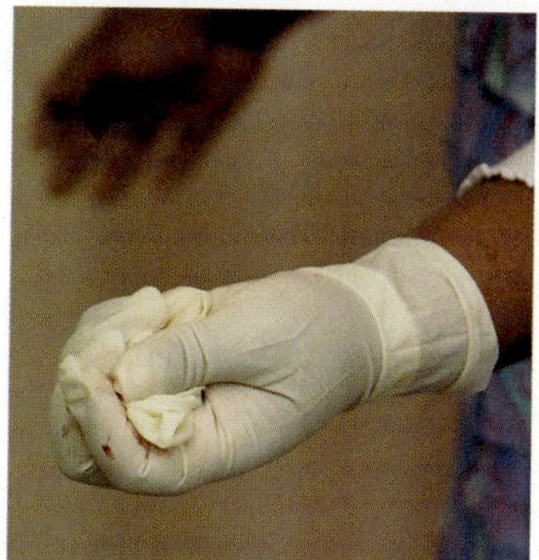

Figure 8-22e ■ Crumple the contaminated inverted glove and hold it in the left hand.

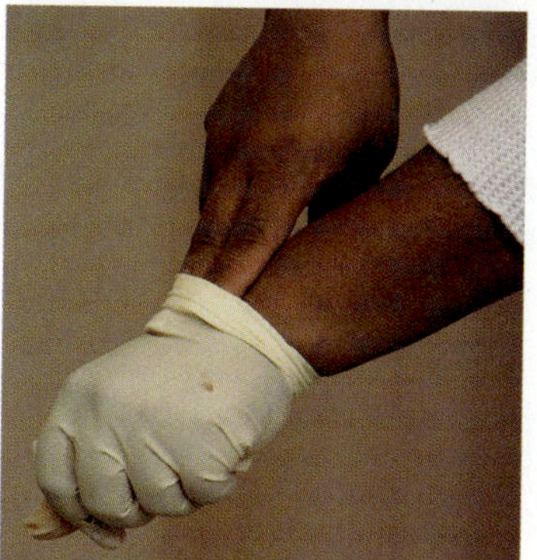

Figure 8-22f ■ Insert two fingers of the ungloved hand between the wrist and under the cuff of the back of the contaminated left glove.

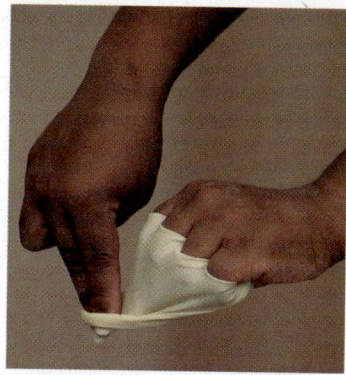

Figure 8-22g ■ Turn the left glove inside out over the fist containing the crumpled other glove.

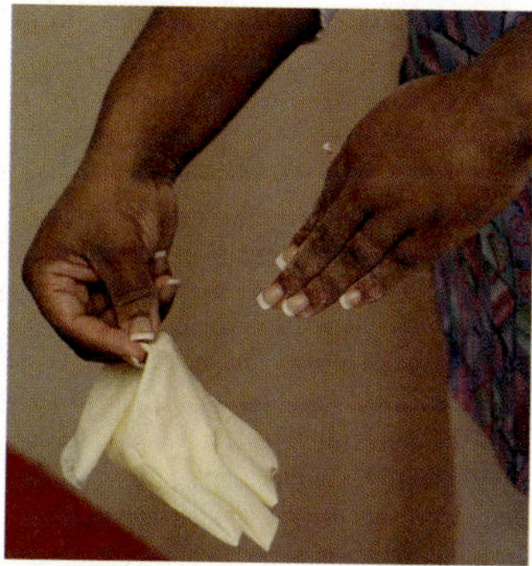

Figure 8-22h ■ The contaminated surfaces of both gloves are inside.

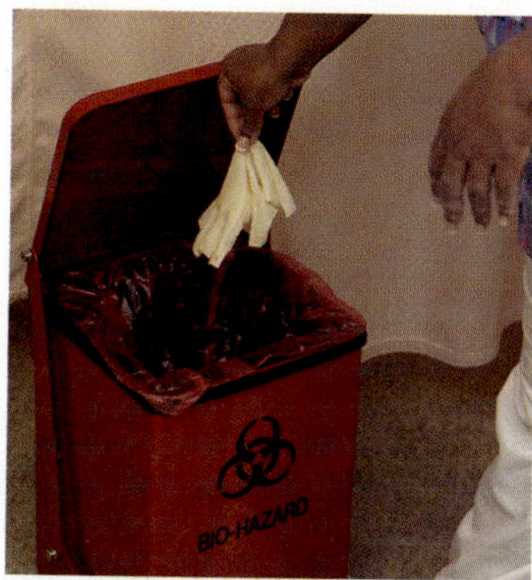

Figure 8-22i ■ Drop the gloves into a biohazard container.

PROCEDURE 8-4

Select, Apply, Remove, and Dispose of Appropriate PPE Following Universal or Standard Precautions

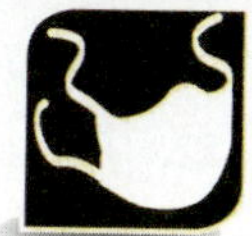

Objective:

To select the appropriate PPE and dispose of contaminated items based on individual procedure or infectious event.

Equipment/Supplies:

- Full set of PPE including gown, gloves, mask, goggles, shoe covers, disinfectant, paper towels, spill kit, laundry container, trash receptacle, and biohazard waste receptacle.

continues

PROCEDURE 8-4 continued

PROCEDURAL STEPS	DETAILS AND/OR RATIONALE
1. If a procedure is ordered, review the provider's orders and the organization's protocol for applying PPE and procedures for the proper disposal of infectious wastes. If involved in an infectious event, follow protocol for handling such events.	Protocols may vary from one facility to another. Some practices follow Standard Precautions while others follow Universal Precautions; always check protocol so you know how to respond.
2. Pull the appropriate PPE, cleaning supplies, or spill kit based on the procedure or infectious event.	This will vary according to the procedure or infectious event.
3. Remove jewelry, lab coat, or any other items that may become contaminated if exposed to bodily fluids.	
4. Wash hands, apply gown, and tie securely. (Figure 8-23a and Figure 8-23b).	Gowns should be worn when ever there is the potential of splash from blood and other bodily fluids.
5. Apply shoe and hair covers, if applicable (Figure 8-23c and Figure 8-23d).	Shoe covers are only necessary when cleaning up infectious wastes on the floor. Hair cover should be worn if there is the potential for splash of blood or other bodily fluids.
6. Apply mask, if applicable (Figure 8-23e)	Masks should be worn when there is a potential for splash of blood or other bodily fluids.
7. Apply safety glasses, if applicable (Figure 8-23f).	Safety glasses should be worn when there is a potential for splash of blood or other bodily fluids.
8. Apply gloves and pull over the cuff of gown to ensure that no skin is exposed (Figure 8-23g).	Gloves should be worn whenever there is potential for contact with blood or other bodily fluids.
9. Enter exposure area, perform procedure, or clean up infectious wastes following the organization's protocol (Figures 8-23h and 8-23i).	
10. Dispose of wastes into the proper receptacles (Figure 8-23j) and transport contaminated instruments and equipment to proper area for cleaning, disinfection, or sterilization.	If your organization follows universal precautions, anything saturated with blood or other potentially infectious material should be placed into a biohazard receptacle; anything not saturated with blood or other potentially infectious material should be placed in regular trash. If practicing standard precautions and BSI, all items contaminated with any blood or bodily fluids should be placed in a biohazard container.
11. Remove contaminated gloves and place in biohazard bag.	Gloves will be most contaminated which is why they are removed first.
12. Remove goggles or face shield and place in biohazard container, if contaminated. (If these items cannot be removed without contaminating hands, apply gloves before removal.)	If these items cannot be removed without contaminating hands, gloves should be worn to reduce further contamination to hands.
13. Remove gown or apron/coverall. Untie the ties and peel the gown away from your neck and shoulder, then turn gown inside out, and roll into a ball. If disposable, place in the biohazard container. If cloth, put in a proper laundry receptacle.	Removing gown by pulling ties and working your hands to the inside of the gown prevents you from touching the front of the gown that may have been contaminated during the procedure or cleanup event.

continues

PROCEDURE 8-4 continued

PROCEDURAL STEPS	DETAILS AND/OR RATIONALE
14. Remove shoe and/or hair covers and dispose of in proper trash receptacle.	
15. Remove mask and place in proper trash receptacle.	
16. Wash hands and put away cleaning supplies.	

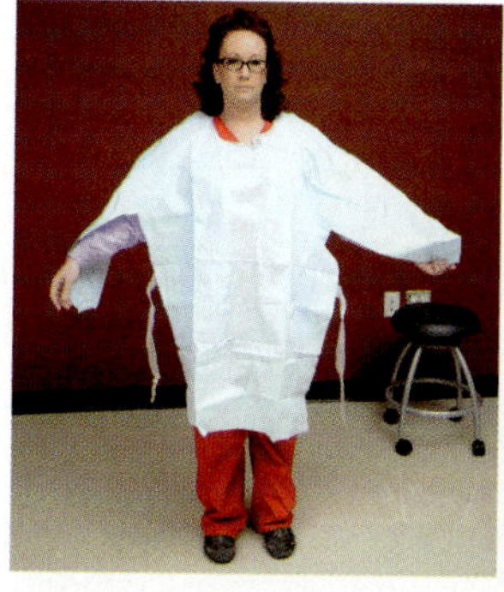

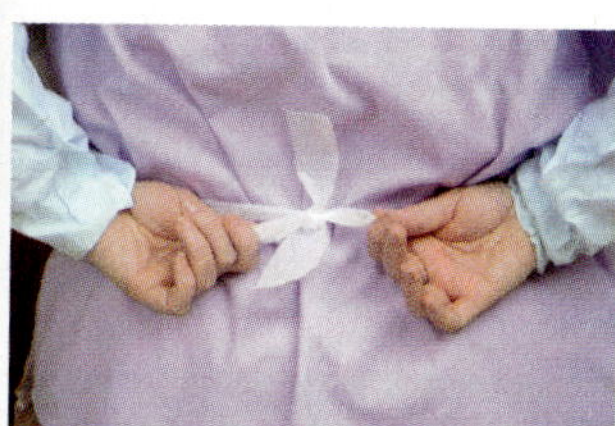

Figures 8-23a and b ■ Apply gown and tie securely, making certain outer garments are complete covered.

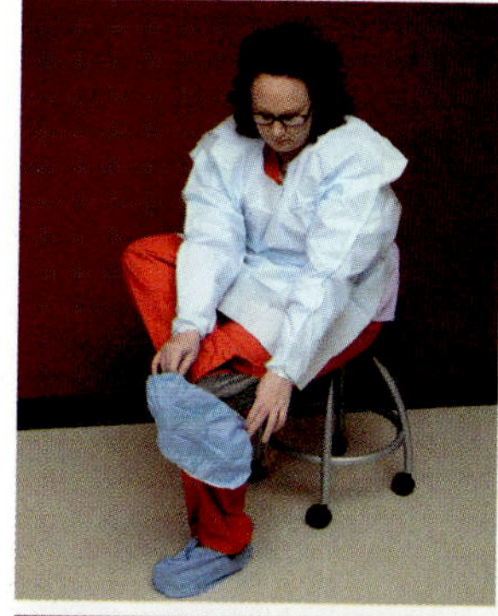

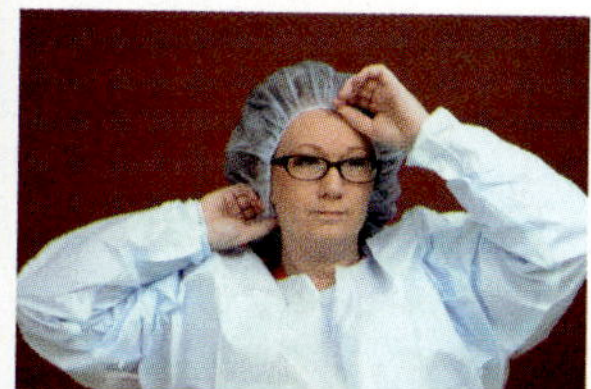

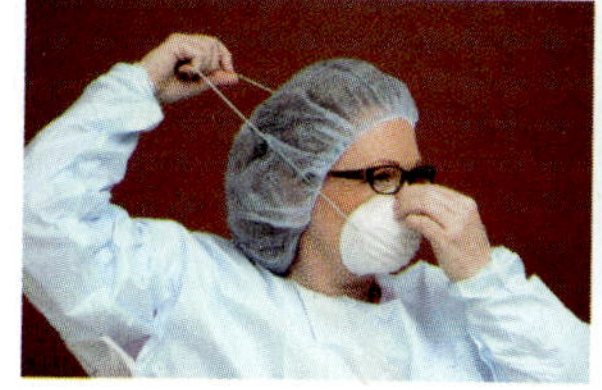

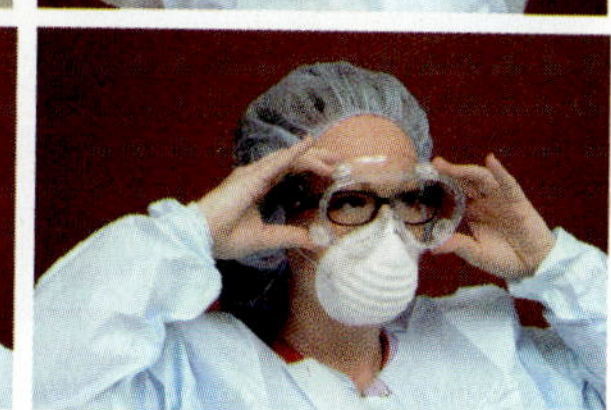

Figures 8-23c, d, e, and f ■ Apply shoe covers, hair cover, mask, and safety glasses, if applicable.

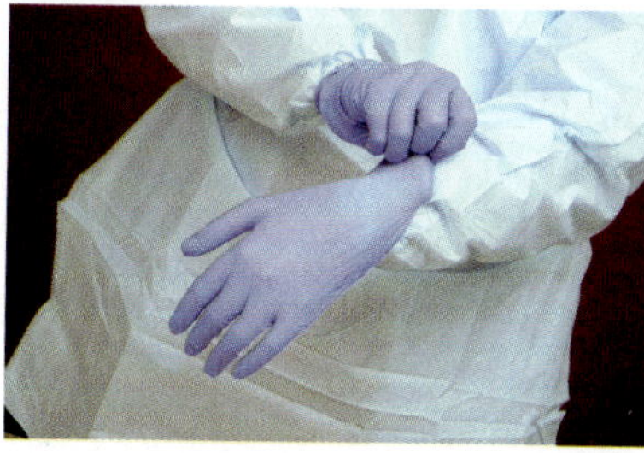

Figure 8-23g Apply gloves and pull over the cuff of gown.

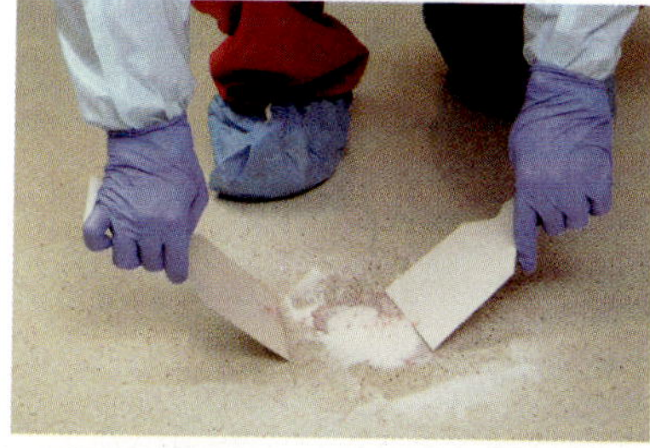

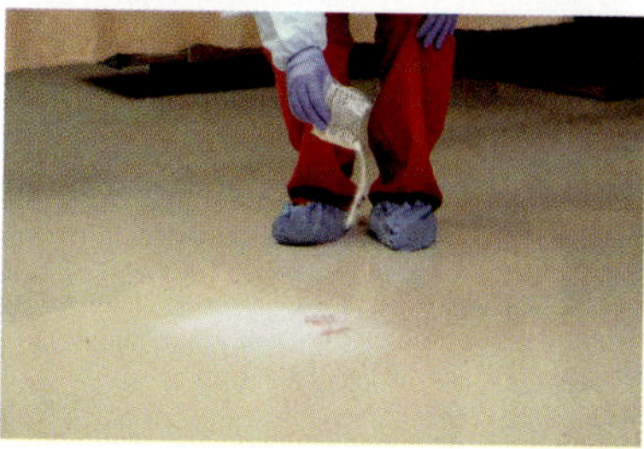

Figures 8-23h and i Perform procedure or clean up infectious wastes following the organization's protocol.

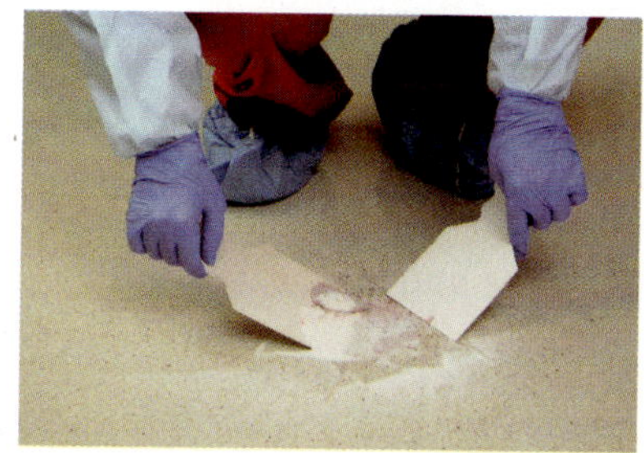

Figure 8-23j Dispose of waste into the proper receptacle.

CHAPTER SUMMARY

- Medical assisting is rewarding but does come with risks such as exposure to diseases as well as laboratory chemicals.
- OSHA and CDC work for our protection and to decrease exposures and prevent the spread of diseases and we should understand the standards, guidelines, and rules from both of these entities.
- Medical assistants should adhere to the OSHA and CDC guidelines, thereby providing the safest environment for ourselves, our patients, coworkers, and society, as well as protecting our practice legally.
- A good working knowledge of the infection cycle, the growth needs of pathogens, types of organisms, and stages of infections is important for us in order to help our patients.
- Medical assistants should understand the difference between inflammation and infection and be able to ascertain when each is happening.
- Medical assistants should be well versed in our body's natural defenses, the various types of immunities, types of vaccines available, and how our immune systems work.
- All health care workers should be able to properly wash their hands, apply alcohol-based gel in lieu of handwashing, and remove contaminated gloves safely.
- In order to protect oneself from biological contamination, medical assistants should utilize PPE whenever appropriate.
- Part of our clinical duties is to properly dispose of contaminated waste according to CDC standards.

CERTIFICATION REVIEW QUESTIONS

1. The branch of science that studies infectious disease is:
   a. demiology.
   b. epidemiology.
   c. pathology.
   d. virology.
2. The stage of infection that produces no identifiable signs or symptoms is the:
   a. incubation stage.
   b. acute stage.
   c. invasion and multiplication stage.
   d. prodromal stage.
3. The destruction of microorganisms before they enter the body is known as:
   a. sterilization.
   b. medical asepsis.
   c. surgical asepsis.
   d. disinfection.
4. Standard Precautions and Transmission-Based Precautions were developed by:
   a. OSHA.
   b. DDC.
   c. CDC.
   d. HHS.
5. Standard Precautions should be observed for:
   a. tears.
   b. saliva.
   c. mucous secretions.
   d. All of these
6. The disease posing the greatest risk to health care workers is:
   a. AIDS.
   b. HIV.
   c. hepatitis C.
   d. Ebola.
7. The primary means of transmitting HIV is:
   a. sharing eating utensils.
   b. through sexual contact.
   c. kissing.
   d. None of the above
8. Barriers used to protect health workers from possible exposure to infectious agents are known as:
   a. safety hoods.
   b. Standard Precautions.
   c. work practice controls.
   d. PPE.

9. Properly disposing of contaminated sharps and body fluids and the use of safety data sheets and spill kits are covered under the title of:
   a. postexposure plans.
   b. PPE.
   c. the cycle of diseases.
   d. biohazard disposal and regulated waste.

10. The terms *direct*, *indirect*, *airborne*, *droplet*, *vertical*, *iatrogenic*, and *inhalation* are words that describe which of the following?
   a. Vectors that carry diseases
   b. Susceptible hosts
   c. Methods of exit and entrance of diseases
   d. Modes of transmission

STUDY RESOURCES

Resources to Test and Reinforce Your Knowledge:	
Certification Review Questions	Take this end-of-chapter quiz
Workbook	• Complete the activities for Chapter 8 • Perform the procedures for Chapter 8 using the Competency Checklists
Resources to Promote Critical Thinking:	
***Solve the Case* Activities**	• Consider these case studies and discuss your conclusions
Learning Lab	• Module 19: Infection Control and Medical Asepsis
MindTap	• Complete Chapter 8 readings and activities

REFERENCES

Centers for Disease Control and Prevention (CDC). (2014). *2014 Hand Hygiene in Healthcare Settings and Clean Hands Save Lives*. Retrieved from http://www.cdc.gov/handhygiene/ and http://www.cdc.gov/handwashing/

Centers for Disease Control and Prevention (CDC). (2014). *2014 HIV/AIDS News and Events, Guidelines and Recommendations*. Retrieved from http://www.cdc.gov/hiv/guidelines/index.html

National Institute of Allergy and Infectious Diseases (NIH). (2012, April 13). *Types of Vaccines*. Retrieved from http://www.niaid.nih.gov/topics/vaccines/understanding/pages/typesvaccines.aspx

United States Department of Labor Occupational Safety and Health Administration (OSHA). (2012). *Bloodborne Pathogen Standards (revised 2012)*. Retrieved from https://www.osha.gov/pls/oshaweb/owadisp.show_document?p_id=10051&p_table=STANDARDS

United States Department of Labor Occupational Safety and Health Administration (OSHA). *OSHA Quick Card—Hazard Communication Safety Data Sheets*. Retrieved from https://www.osha.gov/Publications/HazComm_QuickCard_SafetyData.html

United States Department of Labor Occupational Safety and Health Administration (OSHA). (2012). *OSHA Quick Card—NFPA 704 labeling comparison to OSHA HazCom 2012*. Retrieved from https://www.osha.gov/Publications/OSHA3678.pdf

United States Department of Labor Occupational Safety and Health Administration (OSHA). *OSHA Quick Card—OSHA's Pictograms and Hazards*. Retrieved from https://www.osha.gov/Publications/OSHA3491QuickCardPictogram.pdf

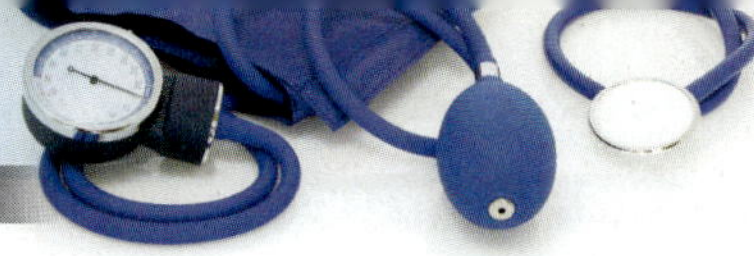

INTRODUCTION

A comprehension of medical and surgical asepsis is essential when preparing trays for surgical procedures, setting up the room for surgical procedures, and cleaning items following the procedure. The medical assistant must be familiar with how to properly clean, disinfect, and sterilize instruments to prevent patients from developing postoperative infections. But that isn't the only reason the medical assistant needs to know how to properly prepare surgical trays. Keeping instruments in prime condition also helps the surgical process to progress more smoothly during procedures because instruments are in good working order. There are a variety of instruments used in ambulatory care settings.

This chapter will introduce the reader to the most common instruments and supplies used in ambulatory care facilities and will discuss how to properly clean, disinfect, and sterilize instruments.

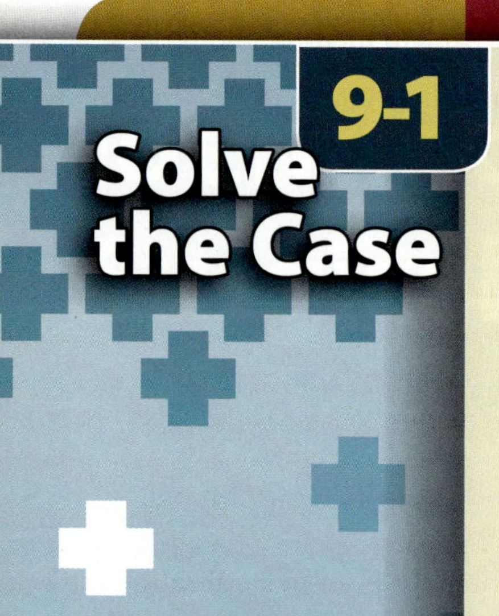

Dr. Rupert has asked you to pull a cyst removal tray for Mrs. Zangmeister's procedure scheduled later today. You pull the only cyst removal tray out of storage and examine it to see if it is ready to go.

1. **Using just your current knowledge, what types of things do you think you will look for as you inspect the the outer wrapping of the tray?**
2. **Would this procedure be a clean or sterile procedure? Explain why you selected the answer you did.**
3. **You notice that there is a very tiny hole in the top of the tray. The tray was stored in a clean air tight container. Since it has been stored the entire time in the air tight container, do you think you need to worry about the tiny hole in the wrapping material? Why or why not?**

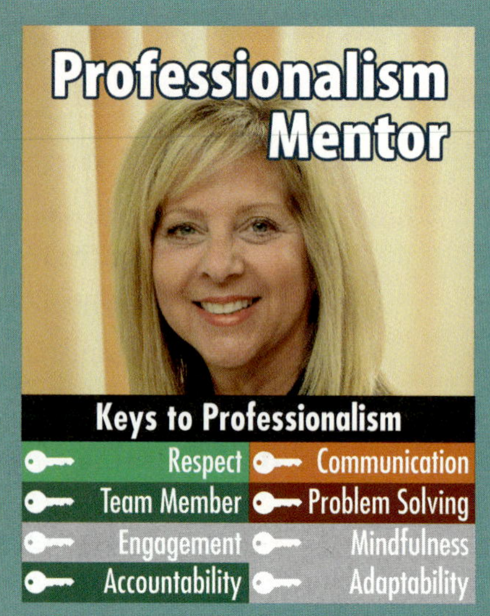

There are a lot of reasons to wash your hands when working in health care. Hopefully you are one of the diligent ones who remembers to foam in and foam out each time you enter an exam room. What would you do if one of your coworkers failed to wash their hands each time they entered and exited an exam room? You know it's the right thing to do and that washing your hands is the best way to prevent the spread of infection. Would you feel comfortable telling her not to forget to use good hand hygiene? In your journal, write down some of the phrases you might use to tactfully remind other health care workers to wash their hands. Describe how the keys identified in this feature box will be necessary to your success in getting your coworkers to change their behavior. ■

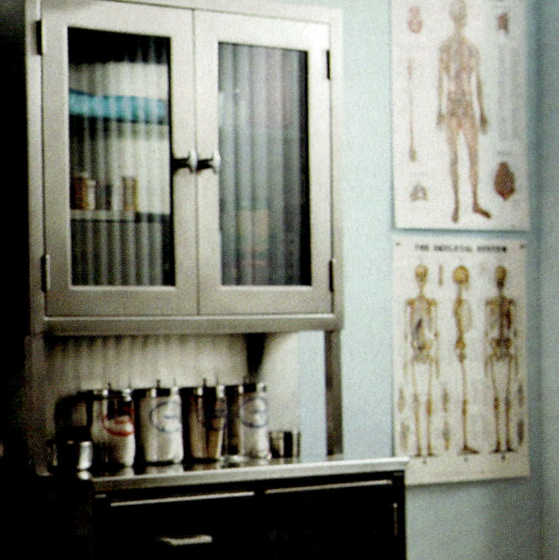

DEVELOPMENTAL OBJECTIVES

After completing this chapter, you should be able to:

1. Correctly spell and define the essential terms.
2. Compare and contrast medical and surgical asepsis and explain how these procedures apply to the ambulatory care setting.
3. Describe the processes of sanitization, disinfection, and sterilization and explain when each method should be used.
4. Prepare items for autoclaving.
5. List the parts of various instruments and explain their functions.
6. Identify common instruments used in ambulatory surgery and explain their uses.
7. List common solutions and supplies used in minor surgery and explain their use.
8. List various methods for closing the skin and explain when each method may be used.
9. Demonstrate how to sanitize, lubricate, and inspect instruments prior to disinfection or sterilization.
10. Demonstrate how to properly disinfect instruments following sanitization.
11. Demonstrate how to properly wrap instruments prior to sterilization and run an automated autoclave.
12. Demonstrate how to apply sterile adhesive strips and remove sutures and staples.

INTRODUCTION

A comprehension of medical and surgical asepsis is essential when preparing trays for surgical procedures, setting up the room for surgical procedures, and cleaning items following the procedure. The medical assistant must be familiar with how to properly clean, disinfect, and sterilize instruments to prevent patients from developing postoperative infections. But that isn't the only reason the medical assistant needs to know how to properly prepare surgical trays. Keeping instruments in prime condition also helps the surgical process to progress more smoothly during procedures because instruments are in good working order. There are a variety of instruments used in ambulatory care settings.

This chapter will introduce the reader to the most common instruments and supplies used in ambulatory care facilities and will discuss how to properly clean, disinfect, and sterilize instruments.

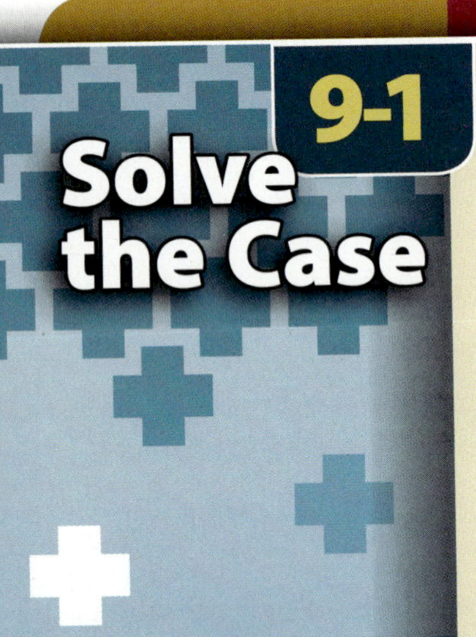

Dr. Rupert has asked you to pull a cyst removal tray for Mrs. Zangmeister's procedure scheduled later today. You pull the only cyst removal tray out of storage and examine it to see if it is ready to go.

1. **Using just your current knowledge, what types of things do you think you will look for as you inspect the the outer wrapping of the tray?**
2. **Would this procedure be a clean or sterile procedure? Explain why you selected the answer you did.**
3. **You notice that there is a very tiny hole in the top of the tray. The tray was stored in a clean air tight container. Since it has been stored the entire time in the air tight container, do you think you need to worry about the tiny hole in the wrapping material? Why or why not?**

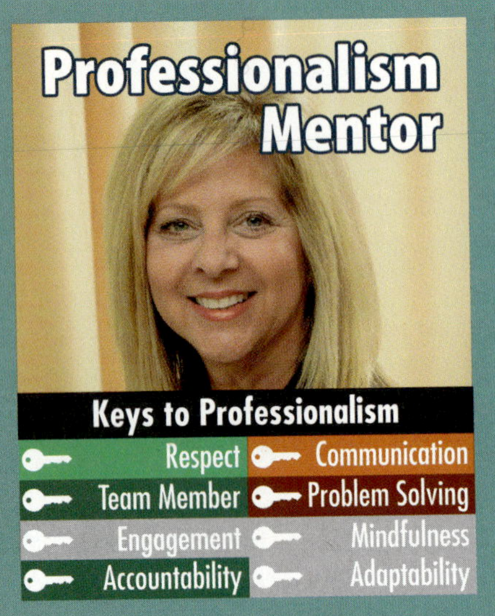

There are a lot of reasons to wash your hands when working in health care. Hopefully you are one of the diligent ones who remembers to foam in and foam out each time you enter an exam room. What would you do if one of your coworkers failed to wash their hands each time they entered and exited an exam room? You know it's the right thing to do and that washing your hands is the best way to prevent the spread of infection. Would you feel comfortable telling her not to forget to use good hand hygiene? In your journal, write down some of the phrases you might use to tactfully remind other health care workers to wash their hands. Describe how the keys identified in this feature box will be necessary to your success in getting your coworkers to change their behavior. ■

9. Properly disposing of contaminated sharps and body fluids and the use of safety data sheets and spill kits are covered under the title of:
   a. postexposure plans.
   b. PPE.
   c. the cycle of diseases.
   d. biohazard disposal and regulated waste.

10. The terms *direct*, *indirect*, *airborne*, *droplet*, *vertical*, *iatrogenic*, and *inhalation* are words that describe which of the following?
   a. Vectors that carry diseases
   b. Susceptible hosts
   c. Methods of exit and entrance of diseases
   d. Modes of transmission

STUDY RESOURCES

Resources to Test and Reinforce Your Knowledge:	
Certification Review Questions	Take this end-of-chapter quiz
Workbook	• Complete the activities for Chapter 8 • Perform the procedures for Chapter 8 using the Competency Checklists
Resources to Promote Critical Thinking:	
***Solve the Case* Activities**	• Consider these case studies and discuss your conclusions
Learning Lab	• Module 19: Infection Control and Medical Asepsis
MindTap	• Complete Chapter 8 readings and activities

REFERENCES

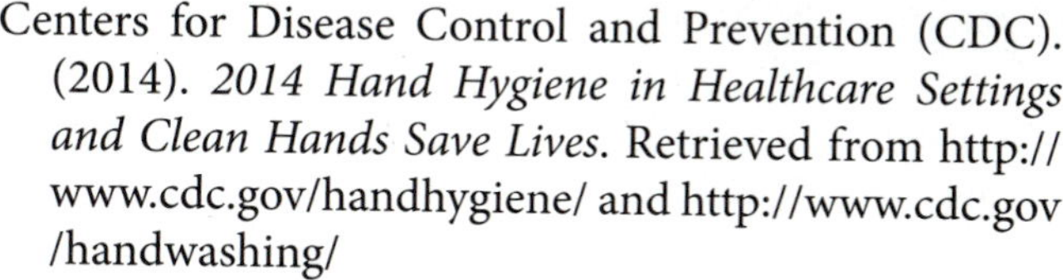

Centers for Disease Control and Prevention (CDC). (2014). *2014 Hand Hygiene in Healthcare Settings and Clean Hands Save Lives.* Retrieved from http://www.cdc.gov/handhygiene/ and http://www.cdc.gov/handwashing/

Centers for Disease Control and Prevention (CDC). (2014). *2014 HIV/AIDS News and Events, Guidelines and Recommendations.* Retrieved from http://www.cdc.gov/hiv/guidelines/index.html

National Institute of Allergy and Infectious Diseases (NIH). (2012, April 13). *Types of Vaccines.* Retrieved from http://www.niaid.nih.gov/topics/vaccines/understanding/pages/typesvaccines.aspx

United States Department of Labor Occupational Safety and Health Administration (OSHA). (2012). *Bloodborne Pathogen Standards (revised 2012).* Retrieved from https://www.osha.gov/pls/oshaweb/owadisp.show_document?p_id=10051&p_table=STANDARDS

United States Department of Labor Occupational Safety and Health Administration (OSHA). *OSHA Quick Card—Hazard Communication Safety Data Sheets.* Retrieved from https://www.osha.gov/Publications/HazComm_QuickCard_SafetyData.html

United States Department of Labor Occupational Safety and Health Administration (OSHA). (2012). *OSHA Quick Card—NFPA 704 labeling comparison to OSHA HazCom 2012.* Retrieved from https://www.osha.gov/Publications/OSHA3678.pdf

United States Department of Labor Occupational Safety and Health Administration (OSHA). *OSHA Quick Card—OSHA's Pictograms and Hazards.* Retrieved from https://www.osha.gov/Publications/OSHA3491QuickCardPictogram.pdf

9

Sterilization Procedures, Instrument Identification, and Surgical Supplies

CHAPTER OUTLINE

Asepsis

Sanitization, Disinfection, and Sterilization

- Sanitization Procedures
- Disinfection Procedures
- Sterilization Techniques

Types of Instruments Used in Minor Surgery

- Identifying the Parts of a Surgical Instrument
- Categories of Instruments

Solutions and Supplies Used for Minor Surgeries

- Common Solutions Used in Minor Surgery
- Common Supplies Used in Minor Surgery
- Common Anesthetics Used in Minor Surgery
- Suture Materials and Other Supplies to Close the Skin

Suture and Staple Removal

ESSENTIAL TERMS

anesthetic
atraumatic needle
autoclave
box lock
disinfection
dissect
endoscopes
fenestrated
handle
jaws
ligature
medical asepsis
minimum effective concentration (MEC)
opened-container life
ratchet
reuse life
sanitization
serrations
shank
shelf life
sterilization
sterilization indicators
surgical adhesive
surgical asepsis
surgical wicks
suture
traumatic needle
ultrasonic cleaner

ASEPSIS

As you learned in Chapter 8, the term *asepsis* means free of germs. **Medical asepsis** refers to the destruction of organisms after leaving the body. Inanimate surfaces that come into contact with bodily fluids or living tissue need to be cleaned and disinfected to avoid the spread of infection. The disinfection of counter tops, mopping or cleaning of floors, and the sanitization of instruments following a procedure are all examples of techniques which employ medical asepsis.

Surgical asepsis is the destruction of all microorganisms prior to a surgical procedure. Sterilization of instruments, setting up sterile fields, and the donning of sterile gloves and gowns prior to a surgical procedure are examples of surgical asepsis. Refer to Figure 9-1 for examples of both medical and surgical asepsis.

Since it is impossible to sterilize the skin's surface, cleaning and using an antiseptic soap as part of surgical asepsis is the procedure most effective in preventing surface microorganisms from entering the surgical incision.

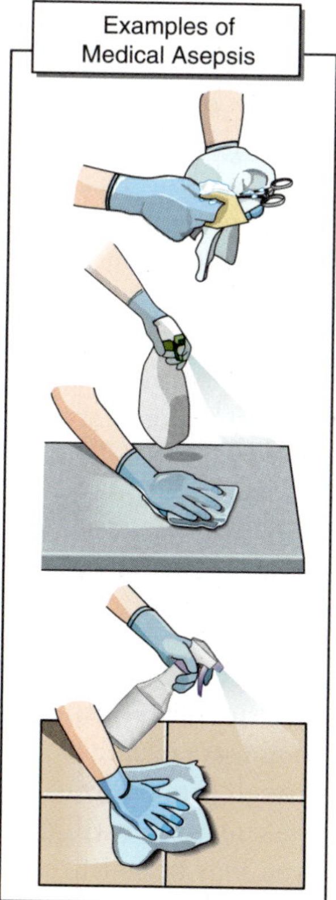

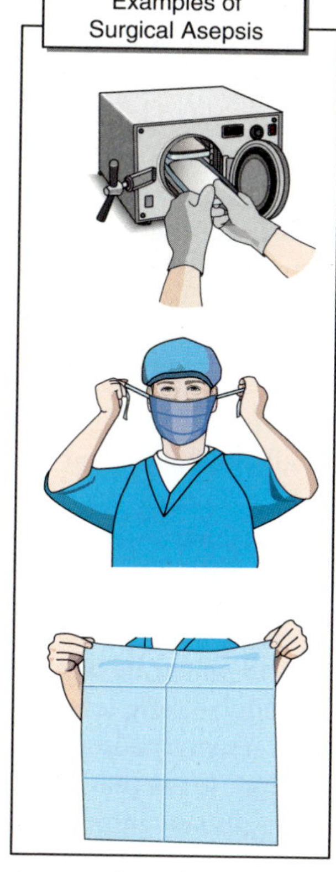

Figure 9-1 ■ Notice the difference in procedures that are considered medical aseptic procedures and procedures that are considered part of surgical asepsis.

SANITIZATION, DISINFECTION, AND STERILIZATION

There are three processes that may be used to prepare instruments and **endoscopes** (illuminated flexible or sometimes rigid tubes used to view body structures or organs) for complete sterilization: sanitization, disinfection, and sterilization. All instruments need to be sanitized prior to disinfection or sterilization. Whether or not the instrument needs to be disinfected or sterilized depends on the type of instrument and how it will be used during the procedure.

Sanitization Procedures

The term **sanitization** means to make sanitary or clean. It is the process by which contaminated instruments are washed and scrubbed to remove potentially infectious materials such as blood, body fluids, and tissue debris. After use, instruments should immediately be placed in a soaking container of distilled water and enzymatic detergent to keep blood and tissue from drying on the instrument. Even though particular instruments from a pack may not have been used, nonvisible body fluids or airborne pathogens may have adhered to the instrument, so they should be treated as though contaminated. Surgical soaps used to sanitize instruments should have a pH relatively close to 7, because acidic or alkaline solutions may cause deposits to form, resulting in damage to the instrument. Utility gloves should be worn to protect the hands from contamination (Figure 9-2). All parts and surfaces of each instrument should be cleansed with a soft brush. Once instruments have been properly scrubbed, they should be rinsed once again using distilled water. Distilled water is chemically pure, which helps prevent instruments from rusting. The instruments should be thoroughly dried following the last rinse with a non-lint-producing material such as muslin cloth and never left to air dry.

Ultrasonic Cleaners

An **ultrasonic cleaner** is a device that cleans instruments by transmitting sound waves through a cleaning fluid. This creates a bubbling effect, loosening debris from the instrument. Using ultrasonic cleaners eliminates the need for manual scrubbing of instruments; however, instruments should be rinsed thoroughly of all visible debris and blood before placing them into an ultrasonic cleaner. Place only like metals together to avoid corrosion. Do not overcrowd the instruments since the ultrasonic vibrations can cause the instrument to tap into each other, which can cause damage. Figure 9-3 shows one type of ultrasonic cleaner.

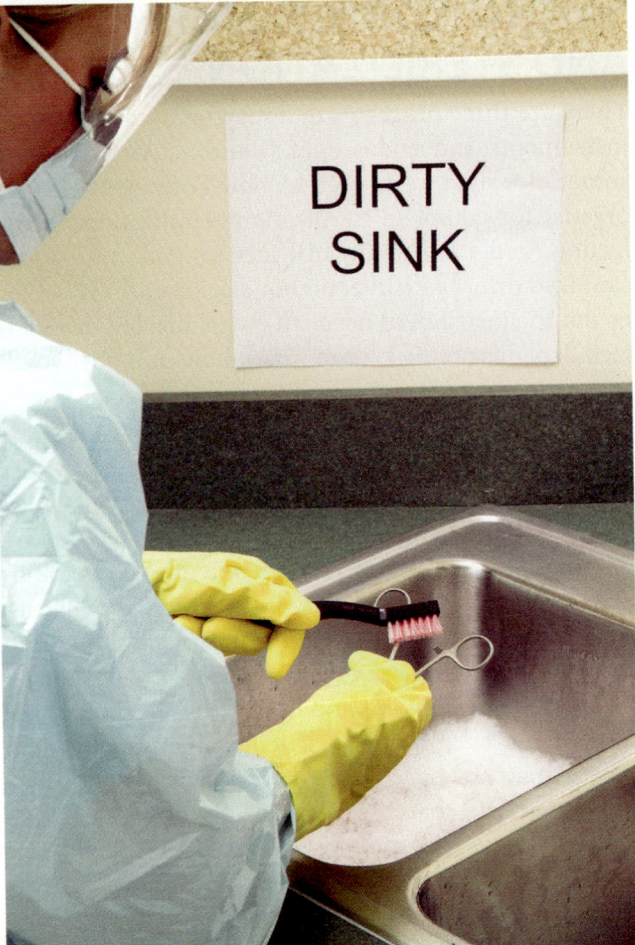

Figure 9-2 ■ Utility gloves help to provide extra protection against sharp instruments.

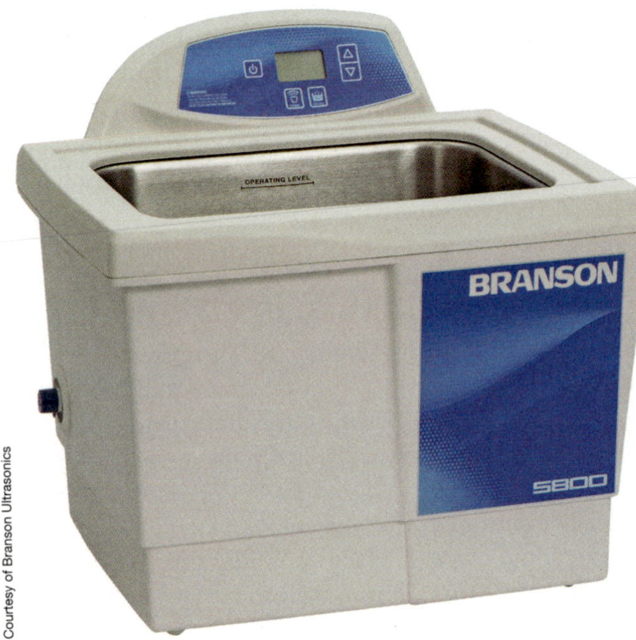

Figure 9-3 ■ The Branson Ultrasonic Cleaner, Model 5800.

Lubricating Instruments

Many manufacturers suggest placing instruments into a lubricating solution following the cleansing process. Instruments are placed into the lubricating solution for 30 to 60 seconds following the cleansing process and dried according to the manufacturer's instructions. Lubricants help to prevent rust and corrosion, help to keep box locks working freely, and maintain the effectiveness of grasping and cutting edges. The instrument should not be rinsed following lubrication because rinsing could remove the lubricant.

Inspecting Instruments

Inspect all instruments for discoloration, defects, and maneuverability prior to sterilizing. Test the sharpness of scissors by cutting into tissue or latex. When cleaning clamps and hemostats, check their serrations, jaw alignment, and box locks for any defects and confirm that the ratchets are secure when closed at each interval. If any defects are found, the affected instruments should be removed from the current supply of instruments and either sent out for repair or discarded. Refer to Procedure 9-1 for instructions on sanitizing and lubricating instruments.

Disinfection Procedures

Disinfection is the use of chemical agents to destroy pathogenic organisms. The majority of disinfectants are not able to kill large numbers of endospores, which are the most resistant of all microorganisms. Disinfection is performed on **inanimate** (nonliving) objects such as counter surfaces, flooring, furniture, and some instruments. Disinfectants are generally not used on the skin because the chemicals in disinfectants can be irritating to the skin and mucous membranes. Chemical disinfectants are used for large instruments, scopes, and items that could be damaged by heat. Sanitization should be performed on an item prior to disinfection.

The level of disinfectant selected is based on the type of instrument and its function. Refer to the following list:

- *Critical items* are instruments or devices that will penetrate or enter sterile tissue. These items require complete sterilization and are usually cleaned by autoclaving or through gas sterilization. Items that are either heat sensitive or will not fit into an autoclave or gas oven may be sterilized through cold sterilization using an FDA-approved sterilant.

- *Semicritical items* are instruments or devices that may come into contact with non-intact skin or mucus membranes and may include items such as ear specula, scopes (laryngoscopes, sigmoidoscopes, cystoscopes, and so on), and diaphragms. These items require an intermediate to high level disinfectant.
- *Noncritical items* are instruments or devices that only touch intact skin; they do not come into contact with mucous membranes or non-intact skin. These items may include items such as stethoscopes, bed rails, blood pressure cuffs, and wheelchairs. Low-level disinfectants may be used on these items.

Levels of Disinfecting Solutions

There are three major levels of disinfecting solutions: low, intermediate, and high. The level or strength of a disinfecting solution is based on both the solution's ability to kill particular types of microorganisms and the numbers of microorganisms that the solution can destroy. Some types of microorganisms are more resistant to particular disinfectants and may require stronger dilutions and longer submersion times. The following is a summary that lists microorganisms in order from most resistant to least resistant:

- Bacterial spores
- Mycobacteria
- Nonlipid or small viruses
- Fungi
- Vegetative bacteria
- Lipid or medium-sized viruses

Examples of disinfectants include isopropyl alcohol, 10% household bleach, idophor germicidal, and glutaraldehyde-based formulas such as Sporicidin, Rapicide, and Cidex Plus. Some of these solutions can be used as a low-level, intermediate-level, or high-level disinfectant based on how long the item is submerged. Some of the high-level disinfectants can be used as sterilants. A sterilant is a high-level liquid disinfectant that has the ability to kill or deactivate all microorganisms and their spores.

Preparing and Storing Disinfectants

Disinfectants may be caustic and cause irritation to skin and other mucous membranes; therefore, medical assistants should always wear gloves and other appropriate PPE (apron/gown, goggles, a mask if splashing is anticipated) and work in well-ventilated areas when using disinfectants.

Three dates that medical assistants must familiarize themselves with when working with disinfecting solutions include the following:

1. **Shelf life**: The amount of time the solution may be stored unopened before losing its potency (the expiration date on the container).
2. **Reuse life**: The amount of time the solution may be used once it has been mixed, prepared, or activated.
3. **Opened-container life**: The amount of time the disinfecting solution may be used once the bottle has been opened.

Disinfecting solutions come in either "ready to use" formulas or as concentrates. Once the solution has been prepared, a label is placed on the outside of the container stating the name and strength of the solution, the date it was prepared, the date it will expire, and the initials of the person that prepared the solution. The solution should be placed in a container with a lid (Figure 9-4) to keep it from evaporating and to keep contaminants out of the solution.

Storing Chemical Disinfectants

Chemical disinfectants may be hazardous in the case of an accidental spill and may also be highly flammable. It is essential that the medical assistant store chemical disinfectants according to the manufacturer's instructions. All chemical disinfectants on the premises should have a Safety Data Sheet (SDS) formerly known as a Material Safety Data Sheet (MSDS) in the SDS manual. The active ingredients in the disinfectant should be included on the SDS form. All hazardous spills must be reported to a supervisor immediately.

Refer to Procedure 9-2 for complete instructions on how to properly chemically disinfect instruments.

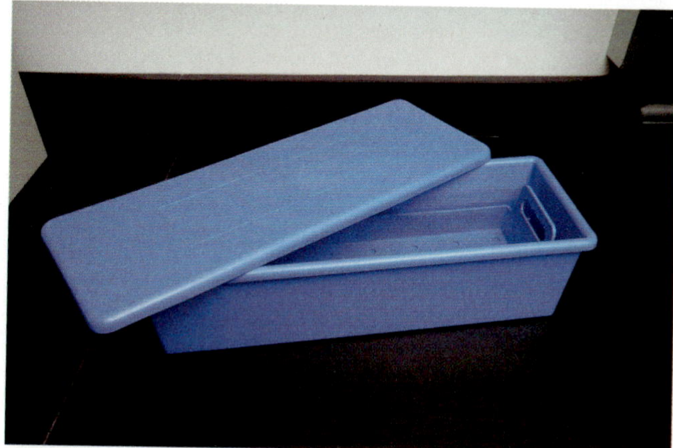

Figure 9-4 ■ An example of a chemical disinfectant container with a lid to keep particles from falling in the solution and contaminating it.

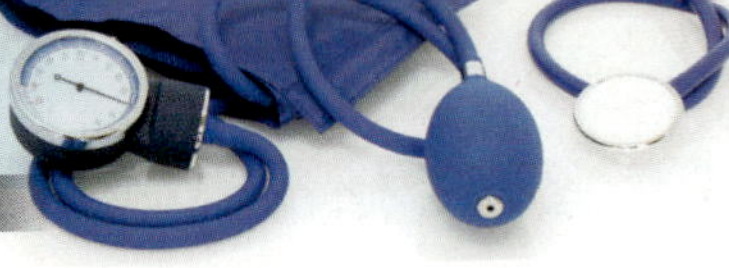

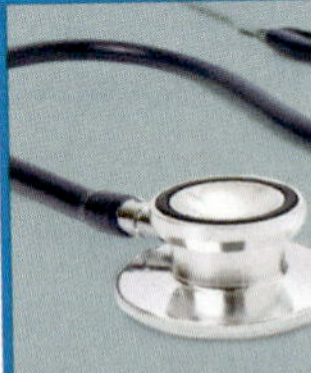

Field Smarts

Many factors can interfere with a disinfectant's ability to destroy microorganisms, including improper dilution ratios, inadequate exposure times, failure to change the solution according to manufacturer's instructions, or placing instruments that are wet directly into the solution. Chemical indicator strips are strips that are used when sterilizing instruments through chemical means to confirm that the necessary environmental conditions needed to achieve complete sterilization have been met. The manufacturers of sterilants have developed strips that are available to test the **minimum effective concentration (MEC)** of disinfecting solutions. The MEC is the concentration of a high-level disinfectant that is necessary to kill bacterial spores. MEC concentration changes after repeated use of a chemical disinfectant. One such solution is Cidexplus® Test Strips. You first place the strip into the solution and hold it motionless for 20 seconds. Remove the strip from the solution and place the side edge on a paper towel for two full seconds. Then place the strip with the indicator pad facing up on a clean paper towel for 5 minutes. The test pad will turn completely red if the solution passes the test; if the solution fails the test, the test pad will turn blotchy or remain its original white color. Figure 9-5 illustrates what the test strip looks like before developing and what it looks like after developing. The test should be performed just prior to placement of the instruments into the solution. The test strip does not tell you if you achieved disinfection or sterilization; it only tells you whether the concentration of the solution is at the desired level.

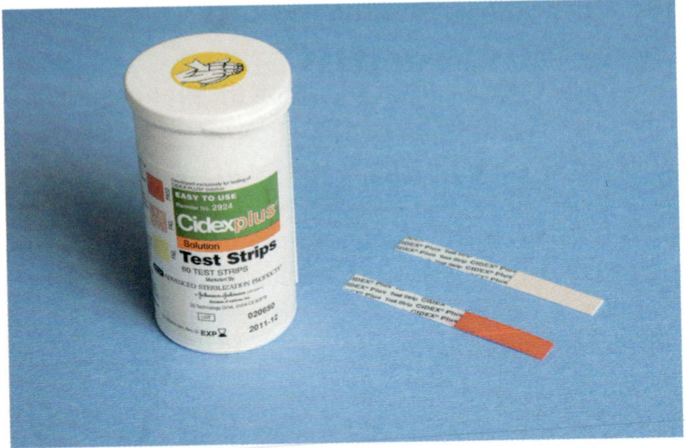

Figure 9-5 ■ Notice what the test strip looks like once it has been developed (red) and what it looks like before developing (white). If there are any splotches or the strip doesn't turn red, it means that the solution has not met the MEC and should not be used.

Sterilization Techniques

Sterilization is the complete destruction of all microorganisms, including endospores, and is the process that should be used on any instrument that will penetrate the skin. There are four basic ways to obtain sterilization of instruments and supplies, but only two of them are practical for most medical clinics: chemical sterilization and autoclaving. Two additional techniques, dry heat and gas sterilization, are discussed here.

Dry Heat Sterilization

Dry heat is not as effective as wet heat and requires a much longer time to completely sterilize items, but it may be used to sterilize articles that may be damaged by wet heat or steam. A common temperature used for dry heat sterilization is 338°F (170°C) for 60 minutes. Dry heat is ineffective against spores and most clinics do not have a dry heat oven.

Gas Sterilization

Some larger health care facilities, such as hospitals and large surgical centers, use gas to sterilize large items such as hospital beds and tables. The gas sterilizers are usually placed in large rooms that can accommodate furniture and the process can take hours for the fumes to dissipate. Ethylene oxide (EtO) is one of the most common gases used for sterilization because of its ability to kill all forms of microorganisms including bacterial endospores. Facilities also choose gas sterilization for products that may become easily damaged by other forms of sterilization. This method of sterilization is also used in manufacturing plants that package sterile needles, sutures, and catheters. Because of the dangers of working with EtO, staff must have specialized training before operating any EtO sterilizers.

Chemical Sterilizing Agents

Chemical sterilizing agents are high-level disinfecting solutions that have the capability to sterilize under the right conditions. Mixed at a stronger ratio and prolonged immersion times are two factors that allow the chemical to sterilize rather than just disinfect. Not all disinfecting chemicals are capable of sterilizing, so the manufacturer's guidance and instructions must be understood and followed.

Autoclaving

Autoclaving, or steam under pressure, is one of the most dependable forms of sterilization and is very cost-effective and practical for use in medical clinics. The physical makeup of an **autoclave** can be compared to that of a pressure cooker. It displaces all the air with steam, which allows for greater pressure (15 pounds of pressure per square inch [psi]) to reach a heat of 250°F to 254°F (121°C to 123°C). The lengthy exposure of steam under pressure kills all microorganisms, including spores. Boiling water can only reach a maximum temperature of 212°F (100°C), which is not high enough to kill endospores. Each autoclave is unique, so one must always read and follow the manufacturer's instructions; however, the general steps for autoclaving are similar from one autoclave to another. Refer to Figure 9-6 for a picture of an autoclave and refer to Procedure 9-4 for how to operate an autoclave.

Wrapping Items to Be Autoclaved

Once instruments have been properly sanitized, inspected, and lubricated, they are ready for sterilization. To maintain sterility after autoclaving, all surgical supplies and instruments are wrapped in an acceptable packaging material; however, there are exceptions.

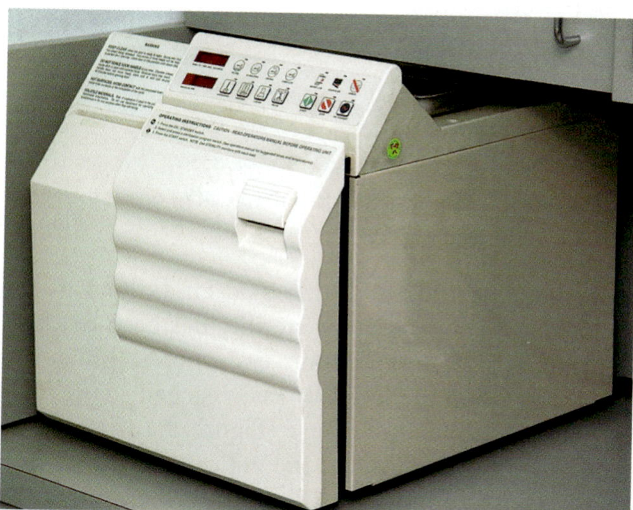

Figure 9-6 ■ An example of a standard desk top autoclave.

Vaginal specula must be sterilized between patients but do not need to be wrapped to maintain sterility unless they are to be used in surgical procedures. Most offices autoclave their specula unwrapped to be used in routine vaginal examinations. All surgical devices and instruments should be wrapped and stored properly to maintain sterility following autoclaving.

Sterilization wraps and packaging must be permeable to steam, yet must still provide an effective barrier against the penetration of microbes and contamination from persons handling the packs prior to use. Specialized products are commercially available.

Types of wraps include the following:

- *Autoclave or sterilization paper* (Figure 9-7): Available in a variety of sizes and cut into squares, this paper is disposable and should not be reused. Autoclave paper is opaque, so the contents of the pack cannot be seen prior to opening, making precise labeling of the package critical. Autoclave wraps are available in various sizes for convenience in wrapping small instruments or large sets of surgical instruments. Exam table paper is not suitable as a sterilization wrap.
- *Sterilization cloth wraps*: Made of woven or unwoven materials, these special cloths come in different sizes and colors and are thicker than autoclave paper, but are still opaque. They are reusable but the cloths should be inspected prior to each use for any thinning of the material, holes, or tears. If any defects are found, the cloth will need to be disposed of or used as cleaning rags.
- *Sterilization pouches* (Figure 9-7): Easy to prepare and made of plastic, paper, or both, these individual pouches usually feature a peel-apart seal on one end of the pouch for easy opening and come in a variety of different sizes. The opposite end

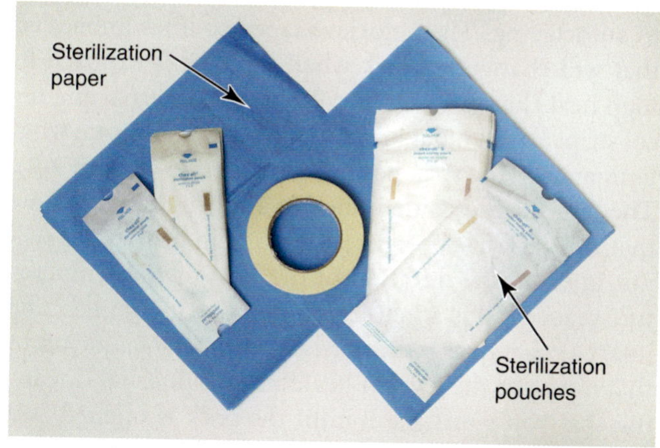

Figure 9-7 ■ Sterilization paper and pouches come in different sizes to accommodate a variety of different instruments.

is open so that the instrument may be inserted into the pouch. Once the instrument is placed in the pouch, the medical assistant will peel off the adhesive strip protector located above the perforation and fold the perforated edge over the adhesive strip, pressing firmly to seal it (refer to Procedure 9-3 for pictures on how to properly load and close the pouch). Another method used to seal the open end is to seal it with a heat sealer. There are also continuous rolls of sterilization pouch material that come in a variety of different sizes and may be cut to desired lengths. Pouches made entirely or partially of plastic provide easy visibility of the contents within the pack. Each pouch includes a sterilization indicator and should be checked for a color change following the autoclaving cycle.

The proper method used to wrap instruments when using autoclave paper or cloth is referred to as the "envelope" or "fanfold" method of wrapping (refer to Procedure 9-3 for a full set of photos on how to wrap instruments using the fanfold method). The pack is wrapped so that it can be opened without contaminating the sterile instruments. Double wrapping is required to facilitate a longer shelf life, better protection of the instruments, and allows for less chance of contamination when opening the pack. Also, when the outer wrapping is opened using proper technique, the inner wrapped sterile package can be placed onto the surgical tray as a controlled bundle.

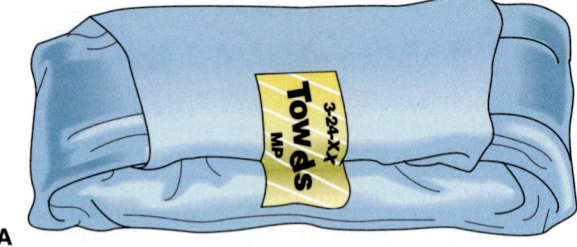

Figure 9-8a ■ Notice how the stripes on the tape are white. That is because the packs have not yet been autoclaved.

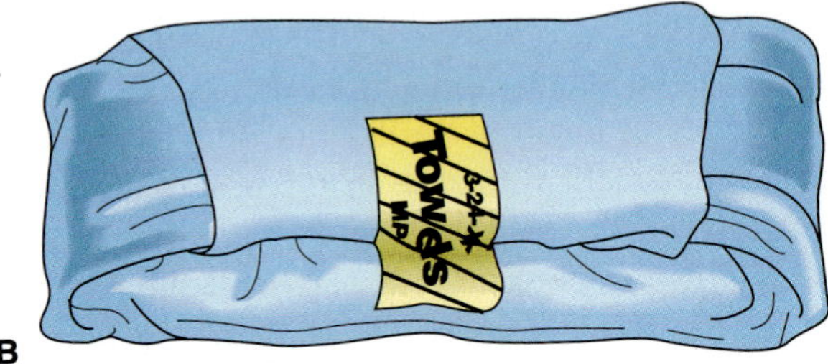

Figure 9-8b ■ Notice how the stripes on the autoclave tape in this picture are black. It's because this pack has been autoclaved.

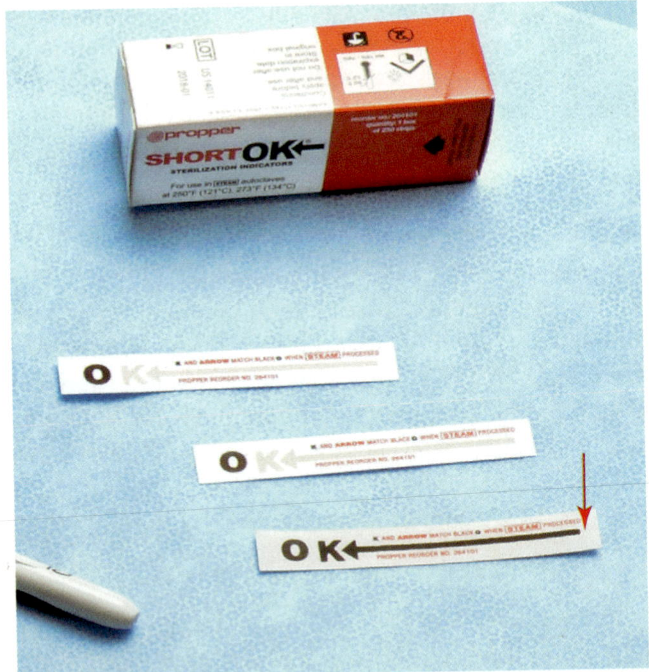

Figure 9-9 ■ The indicator strip turned black once autoclaved, indicating that all parameters have been met for sterilization.

Sterilization Indicators

Sterilization indicators are devices that help in determining whether or not a package has been exposed to the high heat and whether the items inside are sterile. There are two basic types: chemical and biological. Chemical indicators include the autoclave tape used to seal wrapped packs and the small strips of internal chemical indicators that are placed inside each pack prior to autoclaving. The autoclave tape has lines imbedded that will change to black when the tape is exposed to high heat (Figures 9-8a and 9-8b). The internal chemical strips have gradated colored lines that indicate what temperature the strip has been exposed to (Figure 9-9). The tape is an outside indicator and will let you know that the pack has been exposed to high heat, but it will not indicate the duration of the heat or the temperature reached. It is an indicator but not a guarantee. The internal chemical indicator is a bit more reassuring in that it gauges the level of heat, but it is internal (meaning that you won't see it until the pack is opened and ready for use), and the duration of the heat is not indicated. Thus, while both of these methods are useful and should be utilized, the biological indicators are the most dependable to ensure sterility has been reached. Biological indicators contain endospores, which are destroyed when the indicator has reached sterile conditions. Biological indicators (Figure 9-10) are more expensive and require that the indicator be forwarded to a medical laboratory for testing to determine if the spores have been killed. Recommendations are that

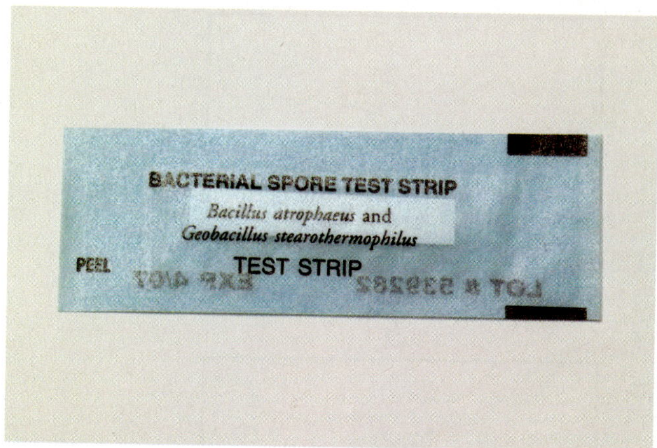

Figure 9-10 ■ An example of a biological indicator.

biological indicators should be used every week or once a month, depending on the frequency of autoclaving.

Labeling

The medical assistant must use a permanent marker (ball-point ink can smudge with moisture) on the package to record three key elements:

1. The name of the item or items
2. The date of sterilization
3. The first initial and last name or initials of the person who prepared the pack for sterilization

Shelf Life

The shelf life or length of time that packs are considered sterile following autoclaving will vary depending on the type of wrapping material used. One must also inspect the pack for any defects, such as moisture, holes, bubbles, or tears, because these defects may be caused by poor wrapping, poor sealing, poor storage, and poor handling of the packs. The general shelf life of double wrapped or items in pouches is anywhere from 3 months to a year, depending on the storage environment. Intact packs carefully stored in closed cabinets or drawers in dry environments will maintain their sterility the longest. A conservative and safe office policy would be to rewrap, resanitize, and resterilize all packs not used within 3 months.

Proper Loading of the Autoclave

The autoclave must be loaded properly, following the manufacturer's instructions, in order for steam to circulate both through and between the packs. Packs should not be crowded and should be placed in a vertical position, separated by at least an inch. Jars should be placed on their sides with their lids removed to facilitate complete sterilization of the contents within the jar. Figure 9-11 illustrates the proper placement of packs and jars in the autoclave.

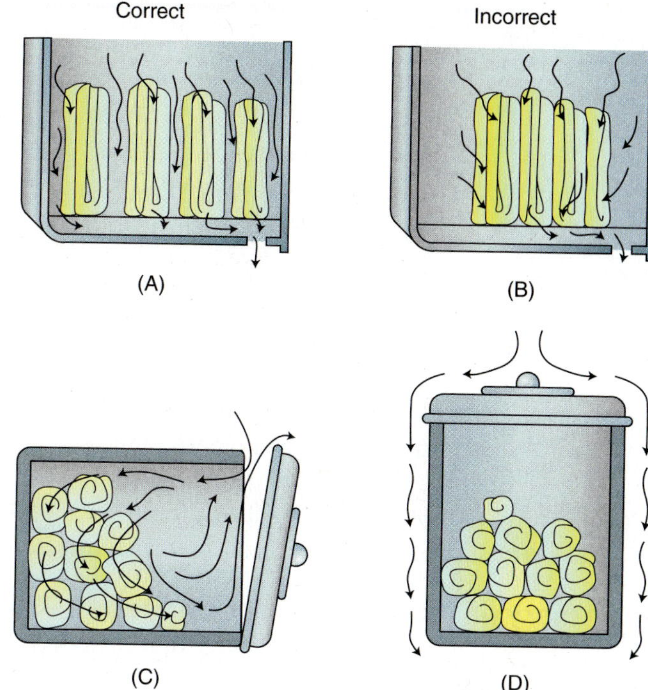

Figure 9-11 ■ (a) The correct way to place packs in an autoclave; (b) how not to place packs in an autoclave; (c) the proper position for a jar in an autoclave; (d) the improper position for a jar in an autoclave.

Maintaining the Autoclave

Because the autoclave is so important in preventing infections, measures must be instituted to ensure proper maintenance. Proper maintenance includes internal and external inspection of the unit, proper cleansing of the unit, and the implementation of a quality assurance program through the use of chemical and biological indicators. Daily maintenance includes the inspection and cleaning of the autoclave's interior and exterior with a damp cloth. The medical assistant should look for any concerns such as frayed electrical cords and problems with the rubber gasket. Weekly maintenance may include a thorough cleansing of the autoclave by running a commercially approved cleanser, such as Omni Cleaner, through the autoclave, following the autoclave manufacturer's instructions as well as the manufacturer's instructions for the cleanser. Offices should also perform weekly spore checks. If the spore test results are positive, another test should be immediately performed prior to the sterilization of any more instruments. If the second spore test comes back positive, the autoclave should not be used again until after it has been properly serviced and the problem resolved.

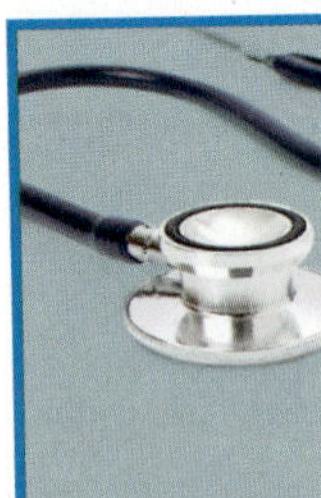

Field Smarts

Always check the following before establishing that a pack is sterile:

1. The sterilization date
2. The sterilization indicator
3. The general condition of the wrapping material to make certain that there are no signs of moisture, holes, or other defects

If there are any concerns that the pack may be contaminated, follow the four "Rs": Remove, resanitize, rewrap, and resterilize.

Summary of Proper Sterilization Steps

The following is a summary of steps that must take place for proper sterilization (Figure 9-12):

- The instrument must be properly sanitized.
- The instrument must be wrapped properly.
- The pack must be loaded into the autoclave properly.
- The pack must be sterilized properly.
- The pack must be stored correctly.

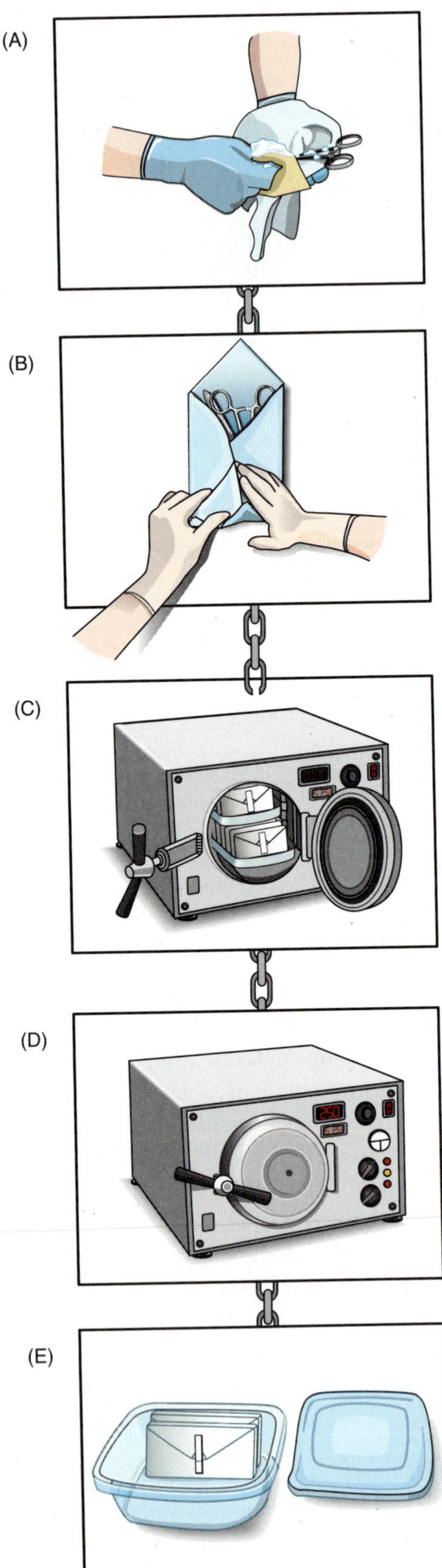

Figure 9-12 ■ An example of the chain of events that must take place in order for sterilization to be achieved. One break in the chain nullifies all other steps. The item will not be sterile.

TYPES OF INSTRUMENTS USED IN MINOR SURGERY

Before medical assistants can become proficient in assisting providers with minor office surgeries, they must first become proficient at identifying instruments that are routinely used during those procedures.

There are literally thousands of instruments used in the health care setting; however, only a small number of those instruments are used to perform minor office surgeries. Surgical instruments are generally made of stainless steel and have a shiny or dull finish, but some instruments are made of plastic and are completely disposable.

Identifying the Parts of a Surgical Instrument

Knowing the different parts of an instrument will assist the medical assistant in determining the instrument's identity and will be useful when performing cleansing and maintenance functions.

- Handles: The **handle** is the part of the instrument that the surgeon uses to hold the instrument. The majority of minor surgical instruments have either

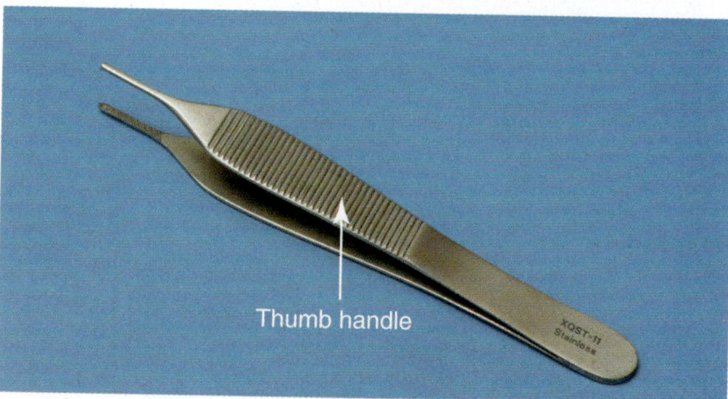

Figure 9-13 ■ Thumb handle.

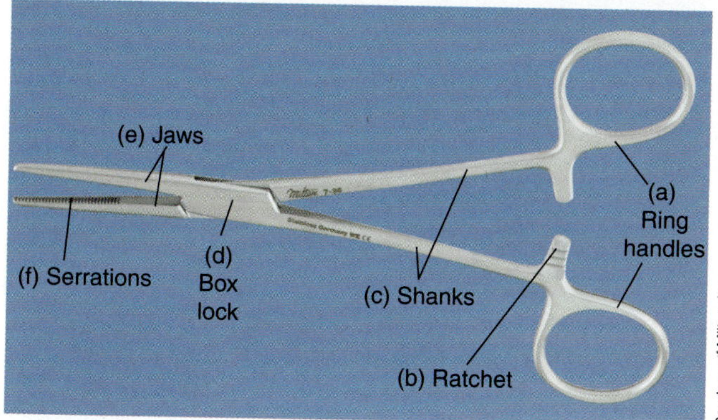

Figure 9-14 ■ The parts of a surgical instrument.

a thumb handle or a ring handle. A thumb handle (Figure 9-13) is held between the index finger and thumb and is opened and closed by pinching and releasing. Instruments with these types of handles, including different types of forceps, are generally used to grasp or pick up items.

- A ring handle (Figure 9-14a) has two rings: one ring is for the thumb and the other ring is for the index finger. Ring-handled instruments contain ratchets, which allow the tips of the instrument to close at varying intervals. Examples of ring-handled instruments include hemostats, needle holders, and Kelly forceps.
- Ratchets: The **ratchet** (Figure 9-14b) of a surgical instrument is centered between the two rings of a ring-handled instrument and is the locking mechanism that tightens or locks the tips of an instrument at varying degrees.
- Shanks: The **shank** (Figure 9-14c) of an instrument connects the handle with the working end of the instrument. The singular term *shank* is used when the instrument has only one shank, such as the shank of a scalpel. The plural *shanks* is used when the instrument is double-sided, such as the shanks of a pair of hemostats or forceps. Shanks are really extensions of the instrument and will vary in length. Instruments with shorter shanks are designed to work in more superficial tissue, while instruments with longer shanks are designed to work in deeper tissue.
- Box locks: The **box lock** (Figure 9-14d) is a special type of hinge found on a variety of ring-handled instruments.

Tips of Instruments

The tip of the instrument will usually indicate its use. Tips can be quite delicate and may be damaged if not handled properly. Because the tips are the part of the instrument that will touch the patient's tissue, they are usually the dirtiest part of the instrument. Because of this, extra care should be taken when sanitizing this portion of the instrument. The following are some examples of different tips found on various types of instruments.

- Jaws: The **jaws** (Figure 9-14e) are the tips of instruments that are used to grasp or clamp items. Some instruments have crevices etched into their tips which are referred to as serrations. **Serrations** (Figure 9-14f) help to improve gripping power when working with tissue that is slippery. Serrations may be found on needle holders, forceps, and hemostats. The jaws of other instruments may be plain or contain varying numbers of teeth, which are used to puncture tissue. Instruments with small teeth are referred to as "mouse-toothed instruments," while instruments with large teeth are referred to as "rat-toothed instruments" (Figure 9-15). Numbers found on instruments that contain teeth identify the number of intermeshing teeth present on the instrument. A tissue forcep is an example of an instrument with jaws that contain teeth.
- Circular blades: The tips of some instruments are in the shape of a loop (Figures 9-16a and 9-16b). These loops are actually blades that are blunt on the outside

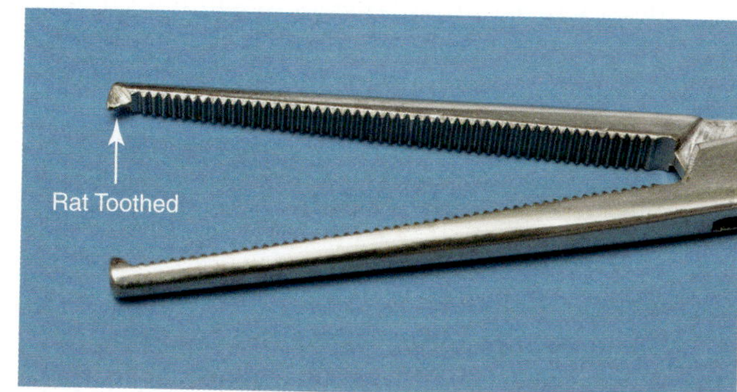

Figure 9-15 ■ An example of an instrument with teeth.

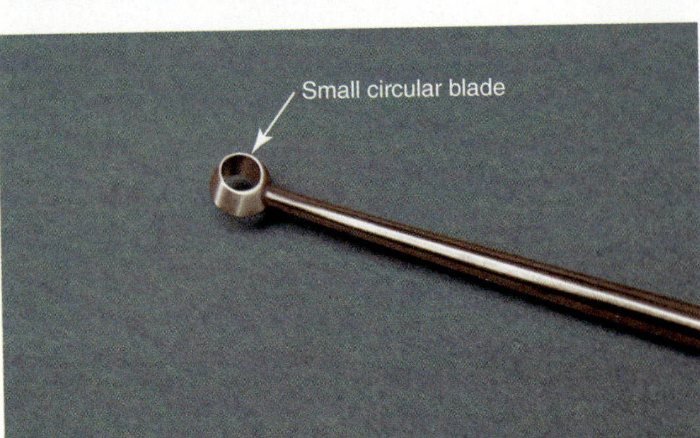

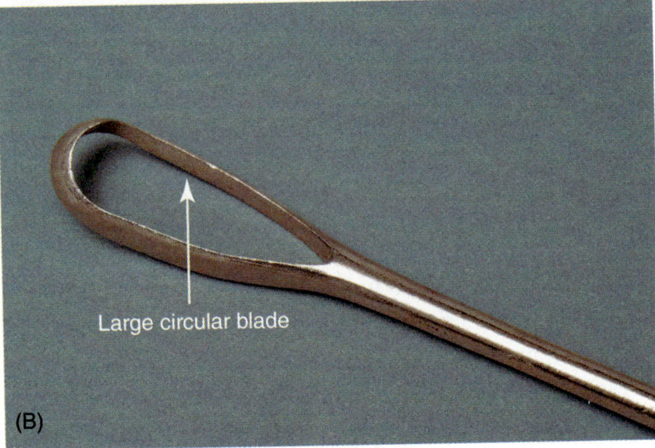

Figure 9-16 ■ Examples of instruments with circular blades.

and sharp on the inside. They are commonly used to remove tissue from a cavity. Examples of circular blades include uterine curettes, cervical curettes, and ear curettes.

- Prongs and hooks: Some instruments have pronged tips (Figure 9-17a) or hooks (Figure 9-17b) that are used to retract, lift, and explore tissue.
- Blades: Blades may be blunt (Figure 9-18a) or sharp (Figure 9-18b), straight or curved, and are used to cut tissue, suture material, and bandaging supplies. Bandage scissors, scalpel blades, and operating scissors (Figure 9-19) are all examples of instruments with tips that contain some sort of blade.

There are many other types of tips found on other types of instruments. Just remember that the tip will most often help to identify the instrument and its use.

Categories of Instruments

Instruments used in minor surgery can be grouped into four major categories:

- Instruments used for cutting and dissecting
- Instruments used for grasping and clamping
- Instruments to improve visualization (dilators)
- Instruments for probing

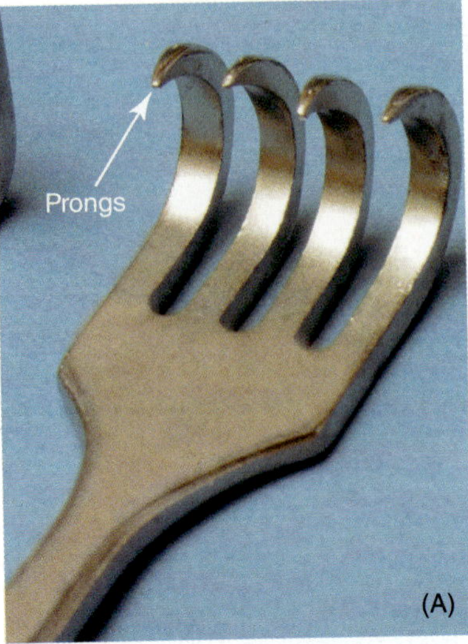

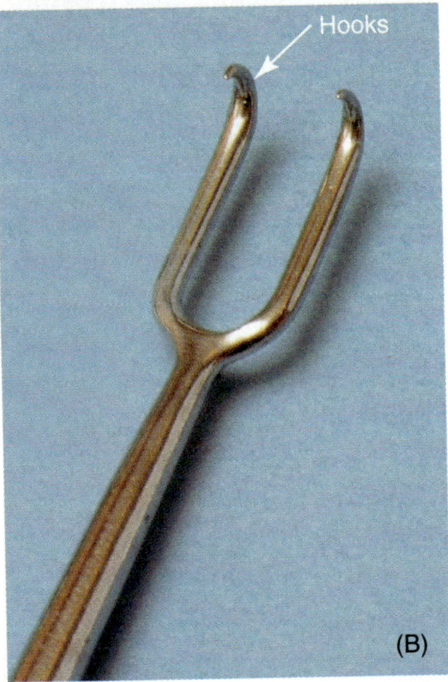

Figure 9-17 ■ Examples of instruments that contain prongs or hooks.

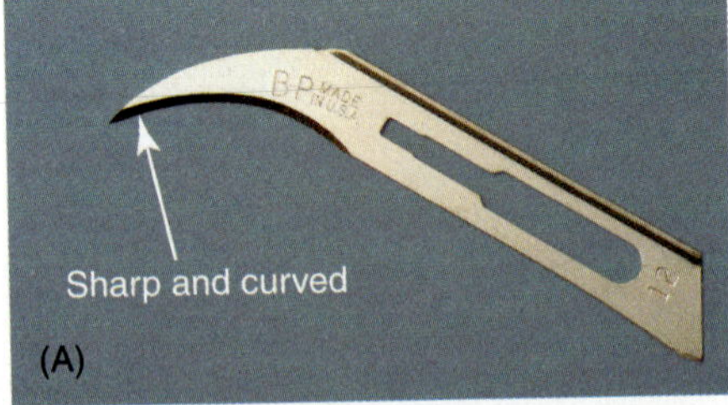

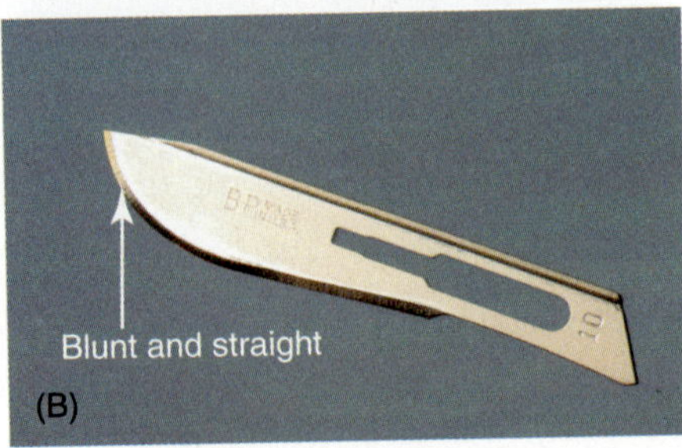

Figure 9-18 ■ Examples of surgical blades.

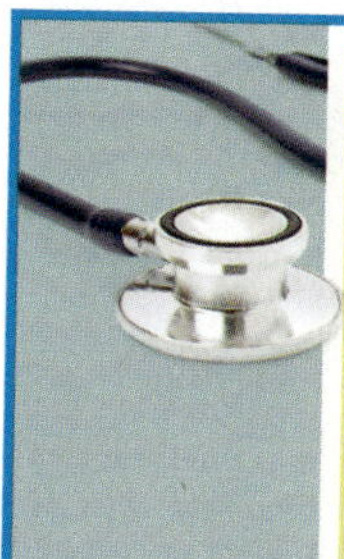

Field Smarts

To check the sharpness of scissor blades, try cutting through a rubber glove or a piece of gauze prior to sterilization. If the blades appear dull, they will probably need to be sharpened.

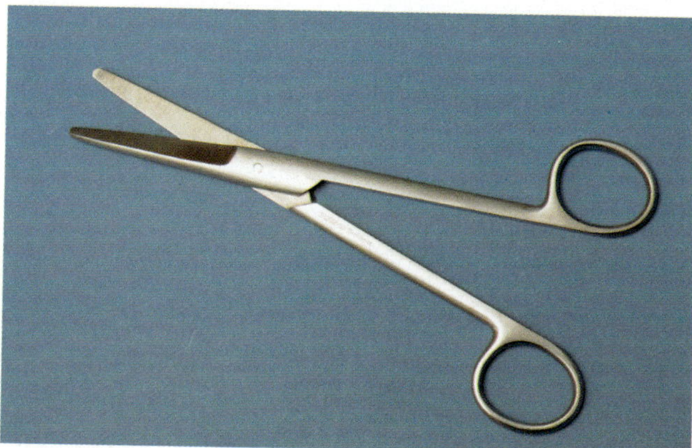

Figure 9-19 ■ Example of a surgical instrument that cuts.

Instruments Used for Cutting and Dissecting

Instruments that are used for cutting and dissecting (see Table 9-1) will usually have sharp edges or tips to cut through skin, tissue, and suture material. The term **dissect** means to cut open or cut apart. Frequently, a surgeon will need to dissect tissue in order to explore for irregular growths or to remove abnormal tissue. Care must be taken when working with these instruments to avoid injuries. Personnel responsible for maintaining these instruments may also be responsible for inspecting the instruments and determining if they need to be sharpened at the time of instrument processing.

Instruments Used for Grasping and Clamping

Instruments that are used for grasping and clamping (see Table 9-2) are primarily used for holding onto tissue and clamping off tissue and blood vessels that may get in the way during a surgical procedure. During the sanitization process, the medical assistant must check to make certain that the locking mechanisms are working correctly on these instruments and that the instruments are lubricated for easy opening and closing.

Instruments to Improve Visualization

It is difficult or even impossible to view certain body structures without the aid of special instruments or devices (see Table 9-3). These instruments are designed to assist the provider in opening structures and moving other structures out of the way in order to provide an opportunity to view organs that cannot be seen externally.

Table 9-1 Instruments Used for Cutting and Dissecting

Name of Instrument (with Example)	Description/Indications
Curettes	Curette comes from the French name *curer*, which means "to clear or clean." It is a surgical instrument that is shaped like a spoon or loop, and is used to scrape and remove tissue from the skin or body cavities. The loop is a circular blade that is sharp on the inside and blunt on the outside so that it doesn't cause damage to the surrounding tissue. There are many different types of curettes. Below are some of the more common forms.
Dermal Curette (Tip)	*Dermal curettes* are used to shave tissue from the skin, such as lesions or melanomas.

continues

Table 9-1 Instruments Used for Cutting and Dissecting *(continued)*

Name of Instrument (with Example)	Description/Indications
Sim's Uterine Curette 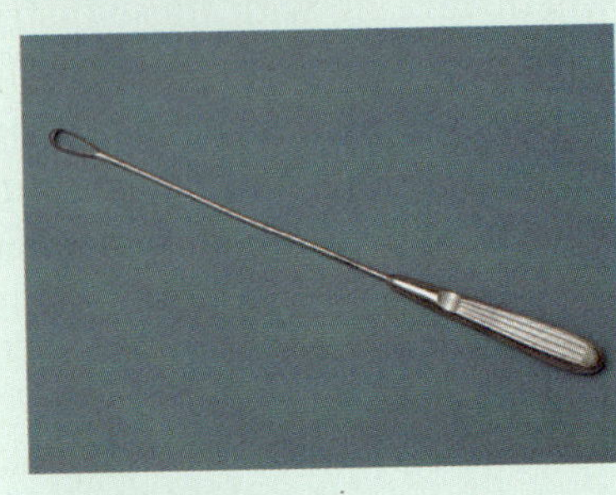 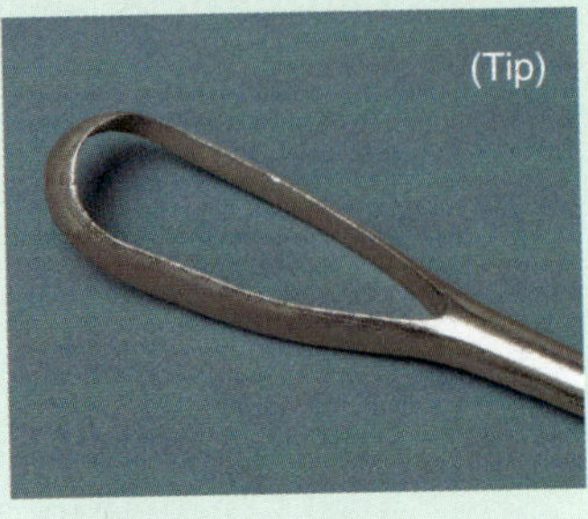	*Uterine curettes* are used to obtain tissue from the endocervical and uterine area for the detection of uterine cancer.
Ear Curette 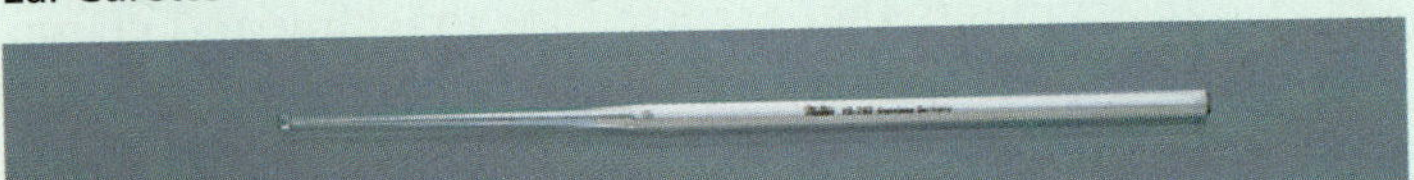	*Ear curettes* are used to remove tissue from the ear, and are especially good for the removal of cerumen, or earwax.
Scalpels and blades	A scalpel or surgical knife is used to make incisions. Typically, the blade is disposable and the handle is reusable; however, the instrument may be completely disposable. Both the handles and the blades come in a variety of sizes and must be matched to fit one another. The numbers on the blade do not match the numbers on the handle; however, only certain size blades fit onto specific handles.
Scalpel handles 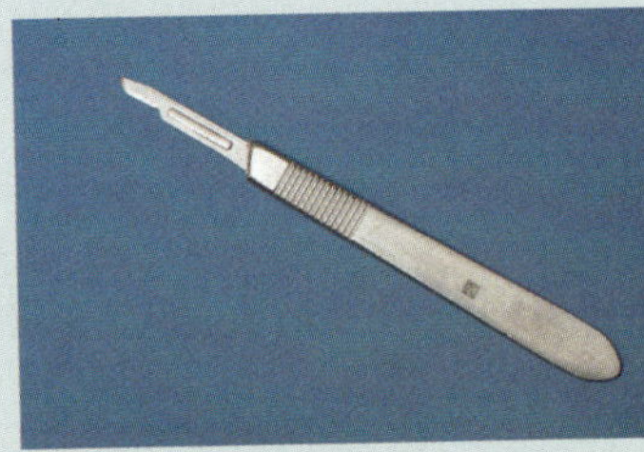 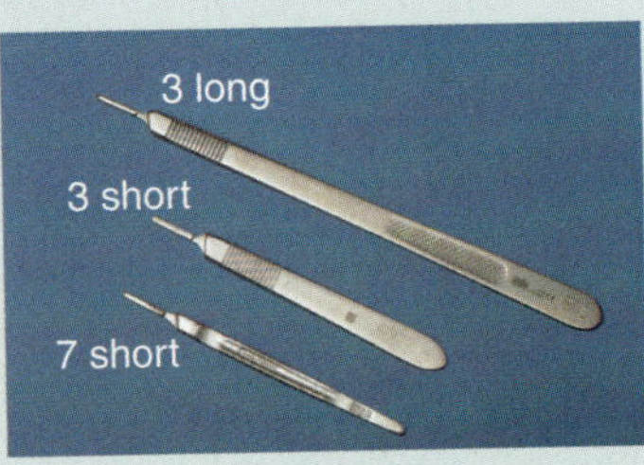	The most popular size handle is the number 3 handle. The number 3L (long) and number 7 handles are used when cutting deeper tissue. The size and shape of the blade is selected based on the type of tissue to be cut. The larger the blade's number, the smaller or finer the blade. Blades range in size from 10 to 25.
Scalpel blades 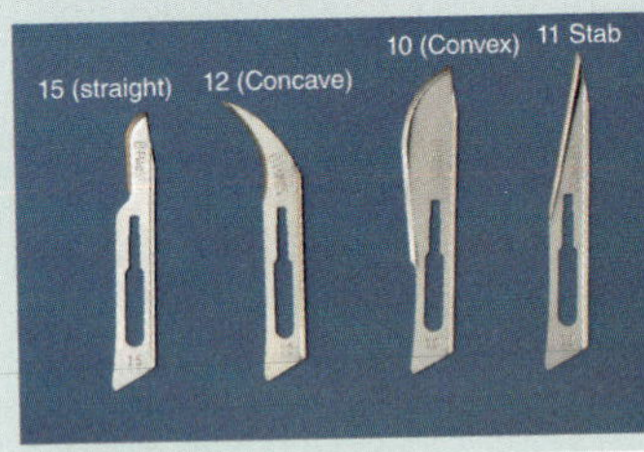	The most common size blades used in minor office surgeries are the numbers 10, 11, and 15. The number 11 blade is often referred to as a stab blade because of its unique point. Blade shapes include the following: *straight* (tip is pointed), commonly used for incision and drainage, *concave* (tip points inward), commonly used to cut fine or delicate tissue, and *convex* (tip points outward), commonly used to extract tissue.
Scissors	The word *scissors* always ends in "s" because each pair of scissors has two blades. Scissors are usually sharp so that they can cut tissue, but come with a variety of options. The blades may be straight or curved and the tips can be sharp or blunt. You may also mix the tips. Tips are described in the following fashion: s/s (sharp/sharp), b/b (blunt/blunt), and s/b (sharp/blunt).
Bandage scissors 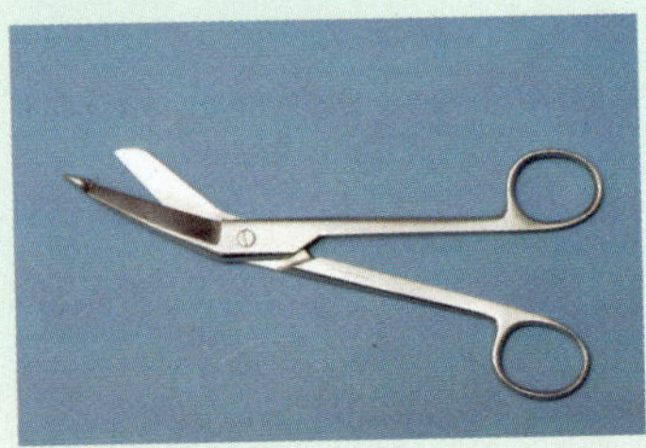	*Bandage scissors* are used for cutting tape, gauze, bandages, and dressings. The blade tip that slips under the dressing is blunt to prevent accidental injury of the patient's skin while cutting the bandage off.

Table 9-1 Instruments Used for Cutting and Dissecting *(continued)*

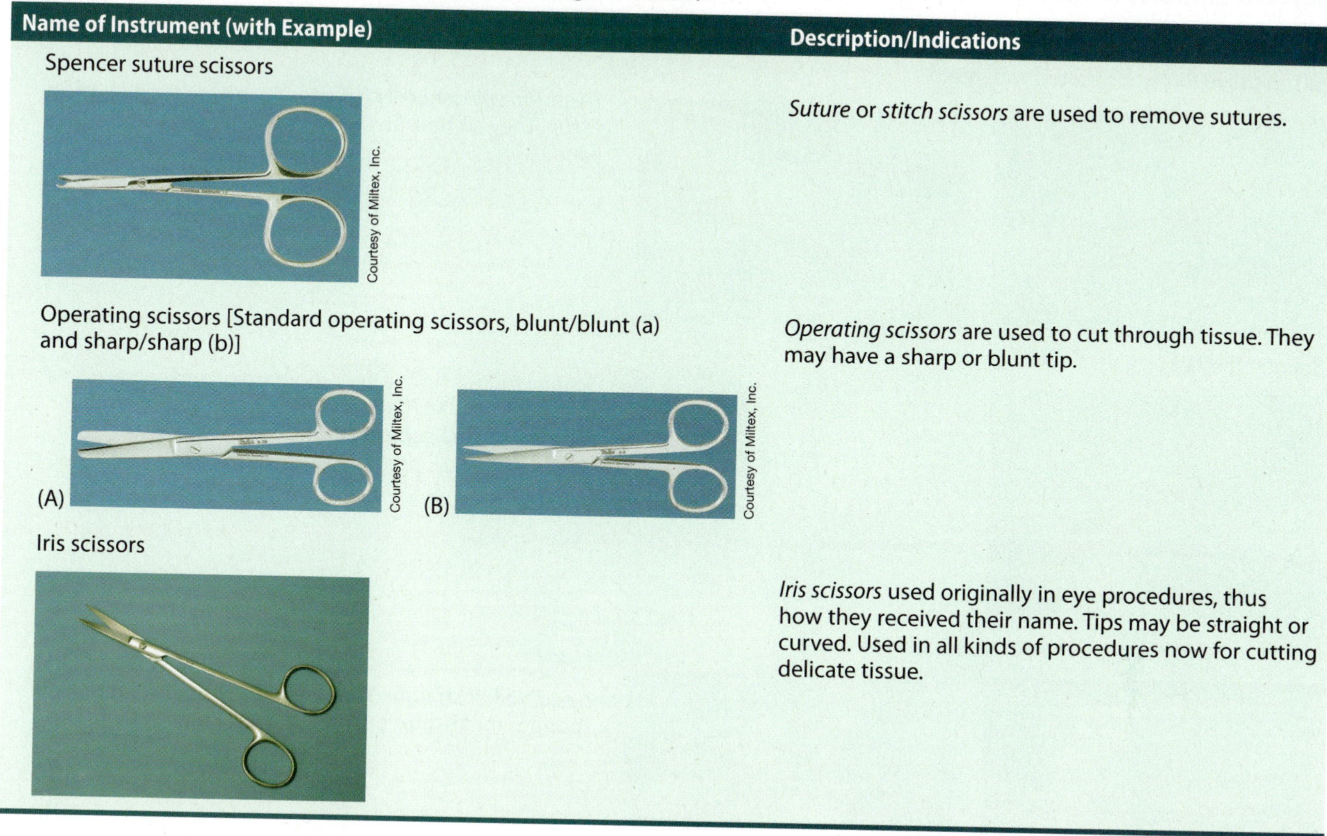

Name of Instrument (with Example)	Description/Indications
Spencer suture scissors	*Suture* or *stitch scissors* are used to remove sutures.
Operating scissors [Standard operating scissors, blunt/blunt (a) and sharp/sharp (b)]	*Operating scissors* are used to cut through tissue. They may have a sharp or blunt tip.
Iris scissors	*Iris scissors* used originally in eye procedures, thus how they received their name. Tips may be straight or curved. Used in all kinds of procedures now for cutting delicate tissue.

Table 9-2 Instruments Used for Grasping and Clamping

Name of Instrument (with Example)	Description/Indications
Forceps 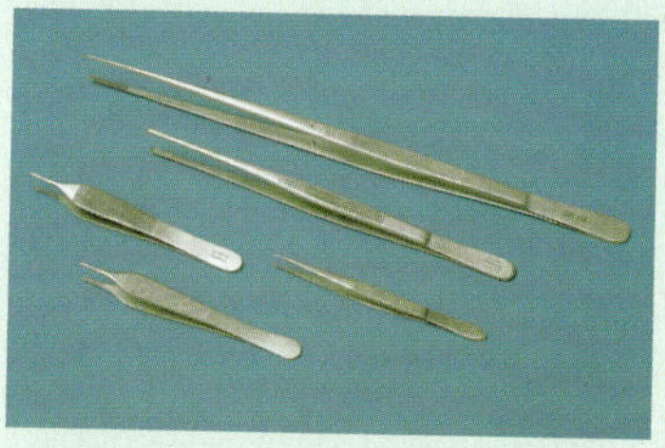	Forceps are used to grasp and hold tissue and other items. The term *forceps* is used for both the singular and plural form of the word. Ring-handled forceps have ratchets to hold the instrument closed at varying tensions. Thumb-handled forceps must be manually squeezed in order to close.
Adson dressing forceps, plain with serrations 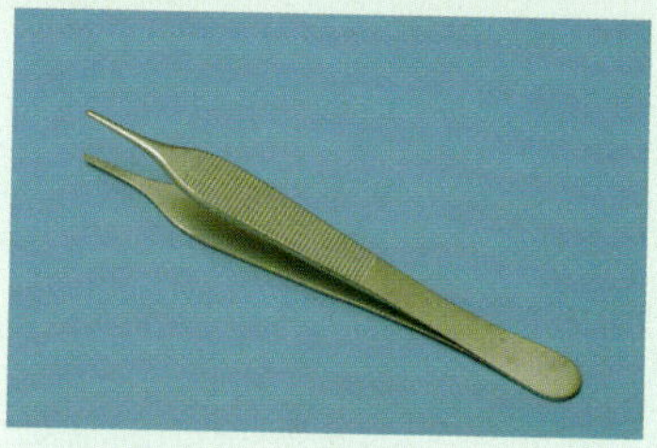 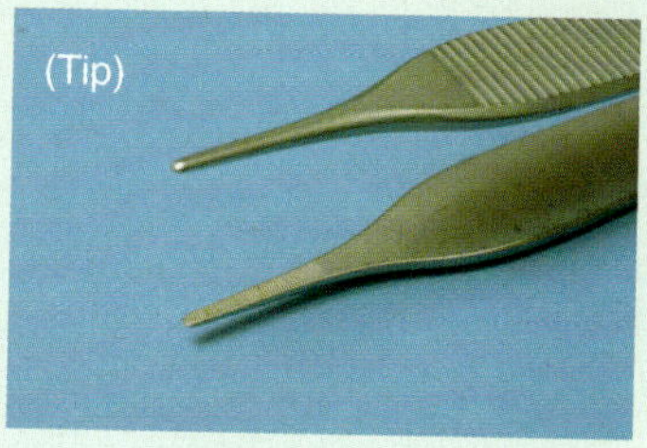 (Tip)	*Thumb* or *dressing forceps* have thumb handles and look like a set of tweezers. They may come with or without serrated jaws. They are used to grab tissue and to pack wounds.
Lucae bayonet forceps 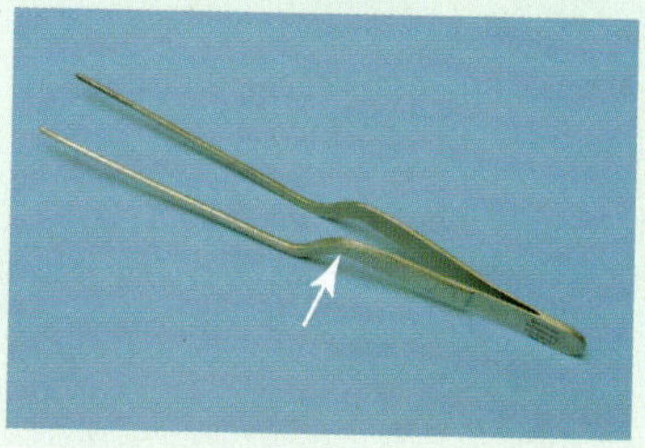	*Lucae bayonet thumb forceps* are used for intrauterine procedures. The offset bayonet handle provides an unobstructed view of confined surgical sites.

continues

Table 9-2 Instruments Used for Grasping and Clamping *(continued)*

Name of Instrument (with Example)	Description/Indications
Adson tissue forceps, serrated with teeth 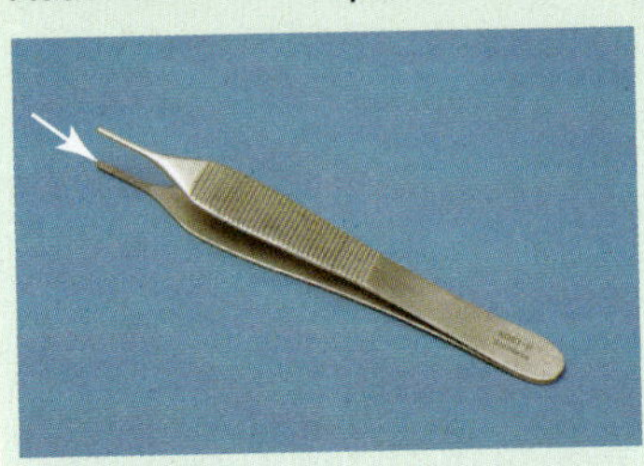 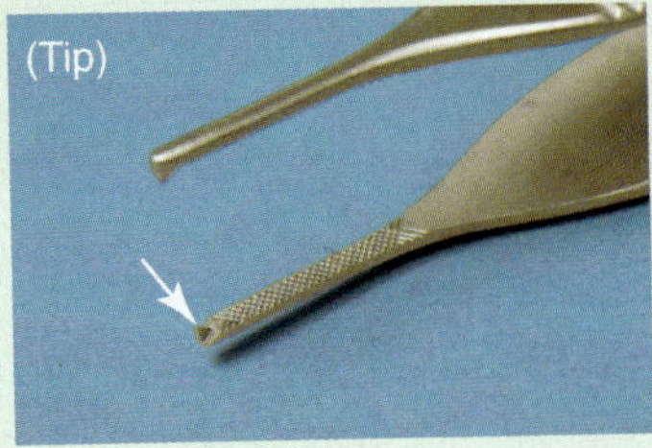	*Tissue forceps* generally have teeth and are used to grasp tissue. They come with either thumb handles or ring handles.
Splinter forceps 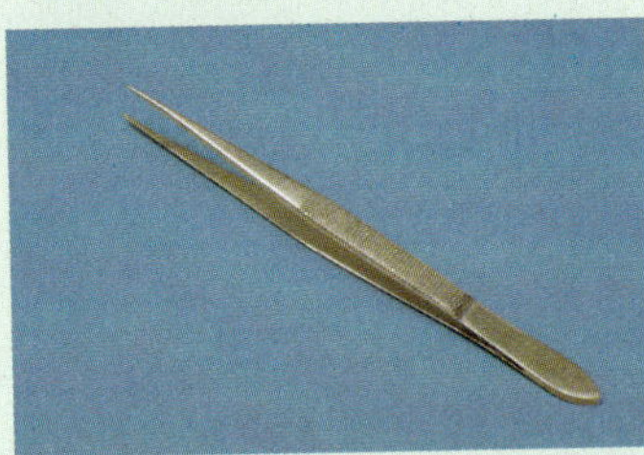	*Splinter forceps* have a very sharp point and come with a variety of handles. They are commonly used to remove splinters or small objects from tissue.
Uterine packing forceps and Forester sponge forceps 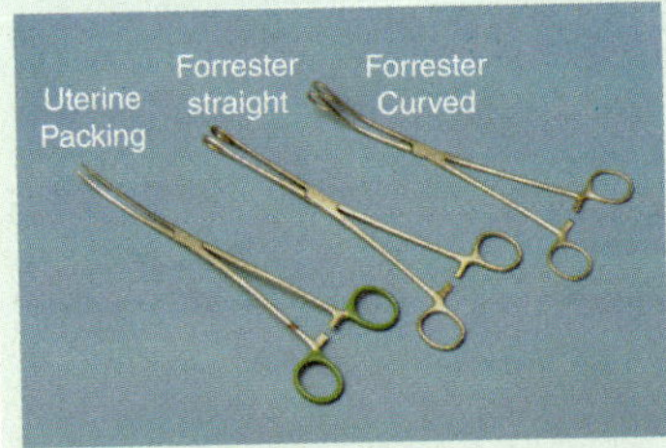 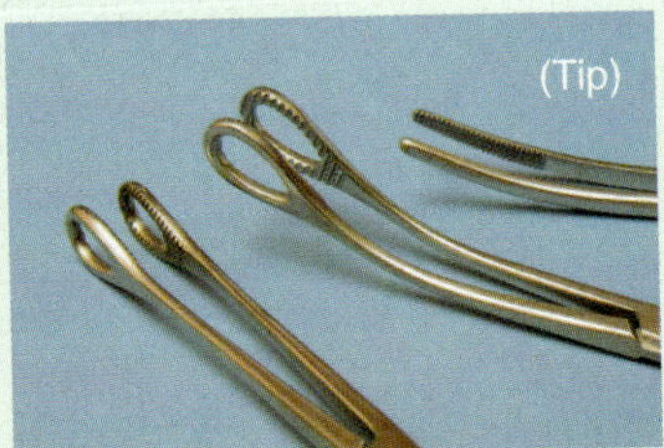	*Sponge forceps* may have large rings or long tips, and may be curved or straight. They are used to apply and remove sponges for absorption and cleaning purposes.
Hemostatic forceps 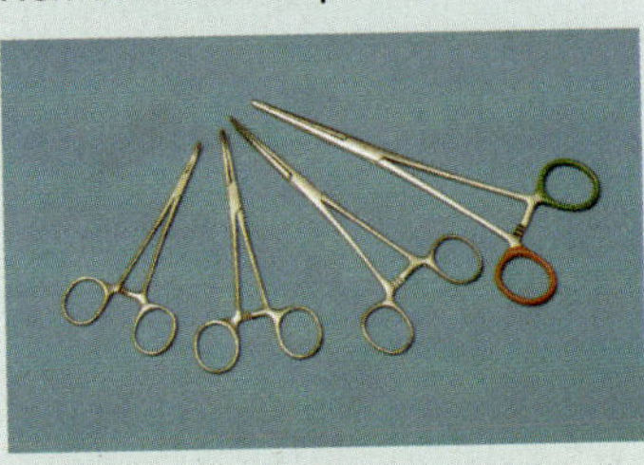	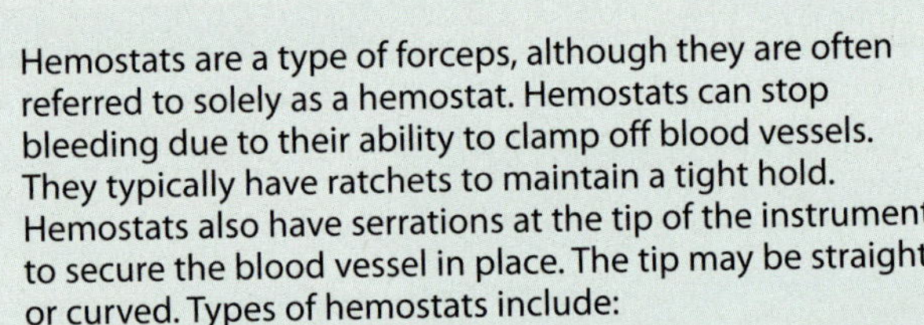 Hemostats are a type of forceps, although they are often referred to solely as a hemostat. Hemostats can stop bleeding due to their ability to clamp off blood vessels. They typically have ratchets to maintain a tight hold. Hemostats also have serrations at the tip of the instrument to secure the blood vessel in place. The tip may be straight or curved. Types of hemostats include:
Mosquito hemostats 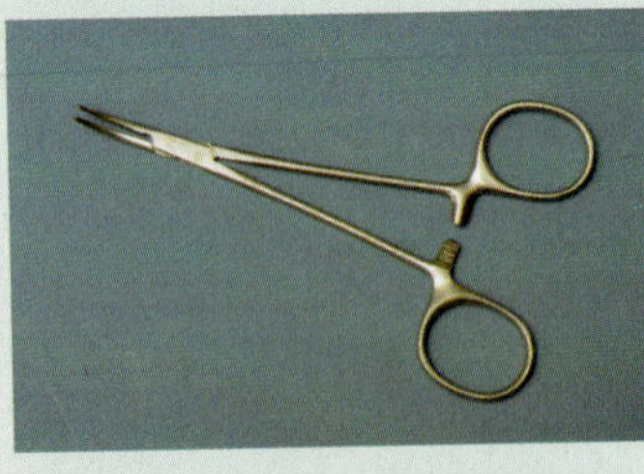 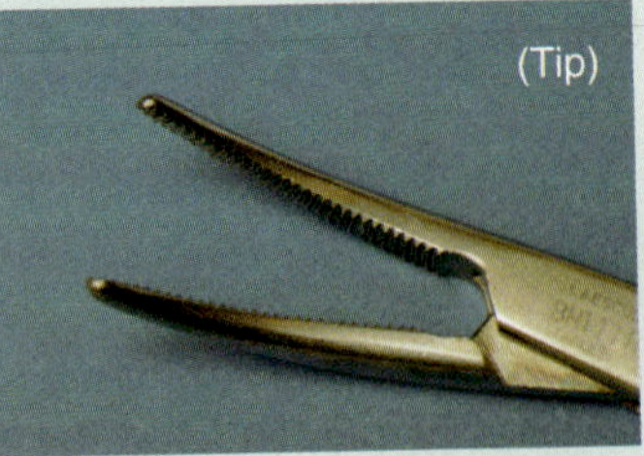	*Mosquito hemostatic forceps* have fine tips with serrations that run the entire length of the tip.
Kelly hemostats 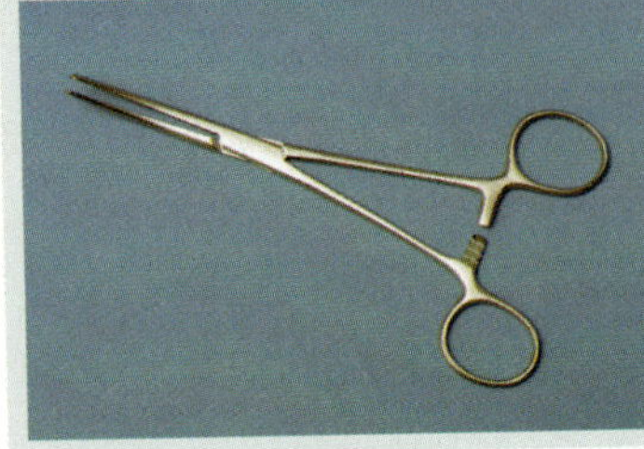 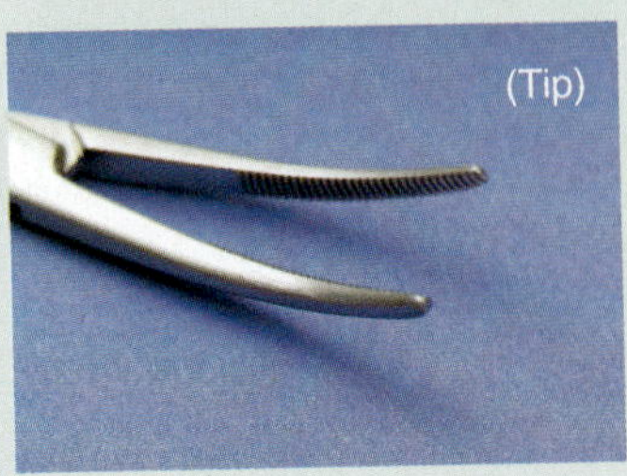	*Kelly hemostatic forceps* have serrations that only run partially up the tip.

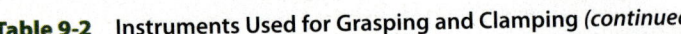

Table 9-2 Instruments Used for Grasping and Clamping *(continued)*

Name of Instrument (with Example)	Description/Indications
Needle holders 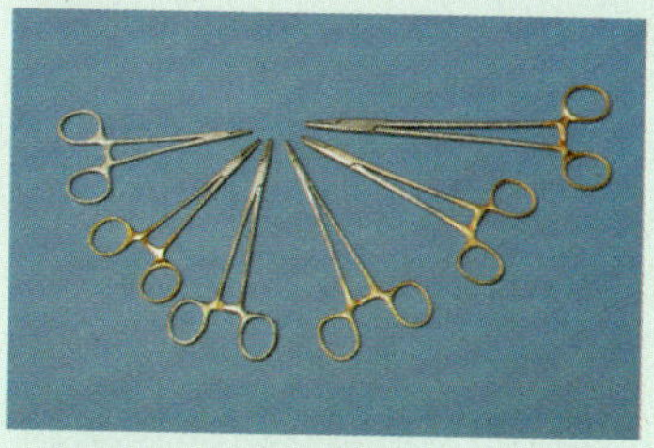	Needle holders are used to grab and firmly hold a needle during the suturing process. The instrument contains ratchets and the tips are serrated.
Needle holder with tip 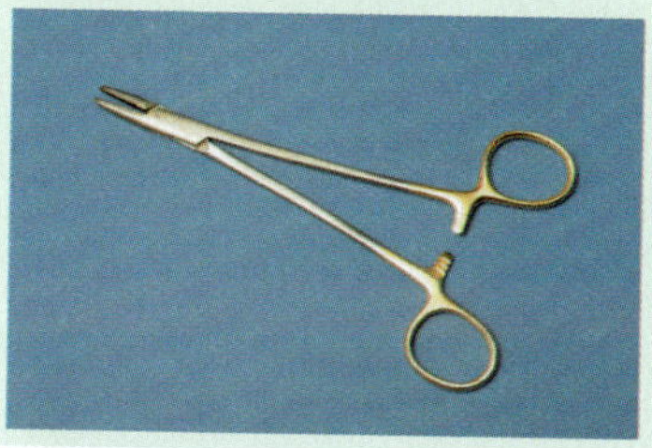 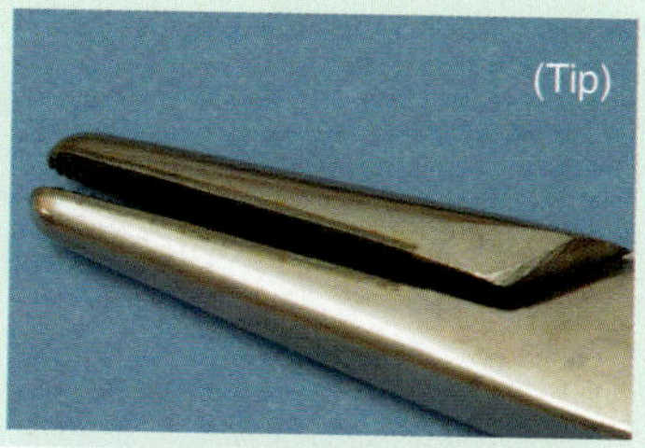 (Tip)	A single needle holder illustrating a close up of the serrated tips.
Towel clamp 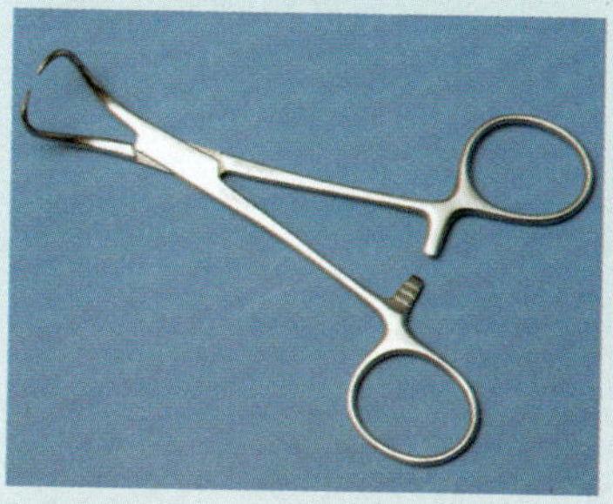 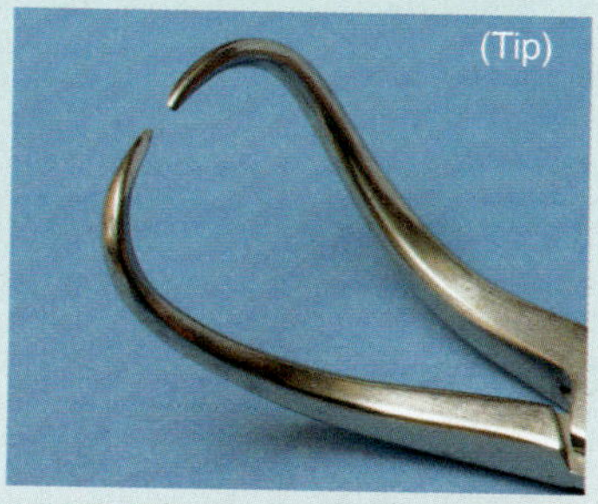 (Tip)	A towel clamp has two sharp tips and is used to hold a sterile towel in place during a surgical procedure. The handles are ratcheted to prevent slippage.

Table 9-3 Instruments to Improve Visualization

Name of Instrument (with Example)	Description/Indications
Dilators	Dilators are double-ended smooth metal rods that have rounded tips and come in varying sizes. The purpose of the instrument is to dilate structures that are constricted, such as the urethra and cervix. Dilators have an array of calibrations ranging from small to large. The provider starts with the very smallest dilator and gradually works up to the dilator that is necessary to relieve the patient's symptoms.
Uterine dilators 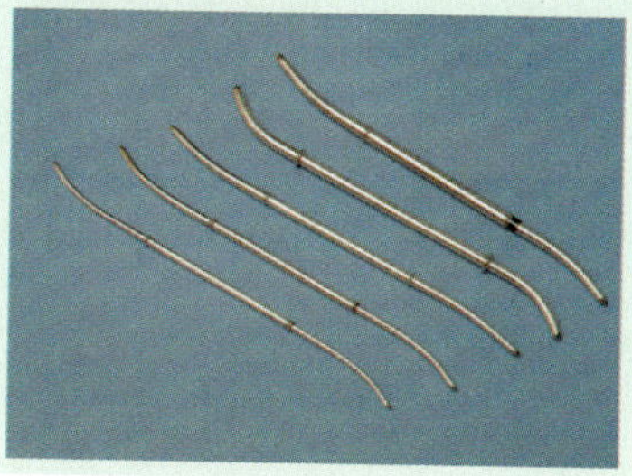	*Uterine dilators* are designed to dilate the cervix, which may be constricted due to a buildup of scar tissue in the area or developmental abnormalities. They are also used to gain access into the uterus for examination purposes.

continues

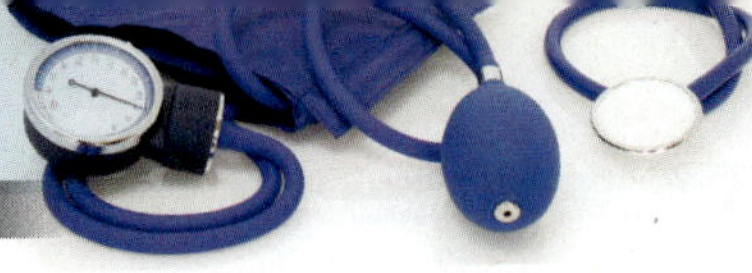

Table 9-3 Instruments to Improve Visualization *(continued)*

Name of Instrument (with Example)	Description/Indications
Urethral dilators 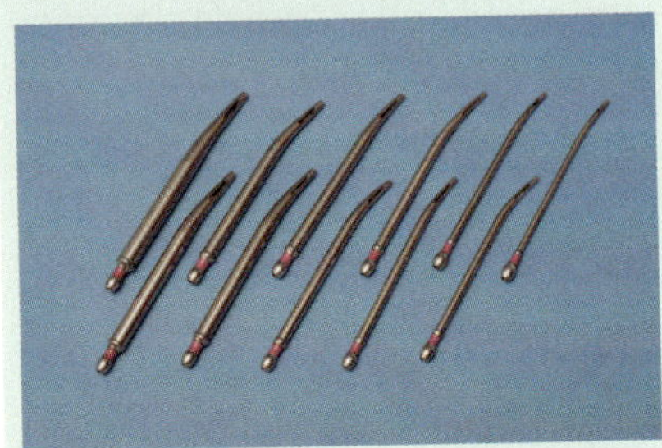	*Urethral dilators* are used to stretch the urethra for the insertion of a scope or to dilate the urethra due to the presence of a stricture.
Probes 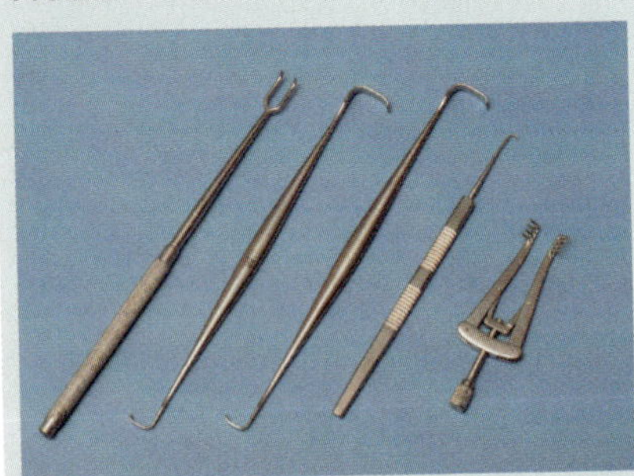	*Probes* are instruments that are used to explore wounds, body cavities, or hidden structures. A sound is a type of probe. It is a long instrument with calibrations that can be used to detect the size and shape of the area that is being probed.
Uterine sound 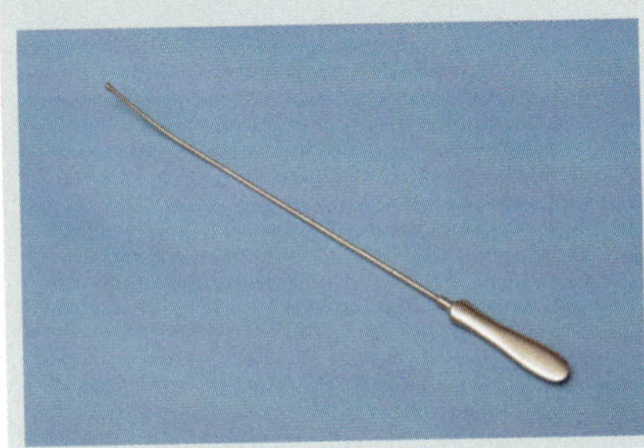 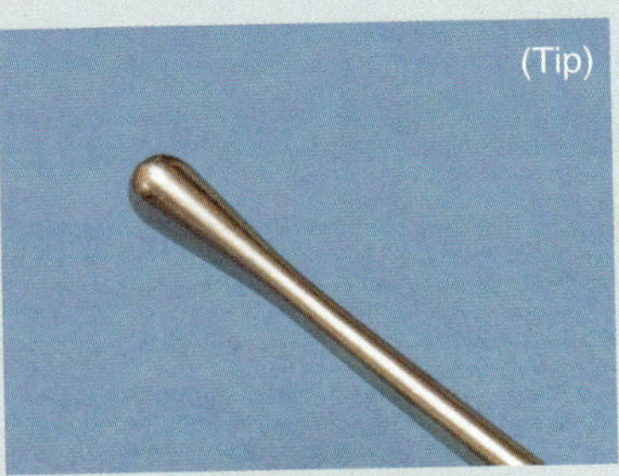 	*Uterine sounds* are designed to facilitate the location of the cervical os, to dilate the cervix, and to determine uterine depth.
Retractors 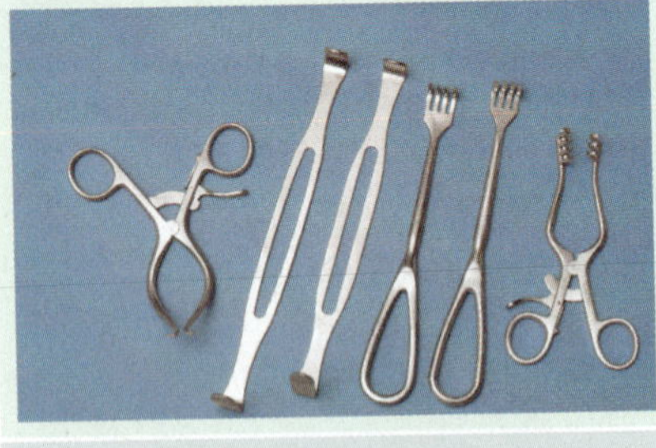 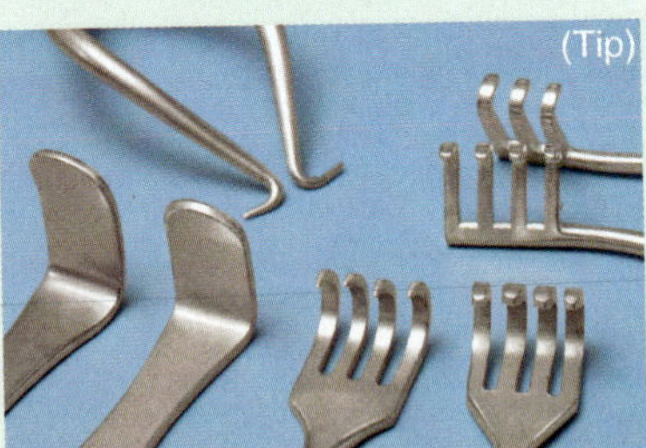 	A *retractor* is an instrument used to pull aside tissue to facilitate better visualization of an area that may be obstructed by other tissue. Retractors come in different sizes with different types of tips made up of single or multiple hooks for separating tissue.
Scopes 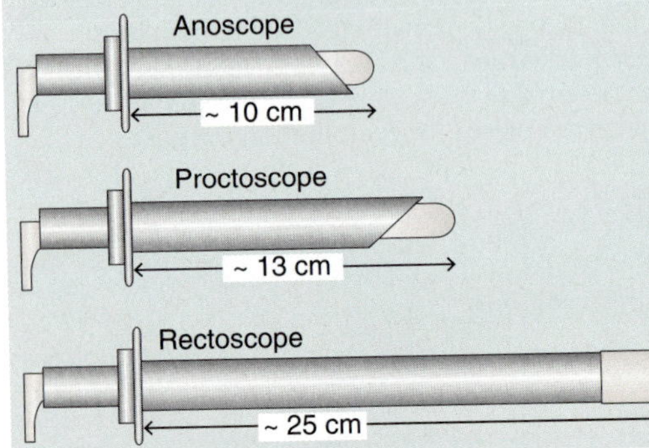 	A *scope* is an illuminated instrument that is used to view an organ or body cavity. These are commonly used in exams, but may also be used during specific surgeries. *Anoscopes* are used to view the anus. *Rectoscopes* are used to view the rectum *Proctoscopes* are used to view the anus and rectum.

Table 9-3 Instruments to Improve Visualization *(continued)*

Name of Instrument (with Example)	Description/Indications
Specula	A *speculum* is an instrument that is used to increase the viewing area of a body cavity for examination purposes. Specula may be metal or plastic and come in various sizes.
Vaginal speculum	*Vaginal specula* are used to open the vagina.
Nasal speculum	*Nasal specula* increase the examination space of the nasal cavity.

SOLUTIONS AND SUPPLIES USED FOR MINOR SURGERIES

Along with instruments, other items are needed to perform minor office surgeries including solutions, drapes, sponges, culture swabs, biopsy containers, packing materials, suture material, and anesthetics. Medical assistants must know what items are necessary for each procedure and at what point each item is used prior to, during, and following the procedure.

Common Solutions Used in Minor Surgery

There are only a few solutions used in minor office procedures which include liquids used to prep the patient's skin and solutions used for irrigating purposes. The two most common solutions used during minor office procedures are sterile iodine and sterile saline.

Table 9-4 lists a variety of liquids that may be used during minor office surgeries and Figure 9-20 shows examples of these solutions.

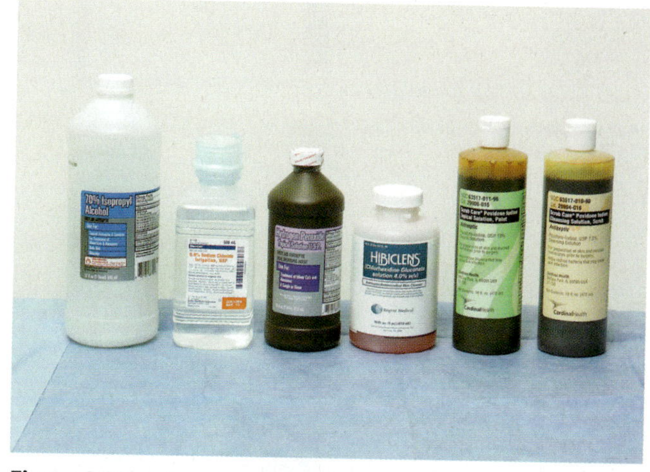

Figure 9-20 ■ A variety of solutions used in minor surgeries.

Table 9-4 Common Solutions Used in Minor Surgery

Solution	Uses in Surgery
Betadine® (povidone-iodine)	For preparation of the skin prior to surgery; this is a skin cleanser that helps reduce bacteria that could potentially cause skin infection
Sterile saline	Used to flush and clean open wounds and to remove foreign particles from wounds
Isopropyl alcohol (isopropanol)	Used as a skin antiseptic; usually available in a 70% solution; also known as rubbing alcohol
Hibiclens® (chlorhexidine gluconate)	May be used as a skin antiseptic or skin cleanser during a surgical scrub; should be used sparingly, may be harsh on tissue if not used as directed
Tincture of benzoin	Used to increase the adhesive capabilities of sterile adhesive skin closures (Steri-Strips®)

Common Supplies Used in Minor Surgery

There is a vast array of supplies that are used throughout surgical procedures. Some supplies will be placed directly on the surgical tray; however, many noninstrument items used during a surgical procedure will be on a side table for easy retrieval. Table 9-5 lists common supplies used for office surgeries and their uses.

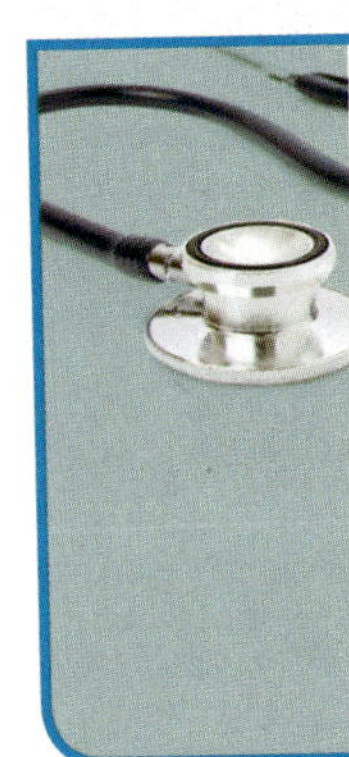

Field Smarts

The contamination of sterile wicks or sterile packing material such as iodoform gauze may result in serious infection to the patient. You must take great measures to ensure the sterility of materials that are placed into an open wound or body cavity.

Table 9-5 Common Supplies Used in Minor Surgery

Name of Supplies	Description/Indications
Nonfenestrated sterile drapes or barriers	Sterile drapes are used to cover the surgical tray and parts of the patient during the procedure. These drapes are usually made of both cotton and polyester and contain a layer of plastic to make them water-resistant. They are available in a variety of different sizes to accommodate their many uses. The majority of surgical drapes will contain a dotted line signifying the outer one-inch border of the drape. This is the area of the drape that may be handled when removing the drape from the package and placing it onto the stand. This border is considered nonsterile.
Fenestrated drapes or barriers	Fenestrated drapes are made of the same materials as nonfenestrated drapes. The term **fenestrated** means to have one or more openings. A fenestrated drape has an opening that is placed over the surgical site once the skin has been prepped. It provides a working area for the provider.
Gauze pads (sponges): 2 × 2, 3 × 3, 4 × 4	Gauze pads or sponges may be used during or following surgical procedures. The pads are used to absorb blood and cleanse and dress wounds.
Sterile gloves, gown, mask, and surgical bonnet 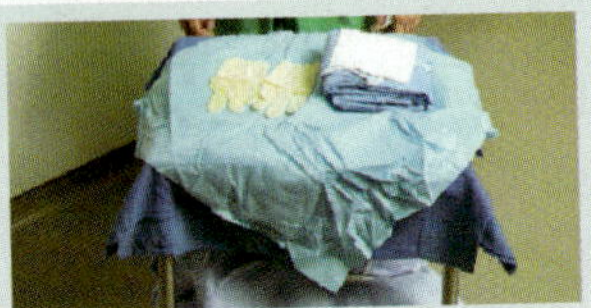	Sterile gloves, a gown, sterile towels, and mask and hair bonnet (not pictured), are set out for the provider to put on prior to the start of the procedure.

Table 9-5 Common Supplies Used in Minor Surgery *(continued)*

Name of Supplies		Description/Indications
Surgical wicks	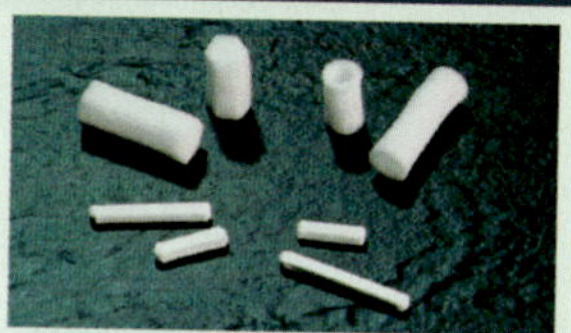	**Surgical wicks** are used to remove small foreign bodies from the eye, ear, or wound. They are also used to instill a minute amount of solution to wounds, as well as to facilitate aspiration and drainage of fluids from wounds that would become infected if such fluids were allowed to lie within the tissue.
Sterile packing material	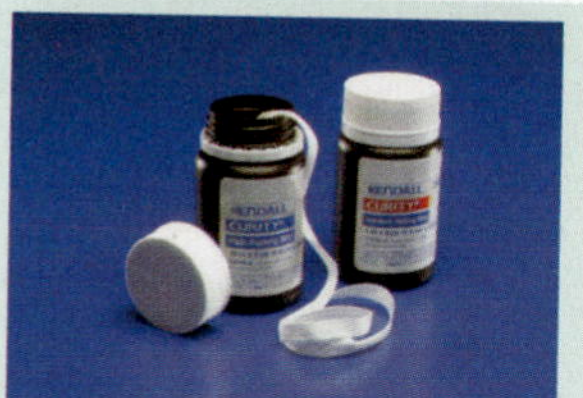	Sterile packing material is usually packaged in long, sterile, cotton strips. The material may be plain or impregnated with a 5% iodoform solution. Iodoform is a crystalline iodine antiseptic that inhibits the growth of microorganisms. Special care must be taken when removing the strips from the container to maintain the sterility of both the strips and the container. The packing material may be used to pack wounds and may also be used to create a surgical wick.
Syringes (a)/needles (b) 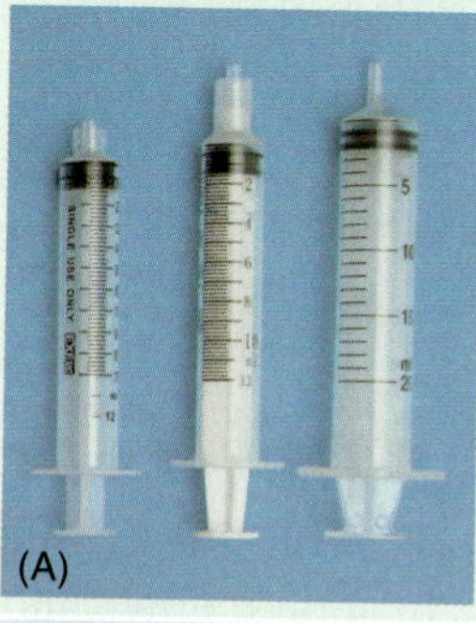 (A)	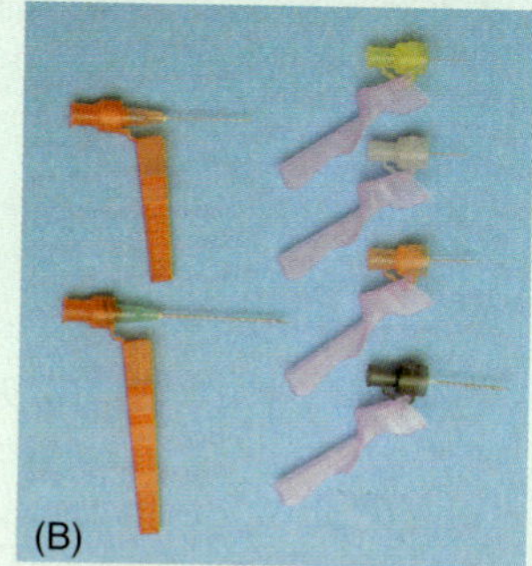 (B)	Sterile disposable needles and syringes are used to anesthetize the surgical area, as well as for irrigation purposes.
Laboratory specimen containers 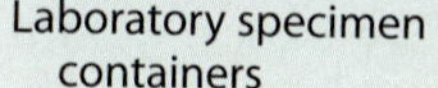	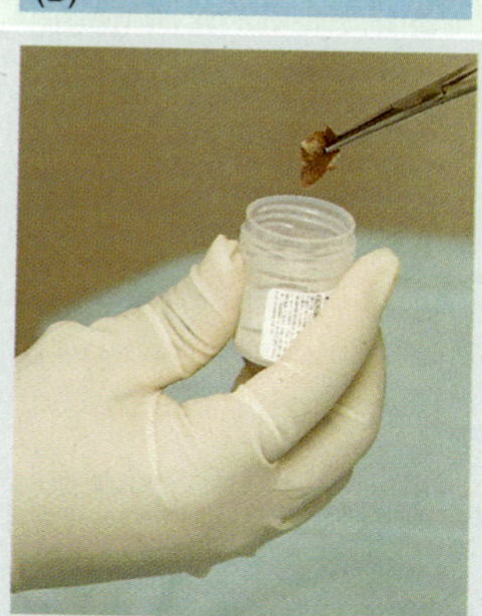	Laboratory specimen containers are filled with a tissue preservative and are used to transport tissue from a biopsy or lesion removal.
Laboratory culture transport tubes	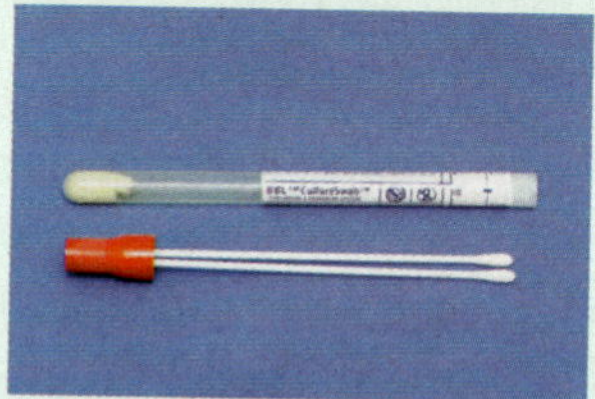	Laboratory culture transport tubes are used when culturing a wound is necessary. They contain a preservative agar and a sterile swab.
Dressings and bandaging supplies	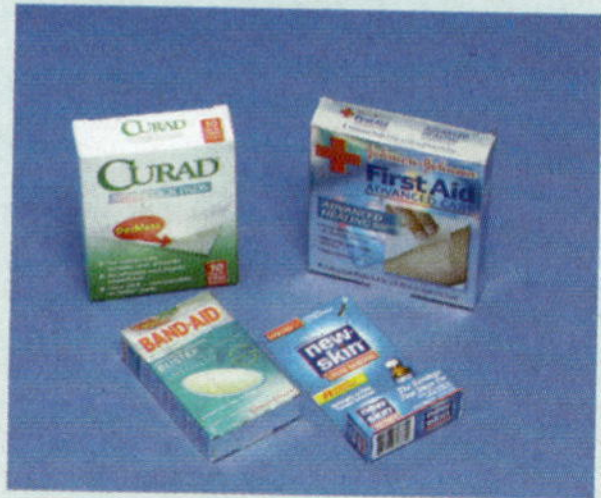	Bandaging supplies are needed to bandage affected areas following surgery.

Common Anesthetics Used in Minor Surgery

An **anesthetic** is used to produce a lack of feeling in patients during a surgical procedure. Anesthetics may be introduced into the body by way of injection, through intravenous routes (veins), topical routes (skin), and through inhalation (respiratory tract). Four types of anesthetics are as follows:

- General anesthetics, which place patients in a reversible loss of consciousness and are used during major surgical procedures.
- Local anesthetics, which are usually administered directly into subcutaneous tissue. Local anesthetics work by blocking sensory pain receptors at the point of injection and in surrounding tissue. Local anesthetics are the most common type of anesthetic used during minor surgical procedures. All synthetic anesthetics end in the suffix "caine" and may contain the additive epinephrine. Epinephrine helps to prolong the effect of the anesthetic. It is also a vasoconstrictor, which helps to reduce the amount of bleeding during the procedure. Manufacturers usually color-code the lettering on the labels of anesthetics according to the name and strength of the medication. Anesthetics with epinephrine may have red lettering or come with a red stripe on the label (Figure 9-21). Epinephrine is not normally used on small appendages such as the fingers, toes, nose, earlobes, or the penis. Because these appendages have a small surface area of tissue, there may be a delay in the blood vessels returning to their original diameter. The prolonged constriction may set the tissue up to become necrotic, thus leading to a sloughing of the tissue. Local anesthetics come in strengths of 0.5 percent, 1 percent, and 2 percent, and are available in vials, cartridges, or ampules. Before setting up a procedure, the medical assistant should ask the provider the following questions:
  - What is the name and strength of the anesthetic desired?
  - Should it contain epinephrine?
- Regional anesthetics are used when a large area of tissue needs to be blocked and requires infiltration of the anesthetic to the surrounding areas. This may be accomplished by using larger amounts of anesthetic or by injecting nerves adjacent to the nerve supplying the surgical site.

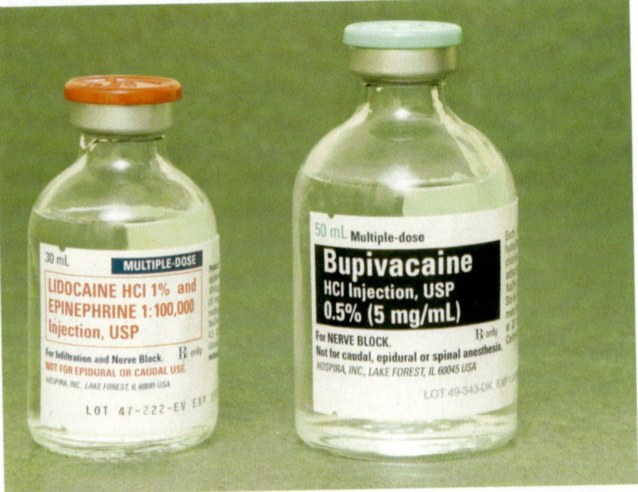

Figure 9-21 ■ Notice how the anesthetic with the red writing on the label contains epinephrine; this is to reduce confusion.

- Topical anesthetics, are applied to the skin and work by deadening surface nerve endings in the areas to which they are applied. They may be applied prior to the introduction of a local anesthetic to reduce the stinging sensation caused by the insertion of the needle. Topical anesthetics may be in the form of liquids, gels, or sprays. Ethyl chloride, also known as "cold spray," is a topical vapor coolant that may be sprayed onto skin to promote a temporary lack of feeling prior to the insertion of the needle. It only lasts for a few seconds, so the provider must work in an efficient manner. Ethyl chloride is flammable and should not be used prior to or during electrotherapy or laser procedures.

Table 9-6 lists examples of different types of anesthetics.

Suture Materials and Other Supplies to Close the Skin

The term **suture** may be used as either a noun or a verb. Used as a noun, it refers to the type of strand or fiber that is used to sew; used as a verb, it refers to the process of sewing. The purpose of a suture is to hold the edges of a wound together until the natural healing process joins the tissue permanently. Suturing promotes faster healing and lessens scaring. The term **ligature** means tying, and is the term that is used when referencing suture material that is used to tie off tubular structures such as the fallopian tubes or vas deferens. The quality of suture material is judged by its tensile strength (the amount of weight necessary to break it divided by its cross-sectional area), its ability to hold a knot, its ability

Table 9-6 Common Anesthetics Used in Minor Surgery

Name of Anesthetic	Description/Indication
Marcaine (bupivacaine)	Long-acting anesthetic Used for local infiltration or nerve blocks
Xylocaine (lidocaine HCL)	Local or regional anesthesia administered by infiltration May contain epinephrine to reduce bleeding through vasoconstriction Most commonly used local anesthetic
Novocaine (procaine HCL)	Oldest injectable anesthetic Used primarily in dentistry Cocaine derivative Has vasoconstriction properties
Carbocaine (mepivacaine HCL)	Injectable local anesthetic Effective for a longer period of time than lidocaine
Epinephrine (adjunct to other anesthetics)	Used as an adjunct to lidocaine Acts as a vasoconstrictor to reduce bleeding
Ethyl chloride	An aerosol product that causes temporary relief from pain by cooling the skin
Nitrous oxide	Administered by inhalation Commonly used during dental procedures Gives a feeling of euphoria

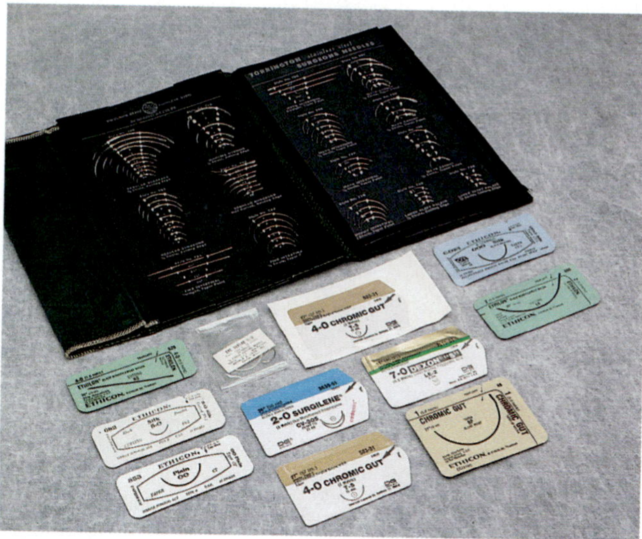

Figure 9-22 ■ A variety of suture packs.

to expand during times of swelling, its ability to recoil to its original size after much handling, and its tissue reactivity. Suture materials and needles (Figure 9-22) are usually selected based on the type of tissue to be sutured and the length of time necessary for healing to take place.

There are two types of suture material: *absorbable,* which is used most often for internal structures, and *nonabsorbable,* which is usually used on external structures; however, nonabsorbable sutures may also be used to tie off certain structures internally. Suture material comes in various sizes and lengths to accommodate the needs of the provider.

Absorbable Suture Material

Absorbable suture material is used when suturing deeper layers of the skin or when suturing structures that are difficult to reach. This type of suture material is absorbed by the body's tissues, and thus does not require manual removal. One of the first absorbable suture materials was referred to as surgical gut or "cat-gut," and was made from tissue taken from sheep intestines. Catgut suture material may be plain or coated with chromium salts, which helps to delay the absorption process and allows more time for healing. Coated catgut suture material is referred to as chromium gut. Today, catgut suture material is rarely used; it has been replaced by synthetic forms of absorbable material that provide much longer absorption rates and cause less irritation (refer to Table 9-7 for examples).

Nonabsorbable Suture Material

Nonabsorbable suture material is the most common type of suture material used in medical office procedures because it is designed for suturing external structures. Examples of nonabsorbable suture material include silk, nylon, dacron, and prolene. Always check the provider's preference prior to setting up the surgical tray.

Table 9-7 Types of Suture Material

Type	Absorbable	Natural/Synthetic	Available Sizes
Polyglycolic acid (Dexon)	Yes	Synthetic	2-0, 3-0, 4-0, 5-0, 6-0
Polyglactin (Vicryl)	Yes (complete after 70 days)	Synthetic	2-0, 3-0, 4-0, 5-0, 6-0
Polydioxanone (PS II)	Yes (complete after 180 days)	Synthetic	2-0, 3-0, 4-0, 5-0, 6-0
Polyglyconate (Maxon)	Yes	Synthetic	2-0, 3-0, 4-0, 5-0, 6-0
Polyamide (Nylon)	No	Synthetic	2-0, 3-0, 4-0, 5-0, 6-0
Polyester (Dacron)	No	Synthetic	2-0, 3-0, 4-0, 5-0, 6-0
Polypropylene (Prolene)	No	Synthetic	2-0, 3-0, 4-0, 5-0, 6-0
Catgut	Yes	Natural	3-0, 4-0, 5-0
Silk	No	Natural	2-0, 3-0, 4-0, 5-0, 6-0

Suture Sizing

Suture sizes are determined by the diameter of the suture. The smallest size typically used in ambulatory care is 6-0 (000000) and is used in cosmetic procedures. Suture sizes 5-0 (00000) and 4-0 (0000) are larger and used primarily on the trunk and extremities. Thick skin may require closure with a size 3-0. Larger diameter sutures (1-0 through 2-0) are generally not used for skin closures.

Suture Needles

Suture needles are used to close wounds and come in a variety of sizes and shapes. **Atraumatic needles** or swaged needles are packaged with suture material fused to an eyeless needle. These types of needles cause less tissue damage than traumatic needles. **Traumatic needles**, or eyed needles, are packaged so that the needle is separate from the suture material, and require the person performing the suturing to thread the needle. Suture needles may be straight or curved, allowing the needle to penetrate deeper tissue. The size and shape of the needle selected is determined by the structure to be sutured. Cosmetic procedures usually require the use of a smaller needle, while noncosmetic structures use larger needles (see Figure 9-23 for a variety of suture needles).

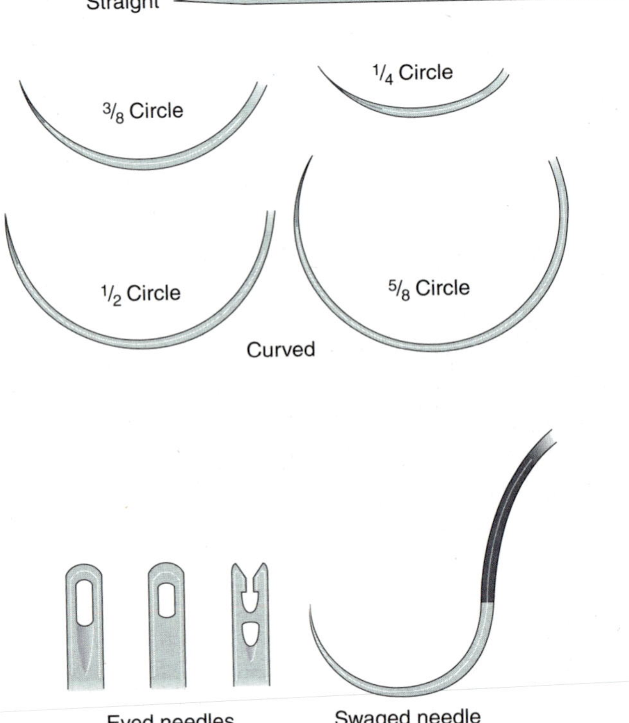

Figure 9-23 ■ Curved and straight suture needles.

Other Supplies Used to Close the Skin

There are other methods that are used to close the skin following surgical procedures or an injury, including the insertion of surgical staples and the application of sterile adhesive skin closures and surgical glues. The method of selection is based on several factors including the age of the patient, the location of the wound, the depth of the wound, and the personal preference of the provider.

Skin Staples

Surgical staples (Figure 9-24) are introduced in the skin by using a surgical stapler. The stapler comes with a cartridge that contains a specific size and number of staples. The stapler may be disposable (designed for one time use) or reusable. The advantages of using staples are that they are quickly inserted, are more economical than sutures, and cause fewer infections because the skin does not have to be handled as much

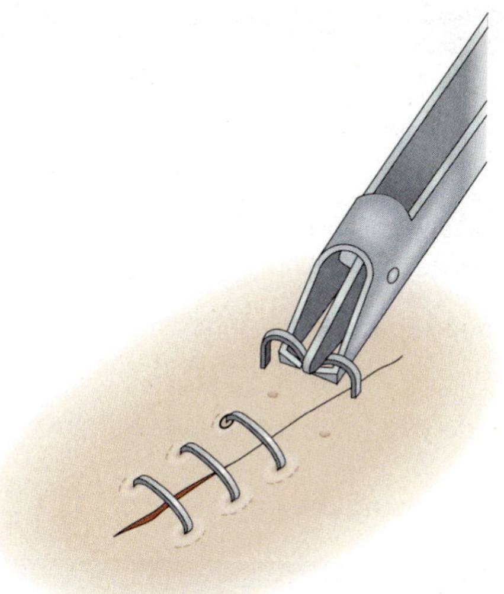

Figure 9-24 ■ An example of surgical staples.

as it does during suturing procedures. The disadvantages of staples may include permanent scars if used inappropriately and imperfect aligning of the wound edges.

Sterile Skin Closures

Medical assistants may be responsible for the application of sterile skin closures. The application of skin closures may be indicated for wounds that are not very deep. The nonallergic adhesive strips are used to approximate the edges of a slightly gaping wound. Benefits of applying adhesive skin closures include the following:

- No local anesthetic needed
- Much more time efficient than applying sutures
- More cost efficient than sutures
- Less scarring
- Reduced risk of infection

Adhesive closures come in a variety of widths and lengths and may be cut with a pair of sterile scissors for exact sizing. Refer to Procedure 9-5 for complete instructions on how to apply sterile adhesive strips.

Surgical Adhesives or Surgical Glue

Surgical adhesives are now used in place of sutures and staples by providers working in trauma, plastic surgery, and pediatrics. The sealants in these products provide the incision site with instant strength usually within a matter of minutes from the time of application.

The benefits of using surgical adhesives include the following:

- Less pain (no anesthetizing needles are necessary)
- Good cosmetic results (no stitch marks)
- Less chance of infection, because a needle is not pulled back and forth through flaps of skin
- No need for a follow-up visit to have sutures or staples removed

A drawback to some surgical glue is the inability to straighten out tissue that was not closed correctly. Some surgical adhesives allow the provider a window of time to make adjustments before the glue hardens. As manufacturers perfect these products, their popularity will increase.

SUTURE AND STAPLE REMOVAL

Patients may have sutures or staples inserted while in the hospital but will often return to their general practitioner's or surgeon's office to have them removed. The medical assistant may be responsible for performing this very important task. It will be important for the medical assistant to examine the wound closely and look for signs of gaping or infection. Examine both the bandage and the suture area following the removal of the bandage. Does the bandage look dirty, tattered, or wet, or does it contain drainage that is consistent with infection? Does the wound look like it is entirely closed, and is there good approximation of the edges of the wound? Are there any signs of infection on the tissue surrounding the wound such as erythema, warmth, or edema? If the bandage appears to be stuck to the wound, the medical assistant may need to saturate the dressing with sterile saline prior to removal. Always pull the edges of the dressing toward the wound. The medical assistant should not remove any sutures or staples until the provider has had an opportunity to inspect the wound area.

The average time spans in which sutures are removed are:

- Scalp: 7 to 10 days
- Face: 3 to 5 days
- Arms and legs: 10 to 14 days
- Trunk: 7 to 10 days
- Joints: 14 days

Refer to Procedure 9-6 for complete instructions on removing sutures and staples.

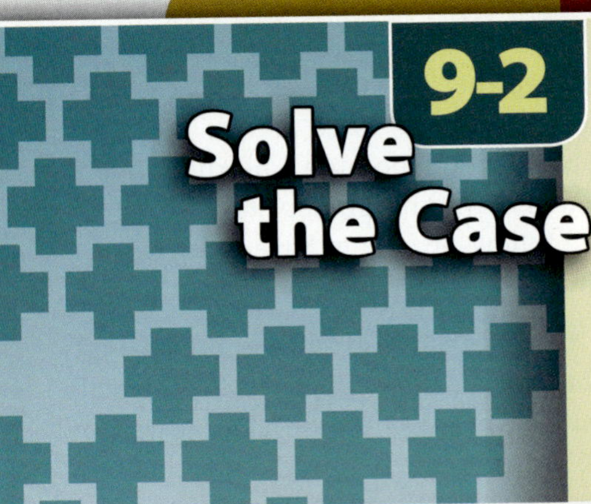

Now that you have read the chapter, refer back to Solve the Case 9-1 and reconsider those questions.

1. **Did you answer them all the same way, or did you change your answers? If you changed any answers, why did you change them?**

The doctor feels like he is going to need to pack the area where the cyst was removed.

2. **What type of packing material do you think the doctor will order?**
3. **Why is sterility so important when using packing material?**

PROCEDURE 9-1

Sanitization and Lubrication of Instruments

Objective:

To properly clean and maintain surgical instruments in order to minimize the risks of post-op infection to the patient and to keep the instruments in excellent working order.

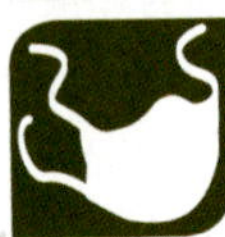

Equipment/Supplies:

- Personal protective equipment (PPE)
- Sink
- Surgical soap or sanitizer
- Utility gloves
- Plastic wash basin (if metal basin used, apply a towel to the bottom)
- Scrub brush
- Distilled water for rinsing
- Waterproof drape
- Muslin cloth or towel
- Lubricating agent (optional)

PROCEDURAL STEPS	DETAILS AND/OR RATIONALE
1. Wash your hands and apply utility gloves.	Utility gloves will protect the medical assistant's hands.
2. Place pre-soaked instruments into basin filled with a solution of warm water and surgical soap.	Pre-soaking the instruments will keep debris from drying on the instrument.
3. Thoroughly scrub each part of the instruments (Figure 9-25). Pay close attention to parts of the instruments that contain crevices, teeth, and serrations.	Microorganisms can hide in hard-to-clean surfaces, such as crevices, teeth, and serrations. It is important to make certain that the whole instrument is properly sanitized or complete sterilization cannot occur.

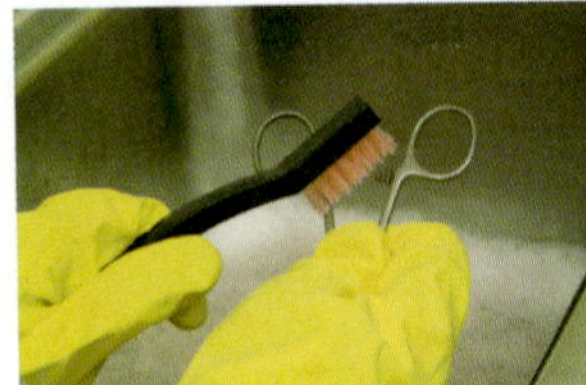

Figure 9-25 ■ The medical assistant must scrub all parts of each instrument, but must scrub especially well where there are crevices, teeth, or serrations.

continues

PROCEDURE 9-1 continued

PROCEDURAL STEPS	DETAILS AND/OR RATIONALE
4. Thoroughly rinse each instrument in distilled water or an approved rinsing solution.	Rinsing in distilled water prevents deposits from building up on the instruments.
5. Place each instrument on a waterproof drape until all instruments have been thoroughly sanitized and rinsed.	Laying the instruments on a towel that is not waterproof will allow the instrument to pick up microorganisms from the surface underneath the towel, causing the instruments to become recontaminated.
6. Dry each instrument with a muslin cloth or comparable material.	Drying instruments with paper products or towels may leave lint on the instrument, which could inhibit sterilization.
7. Inspect each instrument for any defects. Remove any instruments that are damaged.	Instruments that have defects could inhibit complete sterilization and could create problems during the procedure itself.
8. (Optional) Lubricate each instrument, especially on box locks and moving parts (Figure 9-26).	Lubricating instruments helps working correctly.
9. Dry the lubricated instruments according to the instructions found on the lubricant label.	Each manufacturer has its own instructions for using its products.
10. Clean the area using an approved disinfectant.	This cuts down on the number of microorganisms from the previously dirty instruments.
11. Remove utility gloves, hang them upside down (by the finger tips) to dry, and wash hands.	Hanging the utility gloves upside down to dry will assure the water will not enter the gloves and that they are ready for the next use.

Figure 9-26 ■ The medical assistant applies lubricating spray to the box lock of the instrument to keep it functioning correctly.

PROCEDURE 9-2
Chemical Disinfection of Instruments*

Objective:

To properly disinfect instruments that are sensitive to heat or that do not fit into an autoclave.

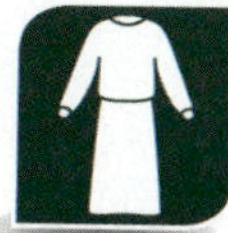

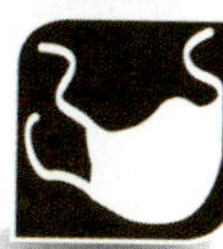

Equipment/Supplies:

- Personal protective equipment (PPE)
- Chemical disinfectant
- Distilled water for rinsing
- An immersion container with lid
- Clean drying cloths
- Clean gloves (for noncritical devices)

PROCEDURAL STEPS	DETAILS AND/OR RATIONALE
1. Choose a room that is well ventilated and clean. Use a fume hood if available.	The fumes from chemical disinfectants can be very irritating to the lungs and toxic to breathe.

* *Notation*: If chemically *sterilizing* surgical scopes or instruments, use sterile water for rinsing, handle only with sterile gloves or sterile transfer forceps, dry with sterile towels and apply to a sterile surgical tray for immediate use, covering immediately with a sterile drape.

continues

PROCEDURE 9-2 continued

PROCEDURAL STEPS	DETAILS AND/OR RATIONALE
2. Check the expiration date of the chemical, its mixing formula and instructions for use, as well as its cautionary information (see SDS).	Using expired chemicals or mixing improperly will negate their effectiveness.
3. Wash your hands, gather the supplies, and apply PPE.	Applying the appropriate PPE will help to protect the medical assistant from possible splashing or inhalation of the chemical.
4. Prepare and pour the solution into an acceptable disinfecting immersion container following the manufacturer's instructions and check the solution with a chemical indicator to confirm it meets the MEC (Figure 9-27).	Mixing proper ratios will help to assure effective disinfecton. If the solution doesn't meet the minimum effective concentration (MEC) level, the instrument will not be properly disinfected.
5. Directly on the chemical container, record the date that the container was opened and activated along with your initials.	The reuse life begins to count down once the container is opened and activated.
6. Place the instrument to be disinfected into the disinfecting tray until the instrument is completely submerged in the disinfecting solution (Figure 9-28). Apply the lid securely on the basin.	If the entire instrument is not submerged, the instrument will not be properly disinfected.
7. Set the timer according to the manufacturer's instructions.	Set the timer so you don't forget about the instrument. Reduced submersion times could inhibit the item from being properly disinfected or sterilized. Increased times could result in damage to the instrument.
8. When the timer goes off, lift the tray out of the disinfecting solution and rinse the item according to manufacturer's instructions.	Adequate rinsing is critical so that all chemical is removed.
9. Dry the instrument with a clean cloth.	Drying the instrument prevents water damage.
10. Clean the area and replace items.	
11. Remove PPE and wash your hands.	

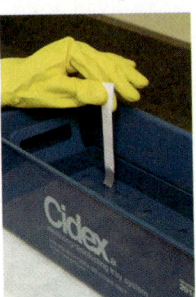

Figure 9-27 ■ The disinfecting solution must be checked to be sure it meets the minimum effective concentration level.

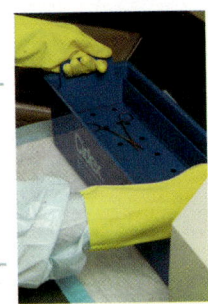

Figure 9-28 ■ The entire instrument must be completely submerged in the solution so that all parts are completely covered by the solution.

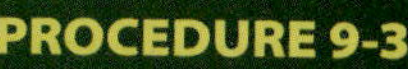

PROCEDURE 9-3

Wrapping Items for Sterilization in an Autoclave

Objective:

To double wrap or package surgical items prior to autoclaving them. Wrapping allows the sterile items to be stored in a drawer or cupboard until they are used.

Equipment/Supplies:

- Sanitized instruments or surgical set of instruments
- Wrapping materials (sterilization paper, muslin cloth, or plastic seal pouch)
- Gauze squares
- Autoclave tape
- Sterilization indicator strip
- Permanent marker

PROCEDURAL STEPS	DETAILS AND/OR RATIONALE
1. Gather the supplies , wash hands, and put on gloves.	Always wash hands and apply gloves before handling sanitized items. This helps to keep the sanitized items as clean as possible.
2. Check the integrity of the wrapping materials for any flaws.	If there are signs of moisture, holes, or tears, the wrapping material should be discarded and replaced with fresh wrapping materials.
3. Check the expiration date on the sterilization indicators.	Sterilization indicators may not be effective if they are expired.
4. Place the items on a clean, dry, flat surface.	A wet surface may compromise the integrity of the wrap.
Wrapping in Paper or Muslin: 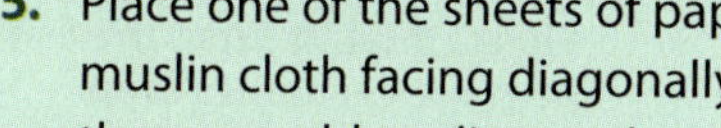	
5. Place one of the sheets of paper or muslin cloth facing diagonally so that they resemble a diamond.	This assists with proper wrapping.
6. Place the sanitized instrument in the center of the paper slightly below the center line. Slightly open instruments with hinges and shield any sharp tips with a piece of gauze. Place a sterilization indicator beside the instrument (Figure 9-29).	The instruments are opened up so that steam is able to penetrate each surface of the instrument. The gauze keeps sharp tips from piercing through the paper. The indicator strip will indicate if conditions were adequate for sterilization to occur within the pack.
7. Take the bottom edge of the paper that is facing you and fold it upward. Fold the top edge of the diagonal back toward you so that there is a flap (Figure 9-30).	The tip of the flap is then easily reached when opening the wrapped item after autoclaving.
8. Fold the right side corner of the wrap toward the center. Fold the tip back toward the right side so that there is a flap (Figure 9-31).	The tip of the side flap is then easily reached when opening the wrapped item after autoclaving.

Figure 9-29 ■ Place the instrument for sterilization in the center of the pack with a sterilization indicator.

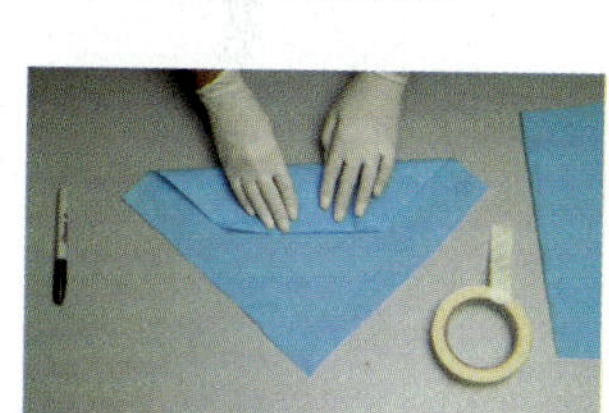

Figure 9-30 ■ Fold the first flap toward the center leaving a small corner turned back on itself.

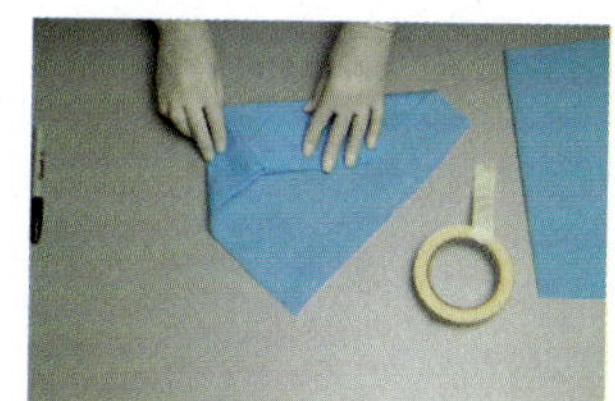

Figure 9-31 ■ Fold one side flap toward the center, leaving a small corner turned back on itself.

continues

PROCEDURE 9-3 continued

PROCEDURAL STEPS	DETAILS AND/OR RATIONALE
9. Repeat step 8 for the other side (Figure 9-32). The item should be snuggly encased, but not tight enough to puncture through the wrap.	The tip of the other side flap is then easily reached when opening the wrapped item after autoclaving. Making sure the items are snuggly wrapped assures they will stay in place.
10. Fold the pack upward from the bottom edge until the article is completely covered, folding the last tip back on itself (Figure 9-33).	This method allows the medical assistant to open the inner wrapped package without contaminating the sterile instruments when setting up a sterile tray.
11. Place the wrapped item onto the center of a second piece of autoclave paper (Figure 9-34). Repeat steps 7 through 9.	Double wrapping provides extra thickness, protection, and ease of opening.
12. The last flap is not folded back on itself, but instead is secured with autoclave tape.	Securing the pack with tape will keep the pack closed. The heat-reactive stripes on the tape will darken when autoclaved, indicating that the package has been autoclaved.
13. Label the pack with the name(s) of the items inside, the date, and your first initial and full last name or initials. (Figure 9-35).	Labeling allows for identification of what is in the pack as well as the date it was sterilized so the pack can be reprocessed if not used within the accepted time frame.
Items in Peel-Apart Pouches:	
14. Label the peel-apart pouch with the name(s) of the items inside, the date, and your first initial and full last name or initials.	Labeling identifies the instrument(s). You can't always determine the exact type of instrument through the plastic, particularly if the tips are covered with gauze.
15. Place instruments in the envelope (handle first).	When opening the pouch, the handle will be accessible first.
16. Pull the backing off of the adhesive strip and bend the adhesive flap downward so that it completely seals the envelope. Apply autoclave tape to the edge of the flap if there are any wrinkles or bumps.	Sealing well is critical for the pack to maintain it sterile properties until opened.

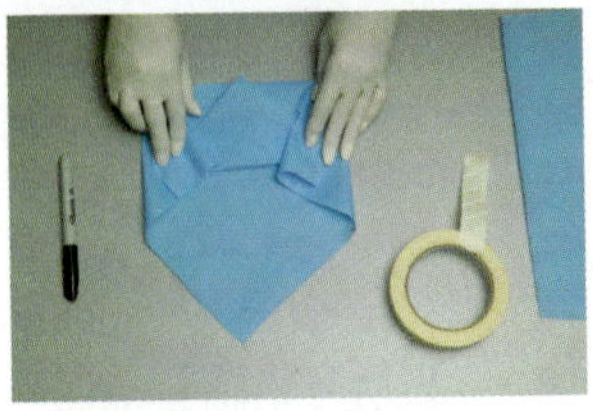

Figure 9-32 ■ Fold the other side toward the center, leaving a small corner turned back on itself.

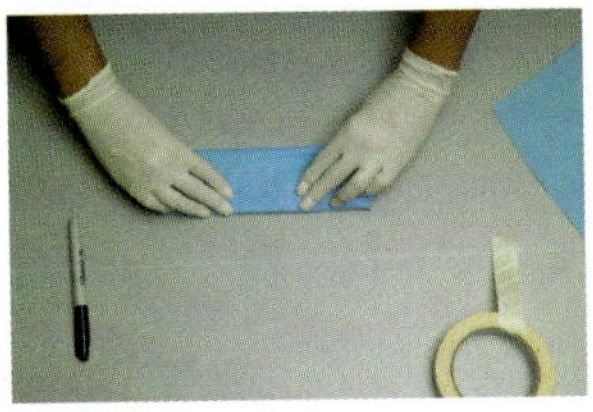

Figure 9-33 ■ Fold the package up from the bottom and secure it.

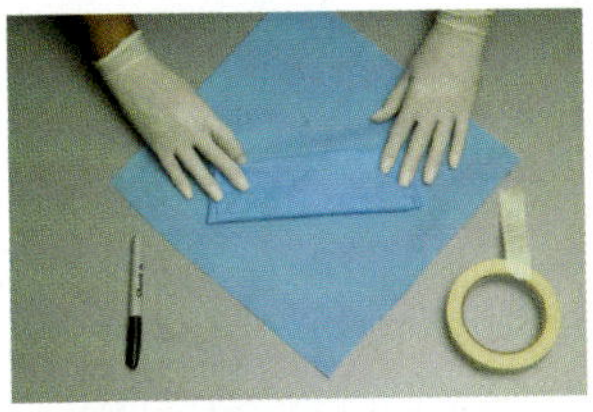

Figure 9-34 ■ Wrap the first package in another wrap.

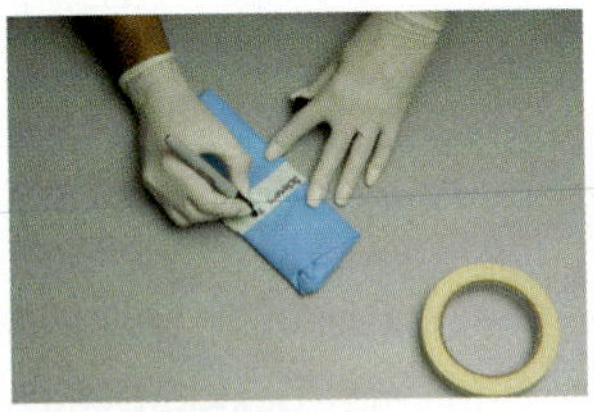

Figure 9-35 ■ Record the name of the instrument, the expiration date, and your first initial and full last name or just initials on the autoclave tape.

PROCEDURE 9-4

Operate an Autoclave

Objective:

To properly operate the autoclave to assure complete sterilization of the items in the pack.

Equipment/Supplies:

- Autoclave
- Packs or items to be autoclaved
- Distilled water
- Pot holder or thermal gloves

PROCEDURAL STEPS	DETAILS AND/OR RATIONALE
1. Wash your hands, apply gloves, and gather the supplies.	Washing your hands and gloving will help to keep items as clean as possible.
2. Arrange the packs on the autoclave trays vertically and separated by at least an inch (Figure 9-36). Jars should be placed on their sides with their lids removed.	Packs must be placed in the autoclave to so that the steam can penetrate all surfaces of each pack. Placing jars on their sides allow the oxygen to escape so the inside of the jar can be sterilized.
3. Check the water level in the autoclave reservoir and add distilled water to the fill-line if needed.	Water is used with each load and must be replaced. Distilled water will decrease mineral build up on the inside of the autoclave.
4. Place loaded trays into the autoclave (Figure 9-37). Make any necessary adjustments to accommodate the proper positioning of the instruments on each tray.	The packs may have slipped during transporting from the autoclave table to the autoclave.
5. Close and latch the door according to manufacturer's instructions.	The door must be adequately sealed in order for the unit to function properly.
6. Select the correct parameters for the type of load you are running.	The settings on the autoclave unit are based on the type of pack you are sterilizing. Wrapped pack, pouches, and so on.
7. Once the load has gone through the complete sterilization cycle the door will automatically vent. Do not open until venting is complete. Once venting is complete, use an oven mitt or pot holder and remove packs from trays.	Venting allows the contents to cool and eventually dry. Using heat-resistant gloves will protect your hands if the machine is still hot.
8. When the items are cool, examine them for tears, holes, or damages of any kind. Make sure the labels are readable and that the stripes on the indicator tape has darkened.	Removing the items before they are completely cool may indicate that they are still damp inside. Labels need to be readable for proper identification. If there are tears or damages to the packs, the sterility cannot be assured. If the tape's indicator stripes are not darkened, perhaps the proper temperature was not reached.
9. Store the items in a clean, closed environment such as a drawer or a cupboard.	This is necessary to maintain sterility of the packs.

Figure 9-36 ■ Place packs vertically on the tray about an inch apart from one another.

Figure 9-37 ■ Place the tray in the autoclave.

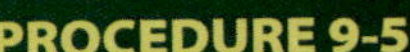

PROCEDURE 9-5

Apply Skin Closures

Objective:

To properly close a wound with adhesive strips.

Equipment/Supplies:

- Skin antiseptic swabs
- Adhesive strips or closures (sized to match the patient's wound)
- Pair of gloves
- Bandaging material
- Biohazard waste container/Trash receptacle
- Patient's chart/EHR

PROCEDURAL STEPS	DETAILS AND/OR RATIONALE
1. Wash your hands and gather the supplies.	Washing hands will reduce number of organisms and gathering supplies will save time.
2. Identify the patient using two identifiers, identify yourself. ***Explain the rationale for performance of the procedure. Show awareness of the patient's concerns related to the procedure being performed.***	Using two identifiers helps to confirm you have the right patient. Explaining the procedure and rationale will help the patient know what to expect and why the procedure is necessary.
3. Inspect the wound and select the size of adhesive strips that best matches the patient's wound.	This will make application of the strips easier and will avoid excess that has to be cut during the procedure.
4. Position the patient so he is comfortable and position the tray for easy access.	The patient will be able to hold still much longer if he or he is comfortable.
5. Clean the tray and apply items to the tray. Avoid contaminating any of the supplies. Supplies include: • 1 pack of skin antiseptic swabs • 1 package of sterile adhesive strips Open all items in a sterile fashion so that they are completely open for easy access.	Because the skin is open, you want to avoid contaminating any of the items that will touch the open skin area to help avoid infection.
6. Wash your hands and apply clean gloves.	Sterile gloves are not necessary as long as you are using swabs and only handling the swab by the handle. You should only be handling strips by the distal tips which shouldn't come into contact with the open portion of the wound.
7. Clean the patient's skin so that the cleansing extends at least 2 to 3 inches (5 to 7 cm) around the wound using sterile antiseptic swabs.	This helps to remove any debris, blood, or skin oils, and helps to prevent infection.
8. Allow the area to completely dry.	The area must be completely dry for best results.
9. Remove the card to which the skin closures are attached using sterile technique. Bend the card at the perforated edge and gently remove the tab. Grasp the skin closure with gloved hands or forceps, lifting straight up. Touch only the edges of the strips.	Touching only the distal edges of the skin closures will prevent any part of the strip touched by your gloved hand or forceps from coming into contact with the open part of the wound.

continues

PROCEDURE 9-5 continued

PROCEDURAL STEPS	DETAILS AND/OR RATIONALE
10. If applying single strips, line the first strip up with the center of the wound (Figure 9-38). Firmly press one end of the strip on either side of the wound to secure it in place.	Starting with the center of the wound helps with approximation of the wound.
11. Gently pull the strip while lining up both edges of the wound so that they come together. (You may need to use the other hand to help oppose the wound edges.)	The wound edges must come together evenly to heal properly and minimize scarring.
12. Once the skin is lined up evenly on both sides, pull the tape to the opposite side while pressing down firmly on the skin.	If the skin is not lined up evenly on both sides, you will not have good wound approximation.
13. Apply the next strip approximately ⅛ inch from the first strip on either side of the first strip.	
14. Perform the same step on the opposite side of the wound (Figure 9-39).	
15. Continue this process until the wound is completely closed.	Going back and forth from the center helps with approximation of the wound.
16. If needed, apply one closure approximately ½ inch away from the strip's edges, running parallel to the wound on both sides of the strips (Figure 9-40).	This helps to secure the adhesive strips to the skin.
17. Make certain that there is good approximation of the wound margins.	If the wound margins are not evenly lined up, the wound margins may not completely close, setting the patient up for infection and scarring.
18. Apply dressing if necessary.	Applying a dressing initially will keep the strips clean and dry. (Patient should remove dressing after a day or two.)
19. Remove gloves and wash your hands.	
20. Give the patient home care instructions. (Instruct patient not to pull the strips off, but to let them fall off on their own. The patient may, however, cut the edges as they curl up.)	It is important for the patient to know how to properly care for the wound and the strips to avoid complications.
21. Place trash in trash receptacle.	

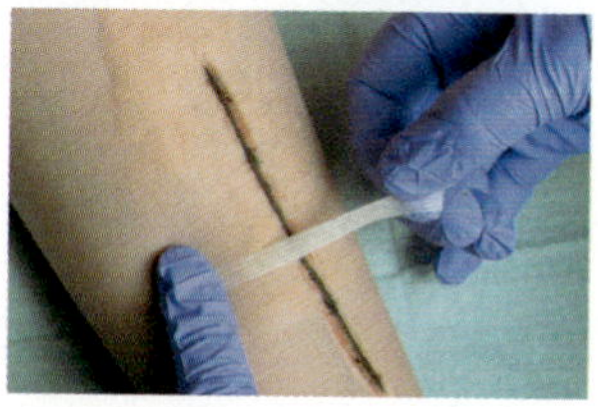

Figure 9-38 ■ The medical assistant places the first strip at the center of the wound.

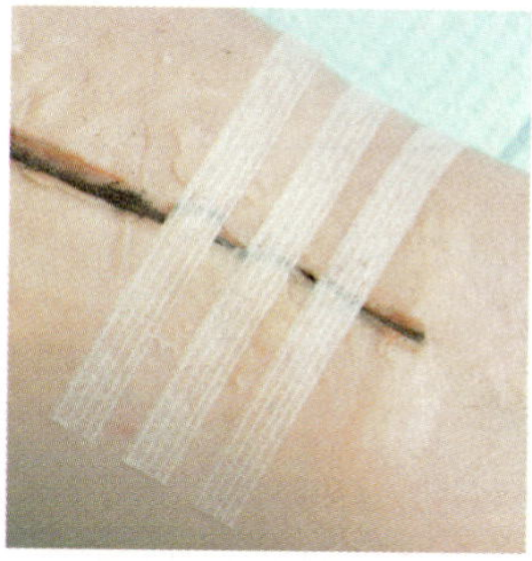

Figure 9-39 ■ Going back and forth from the center helps with approximation of the wound.

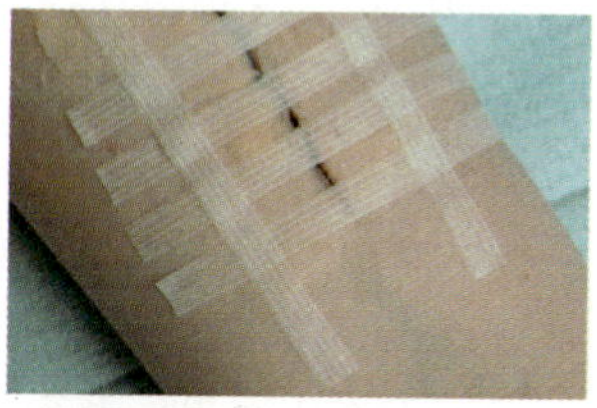

Figure 9-40 ■ Apply one closure approximately ½ inch away from the strip's edges, running parallel to the wound on both side of the strips.

continues

PROCEDURE 9-5 continued

PROCEDURAL STEPS	DETAILS AND/OR RATIONALE
22. Document the procedure in the patient's chart.	Document the date and time, the procedure itself, the location of the procedure, and how many strips were applied. List what type of dressing was applied and any home care instructions given to the patient. Always show the provider's order.

DOCUMENTATION EXAMPLE:

10-12-XX 2:30 p.m.	Steri-strip application x 6 to pt's R. forearm per Dr. Kennedy. Cleaned surrounding area with iodine swabs and applied the strips. Good approximation of wound. Closed spiral dressing applied. Gave pt home care instructions. Pt. to return in 5 days. Pt instructed to call if there are any concerns or complications. C. Brady, CMA (AAMA)------------------------------

PROCEDURE 9-6

Suture or Staple Removal

Objective:

To correctly remove sutures or staples without contaminating internal tissue or causing further injury to the patient.

Equipment/Supplies:

- Suture removal kit (suture scissors and thumb forceps) or staple removal kit (staple remover and thumb forceps)
- Bandage scissors
- Sterile/Clean 4 × 4s for cleansing the skin
- Sterile saline/skin antiseptic
- Examination gloves
- Biohazard waste container/Trash receptacle
- Dressing supplies
- Patient's chart/EHR

PROCEDURAL STEPS	DETAILS AND/OR RATIONALE
1. Identify the patient using two identifiers.	This confirms you have the correct patient.
2. Identify yourself and ***explain the rationale for performance of the procedure. Show awareness of the patient's concerns related to the procedure being performed.***	Explaining the procedure will help the patient know what to expect and why it is necessary. Showing awareness of the patient's concerns illustrates respect and compassion for your patient.
3. Ask if the patient took all of the antibiotic and whether all other home care instructions were followed. ***Incorporate critical thinking skills when performing patient care.***	If the patient didn't take all of their antibiotic, it could lead to infection. The provider should be made aware of this so that he can discuss the importance of taking all medication exactly as prescribed.
4. Examine the outside of the patient's bandage and make a mental note.	A dirty, tattered dressing may indicate that the patient has not been caring for the wound as prescribed.

continues

PROCEDURE 9-6 continued

PROCEDURAL STEPS	DETAILS AND/OR RATIONALE
5. Wash your hands and apply examination gloves.	Washing your hands will help to prevent the spread of organisms. Applying exam gloves helps to protect you from any exudate present on the bandage.
6. Remove the dressing and observe both the inside of the dressing and the wound area for any signs of infection (make a mental note).	Examination of the dressing and the wound addresses any compliance or infection concerns.
7. Discard the dressing into the biohazard container, remove gloves, and wash your hands.	If exudates are present, the dressing should be discarded into biohazard container to prevent the spread of microorganisms.
8. Have the provider observe the wound before starting the procedure.	Removing sutures before they are ready to be removed may result in infection and possible scarring.
9. Once the provider okays the procedure, open supplies including suture removal kit.	You don't want to open supplies until you are sure the procedure is going to take place, otherwise the kit will need to be disposed of (if disposable) or re-sterilized.
10. If sutures are adhered to the bandage, irrigate dressing with sterile water or saline and dry.	If the sutures are adhered to the skin, they will be much more difficult to remove and the procedure will be much more painful to the patient.
11. Cleanse area with a skin antiseptic.	This will remove bacteria and exudates away from the area to lessen the risks of infection.
12. If removing sutures, grasp one side of the first knot with the thumb forceps and gently tug upward on the end of the knot. Using the other hand, work the suture scissors under the knot as close to the skin as possible and cut the suture (Figure 9-41). Pull the knot toward the wound, making certain that no part of the suture that was on the outside goes through the inside of the wound (Figure 9-42).	Do not let any part of the suture that was on the outside of the skin go back through the inside of the skin; it may cause infection.
13. If removing staples, gently grasp the staple with the remover and squeeze the handle of the staple remover until the staple is pinched up and out.	
14. Continue to remove the sutures or staples until all have been removed.	
15. Make sure that the wound still has good approximation and that there is no gapping of the skin (notify the provider if there are any concerns).	If the wound starts to gap at any time during removal, notify the provider before proceeding any further. The wound may not be as healed as originally thought.

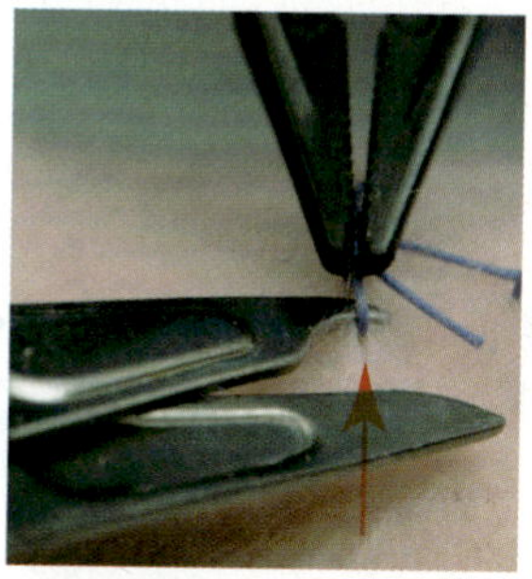

Figure 9-41 ■ The medical assistant cuts the suture as close to the skin as possible on either side of the knot.

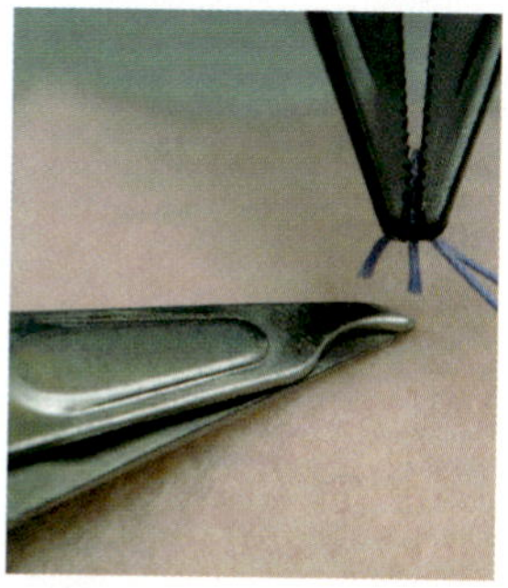

Figure 9-42 ■ Once the knot is cut the medical assistant pulls the suture toward the wound line.

continues

PROCEDURE 9-6 continued

PROCEDURAL STEPS	DETAILS AND/OR RATIONALE
16. Apply antiseptic ointment only if ordered and dress the wound according to the provider's instructions.	In most cases the wound will not need any ointment or dressing; however, if there is any drainage or gapping, the provider may want the area dressed to reduce risks of infection.
17. Remove gloves and wash your hands.	
18. Give the patient any home care instructions and dismiss.	There usually are no home care instructions if the wound is completely closed.
19. Clean the area and dispose of related items in the biohazardous trash receptacle.	
20. Document the procedure.	

DOCUMENTATION EXAMPLE:

12-12-XX 6:30 p.m.	Pt. here to have sutures removed from L. foot. Removed bandage and inspected wound. No exudates on bandage or coming from the wound, ⊝ erythema, ⊝ edema. Dr. Miller inspected wound and gave v/o to remove sutures. Removed all sutures (6 total). Good closure of wound following removal. Dressed site with adhesive bandage. Instructed pt to remove bandage tomorrow and to call with any concerns. Scheduled pt. for a F/U appt. on 2-18-XX Destiny Green, CMA (AAMA)---

CHAPTER SUMMARY

- Asepsis means free of germs. Medical asepsis refers to destruction of organisms after they leave the body. Surgical asepsis is the destruction of all microorganisms prior to a surgical procedure.
- Sanitization means to make sanitary or clean, disinfection is the use of chemical agents to destroy pathogenic organisms, and sterilization is the complete destruction of all microorganisms, including spores.
- Critical items are instruments or devices that will penetrate or enter sterile tissue, semicritical items are instruments or devices that may come into contact with nonintact skin or mucous membranes, and noncritical items are instruments or devices that only touch intact skin.
- There are three major levels of disinfections: low, intermediate, and high.
- Forms of sterilization include autoclaving (most used method and most reliable), dry heat gas sterilization, and the use of chemical sterilants.
- The proper method used to wrap instrument when using paper or cloth is the "fan-fold" method.
- Sterilization or chemical indicators are devices that determine whether or not a package has been exposed to high heat and whether or not the items inside are sterile.
- Summary of proper sterilization includes the following: proper sanitization, proper wrapping, proper loading of packs, proper sterilization technique, and proper storage of sterilized items.
- Parts of an instrument may include the handle, ratchet, shank, box-lock, and tip.
- Tips of instruments may include jaws, serrations, circular blades, prongs and hooks, and blades.
- Categories of instruments include those for cutting and dissecting, those for grasping and clamping, those to improve visualization and those for probing. Instruments used for cutting and dissecting include curettes, scalpels, and scissors. Instruments used for grasping and clamping include forceps,

needle holders, and towel clamps. Instruments to improve visualization include dilators, probes, sounds, retractors, scopes, and specula.

- Typical solutions used during minor surgeries include alcohol, chlorhexidine gluconate, iodine products, tincture of benzoin, and sterile saline.
- Common supplies used in minor surgery include, nonfenestrated and fenestrated drapes, sterile gauze pads, sterile attire, surgical wicks, sterile packing material, syringes and needles, laboratory specimen cups, laboratory culture transport tubes, dressings, and bandage supplies.
- Anesthetics are used to produce a lack of feeling in patients during a surgical procedure.
- Common anesthetics include any of the "caines," ethyl chloride, and nitrous oxide.
- Suture means to sew. There are two categories of sutures: nonabsorbable and absorbable.
- Suture needles include atraumatic and traumatic needles.
- Other supplies to close the skin include skin staples, adhesive skin closures, and surgical adhesives.

CERTIFICATION REVIEW QUESTIONS

1. The type of handle that opens and closes by pinching and releasing is known as a:
   a. ring handle.
   b. thumb handle.
   c. pinch and release handle.
   d. All of the above.

2. What is the part of an instrument that is hinged and found on a ring-handled instrument?
   a. Jaws
   b. Shanks
   c. Box lock
   d. Ratchet

3. What surgical instrument is shaped like a spoon or loop and is used to scrape and remove tissue from the skin or body cavity?
   a. Curette
   b. Surgical spoon
   c. Sound
   d. Forceps

4. Which of the following solutions would not typically be used during minor office surgery?
   a. Sterile saline
   b. Povidone iodine
   c. Isopropyl alcohol
   d. Distilled water

5. Which of the following helps to prolong the effects of an anesthetic agent?
   a. Epinephrine
   b. Norepinephrine
   c. ACTH
   d. Corphrine

6. All of the following are anesthetic agents commonly used in the medical office except:
   a. Xylocaine.
   b. Procaine.
   c. Lidocaine.
   d. ether.

7. Which type of suture material is used in deeper tissues?
   a. Synthetic
   b. Absorbable
   c. Nonabsorbable
   d. Nylon

8. Which of the following suture materials would have the largest diameter?
   a. 3-0
   b. 4-0
   c. 5-0
   d. 6-0

9. You are sterilizing a critical item for a surgical pack. Which form(s) of sterile processing would be acceptable?
   a. Autoclaving
   b. Disinfection
   c. The use of a sterilant
   d. Both a and c

10. The doctor needs a medication that will reduce feeling in the local area and help to control bleeding. Which of the following would be best?
    a. Xylocaine with ether
    b. Xylocaine by itself
    c. Xylocaine with epinephrine
    d. None of the above

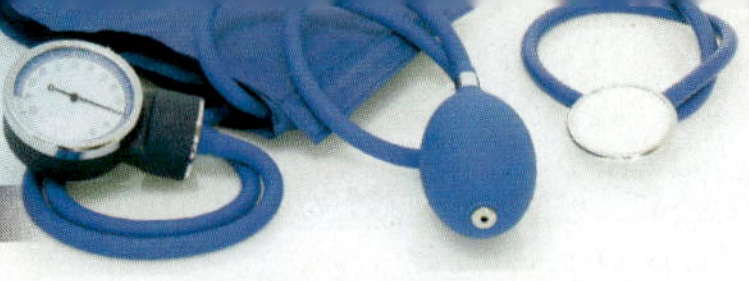

STUDY RESOURCES

Resources to Test and Reinforce Your Knowledge:	
Certification Review Questions	Take this end-of-chapter quiz
Workbook	• Complete the activities for Chapter 9 • Perform the procedures for Chapter 9 using the Competency Checklists
Resources to Promote Critical Thinking:	
***Solve the Case* Activities**	• Consider these case studies and discuss your conclusions
Learning Lab	• Module 19: Infection Control and Medical Asepsis
MindTap	• Complete Chapter 9 readings and activities

REFERENCES

Blesi, M. (2017). *Medical assisting: Administrative and Clinical Competencies*. (8th ed.). Clifton Park, NY: Cengage Learning.

Lindh, W., Pooler, M., Tamparo, C., Dahl, B. & Morris, J. (2014). *Delmar's comprehensive medical assisting: Administrative and clinical competencies*. (5th ed.). Clifton Park, NY: Cengage Learning.

10

Assisting with Minor Office Surgeries and Wound Care Procedures

CHAPTER OUTLINE

Developing a Sterile Conscience

Patient Safety Considerations

Types of Procedures Performed in the Medical Office/Tray Setups

- Procedures That Require No Special Equipment
- Procedures That Require the Use of Special Equipment, Lasers, or Chemicals

Preparing for Office Surgeries

- Setup Procedures
- Once the Patient Enters the Surgical Suite

Performing a Surgical Handwash and Applying Surgical Attire

Assisting the Physician before and during the Procedure

- Pre-Procedure Tasks
- During the Procedure
- At the Conclusion of the Surgery

Wound Care

- Stages of Wound Healing
- Today's Wound Care Philosophy
- Types of Dressings
- Types of Bandage Material
- Wound Care Alternatives

ESSENTIAL TERMS

abscess
aspiration
bandage
closed wound
concentric circle
cryosurgery
debridement
dressing
electrocoagulation
electrodessication
electrofulguration
electrosection
exudate
hyperbaric oxygen (HBO_2) therapy
laceration
laser
open wound
primary dressing
purulent
sanguineous
sebaceous cyst
secondary dressing
serosanguineous
serous
sterile conscience
subatmospheric pressure device

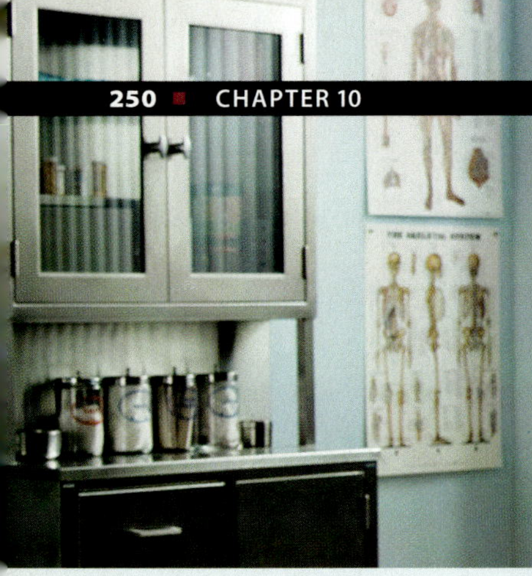

DEVELOPMENTAL OBJECTIVES

After completing this chapter, you should be able to:

1. Correctly spell and define the essential terms.
2. List and describe the different guidelines for developing aseptic technique.
3. Describe how a sterile conscience will help to reduce the patient's risk of developing a postop infection.
4. Describe common surgical procedures performed in ambulatory medicine and list equipment instruments and supplies that should be included for each tray setup.
5. List the three stages of healing and describe interferences that can impede the healing process.
6. Compare and contrast the different types of dressings used in health care and describe when each type would be used.
7. Compare and contrast two different types of alternative treatments used to treat chronic wounds that will not heal.
8. Perform a surgical handwash and apply surgical gloves.
9. Perform sterilization procedures and prepare a sterile field.
10. Apply surgical attire.
11. Remove an old dressing, irrigate the wound, and apply a new dressing.

INTRODUCTION

There are a multitude of tasks that must be completed when preparing for and assisting with minor office surgeries. The procedures for sanitizing, sterilizing, and processing instruments were presented in Chapter 9. This chapter will present important information on preparing patients for surgical procedures, preparing the surgical suite, assisting the physician during the procedure, and setting up surgical trays. Postsurgical and wound care responsibilities are additional topics presented in the chapter.

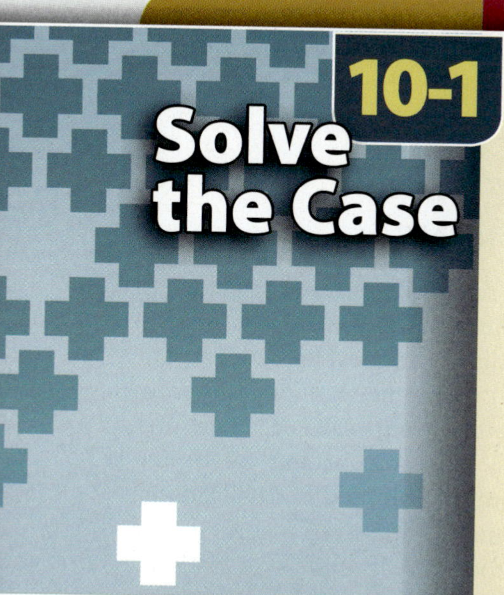

Maria Rodriguez comes into the clinic today to have a boil lanced from her left upper thigh, just below the panty line. She is nervous about pain that may be associated with the procedure and embarrassed at the location of the boil. She asks you if she needs to remove her under garments. She has a heart ailment and was supposed to take a prophylactic dose of antibiotics one hour before arriving for the procedure. When you ask her about it, she states that she took the antibiotic; however, her body language does not match her verbal message.

1. **Based on the patient's symptoms, will she need to remove her undergarments?**
2. **What can you do to institute modesty and make the patient feel less embarrassed throughout the procedure?**
3. **How should you address the prophylactic dose of antibiotics with the patient?**

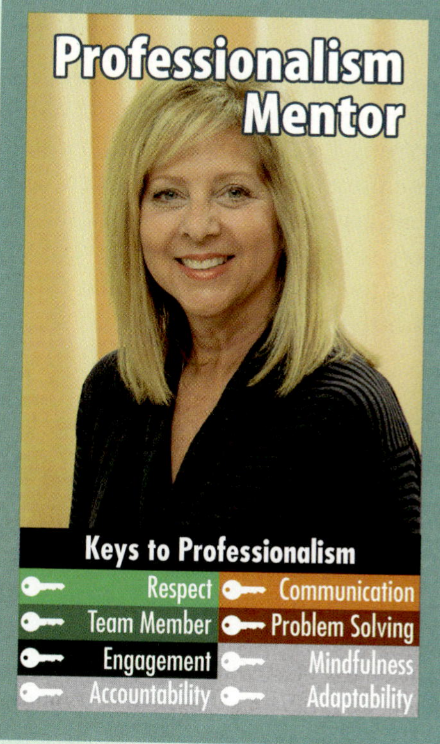

We've all been there, going to the doctor and finding out he is going to perform a procedure you weren't really expecting. That happened to me. Suffering with bursitis in my shoulder, the physician told me a cortisone shot would help. Thank goodness for the medical assistant that day. I'm not afraid of the general-type injection, but one in my shoulder with a long needle seemed scary. As the doctor sprayed a topical numbing spray, the medical assistant held my hand and talked to me about what plans I had for the rest of the day. I know she was trying to take my mind off what was about to happen, and she did. She was honest with me when I asked if it would hurt, the self-confidence she demonstrated in her role to keep me engaged in conversation was apparent as she smiled when it was "all done" and then added "good job," which made me feel as if we were a team that had just crossed the finish line together. She didn't make me feel like I should have acted differently but respected my fears and helped me work through them. Many thanks to that wonderful medical assistant! In your journal describe how the keys listed in this feature box apply to this story. Describe ways you can make the patient feel more at ease when she is nervous about having surgical procedures performed. ■

DEVELOPING A STERILE CONSCIENCE

Chapters 8 and 9 introduced the guidelines for practicing medical and surgical asepsis. This chapter will incorporate those principles and will build on aseptic technique, particularly in the surgical suite.

Surgical technicians must develop a "sterile conscience" in order to be successful in their careers. Medical assistants working in ambulatory surgery should also develop a sterile conscience. A **sterile conscience** is a mind-set of constant vigilance. It is taking ownership for the sterility of items from the time of processing through the termination of the procedure. It involves keeping a watchful eye on the surgical tray, surgical site, and other personnel during the surgical procedure, and putting the patient's best interest above personal interests when sterility is compromised, regardless of the outcome.

In order to develop a sterile conscience, one must know general guidelines for instituting aseptic technique:

1. Remove lab coats and any other clothing that could potentially drag across the field, and pull hair back prior to setting up a sterile tray.
2. Traffic in the suite should be kept to a minimum.
3. Items are either sterile or nonsterile—there is no in-between. If something occurs that makes you question if an item is sterile, treat it as though it is contaminated. ("When in doubt, get it out!")
4. Trays with surgical drapes are only considered sterile if they are at table height or waist level.
5. Handle packs and drapes as little as possible to avoid contamination. Avoid adjusting or moving drapes once in place as this could cause contamination.
6. Do not set up the tray until just before the physician enters the room.
7. Always stand so that your body is at least 12 inches away from the tray when setting up a sterile field, and never reach across a sterile field.
8. The outer 1-inch diameter around any sterile drape is considered nonsterile.
9. Never drop items directly over the field. Stand back 12–18 inches and make certain that there is always a sterile barrier between your hands and the sterile field.
10. Solution containers should be placed at the corner of the tray, and solutions should be poured at a distance of 2 to 6 inches above the solution container. Avoid splashing to prevent strike-through contamination.
11. Always approach a sterile tray or a scrubbed person head-on, and do not walk between two sterile fields. Never leave a sterile tray unattended.
12. Once a sterile item or drape becomes wet, it should be considered contaminated unless there is a waterproof drape underneath.
13. Scrubbed personnel should never allow their hands to drop below their waist and should clasp their hands together when not using them.
14. Avoid talking, coughing, sneezing, or laughing when setting up the surgical tray or assisting the physician.

PATIENT SAFETY CONSIDERATIONS

There are many patient safety concerns associated with surgical procedures other than sterility. Thousands of errors occur each year during surgical procedures. The Joint Commission (JC) is an independent nonprofit organization that accredits health care organizations. Its primary focus is to "promote patient safety and quality of care." The commission modifies its National Patient Safety Goals annually. Patient safety goals should be reviewed annually to ensure compliance. National Patient Safety Goals that apply to the ambulatory surgery environment include the following:

1. Labeling all medications, medication containers (syringes, medicine cups, or basins), or other solutions on and off the sterile field
2. Reducing the risks of surgical fires through staff education and equipment maintenance procedures
3. Using protocol for preventing "Wrong Site," "Wrong Person," and "Wrong Procedure" errors. This standard includes the use of two identifiers when identifying the patient, having the patient mark the site where the surgery is to be conducted, and verifying what procedure is to be performed with the patient immediately prior to the procedure.

TYPES OF PROCEDURES PERFORMED IN THE MEDICAL OFFICE/TRAY SETUPS

In today's world of ambulatory medicine, providers perform quite an array of minor surgical procedures. Many of these procedures only require the use of specific instruments and surgical supplies; however, with the advancement of technology, office surgeries have expanded to incorporate the use of advanced technological equipment, including the use of electrosurgical equipment and lasers. Chemicals may also be used to destroy unwanted growths or cauterize tissue.

The medical assistant should be familiar with equipment and supplies necessary for each procedure. The following section provides general information for common procedures performed in ambulatory care.

Procedures That Require No Special Equipment

Common minor surgical procedures that do not require special equipment include:

- Laceration repairs
- Excision of a sebaceous cyst
- Aspiration of fluid from a joint
- Incision and drainage procedures

Laceration Repairs

A **laceration** is a jagged wound or cut that may be the result of a traumatic injury. Any time the patient presents with a laceration that is gaping, the medical assistant should prepare for a laceration repair.

Whether sutures or other materials such as surgical staples, adhesives, or sterile skin closures will be used depends on the wound itself and preferences of the provider. The medical assistant should check with the provider prior to setting up the tray. The medical assistant should also check the date of the patient's last tetanus shot. If the time since the last shot is more than 10 years, the medical assistant should be prepared to administer the vaccine following an order from the provider.

Excision of a Sebaceous Cyst

A **sebaceous cyst** is a cyst that occurs as the result of a blocked sebaceous gland. Sebaceous glands are responsible for producing sebum, or the oil that helps to keep the skin moisturized. When a patient has a sebaceous cyst, the gland continues to secrete sebum but because the gland is blocked, it forms a capsule and fills with a thick, cheesy-looking, odiferous material. These cysts are usually very painful and become more painful as they grow. Often times the area becomes infected, making their removal much more complicated. Sebaceous cysts are benign and occur frequently on the face, ears, neck, scalp, or back. If the area appears to be infected, the provider may try to drain the cyst and place the patient on antibiotic therapy. Once the infection clears, the provider will then try to completely remove the cyst. Table 10-1 lists items that are necessary for cyst removal.

The medical assistant should be prepared to receive the cyst by holding out a specimen container so that it may be sent out for identification purposes. Patients may be placed on antibiotic therapy following excision to decrease their risk of infection.

Aspiration of Fluid from a Joint

A common type of surgery performed on patients who have arthritis or old sports injuries is joint **aspiration**, or removal of excess fluid that builds up as a result of inflammation. The knee is the most common area of the body where this procedure is performed. The fluid may be sent out for microscopic examination or for culturing purposes. The patient usually receives a combination long-term anesthetic and steroid injection to provide long-term relief. Patients often return in three months to a year to have this procedure repeated, and are placed on antibiotic/anti-inflammatory therapy following the procedure.

Assisting with an Incision and Drainage Procedure

An incision and drainage procedure is routinely performed on patients who have an **abscess** or a localized infection. An abscess walls off a localized infection to keep it from spreading to other areas of the body. Furuncles (which is another name for boils) will also often need to be incised and drained. The provider will lance the area using a sterile scalpel and will place either a rubber Penrose drain or gauze wick into the wound to keep the edges of the wound pulled apart so the wound may continue to drain. The patient's wound is dressed with several sterile 4 × 4s to accommodate the drainage. The patient is usually placed on antibiotics and will return to have the packing material removed at a later date. The medical assistant will instruct the patient on the procedure for changing the dressing.

Table 10-1 includes tray setups for laceration repairs, sebaceous cyst removal, fluid aspirations, and incision and drainage procedures.

Procedures That Require the Use of Special Equipment, Lasers, or Chemicals

Providers may use many other resources to help them perform surgical procedures in the office. The equipment that is used will be based on the type of procedure to be performed, equipment availability, and the provider's preference. The medical assistant will always need to check with the provider for clarification.

Table 10-1 Tray Setups for Laceration Repairs, Sebaceous Cyst Removal, Fluid Aspirations, and Incision and Drainage Procedures

Instruments and Supplies to Be Placed on the Sterile Field	Laceration Repairs	Sebaceous Cyst Removal	Fluid Aspiration from a Joint	Incision and Drainage
Sterile Drapes to set up the Field (If applicable)	X	X	X	X
Needle Holder	X	X		
Scalpel Handle		X		X
Iris Scissors		X		
Surgical Scissors	X			
Dissecting Scissors				X
Tissue Forceps	X			X
Hemostats or Hemostatic Forceps		X	X	X
Two Sterile Cups or Basins	X	X	X	X
Sterile Gauze Pads	X	X	X	X
Items That Start on the Side Table but Are Often Passed to Provider During Procedure	**Laceration Repairs**	**Sebaceous Cyst Removal**	**Fluid Aspiration from a Joint**	**Incision and Drainage**
Scalpel Blades		X		X
Suture Material/Staples/Adhesives	X	X		
Sterile Syringe	X	X	X	X
Sterile Needle(s)	X	X	X	X
Aspiration Needle			X	
Penrose Drain				X
Packing Material		X		
Items Placed on the Side Table	**Laceration Repairs**	**Sebaceous Cyst Removal**	**Fluid Aspiration from a Joint**	**Incision and Drainage**
Those items that will be passed from the side table to the provider during the procedure	X	X	X	X
Appropriate PPE (clean gloves, goggles, masks, and so on)	X	X	X	X
Surgical Attire (gowns, masks, goggles, surgical gloves for provider and MA)	X	X	X	X
Sterile Water or Saline	X	X	X	X
Iodine or Other Appropriate Antiseptic	X	X	X	X
Culture Medium				X
Antibiotic Ointment (only if ordered)	X	X		
Sterile Cotton Tip Applicators	X	X		
Bandage Scissors	X	X	X	X
Sterile Dressing and Bandaging Supplies (gauze, tape, and so on)	X	X	X	X
Formalin or Specimen Containers/Lab Forms	X			
Culture Medium				X
Possible Medications Administered Before, During, or Following Procedure	**Laceration Repairs**	**Sebaceous Cyst Removal**	**Fluid Aspiration from a Joint**	**Incision and Drainage**
Anesthetic (with or without epinephrine)	X	X	X	X
Tetanus Toxoid	X			
Steroid Injection			X	
Disposal Equipment	**Laceration Repairs**	**Sebaceous Cyst Removal**	**Fluid Aspiration from a Joint**	**Incision and Drainage**
Sharp's Container	X	X	X	X
Biohazardous Trash	X	X	X	X
Regular Trash Receptacle	X	X	X	X

Some of the different equipment used during surgical procedures include:

- Electrical surgical/cautery units
- Laser instruments
- Liquid chemicals

Procedures Using Electrical Current

Electrosurgical procedures are performed to destroy benign and malignant lesions, to cut or excise tissue, and to control bleeding. Dermatologists frequently perform these procedures, but other types of providers may also be certified to use electrosurgical equipment. Electrosurgery is useful for treating different types of skin lesions such as skin tags and small angiomas (benign tumors consisting of blood vessels). Types of electrosurgery include electrodesiccation, electrofulguration, electrocoagulation, and electrosection. In **electrodesiccation**, the electrode from the electrosurgical unit touches the skin to stimulate tissue destruction and is frequently performed to treat spider angiomas, warts, and polyps. **Electrofulguration** is used when working with more shallow tissues. The electrode does not touch the skin directly, but instead is held 1 to 2 millimeters away from the skin to produce a sparking sensation. This technique is used to remove polyps and cancer cells. In **electrosection**, the tip of the electrode is shaped like a fine needle, a wire loop, or a triangle and is used to incise or cut tissue for the removal of a specimen. **Electrocoagulation** is used to clot small blood vessels to help control bleeding during minor office procedures. Electrosurgical units (Figure 10-1) come with interchangeable electrodes to help create the proper modality required for the procedure being performed. Table 10-2 lists items that are necessary for electrosurgical procedures.

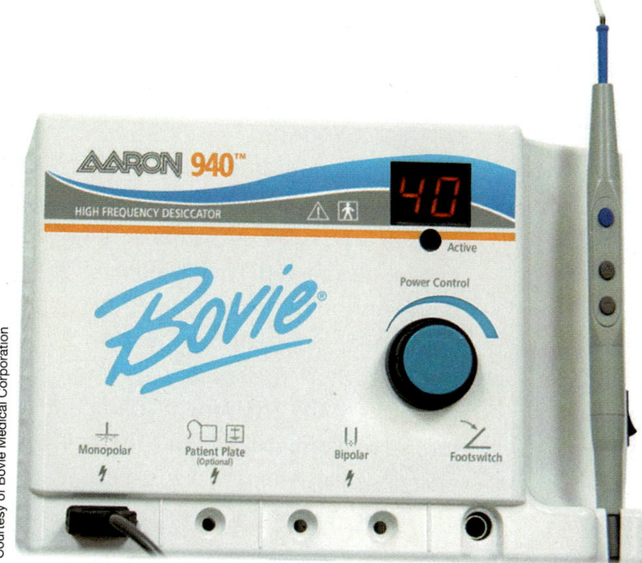

Figure 10-1 ■ The Aaron 940 is an example of electrosurgical equipment.

Table 10-2 Electrosurgical Tray

Items Placed Directly on the Sterile Field	Items Placed on a Side Table
Needle and syringe	PPE
Sterile gauze pads	Antiseptic solution/sterile saline
Cautery needles	Electrosurgical unit
Bovie or cautery pads	Disposable tips
Two sterile cups or basins	Specimen container
	Sterile gloves
	Triple antibiotic cream/ointment
	Gauze/tape
	Biohazard and sharps containers

Laser Procedures

The term **laser** is the acronym for "light amplification by stimulated emission of radiation." Lasers are instruments that use a powerful, high-focused beam of light to remove unwanted tissue and to control bleeding in a variety of invasive and noninvasive procedures. They are also used in many cosmetic procedures. There are many types of lasers, and each laser instrument is designed to perform a specific procedure. Lasers used in minor office procedures are typically designed to destroy old tissue by producing a beam that that can focus directly on its target without hurting surrounding tissue. This technique may be referred to as laser resurfacing and is used to remove the outer layers of skin to help minimize the appearance of wrinkles and fine scars. Lasers can also act as a small scalpel by cutting through tissue in a very precise manner. They may also be used to reattach detached retinas and burn away ulcers. Because lasers are dangerous, health care personnel should follow safe practice standards when exposed to lasers. Safe practices include:

1. Having equipment checked on a regular basis to make certain that it is in good working order; otherwise, the laser could cause severe burns to the patient and persons administering the treatment
2. Posting a special plaque in the entryway of the room where laser is being used to warn those on the outside that the laser is in use
3. Pulling blinds prior to working with lasers to help keep out stray light
4. Removing any items in the way of the beam that could possibly ignite such as paper products and nondisposable sheets and gowns

5. Making sure all personnel (including the provider) wear safety goggles when using laser instruments. The patient should also wear safety glasses when applicable.
6. Having sterile water accessible just in case the heat from the laser causes cloth or paper to ignite.
7. Having patients wear a mouth guard when using lasers in the mouth area to protect their fillings, crowns, and bridges
8. Checking the package insert to determine how the skin should be prepped when working with lasers. If alcohol is used, it should be completely dried to avoid setting off a spark from the lasers.

Assisting with the Laser Procedure

The medical assistant should prepare the area following all of the safety tips above. The laser instrument, gauze, and sterile water should be readily accessible. Responsibilities during the procedure include assisting the provider with the anesthetic and holding the adjoining vacuum hose to clear away vaporized tissue. The medical assistant may also be asked to help control excess bleeding during the procedure. Table 10-3 lists items necessary for laser surgery.

Cryosurgery

Cryosurgery is a procedure in which unwanted tissue, such as skin lesions and warts, is destroyed by freezing the tissue. Cryosurgery, also known as cryotherapy, may involve the use of liquid nitrogen, which is typically stored in a large canister. The liquid nitrogen is usually removed from the large canister and placed into a thermos before taking it into the examination or surgery room. Liquid nitrogen may be used on any lesion on the skin, hemorrhoids, the cervix, and the retina in rare situations. It may also be used to destroy the prostate gland. For smaller skin lesions, the provider may apply liquid nitrogen to the area using a cotton tip applicator. Liquid nitrogen is also available in a pressurized can, which allows the liquid nitrogen to be sprayed over the affected area for easy application.

Patients should be advised that they may feel a little discomfort during the procedure, but the pain usually goes away fairly quickly. The patient may feel a cold sensation followed by a burning sensation while the procedure is being performed. The patient should be informed that more than one application may be necessary.

Table 10-3 Laser Surgery Tray

Items Placed Directly on the Sterile Field	Items Placed on a Side Table
Sterile gauze	PPE
Sterile water (in sterile container)	Anesthetic
	Sterile syringe and needle
	Safety goggles for everyone involved in the procedure.
	Laser instrument/tips
	Biohazardous waste container

PREPARING FOR OFFICE SURGERIES

There are many responsibilities in preparing for patient surgeries. The preparation phase begins days before the surgery to make certain that all necessary supplies and equipment are available and in good working order, and to confirm that patients understand their responsibilities in preparing for the procedure. Patient instructions are usually reviewed during the surgical consultation, but may be reemphasized a few days before the surgery over the phone or through electronic messaging/patient portal. Table 10-4 lists common tasks that should be performed days prior to the procedure.

There are several tasks that will need to be performed the day of the surgery as well (see Table 10-5).

Setup Procedures

Earlier in the chapter you learned what should be included on the surgical tray and side table for particular procedures, but physicians often have their own special preferences for each procedure. You may want to start a surgical procedure card file that lists

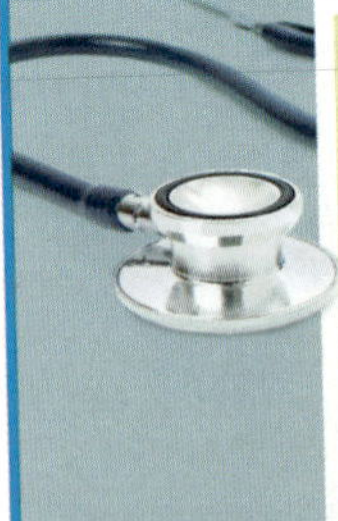

Field Smarts

When using equipment that cannot be sterilized, such as electrocautery units or lasers, the equipment should first be disinfected. Then, sterile barriers should be placed over the equipment before moving it into the area where the surgery is being performed. The equipment should be placed a minimum of 12 to 24 inches away from anything that is sterile. This applies to any surgical procedure in which there is an open wound or incision.

Table 10-4 Tasks to Be Completed Days Prior to the Procedure

Provide the Patient with the Following Instructions	Surgery Room Responsibilities	Insurance Responsibilities
Any fasting or medication instructions	Block off the surgical suite in the appointment scheduler to prevent double-booking.	Notify the insurance company of the anticipated procedure.
Any special preparation instructions (skin cleansing, bowel cleansing, and so on)	Check all equipment to make certain it is in top working order. Check to see if new bulbs or batteries are needed for endoscopes, electrocautery units, and so on.	If necessary, send in pre-certification paperwork.
What clothing and shoes to wear and what not to wear (jewelry, constricting clothing, and so on)	Make certain that all supplies that are necessary for the procedure are in stock and that all instruments or instrument packs are available and in good working order.	Obtain approval from the insurance company well before the procedure is scheduled.
What paperwork, X-rays (radiographs), or insurance information to bring the day of the surgery		
Who should accompany the patient (The patient may not be able to drive following the procedure, may be a minor that needs an adult present, and so on)		

Table 10-5 Tasks to Be Completed the Day of the Surgery

Preparing the Surgical Suite	Once the Patient Arrives
Make certain that the room has been totally cleaned and disinfected or steamed prior to the procedure.	Greet the patient and escort the patient to an examination room.
Gather all necessary supplies including sterile packs, drapes, anesthetic, syringes, suture materials, solutions, bandaging materials, computer with access to patient's electronic health record, and digital X-rays. (If patient record and X-rays are not available in digital format, hard copies should be available.)	If the surgical consent form (Figure 10-2) has not yet been signed, alert the physician. The physician is responsible for explaining the necessity for the procedure, what the procedure entails, risks associated with the procedure, and alternatives in place of the procedure. This process is known as informed consent.
Display X-rays (digitally or in viewbox)	Go over post-op instructions with patient, including wound care instructions, medication instructions, and when to call the office (the patient is more alert before the procedure than following the procedure).
Place all necessary equipment in the room. Make certain that all equipment that will be used during the procedure is completely disinfected and draped if applicable including: electrocautery units, lasers, IV poles, crash trays, and so on.	Have the patient empty the bladder and change into an appropriate gown or other clothing.
Check all equipment to confirm that it is in good working order. (Equipment defects may have developed since the initial inspection.)	Explain what the patient can expect throughout the remainder of the visit.

physician preferences for procedures regularly performed (Figure 10-3).

Before the patient enters the surgical suite, the medical assistant should set up the side table and gather supplies for the surgical tray and skin cleansing. Items should be placed in a logical sequence, usually in the order that each item will be used. Pull in any other necessary equipment such as an electrocautery unit or special laser units. Make certain that the sharps container and both the biohazardous and regular trash receptacles are strategically placed for easy disposal.

Once the Patient Enters the Surgical Suite

Once the patient has signed the consent form, received home care instructions, disrobed for the procedure, and emptied the bladder, it is time to take the patient back to the surgical suite. The patient should be seated and appropriately positioned for the surgery. Select a position that will accommodate access to the site while providing comfort for the patient. The patient's vitals should be taken and recorded in the chart and

CONSENT TO OPERATE

Date __________ Time __________ A.M. P.M.

1. I authorize the performance upon __________
of the following operation __________
to be performed under the direction of Dr. __________
2. The following have been explained to me by Dr. __________
A. The nature of the operation __________
B. The purpose of the operation __________
C. The possible alternative methods of treatment __________
D. The possible consequences of the operation __________
E. The risks involved __________
F. The possibility of complications __________
3. I have been advised of the serious nature of the operation and have been advised that if I desire a further and more detailed explanation of any of the foregoing or further information about the possible risks or complications of the above listed operation it will be given to me.
4. I do not request a further and more detailed listing and explanation of any of the items listed in paragraph 2.

Signed __________
(Patient or person authorized to consent for patient)

Witness __________

Figure 10-2 ■ A sample of a surgical consent form.

Health Coach

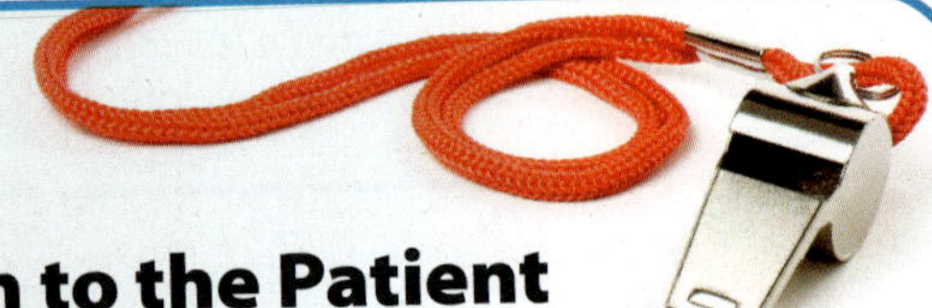

Common Prescriptions Given to the Patient Following a Surgical Procedure

The two most common prescriptions given to patients following a surgical procedure are antibiotics to fight infection and analgesics to assist with pain. Patients should be instructed of the importance of taking all of the antibiotics to prevent post-op infections and should be encouraged to take the analgesic as prescribed on the label for the first few days following the procedure. This will help prevent the patient from getting into pain trouble. Following the first couple of days, the patient should gradually taper down on the pain medication until the patient no longer has to rely on the medication. This will help to prevent the patient from becoming dependent on the medication.

Surgical Items to Be Placed on the Tray	Items to Be Placed on the Side Table or Somewhere Else in the Room	Skin Prep Instructions	Anesthetic	Extra Equipment in the Room	Dr.'s Glove Size and Gown Size
Syringe and needle	Appropriate anesthetic	1. Perform a surgical scrub over the site using concentric circles (one application).	1 or 2% lidocaine or xylocaine without epinephrine	None	Dr. Turner: Glove size: 6 Gown size: S
Scalpel blade and handle	Packing gauze—Iodoform or plain	2. Wet shave only if absolutely necessary.			Dr. Wong: Glove size: 9 Gown size: M
Tissue forceps	Gauze/tape	3. Finish surgical scrub using a new sponge for each application for three solid minutes.			Dr. Winslett: Glove size: 11 Gown size: L
Fenestrated drape	Biohazard/sharps containers	4. Rinse the area with sterile water.			
Penrose drain (up to the physician)	Antiseptic solution (iodine-based)	5. Dry with a sterile towel.			
Dissecting scissors/hemostat	Culture medium	6. Apply iodine antiseptic with sterile applicators (three applications).			
Sterile gauze	Sterile gloves				

Figure 10-3 ■ A surgical procedure card file will help the medical assistant track each physician's specifications.

the site should be exposed for easy access. The surgical light should be angled so that it is directly over the surgical site.

Skin-Prep Procedures

The skin harbors many microorganisms, and can be the trigger that leads to infection. Skin cannot be sterilized, but it should be cleansed in a manner that greatly reduces the number of microbes present. Skin-prep procedures will vary from office to office; however, the following steps are customary for preparing the skin for surgery:

1. Skin should be cleansed with an antimicrobial soap.
2. Skin should be shaved only if absolutely necessary and re-cleansed.
3. Skin antiseptic should be applied to the area (usually an iodine product).
4. The skin antiseptic should be allowed to completely dry before application of the fenestrated drape.
5. Apply the fenestrated drape (a drape with an opening that goes over the surgical site).
6. Waterproof drapes should be placed under the patient before the cleansing begins.

Disposable skin kits (Figure 10-4) include the supplies necessary to perform a skin-prep procedure. Both the surgical soap and antiseptic should be applied using **concentric circles** (circles that start in the center and work their way out to the periphery) as shown in Figure 10-5a. When shaving is absolutely necessary, the skin should be held taut and the razor

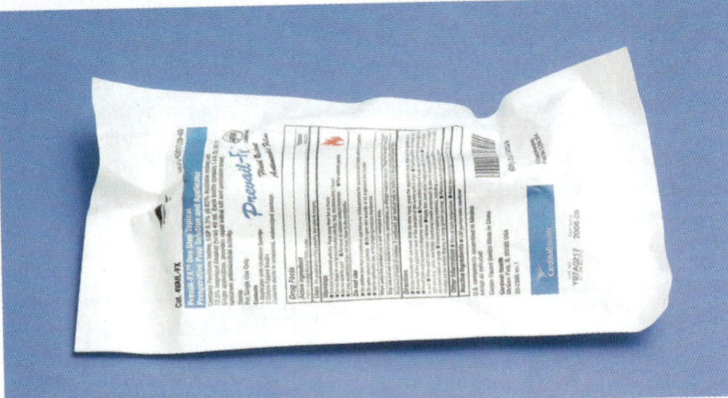

(A)

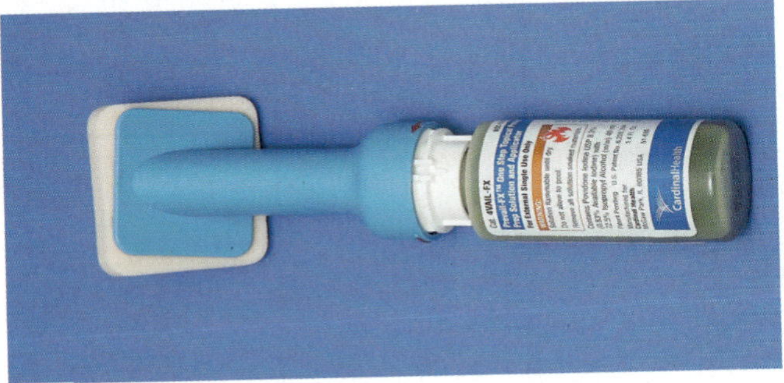

(B)

Figure 10-4 ■ (a) An unopened disposable skin-prep kit; (b) an opened skin prep kit.

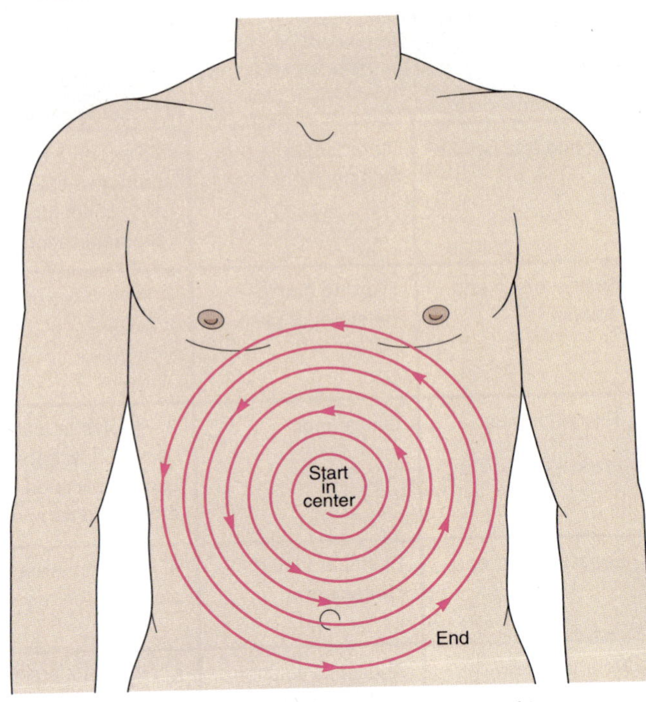

Figure 10-5a ■ When applying surgical soaps or skin antiseptics, apply using concentric circles.

should be angled in the direction that the hair grows (Figure 10-5b). Avoid nicks, as this could expose the patient to infection. Many hospitals and ambulatory surgery centers are now using clippers in place of razors to avoid nicks. Once the skin has been properly cleansed, rinsed, and dried, the antiseptic is applied using sterile sponge forceps or applicator sticks in a series of three applications. Sterile barriers are placed under the site and the patient is instructed to keep the hands under the drape.

New one-step sponge applicator kits are now available that contain chlorhexidine with alcohol or iodophor with alcohol. When such kits are used, the patient receives a special antiseptic soap to use when washing on the morning of the surgery. The medical assistant will observe the skin to make certain it is clean and free of gross contamination. The one-step sponge applicator handle will have a special mechanism for releasing the solution into the sponge. The medical assistant will apply the one-step solution by painting concentric circles over the surgical site for the prescribed amount of applications (usually three). The standard dry time before draping using one-step preps is three minutes. The area dries very quickly because of the alcohol in the mixture.

Refer to Procedure 10-2 for complete instructions on performing skin prep using the one-step procedure.

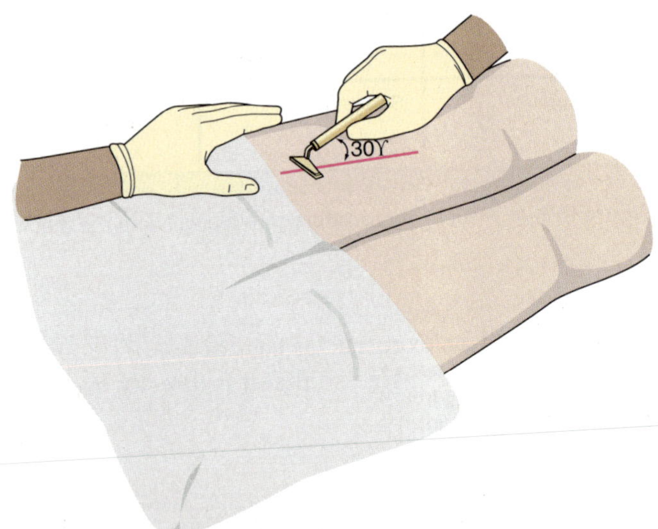

Figure 10-5b ■ Statistics show it is best not to shave unless absolutely necessary. If it is necessary, use a 30° angle and shave in the direction that the hair grows.

Preparing the Mayo Stand and Setting Up the Surgical Tray

The surgical tray is the last item prepared to minimize its exposure to microorganisms. The medical assistant should remove any loose clothing such as a lab coat so that it doesn't drag over the tray. Goggles, hair cover, and a mask should be applied to keep hair, eyelashes and air currents from contaminating the field. The

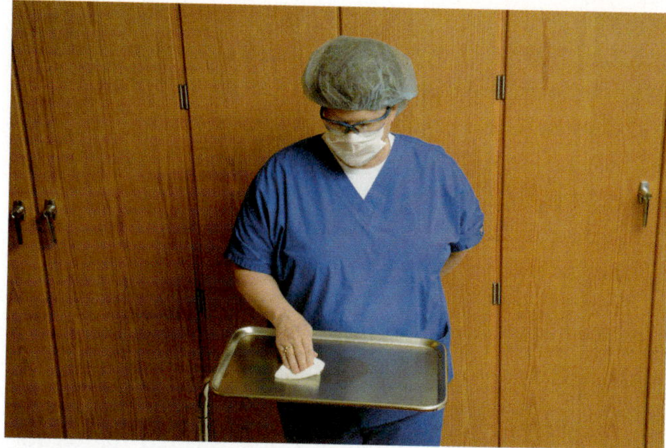

Figure 10-6 ■ When cleaning a Mayo stand, start at the center and work your way toward the outer periphery.

medical assistant should thoroughly wash hands prior to setting up the tray but sterile gloves should not be applied since she will come into contact with items that are nonsterile. The tray should be positioned so that the top of the tray is even with the waist of the preparer. The tray should be cleaned with a disinfectant such as Wexcide or antiseptic wipes starting from the center and working toward the periphery (Figure 10-6). If a sterile barrier is going to be placed on the tray, the medical assistant will remove the drape from the peel-apart package and carefully place it on the tray without contaminating it. The drape's outer 1 inch border is usually marked with a dotted line (Figure 10-7) and identifies the margin of safety between the part of the drape that is considered sterile and the part that is not. The portion of the drape outside the dotted line is the only part of the drape that should be handled when removing it from the pack and placing it on the tray. Special care should be taken to make certain that the drape does not drag over the tray, side table, or come into contact with the medical assistant during removal from the package and placement on the tray. The side of the drape that is facing the medical assistant is the side that will be placed downward on the tray. Refer to Procedure 10-3 for instructions on disinfecting a tray and preparing a sterile barrier.

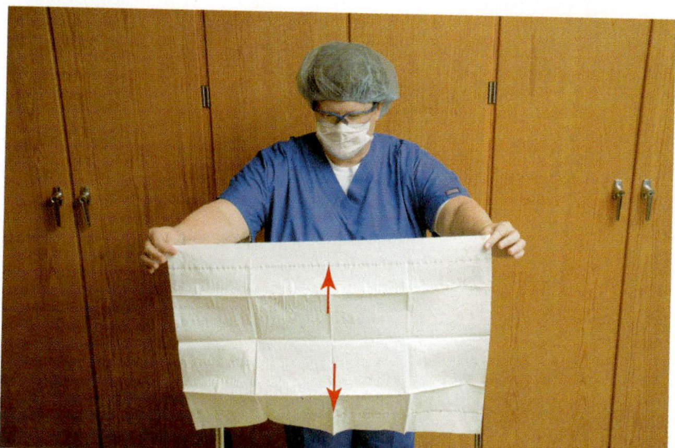

Figure 10-7 ■ The medical assistant should not touch any portion of the sterile drape inside the dotted line.

Placing the Instruments and Other Items on the Tray

Once the Mayo stand has been properly prepared, the instruments and other items are placed onto the tray. Items may be opened singly or collectively, as when using a prepared tray of instruments. When placing items individually onto the field, a sterile drape is initially placed on the field as mentioned above. When opening a prepared tray of instruments, the tray's inner wrap is used as a sterile drape. All packs should be thoroughly examined to confirm the integrity of the wrapping material. The medical assistant should make certain that no moisture, tiny holes, or tears exist anywhere in the wrapping material and that the tape or indicator strip on the wrap has turned the appropriate color. Check to make certain that the pack has not yet reached its expiration date. Any packs that do not fall into the above parameters should be discarded and replaced with a new pack. Once the pack is opened, the sterile indicator strips on the inside of the pack should be checked to make certain that the pack has met the parameters necessary for complete sterilization. Refer to Procedure 10-4 for complete instructions on opening wrapped packs and peel-apart packs and placing them onto the sterile field.

Pouring the Sterile Solution

Sterile solutions generally should not be poured until just before the procedure begins. Two labeled containers are usually placed on the field at the time the tray is prepared. Common solutions used in minor office surgeries are sterile saline and iodine. The names of the solutions, their strengths, and their expiration dates should be checked a minimum of three times prior to use. Once the solution is opened, only the top rim of the bottle should be advanced over the bowl (Figure 10-8). The solution should be poured from a distance of 2 to 6 inches above the field and poured slowly to avoid splash. Either all of the solution should be used, or the remainder that is not used should only be used for nonsterile procedures; once the solution has been opened, it is no longer considered sterile. Refer to Procedure 10-5 for further information on setting up a complete sterile tray and pouring a sterile solution.

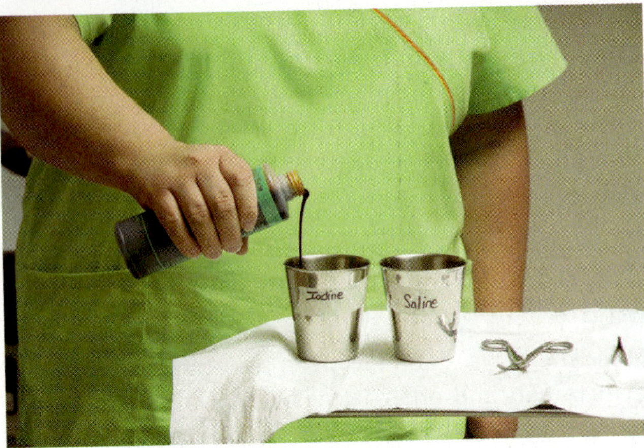

Figure 10-8 ■ When pouring a sterile solution into a sterile container, just advance the top rim of the solution over the container to avoid contaminating the field.

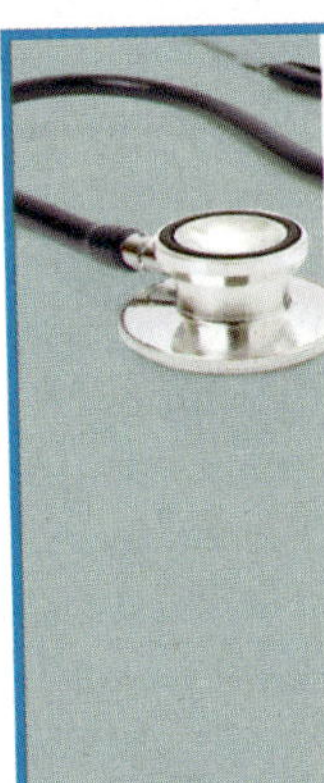

Field Smarts

In the past, health care professionals covered prepared trays with sterile barriers if there was lag time between surgical tray setup and the actual procedure; however, this goes against accepted practices of organizations such as the Association of Perioperative Nurses (AORN). Research indicates that there may be greater risks for contamination when applying and removing drapes. Air currents from the application and removal of the drape may actually pull more microorganisms toward the tray then when the tray is left standing completely still. Shifting of drapes during barrier application and removal may also pose a contamination threat. To reduce the risk of contamination, you should avoid setting up the tray until just prior to the beginning of the procedure.

PERFORMING A SURGICAL HANDWASH AND APPLYING SURGICAL ATTIRE

The medical assistant will only need to perform a surgical handwash and apply surgical attire if working with the physician over the sterile field (see Procedure 10-1). In many minor office surgeries, the physician is the only one that will "scrub in" and apply surgical attire. The medical assistant's duty during these types of procedures is to perform the duties of a circulator. The circulator is the person who circulates throughout the room to give additional items to the physician or to collect items as necessary. The circulator is considered nonsterile and must be careful not to contaminate other surgery personnel or the field.

If the medical assistant is going to scrub in, she should begin by performing a medical aseptic handwash and applying the surgical cap, goggles, and mask. The purpose of applying these items ahead of time is to prevent contaminating the freshly washed hands following the scrub.

The goggles, mask, and cap are not considered sterile, which is why they are applied prior to the surgical scrub. The cap helps to prevent hairs from falling onto the sterile field and the mask prevents air droplets from contaminating the patient or tray. Goggles help to protect the medical assistant's eyes from possible splash.

Surgical sinks, like the one shown in Figure 10-9, are usually very deep to avoid splashing. They are operated with a foot or knee control or an electronic sensor. Scrub brushes are used to cleanse the hands and may be packaged with a surgical soap dispenser that is attached to the brush. Common surgical soaps include Hibiclens and iodine products. The surgical handwash is much more thorough and harsh than a medical aseptic handwash and is designed to eliminate large numbers of microorganisms on the skin by removing dirt, oils, and dead skin cells. Once the scrub is concluded, the hands should be dried with a sterile towel.

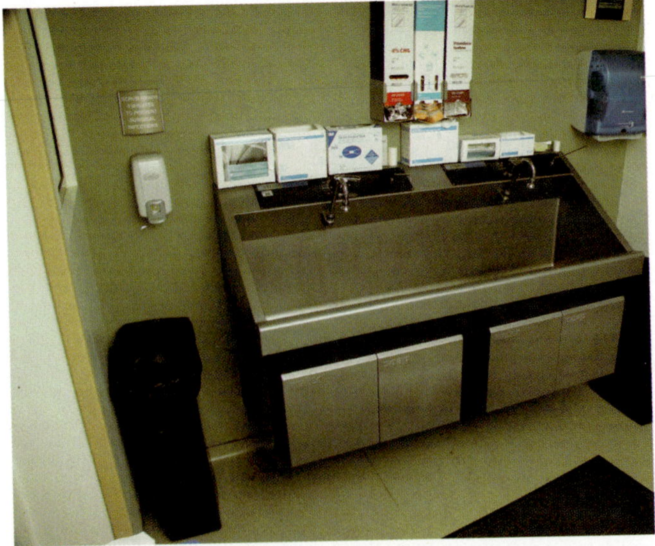

Figure 10-9 ■ The depth of a surgical sink helps to prevent splashing and also decreases risk of accidentally contaminating the hands.

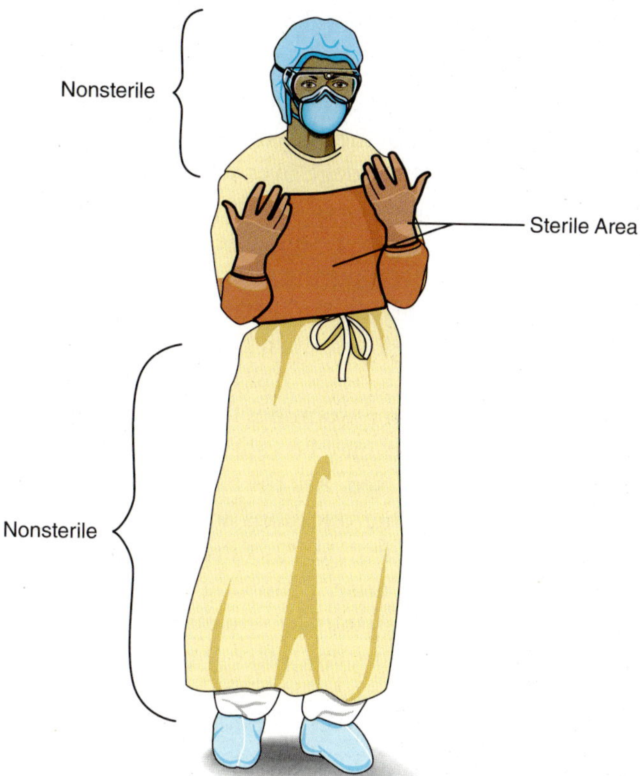

Figure 10-10 ■ This sketch depicts which parts of the surgical attire are considered sterile and which parts are not.

Once the hands are properly cleansed, the gown and gloves are applied. The medical assistant must avoid touching any part of the gown that is considered sterile. Parts of the gown that are considered sterile include the following:

- The front of the gown from the axillary line down to the waist
- The sleeved area of the gown, from the gloved fingers to just above the elbow

Figure 10-10 illustrates which parts of the gown are considered sterile and which parts are not. Refer to Procedure 10-6 for complete instructions on applying surgical attire.

ASSISTING THE PHYSICIAN BEFORE AND DURING THE PROCEDURE

Assisting the physician with related tasks before and during the procedure includes tasks that will vary with each physician. The medical assistant should query physicians before working with them to determine specific preferences.

Pre-Procedure Tasks

The medical assistant will usually have the responsibility of laying out the physician's gloves, gown, mask, goggles, and shoe coverings (if applicable) prior to the procedure and may need to assist the physician with gowning by snapping the gown closed once it has been applied.

Once the physician is situated, the physician will anesthetize the patient. The medical assistant should be prepared to hand the appropriate items to the physician, including the syringe and needle (if not on tray), and be prepared to hold the anesthetic vial for the physician during withdrawal of the medication (Figure 10-11). The assistant should always clean the top of the vial with alcohol and call out the name and strength of the anesthetic, as well as any additives included in the anesthetic before presenting it to the physician.

When presenting the physician with items from peel-apart packages, the medical assistant should peel the packing downward until enough of the item is exposed for the physician to grasp. The packet should

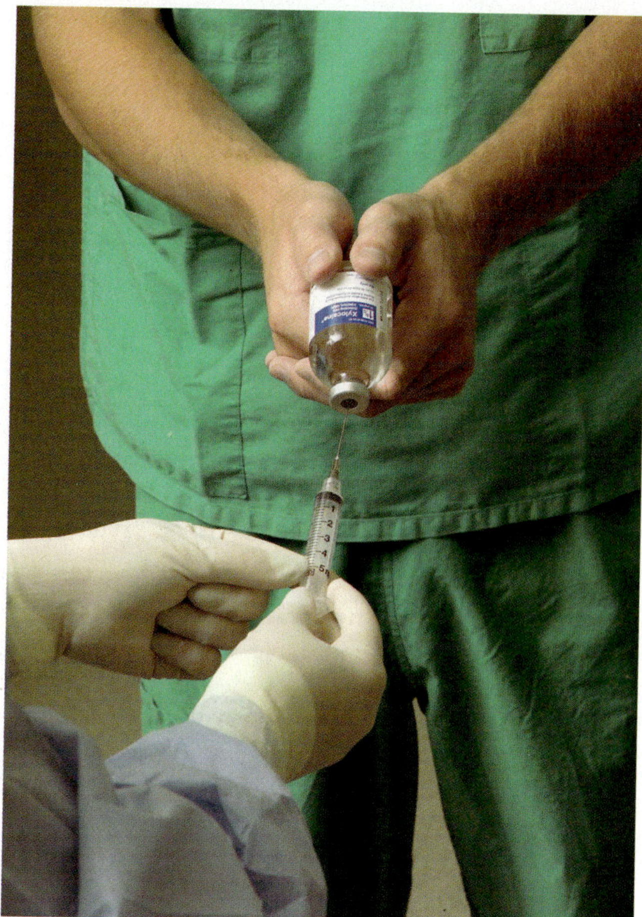

Figure 10-11 ■ The medical assistant may be responsible for holding the anesthetic vial as the physician withdraws the medication.

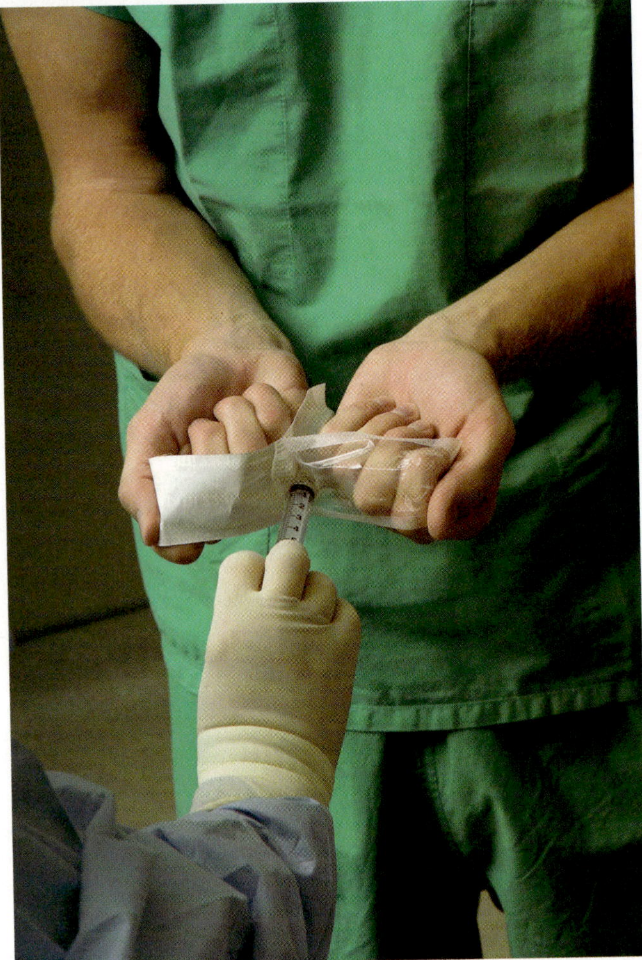

Figure 10-12 ■ This is the proper way to hand the physician contents from a peel-apart pack during a surgical procedure.

be slightly rotated so that it is facing the physician and advanced for easy retrieval (Figure 10-12).

During the Procedure

Once the procedure begins, the medical assistant should wash hands and check in with the patient on a frequent basis to make certain that the patient is comfortable. The medical assistant should be prepared to assist the physician with the following:

1. Handing the physician items that are not on the sterile tray but are on the side table, such as suture material and extra sponges
2. Replacing instruments that may become contaminated during the procedure
3. Using the foot control to open the lid on various trash receptacles and holding the sharps container when necessary (don a pair of clean gloves when handling sharps containers)
4. Receiving patient specimens from the physician (don a pair of clean gloves before accepting any specimens)

At the Conclusion of the Surgery

The medical assistant's role at the conclusion of the surgery is to assist the physician with the removal of surgical attire, to clean the patient's skin, and to apply a sterile dressing and bandage over the surgical wound. The wound is usually closed at this point but may still be vulnerable to infection, so sterile principles should be applied when dressing the site. Once the cleanup and bandaging phases are completed, the medical assistant should remove gloves, wash hands, and retake the patient's vital signs.

Once the physician reexamines the patient following surgery, the caregiver may be called back to assist the patient in getting dressed. Ask the patient and caregiver if they have any further questions and remind them of the next appointment date. Encourage the patient to call if any questions arise. Following the patient's dismissal, the medical assistant should dispose of all trash, and gather instruments and place them in a basin to soak. All linens should be placed in their proper receptacles, and the room should be completely cleaned and disinfected.

The physician is usually the one responsible for documenting the procedure; however, the medical assistant is usually responsible for recording vital sign measurements, skin-prep procedure, type of bandage applied, and home care instructions given to the patient.

WOUND CARE

Wounds may be intentional (as in surgical wounds) or the result of an accident. They are classified as either **closed wounds** (wounds that do not break the skin) or **open wounds** (wounds that do break the skin.) They may be acute (sudden onset, short duration, usually less than 30 days) or chronic (long duration, usually longer than 30 days). Chapter 33 lists different types of wounds and provides first aid instructions on how to treat accidental wounds. The remainder of this chapter will deal specifically with the healing process of an open wound and will list instructions for properly dressing open wounds.

Stages of Wound Healing

The healthy body has internal mechanisms that help to protect skin that has been compromised. Wound healing involves a complex array of events and includes three major stages:

1. First stage (inflammatory stage) (Figure 10-13a): This stage lasts for two to five days following the initiation of the wound. It consists of two different

phases: hemostasis and inflammation. During hemostasis, blood vessels constrict to help control bleeding. Platelets (cells active in blood clotting) and thromboplastin assist in the formation of a blood clot. During the inflammation phase, blood vessels dilate and white blood cells rush to the site to assist in the removal of bacteria and debris from the wound. The entire process stimulates erythema, edema, and warmth to the affected tissue.

2. Second stage (proliferative stage) (Figure 10-13b): This stage follows the first stage, usually lasts anywhere from a couple of days to three weeks, and contains three phases: granulation, contraction, and epithelialization. During the granulation phase, fibroblasts stimulate the release of collagen, which helps to fill in the open wound. Growth cells stimulate the growth of new cells and blood vessels. Angiogenesis, or the formation of new blood vessels, occurs during this phase. During the contraction phase, the edges of the wound contract, which helps pull the wound together. During the epithelialization phase, epithelial tissue starts to form over the wound area, preparing it for closure.
3. Third stage (maturation and remodeling stage) (Figure 10-13c): This stage may last for a couple of weeks up to two years depending upon the severity of the injury. During this stage new collagen forms, resulting in a buildup of scar tissue. The buildup of scar tissue changes the shape of the wound and gives the tissue more strength. Scar tissue is not as sturdy as healthy skin and may become damaged easier than skin that has not been compromised.

Today's Wound Care Philosophy

In 2015, an estimated 6.7 million people suffered from nonhealing wounds according to the Wound Care Awareness website. Wound care management has changed dramatically over the past several years and is a soaring industry. Data from the U.S. Wound Registry states that "the cost of treating chronic wounds exceeds $50 billion annually."

Physicians traditionally believed that it was best to scrub wounds with antiseptics because of their ability to inhibit the growth of microorganisms. The latest studies reveal that cleaning the wound with anything other than normal saline could actually inhibit the healing process. Antiseptics such as iodine products and peroxide are now believed to be toxic to leukocytes and fibroblasts, which are necessary cells for

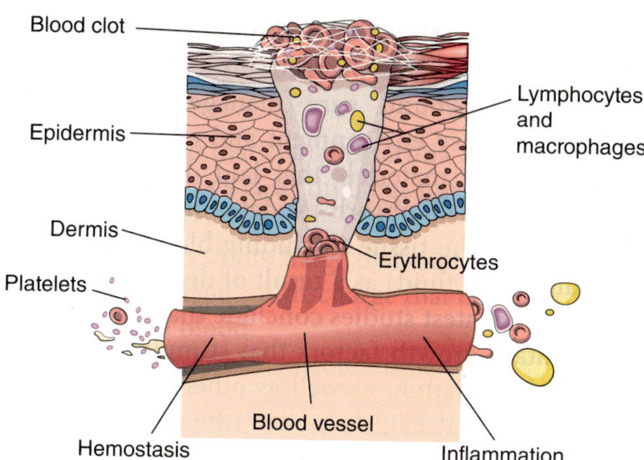

Figure 10-13a ■ Inflammatory stage: The two phases of the inflammatory stage are hemostasis and inflammation. During hemostasis, blood vessels constrict and platelets rush to the site to assist with clot formation. During inflammation, blood vessels dilate and white blood cells gather to assist in the removal of bacteria and debris.

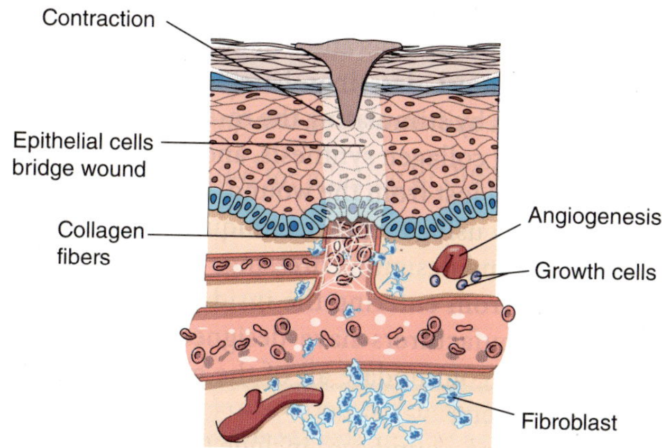

Figure 10-13b ■ Proliferative stage: Fibroblasts stimulate the release of collagen, which helps to fill in the open wound. Angiogenesis (the formation of new blood vessels) occurs, the edges of the wound start to pull together, and epithelial tissue starts to form over the wound.

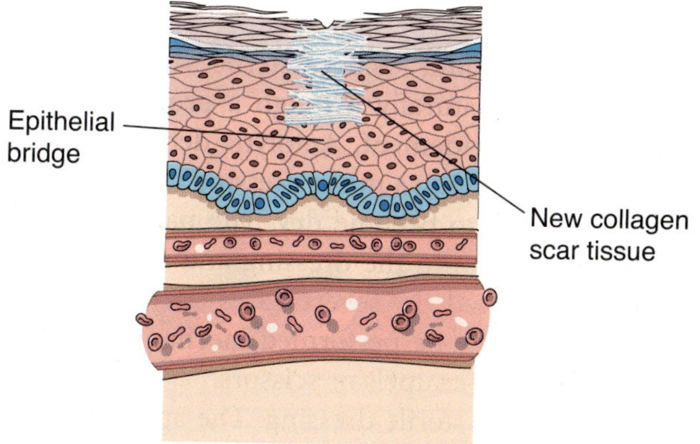

Figure 10-13c ■ Maturation and remodeling stage: New collagen forms, resulting in a buildup of scar tissue. The buildup of scar tissue changes the shape of the wound and gives the tissue more strength.

Guidelines for Bandaging

Bandaging tips include the following:

1. Always place a sterile dressing over an open wound before applying a bandage.
2. Use sterile asepsis when applying a dressing and medical asepsis when removing a dressing.
3. The area should be clean and dry prior to bandage application.
4. Always wrap distal to proximal.
5. Bandages should extend 1 to 2 inches beyond the dressing.
6. Pad bony surfaces and joints to prevent friction.
7. Bandage body parts in their normal positions, slightly flexed to avoid muscle strain or damage.
8. Leave fingers and toes open when applying a bandage to the extremities so that circulation may be evaluated.
9. Check for signs of poor circulation, which include blueness around the nail beds, pallor, skin temperature changes, tingling sensation, and numbness.

Refer to Procedure 10-7 for complete instructions on wound care, including removing an old dressing, irrigating, and applying a new dressing.

Methods of Bandaging

The method of bandaging used is based on the goals for bandaging listed above. Different methods include the following:

- A *circular turn* (Figure 10-16a) is used to anchor a bandage at the beginning or end of a spiral, reverse spiral, figure-eight, or recurrent turn.
- A *spiral turn* (Figure 10-16b) is used when wrapping body parts that are uniform in size. The wrapping material should be wrapped in a spiral fashion by overlapping the previous turn. Each turn should be approximately half to three-fourths of an inch apart.
- A *reverse spiral turn* (Figure 10-16c) is used in order to fit more snugly around the varying contours and dimensions of a limb. Start with a spiral turn and reverse halfway through each turn.
- A *figure-eight bandage* (Figure 10-16d) is used to immobilize a joint or to hold a dressing in place. Start with two circular turns around the hand to anchor the bandage. Roll the gauze diagonally across the front of the joint in a figure-eight pattern, crossing above the joint and then below the joint. Continue until the joint is completely immobilized.

Wound Care Alternatives

Chronic wounds are often difficult to treat. Wounds that do not heal properly may be the result of circulatory problems, diabetes, immune suppression, vasculitis, ischemia, and malignancies. When chronic wounds do not heal, physicians often look for alternative treatments. Two alternative treatments are subatmospheric pressure dressings and hyperbaric oxygen therapy. A **subatmospheric pressure device** (Figure 10-17) uses negative pressure to help close wounds. The physician will start by thoroughly debriding the wound to remove loose or necrotic tissue. Next, the physician will place a piece of sterile foam into the wound, which is sealed with a special adhesive dressing. A hole is cut just slightly above the foam for placement of the tube. Once the pump is turned on, the vacuum will aspirate fluid from the wound, sending it to a receiving canister attached to the unit. The vacuum causes the foam to compress and pull the wound edges together, which helps to promote closure of the

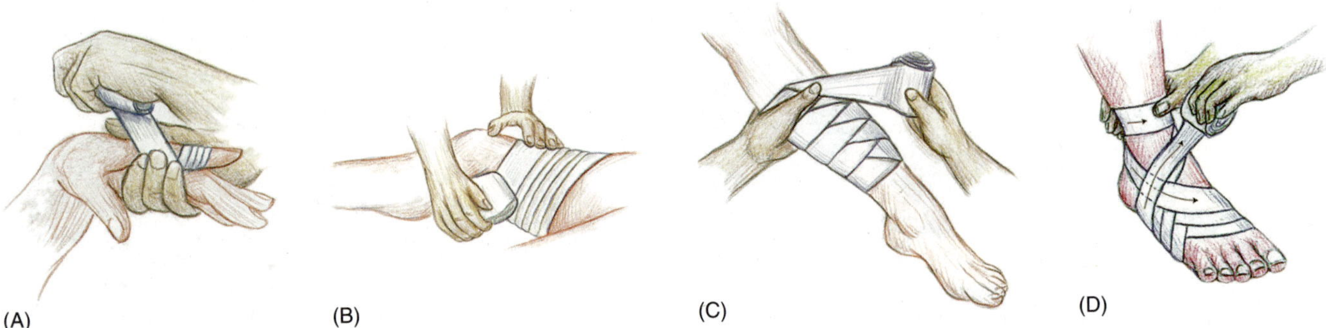

Figure 10-16 ■ Examples of different bandaging techniques: (a) a circular turn, (b) a spiral turn, (c) a reverse spiral turn, (d) a figure-eight turn.

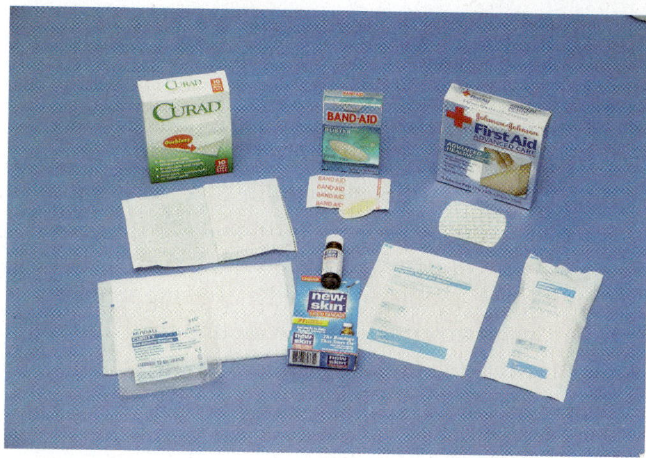

Figure 10-14 ■ Examples of different dressings used in wound care.

4. Encourage patients to change dressings that appear dirty.
5. Avoid ripping or tearing a bandage away from a wound. This could reinjure the site. Instead, soak the bandage with normal saline for several minutes. Always pull a dressing toward the wound when removing.
6. Document the following after removing a dressing: appearance of the dressing, bandage, and wound. Record any unusual drainage and the color of the drainage, and report any unusual odors coming from the area. Terms used for exudates include the following:

   a. **Serous:** Fluid that contains serum. Serous fluid may appear as a clear fluid but sometimes is also yellow.
   b. **Sanguineous**: A discharge that contains blood.
   c. **Serosanguineous**: A discharge that contains both serum and blood.
   d. **Purulent**: A discharge containing pus.

Types of Bandage Material

A bandage and a dressing are uniquely different from one another. A dressing is applied over an open wound and a **bandage** is wrapping material placed over a dressing or closed skin. The selection of bandage material will be based on the goals for bandaging, which may include the following:

1. To hold a dressing in place
2. To immobilize a joint
3. To hold a dressing and to immobilize a joint

Refer to Table 10-6 for a listing of different bandage materials.

Table 10-6 Different Types of Bandaging Material

Kling roller gauze material (Figure 10-15a)	Used quite often to cover a dressing and hold it in place. Does not conform well and may need additional bandaging material to properly cover wound.
Elastic cloth bandage (Figure 10-15a)	An ace bandage or a wrinkled crepe-like bandage that conforms to body shapes and is great for immobilizing joints or covering uneven body surfaces.
Tube gauze (Figure 10-15b)	Long, tube-shaped gauze that fits over a cage-like apparatus Used to cover long, slender parts of the body such as the fingers and toes.

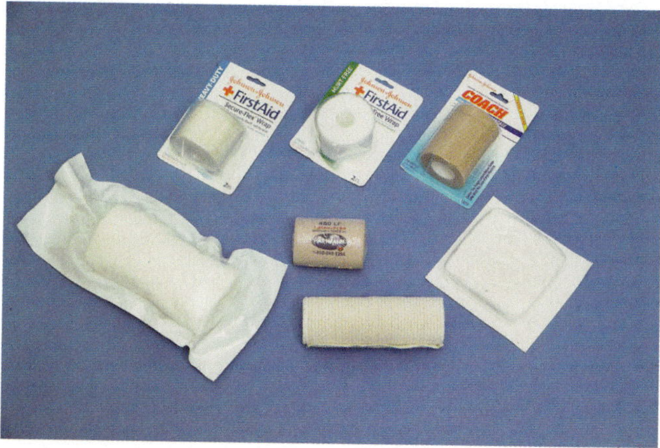

Figure 10-15a ■ Roller gauze material and elastic cloth bandages.

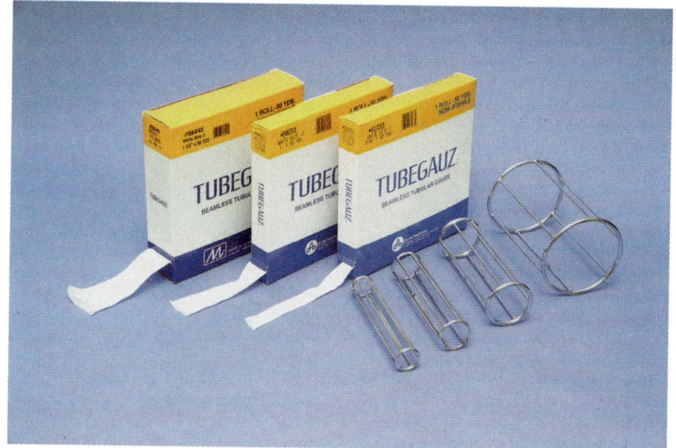

Figure 10-15b ■ Tube gauze with holders.

Guidelines for Bandaging

Bandaging tips include the following:

1. Always place a sterile dressing over an open wound before applying a bandage.
2. Use sterile asepsis when applying a dressing and medical asepsis when removing a dressing.
3. The area should be clean and dry prior to bandage application.
4. Always wrap distal to proximal.
5. Bandages should extend 1 to 2 inches beyond the dressing.
6. Pad bony surfaces and joints to prevent friction.
7. Bandage body parts in their normal positions, slightly flexed to avoid muscle strain or damage.
8. Leave fingers and toes open when applying a bandage to the extremities so that circulation may be evaluated.
9. Check for signs of poor circulation, which include blueness around the nail beds, pallor, skin temperature changes, tingling sensation, and numbness.

Refer to Procedure 10-7 for complete instructions on wound care, including removing an old dressing, irrigating, and applying a new dressing.

Methods of Bandaging

The method of bandaging used is based on the goals for bandaging listed above. Different methods include the following:

- A *circular turn* (Figure 10-16a) is used to anchor a bandage at the beginning or end of a spiral, reverse spiral, figure-eight, or recurrent turn.
- A *spiral turn* (Figure 10-16b) is used when wrapping body parts that are uniform in size. The wrapping material should be wrapped in a spiral fashion by overlapping the previous turn. Each turn should be approximately half to three-fourths of an inch apart.
- A *reverse spiral turn* (Figure 10-16c) is used in order to fit more snugly around the varying contours and dimensions of a limb. Start with a spiral turn and reverse halfway through each turn.
- A *figure-eight bandage* (Figure 10-16d) is used to immobilize a joint or to hold a dressing in place. Start with two circular turns around the hand to anchor the bandage. Roll the gauze diagonally across the front of the joint in a figure-eight pattern, crossing above the joint and then below the joint. Continue until the joint is completely immobilized.

Wound Care Alternatives

Chronic wounds are often difficult to treat. Wounds that do not heal properly may be the result of circulatory problems, diabetes, immune suppression, vasculitis, ischemia, and malignancies. When chronic wounds do not heal, physicians often look for alternative treatments. Two alternative treatments are subatmospheric pressure dressings and hyperbaric oxygen therapy. A **subatmospheric pressure device** (Figure 10-17) uses negative pressure to help close wounds. The physician will start by thoroughly debriding the wound to remove loose or necrotic tissue. Next, the physician will place a piece of sterile foam into the wound, which is sealed with a special adhesive dressing. A hole is cut just slightly above the foam for placement of the tube. Once the pump is turned on, the vacuum will aspirate fluid from the wound, sending it to a receiving canister attached to the unit. The vacuum causes the foam to compress and pull the wound edges together, which helps to promote closure of the

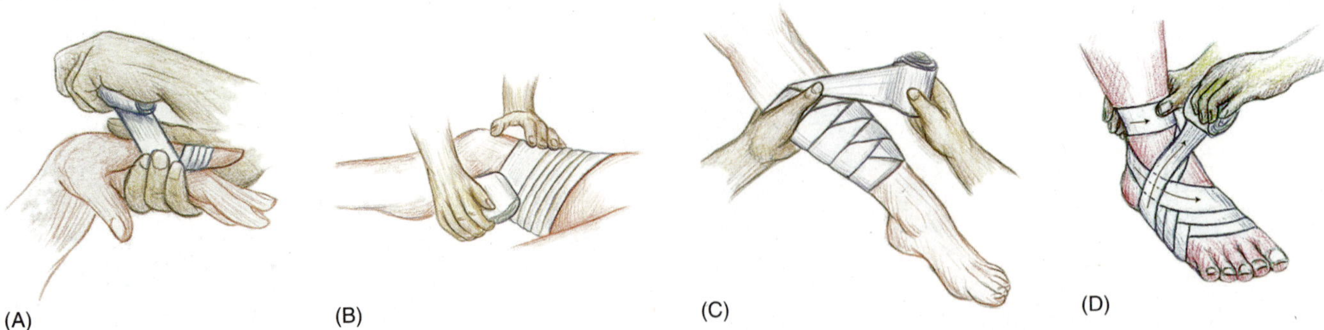

Figure 10-16 ■ Examples of different bandaging techniques: (a) a circular turn, (b) a spiral turn, (c) a reverse spiral turn, (d) a figure-eight turn.

phases: hemostasis and inflammation. During hemostasis, blood vessels constrict to help control bleeding. Platelets (cells active in blood clotting) and thromboplastin assist in the formation of a blood clot. During the inflammation phase, blood vessels dilate and white blood cells rush to the site to assist in the removal of bacteria and debris from the wound. The entire process stimulates erythema, edema, and warmth to the affected tissue.

2. Second stage (proliferative stage) (Figure 10-13b): This stage follows the first stage, usually lasts anywhere from a couple of days to three weeks, and contains three phases: granulation, contraction, and epithelialization. During the granulation phase, fibroblasts stimulate the release of collagen, which helps to fill in the open wound. Growth cells stimulate the growth of new cells and blood vessels. Angiogenesis, or the formation of new blood vessels, occurs during this phase. During the contraction phase, the edges of the wound contract, which helps pull the wound together. During the epithelialization phase, epithelial tissue starts to form over the wound area, preparing it for closure.
3. Third stage (maturation and remodeling stage) (Figure 10-13c): This stage may last for a couple of weeks up to two years depending upon the severity of the injury. During this stage new collagen forms, resulting in a buildup of scar tissue. The buildup of scar tissue changes the shape of the wound and gives the tissue more strength. Scar tissue is not as sturdy as healthy skin and may become damaged easier than skin that has not been compromised.

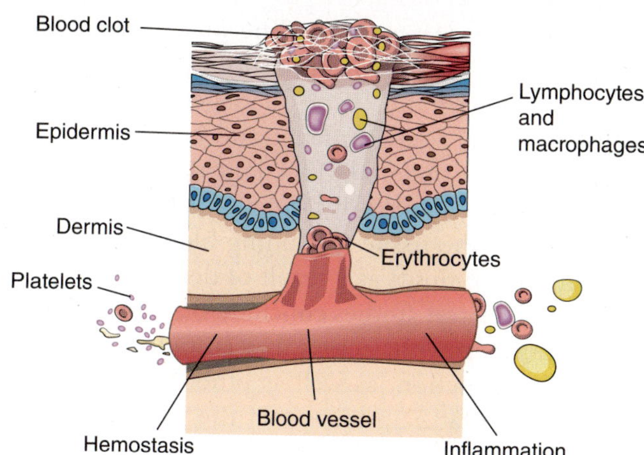

Figure 10-13a ■ Inflammatory stage: The two phases of the inflammatory stage are hemostasis and inflammation. During hemostasis, blood vessels constrict and platelets rush to the site to assist with clot formation. During inflammation, blood vessels dilate and white blood cells gather to assist in the removal of bacteria and debris.

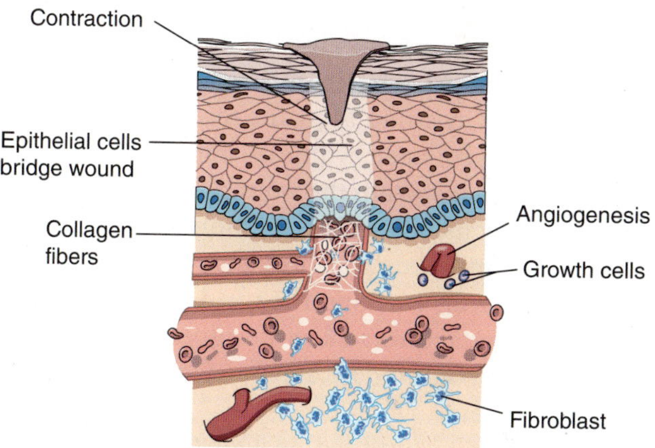

Figure 10-13b ■ Proliferative stage: Fibroblasts stimulate the release of collagen, which helps to fill in the open wound. Angiogenesis (the formation of new blood vessels) occurs, the edges of the wound start to pull together, and epithelial tissue starts to form over the wound.

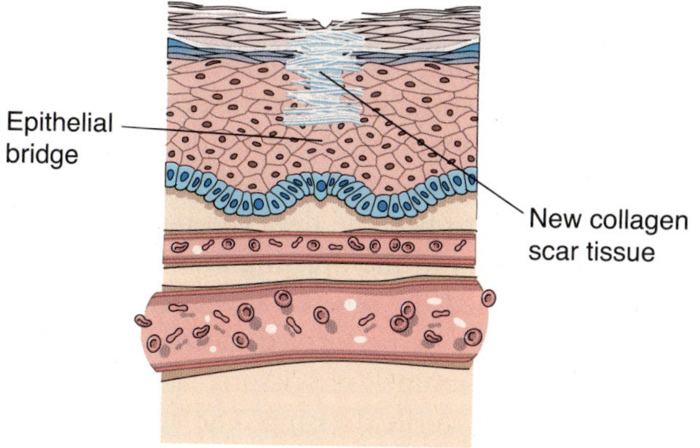

Figure 10-13c ■ Maturation and remodeling stage: New collagen forms, resulting in a buildup of scar tissue. The buildup of scar tissue changes the shape of the wound and gives the tissue more strength.

Today's Wound Care Philosophy

In 2015, an estimated 6.7 million people suffered from nonhealing wounds according to the Wound Care Awareness website. Wound care management has changed dramatically over the past several years and is a soaring industry. Data from the U.S. Wound Registry states that "the cost of treating chronic wounds exceeds $50 billion annually."

Physicians traditionally believed that it was best to scrub wounds with antiseptics because of their ability to inhibit the growth of microorganisms. The latest studies reveal that cleaning the wound with anything other than normal saline could actually inhibit the healing process. Antiseptics such as iodine products and peroxide are now believed to be toxic to leukocytes and fibroblasts, which are necessary cells for wound healing. (However, iodine products are still used to cleanse the skin prior to surgical procedures.)

Traditional wound care management emphasized a clean, dry environment and encouraged the use of dressing materials that laid directly against the wound to help absorb **exudate**, or the fluid that is secreted by the tissue (including blood, pus, dead cells, and tissue fluid) as a result of disease or injury. However, the latest studies conclude that wound exudates contain growth factors that stimulate new cell and vessel formation, as well as other cells involved in immunity that help to protect the wound against infection. Unfortunately, these absorbent dressings not only absorb the exudate but also absorb the healing components within the exudate that are essential for proper healing.

Current guidelines encourage wound care treatments that enhance the body's natural healing process. Three main goals for the treatment of wounds include increased moisture (on the inside of the dressing), warmer temperatures, and control of bacteria. Warm, moist dressings help to speed up the healing process by stimulating the re-epithelialization rate, increasing collagen synthesis, and decreasing the amount of fluid lost from the wound. Bacteria growth is controlled by using aseptic techniques when changing dressings and designing dressings that keep external moisture from entering the inside of the wound. Dressing manufacturers have designed a variety of dressings to accommodate all of the goals of wound care management.

Steps for good wound care include the following:

1. Cleaning and debridement: When the skin is severely damaged, **debridement** (removal of dead tissue) may be necessary. Dead skin can hamper the healing process. Debridement can be accomplished in a variety of different ways. It may be performed through irrigation, or the flooding of the wound with a sterile liquid such as sterile saline. It may be performed naturally through a process known as autolytic debridement. Autolytic debridement is achieved by applying a moist dressing to the wound and allowing it to become dry. The particles from the wound dry onto the dressing and the dressing is gently removed. In severe cases such as burns, debridement may be performed mechanically with the use of sterile scalpels or scissors.
2. Application of a sterile dressing: The application of a sterile dressing helps to keep dirt and bacteria out of the wound, and the special materials and additives within each dressing may help to speed up the healing process.
3. Preventing further injury: It is important for the patient to protect the wound from further injury. The tissue is fragile, and any new injury will destroy the healing that has already occurred and possibly cause more complications.
4. Preventing infection: The patient should be encouraged to wash their hands before and after every dressing change and to never touch an open wound with bare fingers. Giving the patient a set of written instructions for wound care management will help the patient understand how to properly care for the wound and become more compliant.

Types of Dressings

There are several different types of **dressings** available today that help to enhance the healing process. The type of dressing selected will be based on several factors, including the amount of drainage present, whether the wound is acute or chronic, what phase of healing the wound is in, and the physician's preference. These dressings include gauze, hydrocolloids, hydrogels, alginates, collagens, foams, and transparent films. These products are primarily used in hospitals, wound care centers, and in home health care.

Dressings can be classified as either primary or secondary dressings. **Primary dressings** are dressings that lay directly over the wound. These dressings are usually nonadherent and are impregnated with some kind of ointment or water that keeps it from sticking to the wound and helps keep the internal environment moist. **Secondary dressings** are usually placed over primary dressings and assist with absorption of excess wound fluid or exudates from the inside, while keeping outside moisture and bacteria from entering the wound. Adherent dressings are designed to act as a skin substitute and are good for patients with partial thickness burns.

Many of the latest wound care dressings contain multiple layers to create optimal conditions for wound healing. Refer to Figure 10-14 for a picture of various types of dressings.

Applying and Caring for Dressings

Guidelines for applying and caring for dressings include the following:

1. Wash your hands thoroughly before bandaging.
2. Use sterile technique and products when applying dressing to wounds that are open.
3. Use an ointment only if directed to do so by the physician.

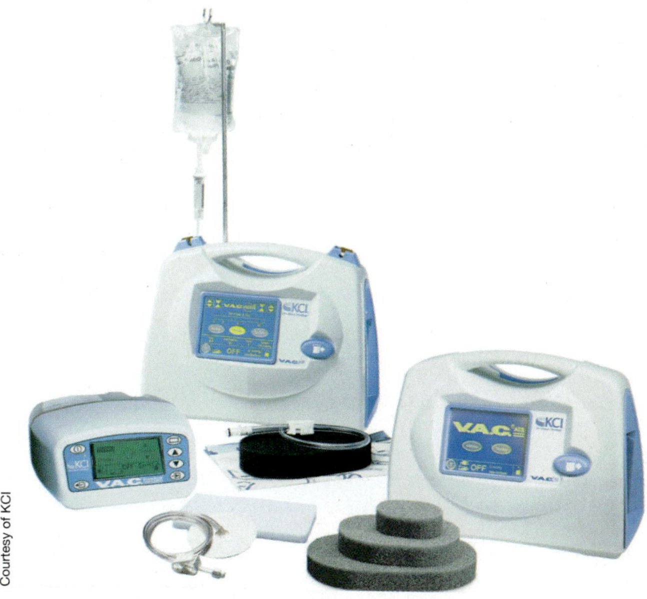

Courtesy of KCI

Figure 10-17 ■ The V.A.C. is an example of a negative pressure wound therapy device.

wound. The negative pressure increases circulation, promotes a moist environment, and reduces the bacterial load.

Hyperbaric oxygen (HBO_2) therapy (Figure 10-18) involves placing the patient into a hyperbaric chamber to treat difficult wounds. The patient undergoes a series of three phases while in the chamber. The first phase, called compression, occurs as oxygen flows into the unit. The second phase, treatment, begins once the chamber has reached the desired oxygen level and continues for the amount of time prescribed. Decompression, the third phase, signifies the termination of the treatment and occurs when oxygen levels are returned to their normal levels.

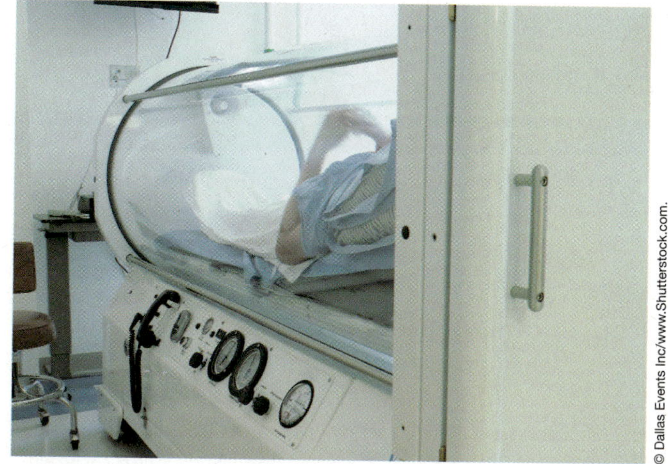

© Dallas Events Inc/www.Shutterstock.com.

Figure 10-18 ■ A hyperbaric oxygen (HBO_2) chamber.

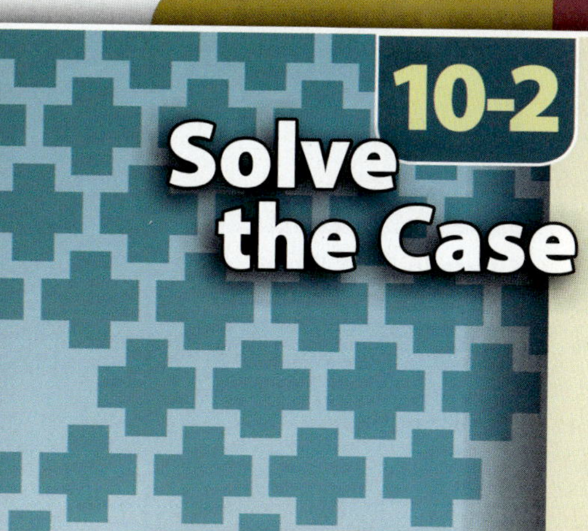

The provider asks you to get patient Maria Rodriguez set up for her procedure. Based on the fact that she is here today to have her boil lanced, answer the following questions.

1. **What procedure does Maria need to have today?**
2. **What items will need to be on the sterile tray and on the side table during the procedure?**
3. **How will you prepare Maria's skin for the surgery?**
4. **What medications do you suspect the provider wants the patient to have when she goes home following the procedure?**

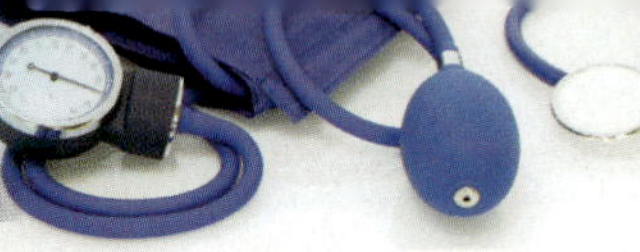

PROCEDURE 10-1

Perform a Surgical Handwash and Apply Surgical Gloves

Objective:

To perform a surgical handwash and apply sterile gloves in an appropriate manner.

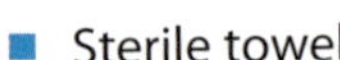

Equipment/Supplies:

- Sterile brush impregnated with antiseptic soap/fingernail cleaner
- Sink/basin
- Sterile towel
- Package of sterile gloves

PROCEDURAL STEPS	DETAILS AND/OR RATIONALE
1. Peel apart a sterile towel without contaminating it and lay the towel on a flat, clean surface close to the area where the handwash is to take place.	Opening the towel ahead of time prevents you from contaminating your hands once they have been scrubbed.
2. Place gloves beside the sterile towel and remove them from the outer wrapper (Figure 10-19). Unfold the pack so that it lies flat. Carefully open each flap of the inner wrapper to expose the gloves without contaminating them. (The gloves should be positioned so that the cuffs are facing you, and the thumbs are pointing outward.)	Same as above.
3. Open the sterile scrub pack containing the impregnated scrub brush and nail cleaner. Do not remove them yet. Place them in the sink area.	
4. Remove all rings and watches and place them in your pockets. Turn on the water using the automatic sensor or foot or knee control and adjust the temperature (should be warm, not hot).	Using a sink with automatic sensors or a foot or knee control will keep you from touching the already dirty sink. Hot water can be damaging to the skin.
5. Rinse your hands under the water, keeping the hands and fingers pointed upward and the arms well above the waist (Figure 10-20).	Hands and fingers should be pointed upward and above the waist throughout the entire procedure to prevent dirt from the upper part of the hands and arms from running back down over the hands.
6. Using just the nail stick and water, clean under each nail (Figure 10-21). Drop the nail stick in the sink and rinse hands.	The undersurfaces of nail beds contain many microorganisms that must be removed before cleansing the hands.

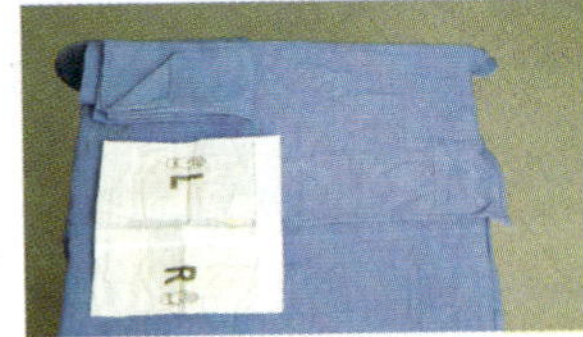

Figure 10-19 ■ The sterile towel and gloves should be laid out just prior to the scrub itself.

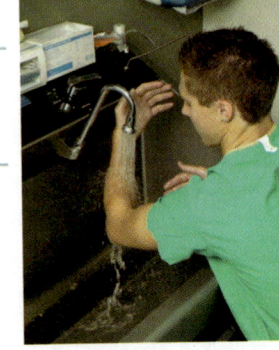

Figure 10-20 ■ When rinsing fingers, hands, and arms, be careful to keep the arms above the waist, and keep fingers pointed in an upward position.

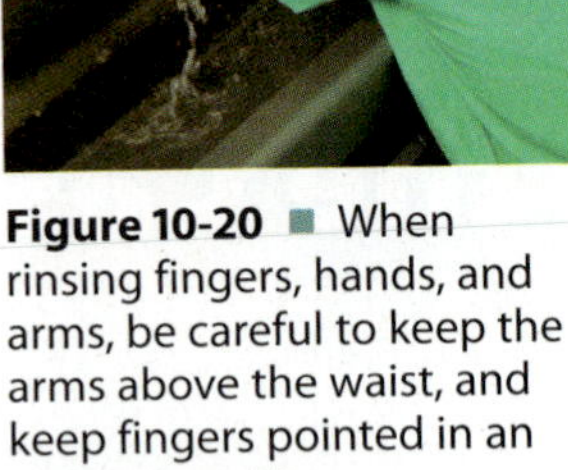

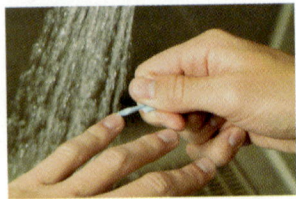

Figure 10-21 ■ Nails harbor many microorganisms and must be cleaned in addition to the skin.

continues

PROCEDURE 10-1 continued

PROCEDURAL STEPS	DETAILS AND/OR RATIONALE
7. Completely wet your hands, wrists, and forearms up to the elbow, keeping hands and fingers pointed in an upward position and well above the waist.	Wetting these areas will assist in the scrubbing process.
8. Obtain the impregnated brush and start the scrub on the palm of the hand (Figure 10-22) and move to the base of the thumb using a circular pattern. Do not go over a section that has already been scrubbed, or you will contaminate it.	Going over a section that has already been scrubbed will contaminate that section.
9. Next, move to the fingers. Scrub each surface of each finger using several vertical strokes from the base of each finger to the nail (there are a total of four surfaces for each finger). Be certain to scrub the skin between the thumb and index finger as well.	Each surface of each finger must be cleansed in order to achieve complete cleansing.
10. Once the fingers are completely scrubbed, turn the hand over and scrub the posterior portion of the hand extending to below the wrists using a circular pattern.	
11. Next, scrub the forearm using a circular pattern from the wrists to slightly above the elbow. Make certain to scrub all four surfaces.	All surfaces from the fingertips to the elbows must be scrubbed to achieve proper cleansing.
12. Rinse both the arm that was just scrubbed and the opposite arm with arms well above the waist and fingers pointed upward. Water should run from the finger tips down the arms and over the elbow. Do not touch any part of the sink while washing or rinsing.	Rinsing both arms allows the soap to be removed from the first arm and re-wets the opposite arm for better lathering. Touching any part of the sink will contaminate the hands or arms.
13. Wash the opposite side using the same steps as the first side. Drop the scrub brush in the sink and rinse thoroughly. The entire length of the scrub will vary between two and six minutes.	Dropping the brush in the sink keeps you from contaminating freshly washed hands. Scrub times will vary because each surgical antiseptic has its own scrubbing directions.
14. Turn off the water using the foot, knee, or sensor control when applicable.	This will prevent contaminating your hands.
15. Pick up the towel in your dominant hand by holding onto the corners. The towel should be several inches away from your body. Using just one side of the towel, start at the fingertips (Figure 10-23) on your nondominant hand and pat dry all the way up to the elbow, making sure that you dry all four surfaces simultaneously. Remember to keep the arms and hands above the waist with fingers pointed upward.	Rubbing the towel back and forth can bring contaminants from the dirtier surfaces (forearms) toward the cleaner surfaces (fingertips).

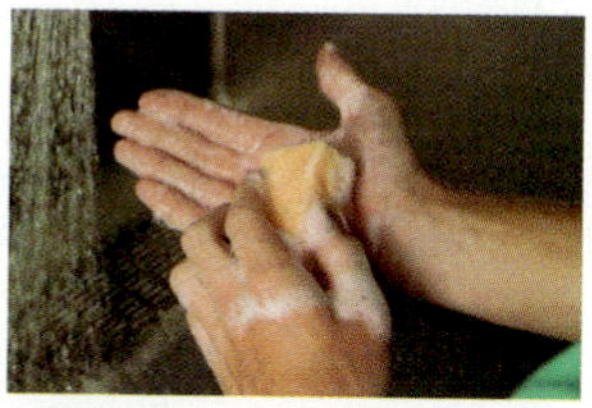

Figure 10-22 ■ Start the scrub on the palm of the hand and work to the base of the thumb using a circular pattern.

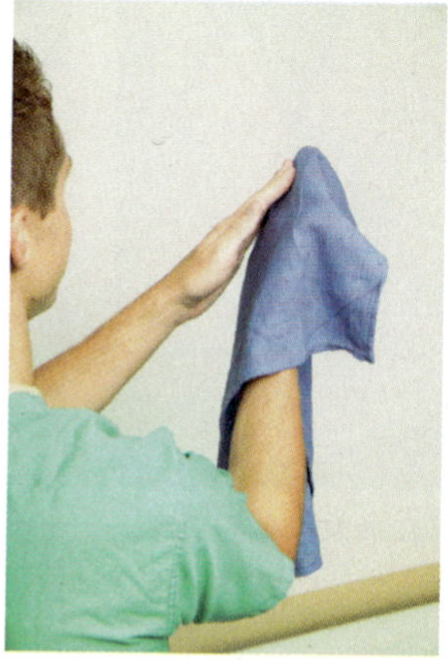

Figure 10-23 ■ Dry hands using a patting motion with a sterile towel starting at the fingertips and working downward. Switch to the opposite side of towel when drying the opposite side.

continues

PROCEDURE 10-1 continued

PROCEDURAL STEPS	DETAILS AND/OR RATIONALE
16. Repeat the same procedure on your dominant hand using the opposite side of the sterile towel.	
17. Once the hands are completely dried, walk to the clean, dry surface where the gloves are laying.	The gloves should be nearby but not directly on the sink so that they are not contaminated by splashing water.
18. Pick up the first glove by the inside cuff using your nondominant hand (Figure 10-24). Lift the glove up and away from the flat surface to avoid dangling the glove across a nonsterile surface. Slide the glove in an upward motion, over the hand (Figure 10-25).	If you do not completely lift the glove upward and away from the counter surface, you may accidentally drag or dangle the fingers over the counter and contaminate the glove.
19. Pick up the second glove with your dominant hand by slipping the four fingers from the gloved hand underneath the cuff of the second glove (Figure 10-26). Make certain that the thumb is facing outward. Slide the glove onto the hand without contaminating either glove.	Remember that sterile items can only touch sterile items. If you touch any part of the sterile glove to your wrist or hand, the glove is contaminated, and you will have to start all over.
20. Leaving your fingers under the cuff, unfold the cuff so that it slides down over the wrist (Figure 10-27). Do not allow the gloved thumb from the opposite hand to touch the inside of the cuff. Repeat the same procedure for the first glove (Figure 10-28).	Allowing the gloved thumb to touch the skin of the opposite hand will contaminate the glove.
21. Examine both gloves for any tears or problems.	The gloves may have become damaged during the application process.

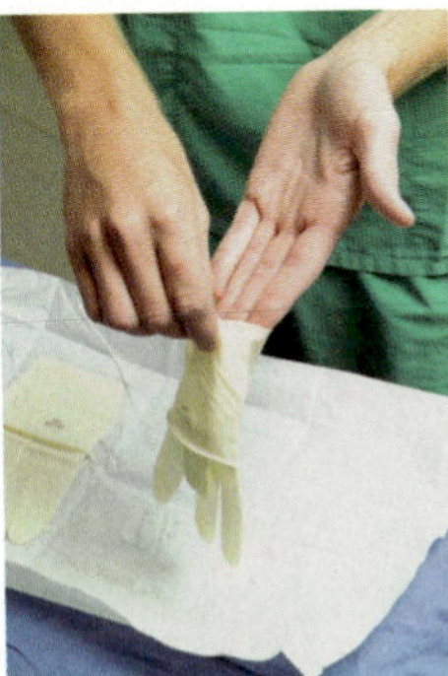

Figure 10-24 ■ Pick up the first glove using your thumb, index finger, and middle finger by grasping the edge of the inside cuff with your nondominant hand.

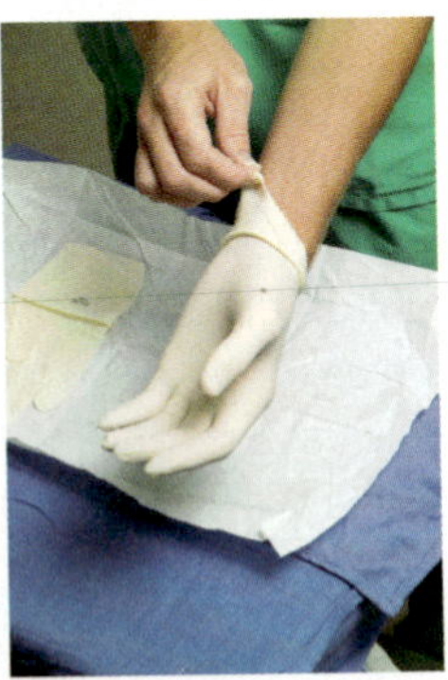

Figure 10-25 ■ Slide the glove onto your dominant hand by pulling the cuff in an upward motion.

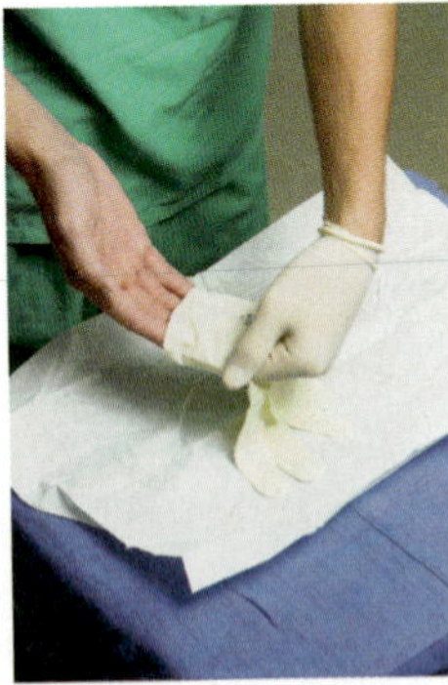

Figure 10-26 ■ Pick up the second glove with your dominant hand by slipping the four fingers from the gloved hand underneath the cuff of the second glove.

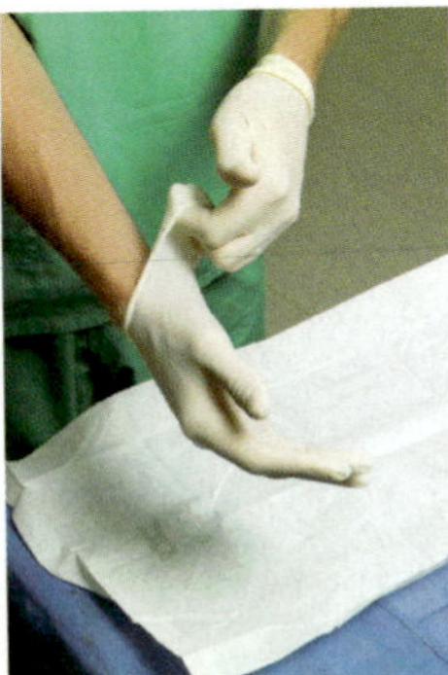

Figure 10-27 ■ Lift up your hand to avoid dangling and with fingers still positioned on the inside of the cuff, roll back the cuff on the nondominant hand over the wrist. Do not allow the gloved thumb from the opposite hand to touch the inside of the cuff.

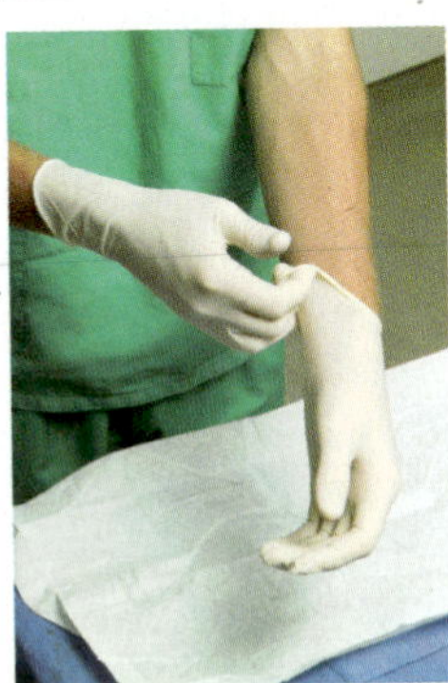

Figure 10-28 ■ Repeat the same procedure for rolling back the cuff for the glove on the dominant hand.

PROCEDURE 10-2

Prepare the Patient's Skin for the Surgical Procedure Using a One-Step Scrub

Objective:

To properly prepare the patient's skin for a surgical procedure using a one-step method (when the patient has cleansed the skin with a special soap the morning of the procedure).

Equipment/Supplies:

- Skin-prep kit
- Sterile gloves
- Sterile drape
- Fenestrated drape

PROCEDURAL STEPS	DETAILS AND/OR RATIONALE
1. Wash your hands and gather the supplies.	
2. Identify the patient using two identifiers. Verify that the patient followed the site cleansing instructions.	Complies with the Joint Commission National Patient Safety Goals and confirms that you have the correct patient.
3. Identify yourself and ***explain the rationale for the performance of the procedure, showing awareness of the patient's concerns related to the procedure being performed.***	Explaining the procedure will help the patient to know what to expect.
4. Expose the surgical site and drape the patient for modesty if necessary. Some facilities ask the patient to mark the area where the surgery is to take place with an "X" before prepping the skin.	Complies with the Joint Commission National Patient Safety Goals.
5. Position the patient for comfort and place absorbent drapes under the area to be cleansed, if applicable.	The pads will keep the surface under the patient from getting wet.
6. Adjust the light so that it illuminates the surgical site (Figure 10-29). Inspect the skin for any gross contamination. If any gross contamination is visible, the skin will have to be thoroughly cleansed before applying the antiseptic cleanser.	If the area has not been properly prepped by the patient, the one-step procedure will not be effective in removing the microorganisms from the skin.
7. Remove absorbent drape and apply sterile drape under the surgical site. Open the skin-prep kit without contaminating the swab or the sponge applicator.	
8. Wash your hands and apply sterile gloves.	Even though the applicator will separate your hands from the sterile tip, you may need to use your other hand for stabilizing as you prep the skin.
9. Remove the swab or sponge, touching only the applicator or handle.	
10. Apply the antiseptic scrub by painting concentric circles over the site (Figure 10-30).	The purpose of the circles is to move the microorganisms from an area of lesser concentration to an area of greater concentration (clean to dirty).

Figure 10-29 ■ Position the light directly over the surgical area.

Figure 10-30 ■ Apply the antiseptic scrub using concentric circles.

continues

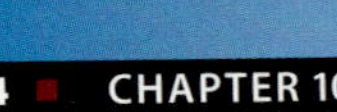

PROCEDURE 10-2 continued

PROCEDURAL STEPS	DETAILS AND/OR RATIONALE
11. Scrub normally lasts anywhere from 30 seconds to two minutes, which equates to about three separate applications with three separate applicators. Follow the physician's orders.	
12. If the physician orders the area to be shaved, pull skin taut and shave in the direction that the hair grows. Remember that shaving is not recommended unless absolutely necessary!	Nicks in the skin can lead to infection.
13. Re-cleanse the skin according to office policy.	
14. Apply fenestrated drape according to the physician's preference (Figure 10-31).	Many physicians prefer to apply the fenestrated drape.
15. Instruct the patient to keep hands below the drapes (when applicable).	Touching the drapes will contaminate them.

Figure 10-31 ■ Apply the fenestrated drape according to the physician's preference.

PROCEDURE 10-3
Disinfect a Surgical Tray and Place a Sterile Barrier on the Tray

Objective:

To clean the surgical tray and apply a sterile barrier using strict aseptic technique.

Equipment and Supplies:

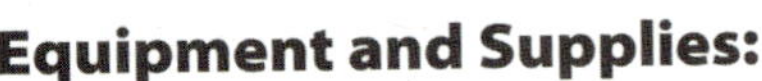

- Mayo stand
- 4 × 4s saturated with disinfectant, but not dripping
- Sterile drape

PROCEDURAL STEPS	DETAILS AND/OR RATIONALE
1. Wash your hands.	
2. Adjust the Mayo stand so that it is right about waist level.	When working in a sterile setting, your hands should always be above your waist.
3. Pick up the 4 × 4s saturated with disinfectant (but not dripping) by only touching the top side of the 4 × 4s. Clean the tray using the bottom side of the 4 × 4s using a circular motion, starting from the center and working toward the periphery, until the whole tray is completely covered (Figure 10-32).	Touching only the top side of the 4 × 4s will keep you from contaminating the side that will clean the tray.
4. Allow the tray to air dry.	
5. Select an appropriate sterile barrier and place it on a clean, dry, flat surface.	

Figure 10-32 ■ Clean the tray using the bottom side of the 4 × 4s using a circular motion until the whole tray is completely covered.

continues

PROCEDURE 10-3 continued

PROCEDURAL STEPS	DETAILS AND/OR RATIONALE
6. Peel back the top flap of the pack, completely exposing the drape. Make certain that the pack is positioned so that the cut corners are facing you.	You want to open it so that it can be removed in a sterile manner.
7. Using your thumb and forefinger, gently pull up one of the top corner edges of the drape without touching any other part of the drape. Lift the drape well above the counter surface and away from you.	If you do not lift the drape well above the counter and out and away from you, you may accidentally contaminate the barrier by dragging the drape over the counter surface or brushing it up against your clothes.
8. Grab the opposing corner so that both corners are now being held along the top edge of the drape. Keep the drape well above your waist and several inches away from your body (Figure 10-33).	Holding the drape well above your waist and several inches away from your body will keep you from contaminating the drape.
9. Pull the drape over the Mayo stand so that the part of the drape that was facing you is lying against the surface of the tray and the part that was facing away from you is now facing upward on the tray (Figure 10-34).	

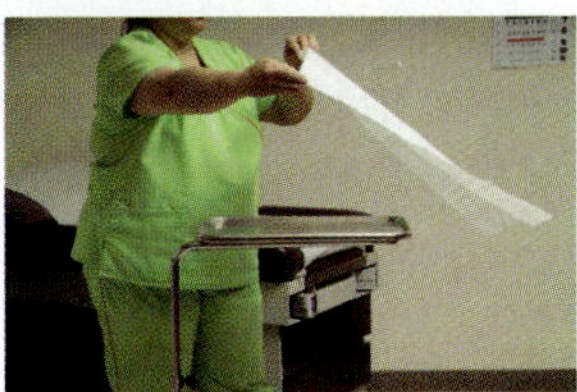

Figure 10-33 ■ Grab the drape so that both corners are now being held along the top edge of the drape. Keep the drape well above your waist and several inches away from your body. (Position drape over the tray.)

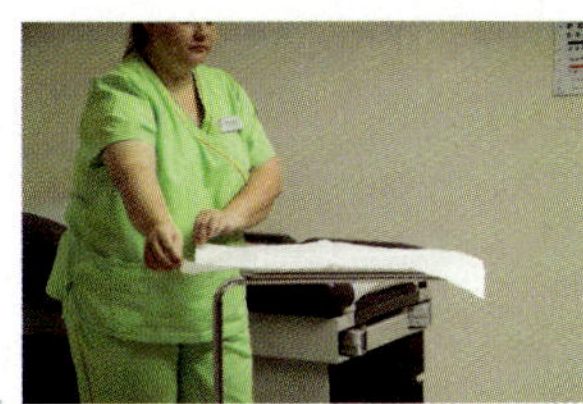

Figure 10-34 ■ Pull the drape over the Mayo stand so that the part of the drape that was facing you is lying against the surface of the tray.

PROCEDURE 10-4
Open Sterile Items and Place Them on the Sterile Field

Objective:
To correctly open and apply items to the sterile field without contaminating the field.

Equipment and Supplies:
- Mayo stand set up with a sterile drape
- Wrapped pair of sterile transfer forceps
- Wrapped single instrument in autoclave paper
- Wrapped gauze in a peel-apart wrapper
- Wrapped tray of instruments

continues

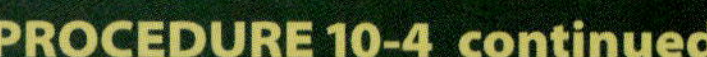

PROCEDURE 10-4 continued

PROCEDURAL STEPS	DETAILS AND/OR RATIONALE
Opening a Sterile Pack and Transferring Items to the Sterile Field Using Sterile Transfer Forceps	
1. Wash your hands.	
2. Place a sterilized pack of transfer forceps on the side table.	The transfer forceps are necessary to move the instrument to the field without breaking sterility.
3. Place the unopened sterilized instrument on the side table, examine the autoclave tape, and make certain that the stripes turned the appropriate color. Check the expiration date and the quality of the wrapper to make certain that the wrap has not been compromised.	
4. Remove the tape from the packet and place it on the side table. Position the pack so that the flap that was taped is facing you.	The tape should be kept in case there are any problems with the pack.
5. Using only your thumb and index finger, grasp the tip of the folded flap that was covered with tape and pull it away from you.	Using more than two fingers to open the flaps may cause you to stray to an area of the flap that is sterile.
6. Using only your right thumb and index finger, grasp the tip of the folded-back flap on the right side and pull it all the way to the right.	
7. Using only your left thumb and index finger, grasp the tip of the folded-back flap on the left side and pull it all the way to the left.	Never reach across a sterile field or wrap. That is why you use the hand that is on the side that is being opened.
8. Using only your dominant thumb and index finger, grasp the tip of the last folded-back flap and pull it toward you without touching anything on the inside of the wrap. The entire instrument should be exposed for easy retrieval later. Check the sterilization indicator in the pack to make certain it turned the appropriate color; if not, remove the pack and get a new one.	
9. Move to the packet containing the sterile transfer forceps. Open the sterile transfer forceps the same way you opened the first pack.	

continues

PROCEDURE 10-4 continued

PROCEDURAL STEPS	DETAILS AND/OR RATIONALE
10. Once the pack is opened, grasp only the handles of the sterile transfer forceps by placing your thumb in one ring and your index finger in the other ring. Do not touch any other part of the instrument. Lift the transfer forceps straight up, keeping the tips facing downward but well above the height of the side table.	Touch only the handles of the instrument so that you do not break sterility. Keeping the tips facing downward will keep the instrument as free from wind currents as possible.
11. Move the transfer forceps to the instrument that needs to be transferred to the sterile field (Figure 10-35). Once you are positioned in front of the sterile instrument, lower the transfer forceps to the sterile instrument and securely grasp the instrument. Lift the instrument well above the height of the side table and approach the sterile tray. Standing a few inches away from the field, gently lower the sterile instrument onto the tray (Figure 10-36). Do not allow your hand to drop below the level of the handle.	
12. Once the instrument has been fully transferred to its appropriate place on the tray, pull the sterile transfer forceps up and away from the field and set them back down on the side table.	Once the instrument has been returned to the side table, it is considered contaminated.
Opening a Peel-Apart Pack	
1. Inspect the package and make certain that the integrity of the wrap has not been altered. Check the control strip to make certain that it turned the correct color. Check the expiration date to make certain that the pack is not expired.	
2. Position yourself so that you are in front of the tray but several inches away from the field.	
3. Grasp both the top edges of the peel-apart pack and carefully peel them apart by rolling the wrap downward on both sides.	
4. Once the wrap has been peeled to the point that the item can be transferred to the field, turn your hands inward and push the pack forward so that the item is just slightly over the field (Figure 10-37). The hands should be well above the field. Gently drop the item onto the field.	Turning your hands inward creates a barrier between your hands and the sterile field. Reaching over the center of the tray sets the tray up for contamination.

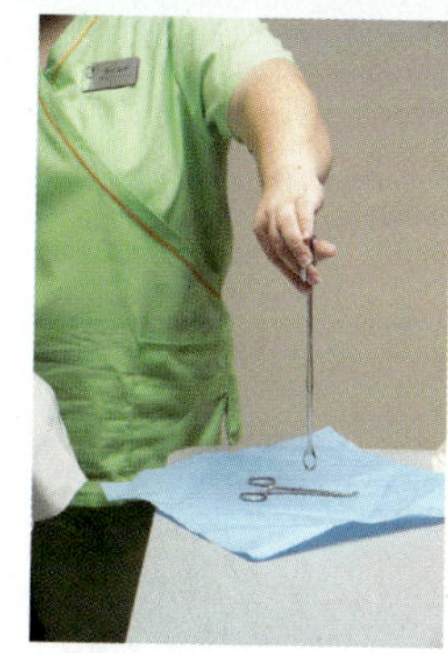

Figure 10-35 ■ Move the transfer forceps to the instrument that needs to be transferred.

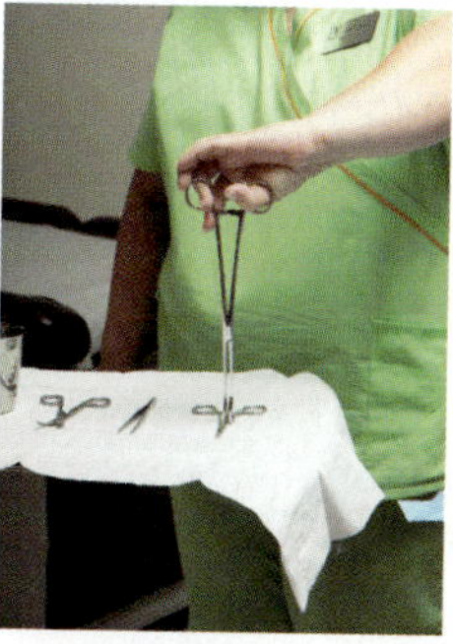

Figure 10-36 ■ Standing several inches away from the field, gently lower the sterile instrument onto the tray. Do not allow your hand to drop below the level of the handle.

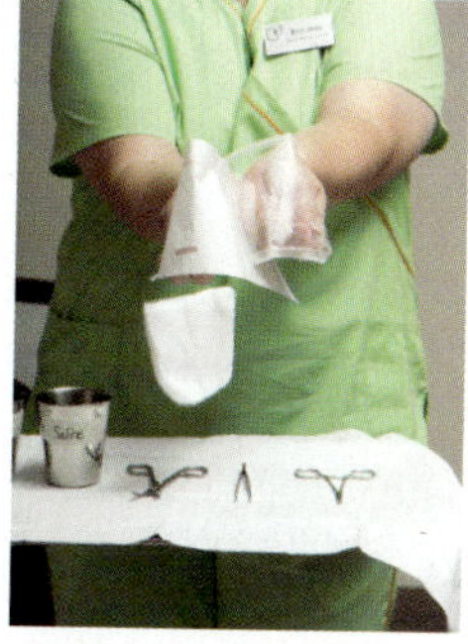

Figure 10-37 ■ Once the wrap has been peeled to the point that the item can be transferred to the field, turn your hands inward and push the pack forward so that the item is just slightly over the field.

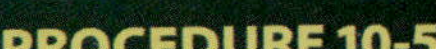

PROCEDURE 10-5

Set Up a Complete Sterile Tray and Pour a Sterile Solution

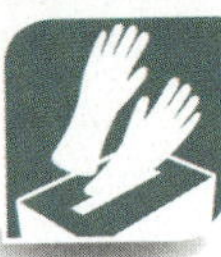

Objective:

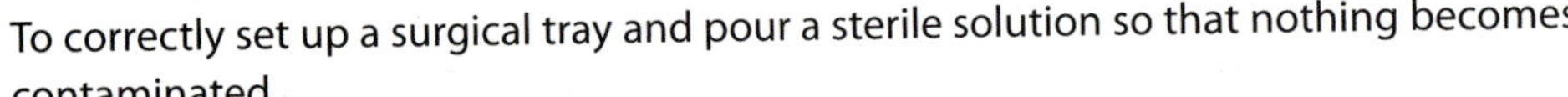

To correctly set up a surgical tray and pour a sterile solution so that nothing becomes contaminated.

Equipment/Supplies:

- Liquid antibacterial soap and sink to perform an aseptic handwash
- One wrapped tray of instruments with liquid basins to pour the sterile solutions into
- Mayo stand
- Small bottle of sterile saline
- Small bottle of sterile betadine
- 4 × 4s saturated with disinfecting solution
- Package of sterile gloves or sterile transfer forceps
- Bottle of alcohol-based hand sanitizer (to cleanse hands before applying surgical gloves)

PROCEDURAL STEPS	DETAILS AND/OR RATIONALE
1. Perform an aseptic handwash using antibacterial soap and water.	Clean hands reduce the spread of microorganisms.
2. Gather the supplies and place them on the side table.	Once you start setting up the tray, you may never turn your back on the tray. You must ensure that the tray does not become contaminated.
3. Properly position the Mayo stand so that it is at your waist level.	Dropping your hands below your waist could cause you to accidentally touch yourself or another object, which could lead to contamination of the sterile tray, especially when wearing sterile gloves to set up the field.
4. Clean the Mayo stand with 4 × 4s that have been saturated with a disinfectant (but not dripping), cleaning in a concentric circular motion.	This will minimize the number of microbes on the stand.
5. Allow the stand to air dry.	
6. Check the instrument pack and make certain that the integrity of the pack has not been compromised.	You do not want to use instruments that are not sterile; doing so will increase the patient's risk of a post-op infection.
7. Check the tape on the outside of the pack to make certain that the stripes turned the correct color and that the pack has not reached its expiration date.	The stripes on the tape should turn a deep black color if the conditions were correct for sterilization to occur inside the autoclave.
8. Pull the tape off of the pack and place it on the side table.	If there is a problem with the pack, the physician will want to know who is responsible.
9. Place the sterile pack on the center of the Mayo stand so that the flap that was taped is facing you.	

continues

PROCEDURE 10-5 continued

PROCEDURAL STEPS	DETAILS AND/OR RATIONALE
10. Using only your thumb and index finger, grasp the tip of the folded flap that was covered with tape and pull it away from you (Figure 10-38).	
11. Using only your right thumb and index finger, grasp the tip of the folded-back flap on the right side and pull it all the way to the right (Figure 10-39).	Reaching over the field to pull back the flap can contaminate the field.
12. Using only your left thumb and index finger, grasp the tip of the folded-back flap on the left side and pull it all the way to the left (Figure 10-40).	Reaching over the field to pull back the flap can contaminate the field.
13. Using only your dominant thumb and index finger, grasp the tip of the last folded-back flap and pull it toward you without touching anything on the inside of the wrap (Figure 10-41).	
14. Repeat steps 10 through 13 for the second layer of wrap. (The inner wrap will become your sterile drape.)	
15. Move to the side table without turning your back on the field.	Never turn your back on the field; you could break sterility without being aware of it.
16. Open the pack of sterile gloves and remove them from the wrapper.	You will need sterile gloves on so that you can arrange items on the field without contaminating it.
17. Open the inner wrapper without contaminating the gloves.	
18. Wash your hands with alcohol-based hand sanitizer following the directions on the bottle.	Using an alcohol-based scrub is very effective against reducing the number of microorganisms and saves time.
19. Apply surgical gloves—remember to hold your hands above the waist.	Dropping the hands below the waist will contaminate the gloves.
20. Approach the field facing forward and stand 12 inches away from the field. Remove the items from the inside of the tray and place them on the sterile field in a logical sequence. Place the basins for the sterile solution on one corner of the stand facing upward.	You may contaminate the field if you are too close to the field. The basins should be on the corner so that you do not have to reach across the field when you set up the field.

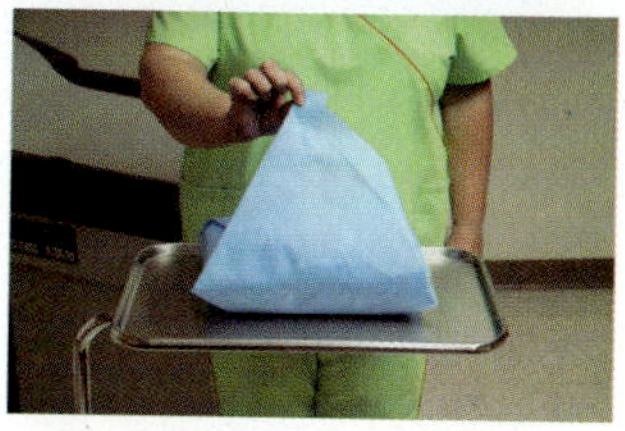

Figure 10-38 ■ Using only your thumb and index finger, grasp the tip of the folded flap that was covered with tape and pull it away from you.

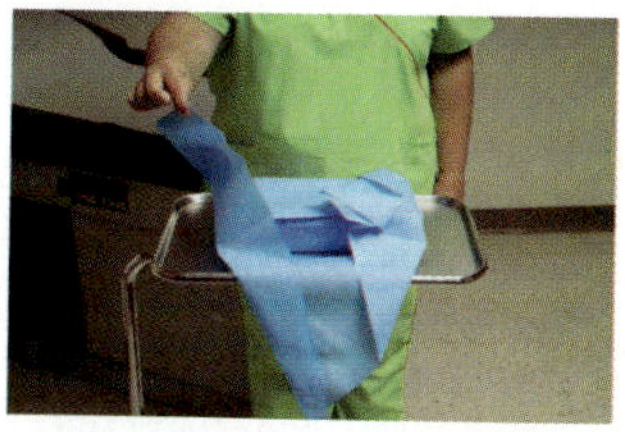

Figure 10-39 ■ Using only your right thumb and index finger, grasp the tip of the folded-back flap on the right side and pull it all the way to the right.

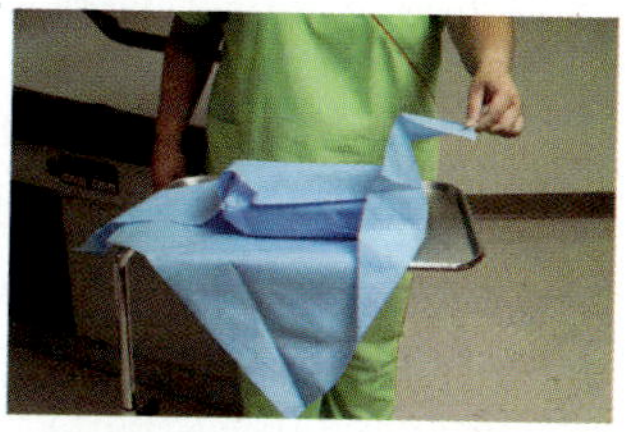

Figure 10-40 ■ Using only your left thumb and index finger, grasp the tip of the folded-back flap on the left side and pull it all the way to the left.

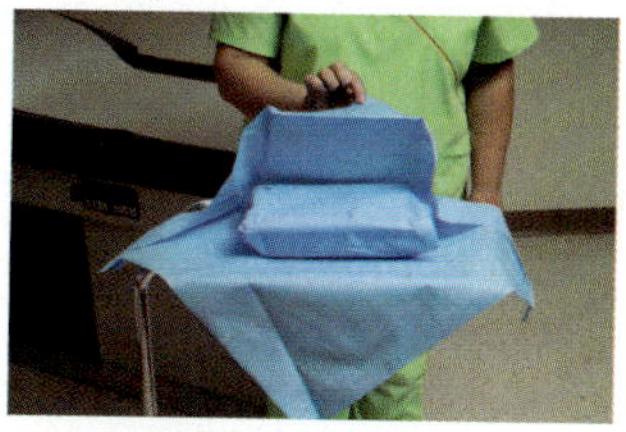

Figure 10-41 ■ Using only your dominant thumb and index finger, grasp the tip of the last folded-back flap and pull it toward you without touching anything on the inside of the wrap.

continues

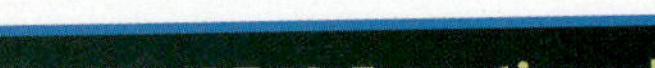

PROCEDURE 10-5 continued

PROCEDURAL STEPS	DETAILS AND/OR RATIONALE
21. Once the field has been totally arranged, remove the sterilization indicator from the inside of the tray and make certain that it is the proper color (Figure 10-42).	You want to make certain now that the conditions on the inside of the pack were ideal for sterilization to occur by checking the inside indicator. If not, a whole new pack will have to be set up.
22. Place the tray that held the instruments onto the side table. Do not turn your body away from the sterile tray as you place the instrument tray on the side table.	Turning your back to the field could cause you to accidentally contaminate the field without being aware of it.
23. Remove gloves and wash your hands with alcohol-based sanitizer.	The gloves will be unsterile once you touch the iodine, so there is no point in keeping them on anymore.
24. Pick up the brand new bottle of iodine and read the label. Make certain that you have the correct solution. Check the label to confirm that the solution has not passed its expiration date.	A new bottle of solution should be used whenever performing a surgical procedure to ensure the sterility of the solution.
25. Pick up the bottle of iodine, palming the label.	Palm the label so that if the solution drips as you pour it, it will not ruin the label. (You may use any remaining solution for nonsterile procedures.)
26. Remove the cap and place it to the side so that the lid is facing upward. Remove the protective seal and place it on the side table.	Never place a lid so that the inside of the lid is downward. This will contaminate the lid for future uses.
27. Move to the tray and approach the corner on which the basins are sitting.	Reaching across the field may contaminate the field.
28. Pour the iodine into the container labeled as iodine, pouring 2 to 6 inches above the field. Be careful not to allow the solution to splash. Fill to the desired level.	You do not want your hand to accidentally touch the bowl into which you are pouring the solution.
29. Repeat steps 24 through 28 with a new bottle of sterile saline, pouring into the container labeled as saline.	
30. If the solutions are not used in their entirety, replace the caps and follow the facility's policy for storing the solutions. Keep in mind that these solutions should not be used for any future surgical procedures.	

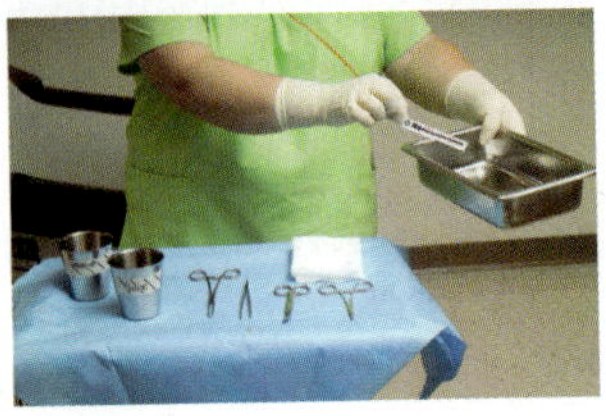

Figure 10-42 ■ Once the field has been totally arranged, remove the sterilization indicator from the inside of the tray and make certain that it is the proper color.

PROCEDURE 10-6

Apply Surgical Attire

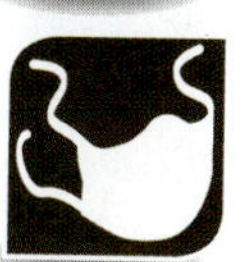

Objective:

To apply surgical attire without contaminating the items that should remain sterile.

Equipment/Supplies:

- Sterile scrub pack (with brush or sponge/antiseptic soap/nail stick)
- Sterile gloves
- Sterile gown pack (with sterile towel)
- Surgical cap
- Goggles
- Mask
- Sink/running water
- Paper towels
- Shoe coverings (if necessary)

PROCEDURAL STEPS	DETAILS AND/OR RATIONALE
1. Gather the supplies.	
2. Remove all rings and watches and perform an aseptic handwash. Do not replace rings or watches following the aseptic handwash.	Rings and watches should be removed to remove the microorganisms underneath.
3. Place a sterile gown pack on a Mayo stand or clean, dry counter surface near the sink. Open the package containing the sterile gown and towel. Sterile gloves may be transferred or dropped onto the field in a sterile manner; otherwise, sterile gloves should be positioned nearby for easy access once the gown is applied (Figure 10-43).	Opening the sterile gown package with the sterile towel and opening the glove package prior to the procedure will keep you from contaminating hands following the procedure.
4. Apply cap, goggles, shoe covers (if needed), and mask.	You apply all nonsterile items before performing a surgical handwash so that you do not contaminate the sterile items following application.
5. Open the sterile scrub pack containing the scrub brush and nail stick.	
6. Follow steps 4 through 16 in Procedure 10-1 for performing a surgical handwash.	
7. Reach down in the sterile package and lift upward on the folded gown by grasping the inside of the gown below the neckline (Figure 10-44).	The inside of the gown is considered nonsterile because it lies against your body.

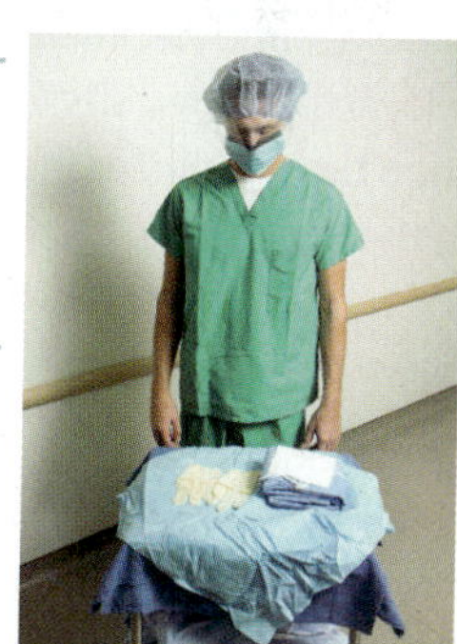

Figure 10-43 ■ Open the sterile gown packet and expose the sterile towel without contaminating it or the other items inside. Sterile gloves may be placed on the tray in a sterile manner.

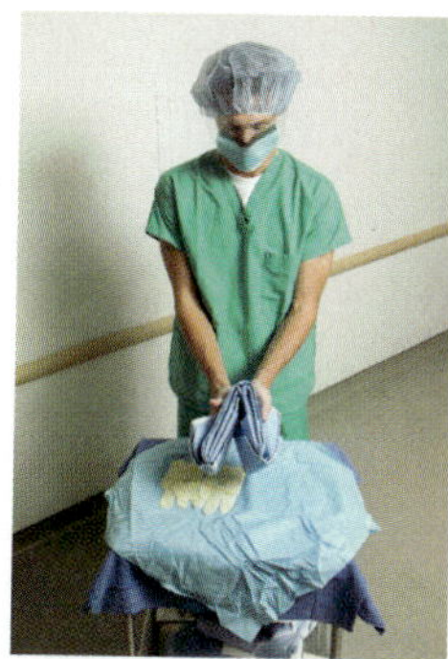

Figure 10-44 ■ Reach down in the sterile package and lift upward on the folded gown by grasping the inside of the gown below the neckline.

continues

PROCEDURE 10-6 continued

PROCEDURAL STEPS	DETAILS AND/OR RATIONALE
8. To provide a wide margin of safety, step away from the table into an area that is unobstructed.	Stepping away from the table or counter will keep you from contaminating the gown when you unfold it.
9. Keeping the inside of the gown toward your body, allow the gown to unfold. Do not touch the outside of the gown with your bare hands.	
10. Keeping the hands well above the waist, simultaneously slip both hands into the armholes (Figure 10-45). Do not allow the hands to extend beyond the cuffs.	Hands should not extend beyond the cuffs to prevent them from contaminating the gown.
11. Have another medical assistant pull the gown up over your shoulders by grasping the inside shoulder and neck seams. Keep the hands within the cuffed sleeves. The gown should then be fastened at the neck and waist level in the back only (Figure 10-46). Do not allow the medical assistant to touch any part of the gown that is to remain sterile.	
12. Using only the outside cuff of your surgical gown from your dominant hand, pick up the glove for your nondominant hand. Lay the glove on the palm side of the outside cuff of the nondominant hand. If correctly positioned, the fingers of the glove should be pointing toward your elbow and the thumb side of the glove should be facing down (Figure 10-47).	Sterile to sterile: Using the outside of the gown to pick up the glove will prevent the glove from becoming contaminated.

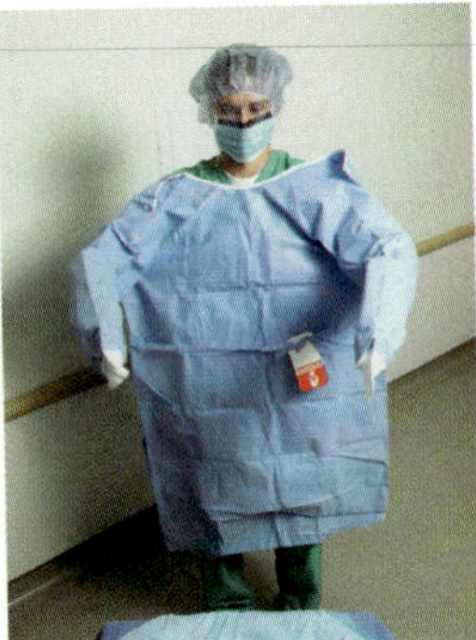

Figure 10-45 ■ Keeping the hands well above the waist, simultaneously slip both hands into the armholes.

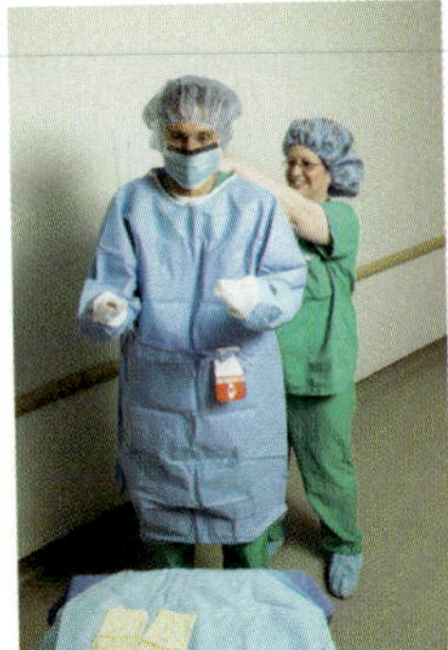

Figure 10-46 ■ Have another medical assistant pull the gown up over your shoulders by grasping the inside shoulder and neck seams (keep hands within the cuffed sleeves). The gown should then be fastened at the neck and waist level in the back only.

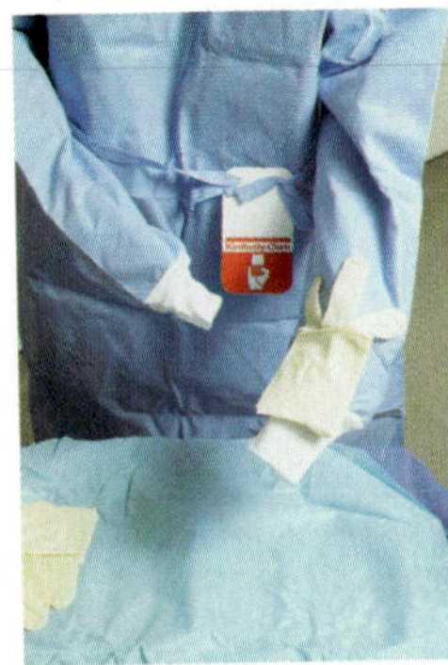

Figure 10-47 ■ Using the outside cuff of your surgical gown from your dominant hand, pick up the glove for your nondominant hand. Lay the glove on the palm side of the outside cuff of the nondominant hand.

continues

PROCEDURE 10-6 continued

PROCEDURAL STEPS	DETAILS AND/OR RATIONALE
13. With both hands still tucked within the inside cuffs of the sleeves, pinch the rolled edges of the glove and stretch the glove up and over the gown cuff while working your fingers out of the cuff and into the glove (Figure 10-48).	If you work your hands through the sleeve before the gloves are on, you will contaminate the gown.
14. Gently slide your fingers into the glove (Figure 10-49).	
15. Pick up the second glove by placing the fingers of the gloved hand under the cuff of the second glove (Figure 10-50).	Picking up the opposite glove by placing your fingers under the cuff will assist you in pulling the glove over the cuff of the gown.
16. Slide the glove over the cuff of the gown on the opposite hand while working your fingers into the glove (Figure 10-51). Make certain both cuffs are folded over stockinette cuffs.	Allowing the fingers to extend beyond the gown before the glove is applied may contaminate the gown.
17. Remember to keep the hands above the waist once gloves are applied (Figure 10-52).	Hands that drop below the waist may result in contamination to the gloves.
18. Pass the cardboard tab to the second medical assistant (Figure 10-53). Grasp the string attached to the cardboard as the medical assistant pulls the cardboard toward the outside. The cardboard will separate from the string.	
19. Pick up the other loose string attached to the front of the gown and tie both strings at the waist and secure (Figure 10-54).	
20. Make sure your hands stay above the level of the waist at all times.	Hands are considered contaminated if they fall below the waist.

Figure 10-48 ■ With both hands, pinch the rolled edges of the glove and stretch the glove up and over the gown cuff while working your fingers out of the cuff of the gown into the glove.

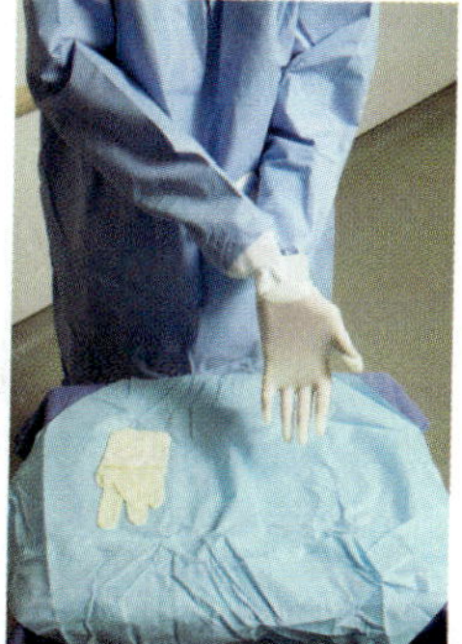

Figure 10-49 ■ Gently slide your fingers into the glove, pulling it over your hand.

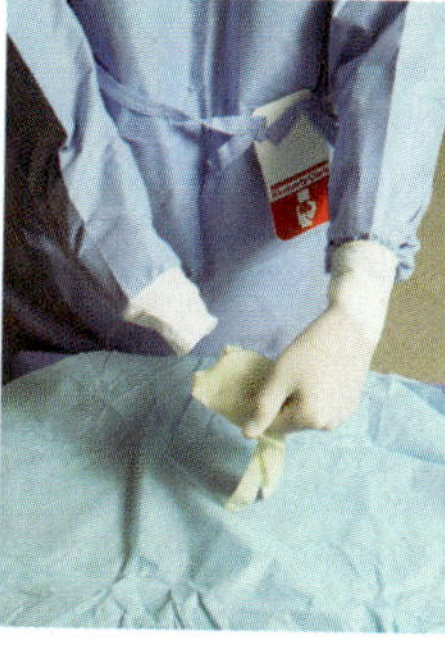

Figure 10-50 ■ Pick up the second glove by placing the fingers of the gloved hand under the cuff of the second glove.

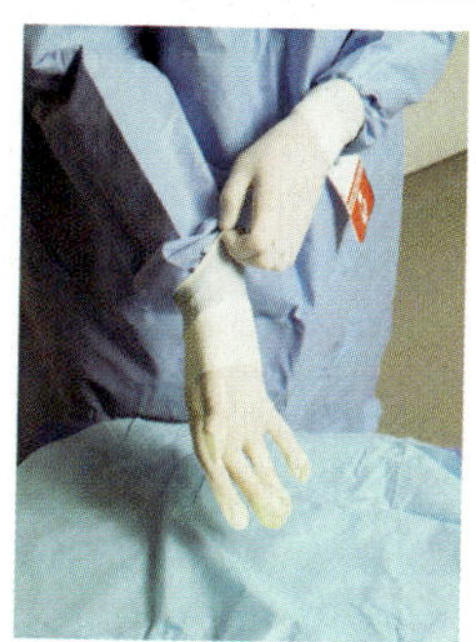

Figure 10-51 ■ Slide the glove over the cuff on the gown on the opposite hand while working your fingers into the glove.

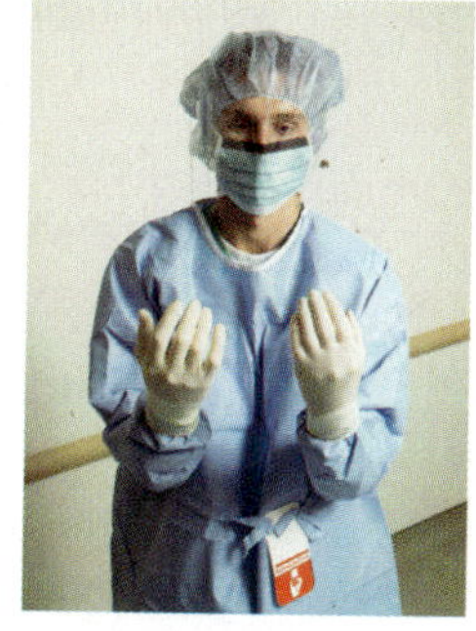

Figure 10-52 ■ Remember to keep hands above the waist once gloves are applied.

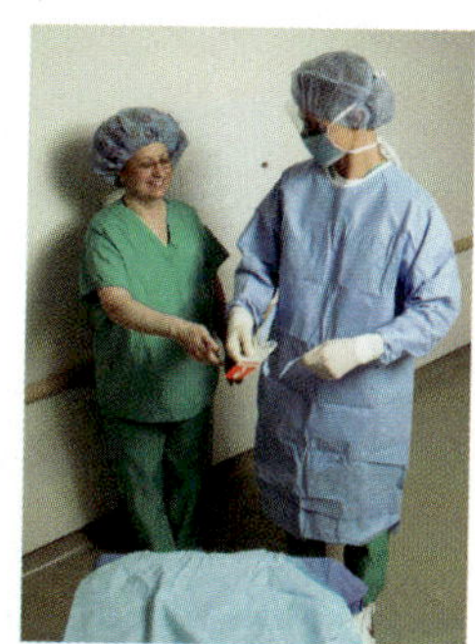

Figure 10-53 ■ Pass the cardboard tab to the second medical assistant.

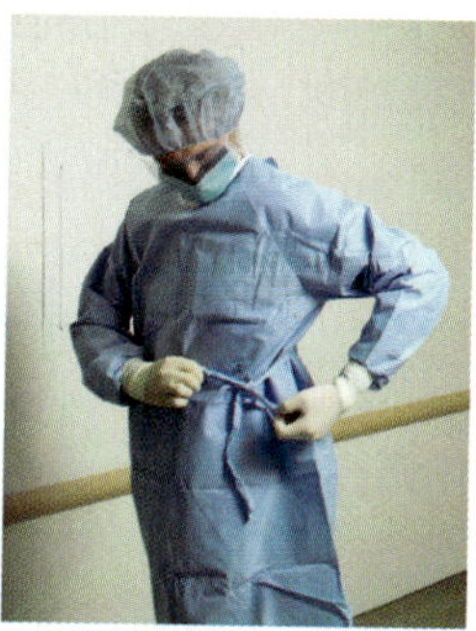

Figure 10-54 ■ Pick up the other loose string attached to the front of the gown and tie both strings at the waist and secure.

PROCEDURE 10-7

Remove an Old Dressing, Irrigate the Wound, and Apply a New Dressing

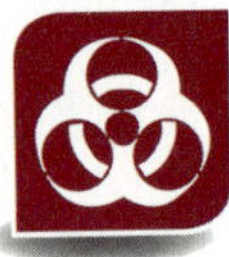

Objective:

To correctly remove an old dressing without contaminating the patient's wound or your gloves and to properly clean the wound and apply a new dressing.

Equipment/Supplies:

- Waterproof pad
- Hand cleanser (alcohol-based)
- Examination gloves
- Sterile gloves
- Sterile basins
- Sterile 4 × 4s
- Sterile water or saline
- 20 mL syringe
- Bandage scissors
- Biohazard container
- Dressing and bandage material
- Patient's chart/EHR

PROCEDURAL STEPS	DETAILS AND/OR RATIONALE
1. Check the patient's chart to determine the type and strength of irrigating solution and dressing to be used, and gather the supplies.	Today's guidelines usually suggest irrigating wounds with sterile saline.
2. Identify the patient using two identifiers.	It is important to know that you have the right patient.
3. Identify yourself.	
4. ***Explain the rationale for performance of the procedure, showing awareness of the patient's concerns related to the procedure being performed.***	Explaining the procedure helps the patient know what to expect.
5. Ask the patient if the patient has had any problems since the surgery and make certain that the patient has been following all home care instructions.	If the patient has encountered problems, the procedure may be postponed.
6. Have the patient expose the area.	
7. Place a waterproof pad under the wound area and position so that the work area is easily assessable.	This is to keep the patient and the patient's clothes dry while irrigating and cleansing the wound.
8. Wash hands using aseptic technique and apply appropriate PPE (nonsterile examination gloves).	The gloves are to protect you from being exposed to exudate when removing the dressing.
9. Inspect the outer covering of the bandage, ***incorporating critical thinking when performing patient care.*** Make a mental note of any concerns. Was the bandage torn, dirty, or wet?	If the bandage material is dirty or tattered, it could indicate that the patient is not following home care instructions, which could lead to infection.

continues

PROCEDURE 10-7 continued

PROCEDURAL STEPS	DETAILS AND/OR RATIONALE
10. Cut the bandage with a pair of bandage scissors along the side of the wound (Figure 10-55). Carefully remove the bandage and dressing by pulling the bandage toward the wound (Figure 10-56).	Pulling the bandage away from the wound could cause the wound to stretch.
11. Inspect the inner portion of the bandage for any drainage or odor. Make a mental note of your findings. Discard the bandage material into a biohazard container.	The physician will not see the bandage material, so if there are any signs of infection on the bandage, the physician will need to be notified.
12. Without touching the wound, look at the wound area and inspect it for any signs of infection, including edema, erythema, drainage, etc. Make a mental note of your findings.	It is important to document any signs of infection for future reference.
13. Remove gloves and wash your hands. Follow office policy regarding having the physician check the wound before redressing.	The gloves were contaminated once they touched the bandage contents.
14. Properly position and clean the Mayo tray with the 4 × 4s containing disinfectant. Allow the stand to air dry.	
15. Place one of the wrapped sterile basins on the center of the Mayo stand. Open using sterile technique.	This basin is for the irrigating solution.
16. Open the peel-apart package containing the sterile 4 × 4s and drop the contents from the packet onto the field.	The sterile 4 × 4s will be used to dry the area once the irrigation is done.
17. Open sterile dressing and place it on the sterile field.	Sterile dressing should be used to cover an open wound to reduce the risk of infection.
18. Open the sterile bandage and place it on the sterile field.	
19. Drop a sterile 20 mL syringe onto the sterile field.	The syringe will be used to irrigate the wound.
20. Pour a small amount of sterile saline into the sterile basin.	Saline will be used to irrigate the wound.
21. Remove the other sterile basin from the side table and place it on the waterproof drape near the wound. Open it in a sterile manner. Instruct the patient not to touch the basin or drape.	This basin should be sterile to protect your gloves when moving the basin during the procedure.

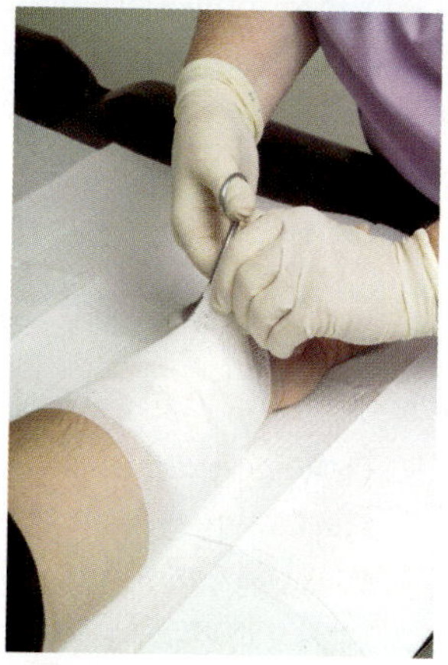

Figure 10-55 ■ Cut the bandage with a pair of bandage scissors along the side of the wound. Carefully remove the bandage and dressing by pulling the corners of the bandage toward the wound.

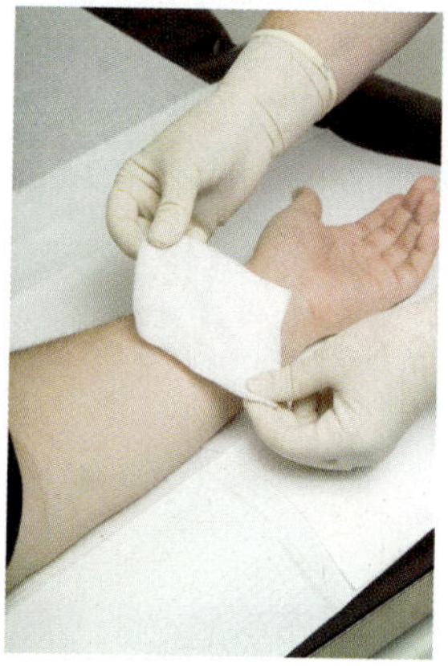

Figure 10-56 ■ Carefully remove the bandage and dressing by pulling the corners of the bandage toward the wound.

continues

PROCEDURE 10-7 continued

PROCEDURAL STEPS	DETAILS AND/OR RATIONALE
22. Thoroughly wash your hands using the alcohol-based sanitizer on the side table.	Hands should always be washed prior to gloving to reduce the risks of contamination.
23. Don a pair of sterile gloves.	Because this is an open wound, sterile gloves should be applied.
24. Arrange items on the tray for easy access.	
25. Draw up irrigating fluid from the basin with the sterile syringe. Irrigate the patient's wound so that the water runs into the basin on the sterile field (Figure 10-57).	You don't want the water to run all over the tray.
26. Dry the wound with sterile gauze.	You do not want to contaminate the area.
27. Open the sterile dressing and place it over the wound (Figure 10-58).	
28. Choose a bandaging technique that best suits the patient's wound.	You want to apply the dressing so that it remains intact.
29. Throw away all trash into proper trash receptacles and give the patient home care instructions and any prescriptions.	The patient must be educated on how to care for the wound for better results.
30. Dismiss the patient and clean the room.	Document the procedure in order to illustrate what was done for the patient.
31. Document the procedure in the patient's chart.	

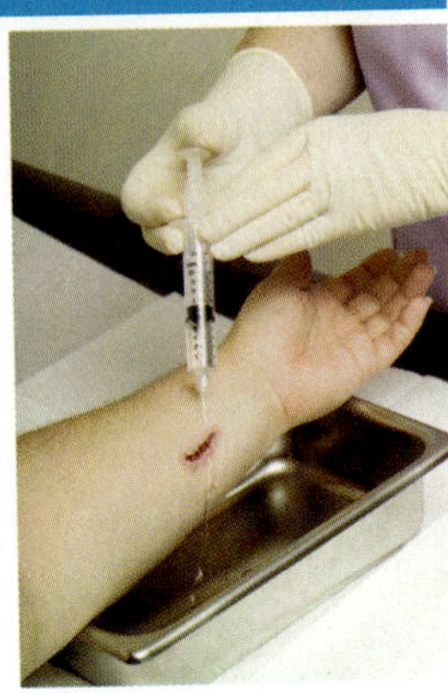

Figure 10-57 ■ Draw up irrigating fluid from the basin with the sterile syringe. Irrigate the patient's wound, according to the physician's orders.

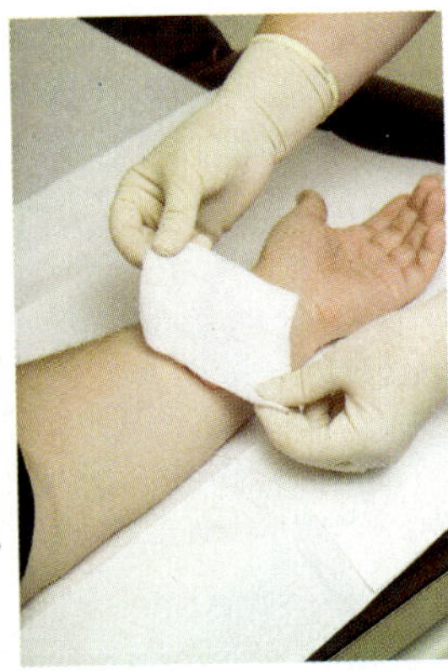

Figure 10-58 ■ Open the sterile dressing and place it over the wound.

DOCUMENTATION EXAMPLE:

04-15-XX 2:30 p.m.	Pt. here for a dressing change following last week's injury to L arm. Pt. states that the she took all of her antibiotic and dressed wound according to home care instructions. Dressing was clean and dry. A small amount of serosanguineous exudate present on the inside portion of the bandage. Negative erythema or edema over the wound area. Irrigated wound with 40 cc of sterile saline. Dried area with sterile gauze. Applied a sterile collagen dressing to the area. Reinstructed pt. on proper wound care. Pt to return next week. Jeanine Ruh, CMA (AAMA) --

CHAPTER SUMMARY

- A sterile conscience is a mind-set of constant vigilance. It is taking ownership for the sterility of items from the time of processing through the termination of the procedure.
- National Patient Safety Goals include labeling all medication containers, reducing the risks of surgical fires through education, and using protocol for preventing "Wrong Site," "Wrong Person," and "Wrong Procedure."
- Tasks that should be completed prior to a surgical procedure include providing instruction in the following areas: fasting and medication instructions, any special preparation instructions such as skin cleansing, proper clothing to be worn the day of the procedure, and instructions of who should accompany the patient the day of surgery.
- Tasks that should be completed the day of surgery include cleaning and disinfecting the room, gathering all supplies for the procedure, putting necessary X-rays on the computer screen or X-ray box, placing necessary equipment in the room, and checking all equipment to make certain it is in good working order.
- Surgical cards or electronic files should be created listing each physician's preferences for particular procedures such as what should be included in particular trays, anesthetic preferences, and glove and gown size.
- The two most common prescriptions given to patients following a surgical procedure include analgesics and antibiotics.
- Skin-prep instructions usually include shaving with surgical clippers (if necessary), cleansing the site with a surgical soap, applying a skin antiseptic such as iodine, and applying a fenestrated drape over the site.
- When setting up the room for a surgical procedure, the Mayo stand should be disinfected, the side table should be set up, the surgical tray should be prepared, and sterile solutions should be poured.
- A surgical handwash should be performed by anyone assisting during the surgery.
- The medical assistant is often responsible for assisting the provider, before, during, and following the procedure.
- Stages of wound care include inflammatory stage, proliferative stage, and maturation and remodeling stage.
- The latest studies reveal that cleaning the wound with anything other than normal saline could actually inhibit the healing process.
- Steps for good wound care include cleaning and debridement, application of a sterile dressing, preventing further injury, and preventing infection.
- A primary dressing is placed directly over the wound, while a secondary dressing is placed over the primary dressing.
- The selection of bandage material will be based on the goals for bandaging, which may include: to hold a dressing in place, to immobilize a joint, to hold a dressing, and immobilize a joint.
- Methods of bandaging include circular turn, spiral turn, reverse spiral, and figure eight.
- Wound care alternatives include subatmospheric pressure dressings and hyperbaric oxygen therapy.

CERTIFICATION REVIEW QUESTIONS

1. All of the following statements apply to the minor surgery setting except:
   a. items are either sterile or nonsterile.
   b. the sterile tray may be set up 30 minutes prior to the start of the procedure.
   c. handling the outside of sterile packs is permissible.
   d. do *not* reach over a sterile field.

2. Which of the following duties should be completed a few days prior to surgery?
   a. Educate the patient about fasting instructions.
   b. Inform the patient about the type of clothing to be worn.
   c. Tell the patient if it will be necessary to have someone to drive the patient home after the procedure.
   d. All of the above.

3. Which of the following statements is true in regards to surgical instruments?
   a. Sterile items can be used more than once, if the procedures are the same.
   b. Surgical instruments can be used for other purposes besides surgery.
   c. A sterile item should not be opened until just prior to use.
   d. A sterile item may be opened 15 minutes prior to the procedure.

4. Which of the following items would not be considered sterile?
   a. Cap
   b. Back of the gown
   c. Goggles
   d. All of the above

5. All of the following are duties of a nonscrubbed medical assistant during a surgical procedure except:
   a. opening lids of trash receptacles.
   b. collecting specimens from the physician.
   c. handling items not on the field to the physician.
   d. handling items that are on the field to the physician.

6. Whose responsibility is it to clean the post-op site and apply a sterile dressing?
   a. Physician
   b. Medical assistant
   c. Patient
   d. None of the above

7. Which of the following solutions is recommended to clean a wound?
   a. Hydrogen peroxide
   b. Iodine
   c. Alcohol
   d. Normal saline

8. Which type of dressing absorbs excess fluid from the wound?
   a. Primary
   b. Secondary
   c. Tertiary
   d. Simple

9. The doctor requests that you give Mr. Mendez two prescriptions following the surgery. They include:
   a. an anesthetic and antibiotic.
   b. an analgesic and antibiotic.
   c. an anesthetic and anticoagulant.
   d. an analgesic and anticoagulant.

10. Which of the following trays requires a Penrose Drain?
   a. Laceration repairs
   b. Excision of a sebaceous cyst
   c. Aspiration of fluid from a joint
   d. Incision and drainage procedures

STUDY RESOURCES

Resources to Test and Reinforce Your Knowledge:	
Certification Review Questions	Take this end-of-chapter quiz
Workbook	• Complete the activities for Chapter 10 • Perform the procedures for Chapter 10 using the Competency Checklists
Resources to Promote Critical Thinking:	
***Solve the Case* Activities**	• Consider these case studies and discuss your conclusions
Learning Lab	• Module 24: Minor Surgery Procedures
MindTap	• Complete Chapter 10 readings and activities

REFERENCES

Bible, J. E., Biswas, D., Whang, P. G., Simpson, A. K., & Grauer, J. N. (n.d.). Which Regions of the Operating Gown Should be Considered Most Sterile? Retrieved September 7, 2015, from http://www.ncbi.nlm.nih.gov/pmc/articles/PMC2635444/

Fife, C., DR, Carter, M., PhD, Walker, D., CHT, & Thompson, B., BS. (2012, January). Wound Care Outcomes and Associated Cost Among Patients Treated in US Outpatient Wound Centers. Retrieved September 07, 2015, from http://www.woundsresearch.com/article/wound-care-outcomes-and-associated-cost-among-patients-treated-us-outpatient-wound-centers-d

Maintaining Asepsis Within a Sterile Field in Surgery. (2009, February 27). Retrieved September 7, 2015, from http://www.infectioncontroltoday.com/articles/2009/02/maintaining-asepsis-within-a-sterile-field-in-sur.aspx

WCAW - Wound Care Awareness Week. (n.d.). Retrieved September 7, 2015, from http://woundcareawareness.com/

Wound Care Treatment & Management. (n.d.). Retrieved September 7, 2015, from http://emedicine.medscape.com/article/194018-treatment

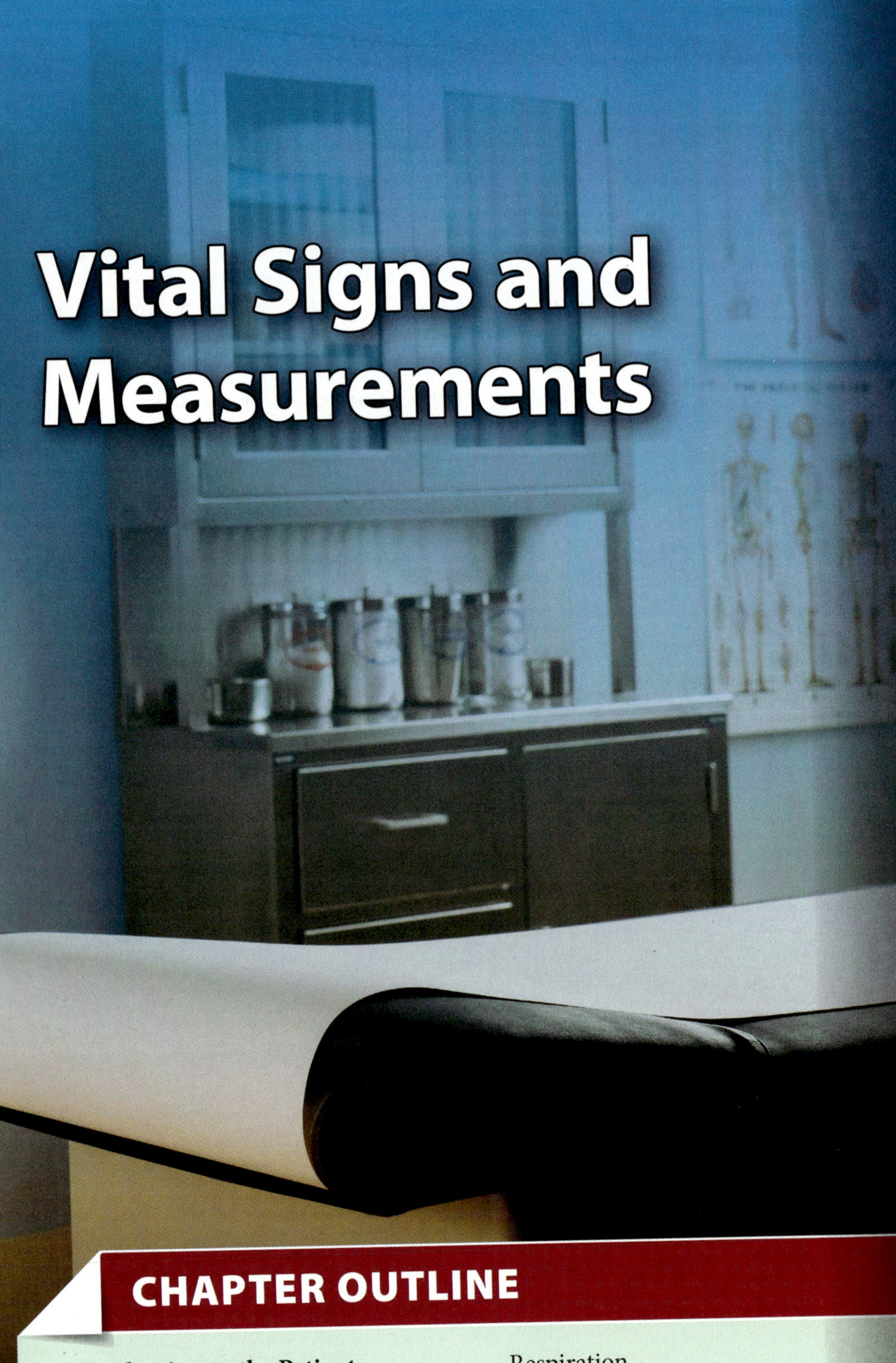

11

Vital Signs and Measurements

CHAPTER OUTLINE

Introduction to the Patient
- Screening the Patient
- The Patient Intake

Height and Weight
- BMI or Body Fat Percentage

Vital Signs
- Temperature
- Pulse
- Respiration
- Blood Pressure
- Electronic Vital Signs
- Pain Assessment
- Pulse Oximetry

ESSENTIAL TERMS

afebrile
arrhythmia
auscultatory gap
baseline
body mass index (BMI)
bradycardia
bradypnea
calipers
Celsius (C)
diastole
diastolic pressure
diurnal rhythms
dyspnea
dysrhythmia
exhalation
expiration
Fahrenheit (F)
febrile
fever
homeostasis
hyperpnea
hypertension
hyperthermia
hyperventilation
hypotension
hypothermia
inhalation
inspiration
Korotkoff sounds
mensuration
metabolism
obesity
orthopnea
orthostatic hypotension
pulse pressure
pulse rate
pulse rhythm
pulse volume
radiate
respiration

continues

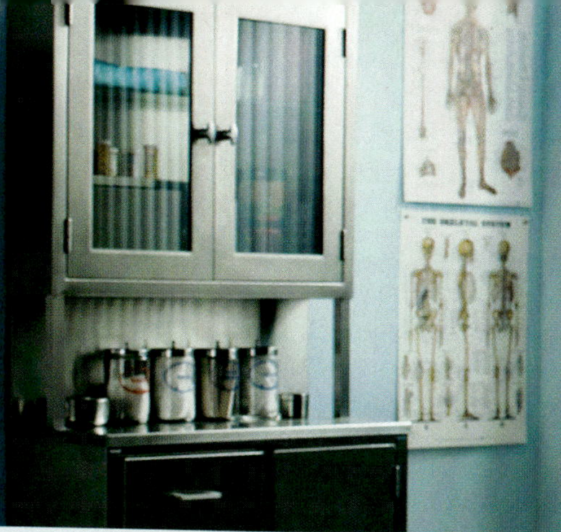

sphygmomanometer
systole
systolic pressure
tachycardia
tachypnea
vasoconstriction
vasodilation
vital signs

DEVELOPMENTAL OBJECTIVES

After completing this chapter, you should be able to:

1. Correctly spell and define essential terms.
2. Explain the purpose for obtaining a height and weight.
3. List the vital signs, the reasons for obtaining them, and the normal ranges for each.
4. Describe the mechanisms that may cause variations in vital signs.
5. List the sites available for obtaining a temperature and the specific reasons for taking measurements at each site.
6. Identify the different pulse points.
7. Define blood pressure and the meaning of systole and diastole.
8. Measure and record temperature, pulse, respiration, blood pressure, and height and weight.

INTRODUCTION

Obtaining accurate **vital signs** is an important role of the medical assistant. Physical changes that occur in the body from one visit to the next may be detected through a change in a patient's vital signs. Vital signs, also known as cardinal signs, include temperature, pulse, and respiration (these three vital signs as referred together as TPR), and blood pressure (BP). Some medical references now include pain assessment as a fifth vital sign. Other measurements that may be taken in addition to vital signs include the patient's height and weight and the patient's oxygen saturation level.

Customarily, all vital signs are obtained during a patient's initial visit to determine baseline readings. Whether or not all vital signs are performed during each subsequent visit will depend on the type of specialty, the provider's preferences, and the patient's symptoms.

Accurate measurements should be taken and the results recorded in the patient's chart. Medical assisting students should practice vital signs regularly to become proficient at these procedures prior to entering the workplace.

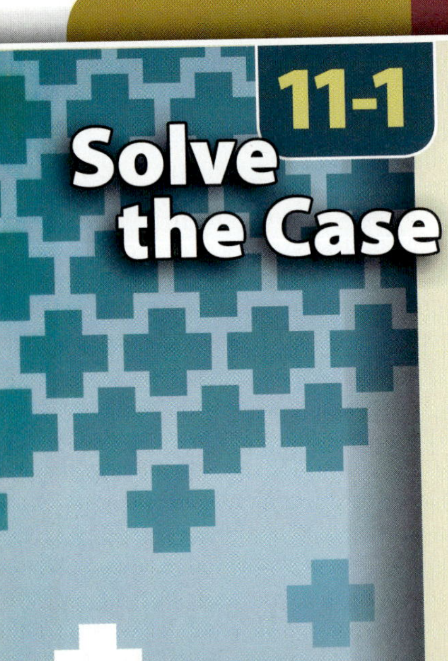

You are working in a family practice office and a regular patient, Mrs. Collins, age 72, walks in complaining of feeling dizzy with a headache. You have assisted with her examinations many times in the past. She appears flushed and irritated. On the way to the examination room, she stumbles slightly. Because she seems weak and dizzy, you decide not to weigh her and to take her vitals in the exam room.

Her BP is elevated (160/102). She seems confused when you ask her about her medications. She was on an antihypertensive medication at the time of her last visit. She took a cab to the clinic for her appointment because she was afraid to drive. No relatives are with her, although her daughter usually accompanies her. Using just your current knowledge, how would you answer the following questions?

1. **How much of a concern is Mrs. Collins' BP?**
2. **Why is the patient's BP such a concern?**
3. **What can you do to help Mrs. Collins feel more at ease?**

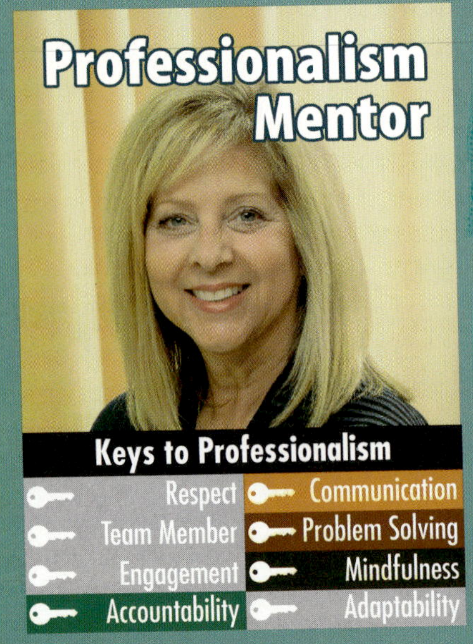

One of the most important skills that a medical assistant can perform in order to demonstrate proficiency is being able to obtain accurate vital signs and various measurements. An experienced medical assistant was attending proficiency testing and was upset when she was asked to repeat a blood pressure because her reading was off. "I was close," she stated, to which the educator replied, "being close is not acceptable." As a medical assistant, you will most likely take blood pressures, pulse rates, temps, or pulse ox readings on a regular basis. Professionalism is not accepting being close, but being accurate. This type of integrity in work ethic is what separates the medical assistant that the physician can trust from the medical assistant that the physician does not have confidence in. The key to success is to be that medical assistant who can always be depended on. ■

INTRODUCTION TO THE PATIENT

The first contact a clinical medical assistant has with the patient occurs when the patient is called from the reception area and taken to the examination room. The medical assistant must be aware of office policies for properly addressing patients in the waiting area.

Most clinics prefer that medical assistants call patients by their title (Mr., Mrs., Miss, Ms.,) and last name, unless patients specifically request to be called by their first name. Some older patients may find it disrespectful to be addressed by their first name by a younger individual. Ask patients directly how they would prefer to be addressed. Record this information in a special area of the patient's chart so that all office staff members will know how to address the patient during future encounters. Most electronic health records (EHRs) have a field for "nickname" where this information can be stored, or an electronic "sticky note" to enter the information.

Screening the Patient

The medical assistant should use all senses during the initial screening process to gather important clues about the patient's health status. The patient should be observed for the following:

- Appearance
- Gait (a person's manner of walking)
- Odors
- Level of awareness
- Emotional state

The medical assistant may make particular observations that the provider may not be able to observe, such as any difficulty the patient experiences while walking from the reception room to the examination room. Patients may express anxiousness or fearfulness to the medical assistant about a particular procedure or examination during the screening process. Sharing this information ahead of time with the provider will assist the provider in knowing how to proceed with the patient.

The Patient Intake

The term *patient intake* describes the process of obtaining vital signs and measurements and conducting a brief patient interview. Information that should be collected during patient intake or the initial screening process may include any of the following:

- Height and weight
- Vital signs
- Reason for the visit (chief complaint) and history of the present illness (The provider may want to do this his or herself.)
- Medication reconciliation
- Drug allergy information
- The patient's medical history

If no specimens are required, allow the patient time to use the restroom prior to examination so he will be more comfortable during the exam. If a urine specimen is necessary, provide the patient with the appropriate supplies and instructions for properly collecting a urine specimen. Store the specimen appropriately until testing can be performed.

The medical assistant should be certain to accurately document all findings collected during the initial screening into the patient's chart.

HEIGHT AND WEIGHT

Measuring the patient's height and weight is often the responsibility of the medical assistant. **Mensuration** is a term that means measurement. Fluctuations in a patient's height or weight could indicate a health disorder or illness; therefore, accuracy and consistency are important. The weight of a patient is usually monitored during each office visit. Height is routinely measured until the patient stops growing, but may be performed on adults for specific types of exams. Height is carefully monitored on female patients during and following menopause. This is largely due the effects that low estrogen levels have on bone density following menopause.

As **obesity** (being 20-30 percent over normal weight) is an increasing problem in the United States, many recommendations on acceptable weights have been explored. Insurance companies and nutritional organizations produce "normal" or desirable weight charts, such as the one seen in Figure 11-1. These do not usually account for body fitness and muscle mass. Body mass index is a better, but not perfect, indicator for weight as it relates to the patient's health. Refer to Procedure 11-1 for instructions on performing height and weight on an adult patient. Refer to Chapter 21 for a procedure on performing these tasks on pediatric patients.

BMI or Body Fat Percentage

Body mass index (BMI) is a numerical correlation between a patient's height and weight. Calculating the patient's BMI may be the responsibility of the medical assistant, and should be documented along with the scale weight. To calculate a patient's BMI, use the following formula:

- Multiply the patient's weight (in pounds) by 703.
- Divide this total by the patient's height (in inches).

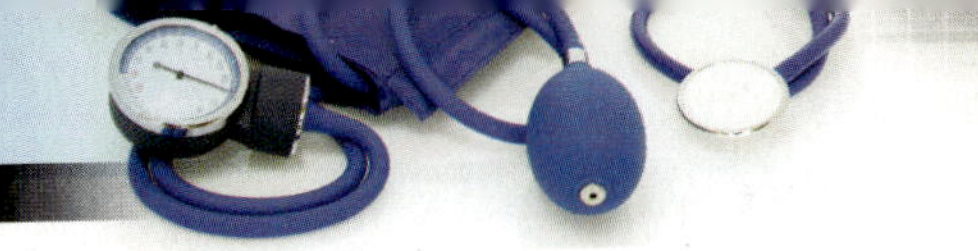

Body Mass Index Table

To use the table, find the appropriate height in the left-hand column labeled Height. Move across to a given weight. The number at the top of the column is the BMI at that height and weight. Pounds have been rounded off.

BMI	19	20	21	22	23	24	25	26	27	28	29	30	31	32	33	34	35	36	37	38	39	40
Height (Inches)																						**Weight (Pounds)**
58	91	96	100	105	110	115	119	124	129	134	138	143	148	153	158	162	167	172	177	181	186	191
59	94	99	104	109	114	119	124	128	133	138	143	148	153	158	163	168	173	178	183	188	193	198
60	97	102	107	112	118	123	128	133	138	143	148	153	158	163	168	174	179	184	189	194	199	204
61	100	106	111	116	122	127	132	137	143	148	153	158	164	169	174	180	185	190	195	201	206	211
62	104	109	115	120	126	131	136	142	147	153	158	164	169	175	180	186	191	196	202	207	213	218
63	107	113	118	124	130	135	141	146	152	158	163	169	175	180	186	191	197	203	208	214	220	225
64	110	116	122	128	134	140	145	151	157	163	169	174	180	186	192	197	204	209	215	221	227	232
65	114	120	126	132	138	144	150	156	162	168	174	180	186	192	198	204	210	216	222	228	234	240
66	118	124	130	136	142	148	155	161	167	173	179	186	192	198	204	210	216	223	229	235	241	247
67	121	127	134	140	146	153	159	166	172	178	185	191	198	204	211	217	223	230	236	242	249	255
68	125	131	138	144	151	158	164	171	177	184	190	197	204	210	216	223	230	236	243	249	256	262
69	128	135	142	149	155	162	169	176	182	189	196	203	210	216	223	230	236	243	250	257	263	270
70	132	139	146	153	160	167	174	181	188	195	202	209	216	222	229	236	243	250	257	264	271	278
71	136	143	150	157	165	172	179	186	193	200	208	215	222	229	236	243	250	257	265	272	279	286
72	140	147	154	162	169	177	184	191	199	206	213	221	228	235	242	250	258	265	272	279	287	294
73	144	151	159	166	174	182	189	197	204	212	219	227	235	242	250	257	265	272	280	288	295	302
74	148	155	163	171	179	186	194	202	210	218	225	233	241	249	256	264	272	280	287	295	303	311
75	152	160	168	176	184	192	200	208	216	224	232	240	248	256	264	272	279	287	295	303	311	319
76	156	164	172	180	189	197	205	213	221	230	238	246	254	263	271	279	287	295	304	312	320	328

www.niddk.nih.gov

Figure 11-1 ■ BMI index and height and weight chart listing statistics for determining a person's BMI.

- Divide this total by the patient's height (in inches) again and then round to the nearest whole number.
- The result is the patient's BMI.

When entering vital signs into the EHR, the BMI automatically populates once the height and weight are entered. There are also several websites available that automatically calculate BMI once the appropriate data is entered.

The Centers for Disease Control and Prevention (CDC) provides ranges for interpreting the BMI outcome:

Less than 18.5	Underweight
18.6–24.9	Acceptable weight
25.0–29.9	Overweight
Greater than 30	Obese

Waist Circumference

Some practices may evaluate waist circumferences to determine obesity. Waist circumference is measured while the patient is in a standing position. A tape measure is placed around the patient's waist just superior to the hip bone.

When using waist circumference to establish excess body fat, the following applies:

- Measurements for a woman greater than 35 inches would be considered excessive.
- Measurements for a man greater than 40 inches would be considered excessive.

Body Fat Calipers

A more accurate procedure for determining body fat is through the use of body fat **calipers** (Figure 11-2). Body fat calipers are devices that measure skinfolds on different parts of the patient's body.

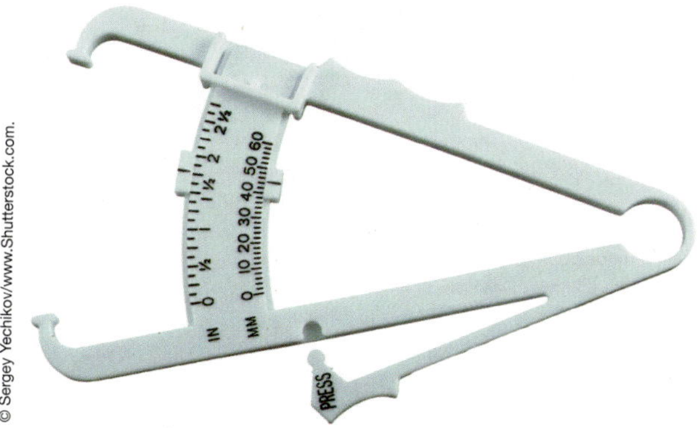

Figure 11-2 ■ Example of a body fat caliper.

VITAL SIGNS

Changes in a patient's health can often be detected through the monitoring of vital signs. Other basic physiological measurements as well as any changes that have occurred since the patient's last medical examination can provide an overall picture of the patient's general state of health.

Temperature, pulse, respiration, and blood pressure (TPR and BP) are standard vital signs taken. Any changes identified during measurement of these vital signs may indicate a health condition or may illustrate the progression of a previously identified medical condition. Obtaining vital signs when the patient is healthy or during an initial visit provides a **baseline** to which future vital signs can be compared.

In addition to TPR and BP, a pain rating may also be obtained from a patient, especially in the hospital environment. Pulse oximetry (a measurement of the oxygen concentration in the blood) is also considered another key indicator of health status, particularly in patients with respiratory complaints or history of respiratory disease.

Temperature

Staying within a particular temperature range is essential for the body to maintain **homeostasis** (a state in which the body's internal conditions are able to remain constant in the midst of changing environments). Tissues and cells in the body function best when the body's temperature ranges between 97°F and 99°F (36.1°C and 37.2°C). Maintenance of a normal body temperature is necessary for an individual to remain in a healthy state.

Structures That Help Regulate Body Temperature

Several structures or organs within the body work together to keep the body's temperature regulated, including the following:

- The hypothalamus: This structure within the brain acts as a thermostat to control body temperature.
- Blood vessels: When the body is hot, **vasodilation** occurs—this is a mechanism in which cutaneous blood vessels dilate (or increase in diameter), allowing more blood to circulate toward the surface of the skin, and causing more heat to **radiate** outward. When the body is cold, **vasoconstriction** decreases the diameter of cutaneous blood vessels, causing blood vessels to sink and trap more heat within the body.
- The integumentary system (skin and pores): This system allows the body to lose heat through perspiration.
- The neuromuscular system: In conjunction with the nervous system, this system works to cause shivering, which helps raise body temperature in frigid conditions.

Heat Produced versus Heat Lost in the Body

To maintain proper body temperature, the amount of heat generated within the body must be balanced with the amount of heat lost from the body. As body temperature rises, certain mechanisms occur to rid the body of excess heat. If body temperature dips too low, the body conserves heat. Table 11-1 shows some causes of heat production along with some causes of heat loss. If the amount of heat produced exceeds the amount lost, **fever** occurs and the patient is considered **febrile**. If the amount of heat lost is greater than the amount of heat generated, hypothermia can occur. A patient with a normal body temperature is said to be **afebrile**.

Normal or average body temperature is approximately 98.6°F (37°C), with allowances for mild fluctuations, as all individuals do not have exactly the same normal body temperature. Variations in temperature may occur as a result of environment, level of activity, and overall health. The time of the day may also influence a temperature reading, due to **diurnal rhythms**. Early morning temperatures taken around 4:00 a.m. tend to be lower than midday readings due to a decrease in metabolism and muscle contractions. Early morning readings can be as low as 96.4°F (35.8°C), while late afternoon and evening measurements taken around 8:00 p.m. may be normal at 99.1°F (37.3°C).

The way a temperature is taken will also affect the outcome; therefore, it is important to document the method by which the measurement was obtained. Rectal temperatures tend to run slightly higher than oral temperatures, but are a more accurate measurement of core temperature. Axillary temperatures run slightly lower than oral temperatures and are generally

Table 11-1 Body Heat Production and Heat Loss

Causes of Heat Production	Causes of Heat Loss
Exercise: causes muscles to contract, generating heat within the body	Perspiration (sweating): heat leaves the body through moisture
Shivering: involuntary response to cold, causing muscle contraction, thus generating heat	Respiration: breathing out moisture containing heat
Metabolism: as nutrients are processed in the body, cells produce energy, which elevates body temperature	Excretion of urine and feces: heat is expelled through fluids in waste materials
Emotions (crying, rage, and anger): increase body temperature	Environmental conditions: exposure to frigid temperatures
Infection: cells produce heat when fighting infections	
Environmental conditions: excessive heat or excessive sun exposure	
Pregnancy and menses: may increase body temperature	

considered less accurate. Tympanic membrane and aural (ear) temperatures typically run higher than oral readings because they are within in a closed cavity.

Temperature Conversion

The majority of medical offices in the United States use the **Fahrenheit (F)** scale to record a patient's body temperature. However, some hospitals and governmental agencies as well as health care centers in other countries use the **Celsius (C)** scale. Use the following formulas when converting between these two scales: When converting from Celsius to Fahrenheit: Multiply the Celsius reading by 9/5 and add 32.

Example:
$C = 36.1 \times 9 = 324.9 \div 5 = 64.98 + 32 = 97°F$

When converting from Fahrenheit to Celsius: Subtract the Fahrenheit reading by 32 and then multiply by 5/9.

Example:
$F = 97 - 32 = 65 \times 5 = 325 \div 9 = 36.1°C$

Most electronic thermometers are able to display both Celsius and Fahrenheit readings.

Methods for Assessing the Body Temperature

Temperatures can be taken in several locations on the body, including the mouth (orally), the armpit (axillary), the rectum (rectally), the ear (aurally or tympanic), and on the skin's surface, such as the forehead (temporal).

Oral Temperature

Temperatures obtained in the mouth or oral cavity are usually obtained using an electronic digital thermometer (Figure 11-3).

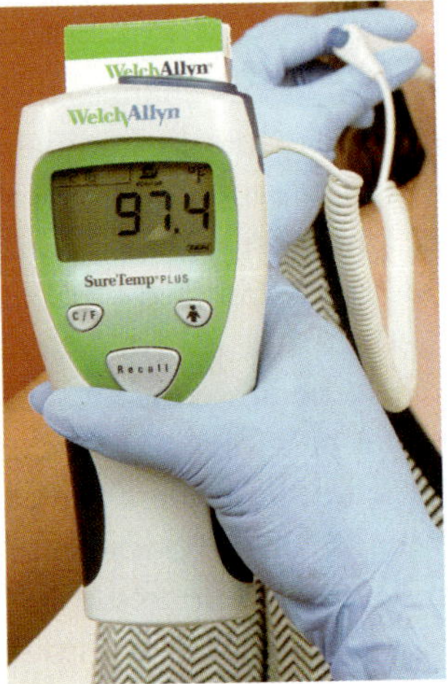

Figure 11-3 ■ Example of an electronic thermometer.

When taking an oral temperature, instruct the patient to refrain from biting down on the thermometer or probe. The blood supply under the tongue beside the frenulum linguae (see Figure 11-24) provides a good environment for temperature measurement. The vascular bed under the tongue is rich in blood supply and the air circulation within the oral cavity is diminished if the patient closes the lips around the thermometer and keeps them closed during the measurement. This ensures a more accurate core body temperature, but can be influenced by multiple factors as discussed next.

Many factors can affect an accurate oral temperature reading such as the following:

- Eating or drinking: Lowers or raises the temperature of the mouth
- Smoking: Elevates temperature in the oral cavity
- Dental problems: Diseased gums or abscesses in the mouth can interfere with obtaining a true body temperature or make it difficult for the patient to hold the thermometer comfortably in the mouth

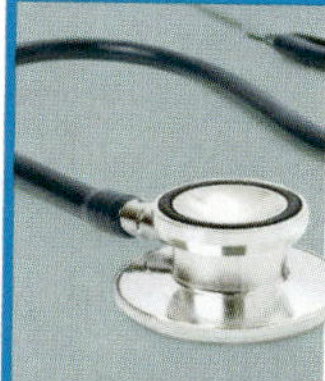

Field Smarts

Normal temperature readings by route:

Oral	98.6°F	37.0°C
Aural	99.6°F	37.7°C
Rectal	99.6°F	37.7°C
Temporal	99.6°F	37.7°C
Axillary	97.6°F	36.3°C

Notice how the aural, rectal, and temporal routes all have the same normal readings. This is because they are all considered core body temperatures because of their depth or proximity to a major artery. Also realize that temperature fluctuations may occur throughout the day. Hormonal activity also influences body temperature. Women who are ovulating will often have higher body temperatures than those that are not.

- Sinus congestion or cold: Inability to breathe through the nose will cause the patient to try and breathe through the mouth, which interferes with the procedure.
- Unconsciousness: An unconscious patient is unable to maintain muscle control to hold the thermometer in the mouth.
- Lack of understanding: Very small children, elderly patients, or non-English-speaking patients may not understand the instructions for holding the thermometer in the mouth, or may not be able to control or coordinate the muscle movement necessary.

Refer to Procedure 11-2 for the detailed steps and rationale for obtaining an oral temperature.

Rectal Temperature

The rectal method is considered one of the most accurate methods for taking body temperature because the rectum is the most closed cavity among all methods and there are fewer variables that can affect the readings. When compared with the oral temperature, rectal temperature readings are approximately 1 degree higher, with a normal reading of 99.6°F (37.7°C). This method of measurement is used most often on younger children (when accuracy is imperative), unconscious patients, and on patients who might not be able to use other methods due to mobility or other health issues. This route is seldom used in the ambulatory health care setting.

Safety is important when taking any temperature, but especially when taking rectal temperatures. When taking a rectal temperature, always hold the thermometer securely and do not allow the patient to move. The sphincter muscles of the rectum may cause involuntary movement of the thermometer, so a firm grip on the thermometer is necessary. Care should be taken to prevent trauma to the fragile mucosa when inserting the thermometer into the rectal cavity. Applying water-soluble lubricant to the thermometer will ease the insertion of the thermometer. Refer to Chapter 21 for details and rationale for obtaining a rectal temperature.

Aural Temperature

Obtaining the body temperature through the ear canal (aural) is one of the most popular methods for taking body temperature. The aural or tympanic membrane thermometer (Figure 11-4) is relatively inexpensive and easy to use. The thermometer is inserted in the ear and a digital result is provided instantly. The thermometer sensor reads the heat emitted from the tympanic membrane (eardrum) as a core temperature.

The aural route may be the preferred route when taking temperature on children, patients who are sleeping or unconscious, and on patients who cannot comply with using the oral method. The following lists conditions in which the aural method should not be used:

- When there is excessive cerumen (ear wax) in the ear
- When there is visible drainage coming from the ear, or the patient complains of ear pain or possible infection
- When the patient has bilateral hearing aids

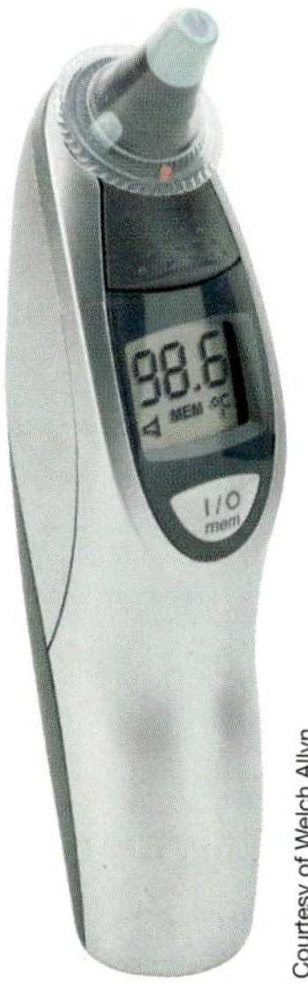

Courtesy of Welch Allyn

Figure 11-4 ■ Thermo-scan tympanic thermometer.

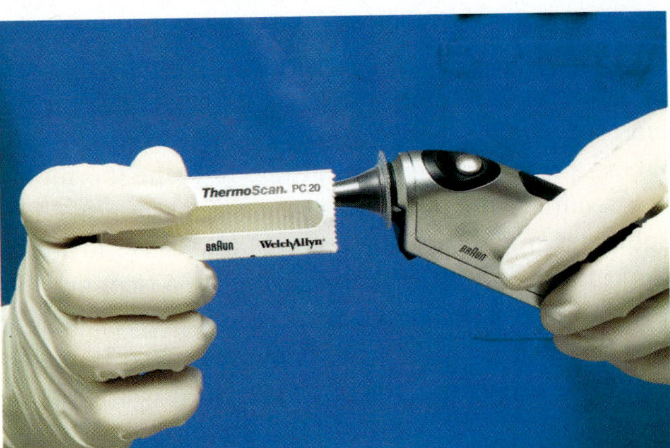

Figure 11-5 ■ Disposable probe covers are used with the tympanic thermometer to prevent cross-contamination.

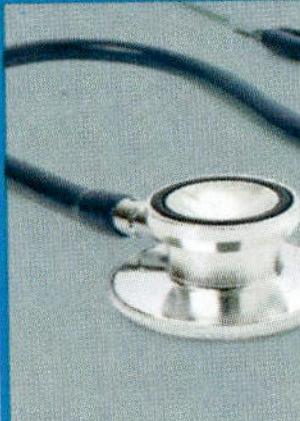

Field Smarts

If the ear canal is not straightened properly or the probe tip is not inserted into right section of the canal while you are taking an aural temperature, the reading will be inaccurate. Another factor that may impact accuracy is the size of the probe tip in comparison to the diameter of the patient's ear canal. If the tips do not match the size of the ear canal, a false reading may occur. Some offices take a reading in each ear and record the higher of the two.

The proper placement of the tympanic membrane thermometer is essential for accuracy. The probe (covered with a disposable ear tip, as seen in Figure 11-5) should be inserted so that there is a tight seal, preventing external air from influencing the reading. The actual probe tip *must* point toward the tympanic membrane. Straightening the canal will assist in providing accurate results. For adults and children above the age of three, straighten the ear canal by gently pulling up and back on the auricle. For infants and children under the age of three, gently pulling the earlobe down and back will straighten the ear canal. Refer to Procedure 11-2 for the detailed steps for performing an aural temperature reading.

Axillary Temperature

The axillary temperature is the least accurate method for obtaining a body temperature and is only used when absolutely necessary. This method is commonly used on young children and those patients who are unable to hold a thermometer in their mouths. The thermometer is placed against the skin under the arm and held in place for the proper amount of time. An average axillary temperature reading is 1 degree lower than an oral temperature reading. Procedure 11-2 lists the steps necessary to obtain an axillary temperature reading.

Temporal Thermometers

The latest technology available for determining core body temperature is the temporal thermometer (Figure 11-6). This device measures the temperature with a gentle stroke over the forehead and to the side over the temple region of the head. Because it is noninvasive and very easy to use, it is ideal for patients of all ages.

Theoretically speaking, the best place to measure core body temperature would be at the center of the heart. A temporal thermometer reads the temperature over the temporal artery, which is connected to the heart by the carotid artery. The carotid artery bifurcates into the temporal and maxillary arteries. Since there is continuous blood flow through this area and the temporal artery lies close to the surface of the skin, it is easy to access and is thought to provide an accurate body temperature reading.

When taking temperature by this method, the thermometer is gently moved over the center of the forehead and across the location of the temporal artery. The sensor scans the infrared heat given off by the blood flowing through the artery. The probe picks up the highest temperature of the area being scanned.

There are some conflicting reports as to the accuracy of this route. Sweating from the skin can cool down the area being measured, which results in an inaccurate measurement. Because of this concern, an additional reading behind the ear below the mastoid process may be taken as well. The site with the highest reading

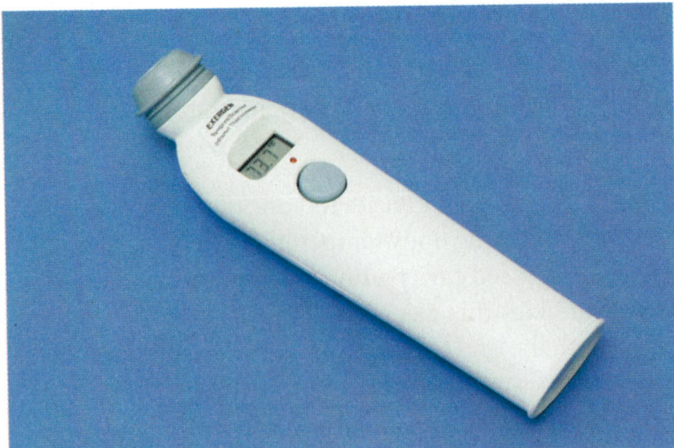

Figure 11-6 ■ New temporal thermometers make it quick and easy to obtain a temperature reading, especially on infants and children.

should be recorded in the patient's chart. Make certain that the forehead and temple region are bare, clean, and dry before using this method. Refer to Procedure 11-2 for a full procedure and figures illustrating landmarks for this method.

Determining Temperature Method

The method chosen to measure temperature will depend on the particular needs of the individual patient and the protocol of the office, which is why medical assistants should be familiar with all methods for taking body temperature.

Fever

Fever, or pyrexia, is a temporary elevation in body temperature and usually results from infection. Fever is not a disease but rather a symptom of disease. Cells that assist with immunity break open and release pyrogens, which reset the body's set-point for temperature. The increase in body temperature helps to destroy pathogens, thus aiding in the patient's recovery. The new temperature set-point tricks the body into thinking it is in a state of hypothermia, which causes shivering and an increase in respiration, heart rate, and muscle tone. This effector response helps to elevate body temperature to the new temperature set-point. Once the pathogens have been destroyed, new cells are released that cause the temperature set-point to return the original set-point. The patient becomes very warm and the body starts to sweat, releasing trapped heat. Because of increased metabolism, infants and young children often spike higher temperatures than adults. Senior adults usually run lower temperatures because of a slower metabolism and may be very sick with elevations of only one or two degrees above normal body temperature.

Fevers may be classified as follows:

- Low-grade: 99.5°F–101°F (37.5°C–38.3°C)
- Moderate: 101°F–103°F (38.3°C–39.4°C)
- High-grade: 103°F–105°F (39.4°C–41.7°C)
- Hyperpyrexia: Greater than 105°F (41.7°C)

High-grade fevers may be complicated by seizures, hallucinations, fast heart rate, and a low fluid volume. High fevers in pregnant patients are also a concern because of possible congenial defects.

Causes of Fever

Commonly, patients who present with a fever have some type of infectious process occurring within the body. Some common causes of fever are as follows:

- Infections: Bacterial, viral, mycobacterial, fungal, parasitic
- Injury: Surgery, crush injuries
- Neoplasms: Lymphoma, leukemia, hepatic carcinoma
- Connective tissue disease: Systemic lupus erythematosus (SLE), rheumatoid arthritis, vasculitis
- Malignant **hyperthermia**: Severe and rapid increase in body temperature
- Heatstroke
- Drug reactions

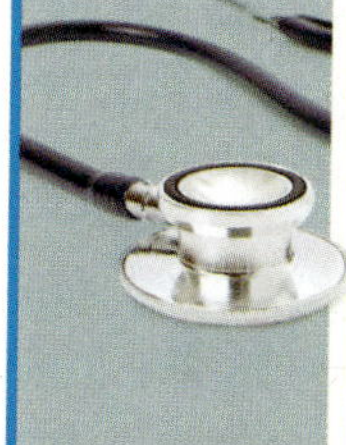

Field Smarts

It isn't necessarily the actual temperature reading associated with the fever but rather the symptoms coinciding with the fever that are of most concern. Some patients with a body temperature of 103°F (39.4°C) may not appear very sickly while other patients with a body temperature of 101°F (38.3°C) may appear very ill. Adult patients and parents of pediatric patients should be educated on the benefits of fever as well as what to watch for in fever patients. Fever is the body's way of fighting microorganisms that invade the body. Microorganisms live best at normal body temperature. Temperature elevations work with the body's immune system to destroy pathogens. Some experts now feel that patients should not take a fever reducer unless the fever climbs above 101°F (38.3°C) because it interferes with the immune response, particularly with vaccinations. Patients should be seen right away when a fever is in combination with listlessness, confusion, sore throat, breathing difficulties, headache and a stiff neck, urinary symptoms, blood in stool, swelling, or a red-hot swollen area of the skin. The reading at which you will bring a patient in for fever will vary according to the age of the patient and the patient's general health.

Table 11-2 Terms That Describe Fever Patterns

Continuous	Fever that remains elevated above the baseline, but does not fluctuate
Intermittent	Fever that comes and goes
Remittent	Fever that has peaks and drops but remains above normal
Lysis	Body temperature gradually returns to normal following a fever
Crisis	Body temperature abruptly decreases to normal, commonly referred to as the fever "breaking"

The Course of a Fever

There are some common terms used to describe the course of a fever. Table 11-2 lists those terms, along with their definitions.

When considering the core body temperature, an elevated temperature or fever is not the only possible outcome. A lowered body temperature, referred to as **hypothermia**, is considered lower than 95°F (35°C). Some common contributors to hypothermia include exposure to cold, decrease in movement (paralysis), excessive alcohol intake, starvation, hypothyroidism, and hypoglycemia. Refer to Chapter 33 to learn more about hypothermia.

Pulse

As the heart contracts, it transports blood out of the ventricles and to the rest of the body. The force of the blood distends the walls of the aorta, creating a pulse that can be felt and evaluated at different points of the body (Figure 11-7). When the pulsation reaches the peripheral arteries, slightly pressing the artery with the pads of the index and middle finger against a nearby bone allows the medical assistant to feel a pulse. The rate, rhythm, and strength of the pulse are all assessed as part of taking pulse measurements. Table 11-3 lists the various sites where a pulse may be felt.

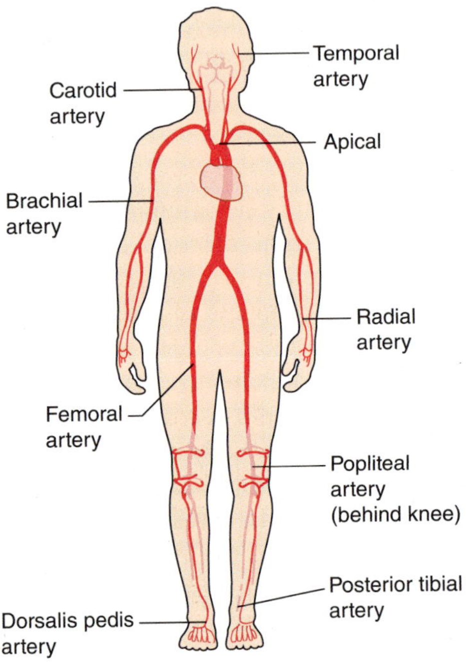

Figure 11-7 ■ There are nine pulse points located on the body where the pulse can be felt and counted.

Pulse Characteristics

When evaluating pulse or heart rate, it is important to not only count the number of times the heart beats per minute, but also to assess the rhythm and strength (volume) of the pulse. Procedure 11-3 provides steps and rationale for obtaining radial pulse and respiration rate.

The **pulse rate** may be measured for 30 seconds and multiplied by two if the intervals between each beat are regular. If the intervals between beats are irregular, or the pulse rate is excessively low or high, pulse rate should be measured for a full minute. Normal rates, which vary in different age groups, are outlined in Table 11-4. Pulse rates normally decline with age. The average range for a healthy adult patient is generally 60 to 100 beats per minute (BPM), and is referred to as a normal sinus rhythm. Many factors can affect pulse rate including the following:

- Gender: The pulse rate in women tends to run a bit higher than the pulse rate of males.
- Level of fitness: Exercise not only improves muscle tone on the outside of the body but the heart as

CRITICAL THINKING CHALLENGE

You work for a pediatrician. A mother calls and says her six-year-old daughter has been sick for the past two days, with a fever ranging between 99°F and 101°F and that her temperature always seems to go up at night. The daughter isn't complaining of any other symptoms, but the mother is concerned because of the night peaks.

1. What kind of information can you share with the mother that may help her feel more at ease?

Table 11-3 Locations of Pulse Sites (in Anatomic Position)

Pulse Site	Description of Location/Indication
Temporal	Located in the temple region of the cranium; mainly used in emergency situations when patient is bleeding profusely from the head. It is also the artery that is involved in measuring temporal temperatures.
Apical	Located at the apex of the heart or at the fifth intercostal (between the ribs) space, just to the left of the midclavicular line. This site can be palpated or can be listened to with aid of a stethoscope and is commonly used to check pulse rate in infants and children up to the age of three.
Brachial	Located in the antecubital space, at the front side of the elbow. Commonly used to measure BP in adults, as a checkpoint for pulse in infants while performing cardiopulmonary resuscitation (CPR), and is the artery that is compressed to control bleeding in the lower arm.
Carotid	Located just laterally to midline of the anterior neck. It is easy to palpate and is used as a checkpoint for pulse when performing CPR both in adults and in children. It is used to help control bleeding from the neck and lower head regions during hemorrhage situations.
Dorsalis pedis	Located on the superior surface of the foot and is often difficult to palpate. It is the site that is routinely used to assess circulation in the foot.
Femoral	Located in the center of the groin region. This artery is used to evaluate circulation in the lower extremities and to control bleeding in the lower leg.
Popliteal	Located on the posterior surface of the knee. May be used for BPs when brachial pulse is not accessible. It is most easily palpated when the knee is slightly bent.
Posterior tibial	Located on the medial aspect of the ankle, posterior to the ankle bone. It is used to evaluate circulation in the feet.
Radial	Located on the radial or thumb-side of the wrist, just superior to the thumb. The radial artery lies over the radius bone. It is the most common site for checking pulse rates in adults.

Table 11-4 Pulse Rates

Patient Population	Average Pulse Rate (BPM)
Newborn to 3 months	80–160
3 months to 2 years	75–160
Toddler (Age 2 to 3 years)	60–140
Children (Age 3 to 10 years)	60–140
Adult (10 and above)	60–100

well. When the heart muscle is strong, it does not have to beat as fast to move blood around the body.

- Emotional status: Emotional states, such as fear and rage, temporarily raise pulse rate.
- Pregnancy: Because of increased metabolism, heart rate increases.
- Fever: Causes an increase in heart or pulse rate.
- Medications: Different medications can elevate or decrease pulse rates.
- Exercise or an increase in activity: Temporarily increases pulse rate.

An excessively rapid heart rate, over 100 BPM, is referred to as **tachycardia** and may be a sign of fever, hemorrhage, dehydration, or heart disease. Vigorous exercise can cause the heart rate to exceed 200 BPM, which is why patients should be examined prior to the start of a strenuous exercise program to make certain that their hearts can handle the increased intensity.

An abnormally slow heart rate, below 60 BPM, is referred to as **bradycardia**. Slow heart rate is often seen in athletes and during times of sleep.

Pulse rhythm refers to the interval timing between measured beats. The intervals between each beat should be consistent and symmetric. Any irregularities are referred to as **arrhythmias** or **dysrhythmias**. Following speculation of an arrhythmia, a provider may order an electrocardiogram (EKG or ECG) to help determine the cause for the irregular rhythm. Refer to Chapter 14 for more information on ECGs.

The **pulse volume**, or strength of the pulse, refers to the amount of blood being discharged from the heart. It should remain consistent and strong. If the amount of blood pumped from the heart to the body is diminished, the pulse will feel *weak* or *thready*. The pulse rate will usually increase to compensate for the lower volume, and would be referred to as *rapid and thready.* This type of pulse is often seen in patients with volume depletion or dehydration. An increase in pulse volume would be termed as a *bounding* pulse. When documenting in the patient record, all characteristics of the pulse should be noted, including rate, rhythm, and volume.

Taking an Apical Pulse

The common location for assessing pulse is in the radial artery; however, when a radial pulse is difficult to palpate, an apical pulse should be performed.

Field Smarts

If you suspect an irregular rate or rhythm after taking a radial pulse, you should follow up by obtaining an apical pulse. This method of obtaining a pulse rate is generally easier to evaluate and more accurate in measurement.

An apical pulse is taken with the aid of a stethoscope. The diaphragm of the stethoscope is placed over the apex of the heart or the fifth intercostal space just to the left of the midclavicular line. Refer to Figure 11-8 for proper placement of the stethoscope when performing an apical pulse.

Apical-Radial Pulse and Pulse Deficit

If a provider orders an apical-radial pulse, two health care workers will take the pulse simultaneously; one counting the radial pulse and the other counting the apical pulse. Subtracting the radial measurement from the apical measurement equals the pulse deficit. For example: If the radial pulse is 72 and the apical pulse is 91, then the pulse deficit is 19 (91 − 72 = 19). This measurement is an indication that the strength of the contractions may not be sufficient enough to force adequate blood to the extremities. A pulse deficit is common in patients with atrial fibrillation. When documenting the results, include both pulse rates and the deficit calculation. Procedure 11-4 provides more information and the rationale in performing an apical pulse assessment.

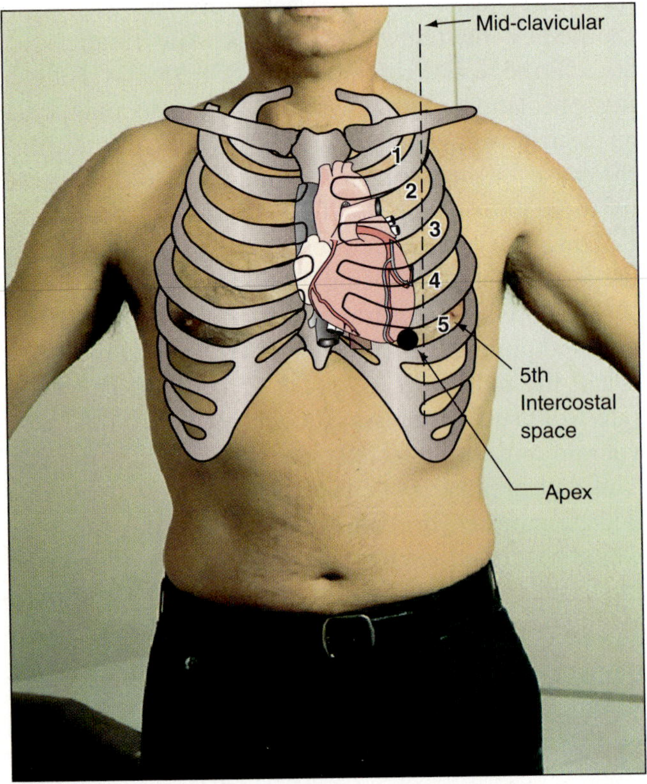

Figure 11-8 ■ Location of the apex of the heart where an apical pulse is counted.

CRITICAL THINKING CHALLENGE

You are having great difficulty locating a patient's radial pulse. You have attempted to count the pulse rate in both wrists but you just can't feel it.

1. **What should you do?**

Respiration

The respiratory system is responsible for the transfer of oxygen (O_2) and carbon dioxide (CO_2) within the body. Essential for life, oxygen is taken into the body and distributed by the circulatory system to be used by all cells. **Respiration**, or the act of breathing, begins with the process of **inspiration** or **inhalation**, bringing air or oxygen into the body. After traveling through the respiratory branches in the lungs, alveoli (microscopic air sacs) transfer the required oxygen to the capillaries. As the blood in the circulatory system distributes the necessary oxygen to the cells, it also transfers carbon dioxide out of the cells and back to the lungs to be removed from the body through **expiration** or **exhalation** (the exhaling of waste products to the outer environment). Figure 11-9 illustrates what happens during the respiration process.

The structure within the brain that controls respiration is the medulla oblongata. When carbon dioxide levels rise in the blood stream, the medulla oblongata is alerted, and it triggers the process of respiration. The diaphragm, through contractions, alters the pressure within the thoracic cavity in the chest, causing involuntary inspiration, or the process of "breathing in." After breathing in, the pressure inside the lungs is now less than the atmospheric pressure. This causes expiration to occur, to balance or equalize the inside and outside pressure. While breathing is often a process done naturally and unconsciously, the body is also able to alter the rate, depth, and pattern voluntarily. Figure 11-10 illustrates the position of the diaphragm during inspiration and expiration.

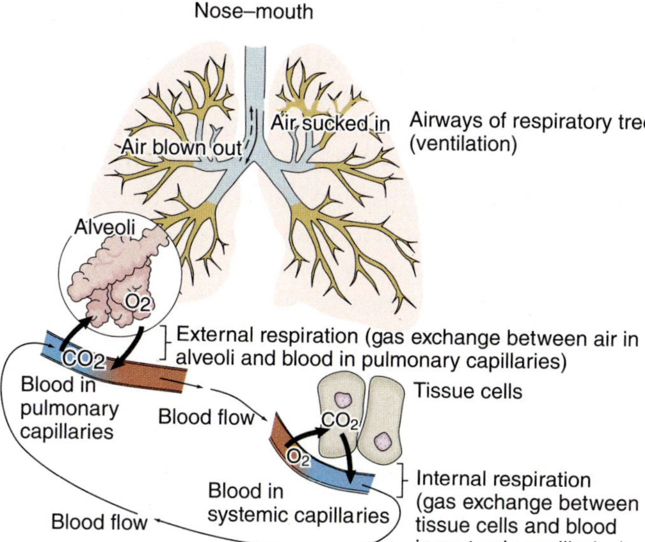

Figure 11-9 ■ What occurs during internal and external respiration.

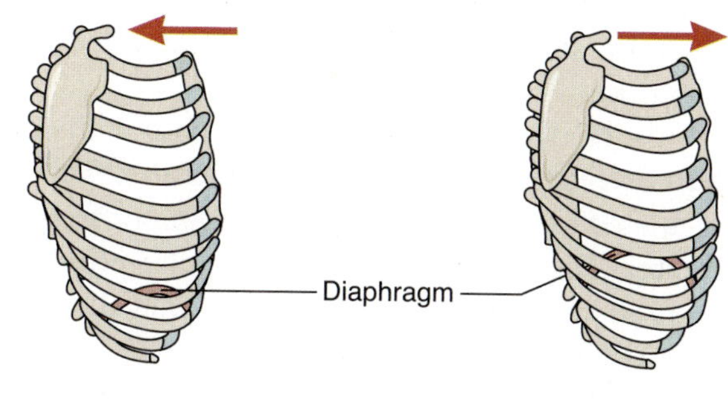

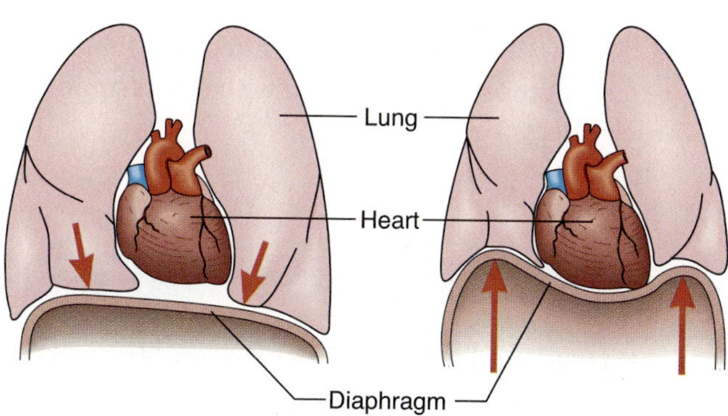

Figure 11-10 ■ The positioning of the diaphragm during inspiration (left) and expiration (right).

Respiratory Rate

The rate of respiration is documented as the number of breaths per minute. Table 11-5 lists the average respiratory rates for different age groups. Note that average respiratory rates decrease with age. Procedure 11-3 details the steps involved in obtaining an accurate respiratory rate.

To obtain an accurate respiratory rate, patients should be unaware that you are measuring their respiration. Remember, breathing can be involuntary or voluntary, and patients may inadvertently or purposefully alter their breathing if they are aware of your actions.

Table 11-5 Average Respiratory Values Measured in Breaths per Minute

Age	Rate
Newborn to 3 months	30–60/min
3 months to 2 years	30–60/min
Toddler (Age 2 to 3 years)	24–40/min
Children (Age 3 to 10 years)	18–30/min
Adult (10 and above)	12–16/min

Factors That Affect Respiration

Like temperature and pulse, there are several factors that affect respiration, including the following:

- Physical activity: Activity normally increases respiration. (Did the patient just climb three flights of stairs?)
- Emotional factors: Emotions such as fear, panic, or rage may temporarily increase respiration.
- Medications: Some medications can cause respiration to either increase or decrease. Respiratory stimulants such as bronchodilators and decongestants cause an increase in respiration, and depressants such as barbiturates and tranquilizers cause a decrease in respiration.
- Age: Respirations typically decrease with age, but may increase if pulmonary disease is present.
- Infectious states: Associated fevers may cause an increase in respiratory rate.

Irregular Breathing Patterns

Patients often experience irregular breathing patterns during respiratory illness or following a life-threatening injury. Table 11-6 lists some of those patterns as well as their characteristics.

Depth during inhalation must also be noted. Three terms used to document depth include the following:

- Shallow, meaning the chest rises minimally
- Normal
- Deep, meaning the chest rises excessively

The depth of inspiration versus expiration will be further evaluated by the provider. A prolonged expiration might indicate obstructive lung disease. Any difficulty noted while breathing should be documented.

The following terms may be used when describing the patient's respiration:

- **Dyspnea** means difficult or labored breathing.
- **Orthopnea** refers to breathing easiest while in a sitting or standing position.

Table 11-6 Irregular Breathing Patterns (Rhythm)

Breathing Pattern	Characteristics
Cheyne–Stokes breathing	A condition in which the patient exhibits deep breathing followed by periods of apnea, normally observed during sleep. Conditions in which this breathing pattern may be observed include heart or lung disease, drug-induced respiratory depression, or brain injury. This pattern is commonly seen prior to death.
Ataxic breathing	Irregular and unpredictable periods of breathing with no specific pattern. This type of breathing may indicate brain damage.
Sighing	Audible exhaling during a long deep breath. While some sighing is normal, frequent and regular sighs should be noted.

- A rapid respiration rate with normal or shallow respirations is referred to as **tachypnea**.
- Rapid and deep respirations are called **hyperpnea** or **hyperventilation**.
- Breathing abnormally slow is referred to as **bradypnea**.

Beyond the basic vital screening, the provider will evaluate the quality of respirations, including any sounds made during respiration. Normally, breathing should be quiet and effortless. Table 11-7 lists some of the breath sounds a provider might observe. Some breath sounds may only be heard with a stethoscope. Others may be obvious during a medical assistant's initial screening of the patient. If the medical assistant hears any unusual sounds coming from the patient's lungs, the provider should be notified right away.

Blood Pressure

A patient's blood pressure (BP) measures the amount of force exerted on the arterial walls as the heart ventricles contract and relax. When documenting BP, it is recorded as a fraction. The phase at which the cardiac ventricles contract (forcing blood from the ventricles into the pulmonary artery and aorta) is referred to as systole. **Systole** occurs when the greatest amount of force is applied to the arterial vessels and is referred to as the **systolic pressure** when measuring BP. The systolic pressure is recorded as the numerator (or top number) when documenting BP. The phase when the cardiac ventricles relax is referred to as **diastole**. The pressure is clearly lower during this phase as the pressure is produced by the recoil of the arteries and is referred to as **diastolic pressure**. The diastolic number is recorded as the denominator (or lower number) of the measurement. The standard unit in which BP is measured is millimeters of mercury (mmHg); however, the unit does not have to be recorded when documenting BPs.

The difference between the systolic and diastolic pressure is referred to as the **pulse pressure**. This can be calculated by subtracting the denominator from the numerator. The normal range for the pulse pressure is between 30 and 50. Table 11-8 lists normal BP ranges for different age groups.

Variables That Can Affect Blood Pressure

There are several variables that can affect BP. Table 11-9 lists several of those factors, along with a description of how each affects BP.

Table 11-7 Breath Sounds and Possible Indications

Breath Sound	Characteristics	Possible Indications
Rales	Usually heard on inspiration intermittently Usually sounds wet Pitch may vary	Local inflammatory process Congestive heart failure (CHF) Pulmonary edema Pneumonia
Rhonchi	Usually heard on expiration, but may also be heard on inspiration Sound may resemble a "honk" or snore	This may indicate some narrowing in the bronchi, and secretions in the larger airways At times, these can clear with coughing
Wheezing	High pitched, almost musical sounds heard during inspiration and/or expiration Can be heard at the mouth and chest	Asthma, chronic obstructive pulmonary disease (COPD), CHF If localized, there may be a partial obstruction, possibly a tumor or foreign body
Stridor	Wheeze-like crowing, heard during inspiration Often louder in the neck region than in the chest	Partial obstruction of larynx or trachea Croup Usually an urgent medical situation
Pleural rub	Creaking sounds similar to crackles but confined to specific area and discrete Usually heard on inspiration and expiration	Inflammation of pleural membranes

Table 11-8 Normal Values of Blood Pressure

Age	Systolic	Diastolic
Newborn to 3 months	60–70 mmHg	
3 months to 2 years	70–74 mmHg	
Toddler (Age 2 to 3 years)	84–113 mmHg	39–69 mmHg
Children (Age 3 to 10 years)	84–123 mmHg	39–82 mmHg
Adult (10 and above)	100–139 mmHg	59–89 mmHg

Equipment Requirements

When measuring BP, it is essential that all equipment used is in good working order and appropriately matched to the size of the patient. The stethoscope is used to listen to different sounds produced within the body, such as a pulsating artery. Figure 11-11 illustrates the different components of a stethoscope and includes the ear pieces, tubing, and chest piece (which may include the bell, diaphragm, or both). Component descriptions include the following:

1. Ear pieces: Should be cleaned with alcohol prior to use and should be positioned so that they point toward the ear canal. The small holes in the end of the ear pieces must transfer the **Korotkoff sounds**, the sounds that are heard during a BP measurement. If the holes are pushed against the sides of the ears, hearing will be difficult, if not impossible.
2. Tubing: Can be either single or double tubing. Tubing transfers the sounds from the chest pieces to the ear pieces. In high-quality stethoscopes with double tubing, sounds may be easier to hear. There is a downside, however. When the tubes touch, extraneous rubbing or tapping sounds may be heard and mistaken for Korotkoff sounds, causing a false reading. Single- or double-tubing stethoscopes are adequate for measuring BP.
3. Chest piece: This is the component in which sounds are transmitted. It may consist of a diaphragm, a bell, or both. The diaphragm is used for high-pitched sounds such as bowel sounds, while the bell is used

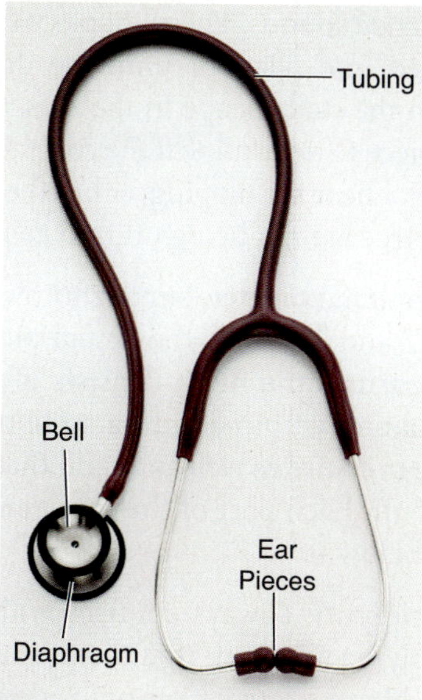

Figure 11-11 ■ Different parts of the stethoscope.

Table 11-9 Variables That Influence BP Readings

Factor	Description
Physiologic changes due to aging	As the patient ages, BP normally increases. Children generally have lower BP than adults. Older adults may have higher BP than younger adults due to a loss of arterial elasticity or occlusion in the arterial walls.
Emotional state	A patient who is anxious or excited may have elevated BP. "White coat hypertension" is often related to anxiety associated with the physician or just being in the medical office.
Medications	Many medications will raise or lower BP, which is why it is essential to obtain a complete listing of all medications the patient is taking including herbs, vitamins, and mineral supplements.
Gender and race	Women's BP fluctuates with life-span changes, puberty, and menopause. Race and heredity will affect BP as well. African Americans tend to have higher BP readings than other races.
Diet and other chemicals	Electrolytes in the diet, such as sodium, can have an impact on BP over an extended period of time. Immediate changes may occur after smoking, consuming caffeine, or using illegal substances such as cocaine.
Exercise	During exercise, BP will temporarily rise.
Positioning of patient	The normal position for taking BP is sitting. If another position is used, such as standing or lying down, it must be noted in the patient record.
Diurnal variances or time of day	During periods of higher metabolism such as when eating or exercising, BP will generally rise. Conversely, when metabolism is at its lowest during periods of sleep, BP will decline.
Inappropriate equipment size	Cuff sizes must be appropriate for the size of the patient. Large adult cuffs should be used on larger patients and pediatric cuffs should be used on children or very small adults. Cuffs that are too small may cause falsely elevated readings, while cuffs that are too large may cause falsely low readings.
Pain or discomfort	Pain or discomfort from a full bladder or constipation may cause BP to rise.

for low-pitched sounds. The chest piece can be rotated until clicked into place or until the desired side is open. With the stethoscope in the ears, tap gently on the chest piece to determine if the correct side is open. If you cannot hear the tapping, either the ear pieces or the chest piece are not being utilized correctly.

The **sphygmomanometer**, similar to those shown in Figures 11-12 and 11-13, is the actual piece of equipment that measures the BP. It consists of an inflatable bladder contained within a cuff, a scale or gauge that measures the pressure as well as a bulb that inflates and deflates the cuff. Each part of the sphygmomanometer is described below:

1. Bladder and cuff: Always confirm with the patient before applying a BP cuff that there is no reason you can't take blood pressure on one side or the other, such as on the side the patient has had a mastectomy or a fistula placed. The cuff should be wrapped securely around the upper arm or thigh and secured with a Velcro fastener. The center or bladder of the cuff should be placed directly over the brachial artery if using the arm for the measurement. Most cuffs have an arrow or another type of symbol that should be pointed directly over the artery being used. It is extremely important to use the appropriate cuff size to ensure an accurate measurement. If the cuff size is too small, a falsely elevated pressure may occur. Conversely, if the cuff is too large, a falsely low pressure may occur. According to the American Association of Family Practitioners (AAFP), a standard-size adult cuff should not be used for any patient whose upper arm is larger than 33 centimeters (cm) in diameter (just over 13 inches). Instead, a large adult cuff should be used. A thigh cuff should be used in patients whose upper arm diameter is larger than 45 cm or 20.4 inches. Figure 11-14 displays different sized cuffs that are used to obtain a BP.
2. Gauge for measurement: May be either an aneroid gauge or a digital readout. The aneroid type becomes more inaccurate with extended use, so gauges will need to be recalibrated on a regular basis by a certified technician. The aneroid gauge has a round scale or dial that is calibrated in millimeters of mercury (mm/Hg), in increments of two. If calibrated correctly, the needle will register zero when the cuff is completely deflated. The cuff contains a section where the aneroid gauge can be attached. This will prevent accidental dropping of the gauge and allows the medical assistant to have a free hand. The millimeter markings are small; therefore, the gauge must be placed so it can be easily read. A digital readout manometer simply displays the reading on a small screen.
3. Bulb: This part inflates and deflates the bladder and cuff. It should be handled with the dominant hand,

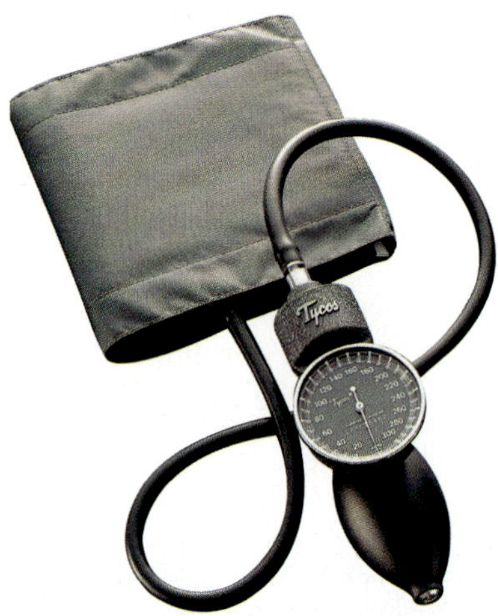

Figure 11-12 ■ An aneroid sphygmomanometer.

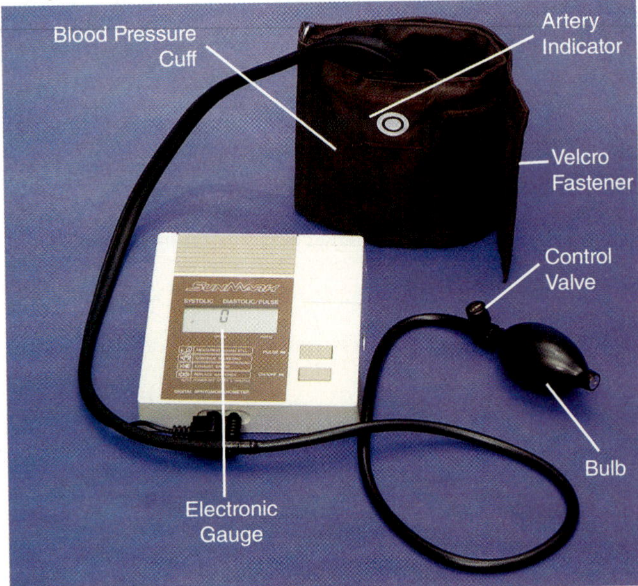

Figure 11-13 ■ A digital sphygmomanometer.

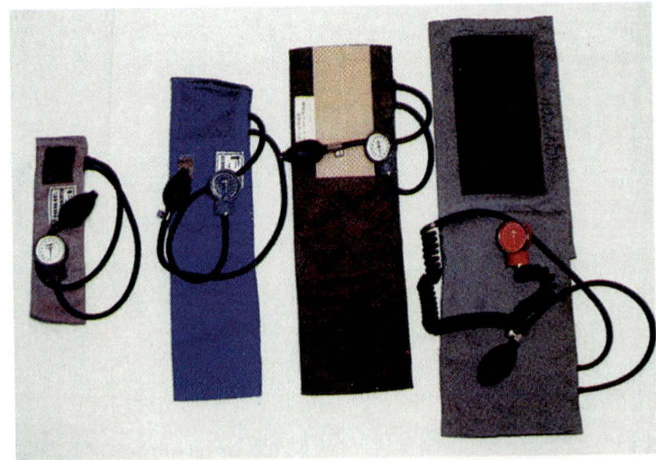

Figure 11-14 ■ The correct size of BP cuff must be used to obtain an accurate reading. From left to right, this photo shows cuffs for pediatric, adult, large adult, and thigh.

allowing the rotation of the control valve with only the thumb and forefinger. This leaves the remainder of the fingers available to compress the bulb to inflate the bladder.

Blood Pressure Classifications

It is important to routinely monitor BPs since **hypertension** (high BP) affects all organs. The eyes, heart, brain, and kidneys may develop pathological changes due to hypertension. In 2014, the Eighth Joint National Committee (JNC 8) recommendations were released to replace the JNC 7 guidelines on BP management. Prior classifications of prehypertension and hypertension were replaced with simplified BP control goals. Any BP under 140/90 is considered controlled for most patients, but a goal of less than 150/90 is used for patients over 60 years old.

Korotkoff Sounds

Correctly hearing and interpreting the sounds during the measurement of a BP involves listening to the different sounds as blood begins to flow back into the brachial artery. Initially, a faint pulsing sound is heard, which gradually increases in intensity. The first sound that is heard is registered as the systolic pressure. This is phase one of the Korotkoff sounds. As the sound intensifies, it takes on a swooshing tone, which is phase two. As pressure is slowly and steadily released from the bladder, the sounds become stronger, signaling phase three. During phase four, the pulsation sounds become softer and more muffled. This distinct change is the diastolic pressure in children. Phase five is when the sounds are totally inaudible, which is the diastolic pressure in adults. The difference between phase four and phase five should normally be only a few mmHg. If the difference between phase four and five is greater than 10 mmHg, then record all three measurements: the systolic, phase four, and phase five (e.g., 162/94/68). It is important to note that occasionally the Korotkoff sounds never disappear. Refer to Procedure 11-5 for a complete list of steps necessary to obtain an accurate BP reading.

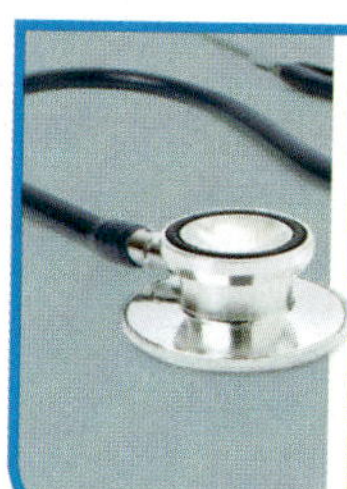

Field Smarts

Terms associated with low BP include **hypotension** (low BP) and **orthostatic hypotension** (BP that drops upon standing).

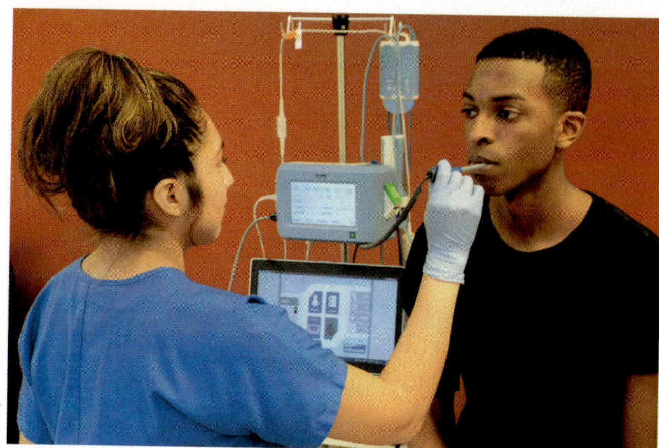

Figure 11-15 ■ The medical assistant is able to get all vital signs using one piece of equipment. Results can be sent electronically to the EHR.

Electronic Vital Signs

As the United States moves toward electronic health records (EHR), manufacturers are developing products that directly interface with the practice's EHR. Many of these devices provide seamless connectivity and make workflow much easier. Figure 11-15 illustrates an electronic piece of equipment that uploads the results of the patient's vital signs into the patient's EHR with just a few clicks of the mouse.

Pain Assessment

The assessment of pain is now being considered as the fifth vital sign. It is often difficult for patients to rate or describe their pain. The medical assistant should provide a measuring tool that will turn a patient's subjective description into a more objective measurable field. One tool that may be used to measure pain is a number scale. Ask the patient to rate the pain using the numbers 0 to 10 (0 represents no pain and 10 represents the worst pain ever experienced). Continuous monitoring of pain during each office visit will show trends in pain and may have a bearing on treatment plans. Another tool that can be used to describe pain is the use of pictures of faces illustrating different emotions. This type of tool is commonly used when working with pediatric patients or patients with language barriers. Refer to Chapter 5 for further explanation on assessment of pain and examples of tools that can be used to measure pain.

Pulse Oximetry

The measurement of pulse oximetry indicates the amount of arterial oxygen (O_2) saturation in the blood. An external probe is attached to an area that has good blood perfusion, such as the earlobe, fingertip, or toe.

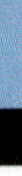
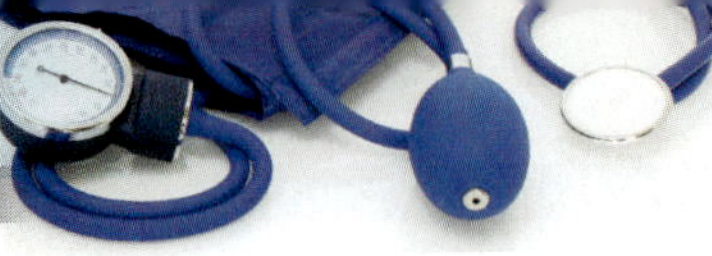

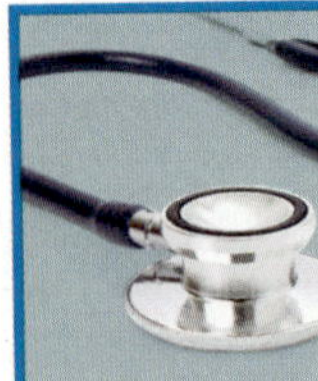

Field Smarts

Auscultatory gap is an occurrence in which Korotkoff sounds diminish and become inaudible (a period of silence) during phase two or phase three of the BP measurement. The sounds later reappear as the BP cuff is deflated. Auscultatory gap is most common in patients with hypertension and in older patients. To make certain that you obtain the correct systolic pressure, try performing BP using the palpatory method. Lifting the arm in the air prior to inflation of the cuff may also help to eliminate this occurrence.

CRITICAL THINKING CHALLENGE

When performing a BP measurement on Mr. Timmons, you obtained a reading of 164/110. Dr. Wong retook the BP and obtained a reading of 190/110. You are frustrated because you pumped the cuff up to 180 but didn't hear anything until 164.

1. **What may be the reason for the discrepancy?**

Depending on the equipment used, the oximeter may calculate oxygen saturation and pulse rate simultaneously. An oxygen saturation of less than 95% implies that oxygen saturation is not adequate and that intervention is necessary. Refer to Chapter 15 to learn more about pulse oximetry.

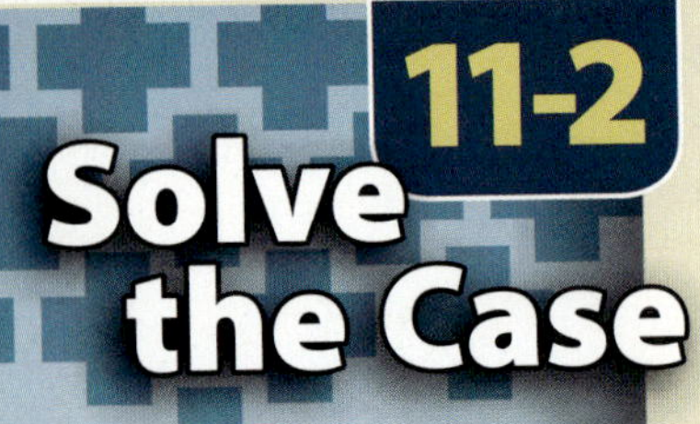

11-2 Solve the Case

Dr. Schwartz has completed his exam of Mrs. Collins and is concerned about her health and home status. During the exam Dr. Schwartz repeated the patient's BP and obtained a reading of (166/102) and an SpO_2 reading of 88. The patient scored well on her stroke assessment test but the doctor is still very concerned about the patient's vital sign ranges. The doctor suspects the patient may have had a transient ischemic attack (TIA) but wants to rule out factors that may mimic the symptoms of a TIA. He asks you to recheck the patient's vital signs, check the patient's blood sugar, perform an ECG, and obtain a rapid PT/INR (prothrombin time/international normalized ratio) on the patient before he prescribes any medications or schedules the patient for a magnetic resonance imaging (MRI) of the brain.

1. **Why do you think the provider performed an SpO_2 reading on the patient?**
2. **What is a normal SpO_2 reading?**

All of the tests you performed come back within acceptable ranges for the patient, however, the patient's BP is now back up to 182/108?

3. **What should be your next step with this patient?**
4. **Is there anyone that should be notified regarding the patient's current status?**

PROCEDURE 11-1

Obtain the Height and Weight of an Adult Patient

Objective:

To accurately obtain and document an adult's height and weight.

Equipment/Supplies:

- Upright scale
- Paper towel
- Patient chart/EHR

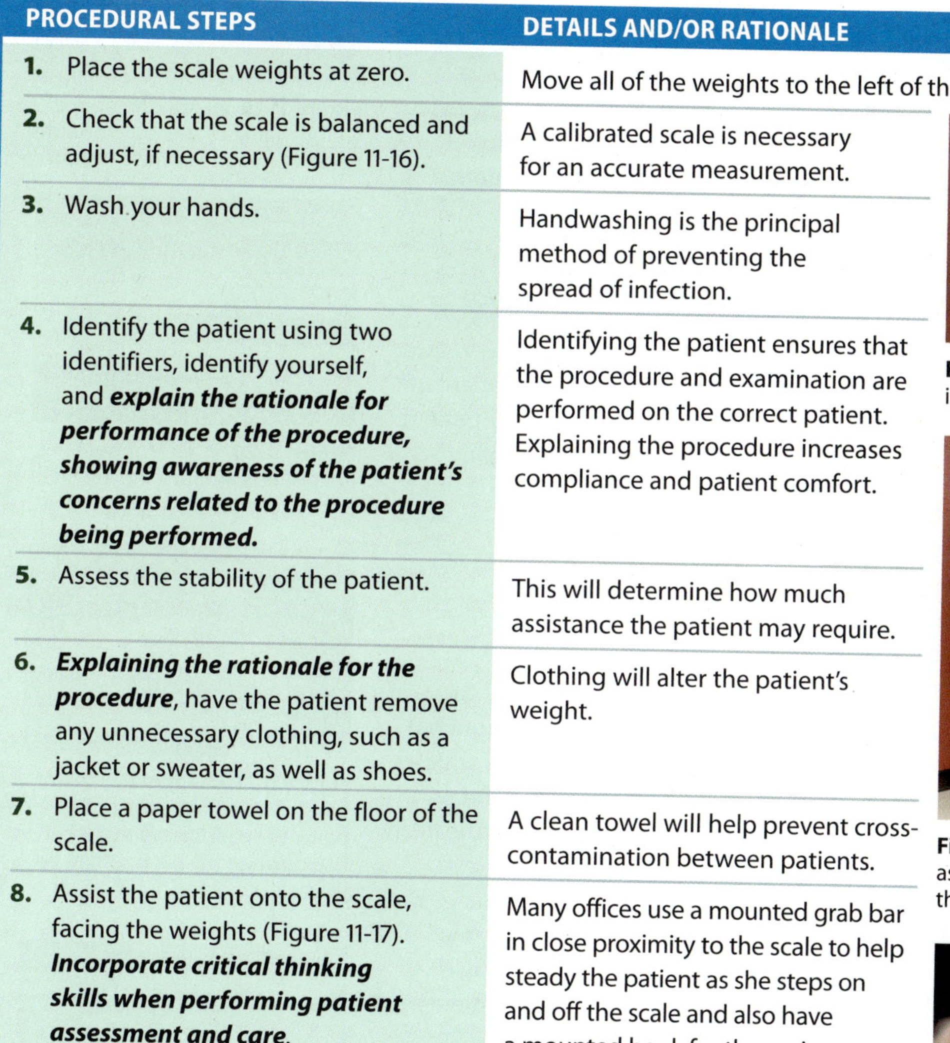

PROCEDURAL STEPS	DETAILS AND/OR RATIONALE
1. Place the scale weights at zero.	Move all of the weights to the left of the scale.
2. Check that the scale is balanced and adjust, if necessary (Figure 11-16).	A calibrated scale is necessary for an accurate measurement.
3. Wash your hands.	Handwashing is the principal method of preventing the spread of infection.
4. Identify the patient using two identifiers, identify yourself, and ***explain the rationale for performance of the procedure, showing awareness of the patient's concerns related to the procedure being performed.***	Identifying the patient ensures that the procedure and examination are performed on the correct patient. Explaining the procedure increases compliance and patient comfort.
5. Assess the stability of the patient.	This will determine how much assistance the patient may require.
6. ***Explaining the rationale for the procedure***, have the patient remove any unnecessary clothing, such as a jacket or sweater, as well as shoes.	Clothing will alter the patient's weight.
7. Place a paper towel on the floor of the scale.	A clean towel will help prevent cross-contamination between patients.
8. Assist the patient onto the scale, facing the weights (Figure 11-17). ***Incorporate critical thinking skills when performing patient assessment and care.***	Many offices use a mounted grab bar in close proximity to the scale to help steady the patient as she steps on and off the scale and also have a mounted hook for the patient to place her jacket and purse.
9. Instruct the patient to stand on the center of the scale and to hold still. Move the lower weight first, then slowly move the upper weight until the scale arrow is balanced (Figure 11-18).	Motion can alter the results of the weight. Remind the patient to remain still during the measurement.

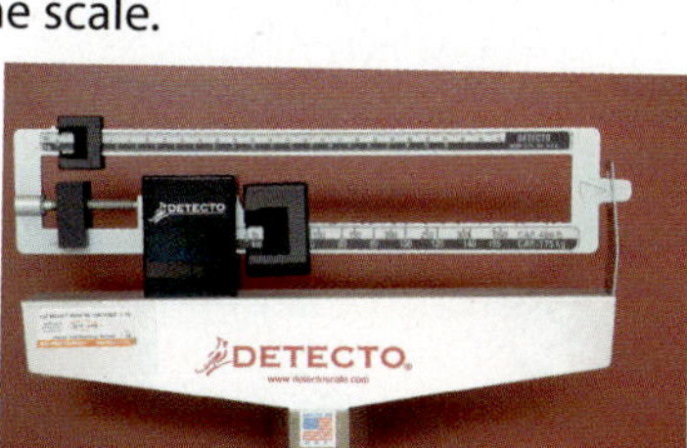

Figure 11-16 ■ The scale is balanced in this picture.

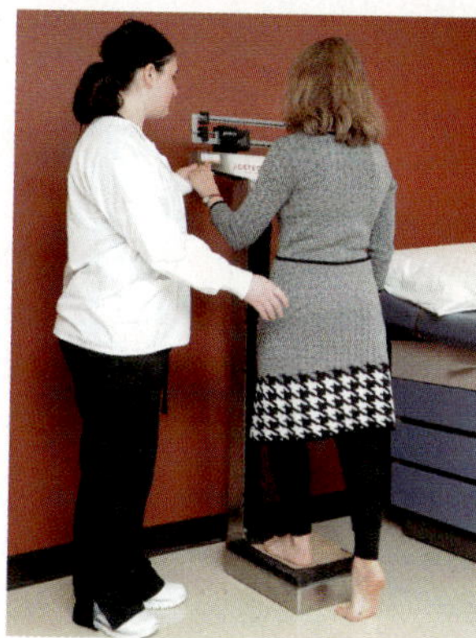

Figure 11-17 ■ The medical assistant assists the patient onto the scale.

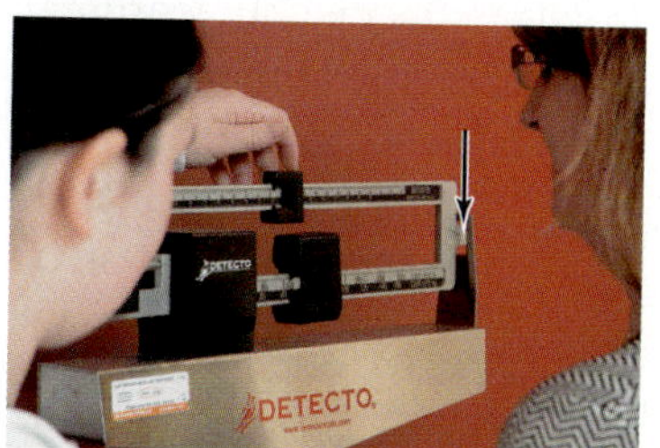

Figure 11-18 ■ The medical assistant moves the lower weight first, then the upper weight until the scale is balanced.

continues

PROCEDURE 11-1 continued

PROCEDURAL STEPS	DETAILS AND/OR RATIONALE
10. Record the measurement by adding the measurement from the lower weight to the measurement from the upper weight (Figure 11-19). (When reading the measurements from the upper bar, the longer calibration markings are pound increments and the shorter line increments are in quarter and half pound increments. The arrows in Figure 11-20 point to 36 ¼, 36 ½, and 36 ¾ pounds.)	
11. Return the weights to zero.	The scale must be balanced to obtain an accurate measurement.
12. Assist the patient off the scale.	Slips and falls may occur when moving off any equipment. Providing assistance will reduce the chance for a mishap.
13. Raise the calibrated height bar to a height that would be greater than the patient's height.	This is performed with the patient off the scale to avoid striking the patient in the head with the height bar.
14. Extend the bar used to measure to a horizontal position.	
15. Assist the patient back onto the scale platform, back toward the measurement tool. Have the patient stand as erect as possible.	
16. Lower the horizontal bar slowly and gently until it reaches the top of the patient's head, forming a 90° angle with the height bar (Figure 11-21).	Continue to hold onto the height bar while the patient steps off the scale to prevent the bar from falling and possibly hitting the patient in the head.
17. Assist the patient off the platform.	This ensures patient safety.
18. Read the height measurement by reading from the top of the bar going down reading it at the junction of the stationary calibration rod and the movable calibration rod (Figure 11-22).	Read the height at the moveable point of the ruler. The markings are measured in ¼ inch increments.
19. Place the measurement bar back to its original position.	
20. Discard the paper towel.	

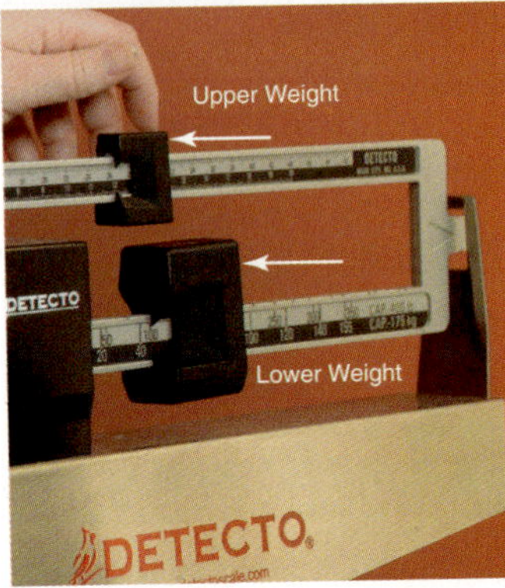

Figure 11-19 ■ Add the upper weight value to the lower weight value to get an accurate weight.

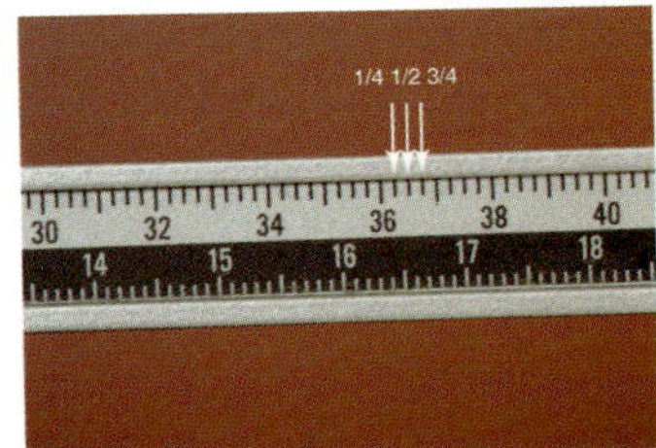

Figure 11-20 ■ The longer lines are pounds and the shorter lines are in quarters and halves.

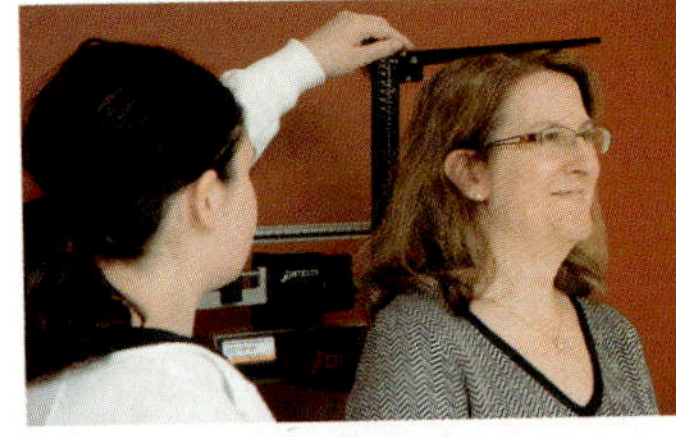

Figure 11-21 ■ Adjust the height bar so it rests on the top of the patient's head. Be sure to push the hair down so the bar is resting on the head itself and not the hair.

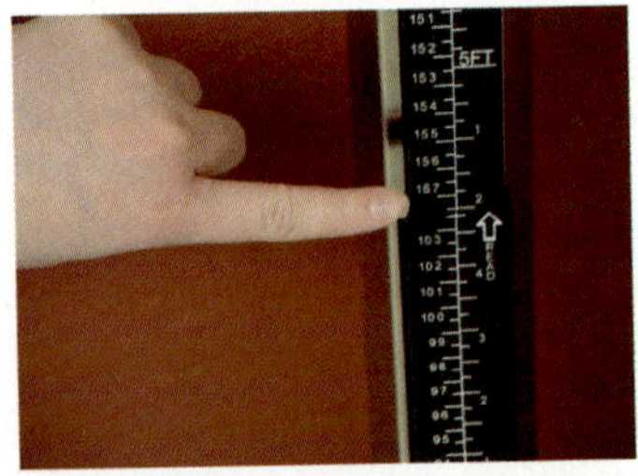

Figure 11-22 ■ A close-up view of the numbers on the height bar used to obtain an accurate height.

continues

PROCEDURE 11-1 continued

PROCEDURAL STEPS	DETAILS AND/OR RATIONALE
21. Document the results in the patient record (if you didn't already). Convert weight into kilograms if necessary. Calculate and record BMI when using a paper chart. ***Reassure the patient of the accuracy of the test results.***	The kilogram measurement may be used in some medication calculations.

DOCUMENTATION EXAMPLE:

12-05-XX 9:35 a.m.	Wt. 135 lbs Ht. 4'11", BMI 27.3, shoes removed. Carla Carlyle, CMA (AAMA)-----------------

PROCEDURE 11-2

Obtain Oral, Aural, Axillary, and Temporal Body Temperatures

Objective:

To obtain and document an accurate oral body temperature, aural body temperature, axillary body temperature, and temporal body temperature.

Equipment/Supplies:

Electronic thermometer (for both oral and axillary methods), aural thermometer, and temporal thermometer.

- Probe covers
- Alcohol pads
- Patient chart/EHR

PROCEDURAL STEPS	DETAILS AND/OR RATIONALE
1. Wash your hands. (Gloving is optional.)	Handwashing is the principal method of preventing the spread of infection.
2. Assemble the equipment.	Having all the necessary supplies ready before obtaining the temperature saves time.
3. Identify the patient using two identifiers, identify yourself, and ***explain the rationale for performance of the procedure, showing awareness of the patient's concerns related to the procedure being performed.***	Identifying the patient ensures that the procedure and examination are performed on the correct patient. Explaining the procedure increases compliance and patient comfort.
4. *Take an oral temperature*	
a. Ask if the patient has ingested hot or cold food or beverages or smoked within the last half hour.	Ingesting hot or cold liquids or foods and smoking can adversely affect the temperature reading making it inaccurate. (Either allow patient to wait or select another method if any of the variables apply.)

continues

PROCEDURE 11-2 continued

PROCEDURAL STEPS	DETAILS AND/OR RATIONALE
b. Make certain that the thermometer is on the appropriate setting (oral or axillary) and cover it with a disposable probe cover (Figure 11-23). ***Incorporate critical thinking skills when performing patient assessment and care.***	It is important to select the correct route setting to obtain an accurate reading.
c. Place the thermometer in the patient's mouth under the tongue to the right or left side of the frenulum linguae (Figure 11-24).	This area of the mouth is highly vascular and gives a more accurate temperature reading.
d. Instruct to the patient not to clench or bite down on the thermometer and to hold the mouth closed and breathe through the nostrils, not through the mouth.	Clenching or biting down on the thermometer may cause improper placement of the thermometer and result in an inaccurate reading.
e. Keep the thermometer in place until a tone or beep is heard.	The beep indicates that the thermometer is ready to be read.
f. Read the digital display (Figure 11-25), remove and discard probe into the trash can, and place electronic thermometer back into the base. ***Reassure a patient of the accuracy of the test results.***	If the thermometer is not recharged, the battery will die.
5. *Take an aural temperature*	
a. Place a clean probe cover over the tympanic probe (Figure 11-26) and make certain the unit is turned on and in the "ready" mode.	A clean probe cover prevents cross-contamination between patients.
b. Straighten the aural canal to best facilitate an accurate measurement (Figure 11-27). (Pull the auricle up and back on adults and children over the age of three. Pull down and back on anyone younger than age three.) ***Incorporate critical thinking skills when performing patient assessment and care.***	The tympanic thermometer relies on obtaining the measurement by having a direct pathway to the tympanic membrane. Thermal energy is radiated by the tympanic membrane.

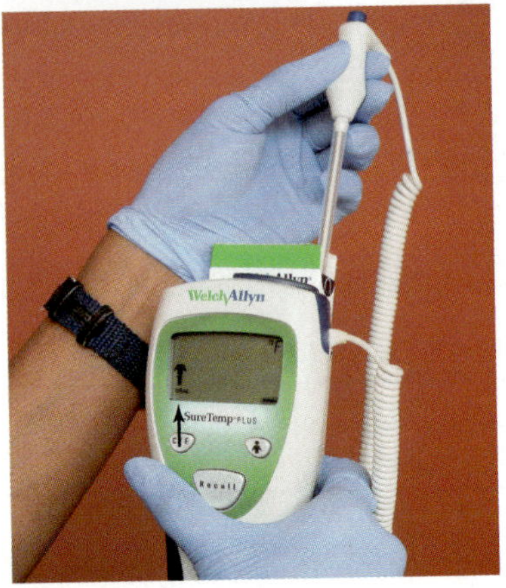

Figure 11-23 ■ Place a clean disposable probe cover on the probe of the electronic thermometer before inserting it into the patient's mouth.

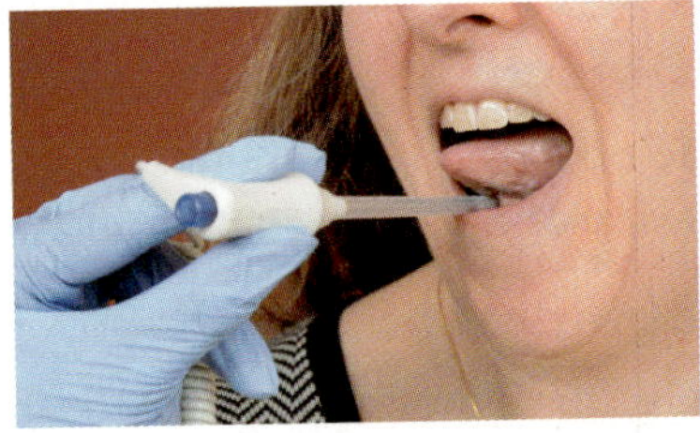
Figure 11-24 ■ Place the thermometer under the patient's tongue and to the side.

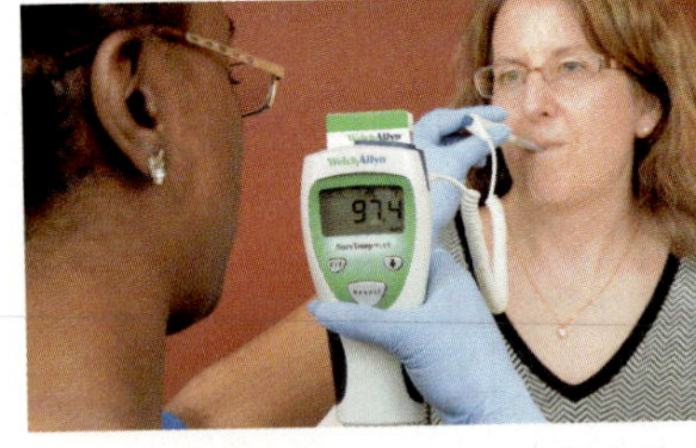
Figure 11-25 ■ Easy-to-see digital readout of the temperature reading.

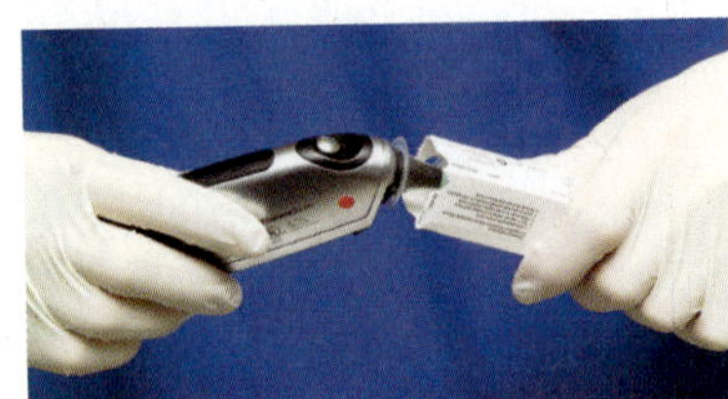
Figure 11-26 ■ Place a disposable probe cover on the tympanic thermometer probe to prevent cross-contamination.

continues

PROCEDURE 11-2 continued

PROCEDURAL STEPS	DETAILS AND/OR RATIONALE
c. Place the covered probe into the patient's ear canal (Figure 11-28), forming a tight seal and pointing the probe toward the eardrum.	The probe must be sealed in the ear canal for the most accurate results. If cool air is allowed to travel into the ear canal, the temperature will register cooler, creating a false reading.
d. Activate the thermometer while having the patient quietly relax.	Pressing the button on the top of the thermometer handle will activate the thermometer.
e. Leave the probe in place until the unit beeps. The temperature will be displayed digitally on the thermometer. ***Reassure a patient of the accuracy of the test results.***	
f. Discard the probe cover in the appropriate waste container. Return the thermometer to storage.	
6. *Take an axillary temperature*	
a. Make certain that the route setting is on axillary (Figure 11-29) and place a new probe cover over the probe.	Using a clean probe cover prevents cross-contamination.
b. Have the patient remove clothing that interferes with the axillary region. Offer a gown or drape for coverage. ***Incorporate critical thinking skills when performing patient assessment and care.***	The thermometer must be placed against the skin, not through the clothing to obtain an accurate reading.
c. Pat the armpit with a dry paper towel if perspiration is present (or have the patient do it).	Perspiration could cause an inaccurate reading.
d. Place the probe tight in the center of the axilla (Figure 11-30).	
e. Instruct or assist the patient in holding the arm tight against the body, holding the thermometer in place until the digital device emits a tone, indicating completion of the reading. ***Reassure a patient of the accuracy of the test results.***	It must fit snuggly in the armpit; air currents will cause an incorrect reading.
f. Remove probe and discard into trash can.	

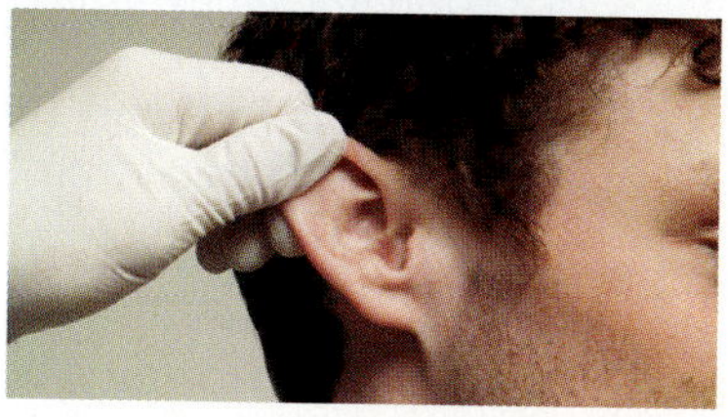

Figure 11-27 ■ The ear canal should be straightened to facilitate easy insertion of the thermometer and to obtain an accurate reading.

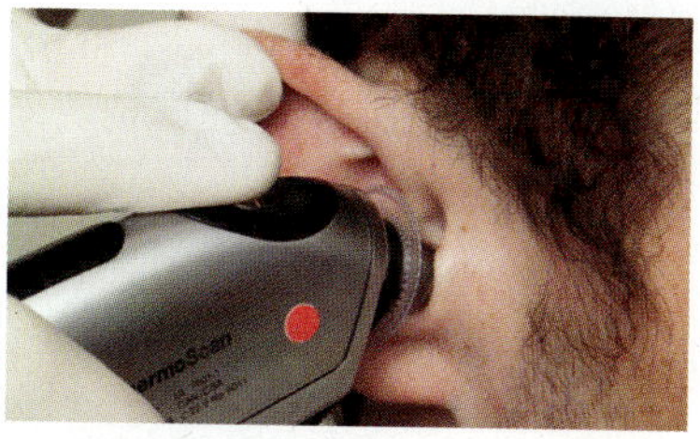

Figure 11-28 ■ Gently insert the probe into the patient's ear canal.

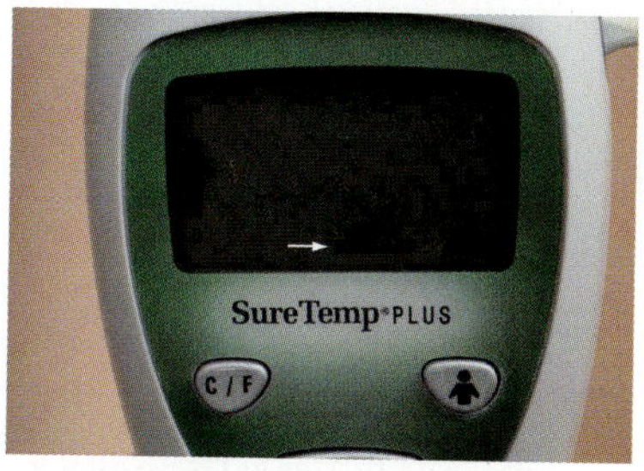

Figure 11-29 ■ When taking an axillary reading, be certain the route setting is on axillary.

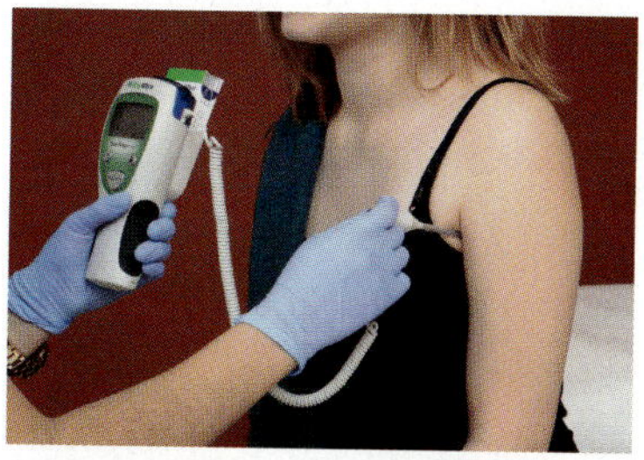

Figure 11-30 ■ The patient holds her arm close to her body as the medical assistant takes her axillary temperature.

continues

PROCEDURE 11-2 continued

PROCEDURAL STEPS	DETAILS AND/OR RATIONALE
7. *Take a temporal temperature*	
a. Clean the thermometer probe with an alcohol swab or place probe cover over the probe and ensure that it is working properly. ***Incorporate critical thinking skills when performing patient assessment and care.***	Keeping the measuring probe clean will help the thermometer to produce accurate readings.
b. Remove hats or scarves on the side of the head that is to be measured and pull hair back if applicable.	The area to be measured must be exposed to the environment. Hats, scarves, and hair can hold heat in, resulting in an inaccurate reading.
c. Check the forehead for perspiration. Wipe dry if perspiration is present.	Perspiration can interfere with an accurate reading.
d. Depress the scan button and place the probe at the midline of the forehead (Figure 11-31). Keep probe flush with the skin and slowly glide the thermometer across the forehead until the probe reaches the hairline on the side of the head over the temporal artery.	Holding the probe flush with the skin will ensure an accurate reading.
e. When the reading is complete, release the scan button, lift the probe from the patient's skin, and check the display for the reading. (Take a second reading behind the ear under the mastoid process if necessary [Figure 11-32].) ***Reassure a patient of the accuracy of the test results.***	Once the scan button is released, the reading will remain in the display window for a short period of time.
f. Clean the probe with alcohol or if using a probe cover, discard in trash receptacle.	
8. Immediately record results on a scrap piece of paper.	You want to record the results immediately so that the reading is fresh in your mind.
9. Return equipment back to its proper location.	
10. Wash your hands and record temperature reading in the patient record.	

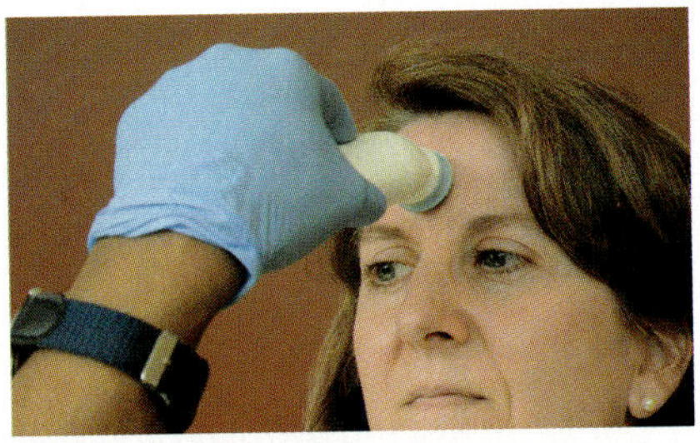

Figure 11-31 ■ The temporal thermometer probe is placed flush with the skin at the midline of the forehead.

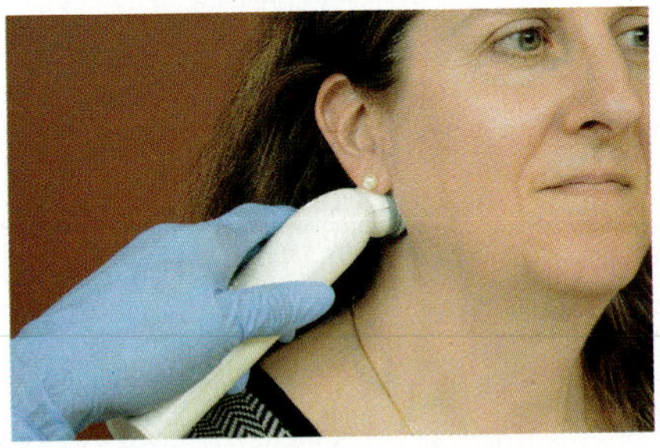

Figure 11-32 ■ A second reading may be taken behind the ear, below the mastoid process.

EHR DOCUMENTATION EXAMPLE:

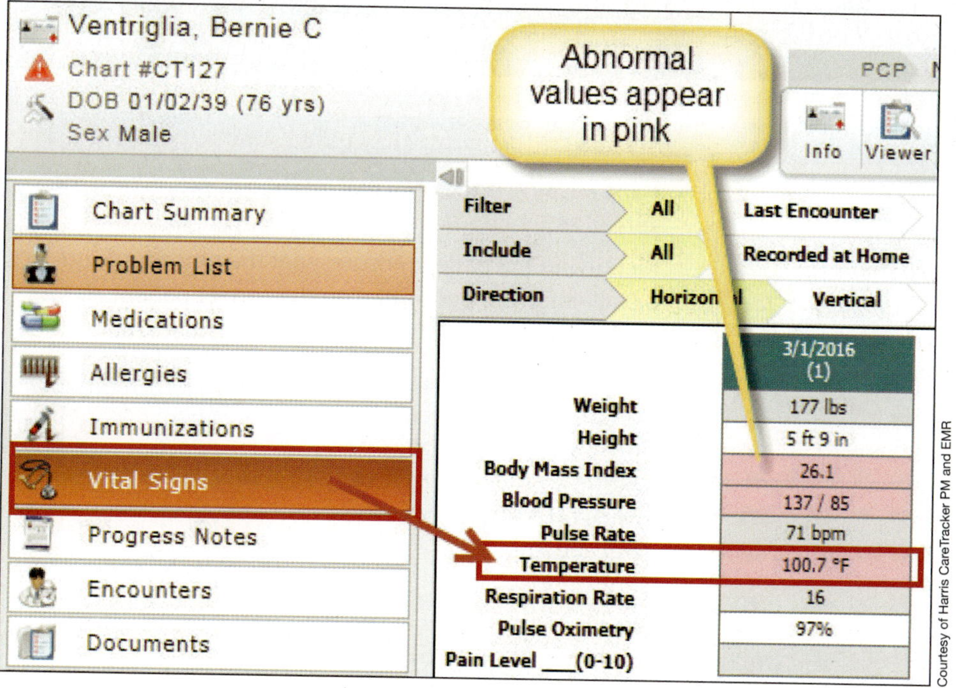

Courtesy of Harris CareTracker PM and EMR

DOCUMENTATION EXAMPLE OF AN AURAL OR TYMPANIC MEMBRANE READING:

11-04-XX 3:00 p.m.	T 99.2°F, TM, L. ear. Cassy Smith, RMA (AMT)--

DOCUMENTATION EXAMPLE OF AN AXILLARY TEMPERATURE READING:

8-7-XX 2:35 p.m.	T 97.4°F Axillary. Lori Moore, CMA (AAMA)--

DOCUMENTATION EXAMPLE OF A TEMPORAL BODY TEMPERATURE:

10-10-XX 10:30 a.m.	T 98.6°F (TA). Kelly Leonard, CMA (AAMA)--

PROCEDURE 11-3

Obtain a Radial Pulse Rate and Respiration Rate

Objective:

To obtain an accurate pulse and respiration rate.

Equipment/Supplies:

- Watch with a second hand
- Patient chart/EHR

continues

PROCEDURE 11-3 continued

PROCEDURAL STEPS	DETAILS AND/OR RATIONALE
1. Wash your hands.	Handwashing is the principal method of preventing the spread of infection.
2. Identify the patient using two identifiers, identify yourself, and ***explain the rationale for the performance of the procedure, showing awareness of the patient's concerns related to the procedure being performed***.	Identifying the patient ensures that the procedure and examination are performed on the correct patient. Explaining the procedure increases compliance and patient comfort.
3. Place the patient in a calm, quiet environment. Allow the patient to relax in a sitting position with the arm in a comfortable location. ***Incorporate critical thinking skills when performing patient assessment and care***.	Anxiety can alter pulse and respiratory measurements. The patient should be calm and quiet.
4. Locate the radial pulse with your second, third, and fourth fingers (Figure 11-33). The hand you use should be opposite from the hand on which you wear your watch. Never use your thumb when measuring the pulse.	The tips of the fingers are very sensitive and able to palpate the pulse easily. The thumb has its own pulse. If you use a thumb for measurement, you may be feeling your own pulse rather than the pulse of the patient.
5. Apply slight pressure onto the radial artery. Increase pressure until the pulse is felt.	Too much pressure will close off the artery so that the pulse cannot be felt. (The amount of pressure will be learned with experience.)
6. Count the number of beats for a minimum of 30 seconds. Multiply this number by two for a full-minute rate.	Fewer than 30 seconds may cause you to miss abnormalities. Pulse and respirations are recorded as beats or breaths per minute so you will need to multiply your reading by two when performing a 30-second check.
7. Note if there are any irregular beats that occur.	If there are any irregular beats noted, count the pulse rate for a full minute.
8. Maintain fingers on the pulse and begin counting respirations (Figure 11-34).	The patient will perceive that you are still measuring pulse. Respirations can be altered by the patient; therefore, it is best if the patient is not aware the measurement is being obtained.
9. Count the number of breaths for 30 seconds. Multiply this number by two for a full-minute rate. ***Reassure the patient of the accuracy of the test results***.	
10. Note any irregular breath sounds.	Extra motions, such as flaring nostrils or pursing lips, as well as other sounds may indicate respiratory disorders. They must be communicated to the provider.
11. Wash your hands.	
12. Document the results of the pulse and respirations in the patient record.	

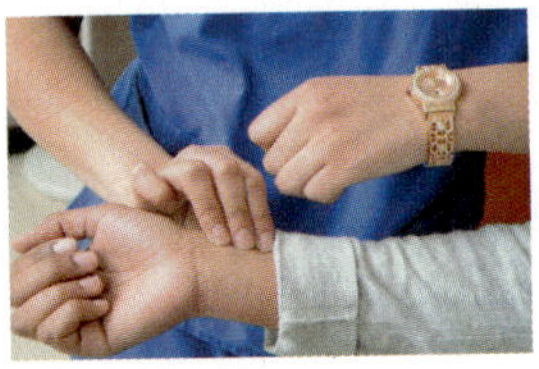

Figure 11-33 The medical assistant measures the pulse using her first, second, and third fingers. If the radial pulse is regular, count for 30 seconds and multiply by two.

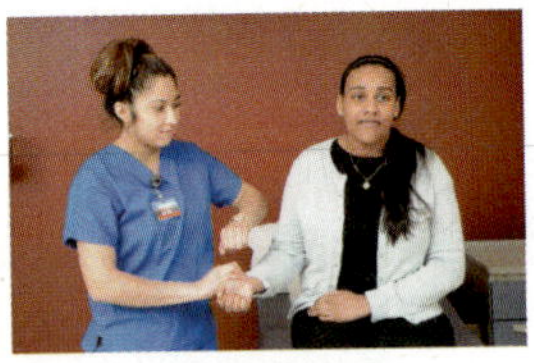

Figure 11-34 ■ The medical assistant maintains fingers on the pulse and begins counting respirations so that the patient is unaware of the respiration measurement.

DOCUMENTATION EXAMPLE:

10-4-XX 9:30 a.m.	P 84 and reg; R 16, unlabored, and reg. Mattie Jones, CMA (AAMA)--------------------------

PROCEDURE 11-4

Obtain an Apical Pulse Rate

Objective:

To obtain an accurate apical pulse reading.

Equipment/Supplies:

- Stethoscope
- Watch with second hand
- Alcohol wipe
- Patient chart/EHR

PROCEDURAL STEPS	DETAILS AND/OR RATIONALE
1. Wash your hands.	Handwashing is the principal method of preventing the spread of infection.
2. Assemble the equipment. Sanitize the stethoscope.	Keeping the stethoscope clean will help reduce risk of cross-contamination.
3. Identify the patient using two identifiers, identify yourself, and ***explain the rationale for the performance of the procedure, showing awareness of the patient's concerns related to the procedure being performed.***	Identifying the patient ensures that the procedure and examination are performed on the correct patient. Explaining the procedure increases compliance and patient comfort.
4. Instruct the patient to expose the chest area by either unbuttoning the shirt or removing clothes from the waist up. If female, provide a gown for privacy. ***Incorporate critical thinking skills when performing patient assessment and care.***	There must be access to the chest region for auscultation of the apical pulse.
5. Remove clothing, gown, or drape covering the left thoracic area.	Attempting to measure the pulse through clothing can cause extraneous noises that may alter the assessment.
6. Place the stethoscope in your ears correctly.	The ear pieces must be pointed in the direction of the ear canal.
7. Locate the apical pulse.	The apical pulse is located at the fifth intercostal space, at the left midclavicular line.
8. After warming the diaphragm of the stethoscope, place it over the apex of the heart (Figure 11-35).	Cold stethoscopes are uncomfortable for the patient. The apex region of the chest often provides the best sound for counting the heart rate.

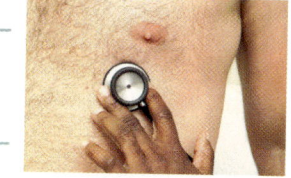

Figure 11-35 ■ The apical pulse can be counted by placing the stethoscope over the apex of the heart.

continues

PROCEDURE 11-4 continued

PROCEDURAL STEPS	DETAILS AND/OR RATIONALE
9. Count the beats for one full minute.	
10. Note any irregularities, along with the quality of sound.	Unusual sounds and patterns of the heartbeat may indicate pathology. This must be communicated to the provider.
11. Remove the stethoscope. ***Reassure a patient of the accuracy of the test results.***	
12. Assist the patient in redressing or draping.	Be aware if there is another examination to follow to prevent the patient from having to undress again.
13. Wash your hands.	
14. Record the results in the patient record.	

DOCUMENTATION EXAMPLE:

4-6-XX 7:45 a.m.	P(ap) 86 and irreg. Cindy Brown, RMA (AMT)--

PROCEDURE 11-5
Obtain a BP Measurement Using the Palpatory Method

Objective:

To accurately obtain a blood pressure (BP) reading.

Equipment/Supplies:

- Sphygmomanometer with appropriate cuff size
- Stethoscope
- Alcohol wipes
- Patient chart/EHR

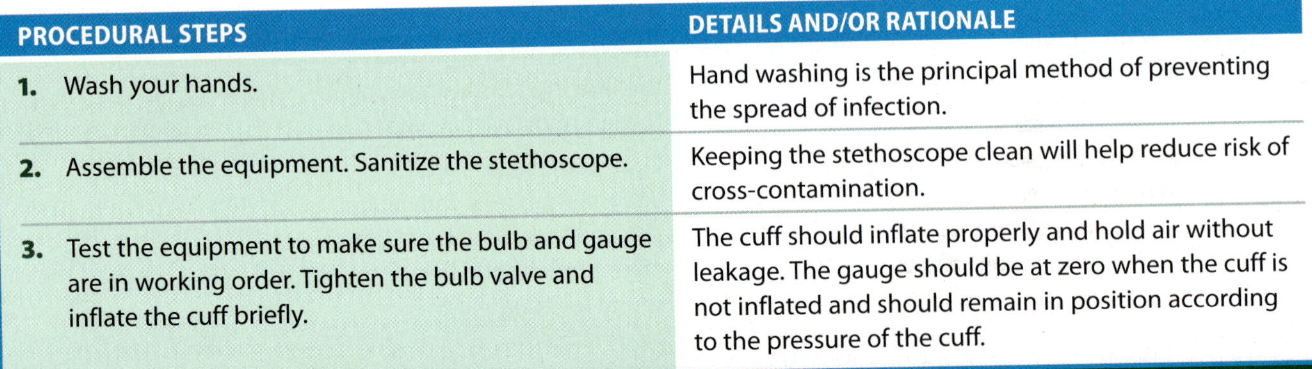

PROCEDURAL STEPS	DETAILS AND/OR RATIONALE
1. Wash your hands.	Hand washing is the principal method of preventing the spread of infection.
2. Assemble the equipment. Sanitize the stethoscope.	Keeping the stethoscope clean will help reduce risk of cross-contamination.
3. Test the equipment to make sure the bulb and gauge are in working order. Tighten the bulb valve and inflate the cuff briefly.	The cuff should inflate properly and hold air without leakage. The gauge should be at zero when the cuff is not inflated and should remain in position according to the pressure of the cuff.

continues

PROCEDURE 11-5 continued

PROCEDURAL STEPS	DETAILS AND/OR RATIONALE
4. Remove any air from the cuff bladder.	This ensures a more accurate reading.
5. Identify the patient using two identifiers, identify yourself, and ***explain the rationale for the performance of the procedure, showing awareness of the patient's concerns related to the procedure being performed***. Ask patient if there is any reason you can't perform blood pressure on one side or the other.	Identifying the patient ensures that the procedure and examination are performed on the correct patient. Explaining the procedure increases compliance and reduces patient anxiety. Taking blood pressure on the side the patient has had a mastectomy or has a fistula could cause problems for the patient.
6. Assess the patient's upper arm diameter to determine if the size of the cuff selected is adequate. ***Incorporate critical thinking skills when performing patient assessment and care***.	An incorrect cuff size will produce inaccurate results.
7. Position the patient in a quiet, comfortable position.	The patient should be calm for the best results. BP can be falsely elevated with increased anxiety or stress.
8. Roll up the patient's sleeve or remove any clothing or garments from the arm that will be used for obtaining the BP.	Tight clothing will hinder the blood flow to the brachial artery.
9. Palpate the brachial artery for a viable pulse (Figure 11-36).	Make a mental note of the location of the strongest pulse.
10. With the patient's palm facing upward, wrap the cuff around the upper arm 1 to 2 inches above the bend of the elbow. The cuff should be snug but not overly tight. The arrow on the cuff, R for right arm and L for left arm, should align with the artery (Figure 11-37). Position the arm so that it is at heart level.	If the cuff is not snug, it could cause an inaccurate reading. If the artery is above the level of the heart, a false low reading might be registered.
11. Adjust the stethoscope so that the sound is coming from the diaphragm side of the chest piece. (Lightly tapping diaphragm with the ear pieces in place will confirm correct side.) Remove the stethoscope tips from your ears.	The side of the chest piece used will vary by office protocol.
12. Adjust the manometer so it is clipped to the cuff and is in clear view.	Clear vision is important for accurate readings. The markings are small so they must be within a readable distance.
13. Hold the bulb in the palm of your dominant hand with the valve between the thumb and first finger. Turn the valve until closed.	Tighten the valve only until it is closed. Over tightening will damage the valve, and difficulty releasing the valve can cause interruption in the procedure.
14. With the other hand, locate the radial pulse.	

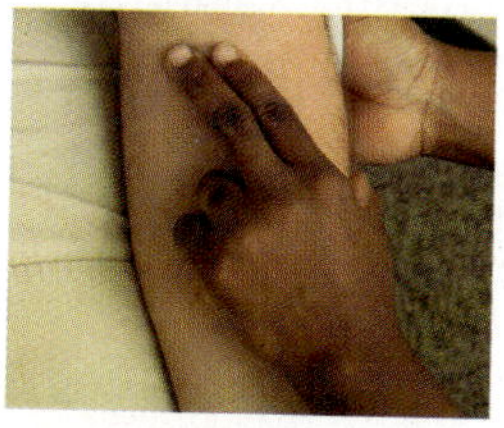

Figure 11-36 ■ Palpate the brachial artery for a viable pulse.

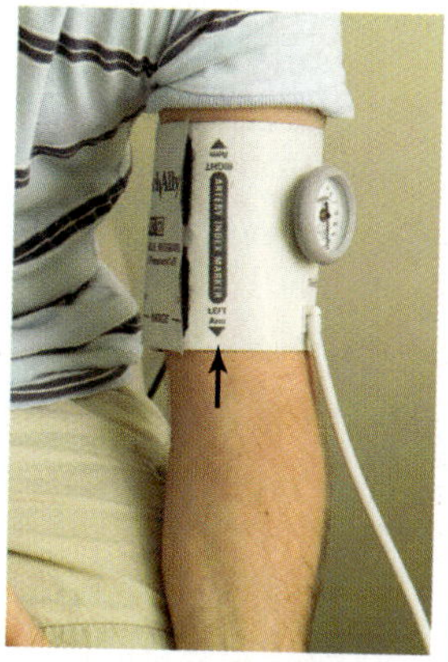

Figure 11-37 ■ The BP cuff should be placed so that the arrow lines up with the artery.

continues

PROCEDURE 11-5 continued

PROCEDURAL STEPS	DETAILS AND/OR RATIONALE
15. Using the bulb, squeeze and inflate the cuff while palpating the radial pulse. Continue until the pulse is no longer felt. Proceed with inflation until the cuff has been inflated 30 mmHg beyond pulse cessation.	As the cuff inflates, the blood flow to the radial artery subsides. The pulse can no longer be felt.
16. Slowly open the valve to release air from the cuff while palpating the radial pulse. Release at 2–3 mmHg per second. Note the pressure on the manometer when the pulse returns.	The reading where the pulse returns is an estimate of the patient's systolic pressure. If the patient already has an office baseline, the palpated BP may not need to be done.
17. Open the valve completely and remove all air from the cuff.	
18. After waiting 30 seconds, prepare to take the BP reading.	
19. Place the stethoscope tips correctly in your ear canals. Place the chest piece over the brachial artery (Figure 11-38). Hold the stethoscope in place with the first two fingers of your hand. Do not hold with your thumb over the chest piece as you may pick up your own pulse. Avoid touching the cuff with the stethoscope. Avoid having the tubing of the stethoscope come in contact with anything.	The thumb pulse may be heard through the diaphragm, confusing the measurement. Any additional sounds will cause confusion. Touching the tubing to anything will create extraneous sounds.
20. Tighten the valve and pump the cuff rapidly up to 20 mmHg above the palpated systolic pressure.	Pumping the cuff 20 mmHg beyond the palpated systolic pressure will keep you out of the auscultatory gap.
21. Begin to release the pressure in the cuff by slowly turning the valve counterclockwise, 2–3 mmHg per second. Observe the manometer carefully. Note the measurement when the first beat is heard. This is the systolic pressure.	The systolic pressure occurs when the blood begins flowing into the brachial artery.
22. Continue to deflate the cuff at this speed. Observe the manometer carefully and note the measurement when the sound ceases. This is the diastolic pressure.	
23. Open the valve completely to deflate the cuff quickly and remove all air from the cuff.	
24. Remove the stethoscope and cuff. ***Reassure the patient of the accuracy of the test results.***	Remove the air quickly after the reading has been made to reduce discomfort for the patient.
25. Wash your hands.	
26. Record the results in the patient record.	

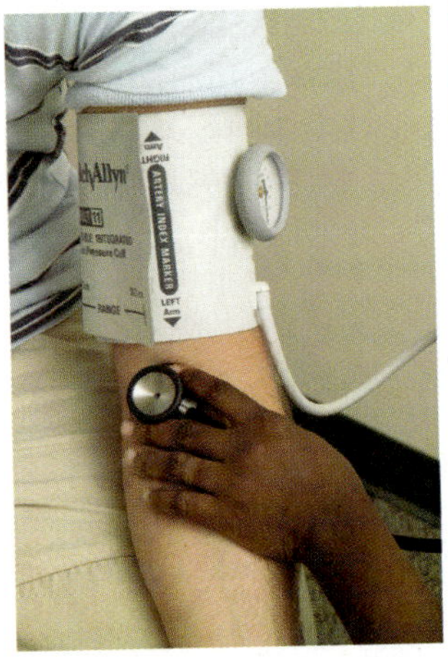

Figure 11-38 ■ Placing the stethoscope directly over the brachial artery makes the BP easier to hear.

EHR DOCUMENTATION EXAMPLE:

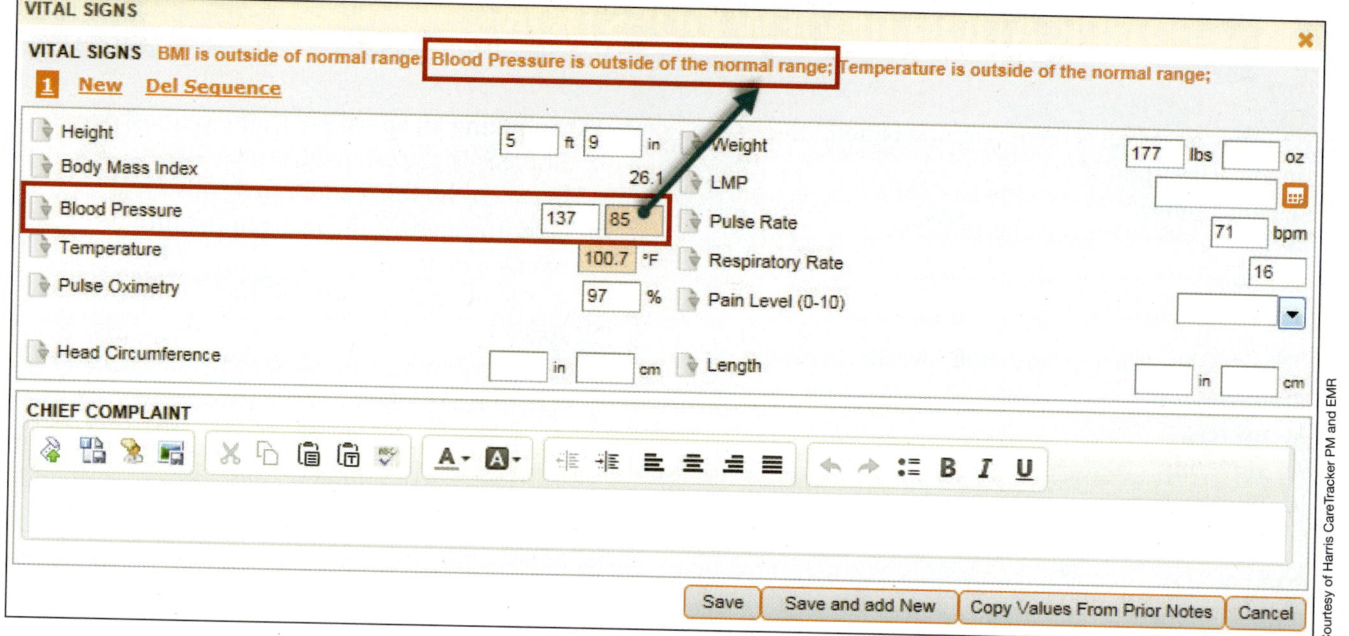

Courtesy of Harris CareTracker PM and EMR

CHAPTER SUMMARY

- Vital signs are important indicators of the patient's health.
- Physical changes that occur in the body from one visit to the next may be detected through a change in a patient's vital signs. Vital signs, also known as cardinal signs, include temperature, pulse, and respiration (these three vital signs as referred together as TPR), and blood pressure (BP).
- The medical assistant should use all senses during the initial screening process to gather important clues about the patient's health status. The patient should be observed for appearance, gait, odors, level of awareness, and emotional state.
- Accuracy in taking and documenting vital signs is imperative to make certain that provider is able to diagnose the patient properly and the patient obtains the proper care.
- Baseline readings are normally taken during the patient's first appointment and evaluated each time the patient returns to the office.
- The medical assistant should be certain to accurately document all findings collected during the initial screening into the patient's chart.
- Any information obtained from speaking with the patient that pertains to the history of present illness or medical history should be recorded appropriately.
- Measuring the patient's height and weight is often the responsibility of the medical assistant.
- Mensuration is a term that means measurement.
- Fluctuations in a patient's height or weight could indicate a health disorder or illness; therefore, accuracy and consistency are important.
- Body mass index (BMI) is a numerical correlation between a patient's height and weight. Calculating the patient's BMI may be the responsibility of the medical assistant, and should be documented along with the scale weight.
- Changes in a patient's health can often be detected through the monitoring of vital signs.
- Other basic physiological measurements as well as any changes that have occurred since the patient's last medical examination can provide an overall picture of the patient's general state of health.
- Temperature, pulse, respiration, and blood pressure (TPR and BP) are standard vital signs taken. Any changes identified during measurement of these vital signs may indicate a health condition or may illustrate the progression of a previously identified medical condition.
- Medical assistants will also record a pain assessment and pulse oximetry.
- Medical assisting students should practice vital signs throughout the entire program.
- Externship sites will be less forgiving of students who struggle in performing vital sign procedures, more than any other procedures performed.

CERTIFICATION REVIEW QUESTIONS

1. During the initial screening of the patient, the medical assistant observes:
   a. appearance.
   b. gait.
   c. odor.
   d. All of the above

2. The causes of heat production include all of the following except:
   a. exercise.
   b. shivering.
   c. perspiration.
   d. metabolism.

3. Which of the following pulse rates would be considered as normal for an adult?
   a. 120 BPM
   b. 40 BPM
   c. 102 BPM
   d. 68 BPM

4. The average respiratory rate for an adult is:
   a. 12–16 per minute.
   b. 30–60 per minute.
   c. 24–40 per minute.
   d. 18–30 per minute.

5. The respiratory rate can be affected by all except:
   a. physical activity.
   b. emotions.
   c. medications.
   d. diet.

6. The pulse pressure when taking a BP indicates the:
   a. difference between the palpable systolic and diastolic pressures.
   b. difference between the palpable systolic and auditory systolic pressures.
   c. difference between the palpable diastolic and auditory diastolic pressures.
   d. difference between the auditory systolic and diastolic pressures.

7. When taking an apical pulse, the stethoscope chest piece is placed in what location?
   a. Between the third and fourth ribs
   b. Over the apex of the heart in the fifth intercostal space
   c. At the midaxillary line of the fifth intercostal space
   d. At the midnipple line between the third and fourth ribs

8. If the medical assistant notices that there is an irregularity when taking a pulse, the pulse should be taken for what additional length of time?
   a. 15 seconds
   b. 30 seconds
   c. 1 minute
   d. 2 minutes

9. What body temperature constitutes a fever?
   a. 97.6°F
   b. 98.6°F
   c. 99.1°F
   d. 99.5°F

10. What organs does hypertension affect?
    a. Eyes
    b. Heart
    c. Kidneys
    d. All of the above

STUDY RESOURCES

Resources to Test and Reinforce Your Knowledge:	
Certification Review Questions	Take this end-of-chapter quiz
Workbook	• Complete the activities for Chapter 11 • Perform the procedures for Chapter 11 using the Competency Checklists
Resources to Promote Critical Thinking:	
***Solve the Case* Activities**	• Consider these case studies and discuss your conclusions
Learning Lab	• Module 11: Vital Signs and Measurements
MindTap	• Complete Chapter 11 readings and activities

REFERENCES

Centers for Disease Control and Prevention. (n.d.). Overweight and obesity. Retrieved May 27, 2015, from http://www.cdc.gov/obesity/adult/defining.html

Ferrari, V. and Heller, M. (2015). *The Paperless Medical Office: Using Harris CareTracker*. Clifton Park, NY: Cengage Learning.

National Center for Biotechnology Information (NCBI). (2014, Feb). 2014 Evidence-Based Guideline for the Management of High Blood Pressure in Adults: Report from the Panel Members Appointed to the Eighth Joint National Committee (JNC8). Retrieved May 27, 2015, from http://www.ncbi.nlm.nih.gov/pubmed/24352797/

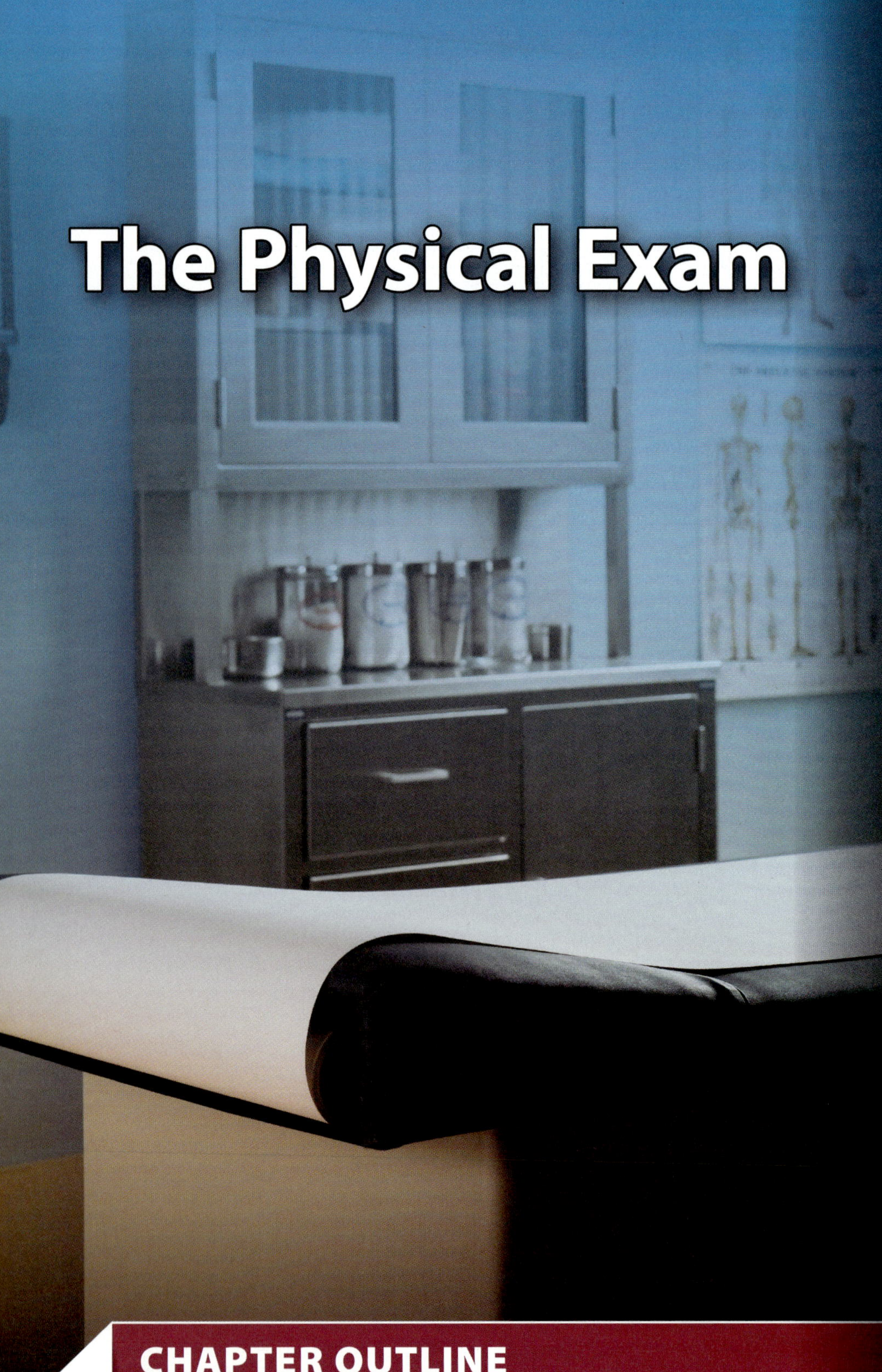

12

The Physical Exam

ESSENTIAL TERMS

auscultation
examination
inspection
manipulation
mensuration
observation
palpation
percussion
posture
tympany
vertigo

CHAPTER OUTLINE

Age-Specific Exams

The Examination Room

Preparation of the Exam Room

Instruments for Examination

Patient Preparation

Patient Positioning and Draping

Patient Assessment

Completing the Visit

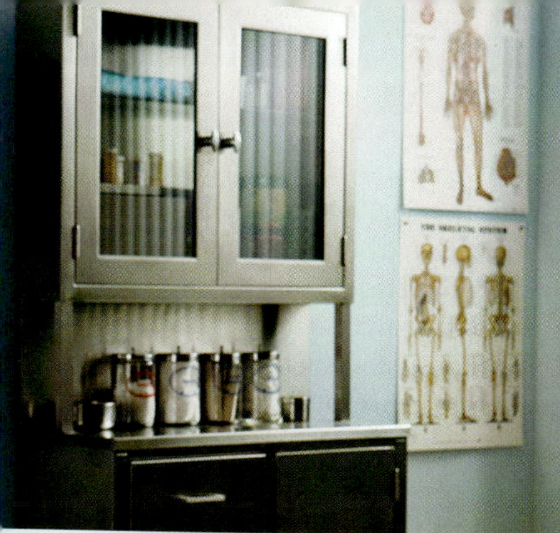

DEVELOPMENTAL OBJECTIVES

After completing this chapter, you should be able to:

1. Correctly spell and define essential terms.
2. Name and discuss the indications for equipment and instruments used by the health team in physical examinations.
3. List and define the six techniques used during the physical examination.
4. Explain the room maintenance and cleaning procedures that are performed by the medical assistant.
5. Explain the various patient positions utilized during the physical examination, including the indications for each.
6. Explain the technique and purpose of draping the patient in each position.
7. List the responsibilities of the medical assistant when assisting the provider with a patient examination.
8. List the medical assistant's responsibilities in completing a patient visit.
9. Assist a provider with the patient exam.

INTRODUCTION

The physical **examination** is a process during which the body is inspected and its systems are evaluated to determine the presence or absence of disease. The medical assistant's role in assisting with the physical exam is multifold and varied in different situations. Preparation of the office environment for the examination often occurs before any patient involvement. Anticipating the needs of both the evaluator (provider) and the patient allows for a professional, efficient, and thorough office visit or procedure. Responding to provider and patient requests is only a small portion of the medical assistant's responsibility. Becoming a professional involves assessing a situation and anticipating solutions.

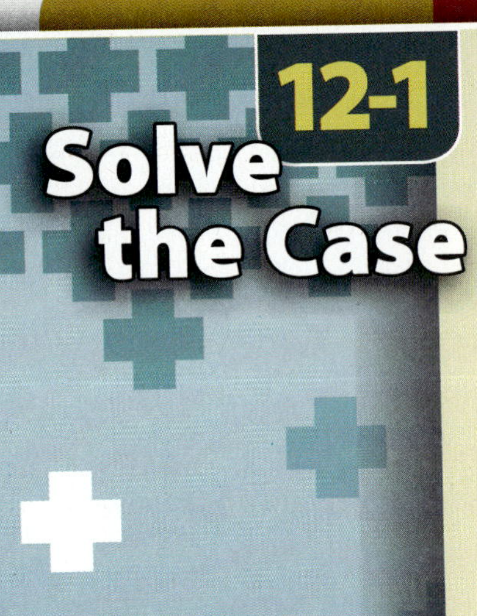

Mr. Choy is a 54-year-old man who presents for a complete physical. He is new to the office and says he doesn't want to be there, but that his wife scheduled the appointment and made him come in. It is obvious that Mr. Choy is very nervous about today's appointment. During the new patient screening you learn that Mr. Choy is a smoker. He also has had some intermittent chest pain over the last few weeks. He has not seen a doctor in at least 20 years. His younger brother recently died of lung cancer.

1. **What types of health risks and preventive care might need to be addressed today?**
2. **How might you address the fear and anxiety that Mr. Choy might have, even if he is not able to voice it?**
3. **What types of preparation can be done in the examination room in anticipation of this visit? What types of equipment/items might you need?**

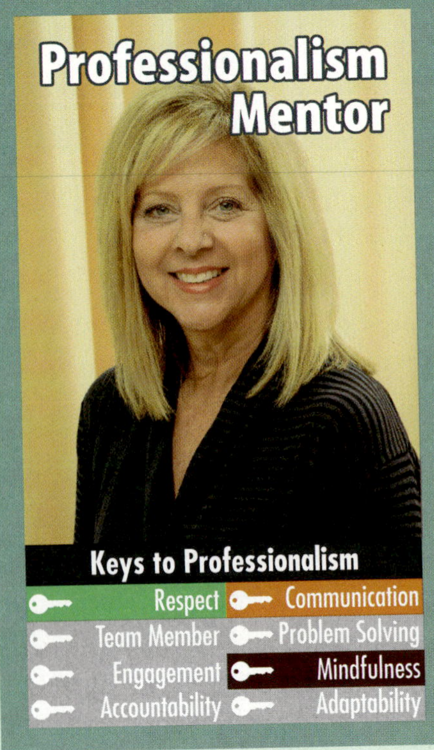

Imagine this scenario: after rooming your patient, they are asked to remove their clothing, put on an exam gown, take a seat on the exam table, and told that their provider will be with them as soon as possible. The patient may be anxious or feeling unwell or most likely both; in addition, the lights are bright, and without their clothing they are probably cold, too. What is your role as the medical assistant in this scenario? You might say your role is to make sure the room is set up appropriately for whatever examination the patient is having. You might also add that your role is to be sure the patient is ready to be seen by the health care provider and draped appropriately. You would be correct with both answers. The key to success in both cases is being *well organized* and *planning ahead,* ensuring that the provider has everything needed when performing a physical examination of the patient. But don't stop there! There are so many things we can do for our patients during the physical exam that make a big difference. Think about what else you could do to ensure that the patient is as comfortable as possible during their examination. In your professional journal, write down two additional measures you would take to go above and beyond for your patient. ■

Assisting with the examination involves all of the senses, and especially includes active listening. The medical assistant provides information to other health providers regarding the patient, serving as a liaison between the patient and the provider. The medical assistant is often the interpreter or reinforcer of important medical information directed toward the patient. The medical assistant's professional role in the physical examination involves being an environmental aide, a compassionate assistant, an informed instructor, an empathetic listener, and a liaison.

AGE-SPECIFIC EXAMS

Specific patient populations may need particular screenings at different intervals; for example, diabetics should have $HbA1_c$ testing done twice a year and should have the following tests performed on an annual basis: dilated eye exams, cholesterol (low-density lipoprotein [LDL]) checks, foot exams, and kidney panels. This is especially important in pay-for-performance organizations. Being familiar with preventive testing guidelines for different ages and immunization management will help the appointment to flow much better and assist providers in meeting meaningful use. Refer to the MindTap resources for Chapter 12 for a listing of preventive testing that should be performed at different age intervals and in specific patient populations. These resources also include a complete listing of immunizations that should be performed throughout adulthood.

EHR Application

Stage 2, Meaningful Use, Core Objective # 12, states that providers should use clinically relevant information to identify patients who should receive reminders for preventive/follow-up care and send these patients the reminders, per patient preference. Patients who do not routinely come in for checkups need to be notified when they are due for screening exams. Most EHR software programs provide reporting tools that can help to identify these patients. The medical assistant may be responsible for running reports and notifying these patients when these tests are due.

THE EXAMINATION ROOM

Preparing the exam room for patient examination and procedures is often the responsibility of the medical assistant. This includes maintaining a clean and prepared examination room. Room temperature must be conducive to examinations. Efficiency of the exam is increased when all instruments and supplies are readily available.

Preparation of the Exam Room

With the continuous flow of patients during a normal office day, the medical assistant must be thorough and efficient in preparing the examination room for each patient's needs. Following the dismissal of each patient, the medical assistant should promptly prepare the examination room for the next patient. The medical assistant should put on the appropriate personal protective equipment (PPE) before cleaning the exam room for protection from infectious body fluids. Guidelines for preparing the exam room include the following:

- Discard all disposable items such as used drapes, gowns, bandaging material, wrappers, and other such items into the proper trash receptacles.
- Place nondisposable gowns and drapes in the laundry bin.
- Place all reusable items in the proper storage area.
- Place the exam table in its proper position and properly arrange all furniture.
- Thoroughly disinfect all counter surfaces and the exam table with an approved disinfectant.
- If the flooring needs tending, clean according to office policy.
- Restock supplies that are running low.
- Spray deodorizer if lingering odors are present. Spray disinfecting spray if the previous patient had a communicable disease.
- Prepare any items necessary for the next patient (adjustments or supply enhancement may be made following the patient interview).

Cleanliness is important to the health and safety of the patient, the provider, and all allied health personnel. Figure 12-1 shows two exam rooms. In which one would you rather be a patient?

Check the schedule to see what the patient is being seen for prior to rooming the patient. If the patient is scheduled for a procedure such as a Pap smear, set up whatever you can before the patient enters the room. If the patient is being seen for transitional care following a hospital visit, make certain that the discharge notes from the hospital visit are available. If the patient had lab tests performed during a previous appointment,

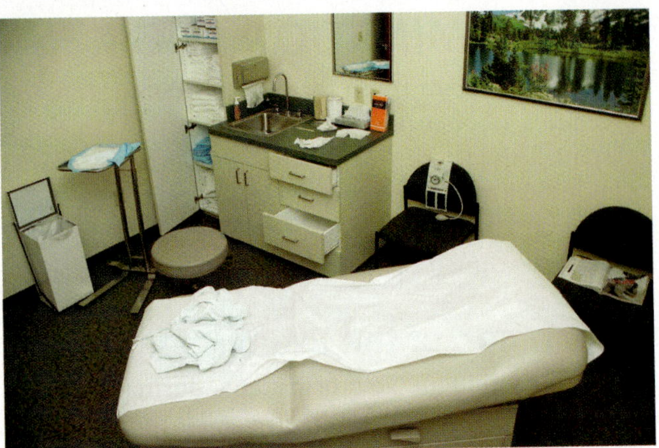

Figure 12-1a ■ An example of an exam room that is not ready for a new patient. There is evidence of the former patient and the room is unclean and unorganized.

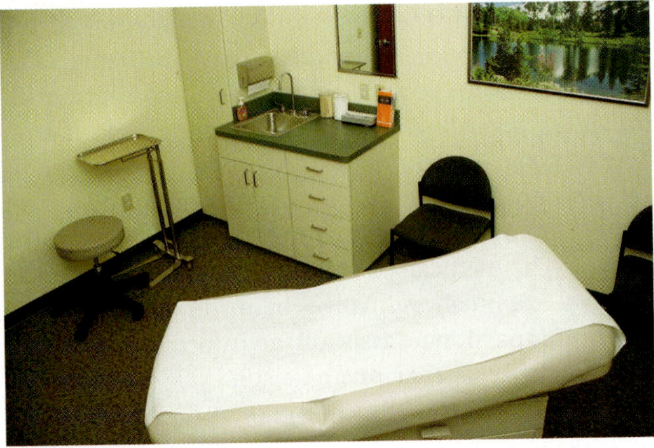

Figure 12-1b ■ An example of a clean and well-organized exam room that is fresh and ready for the next patient.

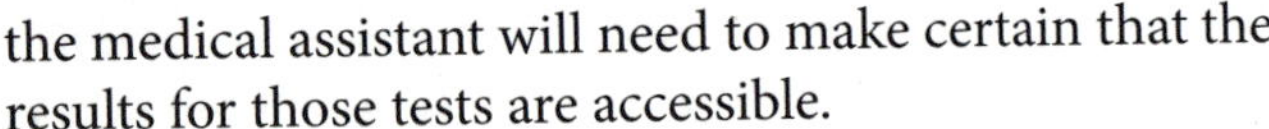

the medical assistant will need to make certain that the results for those tests are accessible.

As you screen the patient, listen carefully to determine if other instruments, trays, or procedures may be necessary based on your latest findings. A good medical assistant is able to anticipate the provider's needs prior to the provider's order. (Caution: Never perform any test or procedure without a direct order from the provider. You can always set up for the procedure as though it is going to happen; however, if the provider doesn't order the procedure, you simply just put the supplies back.) This promotes a smoother patient flow. For detailed instructions and rationale on preparing the exam room, refer to Procedure 12-1.

Instruments for Examination

All examinations require some type of equipment or instruments. A professional familiarizes herself with the different types of instruments and equipment used in each office setting. Equipment and instrument selection will vary with each type of medical practice and each type of procedure or exam. For example, an orthopedic office will use a different selection of instruments than an OB-GYN office. Some instruments, though, are standard within all practices. The figures in Table 12-1 illustrate typical instruments and supplies that are used for a physical exam. In reality, these may vary slightly based on the manufacturer. The medical assistant should have a basic understanding

Table 12-1 Instruments Used in the Typical Medical Examination

Instrument/Supplies	Description/Indications
Basin	Serves several purposes: Used instruments may be placed in the basin to be either cleaned or discarded May hold body fluids, such as emesis May be used to collect fluids during irrigations
Drapes	May be paper or fabric Used for patient privacy and comfort

Table 12-1 Instruments Used in the Typical Medical Examination *(continued)*

Instrument/Supplies	Description/Indications
Gloves 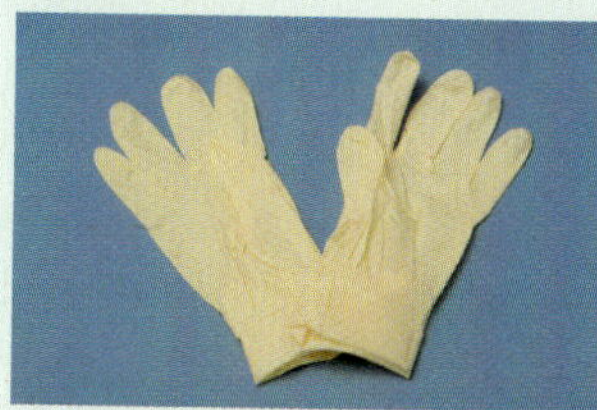	Usually non-latex nitrile, though some may be latex Sterile or nonsterile Different sizes available Learn the different providers' sizes in your facility
Gowns 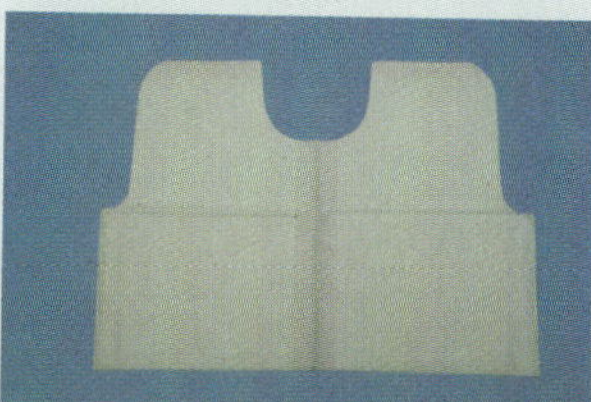	May be paper or fabric May be different lengths Depending on the type of exam, may open to the front or back
Fecal occult blood test 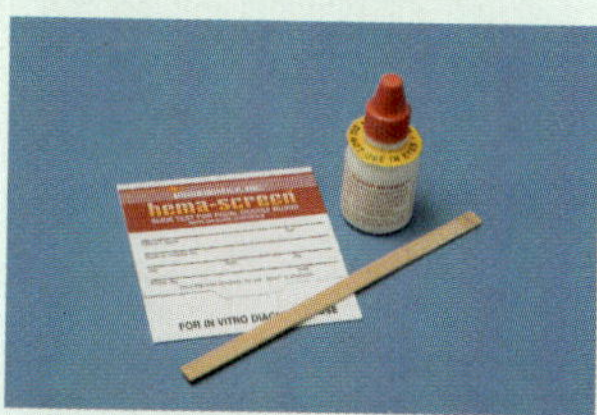	A small cardboard testing card along with a bottle of developer solution Tests for blood in the stool (see Chapter 16)
Lubricants 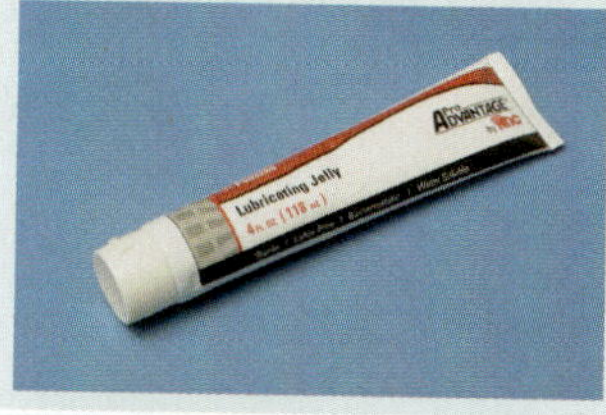	Usually in a tube; nonsterile Used to increase comfort when performing a manual rectal examination or to lubricate certain instruments for insertion into different body cavities
Ophthalmoscope 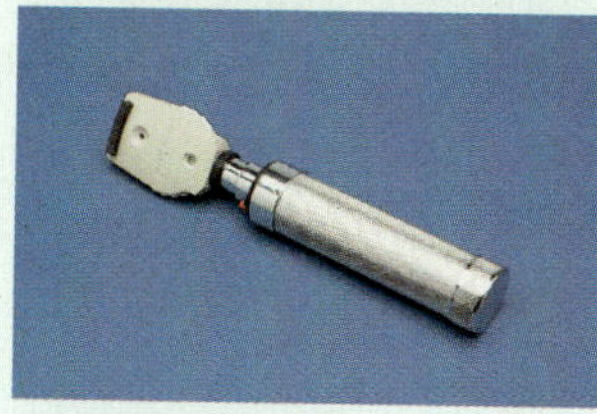	Light source to examine eye interior and optic vessels Maintain functional operation of equipment within the exam room
Otoscope 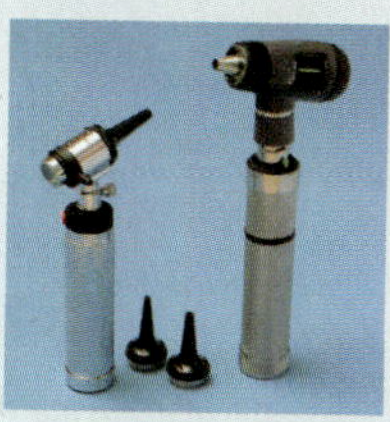	Light source to examine the ear canal and tympanic membranes Ensure that the disposable speculums that attach to the otoscope are stocked for use
Percussion hammer 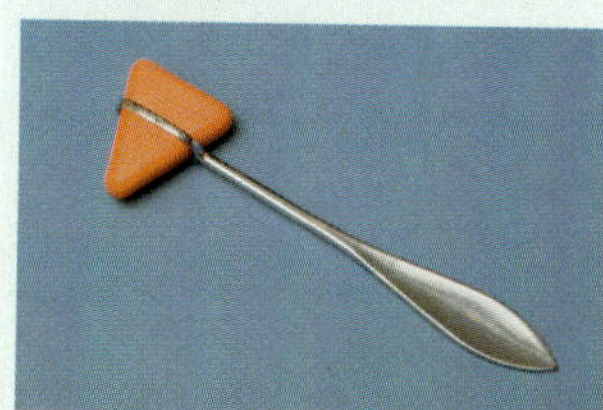	A small triangular hammer made of hard rubber Used to test reflexes during an examination

continues

Table 12-1 Instruments Used in the Typical Medical Examination *(continued)*

Instrument/Supplies	Description/Indications
Cotton or rayon-tipped sterile applicators 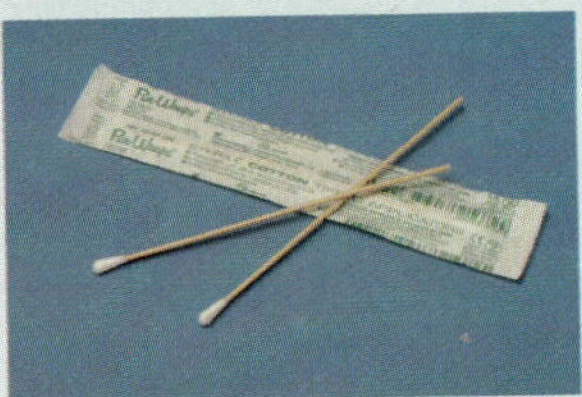	Many specimens will require the use of a sterile applicator, such as wet mount slides and tissue or cell slides (refer to Chapter 27 for further specimen collection requirements)
Various specimen collection kits or containers 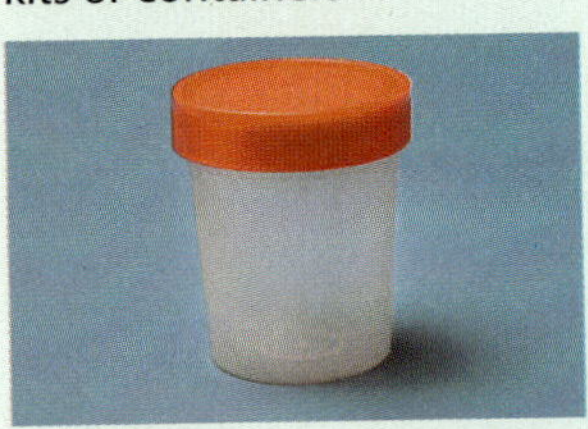	Anticipate which specimens may need to be collected and the specimen collection equipment or supplies needed (refer to Chapters 23 through 28 for more information on specific collection requirements)
Stethoscope 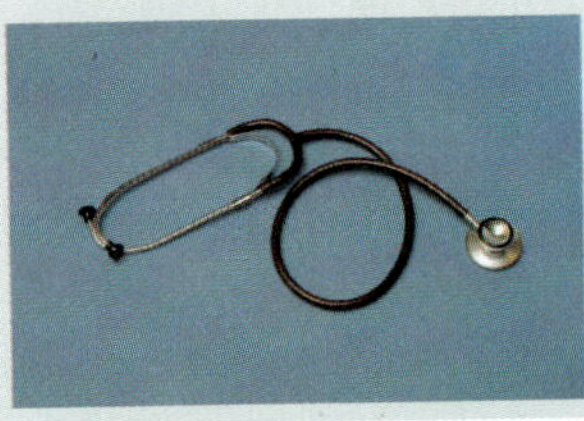	Used for blood pressures and auscultation of body sounds including breath, heart, and bowel
Tape measure 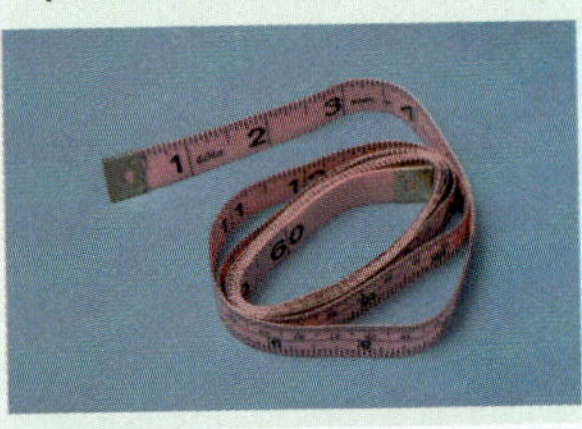	Either in inches or centimeters Used to measure body circumference and length
Neurological pinwheel 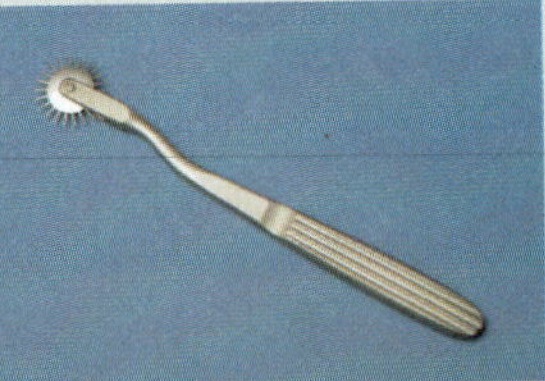	Used to check nerve sensitivity as it is rolled across the skin
Tongue depressors 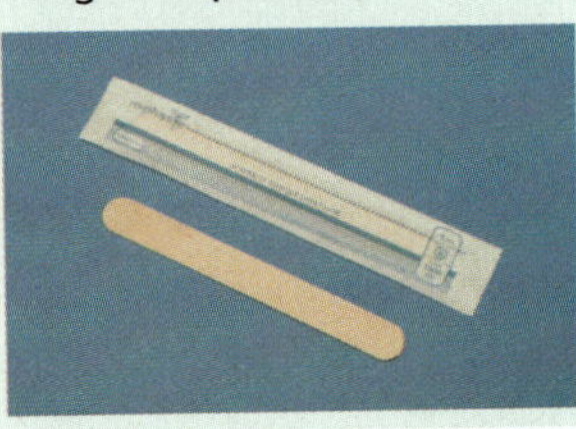	Sterile; used to compress the tongue when inspecting the throat Can also be used during neurological evaluations, such as tracking eye movements
Tuning fork 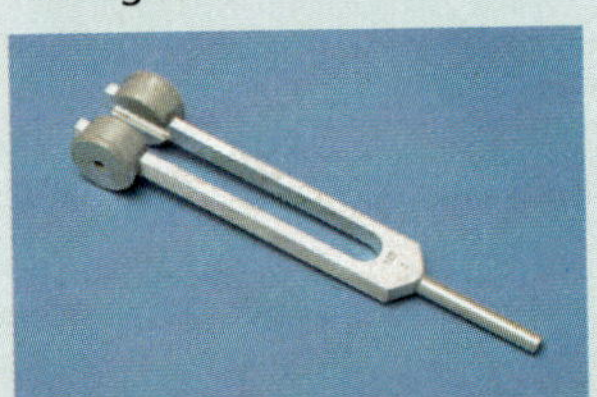	Used to test for bone and air conduction deafness Important in neurological examinations (see Chapter 13)

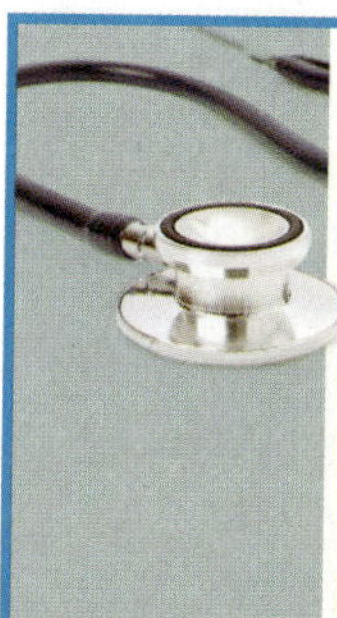

Field Smarts

Patient safety is very important. Take a few moments to periodically sit in the reception room chairs or on the exam table and look for potential dangers—such as frayed electrical cords or sharps containers that are accessible to a curious child. Remember, patients and family members may spend brief periods of time alone in the exam room.

of the function of each piece of equipment or instrument *prior* to the exam. Some equipment is used only rarely. A periodic review of this equipment is essential for the medical assistant to remain proficient in its use and upkeep. Assurance that equipment is functional, including the replacement of batteries, is often delegated to the medical assistant.

In addition to the routine physical exam, other procedures are often performed in the office, usually requiring additional equipment or instruments. Chapter 9 discusses proper identification and maintenance of surgical instruments that are utilized during minor office surgical procedures and Chapter 10 lists different types of instruments and supplies that are needed for various types of procedures.

PATIENT PREPARATION

Preparing the patient for the examination is a key responsibility of the medical assistant. This begins with the initial contact with the patient. Chapter 11 reviews the procedures for obtaining vital signs and performing a brief patient interview. Upon completion of the patient interview, the patient is properly prepped for the examination. Positioning and draping the patient enables the provider to visually and physically assess the patient and determine a diagnosis.

PATIENT POSITIONING AND DRAPING

When preparing the patient for the physical examination or any other procedure, proper positioning and draping will increase access to the patient's body to

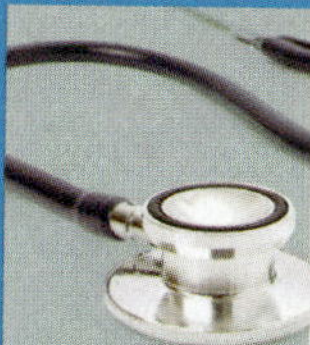

Field Smarts

Another important point is making certain that effective communication between patients and the health care team is completely attainable. The Joint Commission, an independent organization that certifies health care organizations, states that health care organizations need to provide effective, equitable, understandable, and respectful quality care and services that are responsive to diverse cultural health beliefs and practices, preferred languages, health literacy, and other communication needs. If patients are unable to communicate effectively, or fear being discriminated against because of ethnicity, sexual orientation, or socioeconomic status, effective communication will not take place and put the patient at risk of not receiving the best care possible due to communication issues.

facilitate the examination process. Patient comfort and privacy are directly related to correct and thorough positioning. The medical assistant can assist the patient into the position most conducive to the exam while explaining the purpose of this position to the patient. Remember that more than one position may be used during the exam and the medical assistant must be prepared to anticipate position changes in order to provide assistance to the patient and provider.

Always stand next to the exam table when positioning the patient and be aware of movements that may cause the patient to lose balance and fall off the exam table. Provide clear and concise instructions on which direction and what body part the patient is to move. It is important to have the patient roll toward you when changing from a supine position to a prone position to be able to stabilize the patient if she is unbalanced. Assist the patient to an upright position and allow the patient time to recover equilibrium when changing positions (Figure 12-2). Some patients suffer from **vertigo** and can become dizzy or may faint due to changes in posture or head positions.

Providing adequate draping will ensure warmth and allow the patient to feel more dignified and confident.

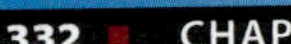

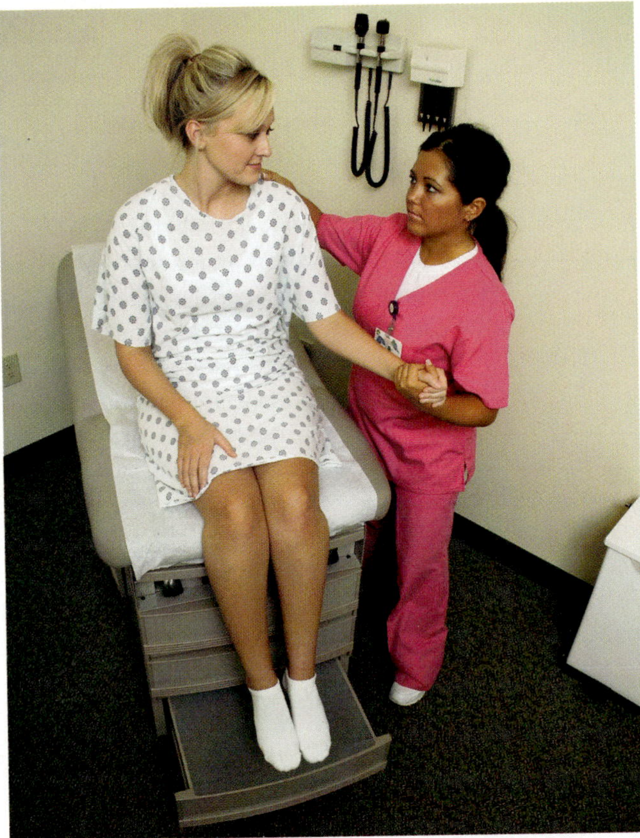

Figure 12-2 ■ The medical assistant helps the patient into a sitting position and makes sure that she is steady before allowing her to step down.

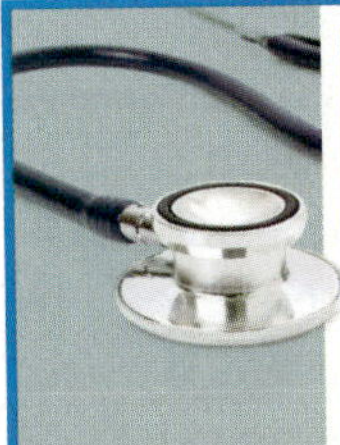

Field Smarts

Remember to provide safety and comfort when positioning your patient. Evaluate the mental and physical status of the patient prior to moving away from the exam table. Physically disabled or mentally impaired patients can easily become injured from a fall if left alone. Continually monitor patients and use safety belts when patients are placed in positions that compromise their safety. Offering your hand to help a patient sit up after lying in a prone position will help the patient who cannot sit up without assistance. Obese or weak patients may need assistance in lifting a leg, whereas patients that suffer from hemiplegia (paralysis on one side of the body) or have had a stroke may need assistance in raising their arms.

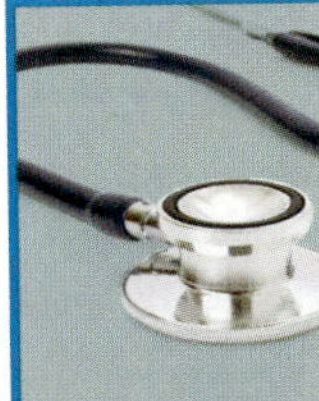

Field Smarts

Remember that the patient is often stressed during an examination. Stress may cause the patient to forget what has been communicated. You should listen carefully to all instructions from the provider in order to "remind" and "reeducate" the patient if needed to ensure better patient compliance after care. Meaningful use guidelines include providing patients with a written clinical summary after their visit. Written information is an excellent supplement to any verbal teaching that was done.

Patient gowns and drapes should be positioned so that only the portion of the body to be examined is exposed. Again, this may change during the examination, and the medical assistant should be prepared to assist and provide adequate draping for the next portion of the exam. Table 12-2 lists the different examination positions, gives a description of each, lists the types of exams the positions are used for, and provides a picture for reference. Procedure 12-2 lists the necessary steps for placing a patient into each of the examination positions.

PATIENT ASSESSMENT

Whether or not the medical assistant will assist the provider during the actual examination will vary according to the following: the patient's physical and mental status, the type of exam that needs to be performed, and the preference of the provider.

Prior to the exam, the medical assistant should screen the patient, obtain vital signs, allow the patient to empty the bladder, and position and drape the patient. This is all completed in a manner that best facilitates the examination or procedure. The provider will assess the status of the patient.

Multiple techniques are employed by the provider during the physical examination. One or all may be used, depending upon the nature of the examination. Table 12-3 explains the six techniques, gives a description of each, and lists examples of what each technique may help to identify.

Table 12-2 Patient Positioning

Position Name	Description/Draping	When Position Is Used
Sitting	Sitting on the side or end of the exam table Drape should be placed squarely over patient's lap	Obtaining vital signs Reviewing medical history Examining the head and neck Evaluating reflexes Listening to cardiac and breath sounds
Supine	Lying flat on the back Drape should be placed lengthwise over the front of the patient	Evaluation of the head, neck, shoulders, chest, abdomen, and extremities Auscultation of abdominal sounds Palpation of thoracic and abdominal regions 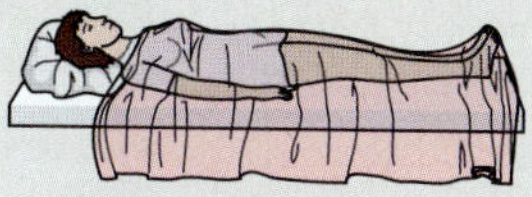
Prone	Lying flat on the stomach Drape should be placed lengthwise over the back of the patient	Examination of the back and vertebrae Exploration of any skin lesions that are present 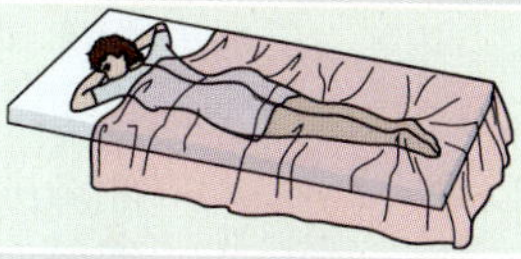
Dorsal recumbent	Lying flat on the back with the knees bent and the soles of the feet flat on the table Drape should be placed lengthwise or diagonally over the patient	Examination of vaginal and rectal areas Insertion of a straight or Foley catheter Examination of the head, neck, thorax, and abdominal areas 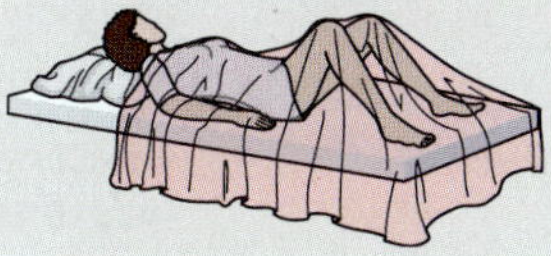
Sims'	Lying on the left side with the left shoulder placed behind the patient while the right leg is flexed and placed in front of the left leg Drape should be placed lengthwise or diagonally across the patient	Examination of the rectum and vagina Rectal temperatures Enemas Flexible sigmoidoscopy 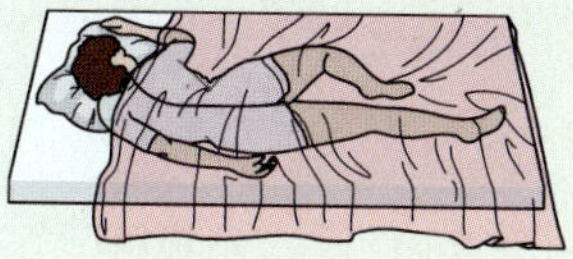
Semi-Fowler's	Lying flat on the back with the head raised to a 45° angle Drape should be placed squarely over the patient	Examination of the head, neck, and upper body Used for patients with respiratory difficulties 45° angle 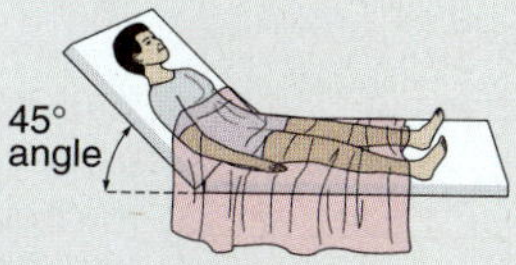
Full-Fowler's	Head of table is brought up to a 90° angle Draping same as semi-Fowler's	Used for patients who cannot sit back at all because of head or neck injuries or breathing difficulties 90° angle 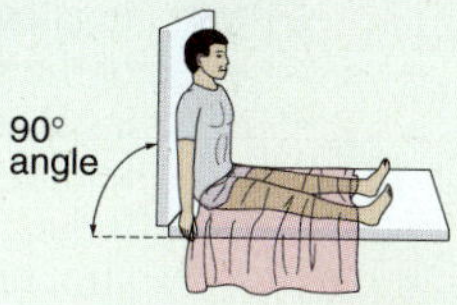
Lithotomy	Lying flat on the back with the knees flexed and the feet in stirrups Drape should be placed squarely or diagonally across the patient	Examination of the genitals and anal area Gynecological exams and Pap smears 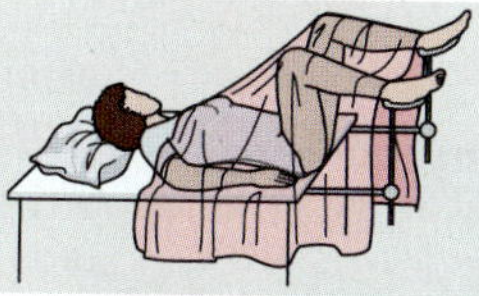
Knee-chest	From the prone position, separate the knees and bring to the chest, raising the buttocks Drape should be placed diagonally across the patient	Examination of the anus and rectum Proctological procedures 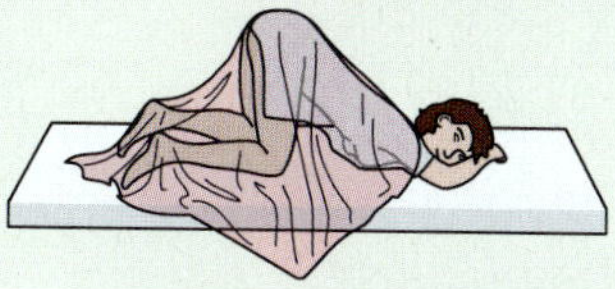
Trendelenburg position	The head of the table should tilt downward toward the floor and the feet should point upward toward the ceiling Drape should be placed lengthwise over the front of the patient	Used for patients that feel faint or are at risk for going into shock 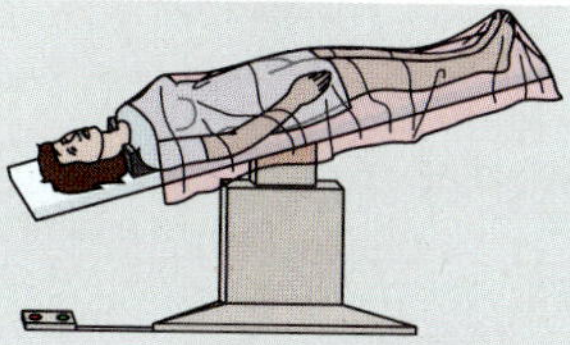
Trendelenburg alternative	The patient's feet and legs are elevated with several pillows or by elevating the foot portion of the table Drape should be placed lengthwise over the front of the patient	Used in place of Trendelenburg when the table is unable to be placed in Trendelenburg position 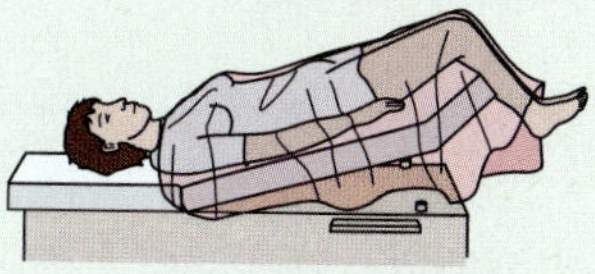

Table 12-3 Examination Techniques Used in the Physical Examination

Technique	Description	Examples of What Might be Evaluated
Inspection	Frequently used to observe the patient for any signs of pathology that might indicate a disease or disorder. This includes observation of physical, mental, and emotional signs.	Skin lesions Scars Body colors such as cyanosis Speech patterns Gait changes Posturing Anxiety 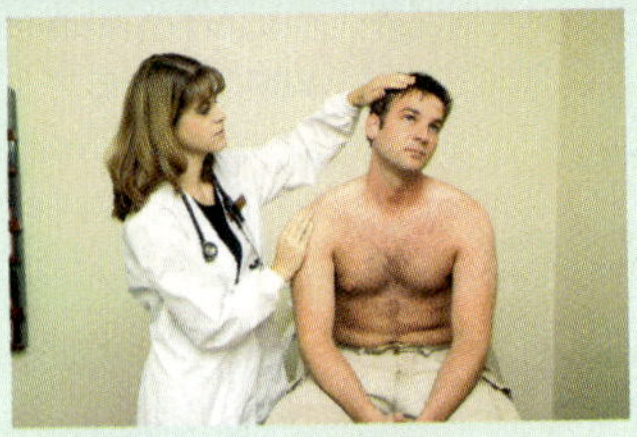
Auscultation	Involves listening skills using a stethoscope. Many parts of the body emit sounds that provide clues to assist with diagnosis and treatment. This is done *before* palpation and percussion for best results.	Lung sounds Heart sounds Bowel sounds 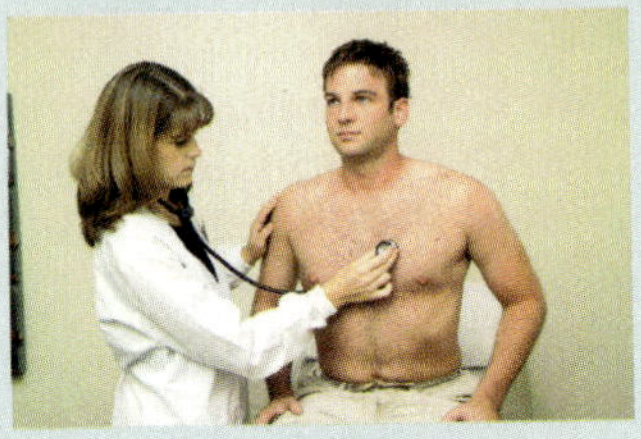
Palpation	Touching the body is one way to evaluate tenderness and pain as well as the location and size of internal organs. Some palpation is light in pressure, whereas some involves deeper pressure.	*Light palpation:* Pain and tenderness Muscle resistance Superficial masses For relaxation *Deep palpation:* Organ enlargement Organ displacement Deep masses 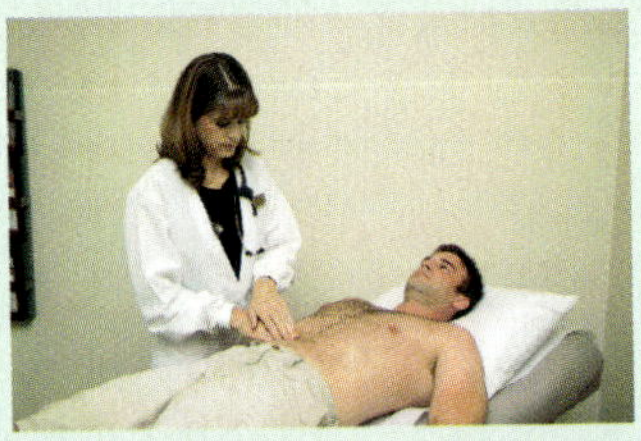
Percussion	Sounds are evaluated by tapping the fingers on the body. Various sounds reverberate over structures to allow determination of the type of structure involved, either solid, liquid, or gas (air). Dullness indicates fluid or a solid structure. **Tympany** (a drum-like sound) indicates air or gas.	Size and location of organs Gas fluids in abdomen Fluids in pleural spaces Liver enlargement 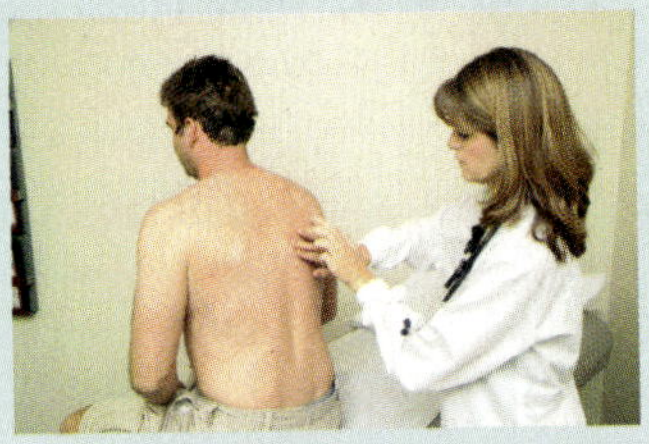
Mensuration	Measurements of different areas of the body, using a tape measure and scales.	Height Weight Length or circumference of a limb Infant chest circumference Infant head circumference 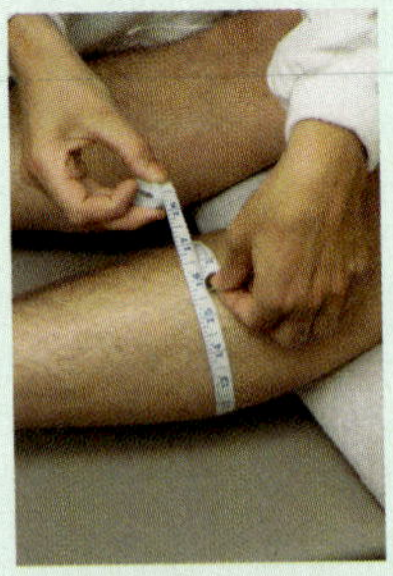
Manipulation	Applying passive movement to a joint while using force.	Range of motion of some joints 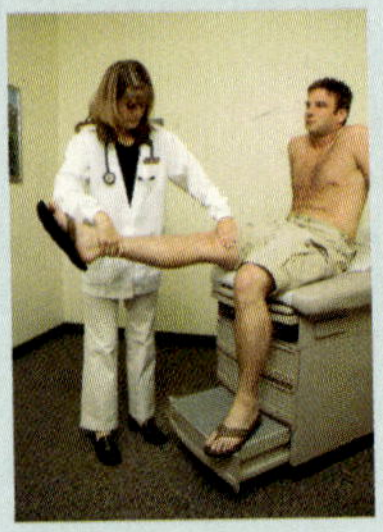

Although the provider performs the actual physical assessment on the patient, the medical assistant will often provide additional assistance to the provider and the patient. Table 12-4 explains the normal sequence of a physical exam. The medical assistant's role in the exam will vary depending upon the patient's mobility and the preference of the provider.

Table 12-4 The Complete Physical Examination Sequence

Comprehensive Exam Section	Examination Techniques	Medical Assistant's Responsibilities	Provider's Responsibilities/ Description of Exam Section
General survey	Inspection	Share with the provider any **observations** (the process of watching or visualizing) noted when assisting the patient to the exam room (the provider doesn't always see the patient walk or the difficulty the patient experienced in removing clothing).	This portion of the exam continues throughout the entire physical. It involves observing the general state of health, to include **posture** (position of the body), gait (the way the patient walks), grooming, odors, facial expressions, speech, and level of awareness.
Vital signs	Auscultation Mensuration	Assist the patient to a sitting position. Obtain temperature, pulse and respiration, and blood pressure. Obtain height and weight.	Vitals are obtained by the medical assistant and repeated by the provider if abnormalities are evident.
Skin	Inspection Palpation	Assist the patient with the gown. Provide adequate lighting in the room.	The skin on the face and upper body is observed. Any discolorations are noted, including patterns, locations, and colors. The hair, hands, and nails are inspected and palpated.
HEENT: Head Eyes Ears Nose Throat	Inspection Palpation	Darken the room for the eye exam. Provide working equipment, including ophthalmoscope, batteries for ophthalmoscope, otoscope, tongue depressors, and speculum for nasal evaluation.	This section includes examination of the head, eyes, ears, nose, and throat. *Head:* scalp, hair, skull, face exam *Eyes:* The provider assesses the physical parts of the eye. *Ears:* Inspects auricles, canals, and ear drums; performs gross hearing screening exam *Nose:* Inspects internal and external nasal cavities; palpates sinuses *Throat:* Inspects mouth, lips, gums, teeth, tongue, tonsils, and palate
Neck	Inspection Palpation	Remove the gown from the neck region.	This evaluation includes palpating and inspecting the cervical lymph nodes. Masses and pulses are felt. The thyroid gland is palpated at this time.
Back	Inspection Palpation	Open the back of the gown to expose the spine and muscles of the back.	The provider will look at and feel the muscles and vertebra of the back. Alignment will be evaluated. Often, the sacral region will be evaluated as well as the range of motion of the lower extremities.
Posterior thorax and lungs	Inspection Palpation Percussion Auscultation	Provide a stethoscope to the provider.	The spine and muscles of the upper back are palpated and inspected. The provider will percuss each side for dullness. Using the stethoscope, breath sounds will be evaluated.
Breasts	Inspection Palpation	Address comfort levels and privacy. The patient's gown may be opened to expose the upper chest area. Replace the gown when completed.	Inspection of the breasts (both genders) occurs, followed by palpation of the breast tissue, axillary nodes, and epitrochlear nodes.
Musculoskeletal (upper body)	Inspection Palpation	Assist the provider as requested.	Range of motion can be evaluated. The hands, shoulders, arms, neck, back, and joints are inspected and palpated.

continues

Table 12-4 The Complete Physical Examination Sequence *(continued)*

Comprehensive Exam Section	Examination Techniques	Medical Assistant's Responsibilities	Provider's Responsibilities/ Description of Exam Section
Anterior thorax and lungs	Inspection Palpation Percussion Auscultation	Provide a stethoscope.	The chest region and breath sounds are evaluated. Voice sounds are also assessed. This is similar to the posterior thorax and lung examination.
Cardiovascular system	Auscultation Inspection Palpation	Assist the patient in transition to the semi-Fowler's position. Lower the patient gown, and provide a drape for comfort and privacy. Provide a stethoscope with a bell attachment and diaphragm.	Jugular and carotid pulsations are inspected and palpated. Using the stethoscope, the carotids are evaluated for bruits.
	Auscultation	Assist the patient to sitting. As the patient leans forward, provide support and security.	While the patient exhales, the provider will listen for murmurs and other abnormalities.
Abdomen	Inspection Palpation Auscultation Percussion	Assist the patient into the supine position. Remove the gown from the abdominal region and drape the area.	The abdomen will be palpated lightly, then more deeply, while being inspected. Bowel sounds will be auscultated. The liver and spleen will be assessed by percussion. The aorta will be palpated, with the pulsations evaluated.
Breasts/axillae	Inspection Palpation	Assist the patient in removing the gown from the breast area. Provide coverage when the exam is complete.	The provider will complete the breast exam in the supine position, to include inspection for dimpling and palpation for masses. The axillary nodes are palpated.
Lower extremities	Inspection Palpation	Provide tools for a neurological exam of the lower extremities. Provide a reflex hammer.	The lower extremity pulses are palpated. Area is inspected for edema, ulcerations, and discolorations. Pitting edema is evaluated. Muscle tone and joint deformities are assessed. Sensations and reflexes are tested.
	Inspection	Allow the patient to sit briefly prior to standing. Assist the patient to a standing position. Provide support with gait if necessary.	The legs are inspected for varicose veins. Muscle tone and alignment is evaluated. The gait may be reexamined at this time.
Nervous system	Inspection	Assist the patient to a sitting or supine position, as requested by the provider.	This section of the examination may be done at various times. It is composed of five components: Mental status Cranial nerves Motor system Sensory system Reflexes
Gynecological exam for women	Inspection Palpation	Prepare tools for examination (see Chapter 17). Assist the patient into the supine position, then place feet in the stirrups. Provide draping for privacy. Put a light in place for the exam. Assist the patient in relaxing for the exam. Assist the patient from the exam table and assist with dressing if needed.	The provider will inspect the external genitalia, vagina, and cervix. A Pap smear will be completed at this time. The uterus and ovaries will be palpated. A rectal exam can be completed at this time.

Table 12-4 The Complete Physical Examination Sequence *(continued)*

Comprehensive Exam Section	Examination Techniques	Medical Assistant's Responsibilities	Provider's Responsibilities/ Description of Exam Section
Prostate and rectal exam for men	Inspection Palpation	Assist the patient into the Sims' position. Provide draping for privacy. Provide an occult blood card if ordered. Have gloves and lubricant available. Assist the patient from the exam table and assist with dressing if needed.	The anal region will be inspected along with the genitalia, if this is not done while the patient is standing. The rectum and prostate are then palpated.

Completing the Visit

Following the physical exam, the provider will leave instructions on what else needs to be completed before the patient can be dismissed. Instructions may be written in the plan section of the progress note or on the patient encounter form.

Procedures that may be necessary before dismissing the patient include the following:

- Performing additional lab or diagnostic testing
- Administering or dispensing certain medications
- Giving any prescriptions or drug samples to the patient and providing instructions on how to take the medication
- Setting up an outside test for the patient
- Completing a referral and setting up an appointment with a specialist
- Providing the patient with home care instructions
- Setting up a new appointment for the patient

After performing any necessary procedures, share the results of the procedure with the provider *before* dismissing the patient. The results may create a change in how the provider wants to proceed. Inform patients of when and how they can receive lab results. Encourage patients to call if they have any other questions. Properly escort the patient to the checkout area and return to the room to prepare it for the next patient.

Refer to Procedure 12-3 for a complete procedure on assisting with the general physical exam.

The medical assistant can be the support that allows for a smooth, successful, and professional patient examination. Compliance with orders and instructions will correlate to the care provided during the exam. From initial preparation of the patient room and equipment and continuing through the patient assessment, the medical assistant must demonstrate a high-level of professionalism, compassion, empathy, assistance, and education for a quality standard of care required in the medical profession.

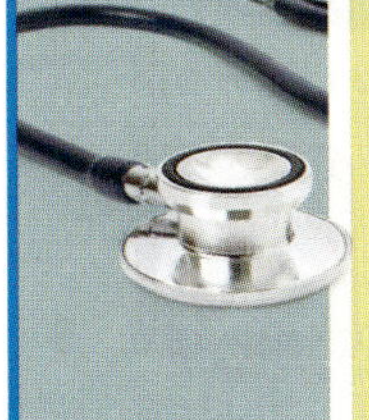

Field Smarts

Be sensitive of the patient's needs and concerns throughout the visit. Take extra time to make certain the patient is properly draped and that you do everything you can to ensure patient comfort. Explaining everything that is going to happen before a procedure or examination begins will help to ease patient anxiety. Encourage patients to alert you if they are uncomfortable or in pain during any part of the exam or procedure so that you can take appropriate responsive measures.

EHR Application

With EHR, the medical assistant can set up a new appointment for the patient directly from the point of care. The appointment screen can usually be accessed in most software programs by going into the main menu and clicking on the "Appointments" icon. Having a clinical staff member set up the appointment will help to ensure that the proper amount of time is reserved for the next appointment and will expedite checkout procedures when the patient leaves.

PROCEDURE 12-1 continued

PROCEDURAL STEPS	DETAILS AND/OR RATIONALE
10. Make one last visual sweep of the exam room to ensure that all equipment and supplies are ready and available for the next patient exam.	A clean, well-stocked exam room reflects positively on the practice.
11. If applicable, activate the room indicator to alert workers that the room is ready for the next patient.	Room indicators may be flags or a light system that can be activated to indicate that the room is ready for the next patient.

PROCEDURE 12-2

Position and Drape the Patient

Objective:

To assist patients into a variety of common positions that are used for various exams and to drape for privacy.

Equipment/Supplies:

- Exam table
- Table paper
- Disposable gloves if necessary
- Patient gown
- Paper or cloth drape

PROCEDURAL STEPS	DETAILS AND/OR RATIONALE
1. Wash your hands and use gloves if necessary, practicing standard precautions.	Handwashing is the principle method of preventing the spread of infection.
2. Prepare the exam room, positioning the table into a low flat position, if applicable.	The room should be ready prior to allowing the patient to enter. Positioning the table low will eliminate the need for climbing. A lowered table allows for better body mechanics.
3. Identify the patient using two identifiers, identify yourself, and ***explain the rationale for performance of the procedure, showing awareness of the patient's concerns related to the procedure being performed.***	It is important to make sure the patient is the correct patient. Educating the patient as to what to expect will encourage patient cooperation.
4. If a gown is to be used, provide this to the patient with instructions on opening in the front or rear. ***Demonstrate the principles of self-boundaries,*** and allow the patient privacy to change into the gown. Provide assistance with gowning if requested.	Depending on the exam, the gown should be worn in a manner that provides exposure for the exam along with the most privacy for the patient.

continues

PROCEDURE 12-1 continued

PROCEDURAL STEPS	DETAILS AND/OR RATIONALE
1. Wash your hands and put on disposable gloves, practicing standard precautions.	This protects the medical assistant when handling contaminated materials. It also provides protection when using disinfectants.
2. Remove any used exam paper and pillow coverings. Discard in an appropriate container.	This prevents any cross-contamination between patients. If body fluids are evident, discard in the biohazard container.
3. Perform disinfection/sterilization techniques, using the designated disinfectant cleaner to wipe the exam table surfaces (Figure 12-3) along with any other trays or countertops that have been used during the previous exam. Always clean from an area of lesser concentration to an area of greater concentration.	Disinfectants will remove contaminants from surfaces and help to prevent any cross-contamination. Cleaning from an area of lesser concentration to an area of greater concentration keeps the medical assistant from pulling microorganisms to an area that was not contaminated or that didn't have as much contamination.
4. Remove gloves, discard, and wash your hands.	Gloves do not need to be worn because you will only be handling clean materials.
5. Place the exam paper on the exam table (Figure 12-4). Replace the pillow cover with a clean or new cover.	Clean paper and pillow covers are needed for each patient to reduce cross-contamination.
6. Check the function of the exam table. Is it at the correct height? If you have an electronic table, make certain that the selection controls are working properly.	If the exam table is not working properly, it could waste time for the both the provider and the patient.
7. Make sure the lighting is effective.	Good lighting is needed for a thorough inspection.
8. If the exam room contains a sink, be sure paper towels or another method for drying the hands are available and functional.	The provider needs all supplies readily available.
9. Make sure all supplies and equipment necessary for the exam are well stocked (Figure 12-5) and placed in a location easily accessible. Have gowns and drapes available. Have gloves for the provider in place. This assists the provider with the examination.	Having supplies readily available saves time.

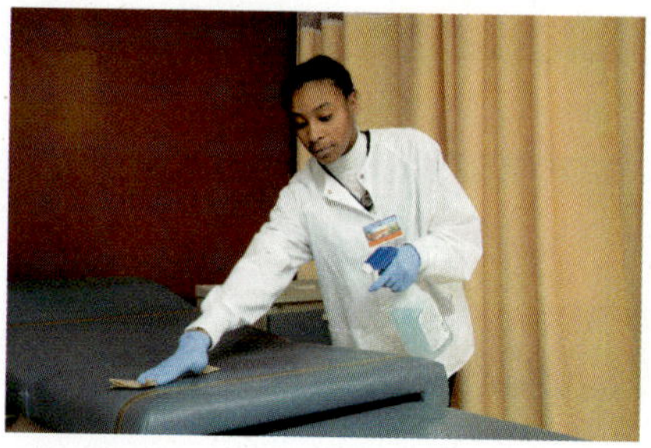

Figure 12-3 ■ The medical assistant cleans the exam table surface, using the designated disinfectant cleaner.

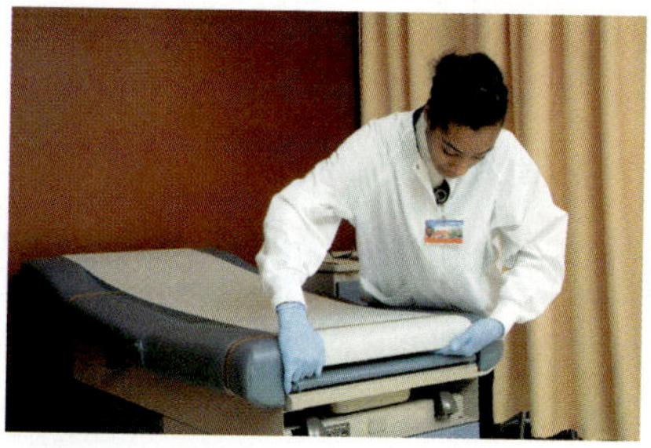

Figure 12-4 ■ The medical assistant places the clean exam paper on the table.

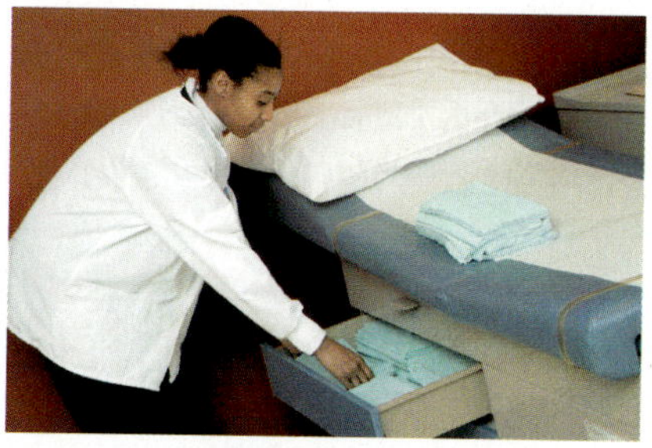

Figure 12-5 ■ The medical assistant makes sure all necessary supplies and equipment are well stocked for the exam.

continues

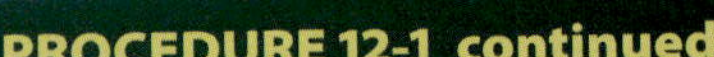

PROCEDURE 12-1 continued

PROCEDURAL STEPS	DETAILS AND/OR RATIONALE
10. Make one last visual sweep of the exam room to ensure that all equipment and supplies are ready and available for the next patient exam.	A clean, well-stocked exam room reflects positively on the practice.
11. If applicable, activate the room indicator to alert workers that the room is ready for the next patient.	Room indicators may be flags or a light system that can be activated to indicate that the room is ready for the next patient.

PROCEDURE 12-2

Position and Drape the Patient

Objective:

To assist patients into a variety of common positions that are used for various exams and to drape for privacy.

Equipment/Supplies:

- Exam table
- Table paper
- Disposable gloves if necessary
- Patient gown
- Paper or cloth drape

PROCEDURAL STEPS	DETAILS AND/OR RATIONALE
1. Wash your hands and use gloves if necessary, practicing standard precautions.	Handwashing is the principle method of preventing the spread of infection.
2. Prepare the exam room, positioning the table into a low flat position, if applicable.	The room should be ready prior to allowing the patient to enter. Positioning the table low will eliminate the need for climbing. A lowered table allows for better body mechanics.
3. Identify the patient using two identifiers, identify yourself, and ***explain the rationale for performance of the procedure, showing awareness of the patient's concerns related to the procedure being performed.***	It is important to make sure the patient is the correct patient. Educating the patient as to what to expect will encourage patient cooperation.
4. If a gown is to be used, provide this to the patient with instructions on opening in the front or rear. ***Demonstrate the principles of self-boundaries,*** and allow the patient privacy to change into the gown. Provide assistance with gowning if requested.	Depending on the exam, the gown should be worn in a manner that provides exposure for the exam along with the most privacy for the patient.

continues

Table 12-4 The Complete Physical Examination Sequence *(continued)*

Comprehensive Exam Section	Examination Techniques	Medical Assistant's Responsibilities	Provider's Responsibilities/ Description of Exam Section
Prostate and rectal exam for men	Inspection Palpation	Assist the patient into the Sims' position. Provide draping for privacy. Provide an occult blood card if ordered. Have gloves and lubricant available. Assist the patient from the exam table and assist with dressing if needed.	The anal region will be inspected along with the genitalia, if this is not done while the patient is standing. The rectum and prostate are then palpated.

Completing the Visit

Following the physical exam, the provider will leave instructions on what else needs to be completed before the patient can be dismissed. Instructions may be written in the plan section of the progress note or on the patient encounter form.

Procedures that may be necessary before dismissing the patient include the following:

- Performing additional lab or diagnostic testing
- Administering or dispensing certain medications
- Giving any prescriptions or drug samples to the patient and providing instructions on how to take the medication
- Setting up an outside test for the patient
- Completing a referral and setting up an appointment with a specialist
- Providing the patient with home care instructions
- Setting up a new appointment for the patient

After performing any necessary procedures, share the results of the procedure with the provider *before* dismissing the patient. The results may create a change in how the provider wants to proceed. Inform patients of when and how they can receive lab results. Encourage patients to call if they have any other questions. Properly escort the patient to the checkout area and return to the room to prepare it for the next patient.

Refer to Procedure 12-3 for a complete procedure on assisting with the general physical exam.

The medical assistant can be the support that allows for a smooth, successful, and professional patient examination. Compliance with orders and instructions will correlate to the care provided during the exam. From initial preparation of the patient room and equipment and continuing through the patient assessment, the medical assistant must demonstrate a high-level of professionalism, compassion, empathy, assistance, and education for a quality standard of care required in the medical profession.

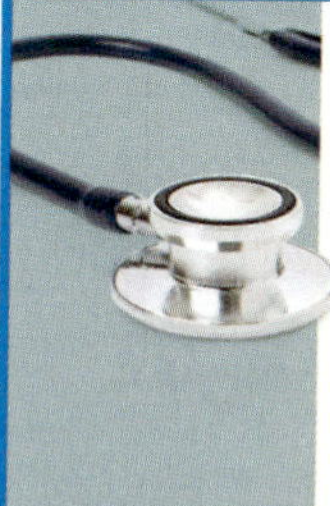

Field Smarts

Be sensitive of the patient's needs and concerns throughout the visit. Take extra time to make certain the patient is properly draped and that you do everything you can to ensure patient comfort. Explaining everything that is going to happen before a procedure or examination begins will help to ease patient anxiety. Encourage patients to alert you if they are uncomfortable or in pain during any part of the exam or procedure so that you can take appropriate responsive measures.

EHR Application

With EHR, the medical assistant can set up a new appointment for the patient directly from the point of care. The appointment screen can usually be accessed in most software programs by going into the main menu and clicking on the "Appointments" icon. Having a clinical staff member set up the appointment will help to ensure that the proper amount of time is reserved for the next appointment and will expedite checkout procedures when the patient leaves.

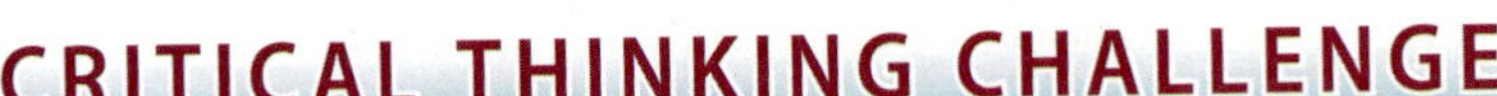

CRITICAL THINKING CHALLENGE

You are assisting the provider during a Pap and pelvic exam. The patient does not verbally state that she is in discomfort but her facial expressions say otherwise.

1. What should you do when you notice the patient is in quite a bit of discomfort during the examination?
2. How might a thorough explanation of what to expect during the procedure assist in improving the patient's mental outlook during the procedure?

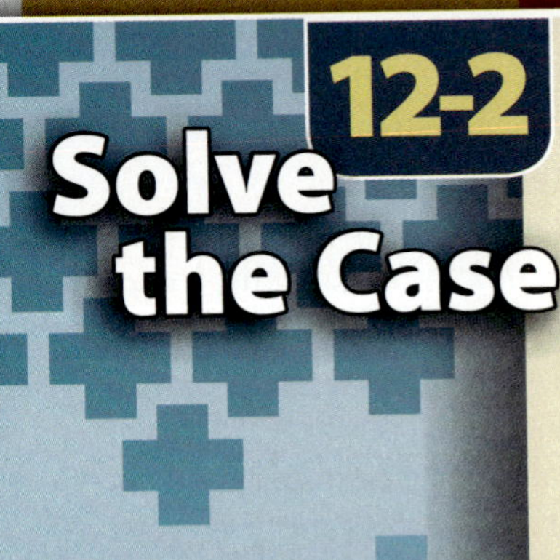

The doctor has ordered an electrocardiogram for Mr. Choy. You learn that Mr. Choy has difficulty breathing when he is in a supine position.

1. **What other position(s) may be suitable for this type of procedure?**
2. **Should you document that the patient was placed in a position other than the supine for this procedure? Why or why not?**

The doctor leaves a note that Mr. Choy is to have a chest X-ray and a chemistry panel before leaving today.

3. **Where specifically would you find these orders?**

PROCEDURE 12-1

Prepare the Examination Room

Objective:

To properly prepare the examination room for a patient coming in for a complete physical exam.

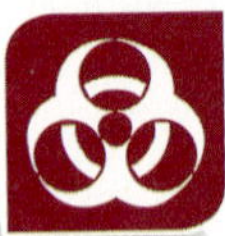

Equipment/Supplies:

- Exam table
- Table paper
- Disposable gloves
- Pillows or support cushions
- Gowns and drapes
- Cleaning supplies
- Lighting
- Disposal containers
- Biohazard containers
- Appropriate instruments and supplies (stethoscope, otoscope, ophthalmoscope, percussion hammer, neurological hammer, pin wheel, hemoccult supplies, lubricant, pelvic exam supplies for a pelvic exam, tape measure, plenty of tissue)

continues

PROCEDURE 12-2 continued

PROCEDURAL STEPS	DETAILS AND/OR RATIONALE
5. Pull out the retractable step to allow the patient to step up and be seated safely on the exam table. Once the patient is seated on the exam table, push in the retractable step and assist the patient into one of the following positions.	A retractable step helps facilitate the patient's ascent to the table surface. If a step is not available, a stool that is wide and provides a stable surface may be used. Retracting the step into the table provides a safer floor space for the provider to move freely around the patient without tripping over the step.
Sitting position: Explain to the patient how to sit. The patient's legs should be flexed, hanging at a 90° angle over the edge of the table. The thighs should be supported on the exam table. Make certain the patient is sitting in a stable manner and be certain the patient is stable. Provide a drape for privacy and comfort. This should cover the lower extremities and lap area.	Using good body mechanics will protect the health of the patient along with the medical assistant. If the patient is unstable, being left alone could result in a fall and injury to the patient. Patient privacy is an essential requirement for patient care. Unnecessary body exposure makes the patient uncomfortable and decreases the chance of patient cooperation and compliance.
Supine position: Ask the patient to sit at the end of the exam table. Have the patient lie back on the exam table and extend the table extension to rest the patient's legs on. Place a pillow under the patient's head and shoulders, for comfort. Place a drape over the torso and lower extremities using lengthwise draping procedure for comfort and privacy.	If the pillow is not placed under both the head and shoulders, excessive flexion of the cervical vertebrae could occur.
Prone position: Ask the patient to sit on the end of the exam table. Have the patient lie back in the supine position and extend the table extension. Instruct the patient to roll toward you and lie on the stomach. Position the patient with the head turned to the side and the arms at the side or above the head. Place a drape on the torso and lower extremities using lengthwide draping procedure for comfort and privacy.	Rolling the patient toward you will provide stability and prevent the patient from falling off the exam table.
Dorsal recumbent position: Ask the patient to sit on the end of the exam table. Have the patient lie back in the supine position and extend the table extension. Ask the patient to bend the knees and place the feet flat on the table. Push the table extension in. Drape the patient using a diagonal draping procedure so that the corner can be easily lifted during the procedure.	Pushing the table extension back in allows more space for the provider to conduct the exam. The diamond or diagonal drape covers the patient and provides easy access for the provider when conducting the exam.

continues

PROCEDURE 12-2 continued

PROCEDURAL STEPS	DETAILS AND/OR RATIONALE
Sims' position: Ask the patient to sit on the end of the exam table. Have the patient lie back in the supine position and extend the table extension. Ask the patient to roll toward you up onto the left side. Instruct the patient to place the left arm behind the body and the right arm in front of the body. Both legs are flexed slightly with the top leg flexed at a more extreme angle. Drape using diagonal draping procedures for comfort and privacy.	Flexing the legs helps to provide easier access to the exam area. The diamond or diagonal drape assists with privacy and provides easy access for the provider during the exam.
Fowler's position: Ask the patient to sit on the end of the exam table. Elevate the head of the exam table to the desired angle (Fowler's is a 90° and semi-Fowler's is a 45°). Drape the patient using a lengthwide procedure for comfort and privacy.	Patients with cardiac or respiratory difficulties are placed in these positions to facilitate easier breathing.
Lithotomy position: Ask the patient to lie in the supine position and pull out the table extension. Extend the stirrups at the end of the exam table and instruct the patient to scoot to the end of the exam table and place the feet in the stirrups; assist the patient, as this is sometimes difficult. Drape the patient with the diamond (diagonal) drape.	Helping the patient place the feet in the stirrups makes it easier. The diamond or diagonal drape provides privacy for the patient and the provider needs only to lift one corner of the drape to conduct the examination.
Knee-chest position: Ask the patient to lie on the exam table in the prone position. Instruct the patient to get on hands and knees and pull the knees as close to the chest as possible. Have the patient turn the head to the side and bend the arms and place them above the head. Drape the patient with the diamond (diagonal) drape.	This can be an uncomfortable and embarrassing position for the patient, so do not place them in this position until the provider is in the room. The diamond or diagonal drape provides privacy for the patient and easy access to the area that is being examined.
6. Instruct the patient not to tuck the drape under or around body parts.	A free-lying drape will allow for small movements and adjustments of the drape to provide maximum coverage.

PROCEDURE 12-3

Assist with the General Physical Examination

Objective:

To assist the provider with all aspects of a complete physical examination.

Equipment/Supplies:

- Examination table
- Table paper
- Gown
- Drape
- Examination equipment/tools
- Patient medical record/pen
- Disposable gloves
- Patient's chart/EHR

PROCEDURAL STEPS	DETAILS AND/OR RATIONALE
1. Prepare the exam room.	
2. Wash your hands and use gloves if necessary, practicing standard precautions.	Handwashing is the principle method of preventing the spread of infection.
3. Prepare a tray with the equipment necessary (Figure 12-6).	Be prepared for what type of exam is being performed. Anticipating the needs of the provider best facilitates the exam and exercises time management.
4. Identify the patient using two identifiers, identify yourself, and ***explain the rationale for performance of the examination to the patient, showing awareness of the patient's concerns related to the examination being performed***.	It is important to make sure you have the correct patient. Educating the patient as to what to expect will relax and comfort the patient.
5. Using the patient record, begin screening the patient and obtain vital signs, height, and weight. ***Incorporate critical thinking when performing patient assessment***.	
6. Allow the patient to use the restroom and collect a specimen if required.	Using the restroom prior to the exam will be more comfortable for the patient and save time in the event the provider wants immediate results or wants to personally examine the specimen microscopically.
7. Prepare a patient for a procedure or treatment by providing a patient gown and drape. Instruct on the proper way to put on the gown. Inform the patient where personal belongings may be placed and request that cell phones and pagers be turned off.	If the patient knows how to properly put on the gown, it will eliminate embarrassment for the patient and also save time.

Figure 12-6 ■ The medical assistant prepares a tray with the necessary equipment for the exam.

continues

PROCEDURE 12-3 continued

PROCEDURAL STEPS	DETAILS AND/OR RATIONALE
8. Place the patient in a sitting position and explain to the patient that you will be alerting the provider that the patient is ready for the exam.	
9. As the provider examines the patient, assist with the exam as necessary. This includes repositioning and draping the patient, active listening, handing equipment to the provider, altering lights as required, ***showing awareness of a patient's concerns***, and chaperoning/reassuring the patient on delicate exams. You may also document items on the patient record as the exam proceeds.	When the medical assistant is present in the room, this provides a secure environment for the patient and protects the provider from false accusations of making improper advances toward the patient.
10. Following the examination, assist the patient in sitting and reorienting.	After lying in a supine or prone position some patients may be dizzy and may need assistance in sitting up. Allow the patient to sit momentarily before moving off of the exam table.
11. Assist the patient from the exam table if needed. Instruct the patient to dress and inform the patient that someone will return to provide further instructions from the provider.	
12. Instruct the patient on any directives the provider ordered. Document instructions in the patient record.	Often the patient will forget what the provider ordered. The medical assistant can reinforce verbally and in writing this information. Copies of lab orders and prescriptions should be placed in the record for any future reference.
13. Accompany the patient to the checkout area and reception area.	Accompanying the patient to the checkout area provides time for additional questions from the patient.

DOCUMENTATION EXAMPLE:

02-13-XX 8:00 a.m.	Patient here for a complete physical today. General concerns include overall fatigue and intermittent joint pain which ranges between 3 and 8 on the pain scale. Pain locations include wrist, shoulders, and knees without radiation. Pt. states that pain is aching in quality and is not relieved by any medications. Pt. states that there is a family history of arthritis. Pain increases during cold or wet weather. Vital Signs: T: 98.6° F, P: 88, R: 16, BP: 130/88. Erin Speck, CMA (AAMA)--

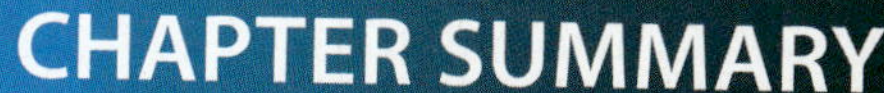

CHAPTER SUMMARY

- The physical examination is done to determine the presence or absence of disease.
- Preparation of the exam room is an important role, and is usually done before the patient even arrives.
- It is important for the medical assistant to anticipate the needs of both the provider and the patient.
- All of the senses are used during assisting with examination.
- Active listening is very important so that the medical assistant can help reinforce instructions and information to the patient.
- The medical assistant's professional role in the physical examination involves being an environmental aide, a compassionate assistant, an informed instructor, an empathetic listener, and a liaison.
- It is the medical assistant's responsibility to clean and stock the exam room and to make sure that all needed supplies and equipment are available to the provider during the exam.
- The medical assistant will also need to place the patient in the correct position for each portion of the exam and may be expected to assist the provider during the exam and obtain and process laboratory specimens.

CERTIFICATION REVIEW QUESTIONS

1. All of the following are examination techniques except:
   a. auscultation.
   b. palpation.
   c. interpretation.
   d. inspection.
2. The lithotomy position is useful in which type of patient exam?
   a. Neuro exam
   b. Pap test
   c. Shoulder exam
   d. Ear exam
3. The Sims' position is used for all of the following except a:
   a. colonoscopy.
   b. pelvic exam.
   c. reflex evaluation.
   d. rectal exam.
4. A patient that is being seen for an abscess on the lower back would be instructed to put the gown on:
   a. open in the front.
   b. open in the back.
   c. both a and b.
   d. None of the above
5. The cleaning and disinfecting of the exam table should be completed how often?
   a. After each invasive procedure
   b. After every patient
   c. When visibly soiled with body fluids
   d. All of the above
6. A patient has the right to privacy and the medical assistant can assist in maintaining the patient's privacy by doing which of the following?
   a. Asking the patient questions in the hallway
   b. Asking the patient questions in the exam room
   c. Asking the patient questions in the reception area
   d. None of the above
7. The provider performs abdominal auscultation, percussion, and palpation with the patient in which position?
   a. Sims' position
   b. Semi-Fowler's position
   c. Supine position
   d. Prone position

8. The patient should be instructed to move in which direction when moving from the supine position to the prone position?
   a. Toward the medical assistant to prevent falling off the table
   b. Away from the medical assistant to prevent the drape from falling off
   c. Toward the end of the exam table to prevent falling off the table
   d. None of the above

9. A male provider will legally require the assistance of a medical assistant in which type of exam?
   a. Performing a Pap smear on a female patient
   b. Performing a rectal exam on a male patient
   c. Performing a throat exam on a female patient
   d. Performing an ear exam on a male patient

10. The equipment used to view the structures of the eye interior and vessels is the:
   a. otoscope.
   b. autoscope.
   c. ophthalmoscope.
   d. stethoscope.

STUDY RESOURCES

Resources to Test and Reinforce Your Knowledge:	
Certification Review Questions	Take this end-of-chapter quiz
Workbook	• Complete the activities for Chapter 12 • Perform the procedures for Chapter 12 using the Competency Checklists
Resources to Promote Critical Thinking:	
***Solve the Case* Activities**	• Consider these case studies and discuss your conclusions
Learning Lab	• Module 21: Clinical Procedures
MindTap	• Complete Chapter 12 readings and activities

REFERENCES

Eligible Professional Meaningful Use Core Measures. (2014, Dec 6). Retrieved from Centers for Medicare and Medicaid: www.cms.gov

13

Eye and Ear Exams and Procedures

ESSENTIAL TERMS

astigmatism
audiologist
audiometer
auricle
cerumen
choroid layer
cones
conjunctiva
fovea centralis
glaucoma
hyperopia
instillation
irrigation
Jaeger chart
lens
myopia
ophthalmic
ophthalmologist
ophthalmoscope
optician
optometrist
ossicles
otic
otorhinolaryngologist
otoscope
oval window
presbyopia
refractive disorder
retina
rods
sclera
Snellen chart
tinnitus
tonometer
tympanic membrane (TM)
tympanometer
visual acuity

15 terms on exam

CHAPTER OUTLINE

Eye and Ear Snapshot
- Eye Anatomy
- Ear Anatomy

Eye and Ear Abbreviation Review

Eye and Ear In-Office and Telephone Screening Tips

Common Diseases or Conditions of the Eyes
- Cataracts
- Macular Degeneration
- Conjunctivitis
- Corneal Abrasion

Common Diseases and Disorders of the Ears
- Neurosensory Hearing Loss
- Conductive Hearing Loss
- Cerumen Impaction
- Ear Infections

Featured Eye Procedures
- Visual Acuity Testing
- Eye Instillation
- Eye Irrigation

Common Eye Medications

Featured Ear Procedures
- Hearing Acuity
- Speech and Word Recognition
- Ear Instillation
- Ear Irrigation
- Miscellaneous Ear Procedures

Common Ear Medications

Common Lab Tests That Coincide with Ear Disorders
- Ear Culture

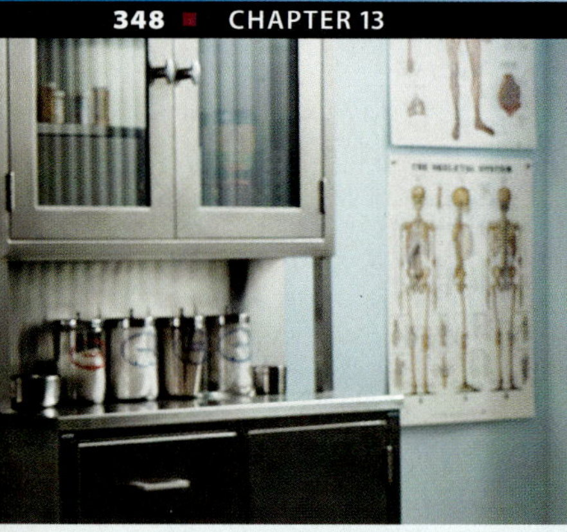

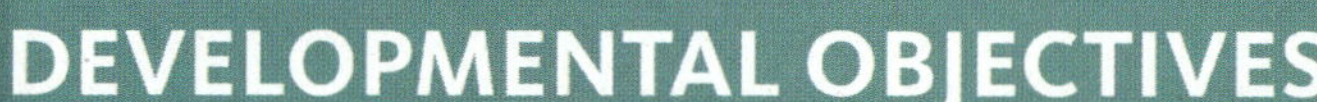

DEVELOPMENTAL OBJECTIVES

After completing this chapter you should be able to:

1. Correctly spell and define the essential terms.
2. List and provide the anatomical locations of the major structures of the eye and ear.
3. Describe the normal functions of the eye and ear.
4. List and use common abbreviations associated with the eyes and ears.
5. Compile a list of common screening questions that should be asked of patients with eye or ear symptoms using established protocols and incorporate critical thinking skills when performing patient assessment.
6. Identify common pathology related to the eye and ear including signs, symptoms, and etiology.
7. Compare structure and function of the eyes and ears over the life span.
8. Analyze pathology for the eyes and ears including diagnostic measures and treatment modalities.
9. Compile a list of common eye and ear medication classifications and conclude how each one acts upon body structures to produce a desired effect.
10. Properly perform visual acuity testing, hearing testing, and ear and eye instillation and irrigation procedures.

INTRODUCTION

As part of a complete physical exam, the medical assistant may be responsible for performing screening tests involving the eye and the ear. Common screening tests performed by the medical assistant include **visual acuity** testing, both near and distance, as well as color vision assessment. A hearing screening may also be performed as part of the physical exam with the use of an **audiometer** (an instrument that measures hearing).

The provider will use the **ophthalmoscope**, an instrument used to examine the internal structures of the eye, and the **otoscope**, an instrument used to examine the ear, during the physical examination. It is the medical assistant's responsibility to make sure both these instruments are in good working order and fully charged prior to the examination.

Some patients may require **instillation** or **irrigation** procedures of the eye and the ear. The medical assistant is often responsible for performing these procedures in the office and providing patients with proper instruction for performing the steps at home.

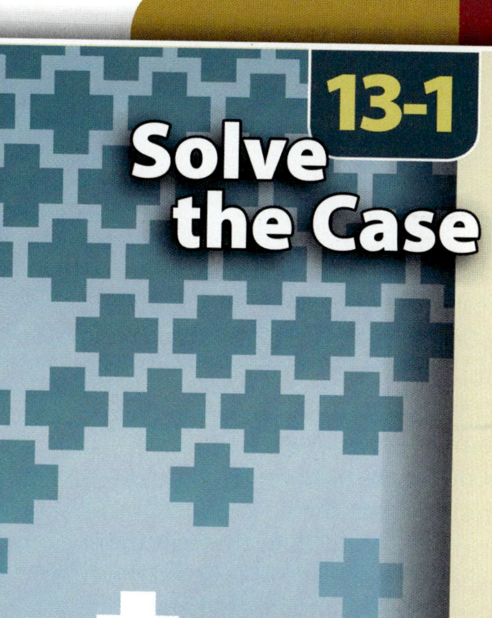

You work for a busy ophthalmology practice. Abda Muhammed, 35-years-old, calls on the phone complaining of "floaters" in her left eye. She goes on to state that even though she has no eye pain, the "floaters" are a real nuisance. Her symptoms came on suddenly this morning and she is leaving for a 14-day trip tomorrow. She states that she really doesn't have time to come in for an appointment and wonders if her condition truly is an emergency or if she can just wait until she gets to her destination and go to an urgent care center. Abda has a history of type 1 diabetes, hypertension, and asthma. With your current level of knowledge, answer the following questions.

1. **Do you feel Abda's symptoms are an emergency?**
2. **Are any of Abda's medical conditions a possible contributor to Abda's symptoms?**
3. **Why is it important for Abda to be seen right away for this condition?**

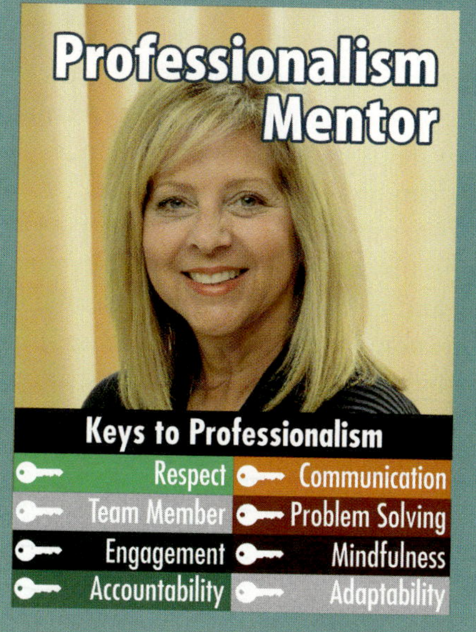

Routine, it is a word that you will hear a lot of when working in the medical field. However, I would be remiss if I did not clarify the necessity of always doing your regular tasks to the best of your ability. As with many routine tests, we hope there are no issues to be discovered, but when there is one, you will want to catch it sooner rather than later. So when you are doing a routine eye exam, or any routine task, remember the physician depends on you to never take short cuts. They trust that you will be vigilant in your data collection no matter how routine it may seem. Many exams are routine until an abnormality is detected and then it turns from routine to something possibly serious. Focus your attention on the details and remember the key to success when doing "routine" tasks such as an eye exam is to never go about a task routinely! ■

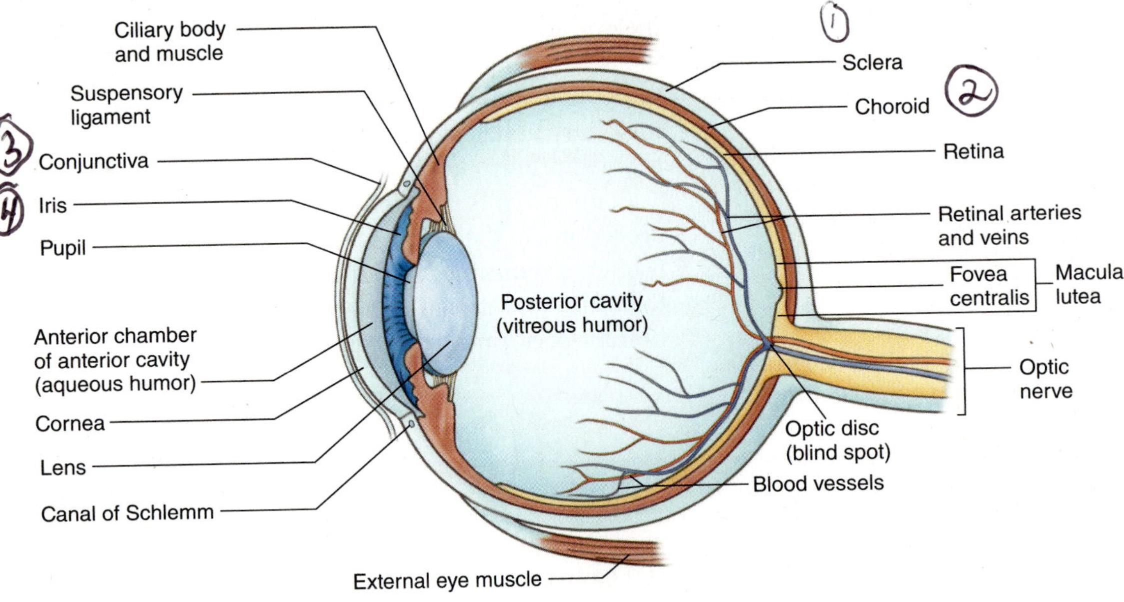

Figure 13-1 ■ Internal view of the eye.

EYE AND EAR SNAPSHOT

Eye Anatomy

The eye is a roughly spherical organ that serves to allow vision. See Figure 13-1 for a diagram featuring the structures of the eye. The eye is covered with three protective layers: The **sclera**, known as the white of the eye, is the outermost lining, followed next by the **choroid layer** or the middle layer. In the anterior eye, the choroid area becomes the cornea, which has a thin layer called the **conjunctiva** overlying it. Light enters the eye via the cornea, a transparent film covering the front of the eye, and then passes through to the anterior chamber, a small fluid-filled area in front of the iris which controls the amount of light entering the eye, and pupil. The iris is the colored part of the eye that surrounds the pupil, the black center.

Light passes through these structures and then through the lens. The **lens** is suspended by ciliary muscles that relax and contract to alter the shape of the lens. These changes cause the passing light to angle and then continue back through the posterior chamber, where the light and the visualized image reach the **retina**, the innermost layer. The **fovea centralis** is an area in the posterior retina where incoming light waves focus, and light, color, and shapes are formed into nerve impulses. These signals travel through the optic nerve and into the brain, where they are processed into our perception of an image.

Specialized cells called **rods** and cones are found in the retina. Rods are sensitive to dim light, whereas **cones** are sensitive to bright light and help differentiate colors.

Ear Anatomy

The outer ear is called the **auricle**, which serves as a mini-satellite dish to catch sound waves and funnel them into the inner ear. Sound waves then pass through the auditory canal until they reach the eardrum, or **tympanic membrane (TM)**. The tympanic membrane vibrates from the incoming sound waves and passes that vibration along to the bones of the middle ear, or **ossicles**. The malleus rests against the TM. The vibrations pass through the malleus and then through the adjacent incus, then stapes. The stapes rests against the membranous **oval window** of the cochlea, a snail-shaped structure of the inner ear. It is within the cochlea that the vibrations are converted into nerve impulses and transmitted via the auditory nerve to the brain, where they are processed as sound.

The inner ear also contains three semicircular canals filled with fluid and hair-like cells that move when the liquid flows over them during motion of the head and body. These hair cells send impulses to the cerebellum of the brain, which helps us to keep our balance. The anatomy of the ear can be seen in Figure 13-2.

General practitioners often examine the patient's eyes during routine physicals and following eye injuries (Figure 13-3) and are trained to treat specific eye conditions. A common instrument used to examine the eye is an ophthalmoscope. A general practitioner is also trained to treat mild disorders of the ear such as ear infections. An otoscope is used to visualize inside the ear. The medical assistant's role during these types of visits will vary but may include asking screening questions prior to the exam, performing visual acuity

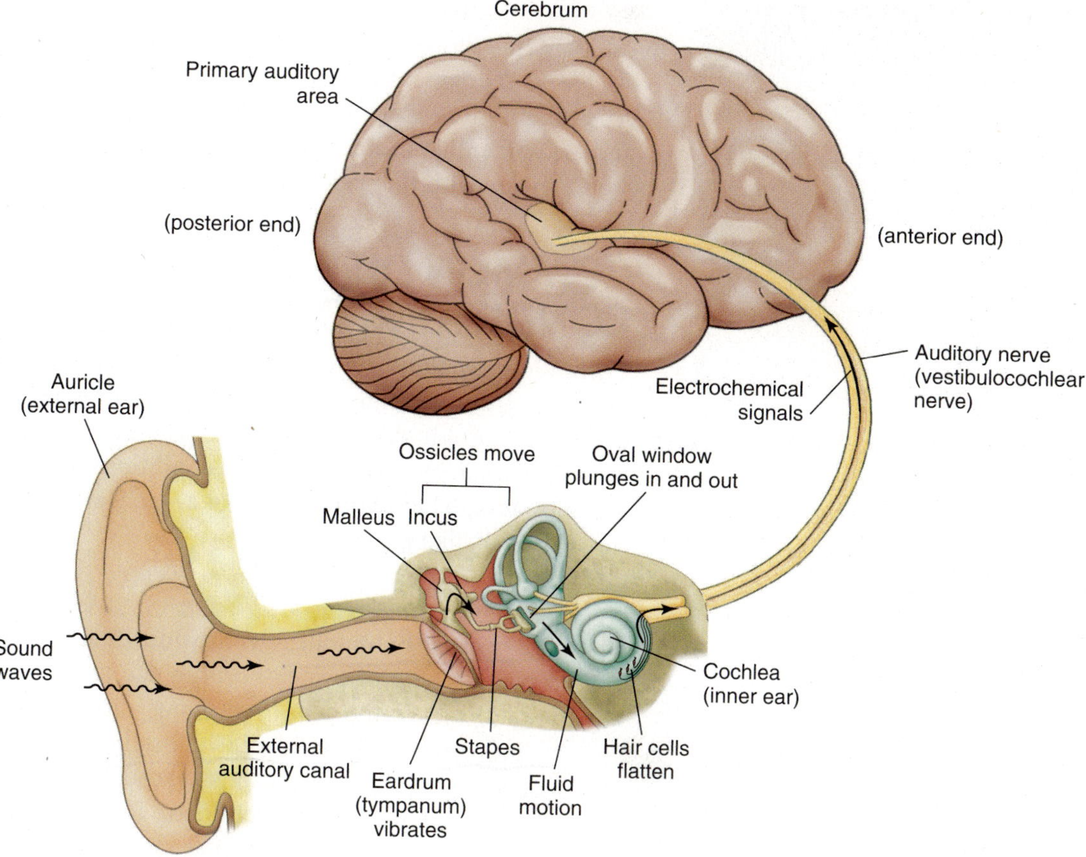

Figure 13-2 ■ Pathway of hearing: sound waves → external ear → auditory canal → eardrum → ossicles (bones of the middle ear) → cochlea → auditory nerve → brain (temporal lobe).

testing, preparing equipment and supplies for the eye exam, assisting the provider during the exam, and performing treatments ordered by the provider such as eye or ear irrigations or the instillation of eye or ear drops.

Often times, the primary care provider will refer a patient to an eye or ear specialist when the patient's condition is beyond the provider's scope of duty:

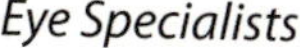

Meet the **Specialists**

Eye Specialists

- **Ophthalmologist:** MD who specializes in the eyes. Able to treat **refractive disorders** (conditions in which the lens and cornea do not bend light correctly, resulting in visual defects), prescribe medications, and perform various types of surgical procedures on the eye.
- **Optometrist**: Not an MD, but a Doctor of Optometry (O.D.). Cannot perform surgery, but can diagnose, prescribe, and treat eye disorders. Can also treat refractive disorders.
- **Optician**: Not an MD and cannot diagnose, prescribe, or treat eye disorders, but is able to fill prescriptions for eyeglasses and contact lenses.

Ear Specialists

- **Otorhinolaryngologist:** A medical doctor who specializes in disorders of the ear is an ear, nose, and throat (ENT) doctor.
- **Audiologist:** A professional trained to identify and treat hearing or balance problems. Must now possess a minimum of a doctoral degree, but does not have to be an MD. These specialists work closely with ENTs and hearing-aid manufacturers and are often responsible for hearing testing and the dispensing of hearing aids and assistive listening devices.

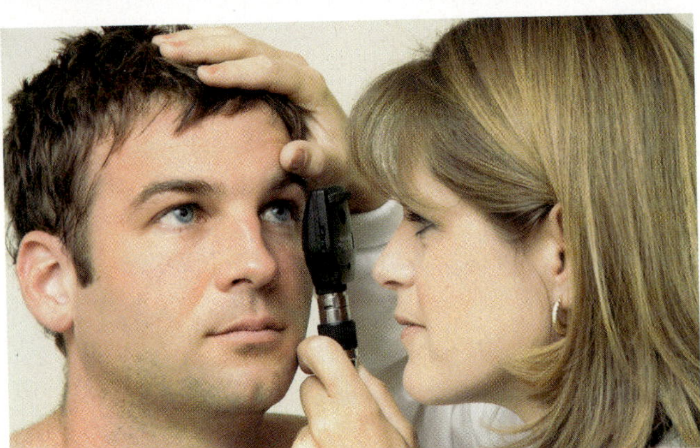

Figure 13-3 ■ A provider uses an ophthalmoscope to examine a patient's eye.

EYE AND EAR ABBREVIATION REVIEW

Medical assistants should be familiar with the abbreviations in Tables 13-1.

EYE AND EAR IN-OFFICE AND TELEPHONE SCREENING TIPS

Medical assistants are often assigned the responsibility of screening patients over the phone or prior to provider examination in the office. The degree of screening will be established by office protocol but, in general, medical assistants should be able to ask a series of questions related to the patient's symptoms. Table 13-2 lists the types of questions that are typically asked during an eye and ear screening, indicating the common procedures that coincide with the patient's symptoms.

Table 13-1 Common Eye and Ear Abbreviations

Eye Abbreviation	Meaning
DVA	Distance visual acuity
NVA	Near visual acuity
OD	Right eye
OS	Left eye
OU	Both eyes
Ear Abbreviation	**Meaning**
AD	Right ear
AOM	Acute otitis media
AS	Left ear
AU	Both ears
ENT	Ear, nose, throat
OE, OM, and OI	Otitis externa, otitis media, and otitis interna
TM	Tympanic membrane

Note: The abbreviations OD, OS, and OU have been placed on the Institute for Safe Medication Practices' (ISMP) "Error Prone Abbreviations" list. These abbreviations should not be used when writing prescriptions or in any other types of medical orders.

COMMON DISEASES OR CONDITIONS OF THE EYES

Common pathology of the eye usually stems from either infection or injury. Infection is usually viral or bacterial. Chronic disease changes of the eye can also be seen, either secondary to other conditions such as diabetes or high blood pressure, or as a stand-alone primary disease, like glaucoma.

Cataracts

The leading cause of blindness worldwide, cataracts are caused by clumping of proteins within the lens, causing a cloudiness of the lens. Symptoms usually start with haziness and increased glare with bright lights and lead to loss of vision. The cause is unknown, though some risk factors have been identified. These include advanced age, ultraviolet radiation from sunlight and other sources, diabetes, hypertension, obesity, smoking, prolonged use of steroid medications, significant alcohol consumptions, family history, and high myopia. Preliminary research shows that use of UV blocking sunglasses, as well as consumptions of antioxidant foods including vitamins C and E and omega-3 fatty acids may help to reduce the risk of cataracts. Cataract surgery is common for advanced cataracts and includes an artificial lens insertion after the damaged lens is removed.

Macular Degeneration

Age-related macular degeneration (AMD) occurs when damage to the macula, an area of the retina, causes blurriness, darkness, or a loss of vision in the center of the visual field. It is usually slow-progressing and does not cause complete blindness, though the loss of central vision makes everyday tasks such as cooking, driving, and reading very difficult. Risk is much higher in patients older than 60, though smoking, family history, and Caucasian race all increase the chances of macular degeneration. There is currently no cure available for AMD, though some vitamin supplements are thought to have some protective benefit.

Conjunctivitis

Conjunctivitis pertains to any infection or inflammation of the conjunctiva. It can be due to bacterial, viral,

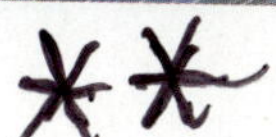

Table 13-2 Patient Screening and Instructions for the Eyes and Ears

Eye Screenings	
Ask the Patient:	• Are you experiencing any visual disturbances, double vision, light sensitivity, excessive tearing, night blindness, drainage, foreign body in eye, blind spots, halos around objects, floaters (little, fiber-like spots) flashes of light, or blood shot eyes? • Do you have a personal or familial history of eye disease? • Do you use contacts and/or eye glasses? Record the date of the patient's last professional eye exam.
For Patients Calling on the Telephone	Patients calling with any of the symptoms above should usually be seen for an appointment, and may often be referred directly to an ophthalmologist or emergency room.
When in the Office:	
Disrobing Instructions	None
Vital Signs	Blood pressure, temperature
Equipment	Ophthalmoscope, Snellen visual acuity chart, occluder, eye tray, cycloplegics (medications that paralyze the ciliary muscle), fluorescein dye, sterile swabs, 4×4s, penlight, irrigating equipment and solutions, and antibiotic drops. **Note:** For patient comfort, dim or turn off lights until provider enters the room.
Possible In-Office Procedures	Visual acuity testing, eye irrigation, eye instillation
Ear Screenings	
Ask the Patient:	• Are you experiencing any hearing deficits, **tinnitus** or ringing in the ear, pain or discharge, buildup of earwax, or a possible foreign body in the ear? • Do you have a history of ear disorders or any recent trauma?
For Patients Calling on the Telephone	Patients calling with any of the symptoms above should usually be seen for an appointment.
When in the Office:	
Disrobing Instructions	None
Vital Signs	Blood pressure, temperature
Equipment	Otoscope, ear tray, ear medication, irrigating equipment and solution (if buildup of cerumen or a foreign body in the ear), audiometer (to measure hearing)
Possible In-Office Procedures	Ear irrigation, ear instillation, audiometry, tympanometry

or allergic causes. Classic presentation is commonly referred to as "pink eye," with a pink coloration of the conjunctiva, along with itching, burning, watering, or thick drainage from the affected eye(s).

Corneal Abrasion

The cornea is very delicate, and even the smallest particle of wood, metal, or other foreign body can scratch the surface, creating a corneal abrasion. Patients are not always even aware of a foreign body in the eye. Symptoms commonly include a foreign body sensation (even if the offending particle is no longer present), along with pain/burning and patients may experience watering of the eye or light sensitivity.

COMMON DISEASES AND DISORDERS OF THE EARS

Hearing loss is the most common disorder of the ear. A hearing loss or defect can be classified as a conduction loss or a nerve loss. Some patients may have a hearing loss from both conductive and nerve defects. This is referred to as a mixed hearing loss. Children should be evaluated periodically to determine if they have any hearing deficits. Hearing deficits can interfere with learning, which causes the child to do poorly in school. Table 13-3 lists some of the problems related to hearing loss.

Neurosensory Hearing Loss

Nerve deafness occurs as a result of damage to the inner ear or the auditory nerve, which blocks the transmission of sound waves to the auditory centers in the brain. Heredity, damage from infectious diseases such as measles or mumps, prolonged exposure to loud noise, tumors, and degeneration due to aging are causes of nerve deafness.

Conductive Hearing Loss

Conduction loss occurs when sound waves cannot reach the middle ear due to impacted cerumen, obstruction of the ear canal due to the presence of foreign bodies or

Health Coach

Featured Disease Spotlight: Glaucoma

Description	**Glaucoma** is a group of diseases that eventually may lead to destruction of the optic nerve, which is the nerve that allows us to see. Many patients with glaucoma have increased ocular pressure, although not all patients with glaucoma experience this increased pressure. According to the Glaucoma Research Foundation, glaucoma is the leading cause of blindness. It also estimates that over 2.2 million Americans have glaucoma, but only half know that they have it.
Diagram	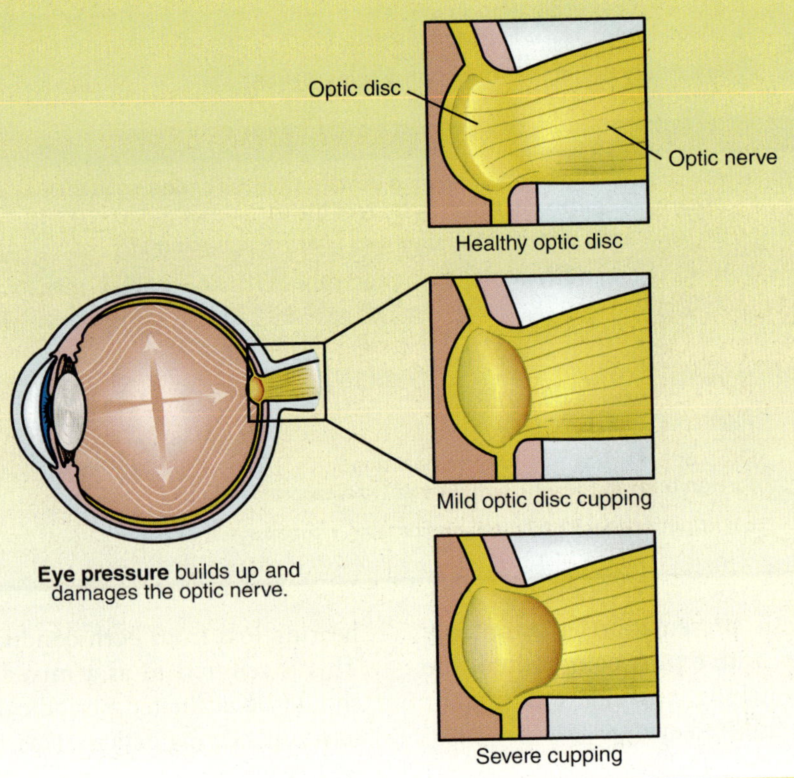
Risk Factors	African American ethnicity, family history of glaucoma, diabetes, age over 60, extreme nearsightedness
Symptoms	Loss of peripheral or side vision; there is usually no pain associated with glaucoma
Diagnostic Testing	Intraocular pressure can be checked using an instrument called a **tonometer**.
Modifying Factors	Regular eye examinations, physical exercise, protecting the eyes from the sun
Treatment	Conventional surgery (trabeculectomy) and procedures such as laser trabeculoplasty help to drain excess fluid from the eye. Medications are usually in eye drop form and aim to decrease the intraocular pressure by either increasing fluid drainage from the eye or by reducing the amount of fluid produced by the eye. There is no known cure.

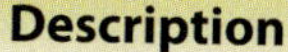

Health Coach

Featured Disease Spotlight: Middle Ear Infections

Description	Infection of the middle ear, typically caused by virus or bacteria
Diagram	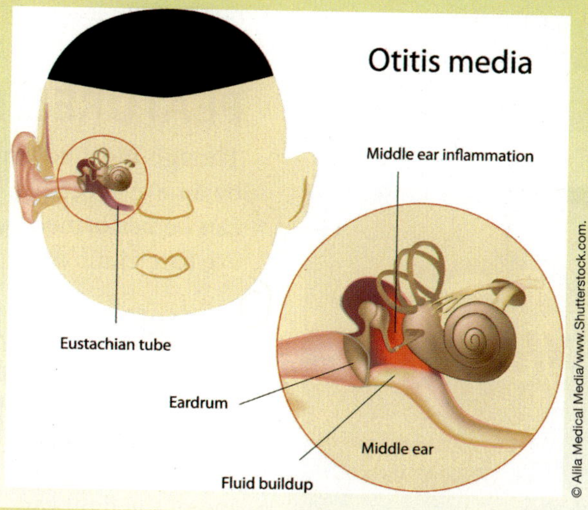
Risk Factors	Family history, exposure to tobacco smoke, not being fully immunized, babies who are bottle-fed while lying down
Symptoms	Pulling at ears, excessive crying, fluid draining from ears, sleep disturbances, fever, headaches, problems with hearing, irritability, difficulty balancing
Diagnostic Testing	**Physical Inspection:** An examiner may diagnose AOM by the appearance of a red, bulging, dull, or retracted eardrum. **Pneumatic Otoscopy:** A puff of air is manually sent into the auditory canal by the examiner while visualizing to be sure the eardrum does not have too much pressure behind it to restrict normal movement. **Tympanometry:** Pressure against the eardrum is measured by a digital device that puffs air into the canal, then measures the movement of the eardrum.
Modifying Factors	To prevent ear infections: • Avoid smoking or exposure to second-hand smoke and do not expose children to second hand smoke • Avoid exposure to air pollutants • Keep yourself and your child up to date with recommended immunizations • Breastfeed your baby for 12 months or more if possible • Bottle feed your baby in the upright position
Treatment	Acute otitis media (AOM) is most often viral and resolves without treatment, though some cases may be caused by bacteria. Bacterial infections are usually treated with the use of antibiotics. Rest, over-the-counter pain relievers such as acetaminophen or ibuprofen, or antipyrine–benzocaine numbing ear drops, may help you or your child feel better.

Table 13-3 Problems Associated with Degrees of Hearing Loss

Degree of Hearing Loss	Associated Problems
Mild	May not hear soft speech.
Moderate	May affect language development, articulation, interaction with others, and self-esteem. The patient usually has difficulty hearing some conversational speech.
Moderate-severe	Difficulty with speech. Does not hear most conversational speech.
Severe	May affect voice quality.
Profound (deafness)	Both speech and language deteriorate.

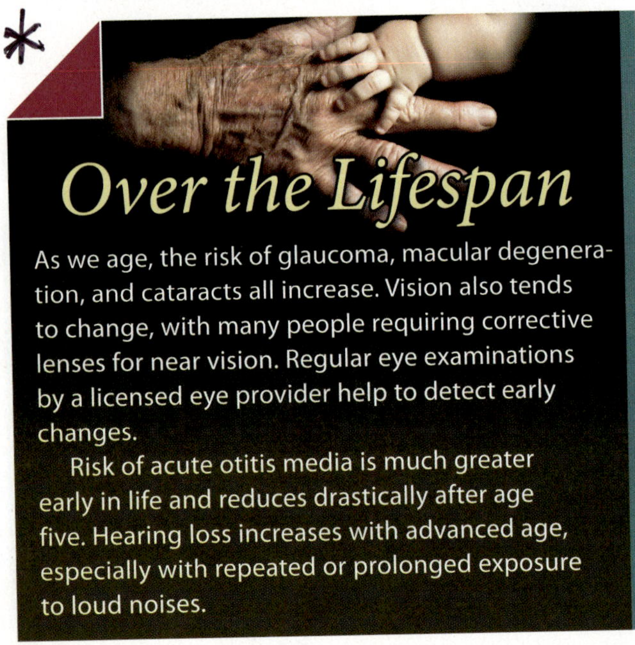

Over the Lifespan

As we age, the risk of glaucoma, macular degeneration, and cataracts all increase. Vision also tends to change, with many people requiring corrective lenses for near vision. Regular eye examinations by a licensed eye provider help to detect early changes.

Risk of acute otitis media is much greater early in life and reduces drastically after age five. Hearing loss increases with advanced age, especially with repeated or prolonged exposure to loud noises.

polyps, or swelling due to otitis media. A scarred tympanic membrane may also cause conduction deafness. This type of deafness is often treatable.

Cerumen Impaction

Obstruction in the auditory canal is most often due to a buildup of excess earwax, or **cerumen**. Specialists discourage use of cotton-tipped swabs for cleaning ears. These tend to just push most of the wax in farther, causing it to build up and form a plug or ball of wax that does not allow the sound waves to pass to the tympanic membrane and middle ear. An impaction sometimes also causes ear pain. It is most often treated with an ear lavage or irrigation (see Procedure 13-8).

Ear Infections

Infections in the ear are quite common and include otitis externa (OE) infection of the outer ear, otitis media (OM) infection of the middle ear, and otitis interna (OI) infection of the inner ear which commonly causes dizziness.

Acute otitis media (AOM) is the most common, especially in babies and small children. The Eustachian tubes in small children tend to lie horizontally and allow fluid to sometimes persist and collect. As they grow, the tubes begin to angle down to the posterior nasopharynx, and fluid tends to drain out of the tubes. Refer to the Health Coach Disease feature on the previous page to learn more about this disease.

FEATURED EYE PROCEDURES

Though most advanced eye procedures are conducted by an eye specialist, several common basic procedures can be performed by medical assistants, whether in an eye care clinic or primary care.

Visual Acuity Testing

Visual acuity testing is a screening procedure used to detect possible errors of refraction. As light enters the pupil, the light rays are bent so they can be focused on the retina. An error of refraction causes improper bending of the light rays, preventing proper focusing on the retina. This type of testing may also be performed on patients following an eye injury to determine if vision has been affected as a result of the injury.

Some refractive errors are caused by a defect in the shape of the eyeball. Refractive errors include the following:

- **Myopia** (nearsightedness): The ability to see only objects that are close up
- **Hyperopia** (farsightedness): The ability to see only objects that are far away
- **Presbyopia**: Farsightedness due to the aging process, caused by loss of elasticity of the lens
- **Astigmatism**: Abnormal curvature of the cornea, which causes blurry vision

Figure 13-4 illustrates the manner in which light rays focus on the retina in refractive errors. Patients with refraction disorders may opt for a variety of treatments including visual devices, such as eyeglasses and contact lenses, or surgical intervention.

Screening Distance Visual Acuity

The **Snellen chart** (Figure 13-5a) is used to test distance visual acuity. This chart is used for adults and school-aged children and consists of different letters in the English alphabet, displayed in decreasing sizes. There are a number of charts that may be used for preliterate children and patients unfamiliar with the English alphabet. The Tumbling E chart consists of the letter

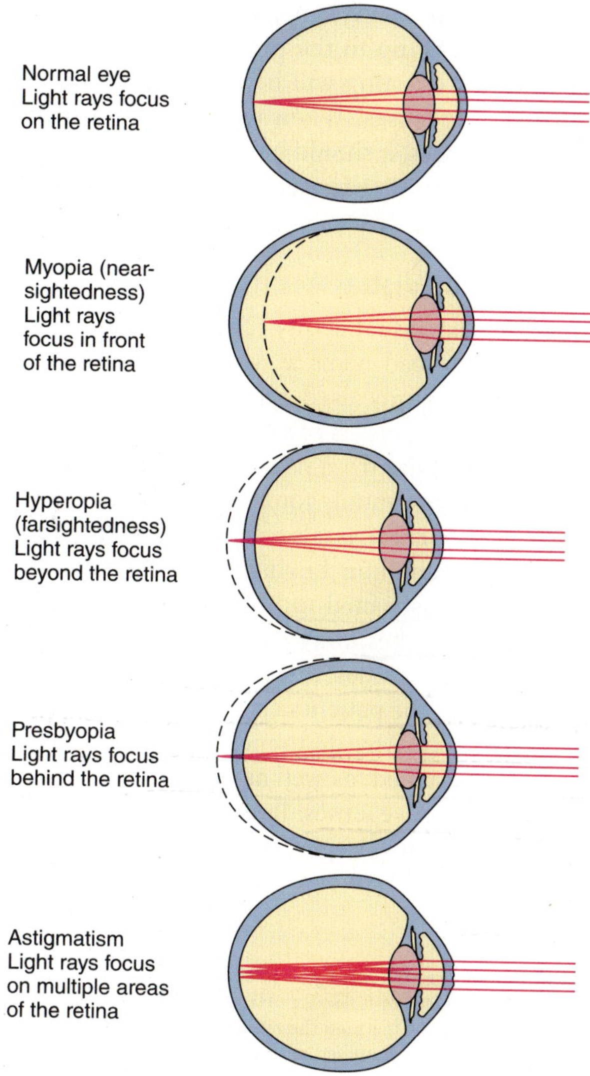

Figure 13-4 ■ Errors in refraction: normal vision, myopia, hyperopia, presbyopia, astigmatism.

"E" arranged in different directions and in decreasing sizes (Figure 13-5b). The patient is asked to describe which direction the open end of the E is facing (toward the top, toward the bottom, toward the left, or toward the right). Children often point in the direction the open end of the E is facing rather than describing the direction. The Landolt C chart is similar to the Tumbling E chart but features a set of circles with different segments missing from each circle (resembling the letter "C"). The patient describes where each missing segment is located. Also available for testing preschoolers aged three to five years are Snellen numbers and picture tests, such as the Allen object recognition chart, the Kindergarten eye test chart (Figure 13-5c) and the LEA chart. The HOTV chart (a chart consisting of the four letters HOTV in descending order) is yet another chart that can be used for patients with limited reading skills. For more information on pediatric visual acuity testing, see Chapter 21.

Performing Visual Acuity Testing

Visual acuity testing should be conducted in a quiet, well-lit area. Adult patients and children aged six and above are placed 20 feet away from the chart during testing, while pediatric patients aged five and below may be placed 10 feet away from the chart. (This will vary depending on the chart that is used.) This distance can be marked on the floor with tape or a painted line. Acuity is measured in each eye separately, usually beginning with the right eye, then the left eye, and then both eyes simultaneously, unless, of course, the patient has poorer vision in one eye; in that case the eye with the poorest vision should be tested first.

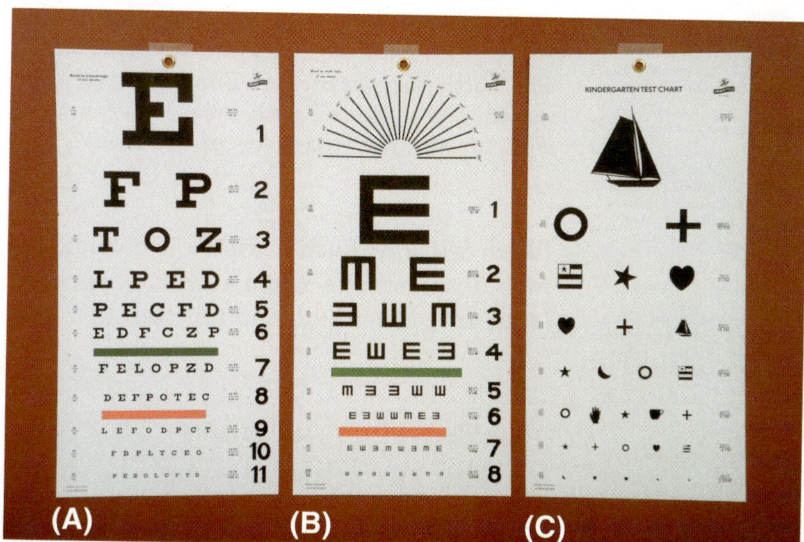

Figure 13-5 ■ (a) A Snellen chart, for screening visual acuity, (b) Tumbling E chart, and (c) Kindergarten eye test chart.

The patient is instructed to cover one eye with an occluder and begin reading downward from the top of the chart. Instructing the patient to keep both eyes open during testing will help to prevent blurring in the eye that is covered with the occluder. The last or smallest line that the patient is able to read without error is generally the line that is recorded for the measurement; however, this may vary in pediatric procedures. The patient should be observed for any signs of difficulty, such as squinting, watery eyes, or leaning forward.

To the left of each line are fractional numbers. The numerator in the fraction represents the distance at which the test is performed. The numerator 20 is used on the standard Snellen chart because the majority of tests are performed at a distance of 20 feet away from the chart. The denominator represents the distance at which patients with normal vision can read the line. If the smallest line the patient can read is the 20/100 line, it means that the patient reads at 20 feet what individuals with normal vision can read at 100 feet. When the test is performed at a distance of 10 feet away from the chart, such as during pediatric testing, the number "10" should be used as the numerator.

The results may be recorded in the patient's chart in the following manner: "R. eye: 20/40," "L. eye: 20/50," and "both eyes: 20/40." When patients wear corrective lenses, it will be up to the provider to determine whether or not the testing will be performed with or without corrective lenses. When testing is performed with corrective lenses, it should be noted as such in the chart. See Procedure 13-1 for step-by-step instructions for performing visual acuity screening on an adult.

Screening Near Visual Acuity

Screening for near visual acuity (NVA) measures the patient's ability to read items at a close distance. The **Jaeger chart**, commonly used for near vision assessment (Figure 13-6), consists of a series of readings with the type ranging in size from newspaper headline print to the small print commonly found in telephone directories. The Jaeger chart is also available in different styles for illiterate and non-English-speaking patients.

The patient is instructed to hold the card at a distance of 14 to 16 inches away from the eyes and continue reading to the smallest line possible. That number is then recorded in the patient's chart. Both eyes should be tested separately. Any differences observed during testing should be noted, as well as whether or not the patient wore corrective lenses. Refer to Procedure 13-2 for instructions on how to perform an NVA screening.

No. 1.
.37M

In the second century of the Christian era, the empire of Rome comprehended the fairest part of the earth, and the most civilized portion of mankind. The frontiers of that extensive monarchy were guarded by ancient renown and disciplined valor. The gentle but powerful influence of laws and manners had gradually cemented the union of the provinces. Their peaceful inhabitants enjoyed and abused the advantages of wealth.

No. 2.
.50M

fourscore years, the public administration was conducted by the virtue and abilities of Nerva, Trajan, Hadrian, and the two Antonines. It is the design of this, and of the two succeeding chapters, to describe the prosperous condition of their empire; and afterwards, from the death of Marcus Antoninus, to deduce the most important circumstances of its decline and fall; a revolution which will ever be remembered, and is still felt by

No. 3.
.62M

the nations of the earth. The principal conquests of the Romans were achieved under the republic; and the emperors, for the most part, were satisfied with preserving those dominions which had been acquired by the policy of the senate, the active emulations of the consuls, and the martial enthusiasm of the people. The seven first centuries were filled with a rapid succession of triumphs; but it was

No. 4.
.75M

reserved for Augustus to relinquish the ambitious design of subduing the whole earth, and to introduce a spirit of moderation into the public councils. Inclined to peace by his temper and situation, it was very easy for him to discover that Rome, in her present exalted situation, had much less to hope than to fear from the chance of arms; and that, in the prosecution of

No. 5.
1.00M

the undertaking became every day more difficult, the event more doubtful, and the possession more precarious, and less beneficial. The experience of Augustus added weight to these salutary reflections, and effectually convinced him that, by the prudent vigor of

No. 6.
1.25M

his counsels, it would be easy to secure every concession which the safety or the dignity of Rome might require from the most formidable barbarians. Instead of exposing his person or his legions to the arrows of the Parthinians, he obtained, by an honor-

No. 7.
1.50M

able treaty, the restitution of the standards and prisoners which had been taken in the defeat of Crassus. His generals, in the early part of his reign, attempted the reduction of Ethiopia and Arabia Felix. They marched near a thou-

No. 8.
1.75M

sand miles to the south of the tropic; but the heat of the climate soon repelled the invaders, and protected the unwarlike natives of those sequestered regions

No. 9.
2.00M

The northern countries of Europe scarcely deserved the expense and labor of conquest. The forests and morasses of Germany were

No. 10.
2.25M

filled with a hardy race of barbarians who despised life when it was separated from freedom; and though, on the first

No. 11.
2.50M

attack, they seemed to yield to the weight of the Roman power, they soon, by a signal

Figure 13-6 ■ When screening for near visual acuity, the patient holds the Jaeger chart 14 to 16 inches from the eyes.

Color Vision Screening

Color vision defect screening is not routinely performed, but may be necessary for people whose jobs involve distinguishing colors, such as pilots, truck drivers, and police and fire personnel. A defect in color vision is commonly referred to as "color blindness," or as color vision deficiency (CVD). This disorder can be inherited, or can be acquired due to eye disease, injury, and certain medications. It can also develop as a result of aging. As a person grows older, the lens of the eye can darken and become yellow, causing problems with distinguishing color. Color vision defects are more common in men. Approximately 8% of males and 1% of females suffer from color vision deficiency.

There are different methods used for color vision screening that use color charts or plates known as pseudo-isochromatic test plates. One method commonly used is the Ishihara method.

The Ishihara Method

The Ishihara method for screening color vision is used to detect color vision deficiency and red-green deficiency. This method uses color plates containing different sized circles. The circles contain primary colored dots, which form a number or a shape against a background of contrasting colored dots (Figure 13-7).

The test consists of 14 plates, but only the first 11 plates are used during the basic screening unless the patient misses any of the first 11 plates; in that case, the remaining three plates are used for testing as well. Additional plates or albums may be purchased for more comprehensive testing.

The Ishihara test should be performed in a quiet area with natural lighting whenever possible. The test should *not* be performed under regular incandescent or fluorescent lighting. A specially designed light booth may be used when natural lighting is not an option. Bright light can cause color distortion, resulting in inaccurate results. The patient is comfortably seated and the medical assistant holds the plates 30 inches away from the patient and at a right angle to the patient's line of vision. The medical assistant will ask the patient to identify the design, shape, or number inside the circle or trace the line within the circle. The patient has approximately three seconds to identify each plate. If the patient is unable to identify particular color plates it may indicate that the patient has a color vision deficiency problem (see Procedure 13-3). The medical assistant will record which plates the patient was unable to identify and share the information with the provider. If a defect is discovered, the patient is generally referred to an ophthalmologist.

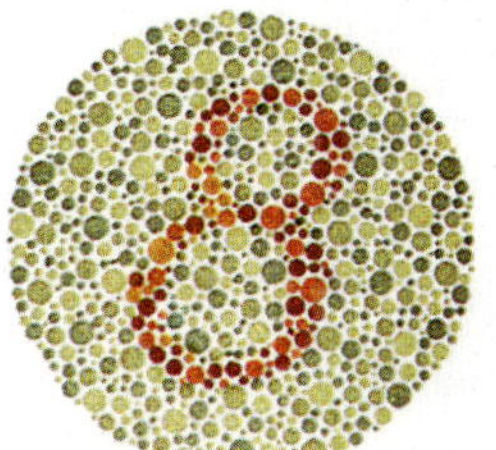

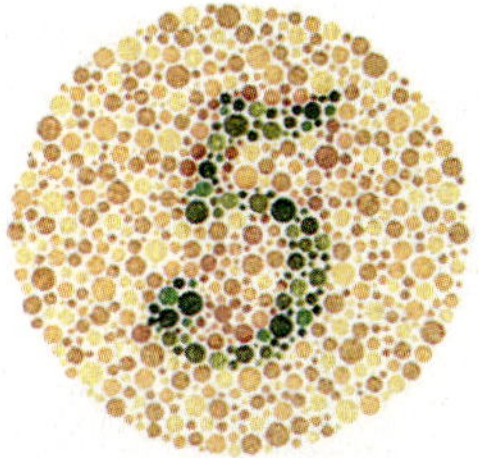

Figure 13-7 ■ Ishihara color plates are used to test a patient's color vision.

Contrast Sensitivity Testing

The measurement of contrast sensitivity provides a screening test for earlier diagnosis and treatment of particular eye diseases. All major eye diseases such as glaucoma, cataracts, macular degeneration, and diabetic retinopathy affect contrast sensitivity. Several charts are now available for evaluating contrast sensitivity.

The Pelli-Robson chart measures contrast sensitivity by defining the faintest contrast the patient can see (Figure 13-8). The chart consists of large letters of a fixed size in varying contrasts.

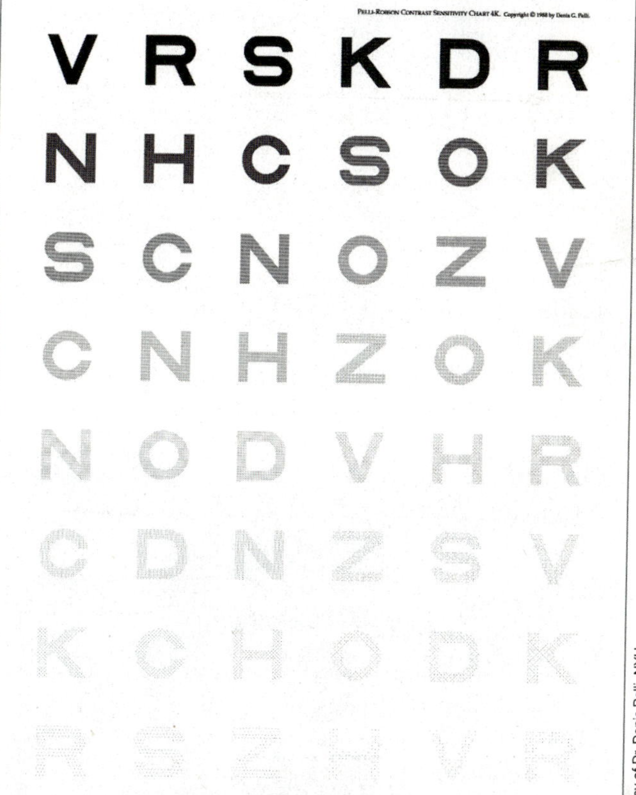

Courtesy of Dr. Denis Pelli, NYU

Figure 13-8 ■ An example of a Pelli–Robson contrast sensitivity chart.

Another contrast sensitivity chart is the Regan chart. This system consists of several charts with different sized letters in low contrast. These charts are similar to the Snellen chart in decreasing levels of contrast.

Instruments for Vision Testing

A vision tester is an instrument that offers simple vision screening in minutes. These testers can perform a variety of tests. The patient simply looks into the tester and the medical assistant displays different visual fields to evaluate both near and distance vision.

The Titmus vision tester is a compact testing device that uses computer-designed optics to screen visual acuity (Figure 13-9). This method can screen patients for all common vision problems and may detect problems that testing with a standard wall chart can miss. The instrument uses a series of test slides (Figure 13-10) that screen the patient for both distance and near visual acuity, muscle balance, peripheral and intermediate vision, and color and depth perception.

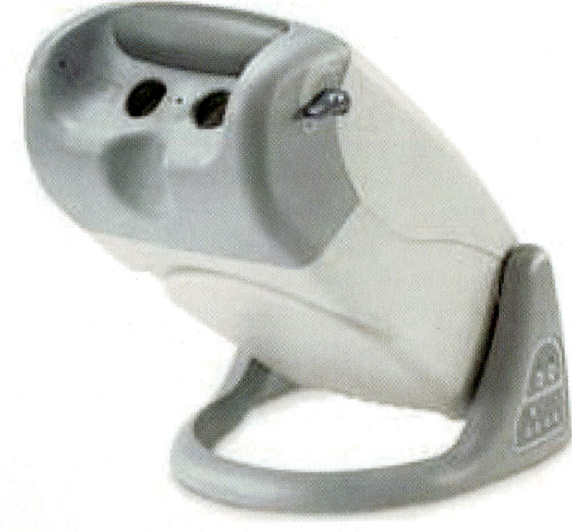
Courtesy of Honeywell International, Inc.

Figure 13-9 ■ Titmus Vision tester.

The testing process takes approximately five minutes to administer. The medical assistant instructs the patient to look into the viewer and stands beside the instrument to change the visual field selection. A visual occluder is incorporated within the viewer for testing each eye separately.

Eye Instillation

Eye instillation is performed for a variety of reasons. Medications are instilled to treat infections and to relieve inflammation, to dilate or constrict the pupil, to anesthetize the eye for examination, and to stimulate circulation in the eye. Some medications or drops are used for a variety of different reasons. It is usually the medical assistant's responsibility to perform instillation and to instruct the patient on proper technique when drops or ointments are to be administered in the home environment.

Medications to be dispensed in the eye come in two forms: sterile drops or sterile ointment. Before instilling drops or ointment in the eye, it is important to make sure the medication is for **ophthalmic** use only. Instructions for performing eye instillation can be found in Procedure 13-4.

Eye Irrigation

An eye irrigation is performed to flush the eye and may be ordered to relieve inflammation, remove foreign particles, cleanse and remove secretions due to infection, and flush out harmful substances such as chemicals. Eyes contaminated from chemicals are usually flushed with water from an eyewash station.

Common solutions used to irrigate the eye include lactated ringer's solution, saline, and water. The pH of tears is approximately 7.1, normal saline is 4.5–7.0, and lactated ringer's solution is 6.0–7.5. Lactated ringer's solution is highly recommended because its pH is closest

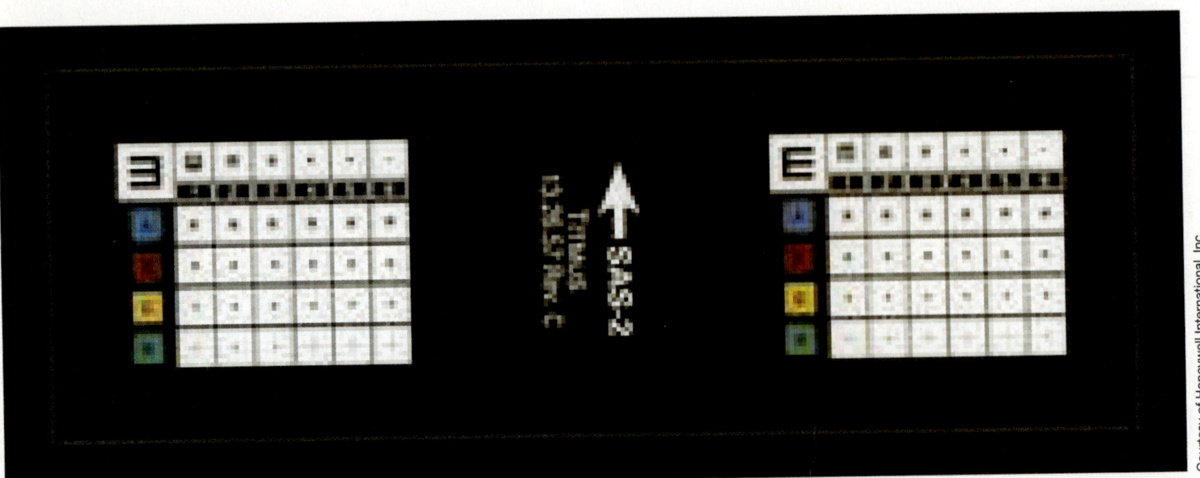

Courtesy of Honeywell International, Inc.

Figure 13-10 ■ Example of test slides the patient sees during Titmus testing.

to the pH of tears. Properly balanced irrigation solutions are commercially available as well. The solution that is ordered will be based on the patient's symptoms and the preference of the provider. Equipment that may be used for eye irrigations includes a rubber bulb syringe or water pick, or a Morgan Lens (a rigid lens that sits on the surface of the eye and under the eyelids and connects directly to an IV line) (Figure 13-11).

Patients should either lie in a supine position or sit up with their face turned to the side of the eye being irrigated. A basin is usually placed underneath the eye to catch the solution. Waterproof pads should be placed over the patient to keep the solution from running onto the patient's clothes. The eyes should be irrigated from the inner canthus (corner) of the eye to the outer canthus, keeping debris or bacteria from reentering the eye. Refer to Procedure 13-5 for a complete procedure for irrigating the eye.

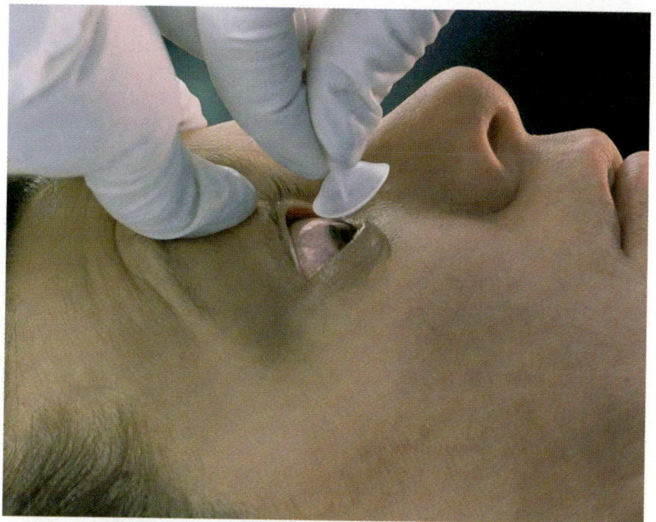

Picture supplied by Mortan, Inc. The Morgan Lens

Figure 13-11 ■ An example of a Morgan Lens that can be used for eye irrigations.

COMMON EYE MEDICATIONS

Eye medications span a variety of pharmaceutical categories. Most are applied topically, in drop or ointment form. It is important that all topical medications administered in the eye be specified on the label as an ophthalmic form of treatment. Refer to Table 13-4 for a list of common eye medications.

FEATURED EAR PROCEDURES

Many basic ear procedures are performed by medical assistants. The following are screening or treatment procedures performed in family practice offices and ENT settings.

Hearing Acuity

Hearing acuity may be performed by an audiologist or a medical assistant. Several methods may be employed to measure hearing acuity. Some are simple gross screenings that use a tuning fork, while others involve the use of a specialized unit known as an audiometer. During any hearing acuity evaluation (see Procedure 13-6), ears are tested one at a time and the ear not being tested should be covered to drown out extraneous sounds.

Gross Hearing Screening

A gross screening is usually performed by the provider during the physical exam. Examples of gross hearing

Table 13-4 Common Eye Medications

Medication Classification	Description	Medication Examples
Alpha-agonists	Used to treat glaucoma	Apraclonidine, brimonidine
Antibiotics (drops)	Drugs used to treat bacterial infections	Bacitracin, Bleph-10, Cortisporin
Antivirals	Treat some specific viral infections, such as influenza	Vitrasert, Zirgan, Viroptic, Herplex, Vira-A
B-Beta blockers	Used to treat glaucoma	Timolol
Carbonic anhydrase inhibitor	Used to treat glaucoma	Brinzolamide
Cholinergic	Used to treat glaucoma	Pilocarpine
Corticosteroids (drops)	Anti-inflammatory drugs used to reduce swelling, irritation, and discharge	Dexamethasone
Combination drugs	Antibiotics and corticosteroids combined into one medication	TobraDex
Monoclonal antibodies	Used to treat macular degeneration	Eylea, Lucentis, Macugen, saffron supplements, and Visudyne used with photodynamic therapy (PDT)
Vitamin/nutritional supplement	Used to treat macular degeneration Used to treat glaucoma	Antioxidants (lutein, zeaxanthin, and vitamins A, C, and E), saffron Gingko

tests include the Weber and Rinne tests described below. The provider stands 1 to 2 feet away from the patient and whispers a series of words or numbers. The patient is asked to repeat the words or numbers. Another gross screening involves holding a ticking wristwatch 4 to 6 inches away from the ear to determine hearing ability. Further testing is indicated if a defect is found upon gross screening.

Tuning Fork Screening

A tuning fork can be used to screen for general hearing. Two common methods known as the Weber test and the Rinne test are performed by the provider.

The Weber test is performed in patients who can hear better in one ear than the other. It involves placing the base of a *vibrating tuning fork* against the crown of the head (Figure 13-12a). The patient is asked where the sound is best heard. Normal hearing is indicated if the sound is heard equally in both ears. A conduction loss is indicated if the patient can hear the sound better in the affected ear, and a sensorineural hearing loss is indicated if the patient can hear the sound better in the unaffected ear.

The Rinne test compares air conduction to bone conduction. During the bone conduction test, the stem of the tuning fork is struck and placed against the mastoid bone behind the ear (Figure 13-12b). The patient is instructed to alert the provider when he can no longer hear the sound. The vibrating tuning fork is immediately moved to the front of the auditory opening for the air conduction test (Figure 13-12c). A patient with normal hearing will be able to hear the sound twice as long by air conduction than by bone conduction. If the patient has a hearing loss caused by a conduction defect, the patient will hear the sound longer during the bone conduction segment of the testing than the air conduction segment. If the patient has a sensorineural hearing loss the patient will hear the sound longer during the air conduction segment of the exam but not for nearly as long as in patients with normal hearing.

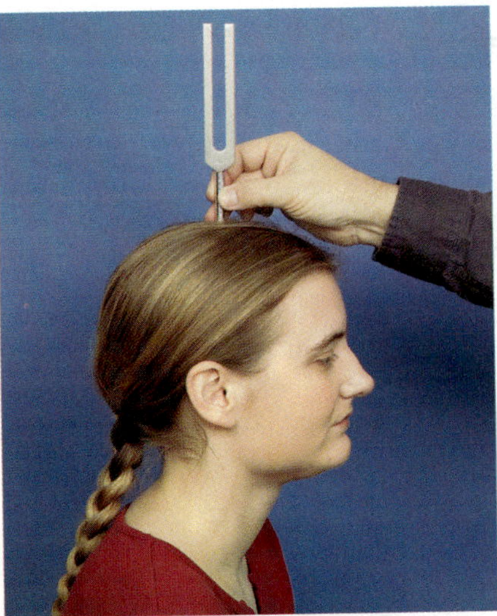

Figure 13-12a ■ During the Weber test, a tuning fork is held against the crown of the patient's head to determine which ear can hear the sound best.

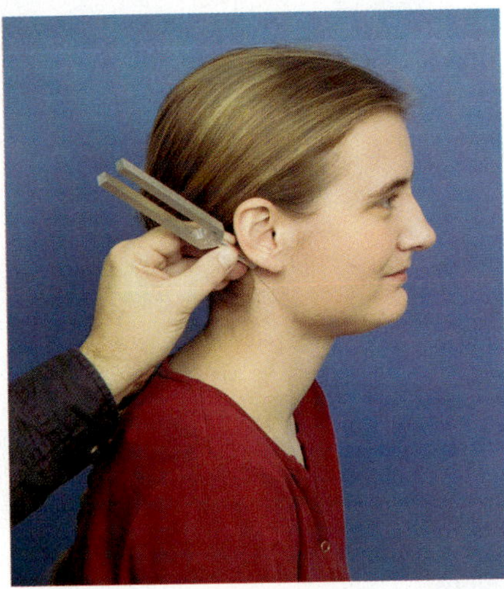

Figure 13-12b ■ During the Rinne test, a tuning fork is placed on the mastoid bone, behind the ear, to determine bone conduction of sound.

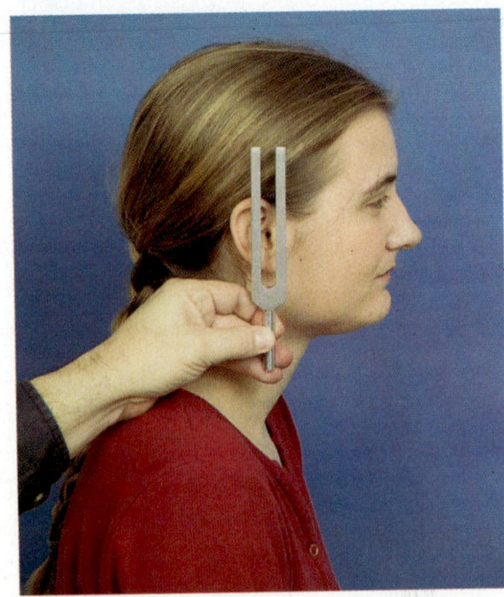

Figure 13-12c ■ During the Rinne test, a tuning fork is held an inch from the patient's ear to determine air conduction of sound.

Pure Tone Audiometry

250 Hz → 8,000 Hz

The **audiometer** is a specialized instrument that measures hearing acuity at different frequencies. It provides information about the extent of hearing loss and which frequencies are involved. Sound amplitude is measured in decibels (dB) and sound frequency is measured in hertz (Hz).

Testing must be conducted in a quiet area so that external noise does not interfere with testing. The patient is seated in a direction facing away from the

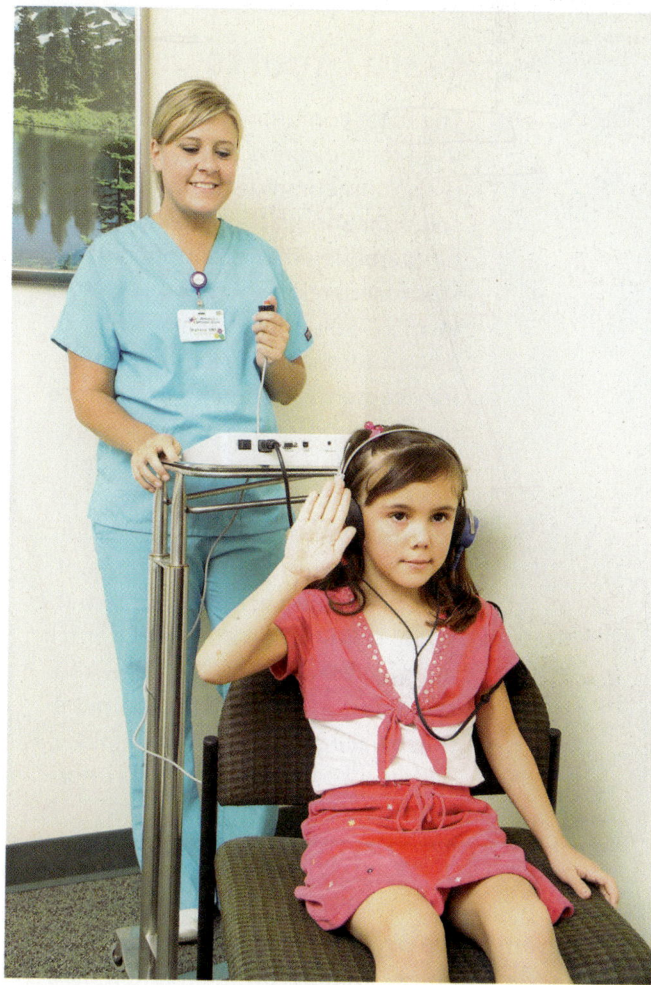

Figure 13-13 ■ The medical assistant tests a patient with an audiometer.

unit and medical assistant. Earphones are placed over the patient's ears. The patient is asked to raise a hand on the side of the head where the sound is heard. The medical assistant adjusts the machine from the lowest frequency of 250 Hz and gradually increases the frequency until the highest pitch or frequency is reached, around 8000 Hz. Each ear is tested separately, and should be tested in an alternating manner so that the patient doesn't pick up on a specific pattern. Once the testing process is completed, an audiogram is produced by plotting the results on a graph. Figure 13-13 shows a patient being tested using an audiometer. This is just one example of an audiometer. Numerous models from several manufacturers are available for use in the medical office. Figure 13-14 shows an example of a manual audiometer commonly used in the medical office.

Speech and Word Recognition

Speech and word recognition testing is done by audiologists to determine if an individual has difficult clearly interpreting speech with varying levels of background

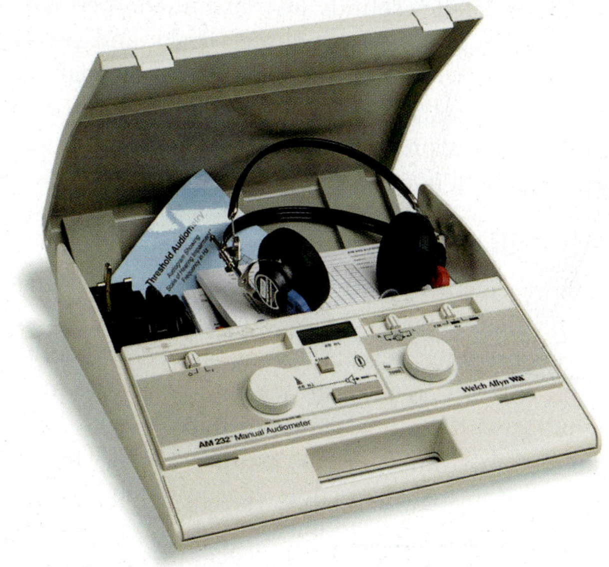

Figure 13-14 ■ An example of a manual audiometer.

noise. This may be done in conjunction with audiometry to determine a functional level of hearing, or to test performance of hearing aids.

Tympanometry

Tympanometry is a procedure used to determine whether or not the middle ear is transmitting sound waves. This procedure is useful in diagnosing middle ear infections that commonly cause hearing loss in children.

The **tympanometer** is an electronic device with an attached probe that is placed snugly in the patient's ear (Figure 13-15). Pressure is applied in the ear canal

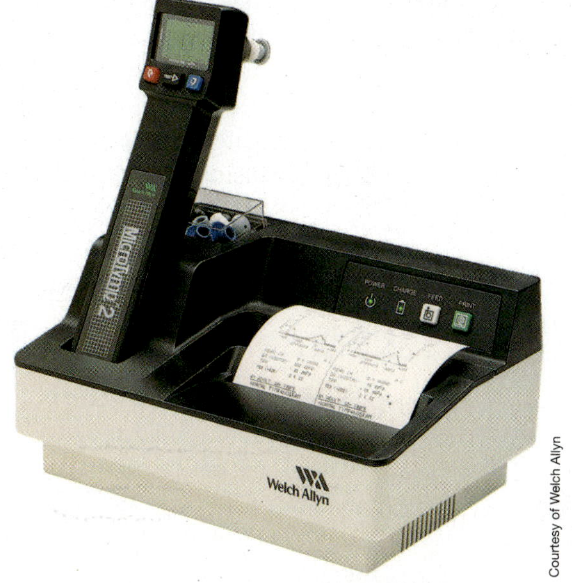

Figure 13-15 ■ An example of a tympanometer. This model tests in one second and prints results that can help the provider diagnose otitis media and other middle ear conditions.

while low-frequency sounds are transmitted. A recording or tympanogram is produced. Peaks and waves are measured to determine possible abnormalities in the middle ear. In a normal ear, the eardrum will vibrate due to the pressure. If fluid is present in the ear, the eardrum will not move.

Ear Instillation

Liquids are instilled into the external auditory canal to treat infections, to relieve pain, and to soften impacted cerumen for easier removal. The medical assistant will usually perform the instillation and must be familiar with ear anatomy to ensure correct delivery of the medication (see Procedure 13-7). The ear canal forms an S-shaped curve as it leads inward and it must be straightened to ensure that the medication reaches the tympanic membrane. The medical assistant must be sure that the medication is for **otic** use before instillation.

Ear Irrigation

Ear irrigation, or lavage, involves washing the external ear canal with a stream of solution. This procedure (see Procedure 13-8) is performed to dislodge a foreign object, cleanse the ear canal, remove impacted cerumen, or reduce inflammation. Impacted cerumen may be softened with mineral oil or hydrogen peroxide prior to removal. An irrigation is contraindicated if the tympanic membrane is perforated, as this could cause an irritation or infection of the middle ear.

Different types of irrigating systems include the following:

- Pomeroy syringe: A metal syringe that is filled with irrigating solution. The tip of the syringe is placed in the ear canal and the plunger is depressed to push the fluid into the ear.
- Waterpik system: The oral irrigator can be converted into an ear irrigator by using the proper tip for ears.
- Electronic ear irrigator (Figure 13-16): There are several of these systems on the market; they come equipped with pressure controls and suction equipment to remove debris as it is dislodged. These irrigators are designed so that the stream of solution is directed toward the roof of the ear canal to prevent damage to the eardrum.
- Elephant ear wash: This device is convenient and easy to use. It consists of a spray bottle with tubing attached to a nozzle. The bottle is filled with warm water and as the medical assistant pumps the trigger, it sprays the water into the ear with enough pressure to clean the ear, but doesn't cause discomfort or damage.

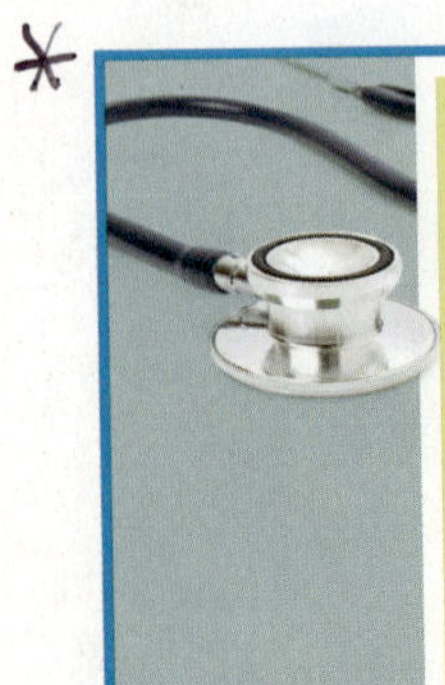

Field Smarts

When performing an ear instillation or irrigation on an adult or child above the age of three, the ear canal can be straightened by pulling up and back on the auricle. For children under the age of three, the auricle should be pulled down and back.

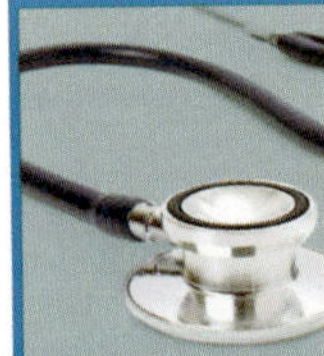

Field Smarts

The most common irrigation solution used for the ears is water. Saline is also sometimes used. Irrigation solutions should be warmed to body temperature whenever possible (approximately 99°F to 100°F) (37°C to 38°C). Solutions that are cooler or warmer than body temperature may cause the patient to experience dizziness and/or nausea. Extremely hot or cold solutions can damage the eardrum. Use a thermometer to test the temperature of the solution before administering the treatment. When irrigating with saline, place the saline solution in a bowl and warm it in the microwave. Always check the temperature after removal from the microwave to make certain it falls within acceptable parameters prior to irrigation

Miscellaneous Ear Procedures

Though the most commonly performed procedures in primary care are listed above, many others exist. The following procedures are not typically performed by a medical assistant.

Tympanostomy

Tympanostomy is a very common procedure performed by ENT specialists. It involves making a hole in the tympanic membrane to let fluid drain out from

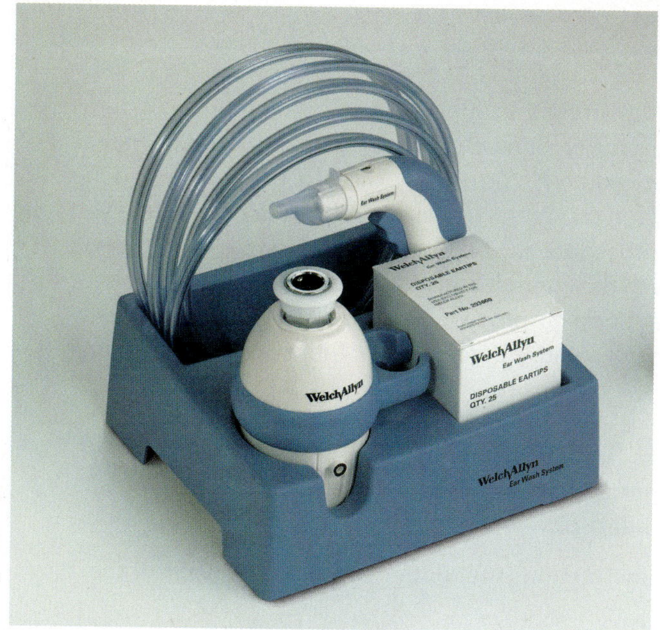

Courtesy of Welch Allyn

Figure 13-16 ■ An electronic ear irrigator.

the middle ear. It is most often performed in children with recurrent middle ear infections, and many times involves the placement of tympanostomy tubes, which keep the hole open for 1–2 years while the Eustachian tubes change their angle as the child grows. Most tubes fall out eventually on their own, though other types need to be removed in another procedure.

Foreign Body Removal

Foreign bodies are commonly found in ears. These are varied in younger patients and include many household or food items such as small toys, marbles, beans, and so on. Pieces of hearing aids and cotton from the tip of a cotton swab are more common in adults. Foreign objects can be removed with a small tool, such as a cerumen scoop, or alligator forceps. Other times, an object may be removed with irrigation, or the use of suction.

COMMON EAR MEDICATIONS

Medications for ear ailments can be in oral form, or topical drops applied directly into the ear canal. Table 13-5 lists some examples.

COMMON LAB TESTS THAT COINCIDE WITH EAR DISORDERS

Laboratory tests are not very common for ear pathology. Microbiology testing such as an ear culture may be ordered in some practices.

Ear Culture

A culture swab may be obtained of drainage from the auditory canal. This can help identify the pathogen of an active infection. A primary microorganism can then be tested further for resistance to potential treatments. Many providers will treat presumptively without obtaining a culture, while others make it routine practice.

Table 13-5 Common Ear Medications

Medication Classification	Description	Medication Examples
Antibiotics (drops)	Drugs used to treat bacterial infections in the form of ear drops. Commonly used for external infections of the ear.	Ofloxacin, Cortisporin otic
Antibiotics (orals)	Drugs used to treat bacterial infections in the form of an oral medication	Amoxicillin, azithromycin, cefdinir, ceftriaxone
Antifungal (drops)	Drugs used to treat fungal causes of ear infection	Acetic acid
Corticosteroids (drops)	Drugs used to treat ear inflammation, reduce swelling, irritation, and discharge	Fluocinolone
Combination antibiotic–corticosteroid drops	Drugs that are both an antibiotic and corticosteroid combined into one medication	Ciprofloxacin–hydrocortisone, acetic acid–hydrocortisone, ciprofloxacin–dexamethasone

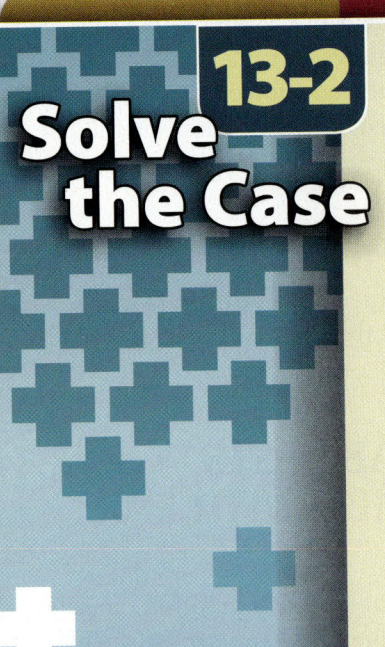

You were able to get Abda Muhammed an appointment for this morning. It turns out that Abda has a small tear in her retina. Dr. Munsey decides the patient needs to have a scleral buckling procedure. Unfortunately, this procedure can't be done until tomorrow morning. When the doctor leaves the room, the patient tells you she is very upset that the procedure can't be performed today and that this is interfering with her trip. Go to the Internet and look up educational materials for patients who have a scleral buckling procedure. Make certain that the educational materials include the following: a description of the procedure and home care instructions following the procedure.

1. **What is the purpose of a scleral buckling procedure?**
2. **Why is it so important for the patient to have the procedure now instead of following her trip?**
3. **List basic home care instructions that patients should follow after the procedure.**

Following the procedure, the doctor orders one drop of Tobradex (ophthalmic) four times a day and one drop of atropine (ophthalmic) two times a day.

4. **What is the purpose of these two medications?**

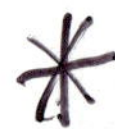

PROCEDURE 13-1
Snellen Chart Visual Acuity Testing

Objective

To screen for distance visual acuity.

Equipment/Supplies

- Snellen eye chart
- Occluder
- Alcohol wipes

PROCEDURAL STEPS	DETAILS AND/OR RATIONALE
1. Wash your hands and assemble the equipment. Clean the occluder with an alcohol wipe and allow it to air dry.	The occluder should be cleaned before and after testing to prevent patient-to-patient cross-contamination.

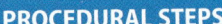

continues

PROCEDURE 13-1 continued

PROCEDURAL STEPS	DETAILS AND/OR RATIONALE
2. Identify the patient using two identifiers, identify yourself, and ***explain the rationale for performance of the procedure, showing awareness of the patient's concerns related to the procedure being performed***. If the patient wears contact lenses, testing should be conducted with contacts. If the patient wears glasses, testing may be conducted both with and without glasses.	Having the patient remove contacts would be very burdensome so most providers (unless working for an ophthalmologist) will not require an exam without correction in this instance.
3. In a well-lit area, instruct the patient to stand at the mark placed 20 feet from the eye chart. Ask the patient to cover the left eye with the occluder (Figure 13-17). Ask the patient to read the chart aloud (keeping both eyes open), beginning with the 20/200 line or with one of the several lines above the 20/20 line.	Closing the eye covered by the occluder can cause squinting in the eye being tested and may also cause the eye covered by the occluder to become blurry before it is tested. Beginning the testing with one of the higher lines helps the patient get into a routine and feel confident about the testing.
4. Stand next to the chart and point to each line during testing (Figure 13-18).	Pointing to the line being read helps to narrow the field of vision to one row at a time.
5. Record the results as the last line the patient can read without errors. Acuity is recorded as a fraction as follows: R. eye 20/10, L. eye 20/30, both eyes 20/20.	The medical assistant must pay close attention while the patient is reading to ensure accurate results.
6. ***Incorporating critical thinking skills when performing patient assessment,*** observe the patient during the screening for signs of difficulty such as squinting, watering of the eyes, or repositioning of the head.	Any of these signs could indicate a vision problem. If the patient squints or leans forward, it could change the outcome of the test.
7. After screening the right eye, repeat the procedure for the left eye and then with both eyes.	
8. Clean the occluder with alcohol, wash your hands, and document results in the patient's chart.	Occluder must be cleaned after each use to prevent cross-contamination.

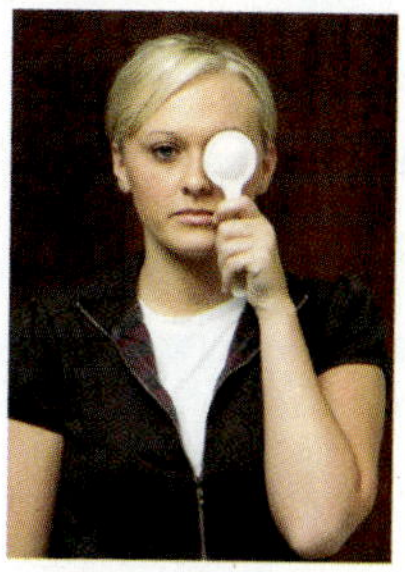

Figure 13-17 ■ The patient covers her left eye with an occluder.

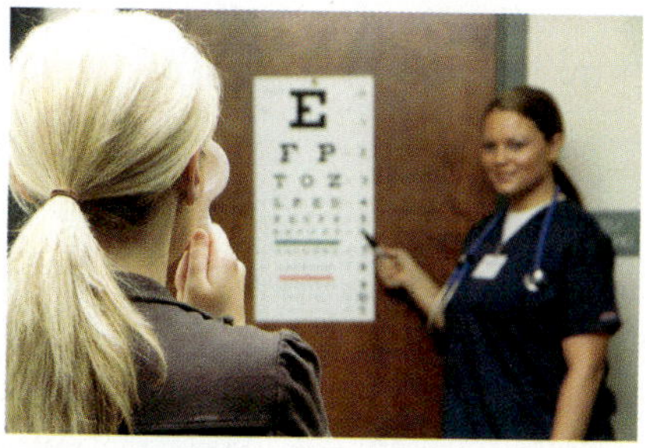

Figure 13-18 ■ The medical assistant points to the line the patient is to read.

DOCUMENTATION EXAMPLE:

08-12-XX 1:10 p.m.	Snellen visual screening per Dr. Kelly. R. eye 20/10, L. eye 20/30, both eyes 20/20. Patient was observed squinting during testing of both eyes. Lillian Kelly, CMA (AAMA) ------------------

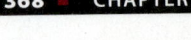

PROCEDURE 13-2

Screen Near Visual Acuity

Objective

To screen near visual acuity.

Equipment/Supplies

- Jaeger near visual acuity chart
- Occluder
- Alcohol wipes

PROCEDURAL STEPS	DETAILS AND/OR RATIONALE
1. Wash your hands, assemble the equipment, and clean the occluder with an alcohol wipe.	Hands must be washed before and after each patient to prevent cross-contamination. The occluder must be cleaned before and after each patient for the same reason.
2. Identify the patient using two identifiers, identify yourself, and ***explain the rationale for performance of the procedure, showing awareness of the patient's concerns related to the procedure being performed***.	A clear explanation of the procedure will ensure accurate test results.
3. With the patient in a sitting position, instruct the patient to hold the card approximately 14 inches from the eyes (Figure 13-19).	This is the distance at which a person with normal vision is able to read small print.
4. Instruct the patient to cover the left eye with the occluder and read the chart (out loud) with the right eye.	Each eye should be tested separately for accurate results.
5. Record the results as the last line the patient can read without errors.	
6. Repeat the procedure for the left eye and both eyes together. The patient should be tested with and without corrective lenses, if worn. (Do not have the patient remove contacts.)	
7. Wipe the occluder with an alcohol wipe.	The occluder should be cleansed with alcohol to prevent patient-to-patient cross-contamination.
8. Wash your hands and document results in the patient's chart.	

Figure 13-19 ■ The patient's near visual acuity is assessed using the Jaeger chart.

DOCUMENTATION EXAMPLE:

11-08-XX 12:30 p.m.	Jaeger near visual acuity screening per Dr. Price. R. eye, No. 10 (2.25M), L. eye, No. 7 (1.5M), both eyes, No. 6 (1.25M) with corr. Lillian Kelly, CMA (AAMA)----------------------------

PROCEDURE 13-3

Ishihara Test for Color Vision

Objective

To assess a patient's color vision.

Equipment/Supplies

- Ishihara plates

PROCEDURAL STEPS	DETAILS AND/OR RATIONALE
1. Wash your hands and assemble the equipment.	Hands must be washed before and after each patient contact to prevent the possible spread of infection.
2. Identify the patient using two identifiers, identify yourself, and ***explain the rationale for performance of the procedure, showing awareness of the patient's concerns related to the procedure being performed***. The test should be conducted in a room illuminated by daylight.	Direct sunlight or harsh electric light can distort the color plates.
3. Starting with the practice plate as an example, hold the plate 30 inches from the patient and at a right angle to the patient's field of vision (Figure 13-20). Instruct the patient to identify the number formed by the colored dots. Patient should only have three seconds to read each line.	**Figure 13-20** ■ The patient's color vision acuity is tested using Ishihara plates.
4. Repeat the procedure with all plates. *Note*: Lines will have a winding line that the patient will need to trace rather than a number to read. Record the results after each plate.	List the plate number and the number identified by the patient. Example: Plate 4:12. If a patient can't identify the plate, results would be recorded with an "X," such as Plate 6:X, or just list the plates that the patient could not identify correctly.
5. Protect the plates from light when not in use.	Exposure to direct sunlight can cause fading of the color plates.
6. Wash your hands and document results in the patient's chart.	

DOCUMENTATION EXAMPLE:

01-11-XX 11:30 a.m.	Ishihara color vision screening per Dr. Bell. Plate 4:X, all other plates correctly identified, Jacob Heller, CMA (AAMA) --

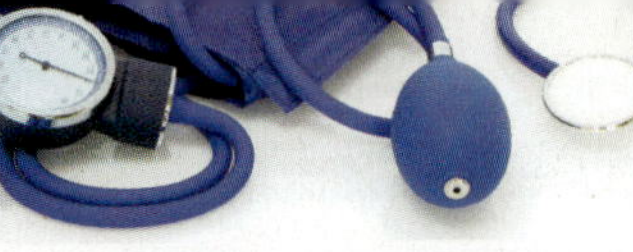

PROCEDURE 13-4

Eye Instillation

Objective

To instill liquid or ointment ophthalmic medication into the eyes to treat infection, anesthetize the eye prior to a procedure, soothe eye irritation, or dilate the pupils for examination.

Equipment/Supplies

- Disposable gloves
- Gauze
- Disposable eye dropper (if applicable)
- Disposable ophthalmic medication
- Tissues

PROCEDURAL STEPS	DETAILS AND/OR RATIONALE
1. Wash your hands and assemble the equipment. If the medication has been refrigerated, it must come to room temperature before instilling.	Bringing the medication to room temperature before instilling is more comfortable for the patient.
2. Check medication against the provider's orders and look for the word *ophthalmic* on the label. Check the expiration date and check the label three times before administration.	Sometimes, the same medication comes in different forms. Never instill a medication into the eye that is not intended for ophthalmic use. Check the label when taking the medication from the shelf, before withdrawing the medication, and before administering.
3. Identify the patient using two identifiers, identify yourself, and ***explain to the patient the rationale for performing this procedure, showing awareness of the patient's concerns related to the procedure being performed***.	
4. Wash your hands and apply gloves.	Gloves help to keep hands from becoming contaminated during procedure.
5. Place the patient in a sitting or lying position and prepare the medication. For eye drops, withdraw the medication into a sterile dropper. For eye ointment, remove the cap from the tube.	Do not allow the dropper to touch anything other than the solution inside the bottle and do not touch the tip of the ointment tube to the eye or the tip will be contaminated.
6. Instruct the patient to look up at the ceiling. With your fingers over a tissue, gently pull down on skin to expose the lower conjunctival sac (Figure 13-21).	Looking up discourages the patient from blinking when drops are instilled.
7. Instill the correct number of drops into the center of the lower conjunctival sac or place a thin line of ointment along the lower surface of the eyelid. *Do not touch the tip of the medication applicator to the eye.*	If the tip of the eyedropper or the tip of the ointment tube touches the eye, it is considered contaminated.

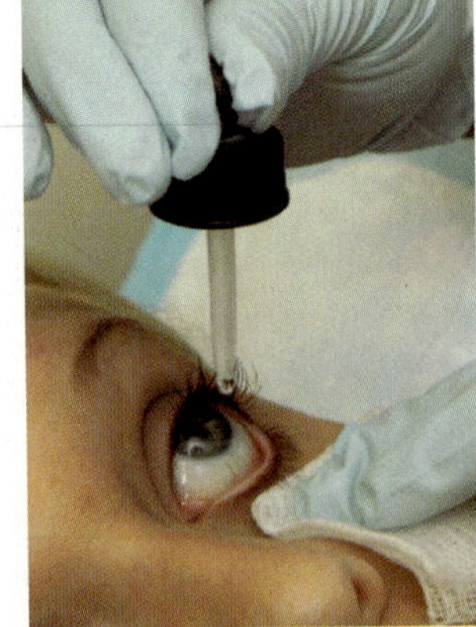

Figure 13-21 ■ The patient looks up as the medical assistant instills eye drops.

continues

PROCEDURE 13-4 continued

PROCEDURAL STEPS	DETAILS AND/OR RATIONALE
8. Instruct the patient to close the eye and roll the eyeball around.	Rolling the eye helps to evenly distribute the medication.
9. Dab excess solution from the eyelid with gauze.	Dabbing removes any excess medication.
10. *Do not return any unused medication to the bottle.* Discard the unused medication, and return the dropper to the bottle without touching the dropper to the outside of the bottle.	Touching the outside of the bottle with the dropper will contaminate it. Unused solution should not be returned to the bottle as the remaining medication will be contaminated. (Most solutions today are squeezable bottle in which a dropper is not necessary.)
11. Discard used equipment and supplies.	
12. Remove gloves and wash your hands.	Hands must be washed after removing gloves to remove any contamination from inside the gloves.
13. Record the procedure in the patient's chart.	

DOCUMENTATION EXAMPLE:

12-14-XX 12:15 p.m.	Visine, 2 gtt R. eye per Dr. Gamble. Pt. tolerated procedure well. Pt. to RTO in 10 days. C. Wesson, CMA (AAMA) --

PROCEDURE 13-5

Eye Irrigation

Objective

To flush the eye with solution to remove a foreign object, soothe irritation, apply an antiseptic, or cleanse drainage from the eye.

Equipment/Supplies

- Disposable gloves
- Sterile irrigation solution
- Water pick
- Basin
- Disposable towel or impervious drape
- Gauze
- Towel

PROCEDURAL STEPS	DETAILS AND/OR RATIONALE
1. Wash your hands and assemble the equipment. Note: if both eyes are to be irrigated, separate supplies will be needed for each eye.	Separate supplies are used to prevent cross-contamination.

continues

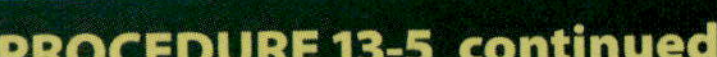

PROCEDURE 13-5 continued

PROCEDURAL STEPS	DETAILS AND/OR RATIONALE
2. Identify the patient using two identifiers, identify yourself, and ***explain to the patient the rationale for performing this procedure, showing awareness of the patient's concerns related to the procedure being performed.***	
3. Place the patient in a sitting or supine position with the head turned toward the affected eye.	This position allows for solution to flow from the affected eye into a basin and avoids cross-contamination from one eye to the other.
4. Check the expiration date of the solution and check the label three times. Note: Solution should be warmed to body temperature (99°F or 37.2°C).	Warming the solution to body temperature makes the procedure more comfortable for the patient.
5. Place a towel on the patient's shoulder and place a basin beside the affected eye. Wash your hands again and apply gloves.	The towel protects the patient's clothing. This position allows the solution to easily flow into the basin.
6. Cleanse the eyelid from the inner to outer canthus with moistened gauze. Discard the gauze after each cleansing.	Cleansing removes any debris or discharge from the eyelid.
7. Prepare a water pick with irrigating solution and hold the eye open with the index finger and thumb.	The patient will have a tendency to close the eye if it is not held open.
8. Rest the bulb of the water pick on the bridge of the patient's nose. Be careful not to touch the eye or conjunctiva with the tip of the water pick.	Touching the eye will cause contamination of the water pick.
9. Instruct the patient to stare at a fixed spot and open the water pick valve, allowing the solution to flow along the lower conjunctiva from the inner to outer canthus and into the basin (Figure 13-22).	Allowing the solution to flow from the inner to outer canthus eliminates cross-contamination from one eye to the other.
10. After irrigation is complete, dry the eyelid and eyelashes from the inner to outer canthus with gauze.	Drying the eyelid removes excess irrigating solution.
11. Discard supplies in an appropriate container.	
12. Remove gloves, wash your hands, and document the procedure in the patient's chart.	

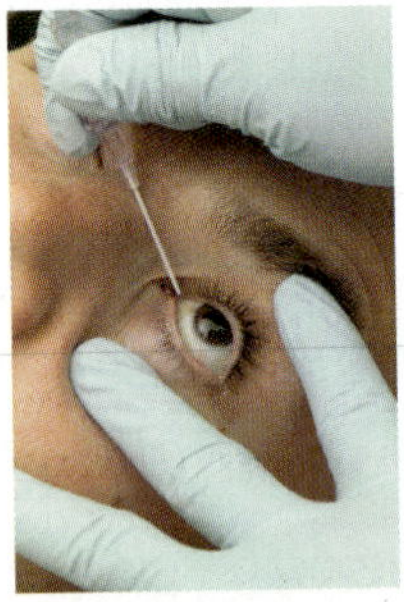

Figure 13-22 ■ The medical assistant performs an eye irrigation using a water pick.

DOCUMENTATION EXAMPLE:

05-22-XX 2:30 p.m.	Eye irrigation, 600 mL normal sterile saline, L. eye per Dr. Black. Return solution clear. Pt. tolerated procedure well. J Barnes, CMA (AAMA) --

PROCEDURE 13-6

Hearing Acuity Testing

Objective

To test a patient's hearing, to determine and define hearing deficits.

Equipment/Supplies

- Audiometer with headphones
- A quiet, ideally soundproof room

PROCEDURAL STEPS	DETAILS AND/OR RATIONALE
1. Review the provider's order, wash your hands and assemble the equipment.	Washing hands helps to cut down on risks of patient contamination. Assembling equipment ahead of time makes the procedure run much more efficiently.
2. Identify the patient using two identifiers, identify yourself, and ***explain to the patient the rationale for performing this procedure, showing awareness of the patient's concerns related to the procedure being performed***.	Identifying the patient using two identifiers helps to insure you have the correct patient. Explaining the test and rationale helps patient perform better during testing.
3. Seat the patient in a comfortable chair in a quiet, soundproof room. Provide headphones to the patient to place over the ears.	Placing the patient in a room with little outside sound assists in attaining accurate results.
4. Instruct the patient to raise the left hand if a sound is heard in the left ear, and the right hand if a sound is heard in the right ear. (Do not allow patient to see you pressing the buttons.)	If patient observes you pressing the buttons they may say they hear something when they really don't.
5. Record your findings on a special graphing form or in the patient's chart.	

DOCUMENTATION EXAMPLE:

05-22-XX 2:30 p.m.	*Audiometry testing per Dr. Dorado. Results for both ears fell in the normal range. Graphing results available in "Results" section of chart. G. Parsons, CCMA --------------------*

PROCEDURE 13-7

Ear Instillation

Objective

To instill a solution or medication to treat infection, relieve pain, or soften cerumen for removal.

Equipment/Supplies

- Disposable gloves
- Otic solution or medication
- Sterile ear dropper (If applicable)
- Gauze squares
- Cotton balls

continues

PROCEDURE 13-7 continued

PROCEDURAL STEPS	DETAILS AND/OR RATIONALE
1. Wash your hands and assemble the equipment.	Washing your hands helps to reduce the risks of infection and assembling the equipment helps to save time during the procedure.
2. Identify the patient using two identifiers, identify yourself, and ***explain to the patient the rationale for performing this procedure, showing awareness of the patient's concerns related to the procedure being performed***.	Identifying the patient with two identifiers helps to confirm that you have the correct patient. Explaining the procedure helps the patient know what to expect during the procedure.
3. Check the medication against the provider's orders and check the medication three times. Check the expiration date of the medication and verify that the medication is for otic use.	Checking the medication three times reduces the chances for error. Some medications come in different forms. Never instill a medication into the ear that is not intended for otic use.
4. Instruct the patient to lie with affected ear up or to sit with head slightly tilted toward the unaffected ear. Place a towel on the patient's shoulder of the affected side.	Tilting the head improves the flow of medication into the ear.
5. Apply gloves.	
6. Grasp the top of the ear and pull up and back for adults, or grasp the earlobe and pull down and back for children under three (Figure 13-23).	Pulling on the ear straightens the canal for easier flow of the solution.
7. Instill the prescribed amount of medication into the ear canal by depressing the rubber bulb of the dropper. *Do not touch the tip of the dropper to the ear.*	Touching the ear with the dropper will contaminate the dropper.
8. Instruct the patient to keep the head tilted toward the unaffected side for approximately five minutes.	Keeping the head tilted distributes the medication and prevents it from leaking out.
9. Insert a slightly moistened cotton ball into the ear canal (per the provider's orders) and instruct the patient to leave it in place for 15 minutes.	Moist cotton will not absorb medication and will prevent leakage of the medication when the patient is ambulatory.
10. Dispose of used equipment and supplies.	
11. Remove gloves and wash your hands.	
12. Document the procedure in the patient's chart.	

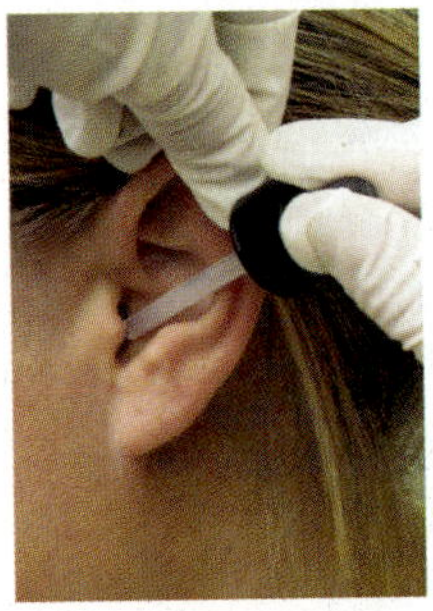

Figure 13-23 ■ Eardrops are instilled into the ear canal.

DOCUMENTATION EXAMPLE:

12-20-XX 10:15 a.m.	3 gtts of Auralgan administered to left ear per Dr. Emily White. Patient states the pain is a little better. A. Price, RMA (AMT) --

PROCEDURE 13-8

Ear Irrigation

Objective

To flush the ear with solution to remove excess cerumen or a foreign object from the ear canal.

Equipment/Supplies

- Disposable gloves
- Irrigation device
- Sterile irrigation solution warmed to body temperature/basin
- Ear or emesis basin for return solution
- Towel or impervious pad to protect patient's clothing
- Gauze squares
- Otoscope

PROCEDURAL STEPS	DETAILS AND/OR RATIONALE
1. Wash your hands and assemble the equipment and supplies. Check the name and strength of irrigation solution as well as the expiration date. (Label should be checked 3x.)	Washing hands helps to cut down the risks of cross contamination and infection. Use of outdated solution may not result in desired results.
2. Identify the patient using two identifiers, identify yourself, and ***explain to the patient the rationale for performing this procedure, showing awareness of the patient's concerns related to the procedure being performed***.	Explaining the procedure will assist the patient in knowing what to expect. (Let patient know she may feel a little lightheadedness or dizziness and to alert you if she feels pain during the procedure.)
3. Place the patient in a sitting position with the head tilted to the affected side.	Tilting the head promotes better drainage of solution out of the ear canal.
4. Place a towel or impervious drape over the patient's shoulder and instruct the patient to hold an ear or emesis basin under the affected ear and against the neck.	This will help to prevent the solution from running down the patient's neck and onto clothing.
5. Apply gloves and pour sterile irrigating liquid into sterile/clean basin.	
6. Fill irrigating syringe or device with warmed irrigating solution (around 99 degrees F [37.2 degrees C] to 100 degrees F [37.8 degrees C]). If using syringe expel any air at the top of syringe.	Pushing air into the ear may cause damage to internal ear structures and feel uncomfortable to patient.
7. Gently pull the top of the ear up and back in adults and down in back in children three and under.	This straightens the ear canal.
8. Insert the tip of the irrigation syringe or device into the ear canal. Aim the irrigation solution so it flows up toward the roof of the ear canal (Figure 13-24).	Allowing the solution to flow directly toward the tympanic membrane can be painful and can cause injury.
9. Continue the process until the desired effects are obtained.	

Figure 13-24 ■ The medical assistant squeezes on the bulb and directs the flow of the solution toward the roof of the ear.

continues

PROCEDURE 13-8 continued

PROCEDURAL STEPS	DETAILS AND/OR RATIONALE
10. Dry the outer ear and if office protocol, check the inner ear with an otoscope to determine removal of foreign matter.	You want to make certain that the canal is clear.
11. Remove the towel from patient's shoulder and ear basin and have the patient lie on the affected side with towel under her head on the exam table.	This allows for any remaining solution to drain out.
12. After five to ten minutes, have provider check ear for clearance of debris.	
13. Remove gloves and wash your hands.	
14. Document the procedure in the patient's chart. (Make certain you summarize what was in the return basin.)	

DOCUMENTATION EXAMPLE:

12-20-XX 10:15 a.m.	Right ear flushed with warmed water as ordered by Rick Lopez, ANP. Large return of cerumen. Tympanic membrane clearly visualized. Patient reports notable improvement in hearing. Procedure tolerated well. A. Price, RMA (AMT) --------------------------------------

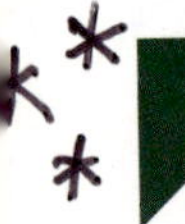

CHAPTER SUMMARY

- The eye is a spherical organ that serves to allow vision. The three layers of the eye include the sclera (outermost layer), choroid (middle layer), and retina (inner layer). The lens contracts and relaxes to alter the shape of the eye. Rods and cones are found in the retina and allow us to see in dim light (rods) or to see in bright light or in color (cones).
- The outer ear is the auricle it helps to draw sound waves into the ear. The tympanic membrane is the ear drum and vibrates the sounds and passes them to middle ear or ossicles. In the cochlea of the inner ear is where vibrations are converted to nerve impulses and transmitted to the brain, where they are processed as sound.
- Eye specialists include an ophthalmologist, optometrist, and optician. Ear specialists include otorhinolaryngologist (ENT) and audiologist (hearing specialist).
- Common diseases of the eye include macular degeneration (damage to the macula causing loss of central vision), conjunctivitis (pink eye), cataracts (clumping of proteins within the lens), corneal abrasion (scratch in the cornea), and glaucoma (increased ocular pressure in the eye).
- Common disorders of the ear include neurosensory hearing loss (damage to the inner ear or auditory nerve), conductive hearing loss (obstruction of the ear canal), cerumen impaction (wax buildup) and otitis externa (infection of the outer ear), otitis media (infection of the middle ear), and otitis interna (infection of the inner ear).
- Visual acuity testing detects possible errors of refraction and is done for both near and far vision. Common screening devices include the Snellen eye chart (adults), the tumbling E chart (preliterate and patients unfamiliar with English alphabet), Landolt C (similar to tumbling E chart), and the Snellen numbers and picture tests and LEA and HOTV chart. Acuity tests are usually performed at a distance of 20 feet; however, some pediatric charts require the patient to be 10 feet away from the chart. The Jaeger chart is used for near visual acuity testing and Ishihara testing is performed for color screenings. The Pelli–Robson chart measures contrast sensitivity and is an early detector of major eye diseases.

- A common instrument that measures vision is the Titmus vision tester (compact testing device).
- Eye instillation is a procedure in which drops or ointment are placed in the eye. Eye irrigation is a procedure that flushes the eye to remove debris or harmful substances.
- Featured ear procedures include hearing acuity tests (measures patient's ability to hear), Weber test, and Rinne test (tests that can be done by the provider with a tuning fork to measure hearing), speech and word recognition testing (determines how clearly speech can be interpreted with varying degrees of background noise), and tympanometry (a test which detects if the middle ear is transmitting sound waves).
- Ear instillation is a procedure in which drops are placed in the patient's ear and ear irrigation flushes the ear to remove cerumen and other debris.

CERTIFICATION REVIEW QUESTIONS

1. The leading cause of blindness world-wide is known as:
   a. stye.
   b. glaucoma.
   c. presbyopia.
   d. cataract.
2. A specialized instrument that measures hearing acuity at different frequencies is the:
   a. tuning fork.
   b. tympanometer.
   c. audiometer.
   d. Rinne tester.
3. Which of the following charts is commonly used to assess distance visual acuity in the adult?
   a. Snellen
   b. Jaeger
   c. Ishihara
   d. Tumbling E
4. Which of the following is an example of a gross hearing test?
   a. Rinne test
   b. Audiometry
   c. Weber test
   d. Meniere's test
5. What is the proper way to position the ear when performing an ear instillation in a child under the age of three?
   a. Up and back
   b. Down and back
   c. Up and forward
   d. Down and forward
6. What chart(s) may be used to determine visual acuity in a preschooler?
   a. Tumbling E chart
   b. Landolt C chart
   c. Allen object recognition chart
   d. All of the above
7. The instrument that the provider uses to examine the ear is the:
   a. otoscope.
   b. auroscope.
   c. ophthalmoscope.
   d. tympanoscope.
8. Which of the following diseases eventually lead to destruction of the optic nerve?
   a. Macular degeneration
   b. Cataracts
   c. Glaucoma
   d. Conjunctivitis
9. Irrigating solutions of the ear should be:
   a. brought to room temperature before using.
   b. brought to body temperature before using.
   c. 110–120°F before using.
   d. 70–80°F before using.
10. If a patient complains of pain during an ear irrigation you should:
    a. tell the patient that the test is necessary and ask them to tolerate the irrigation for as long as possible.
    b. stop the procedure and tell the patient to reschedule for another appointment when their ears aren't so sensitive.
    c. stop the procedure and ask the patient for specifics so that you can discuss with the provider how to move forward.
    d. None of the above

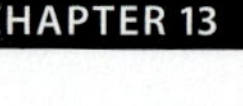

STUDY RESOURCES

Resources to Test and Reinforce Your Knowledge:	
Certification Review Questions	Take this end-of-chapter quiz
Workbook	• Complete the activities for Chapter 13 • Perform the procedures for Chapter 13 using the Competency Checklists
Resources to Promote Critical Thinking:	
***Solve the Case* Activities**	• Consider these case studies and discuss your conclusions
Learning Lab	• Module 14: Nervous, Sensory and Integumentary Systems
MindTap	• Complete Chapter 13 readings and activities

REFERENCES

Facts about Age-Related Macular Degeneration. (2013, July). Retrieved from https://www.nei.nih.gov/health/maculardegen/armd_facts

Otitis Externa. (2014, December 29). Retrieved May 5, 2015, from http://emedicine.medscape.com/article/994550-overview

Scleral Buckling (Aftercare Instructions). Care Guide. (n.d.). (2015, October 4). Retrieved from http://www.drugs.com/cg/scleral-buckling-aftercare-instructions.html

14

Cardiovascular Exams and Procedures

CHAPTER OUTLINE

Cardiovascular System Snapshot
- Heart Anatomy
- Blood Vessels
- Cardiovascular Physiology
- Cardiac Conduction System

Cardiovascular Abbreviation Review

Cardiovascular In-Office and Telephone Screening Tips

Common Cardiovascular Diseases
- Cardiac Arrhythmias
- Coronary Artery Disease
- Other Cardiovascular Conditions

Featured Cardiovascular Procedures
- Electrocardiograms
- Holter Monitor
- Miscellaneous Cardiovascular Procedures

Common Cardiovascular Treatments and Medications

Common Lab Tests That Coincide with Cardiovascular Disorders

ESSENTIAL TERMS

amplitude
arrhythmia
artifact
arthrectomy
atherosclerosis
augmented lead
baseline
bipolar leads
cardiac ablation
cardiac catheterization
cardiac cycle
cardiac pacemaker
cardiologist
cardiothoracic surgeon
cardiovascular surgeon
cardioversion
coronary artery bypass graft
coronary artery disease
defibrillation
depolarization
dobutamine stress test
echocardiography
electrocardiogram (ECG or EKG)
electrocardiograph
electrodes
electrolyte
electron beam CT scan
Holter monitor
interval
isoelectric line
lead
noninvasive heart scan
normal sinus rhythm
percutaneous transluminal coronary angioplasty (PTCA)
precordial leads
repolarization
rhythm strip
segment
standardization
stress echocardiography
stylus
treadmill stress test

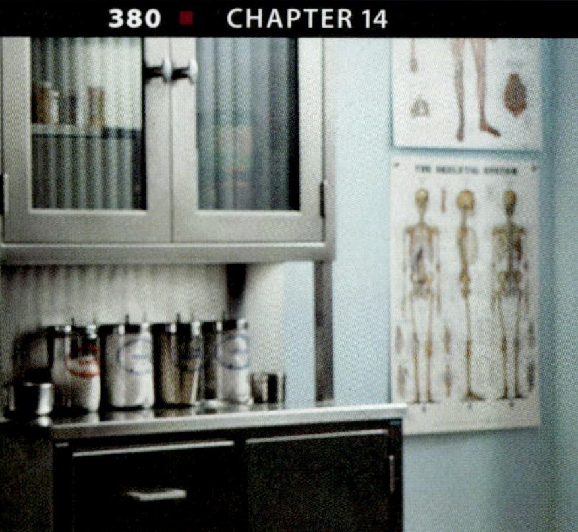

DEVELOPMENTAL OBJECTIVES

After completing this chapter you should be able to:

1. Correctly spell and define the essential terms.
2. List and provide the anatomical locations of the major structures within the cardiovascular system.
3. Describe the normal functions of the cardiovascular system.
4. List the major arteries that supply the heart with its blood supply and analyze how these arteries become diseased throughout the years.
5. Trace the blood's circulation through the heart and explain what occurs when the heart is weakened by disease or injury.
6. Describe the heart's electrical conduction system and list factors that can interfere with the conduction of electrical current through the heart.
7. Identify and use common cardiovascular abbreviations.
8. Compile a list of common screening questions that should be asked of patients with cardiovascular symptoms using established protocols and incorporate critical thinking skills when performing patient assessment.
9. Identify common pathology related to the cardiovascular system including signs, symptoms, and etiology.
10. Compare structure and function of the heart across the life span.
11. Analyze pathology for the cardiovascular system including diagnostic measures and treatment modalities.
12. Label each wave of the ECG cycle and describe the heart's action during each phase of the cardiac cycle.
13. Compare and contrast different types of ECG machines.
14. Describe the physical makeup of ECG paper, and state the functions of electrolytes and electrodes.
15. List the 12 leads of an ECG and their marking codes, and compare voltage paths for the limb and augmented leads.
16. Identify common artifacts found on the ECG tracing and choose appropriate steps to correct them.
17. Compile a list of common cardiovascular medication classifications and conclude how each one acts upon body structures to produce a desired effect.
18. Prepare the patient and perform an ECG and Holter Monitor testing.

INTRODUCTION

Approximately 84 million people in the United States have cardiovascular disease (CVD). Heart disease is the leading cause of death for both men and women. One out of every three deaths that occurs in this country is a result of heart disease.

The Center for Disease Control and Prevention (CDC) Survey estimates that one out of three adults has hypertension or high blood pressure (a risk factor of heart disease) and only around 47% of these individuals have their hypertension under control. There are a host of other risk factors that contribute to heart disease, many of which are modifiable.

The costs of treating patients with heart disease have soared over the last several years, to almost $400 billion per year. Further statics illustrate that 3.7 million patients go to the hospital for heart disease each year and 12.4 million people visit their provider for heart

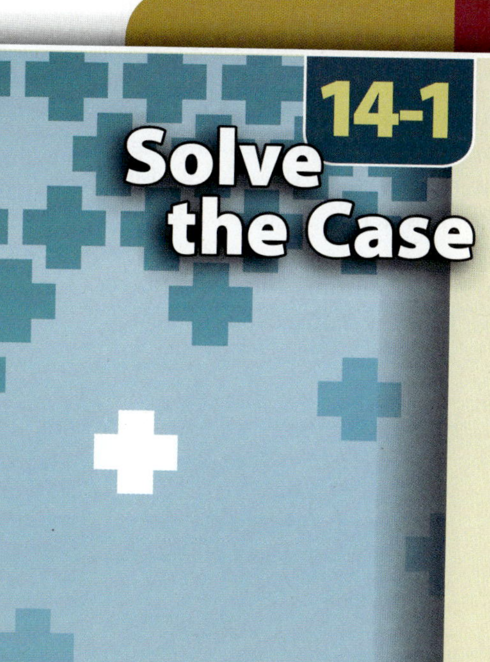

Mr. Kyle Duncan is a 55-year-old patient who has multiple health problems. He was diagnosed with insulin-dependent diabetes mellitus (IDDM) at the age of 25 and was diagnosed with end-stage renal disease (ESRD) three years ago. He now performs peritoneal dialysis in his home. Mr. Duncan recently had a stress test that revealed possible blockages in his coronary arteries. The stress test was part of a battery of tests performed for prekidney transplant assessment. As a result of the stress test, Dr. Dorado (Mr. Duncan's cardiologist) ordered a heart catheterization and the patient is here to obtain the results. In order to be considered for heart transplant, Mr. Duncan must pass the heart health portion of the preassessment testing, or preoperative cardiac clearance.

1. **What might Mr. Duncan be concerned about as he waits for the provider to go over the heart catheterization results?**
2. **If Mr. Duncan does have coronary blockages, do you think that his chances for transplant are over?**
3. **Do you know of any treatments available to patients with coronary artery blockages?**

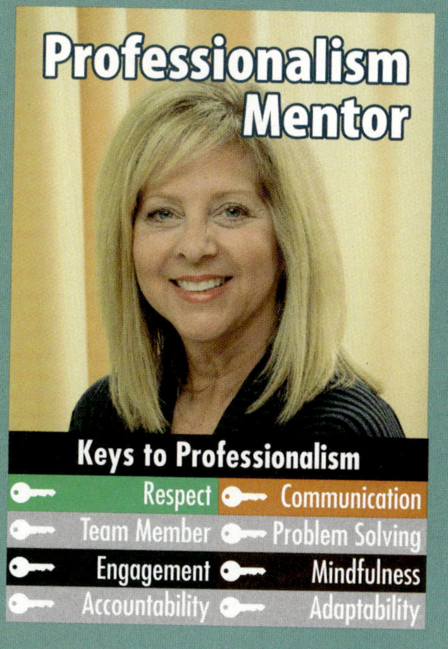

Obtaining a diagnosis of cardiovascular disease can be devastating. Can you imagine how you would feel if you received a similar diagnosis? An important key that should be instituted when working with a patient newly diagnosed with heart disease is *respect*, specifically the *compassion* element of respect. The patient will need someone to listen to their fears or concerns once the provider exits the room. For patients lacking courage to speak, a pat on the shoulder, a squeeze of the hand, or even a hug can go a long way. Another element of respect is *empathy*. Empathy is displayed when you take extraordinary measures to keep the patient covered during a 12-lead ECG or when you communicate each step you will perform during a procedure, so the patient isn't startled and knows what to expect. Sometimes it's the little things we do for our patients that make the biggest difference. ■

disease annually. With these kinds of statistics, the need for cardiac education and cardiac screenings is essential.

Two procedures that help to monitor heart health are the electrocardiogram and Holter monitoring. The medical assistant is usually the health care professional responsible for performing or setting up these tests in the provider's office. Precise skills and knowledge are essential when performing all forms of cardiac testing.

CARDIOVASCULAR SYSTEM SNAPSHOT

The cardiovascular system is composed of the heart and blood vessels and has four major functions:

- Transporting nutrients, gases, and waste products around the body
- Protecting the body from infection and blood loss
- Maintaining thermoregulation (body temperature regulation)
- Fluid balance

Heart Anatomy

The heart is a muscular pumping organ that is located within the mediastinum. Two-thirds of the adult heart lies to the left of the midline. The *apex* (is the rounded tip at the the bottom of the heart) lies just above the diaphragm. The *base* (the top of the heart) is approximately at the level of the third rib. A normal adult-sized heart is often compared to the size of a person's closed fist. The heart is comprised of four chambers: two upper chambers known as the right and left *atria* and two lower chambers known as the left and right *ventricles*. The heart is separated in the middle by a structure called a *septum*. Refer to Figure 14-1 for a diagram of the heart.

There is an outer layer surrounding the heart called the *pericardium*. This layer is composed of tough

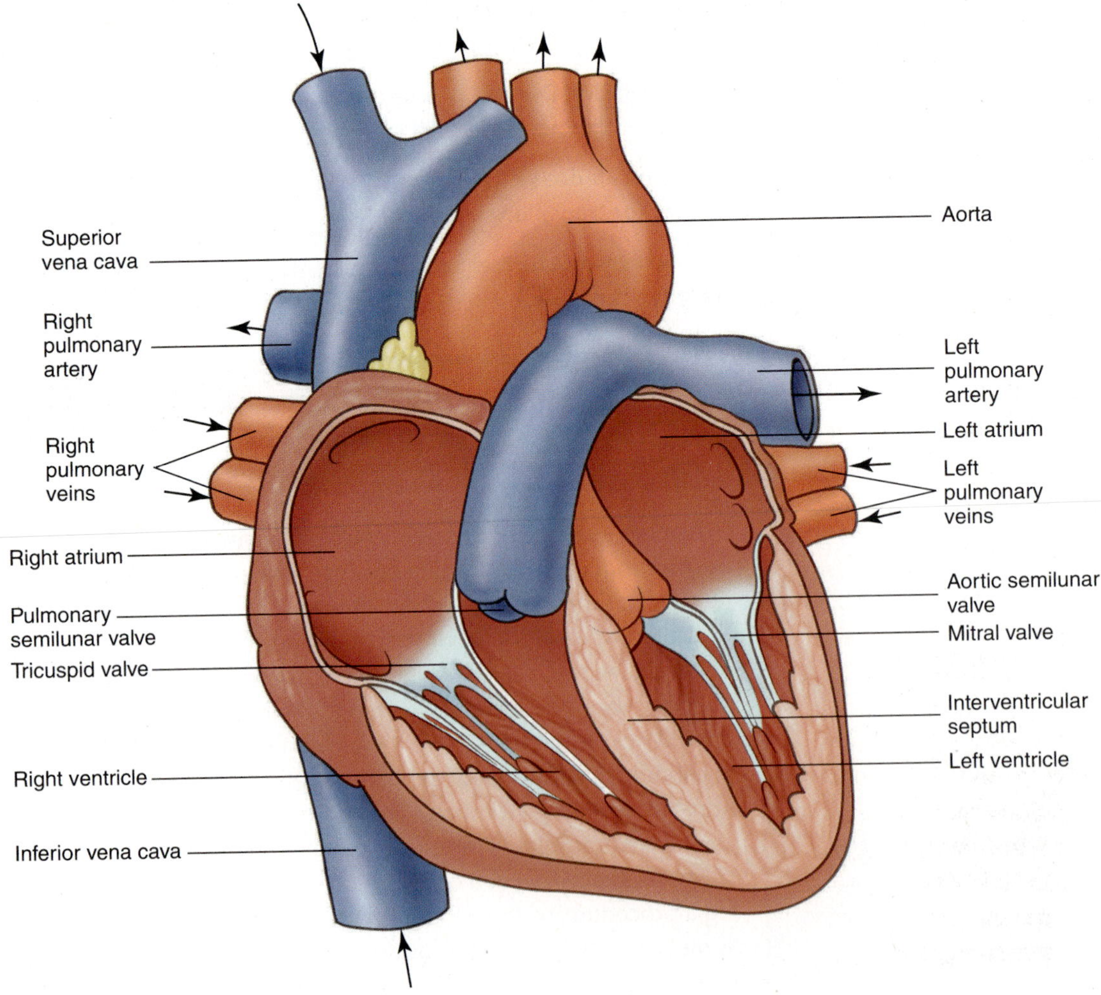

Figure 14-1 ■ The major anatomical structures of the heart.

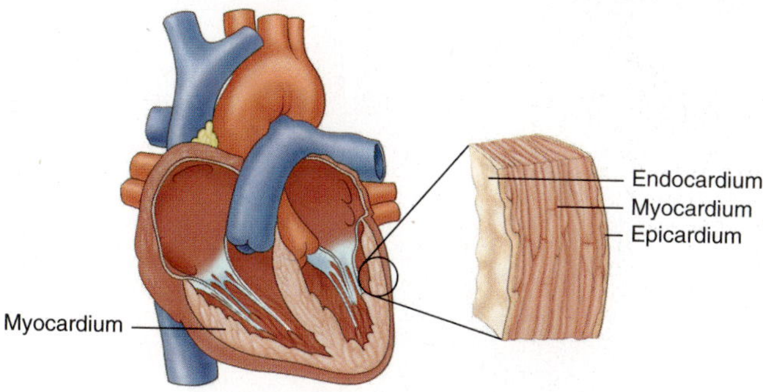

Figure 14-2 ■ The different layers of the heart.

fibrous connective tissue and serves to prevent the heart from overstretching as well as providing a small layer of fluid to allow the heart to contract more freely. Within the heart there are three primary layers of tissues. The heart contains specialized cardiac muscle, which is not found anywhere else in the body. The *epicardium* is the smooth outer layer of the heart. The main coronary arteries are located on the surface of the epicardium. The thick middle layer is called the myocardium. The *myocardium* is composed of specialized cardiac muscle cells and is responsible for the contraction of the heart muscle. The inner layer is the *endocardium* and is composed of thick connective tissue as well as stretch sensors, which are only now being understood. Refer to Figure 14-2 for an illustration of the layers of the heart.

Blood Vessels

There are three types of blood vessels: arteries, veins, and capillaries. *Arteries* are thick, muscular-walled vessels under high pressure, and their function is to carry oxygenated blood from the heart to the body's tissues. One way to remember the function of arteries is to associate "a" with away. *Veins,* in contrast, carry oxygen-poor blood back to the heart and are low-pressure circuits. The largest two veins in our bodies are the superior vena cava (SVC) and the inferior vena cava (IVC). The SVC drains blood from the head and neck. The IVC collects blood from the rest of the body. The pulmonary veins carry oxygenated blood from the lungs to the heart. *Capillaries* are tiny blood vessels that allow for exchange of nutrients, oxygen, waste products, and carbon dioxide between blood and body tissues. The capillaries are often referred to as the connecters between the arteries and the veins.

The heart has its own circulatory network that supplies the tissues of the heart with oxygen. The *coronary arteries* consist of the following:

- *Right coronary artery* (RCA) divides into the right marginal artery and posterior descending artery. The RCA supplies blood to the majority of the right side of the heart as well as the bottom portion of both ventricles and the back of the septum.
- *Left coronary artery* (LCA) supplies the majority of blood to the left side of the heart and the front of the septum. This supplies the strongest portion of the heart through the left anterior descending (LAD) and left circumflex (LCX) arteries. Blockages at the LCA or early LAD are often referred to as "widowmakers" because they can be so deadly.
- *Collateral circulation* is a network of tiny blood vessels that only open in a crisis situation. When the coronary arteries become severely occluded, these vessels enlarge, allowing blood to flow around the occluded vessel or to another blood vessel nearby.

The *coronary veins* take the deoxygenated blood and waste from the heart and return them to the right atrium. Refer to Figure 14-3 for a sketch of the coronary arteries and refer to the "Featured Diseases" section of the chapter to learn more about coronary artery disease.

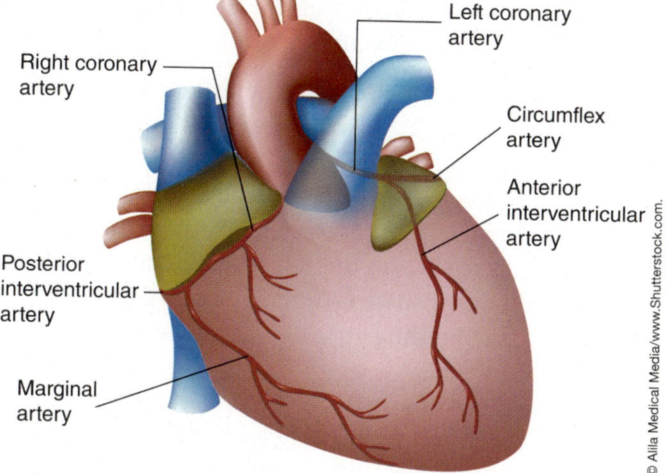

Figure 14-3 ■ The major arteries that supply the heart with oxygen.

Cardiovascular Physiology

The blood flow of the heart is an important concept for better understanding of the abnormalities that can occur in this vital organ. Oxygen-poor blood returns from the body's tissues to enter the *right atrium* (RA) via the superior and inferior vena cava. This blood then travels through the *tricuspid valve* into the *right ventricle* (RV). Within the ventricle, the blood is forced into pulmonary circulation through the *pulmonic valve* and into the *pulmonary artery* (PA). At this point the blood enters the lungs and fills the alveolar capillaries. The blood becomes oxygenated and carbon dioxide is released through the pulmonary system (lungs). This oxygenated blood then moves into the *left atrium* (LA) through the pulmonary veins. The blood from the LA is propelled through the *mitral valve* into the *left ventricle* (LV). The LV is the workhorse muscle of the heart. The LV forces blood through the *aortic valve* and into the aorta into a vast network of arteries in the body. This force produces the systolic pressure (high number) of blood pressure readings while the muscular recoil of the arteries maintains the diastolic pressure (lower number). Refer to Figure 14-1 for a diagram of the structures mentioned in this section.

Cardiac Conduction System

The heart's intrinsic conduction system is responsible for the electrical activity that controls all cardiac function. Specialized cells and fibers referred to as nodes or bundles are located under the endocardium. An understanding of the conduction system is essential for the comprehension of cardiac physiology. Refer to Figure 14-4 for a diagram of the heart's electrical system, which is described in more detail below:

- The *sinoatrial* (SA) *node* is the primary pacemaker of the heart. The SA node generates impulses through the muscle fibers of the atria. This electrical impulse is referred to as **depolarization**, which causes myocardial contraction. Sodium and calcium ions rush into the cell at this point to change the cell to a positive charge. This charge travels to the surrounding atria as well as the internodal pathways.
- *Internodal pathways* receive the electrical activity from the SA node and deliver it to the *atrioventricular* (AV) *node*. It is located in the right atrium (RA) above the tricuspid valve.

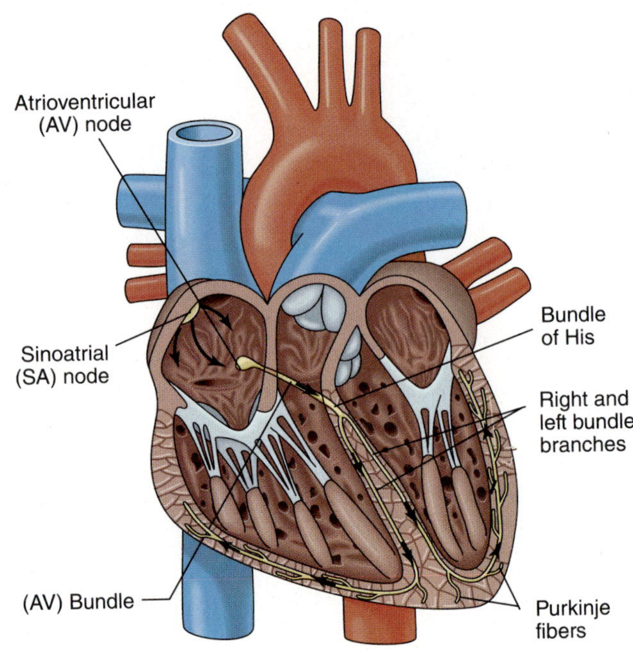

Figure 14-4 ■ The electrical conduction system of the heart.

- *AV junction* is where the AV node meets the bundle of His, which branches into a right and left bundle branch.
- The *bundle branches* conduct electricity to the *Purkinje fibers*, which deliver electricity to the ventricles.
- The final part of one cardiac cycle or one heartbeat is the resting phase called **repolarization**. The cell is then returned to a negative state.

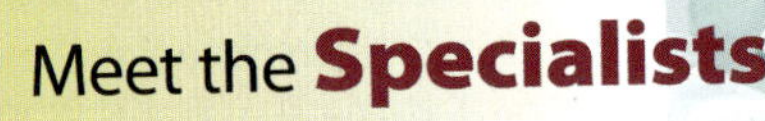

Meet the **Specialists**

Specialists who treat cardiovascular disorders include the following:

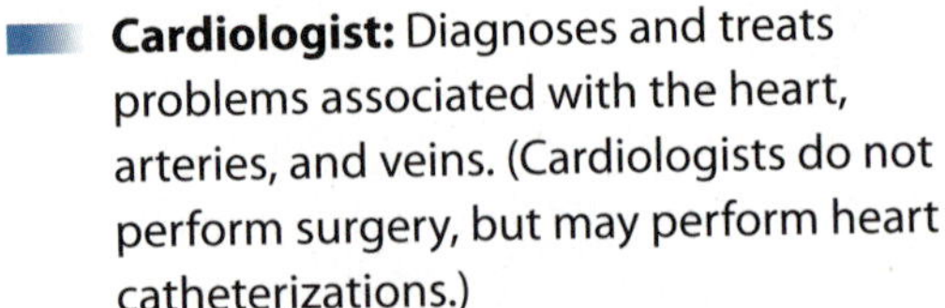

- **Cardiologist:** Diagnoses and treats problems associated with the heart, arteries, and veins. (Cardiologists do not perform surgery, but may perform heart catheterizations.)
- **Cardiovascular Surgeon:** Performs procedures on the heart and great vessels of the heart.
- **Cardiothoracic Surgeon:** Performs procedures on patients with diseases affecting organs of the heart and lungs.

Table 14-1 Common Cardiovascular Abbreviations

Abbreviation	Meaning	Abbreviation	Meaning
AAA	Abdominal aortic aneurysm	MUGA	Multiple-gated acquisition (scan)
ACS	Acute coronary syndrome	MVP	Mitral valve prolapse
Afib	Atrial fibrillation	NSR	Normal sinus rhythm
AICD	Automatic implantable cardioverter-defibrilator	PAC	Premature atrial contraction
AMI	Acute myocardial infarction	PAD	Peripheral artery disease
AS	Aortic stenosis	PTCA	Percutaneous transluminal coronary angioplasty
ASHD	Arteriosclerotic heart disease	PVC	Premature ventricular contraction
CABG	Coronary artery bypass graft	PVD	Peripheral vascular disease
CAD	Coronary artery disease	RBBB	Right bundle branch block
CHF	Congestive heart failure	SBE	Subacute bacterial endocarditis
ECG, EKG	Electrocardiogram	STEMI	ST segment elevation myocardial infarction
ECHO	Echocardiogram	SVT	Supraventricular tachycardia
HTN	Hypertension	TEE	Transesophageal echocardiogram
JVD	Jugular venous distention	VF	Ventricular fibrillation
LBBB	Left bundle branch block	VSD	Ventricular septal defect
MR	Mitral regurgitation	VT	Ventricular tachycardia

CARDIOVASCULAR ABBREVIATION REVIEW

Table 14-1 features common abbreviations used in cardiovascular specialties. Medical assistants should be familiar with these abbreviations.

CARDIOVASCULAR IN-OFFICE AND TELEPHONE SCREENING TIPS

Medical assistants may have the responsibility of screening patients over the phone and prior to provider examination. The depth of screening will be established by office protocol, but in general, medical assistants should be able to ask a series of questions related to the patient's symptoms. Table 14-2 lists the types of questions that are typically asked when patients complain of cardiac symptoms and lists common actions that should be offered when screening over the phone. The table also lists common procedures that may be ordered when the patient comes into the office.

Important Note: Medical assistants should never perform any procedure unless directed to do so by the provider; however, they can set up various equipment and supplies to help save time in the event that testing is ordered.

Provider's Call

Patients calling on the phone, with a history of angina, may be instructed to take up to three nitroglycerine tablets five minutes apart. If the pain does not subside, the patient should be encouraged to call the EMS. Patients with no history of angina may be directed to slowly chew up one 325 mg, or four 81 mg aspirin while waiting. This is especially useful if started within 30 minutes of the onset of pain. *(Of course, never give any medication instructions without checking medication allergies and without a direct order from the provider.)*

COMMON CARDIOVASCULAR DISEASES

There are many conditions that affect the cardiovascular system. In this section, we will describe some of the most common conditions that affect the heart.

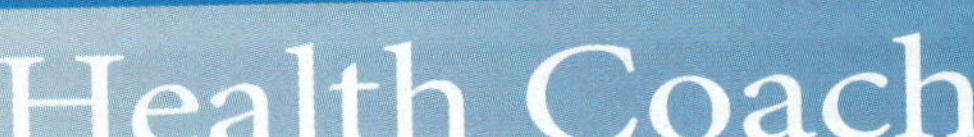

Health Coach

Featured Disease Spotlight: Coronary Artery Disease (CAD)

Description	Coronary artery disease is a condition in which the coronary arteries become sclerotic (hardened) and narrow due to a condition known as **atherosclerosis**; a buildup of cholesterol, calcium, and other substances. Over time plaque buildup reduces the diameter of the arteries (occlusion) (Figure 14-5), making it difficult for blood to flow freely to the myocardium. Eventually, as blood hits the plaque during myocardial contraction, the plaque may break open exposing the cholesterol core inside, promoting a blood clot to form. The increased reduction of blood flow may lead to myocardial infarction or heart attack.
Diagram	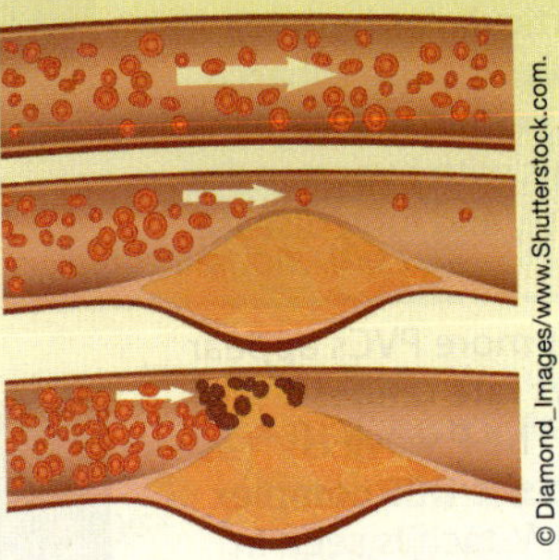 **Figure 14-5** ■ Plaque from atherosclerosis builds up in the coronary arteries.
Risk Factors	Familial history, high cholesterol, diabetes, hypertension, obesity, tobacco use (all forms), high-fat diets, sedentary lifestyle, and stress.
Symptoms	*Angina pectoris* (chest pain during exertion); heart palpitations; shortness of breath (especially during exertion), radiating pain to the jaw, neck, back, or arms (especially left sided); irregular heart beat; and cardiac arrest. Keep in mind, some persons may have no symptoms, while others may have one or any combination of symptoms listed.
Diagnostic Testing	*Blood Tests*: Can be an early detector of coronary artery disease. The most common blood test is the *lipid panel*, which detects cholesterol levels in the blood including *total cholesterol* (normal range is 0–199 mg/dL); *high-density lipoprotein (HDL)* (good cholesterol) (normal range is 40–60 mg/dL); *low-density lipoprotein (LDL)* (bad cholesterol) (normal range is 0–99 mg/dL). Though providers may still use triglyceride levels, VLDL levels, and LDL/HDL ratios to estimate the patient's risk for coronary artery disease, newer tools have been endorsed by the American College of Cardiology and American Heart Association. These calculators use HDL and total cholesterol as well as age, sex, race, history of diabetes, history of hypertension, blood pressure, and smoking history to assess the patient's 10-year and lifetime risk of atherosclerotic cardiovascular disease. *Stress Echocardiography*: Ultrasonic pictures of the heart taken at rest and during high-levels of stress. Stress on the heart may be created through walking on a treadmill or administration of drugs that cause heart rate to increase. *Cardiac Catheterization*: A long catheter is threaded either from the groin region (femoral artery) or arm region (brachial artery) with the assistance of an X-ray camera (fluoroscopy). Iodine dye is injected into the coronary arteries once the catheter reaches its destination. Pictures are taken and reviewed for occlusion or blockages. *Electron Beam CT Scan (EBCT)*: This test takes images of the heart between beats detecting calcium deposits associated with atherosclerosis. The test is so sensitive that it can detect coronary occlusions less than 20%. This allows for early intervention before surgical intervention is necessary. Often the results will be reported with a calcium volume score.

continues

Table 14-3 Common Arrhythmias *(continued)*

Condition	Description	Illustration
Atrial fibrillation (AF or A-Fib)	Rapid, disorganized atrial signals that lead to a disorganized, rapid ventricular heart rate ranging from 110 to 180 BPM. The P waves are small and irregular, and cannot be differentiated. This arrhythmia can appear in healthy individuals as well as in those with mitral valve disease, rheumatic heart disease, hypertension, and coronary artery disease.	
Premature ventricular contractions (PVCs)	Occurs on the ECG tracing before a normally conducted beat. They are characterized by a beat that comes early in the cycle, the absence of the P wave, and a wide QRS complex. Following a PVC, there is an identifiable pause before the next normal cycle. This particular arrhythmia can be found in individuals who use tobacco, alcohol, caffeine, and certain medications as well as in individuals with hypertension, coronary artery disease, and lung disease with hypoxia.	Normal Normal PVC PVC
Ventricular tachycardia (VT or V-tach)	Occurs when three or more PVCs appear in a row and the heart rate ranges from 150 to 250 BPM. The P wave is indistinguishable and the QRS complex is wide and distorted. V-tach is seen in individuals with both acute and chronic heart disease, coronary artery disease, and as a result of a myocardial infarction. This arrhythmia is life threatening and can deteriorate into ventricular fibrillation and cardiac arrest.	
Ventricular fibrillation (VF or V-fib)	The most serious of the cardiac arrhythmias. It is characterized by uncoordinated beats that cause a quivering or twitching of the ventricles. No blood is being pumped out to the tissues of the body, which will lead to death if not rapidly identified and corrected. V-fib is common during an acute myocardial infarction and is also seen in patients with existing cardiac disease. This arrhythmia can cause sudden death and an attempt to correct it must be initiated immediately.	

Defibrillation

Defibrillation is defined as reversing fibrillation of the heart muscle by physical, electrical, or chemical means to a life-sustaining rhythm. A device known as a *defibrillator* is used to deliver electrical shocks to the heart through pads or electrodes placed on the chest wall. The purpose of the electrical shock is to convert a cardiac arrhythmia back to a normal sinus rhythm. This process is known as **cardioversion**. Many ambulatory care facilities keep a defibrillator on a crash cart for easy and quick access during an emergency. It is the medical assistant's responsibility to routinely check the defibrillator to make sure it is in good working order.

Coronary Artery Disease

Coronary artery disease is the number one killer of adults in the United States and affects more than 15 million people annually. Refer to the Health Coach Disease Feature to learn more about this disease.

Health Coach

Featured Disease Spotlight: Coronary Artery Disease (CAD)

Description	Coronary artery disease is a condition in which the coronary arteries become sclerotic (hardened) and narrow due to a condition known as **atherosclerosis**; a buildup of cholesterol, calcium, and other substances. Over time plaque buildup reduces the diameter of the arteries (occlusion) (Figure 14-5), making it difficult for blood to flow freely to the myocardium. Eventually, as blood hits the plaque during myocardial contraction, the plaque may break open exposing the cholesterol core inside, promoting a blood clot to form. The increased reduction of blood flow may lead to myocardial infarction or heart attack.
Diagram	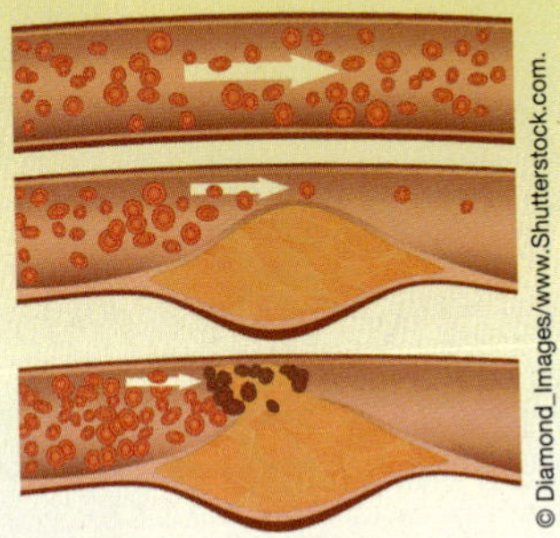 **Figure 14-5** ■ Plaque from atherosclerosis builds up in the coronary arteries.
Risk Factors	Familial history, high cholesterol, diabetes, hypertension, obesity, tobacco use (all forms), high-fat diets, sedentary lifestyle, and stress.
Symptoms	*Angina pectoris* (chest pain during exertion); heart palpitations; shortness of breath (especially during exertion), radiating pain to the jaw, neck, back, or arms (especially left sided); irregular heart beat; and cardiac arrest. Keep in mind, some persons may have no symptoms, while others may have one or any combination of symptoms listed.
Diagnostic Testing	*Blood Tests*: Can be an early detector of coronary artery disease. The most common blood test is the *lipid panel*, which detects cholesterol levels in the blood including *total cholesterol* (normal range is 0–199 mg/dL); *high-density lipoprotein (HDL)* (good cholesterol) (normal range is 40–60 mg/dL); *low-density lipoprotein (LDL)* (bad cholesterol) (normal range is 0–99 mg/dL). Though providers may still use triglyceride levels, VLDL levels, and LDL/HDL ratios to estimate the patient's risk for coronary artery disease, newer tools have been endorsed by the American College of Cardiology and American Heart Association. These calculators use HDL and total cholesterol as well as age, sex, race, history of diabetes, history of hypertension, blood pressure, and smoking history to assess the patient's 10-year and lifetime risk of atherosclerotic cardiovascular disease. *Stress Echocardiography*: Ultrasonic pictures of the heart taken at rest and during high-levels of stress. Stress on the heart may be created through walking on a treadmill or administration of drugs that cause heart rate to increase. *Cardiac Catheterization*: A long catheter is threaded either from the groin region (femoral artery) or arm region (brachial artery) with the assistance of an X-ray camera (fluoroscopy). Iodine dye is injected into the coronary arteries once the catheter reaches its destination. Pictures are taken and reviewed for occlusion or blockages. *Electron Beam CT Scan (EBCT)*: This test takes images of the heart between beats detecting calcium deposits associated with atherosclerosis. The test is so sensitive that it can detect coronary occlusions less than 20%. This allows for early intervention before surgical intervention is necessary. Often the results will be reported with a calcium volume score.

continues

Table 14-1 Common Cardiovascular Abbreviations

Abbreviation	Meaning	Abbreviation	Meaning
AAA	Abdominal aortic aneurysm	MUGA	Multiple-gated acquisition (scan)
ACS	Acute coronary syndrome	MVP	Mitral valve prolapse
Afib	Atrial fibrillation	NSR	Normal sinus rhythm
AICD	Automatic implantable cardioverter-defibrilator	PAC	Premature atrial contraction
AMI	Acute myocardial infarction	PAD	Peripheral artery disease
AS	Aortic stenosis	PTCA	Percutaneous transluminal coronary angioplasty
ASHD	Arteriosclerotic heart disease	PVC	Premature ventricular contraction
CABG	Coronary artery bypass graft	PVD	Peripheral vascular disease
CAD	Coronary artery disease	RBBB	Right bundle branch block
CHF	Congestive heart failure	SBE	Subacute bacterial endocarditis
ECG, EKG	Electrocardiogram	STEMI	ST segment elevation myocardial infarction
ECHO	Echocardiogram	SVT	Supraventricular tachycardia
HTN	Hypertension	TEE	Transesophageal echocardiogram
JVD	Jugular venous distention	VF	Ventricular fibrillation
LBBB	Left bundle branch block	VSD	Ventricular septal defect
MR	Mitral regurgitation	VT	Ventricular tachycardia

CARDIOVASCULAR ABBREVIATION REVIEW

Table 14-1 features common abbreviations used in cardiovascular specialties. Medical assistants should be familiar with these abbreviations.

CARDIOVASCULAR IN-OFFICE AND TELEPHONE SCREENING TIPS

Medical assistants may have the responsibility of screening patients over the phone and prior to provider examination. The depth of screening will be established by office protocol, but in general, medical assistants should be able to ask a series of questions related to the patient's symptoms. Table 14-2 lists the types of questions that are typically asked when patients complain of cardiac symptoms and lists common actions that should be offered when screening over the phone. The table also lists common procedures that may be ordered when the patient comes into the office.

Important Note: Medical assistants should never perform any procedure unless directed to do so by the provider; however, they can set up various equipment and supplies to help save time in the event that testing is ordered.

Provider's Call

Patients calling on the phone, with a history of angina, may be instructed to take up to three nitroglycerine tablets five minutes apart. If the pain does not subside, the patient should be encouraged to call the EMS. Patients with no history of angina may be directed to slowly chew up one 325 mg, or four 81 mg aspirin while waiting. This is especially useful if started within 30 minutes of the onset of pain. *(Of course, never give any medication instructions without checking medication allergies and without a direct order from the provider.)*

COMMON CARDIOVASCULAR DISEASES

There are many conditions that affect the cardiovascular system. In this section, we will describe some of the most common conditions that affect the heart.

Table 14-2 Patient Screening Instructions for the Cardiovascular System

Ask the Patient	• Are you experiencing any difficulty breathing; shortness of breath; chest pain or pressure; radiation of pain to the arms, neck, or jaw; heart palpitations; nausea or vomiting; swelling in the hands or feet or fainting episodes? • Do you have any history of cardiovascular disease? • When pain is involved, describe the pain (stabbing, sharp, or dull). Is the pain continuous or intermittent? Rate the pain on a scale from 1 to 10. • List what makes symptoms better or worse. • List duration of symptoms.
For Patients Calling on the Telephone	Chest pain patients are usually encouraged to call the EMS to be on the safe side. However, the provider's call box featured on the previous page lists some instructions that may be given to patients while they are waiting on the EMS.
When in the Office	
Disrobing Instructions	Have the patient remove all clothing from waist up and to put a gown on so it opens in the back.
Vital Signs	Take and record all vital signs.
Equipment	Patients should be placed in a room designated to handle emergencies such as the cardiac bay, trauma room, and so on. Equipment you will need includes an ECG unit, pulse oximeter, oxygen and mask or nasal cannula, AED, crash cart, and IV materials.
Possible Procedures	ECG, pulse oximetry, defibrillation, and CPR.

Cardiac Arrhythmias

Cardiac **arrhythmias**, sometimes referred to as *dysrhythmias*, are irregularities in the heart's rhythm. They can be caused by either physiological or pathological interruptions in the orderly discharge of electrical impulses from the SA node or any other conductive tissue of the heart.

The medical assistant should be able to recognize basic arrhythmias so that the proper steps can be taken. The normal cardic cycle includes a P wave, QRS complex, and a T wave. The sequence should repeat itself in a continuous, even pattern. Any extra beats, abnormal heart rates, or abnormal rhythms are considered arrhythmias. Refer to the ECG section for an in-depth look at the cardiac cycle. **Normal sinus rhythm** is the term used to describe an ECG that falls within normal limits (WNL). The normal adult heart rate ranges from 60 to 100 beats per minute (BPM). *Sinus bradycardia* is the term used to define a regular heart rate below 60 BPM, while *sinus tachycardia* refers to a regular heart rate above 100 BPM.

Some common arrhythmias are described in Table 14-3.

Table 14-3 Common Arrhythmias

Condition	Description	Illustration
Premature atrial contractions (PAC)	Usually considered benign. Commonly occur in patients who smoke, take in caffeine, or use other stimulants.	P wave R wave
Paroxysmal atrial tachycardia (PAT)	One of the most common arrhythmias; usually occurs suddenly with a heart rate ranging from 130 to 250 BPM. Usually lasts for a few seconds and returns to pre-PAT status.	

Featured Disease Spotlight: Coronary Artery Disease (CAD) *continued*

Modifying Factors	Diet and exercise are two of the most important therapies for both lowering cholesterol and maintaining heart health. The American Heart Association states that you should exercise at least three to five times per week for a minimum of 30 minutes per session. Fat intake should be less than 27% of your total caloric intake (< 60 grams of fat per day in adults) with no more than 6% of calories from saturated fat. Increase fruit and vegetable intake, cook foods in canola or olive oil (when oil is required), increase garlic intake, avoid lots of red meat, and eat one or two servings of seafood per week. Other prevention and maintenance tips include; smoking cessation, controlling high blood pressure, controlling blood sugar, and taking a low dose of aspirin daily, which has been proven to lower risks of heart attack.
Drug Therapy	*Aspirin*: Acts as an anticoagulant by helping to prevent clots from forming *Beta Blockers*: Help to lower blood pressure and heart rate which aids in prevention of heart attacks. These drugs also lower the demands on the heart. *Calcium Channel Blockers*: Decrease blood pressure, heart rate, and dilate coronary arteries. *Angiotensin-Converting Enzyme (ACE) Inhibitors*: Reduces blood pressure, increases blood flow, and is especially useful with patients suffering from diabetes, cardiomyopathy, or prior myocardial infarction. Latest findings show that this drug helps in reducing the number of cardiac events. *Statins:* Lower lipid levels in the blood. Benefits of statins include a reduction of plaque in the coronary arteries, and a reduction of the progression of CAD.
Invasive Therapy	*Percutaneous Transluminal Coronary Angioplasty (PTCA)*: This procedure is similar to a heart catheterization but provides both diagnostic and therapeutic benefits. A very thick, sturdy catheter with a balloon is guided through the coronary arteries. Once the blockage is found the balloon is inflated and the artery widens. The balloon is removed; however, the plaque now is flattened against the arterial walls allowing blood to flow more freely. A **stent** (Figure 14-6) is often inserted during PTCA to decrease risks of the arteries collapsing after angioplasty. 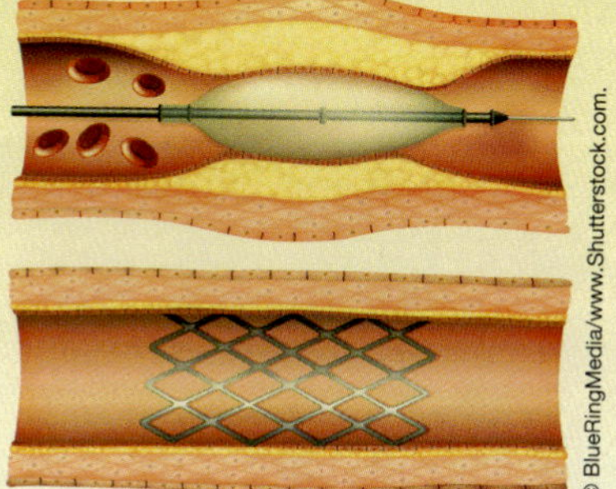 © BlueRingMedia/www.Shutterstock.com. **Figure 14-6** ■ A stent helps to prevent the artery from re-occluding. *Arthrectomy*: In cases in which PTCH is not a solution due to calcification or other factors, an arthrectomy may be the answer. In this procedure the fat is removed by cutting it or burning it with a laser. Not everyone is a candidate for this procedure. Coronary Artery Bypass Graft (CABG): This procedure is performed in severe blockages. An artery or vein from another part of the body is connected or graphed to the blocked artery/arteries so that blood is rerouted around the blockage. This is the most common open heart procedure performed today.

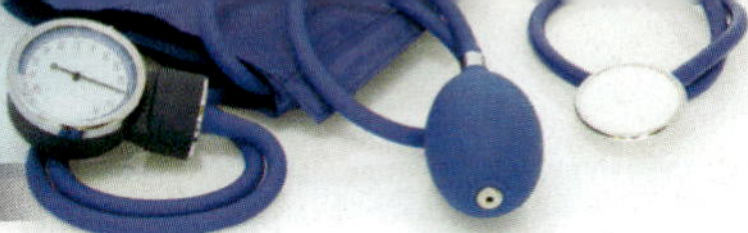

Table 14-4 Other Common Cardiovascular Conditions

Condition	Description
Aneurysm	The thinning and ballooning of an artery. May lead to a rupture and internal bleeding. Common sites include the brain and aorta.
Angina pectoris	Severe chest pain episode due to constriction of the coronary arteries and *ischemia* (reduction of blood flow to the myocardium). The pain usually worsens as ischemia increases.
Congestive heart failure	A condition in which the heart weakens and is no longer able to adequately pump blood and other fluids around the body. This causes a backup of fluid resulting in congestions in areas where the backup occurs. There are two types of failure: *Left-sided failure*, which causes *pulmonary edema* (a buildup of fluid in the lungs). *Dyspnea* (difficulty in breathing) may be a symptom of this condition. *Right-sided failure* causes a buildup of fluid throughout the rest of the body. Symptoms usually include *edema* or swelling in the feet and ankles; however, progressed symptoms may involve the GI tract, liver, and arms.
Heart murmur	A condition in which the heart valve (any of the four) is not completely closing, or there is a hole in the septum allowing turbulent blood flow. This turbulent blood flow results in different murmur sounds, which are differentiated by location and severity. Murmurs are often fine without any intervention but occasionally the need for surgical intervention is necessary in severe cases.
Hypertension	Elevated blood pressure due to array of factors including smoking, obesity, lack of exercise, excessive sodium in the diet, stress, aging, and familial disease. Elevated blood pressure causes the heart to work harder leading to further complications. Refer to Chapter 11 for more information on hypertension.
Myocardial infarction (MI)	Total blockage of a coronary artery/arteries causing blood flow to cease to the tissue nourished by the artery. This can lead to an infarct or death of the affected tissue. In cases where substantial tissue is involved, this may lead to death. An MI is also known as a heart attack.
Thrombus	A blood clot attached to the inside of an artery. More of a concern when it involves a deep vein or artery. The clot can cause a complete restriction of blood to the area or the clot may dislodge and become an *embolus* that moves to a critical vessel of the body such as the pulmonary artery, coronary artery, or cerebral artery.

Other Cardiovascular Conditions

Cardiovascular specialty practices also see patients with many other conditions besides arrhythmias and coronary artery disease. For information on some of these other conditions refer to Table 14-4.

FEATURED CARDIOVASCULAR PROCEDURES

Medical assistants often have the responsibility of performing cardiovascular procedures, setting up outside procedures (procedures not performed in the office),

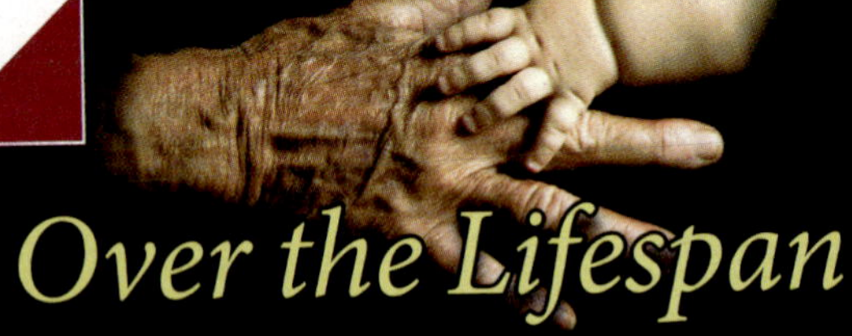

Over the Lifespan

As the body ages, arteries that were elastic and pliable lose elasticity, dilate, and elongate. This causes the heart to work harder to force blood around the body, which increases arterial pressure. Hypertension accelerates damage to the arteries by creating microscopic tears and the buildup of scar tissue. The scar tissue may allow substances such as fat and cholesterol to easily lodge in the damaged tissue, eventually turning into plaque, resulting in a reduction of blood volume to other organs. Clot formation increases the patient's risk of heart attack, TIAs, and stroke. Smoking, a sedentary lifestyle, poor dietary choices, and even some medications can accelerate this process. Over time, the decrease in blood flow may result in irreversible damage to the heart, kidneys, and brain.

Changes may also occur in the electrical tissue of the heart. As the heart ages, fibrous tissue and fat deposits often develop along the electrical pathways of the heart, resulting in a loss of cellular function and a slower heartbeat. Valves in the heart oftentimes thicken over the years, resulting in stiffening, which may lead to heart murmurs in the elderly patient.

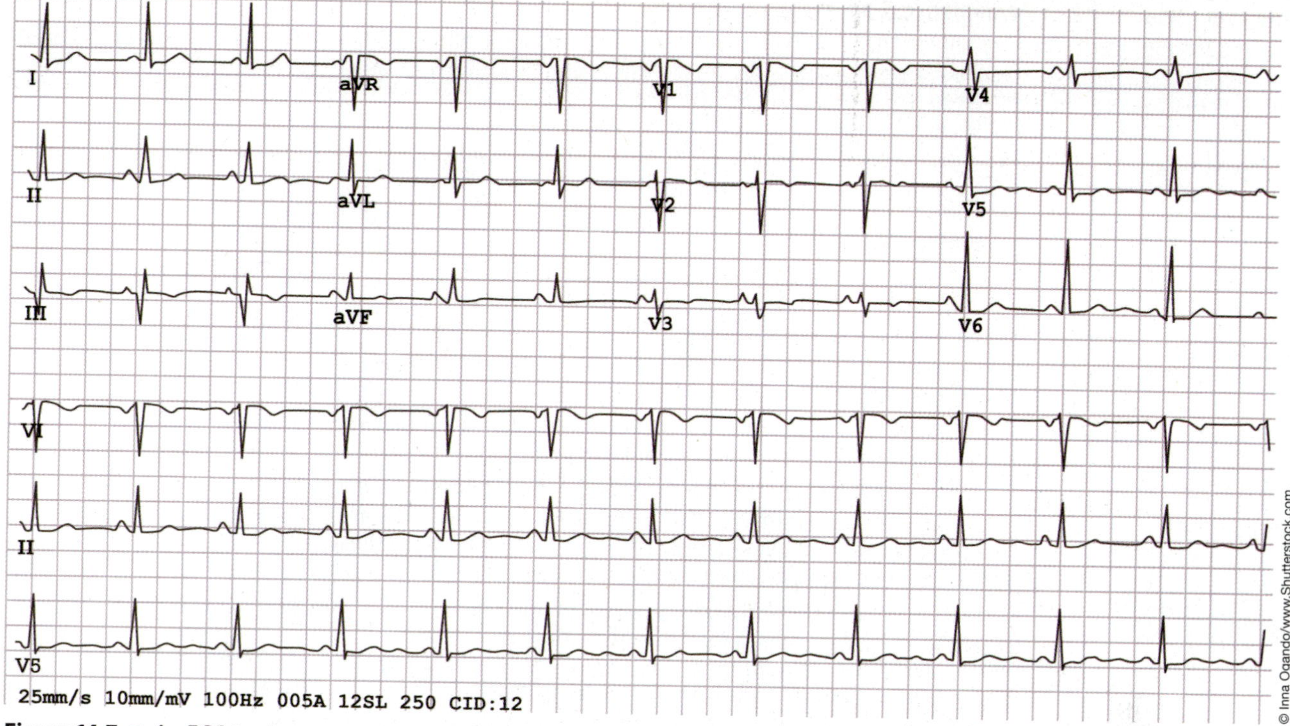

Figure 14-7 ■ An ECG tracing.

and educating patients about healthy heart choices. There are a variety of tests that are performed to help in the diagnosis of cardiovascular conditions. This section will focus on procedures routinely performed by medical assistants.

Electrocardiograms

The **electrocardiogram (EKG or ECG)** (Figure 14-7) is a safe, noninvasive, and painless diagnostic tool that can be quickly and easily performed in the provider's office. It provides valuable information concerning the patient's heart health as it measures the amount of electrical activity produced by the heart and the time required for the impulses to travel through the heart with each heartbeat.

Although the ECG cannot predict a future myocardial infarction (heart attack), it can detect damage caused by a previous event and by *ischemia*, a temporary lack of blood flow to the heart. An ECG can also evaluate cardiac *arrhythmias* (abnormal heart rhythms), detect if there is an electrolyte imbalance, detect adverse effects resulting from hypertension, and follow the heart's response to medication.

The medical assistant is usually the health care professional responsible for performing the ECG in the provider's office. Precise skills and knowledge are essential when performing all forms of cardiac testing.

Cardiac Cycle

A **cardiac cycle** is the events that occur from the initiation of one heart beat to the onset of the next heart beat. One cardiac cycle occurs every 0.8 seconds. The contraction phase of both ventricles is called *systole* and lasts about 0.28 seconds. Following systole, the ventricles relax and this phase is referred to as *diastole*, duration about 0.52 seconds. An electrocardiogram (ECG or EKG) is the graphic representation of the cardiac cycle. The tracing on the ECG represents the cycle of electrical conduction only, not the mechanical activity of the heart.

ECG Waveforms

A waveform (Figure 14-8) refers to a positive (upright deflection) or negative (downward deflection) from the isoelectric line. The **isoelectric line** is the straight

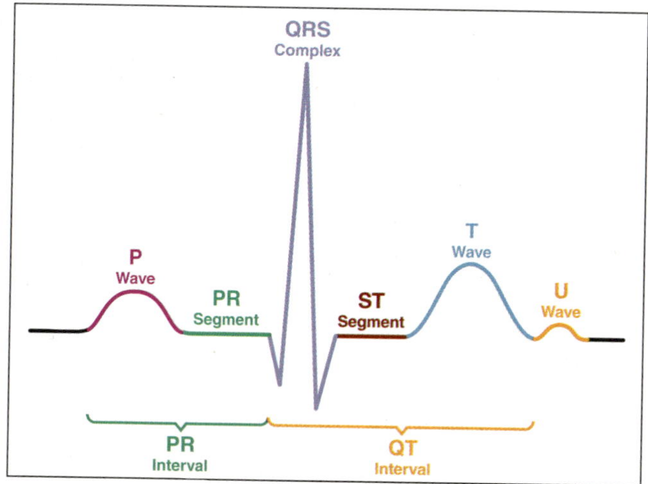

Figure 14-8 ■ A sketch of an ECG waveform. Notice the difference between waves, segments, and intervals.

Table 14-5 Waveforms of a Complete Cardiac Cycle

Wave, Segment, or Interval	Physiology	Approximate Time Interval
P wave	Depolarization of the left and right atria	0.06–0.1 seconds
PR segment	Represents the conduction time of the atrioventricular node, down the bundle of His and through the bundle branches. (Begins with the end of the P wave and finishes with the start of the Q wave.) Not really significant in disease.	Not relevant with segments
PR interval	Time interval from SA node through internodal pathways to the ventricles. (Begins with the start of the P wave through the start of the QRS complex.) An increase in the length could indicate a heart block; a decrease in length could indicate Wolf Parkinson White syndrome.	0.12–0.2 seconds
QRS wave or complex	Conduction of impulse from the bundle of His through the ventricles; represents ventricular depolarization. Widening may suggest a ventricular escape rhythm disorder or a bundle branch block.	0.13 seconds
ST segment	The time at which the entire ventricle is depolarized; end of the S wave to the beginning of the T wave. An elevation may indicate a myocardial infarction or pericarditis; a depression may indicate ischemia.	Not relevant with segments
QT interval	The total time from ventricular depolarization to complete repolarization; Begins at the start of the Q wave and ends at the end of the T wave. An increase in length predisposes the patient to an increased risk of tachycardia arrhythmias such as V-tach.	0.38–0.42 seconds
T wave	Resting phase of cardiac cycle called ventricular repolarization. This can be peaked in hyperkalemia.	Not relevant
U wave	Seldom seen and not really mentioned in most texts today. Its origin is unknown. May be seen in patients with hypokalemia or in patients with bradycardia.	Not relevant
PQRSTU cycle	A complete cardiac cycle	

line seen on the ECG strip. The waveforms produced on the ECG graphing paper correlate with the heart's electrical activity. The provider will review each waveform for abnormalities and will even be able to target the location of the heart affected. In order to identify these waveforms, it is first important to understand some basic terminology.

- **Baseline**: This is a flat, horizontal line separating ECG cycles. The baseline (or isoelectric line) is used as a reference point when centering the tracing. The waves will deflect positively or negatively from the baseline. A positive deflection is characterized by an upward deflection above the isoelectric line as the electrical signal moves toward the electrode. A negative deflection is characterized by a downward deflection below the isoelectric line as the electrical signal moves away from the electrode.
- **Segment**: This is the space between two waves.
- **Interval**: This includes a combination of one or more waves and a segment. This represents the length of a wave.

Table 14-5 lists the wave forms, segments, and intervals of a complete cardiac cycle and depicts the physiological aspects associated with each wave. Although medical assistants will not be interpreting ECGs, knowing the significance of each section of the wave helps determine the importance of a good quality tracing.

ECG Equipment and Supplies

The ECG machine or **electrocardiograph** is a device that plots the electrical potential on the skin that generates a record of the electrical current going through the heart. The ECG usually consists of the unit itself and a cable with ten color-coded wires (Figure 14-9). One side of the cable connects directly to the ECG unit while the other side (containing the ten separate wires) connects to **electrodes** attached to the patient's skin. The American Heart Association standardizes wire colors and codes used for heart monitoring equipment manufactured in North America. Table 14-6 depicts the colors of each wire, their abbreviations, and the location associated with each wire.

Multichannel ECG Unit

The multichannel ECG unit can record multiple leads at the same time. The 12-lead tracing is produced quickly

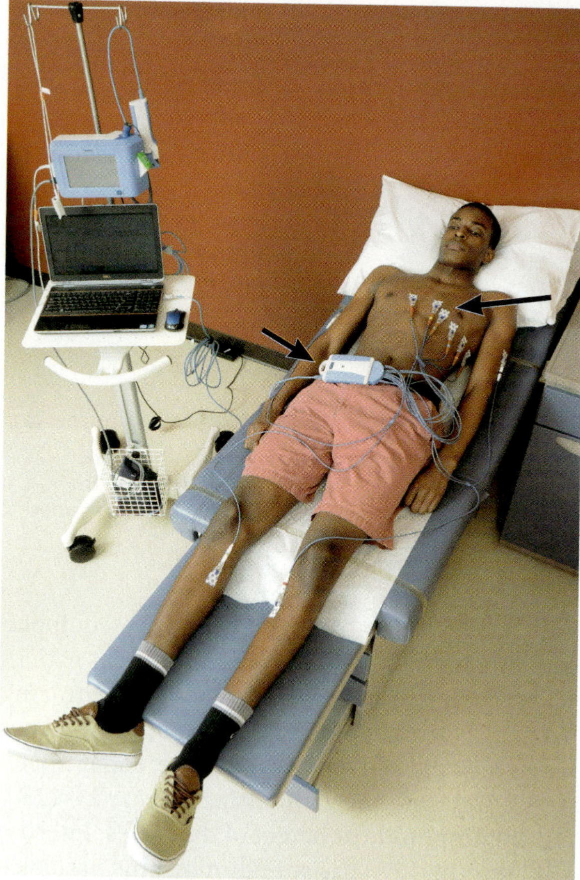

Figure 14-9 ■ An ECG unit with a patient cable. Notice the different colors on the cable wires.

Table 14-6 Wires, Abbreviations, and Color Codes

Location	Abbreviation	Color
Right arm	RA	White
Left arm	LA	Black
Right leg	RL	Green
Left leg	LL	Red
Chest	V1	Brown/red
Chest	V2	Brown/yellow
Chest	V3	Brown/green
Chest	V4	Brown/blue
Chest	V5	Brown/orange
Chest	V6	Brown/purple

on a special 8.5 × 11 inch piece of paper that fits easily into the patient's chart and requires no mounting. The three-channel machine is most commonly used in the provider's office and records three leads simultaneously; however, some units can run a variety of combinations, including 3, 4, 6, or 12 leads all at the same time. Figure 14-10A shows an example of a multichannel electrocardiograph. Many of these units have interpreting capabilities, which provide instantaneous results. Figure 14-10B features an ECG tracing with interpretation. Even though many units have interpretation capabilities, a provider must confirm the findings.

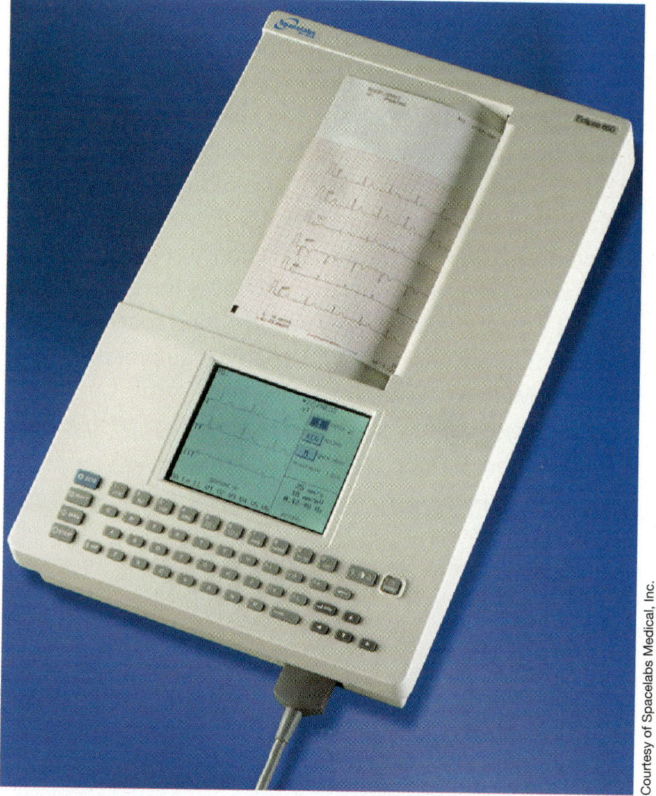

Courtesy of Spacelabs Medical, Inc.

Figure 14-10A ■ Portable Eclipse 850 ECG.

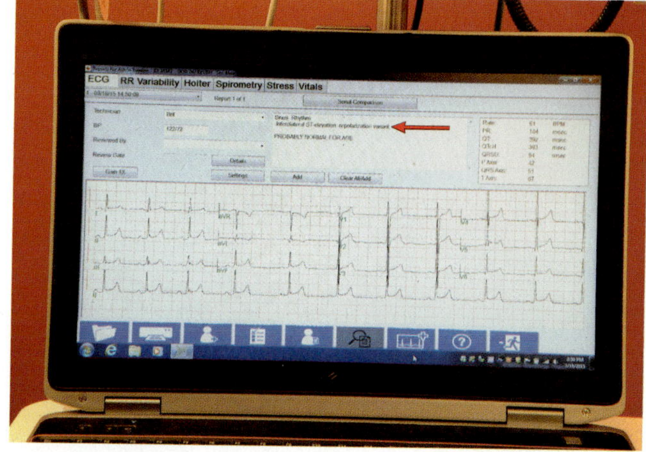

Figure 14-10B ■ An example of an electronic ECG with interpretation.

EHR Application

Web-Enabled Electrocardiograph Equipment

Manufacturers of medical equipment are teaming up with EHR software developers to create diagnostic digital solutions that interface with one another. Diagnostic equipment, such as electronic vital sign equipment, pulse oximeters, pulmonary function units, and electrocardiographs are now able to be linked directly with the practice's EHR software. This function alleviates the need to scan the information into the EHR, which saves a great deal of time and reduces potential errors from scanning diagnostic reports into the wrong electronic charts. It also saves the establishment a great deal of money in purchasing specialized paper that will only work with specific equipment.

The Midmark IQ system (Figure 14-11) features an all-in-one solution which includes the IQecg®, IQspiro®, IQvitals, and IQ Holter, which all fit onto one cart.

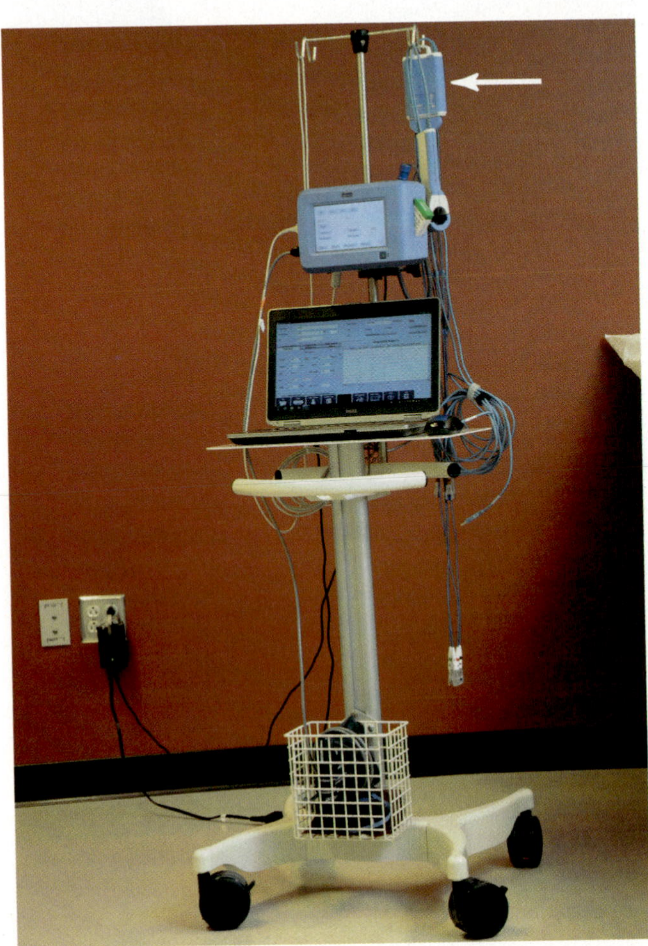

Figure 14-11 ■ The arrow points to the Midmark IQecg®.

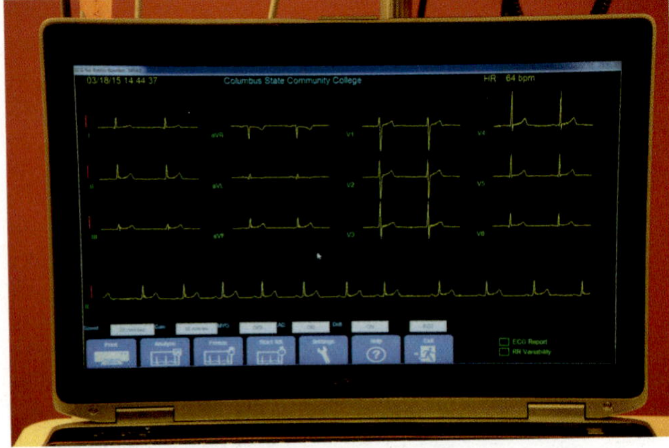

Figure 14-12 ■ (a) The paper speed is set on 50 mm/sec. (b) The sensitivity control is set on 10, which will cause the standardization to be 10 mm high. (c) The AC Filter was turned on for this ECG.

Many of the latest electrocardiographs are equipped with alphanumeric keypads to enter pertinent patient data and a lighted display monitor to view the tracing and particular settings. Menu options allow the user to change various settings such as the paper speed (Figure 14-12A) and the gain setting (Figure 14-12B), which is the amplitude or height of the waves. Internal filters (Figure 14-12C) assist in diminishing variables that can interfere with the electrocardiogram, such as somatic tremors (shivering or shaking from the patient) and electrical interference coming from other equipment. Today's ECG technology allows users to store data, print a copy of the ECG, or transmit the ECG electronically to the patient's electronic medical record.

In addition to the ECG unit, specialized paper is needed to record the tracing when a hard copy is required, along with electrodes and some form of electrolyte.

ECG Paper

Special paper is required for recording a hard copy of an ECG. The color of the graphing lines on the ECG paper may be red, black, or blue, depending on the manufacturer of the paper. The paper is covered by a white plastic or wax coating. As the heated **stylus** (the wire that produces the tracing) moves in response to the patient's heartbeat, it melts the plastic, resulting in a tracing.

The ECG paper is imprinted with two sets of squares. Each small square is 1 mm high and 1 mm wide, while each large square is 5 mm × 5 mm, and consists of 25 small squares (Figure 14-13). Each large square is outlined in darker ink for easy counting. Each small square is equal to 0.04 seconds and each large square is equal to 0.2 seconds. The vertical

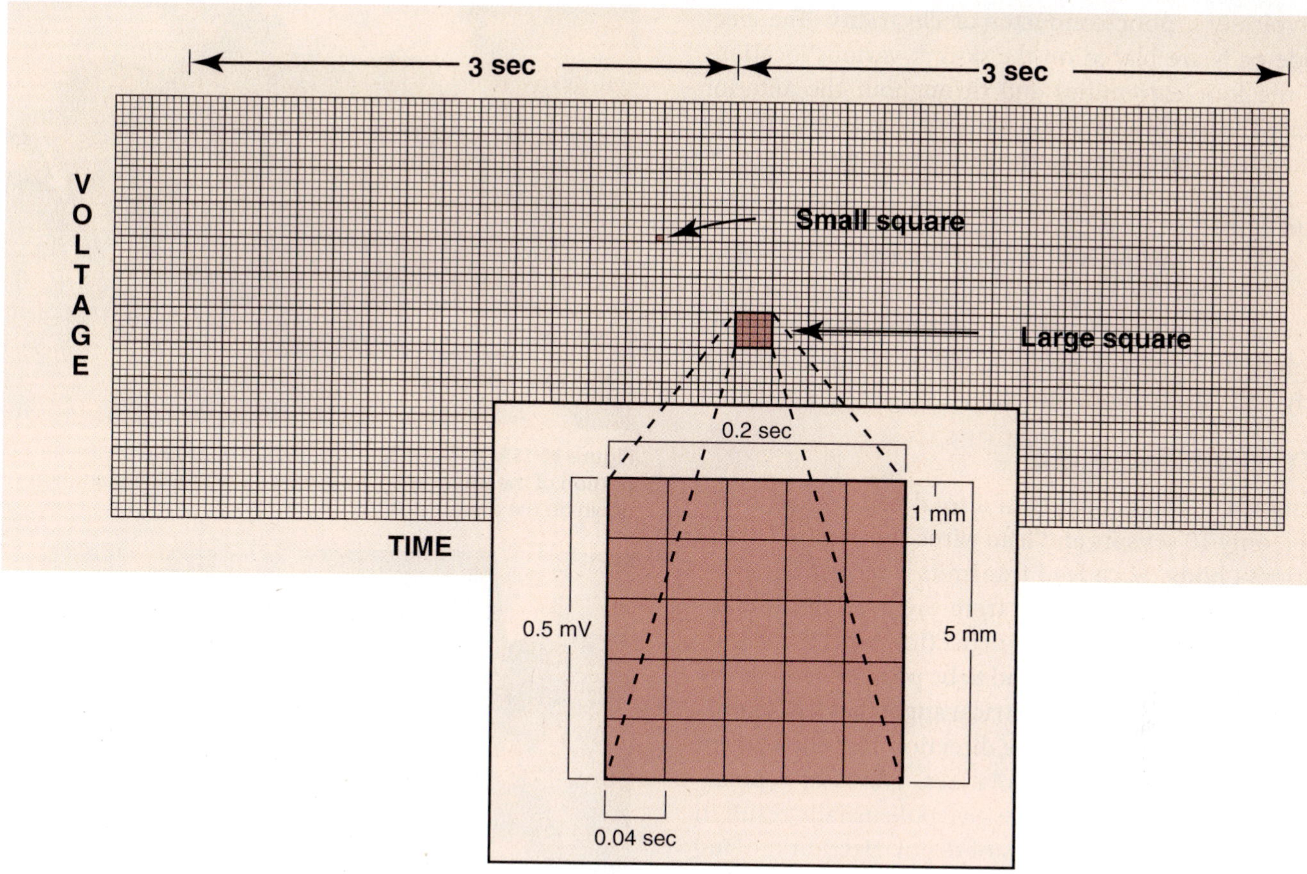

Figure 14-13 ■ ECG graph paper illustrating the size of the small and large squares used to measure the time and voltage of heartbeats.

lines measure the **amplitude** or how high the complex deflects, and the horizontal lines measure the timing of the impulses. After the recording is produced, the provider is able to count the number of squares on the paper and perform a calculation to determine the time it takes for each deflection and the amount of voltage or cardiac electrical activity present. These calculations assist the provider in determining various heart abnormalities. As electrocardiograph units are replaced with computerized models that connect directly with the EHR, there will be no need for ECG paper.

Paper Speed

The ECG paper normally runs through the machine at a rate of 25 millimeters per second (mm/sec). If the heart rate is elevated and the complexes are spaced too closely together for an accurate interpretation, the paper speed may be increased to 50 mm/sec, which will spread the complexes farther apart. The change in paper speed is usually automatically indicated at the top or bottom of the tracing. Even though fully digital ECGs do not use "paper," the speed at which the ECG is displayed must still be controlled. Settings within the computer will allow you to make necessary adjustments.

Electrodes and Electrolyte

Electrodes, also known as sensors, are attached to the patient and designed to detect electrical activity coming from the heart. The majority of electrodes are disposable self-adhesive pads (Figure 14-14) made of conductive material that contains an **electrolyte** solution that helps conduct the electrical current. The skin

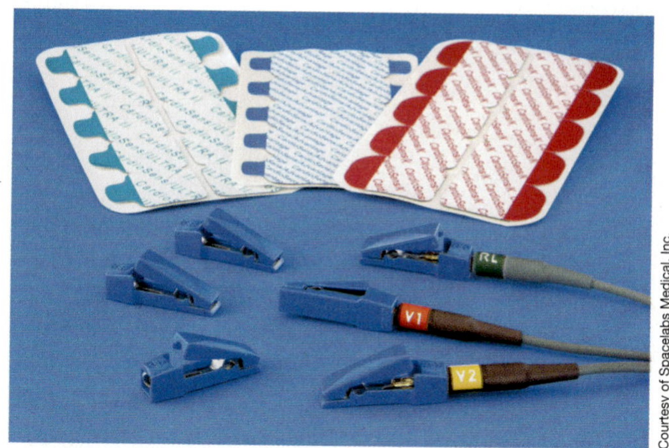

Courtesy of Spacelabs Medical, Inc.

Figure 14-14 ■ Example of different electrode pads and clips.

is typically a poor conductor of electricity. The electrode pads are placed on the skin at various locations on the four extremities and throughout the anterior chest. The impulses are transmitted from the electrodes through the lead wires to the ECG machine.

Skin Prep

In order to get the best tracing possible, sites where electrodes are to be placed should be cleansed with alcohol and abraded with gauze until the skin turns slightly pink prior to applying the electrodes. Particularly hairy areas should be shaved.

ECG Lead Placement

A standard ECG consists of a total of 12 leads; however, only 10 sensors and lead wires are attached to the patient's body. Each **lead** transmits a recording of the electrical impulses coming from the heart at different angles. What influences a deflection within the cardiac cycle of a particular lead to be positive or negative is contingent on the geometrical angle that the heart is being viewed from, and the direction that the current is flowing as the heart depolarizes. Waves of depolarization moving toward a positive pole usually result in a positive deflection; waves of depolarization moving away from a positive pole usually result in a negative deflection. If a particular lead produces a deflection other than what is anticipated, it could indicate heart pathology or a problem with the placement of the electrodes.

The limb electrodes are placed on the fleshy, nonbony part of the patient's upper arms (Figure 14-15A) and lower legs (Figure 14-15B). The tabs on the electrodes should be pointing downward on the arms and upward on the legs to reduce tension or pulling on the electrodes. Electrode tabs on the chest should also be facing downward and placed on the wall of the chest at the appropriate spaces.

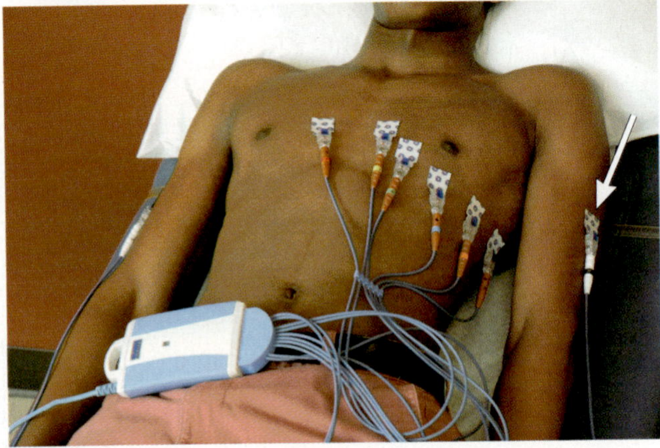

Figure 14-15A ■ The electrodes should be placed on the fleshy portion of the upper arms. Notice how the tabs are pointing down on the arms.

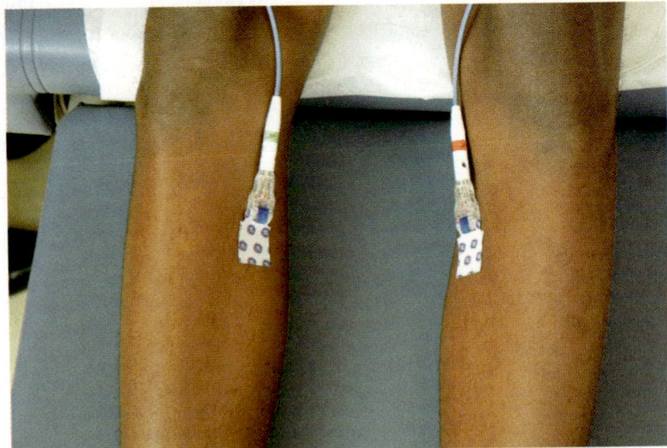

Figure 14-15B ■ The electrodes should be placed on the inside fleshy portion of the lower legs. Notice how the tabs are facing upward.

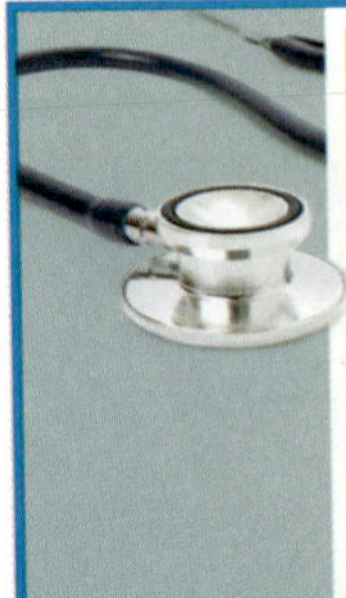

Field Smarts

When working in an office that operates more than one ECG unit, make certain that your electrodes correspond with the unit you are using. Using electrodes that are manufactured for a different unit can cause a poor tracing. Also, it is important to make certain that the alligator clips, located at the distal tips of the lead wires, are free of lint and other particles that could interfere with the tracing.

Standard Limb Leads

Leads I, II, and III are known as the "standard limb leads" and are often referred to as **bipolar leads** because they record the electrical activity from two limb electrodes at the same time.

These leads measure the electrical activity of the heart between a negative (–) pole and a positive (+) pole. Lead I records the difference in voltage between the RA (– pole) and LA (+ pole); lead II records the difference in voltage between the RA (– pole) and LL (+ pole); and lead III records the difference in voltage between the LA (– pole) and LL (+ pole). *Note*: The RL wire is used as a reference point or ground wire and is not part of the recording even though an electrode is placed on the right leg.

Augmented Leads

The next three limb leads—aVR, aVL, and aVF—are known as the **augmented leads** and referred to as unipolar because only a single positive electrode is referenced against a "null point" (a point with little or no significant electronic variation) between the remaining limb electrodes. The aV stands for *augmented voltage* and is referred to as augmented because the electrical impulses from these three leads are very small and the ECG machine must augment or increase their size to make them readable. The last letter in each of the augmented leads is an abbreviation that relates to the positive pole or electrode used in each lead. Lead aVR (right arm) records the difference in voltage between the RA (the + pole) and a midpoint between the LA and LL (the negative reference point). Lead aVL (left arm) records the difference in voltage between the left arm (+ pole) and a midpoint between the RA and LL (negative reference point). Lead aVF (foot or left leg in this case) records the difference in voltage between the left leg (+ pole) and a midpoint between RA and LA (negative reference point).

Figure 14-16 illustrates the pathways of impulses for the bipolar leads and augmented leads.

Chest or Precordial Leads

The chest or **precordial leads** are the last six leads of the standard 12-lead ECG and do not require any amplification because of how close they are to the heart. These leads are also unipolar and are designated as leads V1 through V6. Correct placement of the chest electrodes is crucial to obtaining an accurate reading. The precordial leads record the electrical activity from a null or midpoint within the heart to one of the six landmarks on the chest wall where an electrode is placed. Anatomical placement of chest electrodes is as follows:

- V1: Fourth intercostal space at the right margin of the sternum
- V2: Fourth intercostal space at the left margin of the sternum
- V3: Midway between V2 and V4 on the 5th rib
- V4: Fifth intercostal space at the midclavicular line
- V5: Same horizontal level as V4 at the left anterior axillary line
- V6: Same horizontal level as V4 and V5 at the left midaxillary line

Figure 14-17 illustrates the correct positioning of the chest electrodes.

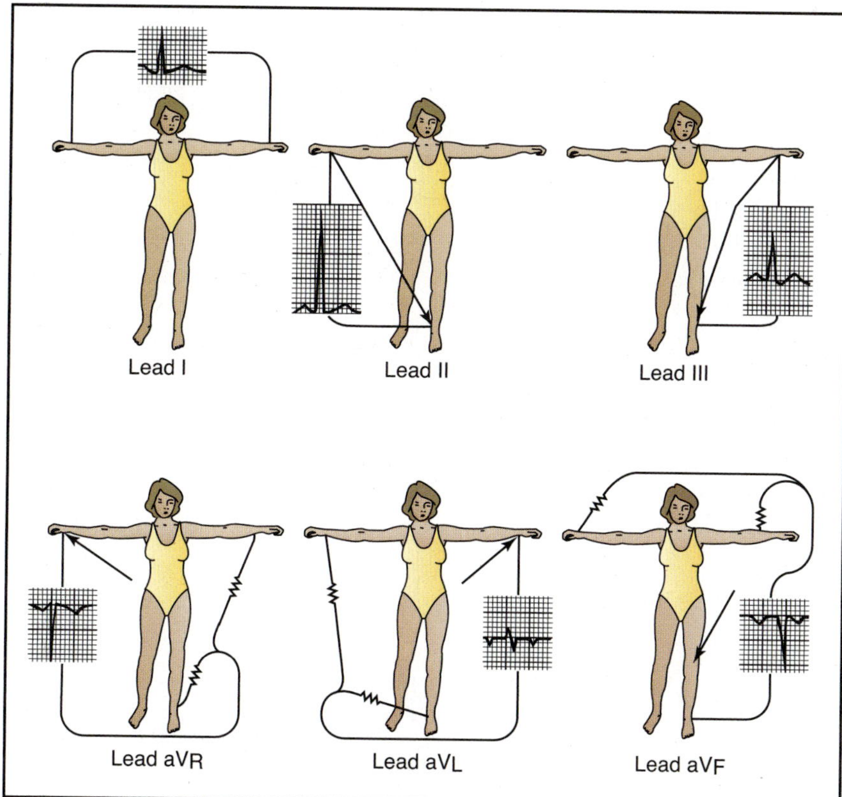

Figure 14-16 ■ Lead placement and the pathways of impulses for bipolar and augmented leads. The arrows are pointing to the positive electrodes or poles.

Figure 14-17 ■ The proper position of the chest electrodes on a 12-lead ECG.

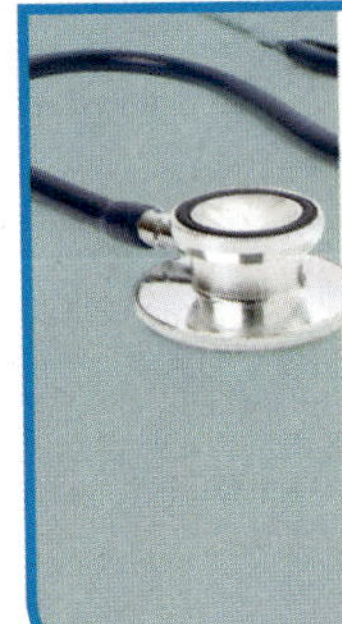

Field Smarts

Placing V1 and V2 one intercostal space too high may make it appear that the patient had a previous myocardial infarction. Proper placement of electrodes is essential for an accurate reading.

Lead Marking Codes

All leads must be marked for identification and mounting purposes. The majority of today's models will automatically mark each lead and will print the actual name of the lead at the top of the ECG tracing toward the beginning of each lead. The first three limb leads are identified with roman numerals, the augmented leads begin with a lower case a, and the chest leads all begin with the letter V or C. Refer to Table 14-7 for lead markings typically seen on a standard ECG.

Rhythm Strip

In a **rhythm strip**, which is a separate 12-inch recording of a particular lead, lead II generally appears at the bottom of a standard 12-lead ECG. A rhythm strip assists the provider in detecting abnormalities in the patient's heart rhythm that may not be detectable in the standard leads due to the shorter representations of each lead. Refer to Figure 14-10B for an example of a rhythm strip.

Table 14-7 Typical Markings on a Standard Electrocardiogram

Lead I	aVR	V1 or C1	V4 or C4
Lead II	aVL	V2 or C2	V5 or C5
Lead III	aVF	V3 or C3	V6 or C6

Do you notice how Lead II runs the entire width of the paper at the bottom of the ECG?

Standardizing the ECG

To ensure that the ECG machine is working properly, a **standardization** mark is made at the beginning of each lead, or group of leads when using a multichannel unit. This function is assurance that the electrocardiograph is measuring the impulses properly. According to universal standard, 1 millivolt (mV) of cardiac activity will deflect the stylus 10 mm high, which is ten small or two large vertical squares on the ECG paper.

The sensitivity control, also referred to as "gain" on many units, controls the size of the standard and amplitude of the heart beat and is normally set on the number "10" or "1" depending on the particular unit. At the beginning of the ECG, the automatic electrocardiograph will place 1 mV of electricity into the unit, triggering the stylus to move 10 mm high. This process mimics normal heart activity. If the standardization extends above or below 10 mm while on this setting, the medical assistant should seek technical assistance. The amplitude of the waves may be adjusted for abnormally large or abnormally small beats by changing the sensitivity or gain setting. Figure 14-18 shows examples

(A)

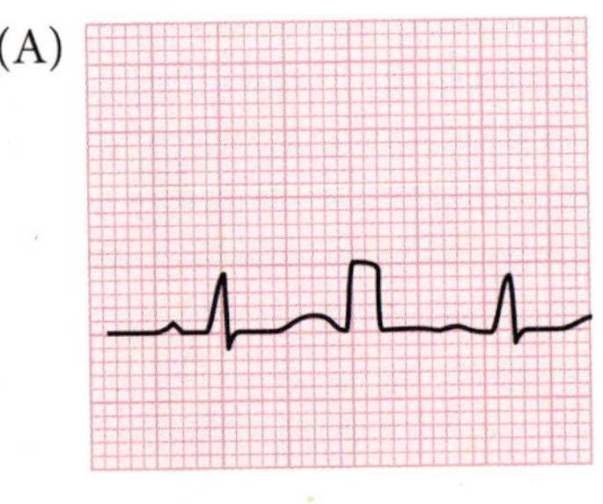

(B)

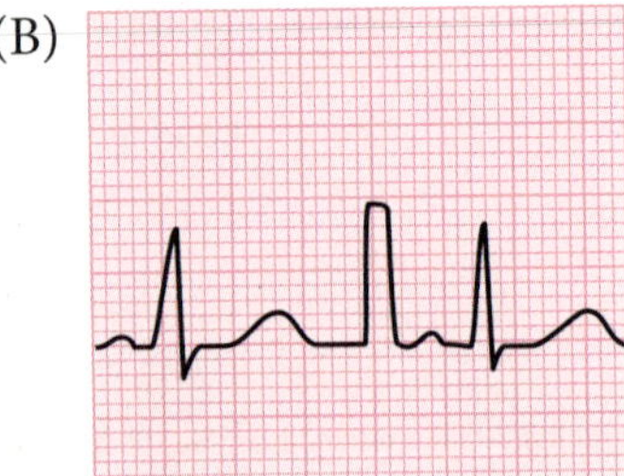

(C)

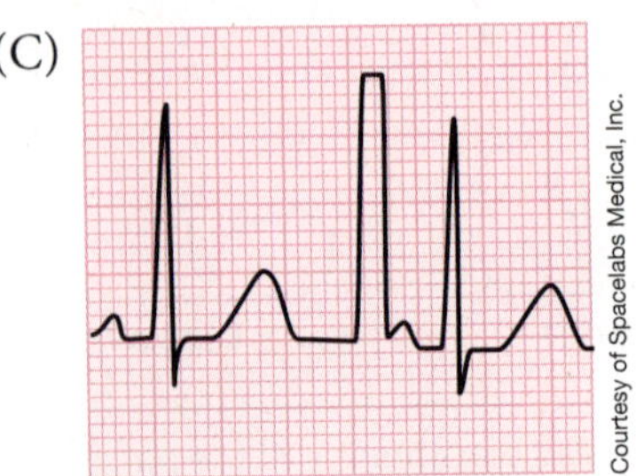

Courtesy of Spacelabs Medical, Inc.

Figure 14-18 Example of standardizations at different settings: (a) 5 mm high; (b) 10 mm high (normal); and (c) 20 mm high.

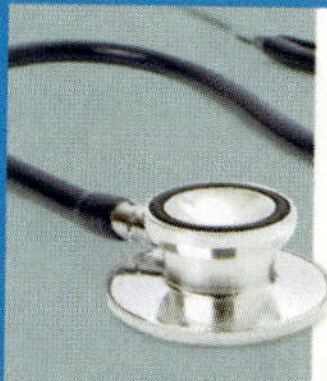

Field Smarts

When performing an ECG, if the patient's R waves are large and deflecting outside of the graphing lines on the ECG paper, you may need to either manually lower the baseline, or decrease the sensitivity control or gain to "5" or "½." This will cause the stylus to move half as high (5 mm). If waves are too small and difficult to read, you may need to increase the sensitivity to "20" or "2," which will double the size of the impulse; the stylus will deflect 20 mm high. Always perform a standardization when changes are made to the sensitivity so that the practitioner is aware of the change. Record a standardization when you return the sensitivity back to its original setting.

of the standardization mark when the sensitivity is set at 5, 10, and 20 mm. Refer back to Figure 14-12b to see what the gain setting looks like on an ECG unit.

Performing the Resting 12-Lead ECG

When performing a standard resting 12-lead ECG, no matter what type of ECG unit is used, the placement of electrodes, instructions for patient preparation, lead wire connections, and troubleshooting to correct artifacts are basically the same. Although the steps are similar, each machine may vary slightly so it is important for the medical assistant to become familiar with the particular unit that is used within the practice. If the practice uses two units, the medical assistant should become familiar with both. Procedure 14-1 lists the steps for performing an ECG using a multichannel unit.

Artifacts

In order for a provider to accurately interpret an ECG tracing, it must be performed correctly and be free of **artifacts** or unwanted interference. If an artifact appears, the medical assistant should know how to locate the source and correct it. The most common types of artifacts are listed in Table 14-8.

Table 14-8 Common Artifacts That Appear on an ECG Tracing

Type of Artifact	Potential Causes	Correction Techniques	Picture of Artifact
Somatic tremor	Muscle Tremors: *Voluntary:* Occur when the patient moves, talks, coughs, etc. *Involuntary:* Occur as a result of a physical condition, such as Parkinson's disease.	Fully explain the procedure to the patient and make the patient as comfortable as possible. Place a pillow under the patient's head, and make sure the room is warm enough. Check to see if there is a filter on the unit for somatic or muscle interference; if there is, make the appropriate adjustments. Have patient place hands under the buttocks to help control involuntary shaking.	
Wandering baseline	The electrode wire is not securely attached to the electrode. The alligator clip that is attached to the electrode is not correctly positioned. The patient may be wearing body creams, lotions, or oils.	Clips and lead wires should be firmly attached to the electrodes. The patient cable should not dangle or pull on the electrode. Follow manufacturer's instructions for proper placement of the clip. Clean the area with alcohol where the electrode will be placed to remove any skin products.	
Interrupted baseline	A broken patient cable wire. The lead wire becomes detached from the electrode.	Replace the wire. Be sure the wire is securely attached to the electrode.	
AC interference	Most of today's units have internal filters that filter out AC	Check to make certain that the filter for AC is depressed or activated.	

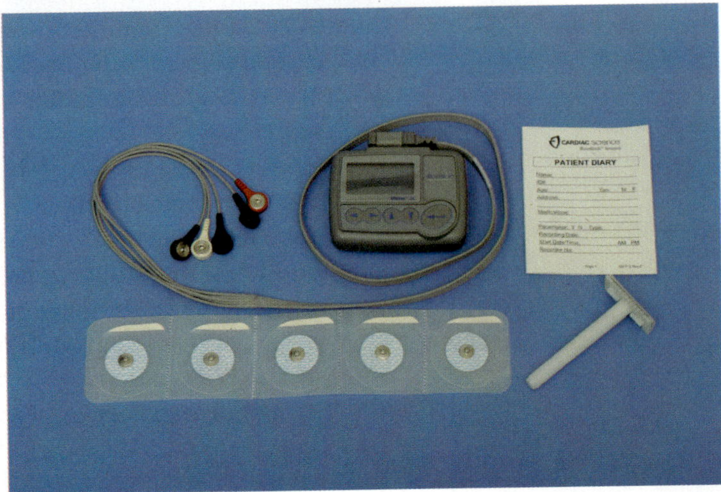

Figure 14-19 ■ Picture of a Welch Allyn HR-100 Holter Recorder with patient cable.

Holter Monitor

The **Holter monitor** (Figure 14-19) is a portable ambulatory heart monitoring device that continuously looks at a patient's heart over a prolonged period of time (usually 24 hours but may be longer in some instances). Monitoring is useful for patients who experience sporadic cardiac symptoms, such as fatigue, chest pain, dizziness, and fainting or syncope. The patient depresses an event button when irregular symptoms occur and records those symptoms in a special diary. The cardiologist then compares the symptoms with the tracing made at the time of the event. This assists in the diagnosis of sporadic arrhythmias that may not show up during routine ECG testing.

The Holter monitor is a battery-operated recorder that uses a digital memory card to record the tracing. It may be placed in a pouch and worn around the patient's waist with a belted fastener or strapped in place over the patient's shoulder. Newer smaller models are placed in a small pouch and fastened around the patient's chest, making it much easier for the patient to move around. A total of four or five electrodes (depending on the unit) are placed on the patient's chest at different locations (Figure 14-20); these locations are different from the locations for chest electrodes on a standard 12-lead ECG. The electrodes are usually made of foam, contain electrolyte, have an adhesive backing, and a snap on the front where the wires attach to the electrodes. The medical assistant's duties include preparing the patient, explaining the procedure, attaching and removing the monitor, and stressing to the patient the importance of keeping an accurate and complete activities diary. The patient should be advised to maintain usual daily activities, with the exception of swimming, showering, or taking a bath while wearing the monitor.

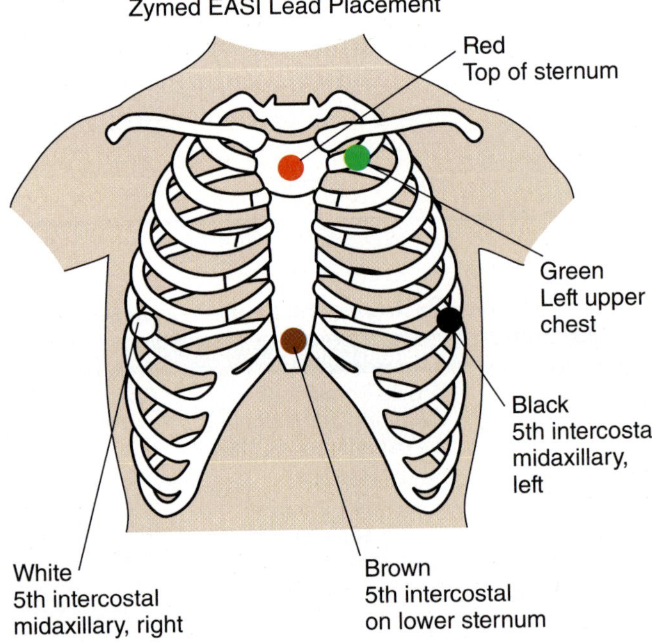

Figure 14-20 ■ Electrodes must be properly placed according to the manufacturer's directions to ensure an accurate tracing.

Skin lotions and oils as well as chest hair will need to be removed prior to application of the leads. The chest is normally abraded with gauze squares or a special prep kit to ensure that sites are free of all dirt and oils. The chest should be thoroughly dried before application. Once the electrodes are properly applied, they are connected to the monitor by lead wires. All lead wires must be securely attached to the electrodes to prevent an interruption in the tracing. Once the patient is connected, the monitor must be checked to ensure that it is working properly. One end of the test cable is attached to the monitor and the other end is connected directly to the ECG machine. A short baseline reading

Health Coach

Holter Monitor Patient Pointers

It is important that the patient be given guidelines to follow to ensure an accurate recording. During the 24-hour monitoring period, a complete and accurate activity diary must be maintained. All activities and changes in emotional state should be noted in the diary along with the time of their occurrence. Figure 14-21 is one example of a diary page used along with the Holter monitor.

If the patient experiences any symptoms such as shortness of breath, chest pain, dizziness, or palpitations during the monitoring period, this should be recorded in the diary along with the time of the occurrence. Some monitors are equipped with an event button or marker that can be used when the patient experiences unusual symptoms. When the patient depresses the button, the monitor automatically places a mark on the recording that alerts the person interpreting the tape to look for an abnormality.

Once the 24-hour monitoring period has ended, the patient is instructed to return to have the monitor removed. The recording is then evaluated by a special Holter scanning device or by computer. The analysis is usually performed in a hospital ECG department. The provider usually receives a written report within 24 hours. The report will include sample printouts of any abnormalities. Refer to Procedure 14-2 for instructions on Holter monitor placement.

Basic Instructions Given to Holter Monitor Patients

- Keep the monitor dry at all times (no bathing, showering, or swimming).
- Avoid activities that cause excessive perspiration.
- Avoid using electrical appliances such as an electric shaver, electric toothbrush, or hair dryer. Using these items may cause electrical interference.
- Avoid magnets, metal detectors, and areas with high voltage. Do not sleep under an electric blanket during the monitoring period.
- Immediately depress the event marker when related symptoms are present.
- Avoid touching or moving any of the electrodes.
- Do not handle or remove the monitor from its pouch, unless instructed to do so at the end of the monitoring period.
- List all activities such as going up and down the stairs, exercise, smoking, bowel movements, sexual activity, meals (what you consumed, including beverages), medications consumed, and sleep patterns that occur during the monitoring period.
- List any extreme emotional states such as anger, stress, etc.

Geriatric patients may need help from caregivers or family members when documenting their activities.

is recorded to check for correct wave activity and the presence of artifacts. Any artifacts or problems with the unit should be remedied before the patient leaves.

Miscellaneous Cardiovascular Procedures

Various equipment and techniques are available to diagnose cardiac problems in addition to the ECG. Most are noninvasive, painless, and require little or no patient preparation. The majority of these procedures can be performed on an outpatient basis.

Treadmill Stress Test

Providers often order a treadmill stress test for patients who have possible cardiac symptoms but do not show any abnormalities on the standard ECG as well as for patients who are just starting a rigorous workout program who may be at risk for complications. During exercise on a treadmill, a heavier workload is placed on the heart, stimulating abnormalities to appear that wouldn't have appeared without the extra load on the heart. The **treadmill stress test** is a noninvasive procedure during which the patient walks on a treadmill while connected to an ECG machine. Chest electrodes connected to an ECG machine are placed on the patient prior to the procedure and the speed of the treadmill is gradually increased until the patient can no longer tolerate the exercise. In rare instances, myocardial infarction and serious arrhythmias may occur during testing. For that reason, the patient is closely monitored by a physician during the procedure. The medical assistant usually takes blood pressure readings before,

HOLTER MONITOR DIARY

During the Holter monitoring period it is important to keep a diary of activities that you perform as well as symptoms you experience. This diary will assist the physician in comparing changes that occur on the ECG with the activity you were performing when the changes occurred.

The following is information that should be listed on the diary record:

- **Date:** Because the monitoring period can be anywhere from 24 to 72 hours, it will be important to list the date your symptoms occur.
- **Time:** Record the time for all activities you perform or symptoms you experience. This will assist the physician in matching this information up with changes that occur in the tracing.
- **Activities or Events:** Record any strenuous activity or activities that can cause changes in your metabolic rate including: walking, exercise, bowel movements, eating, sexual activity, etc.
- **Symptoms:** Record any unusual symptoms that you experience during the testing period such as: shortness of breath, racing heart, dizziness, chest pain, etc. List the activities you were performing when the symptoms began. *(Remember to click on the event button on your monitor when symptoms occur.)*

DATE	TIME	ACTIVITY	SYMPTOMS

Figure 14-21 ■ An example of a patient diary page for Holter monitoring.

during, and following the procedure. If the patient experiences any unusual symptoms, such as chest pain, shortness of breath, or extreme fatigue, the physician will terminate the test. Figure 14-22 shows an example of a patient being analyzed during a treadmill stress test.

Dobutamine Stress Test

The provider may order the **dobutamine stress test** for patients who are unable to exercise on a treadmill due to physical limitations or age. The drug dobutamine is injected intravenously into the patient, causing the heart rate to increase and simulating exercise. The ECG is recorded and blood pressure readings are monitored in the same manner as the treadmill stress test.

Echocardiography

Echocardiography is defined as a noninvasive diagnostic test that uses ultrasound to visualize internal cardiac structures. This method allows for visualization of all heart valves and assessment of heart chamber size.

The patient is placed in a supine position and electrodes from a standard 12-lead ECG are placed on the patient's extremities. Chest electrodes are not used during the procedure. A transducer is placed against the

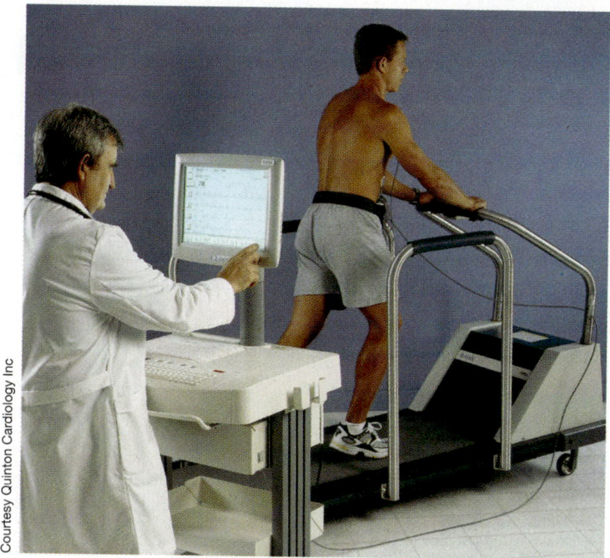

Courtesy Quinton Cardiology Inc

Figure 14-22 ■ A cardiac stress test.

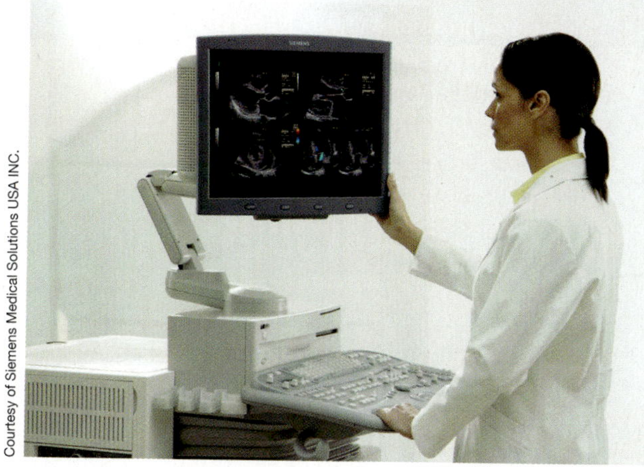

Courtesy of Siemens Medical Solutions USA INC.

Figure 14-23 An example of an echocardiograph machine.

patient's skin and moved over different areas of the chest wall. Sound waves that bounce off the structures of the heart cause echoes to be sent back to the transducer. The echoes are then converted by the ultrasound machine into images that can be examined by a computer and transformed into photographs and films of the heart and its related structures. Figure 14-23 shows an example of an echocardiograph machine.

Cardiac Catheterization

Cardiac catheterization is a specialized procedure that allows for visualization of the coronary arteries. This diagnostic procedure allows the provider to determine if there are any blockages present and the amount of occlusion in each artery. Symptoms may or may not be present with coronary occlusion and many patients deny symptoms even when an artery is almost completely occluded.

During cardiac catheterization, a tiny plastic tube or catheter is threaded through a major vessel, usually the femoral artery, and passed into the heart. Once the catheter is in place, a contrast medium is injected into the heart, which produces a clear image of the coronary arteries, allowing the provider to determine the presence of any blockages. Blood pressure and cardiac output may also be measured during the procedure. If a blockage is detected, a procedure known as angioplasty or "balloon" surgery can be performed at the same time. A device known as a stent can also be placed inside the artery to hold it open and permit blood to flow freely.

Noninvasive Heart Scan

A new **noninvasive heart scan** is available to evaluate and measure plaque in the coronary arteries by determining the amount of calcium present. The amount of calcium in a coronary artery can indicate the amount of plaque buildup. The heart scan can detect calcium deposits before the patient develops cardiac symptoms (chest pain or shortness of breath). If plaque buildup is detected early, treatment can be initiated before the plaque completely occludes the coronary artery or breaks loose, causing a heart attack.

The noninvasive heart scan is open, painless, and fast. No needles or contrast media are used and the patient does not even have to get undressed. The scan is 95% to 99% accurate and gives the provider an individualized report for each patient with suggestions for clinical follow-up.

COMMON CARDIOVASCULAR TREATMENTS AND MEDICATIONS

There are a variety of treatments in the form of procedures and medications that treat cardiovascular conditions. Some cardiovascular treatments were already featured in the Health Coach Disease Feature earlier in the chapter. Others can be found in Table 14-9.

There are also several medications used in the treatment of cardiovascular disorders. Table 14-10 features some of the most common cardiovascular medications.

COMMON LAB TESTS THAT COINCIDE WITH CARDIOVASCULAR DISORDERS

Several lab tests can be performed to evaluate specific cardiovascular disorders. Table 14-11 features some of the common lab tests that coincide with cardiovascular disease.

Table 14-9 Common Cardiovascular Treatments

Procedure	Description
Arthrectomy	A procedure to remove fat from the coronary arteries by cutting or burning it out with a laser.
Coronary artery bypass graft (CABG)	This procedure is performed in patients with severe blockages. An artery or vein from another part of the body is connected or graphed to the blocked artery/arteries so that blood can flow around it. This is the most common open heart procedure performed today.
Cardiac ablation	A procedure that destroys electrical tissue in the heart that causes an abnormal rhythm. Often performed through a catheter, but sometimes is performed during open heart procedures.
Cardiac pacemaker	A small device placed in the chest or abdomen to help control arrhythmias. Small electrical pulses are used to stimulate the heart to beat at a normal rate.
Cardioversion	A procedure or medication that reverses a cardiac arrhythmia. A small electrical shock may be used to shock the heart back into a normal rhythm. An antiarrhythmic may also be used to reverse an arrhythmia.
Percutaneous transluminal coronary angiography (PTCA)	A minimally invasive procedure to open coronary arteries that are occluded. A very thick, sturdy catheter with a balloon is guided through the coronary arteries. Once the blockage is found the balloon is inflated and the artery widens. The balloon is removed; however, the plaque is now flattened against the arterial walls allowing blood to flow more freely.

Table 14-10 Common Cardiovascular Medications

Medication Classifications	Description	Medication Examples (Trade Names)
Antianginals	Drugs used to treat angina, usually referred to as vasodilators. These drugs are used to open up blocked coronary blood vessels.	Nitro-Bid, Nitrostat, and Nitrogard (all of which are nitroglycerins), Ranexa, Isordil, and Imdur
Antiarrhythmics	Drugs used in patients with arrhythmias to help the heart attain a normal rhythm.	Tambocor, Procanbid, Cardarone, Betapace, Toprol, and Calan
Anticoagulants	Drugs used to prevent the blood from clotting. Often used in patients who have had previous heart attacks, strokes, or blood clots.	In Hospital: Heparin and Lovenox Home Therapy: Coumadin, Pradaxa, Eliquis, and Xarelto
Antihypertensives	Drugs used to treat hypertension or high blood pressure. Refer Health Coach Feature 15-1 for different classifications of antihypertensives.	Lopressor or Toprol, Corgard, Procardia, Calan, Altace, and Vasotec.
Antiplatelet	Drug (platelet aggregation inhibitor) used to decrease the risk of stroke or heart attack by helping to prevent clot formation. May be used in conjunction with aspirin therapy.	Aspirin, Plavix, Aggrenox, and Ticlid
Cardiotonics	Drugs that strengthen the heart in patients with heart failure. Categories include: Ace inhibitors and Angiotensin II receptor blockers; Beta blockers and vasodilators.	Digoxin, Toprol, Levophed, Amrinone, Dobutamine, Capoten, Altace, and Cozaar
Cholesterol-lowering drugs	These are drugs that lower cholesterol levels in the blood. The most common of these are the statins, however, other drugs in this category include: niacin, bile-acid resins, fibric acid derivatives, and cholesterol-absorption inhibitors. We will just feature the statins here as they are the most efficient and reduce mortality and risk.	Examples of statins: Lipitor (atorvastatin), Lescol (fluvastatin), Mevacor (lovastatin), Zocor (simvastatin), and Crestor (rosuvastatin)
Diuretics	Drugs used to remove excessive fluid from the body. Often used to treat hypertension and in the treatment of congestive heart failure. Common types include: thiazides, loop diuretics, and potassium-sparing agents.	Diuril, Microzide, Thalitone, Bumex, Lasix, and Midamor.
Vasodilators (see antianginals)		

Table 14-11 Common Lab Tests That Coincide with Cardiovascular Disorders

Test	Clinical Significance
Brain natriuretic peptide (BNP)	BNP is a hormone made by the heart and tends to increase in patients with heart failure. BNP levels increase as heart failure worsens and decreases as heart failure lessens. This level is sometimes tested to check the effectiveness of drug therapy.
Cardiac enzymes (troponin, myoglobin, creatine kinase CK-MB, and lactate dehydrogenase (LDH))	Measures enzymes and proteins associated with heart muscle injury. Often ordered in the ER to diagnose a heart attack. Used to check for injury following bypass surgery and determine if cardiac interventional procedures are successful.
Basic metabolic panel (BMP)	Gives the provider information about acid/base balance, glucose level, electrolyte balance (very important in heart function), and kidney health.
Lipid panel/liver panel	A lipid panel is a blood test, which detects cholesterol levels in the blood including total cholesterol, HDL, LDL, triglycerides, and VLDL. For more specifics on this test, refer to the Featured Disease Spotlight found earlier in the chapter. A liver panel is often performed on patients taking statins. Statins can cause changes in liver function.
Prothrombin time (PT)/international normalized ratio (INR)	Used to test the effectiveness of the anticoagulant warfarin (Coumadin). Normal therapeutic INR level usually runs between 2.0 and 3.0. Patients running below this range are at higher risk of developing a clot. Patients running above this value are at a higher risk of bleeding internally.

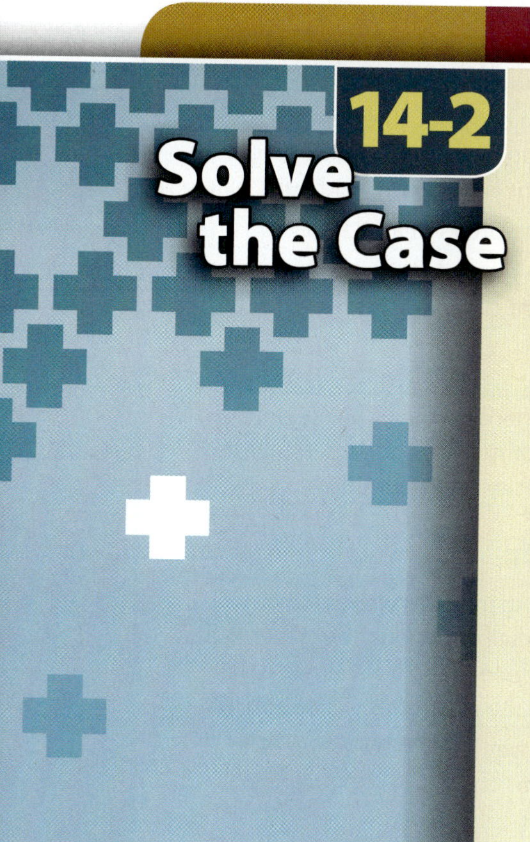

Review the following notes from Mr. Duncan's visit with Dr. Dorado:

Patient Symptoms: Patient complains of intermittent shortness of breath and swelling in feet and legs. Patient doesn't feel peritoneal dialysis is effective. ***Current Medications*** include: Levothyroxine sodium oral tabs (100 mcg), Sensipar oral tabs (30 mg), Toprol oral tabs (25 mg), Lasix (40 mg), Crestor oral tabs (10 mg), and NovoLOG Mix 70/30 (after meals). Today's ***Vital Signs*** include a BP of 186/96, a pulse rate of 94, and respiration of 20. ***Patient's height*** is 6′ 2″ and ***weight*** is 245 pounds. ***Assessment Information***: Dr. Dorado tells Mr. Duncan that he has major blockages in three coronary arteries and will need to have open heart surgery to repair the arteries. The doctor doesn't make any promises that Mr. Duncan can still be considered for transplant but does state that another assessment can be performed six months following surgery. He also tells Mr. Duncan that he believes he is in the beginning stages of heart failure but is hopeful this will improve following surgery. **Provider's Plan** includes the following: Set patient up for a surgery consult with Dr. Thomas Ruppert, provide educational materials on the CABG procedure, provide patient with a new Rx for Toprol 50 mg per day, and add an Rx for Lasix 40 mg.

1. **Based on the patient's symptoms and the doctor's diagnoses, what may be causing the patient's shortness of breath and swelling in the legs?**
2. **Which of Mr. Duncan's medications helps to control his hypertension and why do you believe the doctor doubled this medication?**
3. **What is Lasix and why do you believe the doctor added this medication to the patient's drug list?**
4. **Go to the Internet and look up educational materials for the newly prescribed medications the patient is to take as well as the surgical procedure the patient is to have. Role-play with a classmate discharging the patient and going over educational materials.**

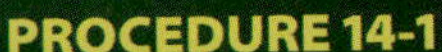

PROCEDURE 14-1

Perform a Standard 12-Lead Electrocardiogram with a Multichannel Unit

Objective:

To record an accurate tracing of the electrical activity of the patient's heart, free from artifacts and interference.

Equipment/Supplies:

- Table with pillow and drape
- Patient gown/Cape
- Alcohol
- Cotton balls/Gauze Pads
- Tissues
- Razor
- Machine with patient cable
- Disposable electrodes
- ECG tracing paper if applicable
- Mounting form (if applicable)
- Patient's chart/EHR

Note: *ECG machines vary from one manufacturer to another. Follow the specific instructions for the unit you currently use.*

PROCEDURAL STEPS	DETAILS AND/OR RATIONALE
1. Perform the ECG in a quiet, warm, and comfortable room away from other electrical equipment.	Electrical equipment can cause AC interference, resulting in a poor tracing. The patient will be more comfortable if the patient is in a warm and quiet place.
2. Wash your hands and assemble all equipment.	Clean hands prevent the spread of infection.
3. Identify the patient using at least two identifiers, identify yourself, and ***explain the rationale for the performance of the procedure*** and why it is important not to move or talk during the tracing.	An informed patient is a relaxed patient. Any movement by the patient can cause interference on the tracing.
4. ***Show awareness of a patient's concerns related to the procedure being performed.***	Patients may feel apprehensive about having an ECG due to misinformation or may be concerned that the wires are putting electricity into their body.
5. ***Intervene on behalf of the patient regarding issues/concerns that may arise.***	
6. Instruct the patient to remove all clothing from the waist up and to expose the lower legs. Provide drape and cape and instruct patient to put the cape on so it opens in the front.	Capes should be offered to males as well as females because some males are self-conscious about their breast tissue. Having the cape open to the front allows easier access to the skin where the electrodes will be applied.
7. Prep the patient's skin by scrubbing the areas where the electrodes are to be placed with alcohol and drying with a 4 × 4 gauze pad until the skin turn slightly pink. (Dry shave areas on men that are particularly hairy.)	The patient's skin must be clean, dry, and free from lotions and powders for good conductivity between the skin and the electrode. Excessive hair may also interfere with recordings.
8. Place the limb electrodes on the fleshy part of the upper arm and the inner part of the calf midway between the knee and the ankle (Figure 14-24). (Electrode tabs on the arms should be facing downward, electrode tabs on the legs should be facing upward.)	Placing the electrodes over large muscles or bones may cause interference.

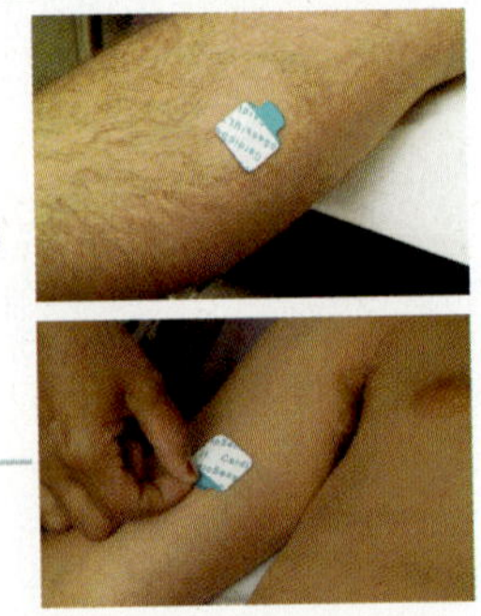

Figure 14-24 ■ Disposable electrodes should be attached to the fleshy parts of the arms and legs on the patient.

continues

PROCEDURE 14-1 continued

PROCEDURAL STEPS	DETAILS AND/OR RATIONALE
9. Place all six chest electrodes in the correct positions on the chest by counting down the correct intercostal spaces and locating the proper landmarks (Figure 14-25). Do not trust your eyes alone. (Electrode pad tabs should be facing downward for all chest electrodes.)	Correct lead placement is essential for an accurate tracing.
10. Securely connect all lead wires to the corresponding electrodes following the body's natural contour. Be sure that lead wires are pointed downward on the legs and upward on the arms and chest. (Confirm that leads are not pulling upward once the wires are connected. If they are, make the proper adjustments.) The patient cable should lie over the patient's abdomen.	Placing the leads onto the chest following the body's natural contour will help to prevent the wires from becoming tangled. If the leads are pulling upward from the skin, you will not get an accurate tracing.
11. Connect the patient cable to the machine and turn machine to the "ON" position. Enter the patient's data into the unit by using the keypad. Requested information may include the patient's name, age, gender, height, weight, and any cardiac medications currently being taken.	Depending on the type of machine used, allow sufficient time for the machine to warm up. Different factors can affect the reading so knowing this information will assist the provider in determining why abnormalities may be present.
12. Press the auto run button on the machine and allow the tracing to be recorded. Observe the standardization mark for accuracy.	The standardization mark should measure 10 mm high if the settings are correct and the unit is working properly.
13. Observe the tracing for problems or artifacts. ***Incorporate critical thinking skills*** when a problem is identified. Determine if any changes are needed with regard to the amplitude of the beats (gain or sensitivity control) or the heart's rhythm (paper speed).	Artifacts or other problems must be corrected to ensure a clear tracing that can be adequately measured.
14. Allow the provider to briefly scan the tracing before disconnecting the patient from the machine.	This eliminates the need to reconnect the patient should the provider request a longer tracing or a repeat of a specific lead.
15. Disconnect the lead wires and remove the electrodes from the patient.	Disconnecting the lead wires before removing the tabs can prevent damage to the equipment.
16. Clean the equipment following manufacturer's guidelines. Replace tracing paper as needed.	Be courteous to your coworkers. Never leave a machine unclean or without sufficient paper for the next tracing.
17. Wash your hands and document the procedure.	Hands must be washed before and after each procedure to prevent the spread of organisms from one patient to the next.
18. Place the tracing in the patient's chart or upload into the patient's EHR.	

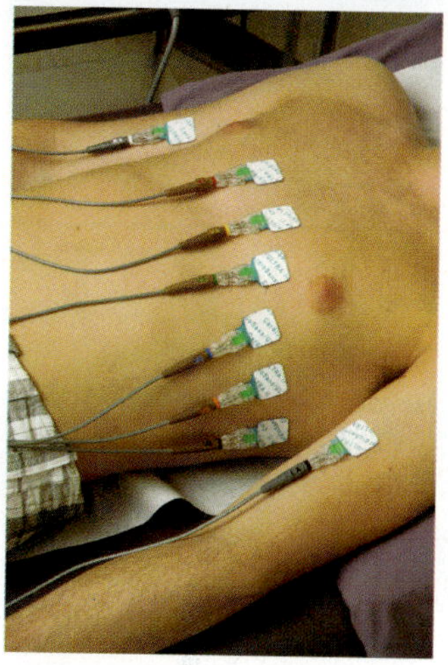

Figure 14-25 ■ Proper chest electrode placement.

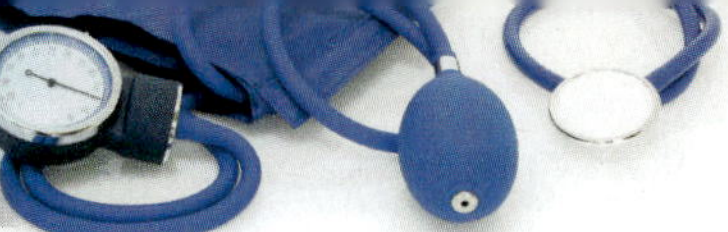

DOCUMENTATION EXAMPLE:

Zotto, Adam	Last Appt: 4/27/2015 - Established Patient Sick, Amir Raman, NVFA	Next Appt: 6/1/2015 - Established Patient Sick, Amir Raman, NVFA	
DOB (Age): 01/02/48 (67) Sex: M		Vitals: 7 Medications: 3 Allergies: 0 Diagnosis: 3	
Order # [Generates upon completion]		Status: Open	Mark Order Inactive
Order Type	Lab / Diag. Imaging / (●) Procedure	Due Date	- Select - 06/01/2015
Ordering Physician	Raman, Amir	Coll. Date & Time	06/01/2015 01 : 00 : 00 PM
Facility	- Select -	Time of Day	- Select -
Copy Result To	Alfred P Peretti	Frequency	(●) Single Order / Repeat...
Diagnosis	Unspecified Essential Hypertension (4...	Patient Notes	12 Lead EKG. Patient tolerated well.. Results sent to Dr. Amir's task box.
ABN given to Pt	Yes / (●) No		172 characters remaining.

PROCEDURE 14-2

Apply the Holter Monitor

Objective:

To correctly apply a Holter monitor and properly educate the patient on how to care for the monitor and electrodes, and instruct the patient on what events need to be written in the event journal or diary.

Equipment/Supplies:

- Alcohol swabs
- Razor
- Abrasive pads
- Compound benzoin tincture swabs
- Disposable electrodes
- Holter monitor/memory card
- Carrying case with belt clip or Lanyard
- New battery or batteries (usually one or two AA batteries)
- Carrying case
- Patient activity diary
- Patient's chart/EHR

Note: *Holter monitors will differ slightly depending on the specific unit. Check the manufacturer's instructions for the unit you currently use and for the proper placement of electrodes on the patient's chest.*

PROCEDURAL STEPS	DETAILS AND/OR RATIONALE
1. Wash your hands and assemble the equipment and read manufacturer's instructions. Check expiration date on electrodes. Make certain memory or flash card is in the recorder and place a new battery in the monitor following polarity diagram that came with your unit. Refer to Figure 14-20 for a sample diagram.	If electrodes have passed their expiration date, the electrolyte may be dried out, which may cause problems during the tracing. A new battery will ensure efficient power throughout the entire monitoring period.
2. Complete necessary forms and set up the patient diary by entering required information.	

continues

PROCEDURE 14-2 continued

PROCEDURAL STEPS	DETAILS AND/OR RATIONALE
3. Identify the patient using at least two identifiers, identify yourself, and ***explain the rationale for the performance of the procedure***. Instruct the patient to disrobe from the waist up and to put a gown on so it opens in the front.	Explaining the procedure will assist the patient in knowing what to expect throughout the application.
4. ***Show awareness of a patient's concerns related to the procedure being performed.***	Patients may feel apprehensive about having the procedure due to misinformation or may be concerned that the wires are putting electricity into their body.
5. If applicable, ***intervene on behalf of the patient regarding issues/concerns*** that arise when explaining the procedure.	The patient may be concerned what the results will reveal. Always keep the provider in the loop.
6. Prep the patient's skin: Dry shave hair, if necessary, and rub the area of skin where electrodes will be placed with an alcohol swab. Next, abrade the skin with dry gauze or prepackaged pads (Figure 14-26).	Clean, abraded skin provides better contact with the electrodes.
7. If applicable, spread a small amount of compound benzoin tincture over the area in which each electrode will be placed.	Using compound benzoin tincture will help the electrodes adhere better to the skin.
8. Remove the electrodes from the package and study the manufacturer's electrode placement diagram to see which electrode/wire will be placed on the chest first, second, third, and so on. Attach the lead wires to the electrodes in the order they will be applied to the chest.	Attaching the wires in the order the electrodes will be applied to the chest will help to prevent the wires from becoming tangled.
9. Peel the backing from the electrode and check to make certain the electrolyte is moist. Correctly place disposable electrodes on the proper landmarks of the chest one at a time until all electrodes have been placed on the chest	If the pads are dried out, it will result in a poor tracing.
10. Be sure the electrodes adhere firmly to the skin by applying gentle pressure around the outer border of each electrode. (Avoid pressing on the center of the electrode pad as this may cause the electrolyte gel or solution to seep from the pad.)	Good contact with the skin provides an accurate tracing.

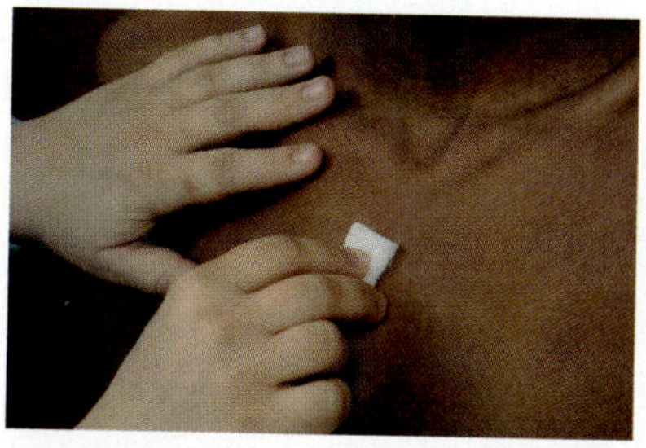

Figure 14-26 ■ The MA is prepping the patient's skin with a gauze pad after cleaning with alcohol.

continues

PROCEDURE 14-2 continued

PROCEDURAL STEPS	DETAILS AND/OR RATIONALE
11. Make a stress loop (Figure 14-27) for each electrode and wire and reinforce the electrodes to the skin with a piece of nonallergenic tape if necessary (Figure 14-28).	Reinforcing the electrodes with tape helps the electrodes stay on more securely.
12. Connect the patient cable to the patient input connector on the monitor and turn on the unit following manufacturer's instructions.	
13. Review the waveform on the LCD advancing through each channel to verify proper connection. (Follow manufacturer's instructions for this process.) ***Incorporate critical thinking skills*** when a problem is identified.	Verifying the waveform on each channel will confirm that the Holter is working properly.
14. Make certain that the date and time are set correctly; if not, make necessary adjustments.	If the date and time are incorrect, it will not match the patient's diary entries.
15. Note the start time on the Holter explanation sheet and in the patient's diary. Show the patient the location of the event button and explain what should be recorded in the diary and how to care for the monitor. Refer to Health Coach (Holter Monitor Patient Pointers) for a full list of instructions that should be shared with each patient.	An accurate diary relates patient symptoms with cardiac activity. Proper care of the monitor is essential for the monitor to function properly.
16. Specify the exact time the patient should return to the office for removal of the monitor. (The latest models will automatically stop recording after the 24-hour period is completed.) The patient should be instructed how to remove the electrodes and secure the monitor for safe keeping.	The monitor should be removed shortly after completion of the study.
17. Insert recorder in the pouch and secure the pouch to the patient's body using the belt (Figure 14-29) or lanyard provided by the manufacturer.	
18. Dismiss the patient and wash your hands and document the procedure in the patient's chart.	

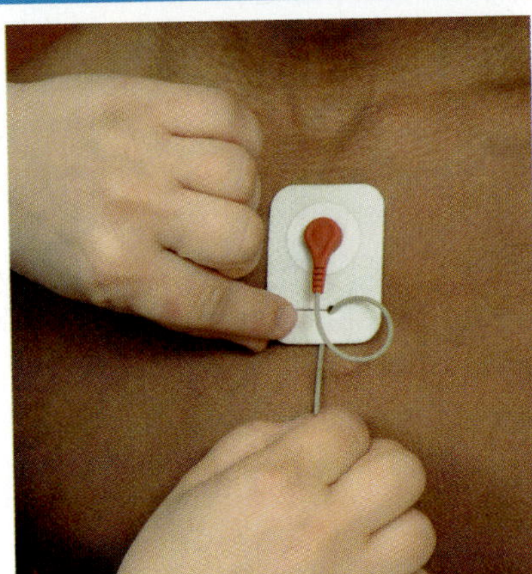

Figure 14-27 The medical assistant makes a stress loop to reduce pulling on the monitor as the patient moves.

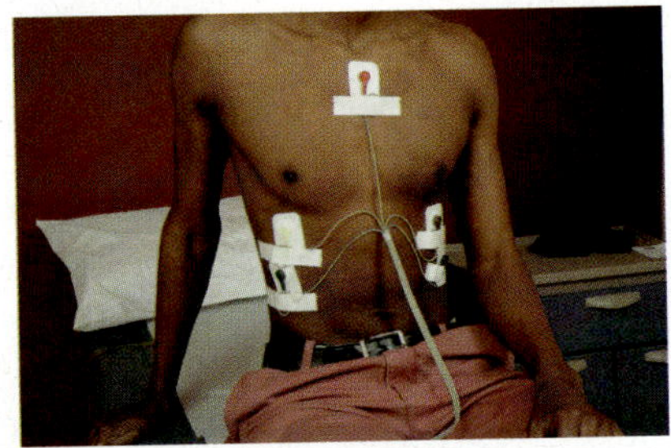

Figure 14-28 Placement of the electrodes on the chest for Holter Monitoring. Remember to follow the manufacturer's instructions because placement will vary from manufacturer to manufacturer.

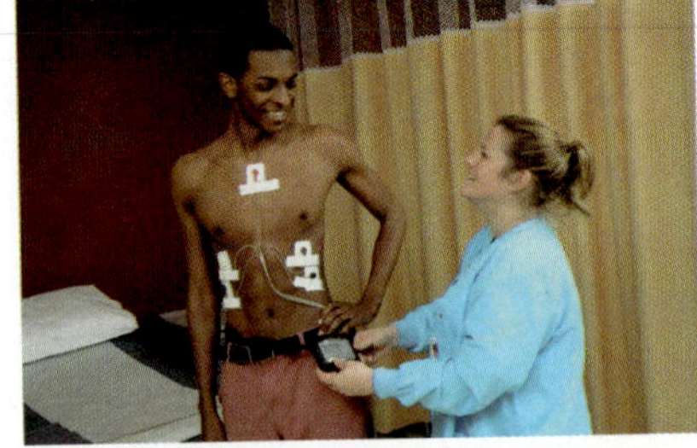

Figure 14-29 The Holter Monitor is secure in the pouch and strapped to the patient's waist.

DOCUMENTATION EXAMPLE:

09-03-XX 9.30 a.m.	Holter monitor application per Dr. Beavers. Positive waveforms on each channel. Instructed patient on proper management of unit and items to enter in activity diary. Pt. instructed to return at 9:30 a.m. on 09-04 for monitor removal. Lillian Kelly, CMA (AAMA) ------------

CHAPTER SUMMARY

- The cardiovascular system is composed of the heart and blood vessels and has four major functions: transporting nutrients and wastes around the body, protecting the body from infection and blood loss, maintaining thermoregulation, and fluid balance.
- The heart has four chambers: two upper chambers known as the left and right atria and two lower chambers known as the ventricles.
- The heart has three layers: the endocardium (contains the heart's electrical system), the myocardium (middle muscular layer, responsible for contractions), and the pericardium (outer layer of the heart and tissue that makes up the pericardial sac).
- There are three types of blood vessels in the body: arteries carry oxygenated blood away from the heart and to the body's tissues, veins carry blood low in oxygen and high in CO_2 toward the heart, and capillaries connect arteries to veins and are where the exchange of gases takes place.
- The coronary arteries supply the heart with its oxygen and the coronary veins take deoxygenated blood and wastes from the heart and return it to right atrium.
- Normal blood flow through the heart: S & I vena cava → right atrium → tricuspid valve → right ventricle → pulmonic valve → pulmonary artery → lungs → pulmonary veins → left atrium→ mitral valve → left ventricle → aortic valve → aorta → arteries throughout the body.
- The cardiac conduction system controls all cardiac function and flows in the following direction: SA node (the heart's pacemaker) → internodal pathways → AV node → AV junction → bundle of His → L and R bundle branches→ Purkinje fibers
- Depolarization is the discharge of electricity which causes myocardial contraction and repolarization is considered the resting phase of the cardiac cycle.
- Common cardiovascular diseases include cardiac arrhythmias (an irregularity of the heart's rhythm. Refer to Table 14-3 for common arrhythmias) and coronary artery disease. Other common cardiovascular conditions can be found in Table 14-4.
- Featured cardiovascular procedures include the electrocardiogram (a test that checks the heart's electrical activity and Holter monitor testing (a 24- to 72-hour recording device that checks electrical heart function for a specific amount of time).
- A cardiac cycle is the events that occur between the origin of one heart beat and the beginning of the next heart beat. An ECG is a graphic representation of the cardiac cycle.
- A waveform refers to a positive or negative deflection from the isoelectric line. A waveform represents the following: P wave (atrial depolarization), QRS complex (ventricular depolarization), T wave (ventricular repolarization), and U wave (seldom seen).
- ECG equipment and supplies include the electrocardiograph, electrodes or sensors, and ECG paper.
- Standard Limb Leads: Leads I, II, and III; often referenced as bipolar leads because they record the electrical activity from two limbs at the same time. Lead I (RA-LA), Lead II (RA-LL), and Lead III (LA-LL). Augmented Leads: aVR (LA and LL)-RA, aVL (RA and LL)-LA and aVF (LA and RA) -LL.
- A rhythm strip is a separate 12-inch recording of lead II to check for any arrhythmias.
- A standardization is a mark made at the beginning of each lead to make certain that the unit is functioning properly. Normal standardization is 10 mm high.
- An ECG artifact is unwanted interference that can occur on an ECG tracing. Types of artifacts include somatic tremors, wandering baseline, interrupted baseline, and AC interference. See Table 14-8 for specifics.
- Other cardiac testing includes the treadmill stress test, dobutamine stress test, echocardiography, cardiac catheterization, and a noninvasive heart scan.
- Cardiovascular treatments include cardiac ablation, cardiac pacemaker, cardioversion, and percutaneous transluminal coronary angiography. Specifics for these procedures can be found in Table 14-9.
- Common cardiovascular medications include antianginals, antiarrhythmics, anticoagulant, antihypertensives, antiplatelets, cardiotonics, cholesterol-lowering drugs, diuretics, and vasodilators. Refer to Table 14-10 for specifics.
- Common lab tests to detect cardiovascular disorders include brain natriuretic peptide (BNP), cardiac enzymes, basic metabolic panel, liver/lipid panels, and prothrombin time/INR. Refer to Table 14-11 for specifics.

CERTIFICATION REVIEW QUESTIONS

1. The upper chambers of the heart are known as the:
   a. atria.
   b. ventricles.
   c. aorta.
   d. vena cava.
2. The pacemaker is the:
   a. SA node.
   b. AV node.
   c. Bundle of His.
   d. Purkinje fibers.
3. As aging occurs the coronary arteries become:
   a. more elastic and pliable.
   b. shortened and less pliable.
   c. less elastic and dilated.
   d. more elastic and elongated.
4. Patients calling on the phone with chest pain should be instructed to:
   a. come in for an appointment.
   b. take an aspirin and call back if the pain does not resolve.
   c. have someone drive the patient to the hospital.
   d. have the patient or someone else in the home call the EMS.
5. Contributors to coronary heart disease include which of the following?
   a. Familial history
   b. High cholesterol
   c. Obesity
   d. All the above
6. A patient with left-sided heart failure may exhibit which of the following symptoms?
   a. Shortness of breath
   b. Swelling in legs
   c. Swelling in the feet
   d. Swelling in both the legs and feet
7. The P wave in a cardiac cycle represents:
   a. atrial depolarization.
   b. atrial repolarization.
   c. ventricular depolarization.
   d. ventricular depolarization.
8. The wire color for Lead V4 is:
   a. brown/yellow.
   b. brown/blue.
   c. brown/green.
   d. brown/purple.
9. Which of the following is responsible for helping to conduct electricity during an ECG?
   a. Electrode
   b. Electrode wire
   c. Electrolyte solution on the electrode
   d. Patient cable
10. If the waves on an ECG are so large they are deflecting off the graphing paper, you should do what?
    a. Increase the sensitivity to 20
    b. Increase the paper speed to 50 mm/sec
    c. Decrease the sensitivity to 5
    d. Decrease the paper speed to 10 mm/sec

STUDY RESOURCES

Resources to Test and Reinforce Your Knowledge:	
Certification Review Questions	Take this end-of-chapter quiz
Workbook	• Complete the activities for Chapter 14 • Perform the procedures for Chapter 14 using the Competency Checklists
Resources to Promote Critical Thinking:	
***Solve the Case* Activities**	• Consider these case studies and discuss your conclusions
Learning Lab	• Module 23: Cardiology and Radiology
MindTap	• Complete Chapter 14 readings and activities, including medical terminology and patient navigation study tools.

REFERENCES

Centers for Medicare & Medicaid Services (CMS). (n.d.). *2014 Clinical Quality Measures (CQMs) Adult Recommended Core Measures*. Retrieved September 21, 2014, from http://www.cms.gov/Regulations-and-Guidance/Legislation/EHRIncentivePrograms/Downloads/2014_CQM_AdultRecommend_CoreSetTable.pdf

Ehrlich, A., & Schroeder, C.L. (2013). *Medical terminology for health care professionals* (7th ed.). Clifton Park, NY: Cengage Learning.

Heart Disease by the Numbers: Facts, Statistics, and You. (n.d.). Retrieved September 21, 2014, from http://www.healthline.com/health/heart-disease-infographic

Heart Disease Facts. (2014, August 18). Retrieved September 21, 2014, from http://www.cdc.gov/HeartDisease/facts.htm

High Blood Pressure Facts. (2014, July 7). Retrieved September 21, 2014, from http://www.cdc.gov/bloodpressure/facts.htm

Senisi Scott, A., & Fong, E. (2014). *Body structures and functions* (12th ed.). Clifton Park, NY: Cengage Learning.

Singh, V. N. (n.d.). Heart Disease: Get Facts, Statistics and Prevention Tips. Retrieved on September 21, 2014, from http://www.emedicinehealth.com/coronary_heart_disease/article_em.htm

What Is High Blood Pressure? (n.d.). Retrieved September 21, 2014, from http://www.heart.org/HEARTORG/Conditions/HighBloodPressure/AboutHighBloodPressure/What-is-High-Blood-Pressure_UCM_301759_Article.jsp

15

Pulmonary Examinations and Procedures

ESSENTIAL TERMS

bronchoscopy
carcinogen
cardiothoracic surgeons
chest CT
dyspnea
hypoxic
induration
inhalers
Mantoux skin test (PPD testing)
metered-dose inhaler (MDI)
nebulizer
oxygen saturation
peak expiratory flow (PEF)
peak flow meter
pleural effusion
pulmonary function testing
pulmonologist
pulmonology
respiratory therapists
sleep apnea
spirometer
spirometry
sputum
thoracentesis
tuberculosis (TB)
vital capacity (VC)

CHAPTER OUTLINE

Respiratory System Snapshot
- Lung Anatomy
- Pulmonary Physiology

Pulmonary Medical Abbreviation Review

Respiratory In-Office Screening and Telephone Screening Tips

Common Respiratory Diseases
- Contagious Infections
- Tuberculosis
- Lung Cancer
- Emphysema

Featured Pulmonary Procedures
- Pulmonary Function Testing
- Peak Flow Testing
- Pulse Oximetry Testing
- Sputum Collection
- Miscellaneous Pulmonary Procedures

Common Pulmonary Treatments and Medications
- Nebulizers
- Inhalers
- Oxygen Administration

Common Lab Tests That Coincide with Respiratory Disorders

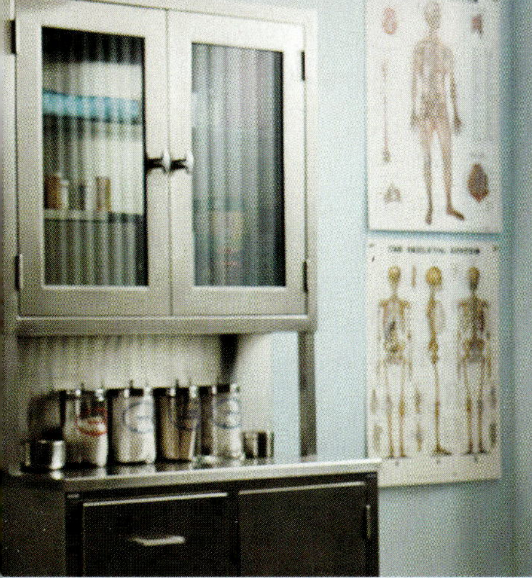

DEVELOPMENTAL OBJECTIVES

After completing this chapter, you should be able to:

1. Correctly spell and define the essential terms.
2. List and provide the anatomical locations of the major structures within the respiratory system.
3. Describe the normal functions of the respiratory system.
4. List and use common abbreviations associated with the respiratory system.
5. Describe the types of respiratory specialists and what their roles are in patient care.
6. Compile a list of common screening questions that should be asked of patients with respiratory symptoms using established protocols and incorporate critical thinking skills when performing patient assessment.
7. Create a plan describing how to respond during a respiratory emergency.
8. Identify common pathology related to the respiratory system including signs, symptoms, and etiology.
9. Compare the structure and function of the respiratory system across the life span.
10. Analyze pathology for the respiratory system including diagnostic measures and treatment modalities.
11. List and describe the different values associated with pulmonary function testing and explain what "personal best" means when comparing results from one individual to another.
12. Describe the role of the medical assistant during pulmonary function testing and explain how this role assists the patient in obtaining the best result possible.
13. Describe the Asthma Action Plan, including how zones are determined for each patient and what benefit this has on patient treatment outcomes.
14. Explain the purpose of pulse oximetry testing and record the average SpO_2 range for healthy individuals.
15. Provide solutions for resolving each factor that can interfere with pulse oximetry testing.
16. List five types of procedures and three types of laboratory tests that aid in diagnosing respiratory disorders.
17. Demonstrate how to effectively coach a patient on why and how to quit smoking (smoking cessation).

INTRODUCTION

The pulmonary system is also referred to as the respiratory system. It includes all the essential organs and processes for breathing, taking oxygen into the body, and excreting carbon dioxide from the body. It is also responsible for our ability to speak, sing, and make other vocalizations. Regulations of the oxygen and carbon dioxide levels help to maintain homeostasis by regulating the pH of the body as well.

Respiratory health is vitally important to the patient's overall health. If the patient has a breathing disorder, it affects other major organs including the heart and brain. Respiratory conditions that severely obstruct breathing can result in death. The medical assistant must be able to identify life-threatening encounters and institute measures to sustain breathing.

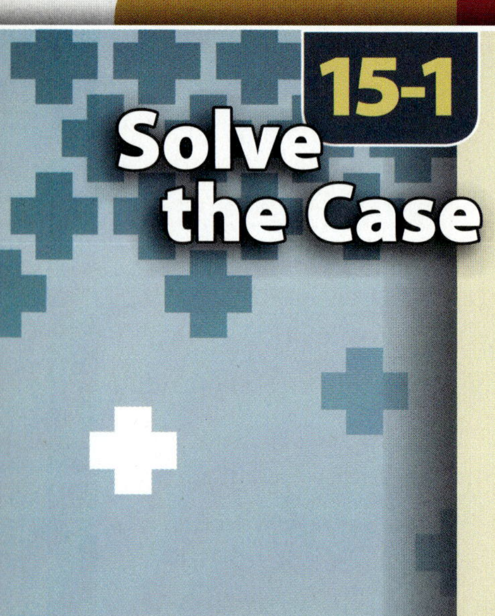

Ms. Calhoun is a 35-year-old woman with five days of steadily worsening cough and chest congestion. She is having trouble sleeping due to the cough. With the use of an OTC nighttime cough syrup, she is able to sleep one to two hours at a time. Her coughing fits are not productive of sputum and her chest feels tight. She typically smokes ½ pack of cigarettes per day, but "can't even smoke" since her cough has gotten so bad. She denies any fever. She had asthma "as a child," but has not used an inhaler since she's been out of high school. She does not appear to be in severe respiratory distress.

1. **What preliminary vital signs should a medical assistant obtain from Ms. Calhoun?**
2. **What kind of a role does Ms. Calhoun's smoking habit play, if any, in her current illness?**
3. **What kind of treatments do you think might be helpful for Ms. Calhoun?**

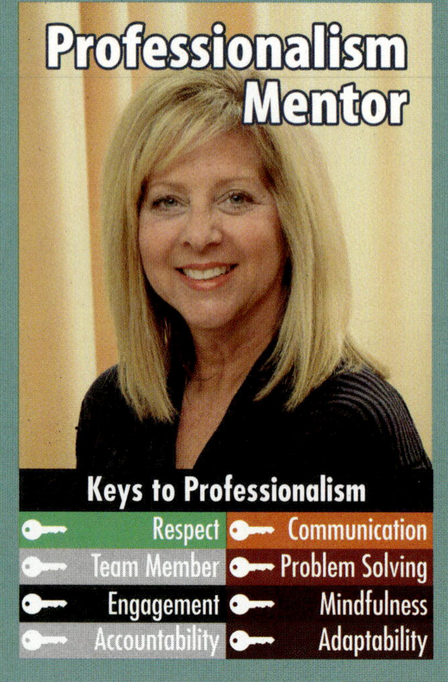

Imagine trying to breathe through a straw for an hour. That might be how your patient with severe pulmonary problems feels when trying to breathe. Consider this: a medical assistant was administering a pulmonary function test to a patient with severe COPD. After several attempts, the patient seemed frustrated and breathless and took his nose clips off, unable to continue the test. The medical assistant, recognizing the patient's increasing frustration, decided to do the test in increments so that the patient could rest in between. While it may have taken a little longer to get the test done, this collaborative effort between the patient and medical assistant resulted in the patient being able to finish the test and keep his composure. By being flexible with the testing plan, the medical assistant was able to get the test completed and the results to the physician while keeping the patient from having a miserable experience. Imagine how relieved the patient was to get through the exam without feeling like he was breathing through a straw the entire time. The medical assistant demonstrated his professionalism by taking a tough experience and turning it into a positive one for his patient. ■

RESPIRATORY SYSTEM SNAPSHOT

The respiratory system is comprised of all body parts that help us to breathe. It has three major functions:

- To obtain necessary oxygen to fuel the body's cells
- To excrete carbon dioxide waste products from the body
- To enable vocalization

Lung Anatomy

The body has two lungs, contained within the rib cage. Each lung is divided into lobes. The right lung has three lobes, while the left has only two (Figure 15-1). The heart fits snugly between the lungs. Lung tissue is firm and spongy. The lungs are surrounded by a protective layer called the pleura. A very small space exists between the lungs and the pleura and is referred to as the pleural space. Under normal conditions, this space is minimal, with the pleura lying directly on the lung surface. The lungs expand and shrink as they fill with air and then empty, though complete emptying never occurs.

Air enters the body through the mouth and nose and then passes between the pharynx and lungs via the larynx and trachea. The trachea is a hollow tube reinforced with cartilaginous rings to keep it open. The trachea divides into two primary bronchi. Each primary bronchus leads to one lung, before branching into smaller and smaller airways called bronchioles. At the end of each bronchiole is a grape-like cluster of small sacs called alveoli. Millions of alveoli are contained within the lungs. Refer to Figure 15-2 for a diagram of the respiratory system.

Pulmonary Physiology

Air is taken in through the nose and mouth and passes down the throat (or pharynx). The mucosal tissue and saliva in the nose and mouth help to warm and moisten the incoming air and can also trap particles, such as dust. It is here at the base of the pharynx that both the esophagus and trachea begin. A mucosal flap called the *epiglottis* typically stays open to allow air to enter the lungs. The swallowing reflex causes involuntary closure of the epiglottis over the trachea to divert food into the esophagus.

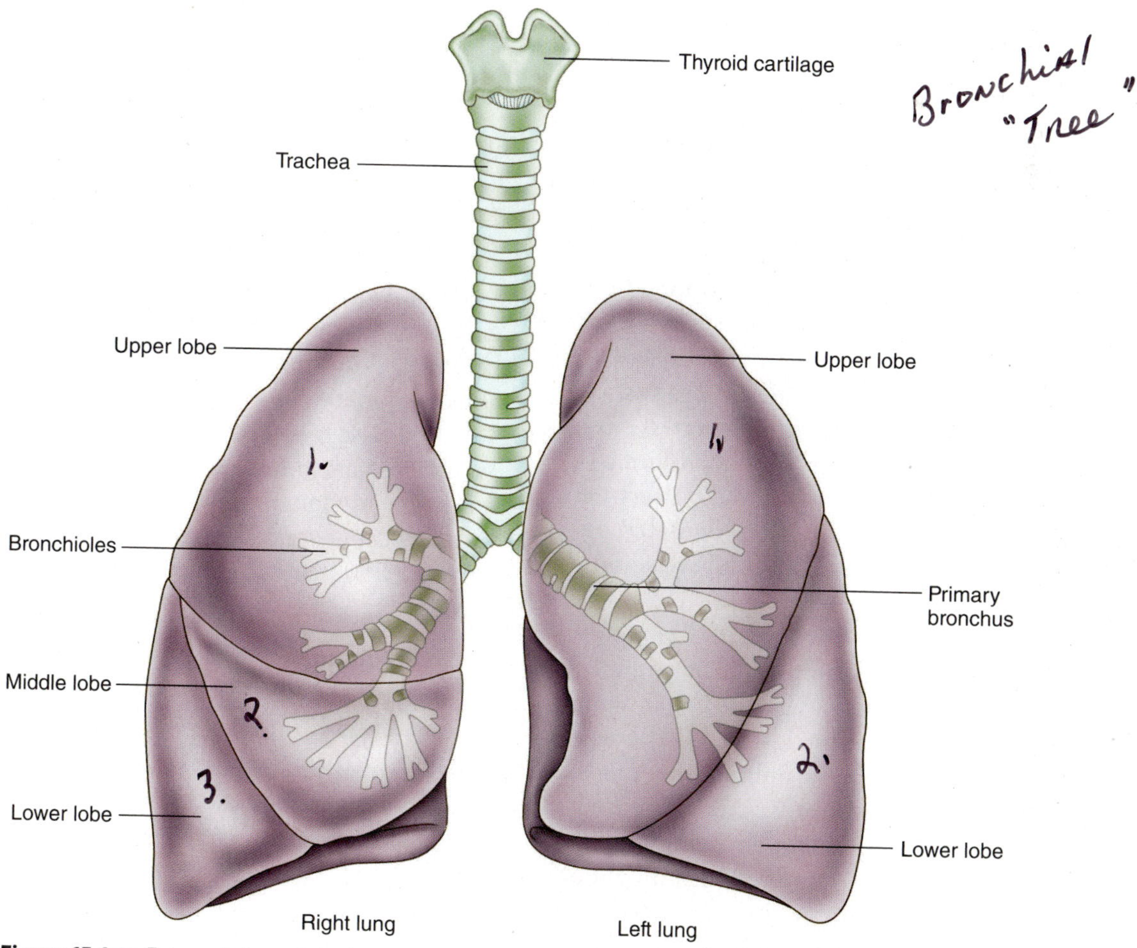

Figure 15-1 ■ External view of the lungs. Note the three lobes of the right lung and the two lobes of the left lung.

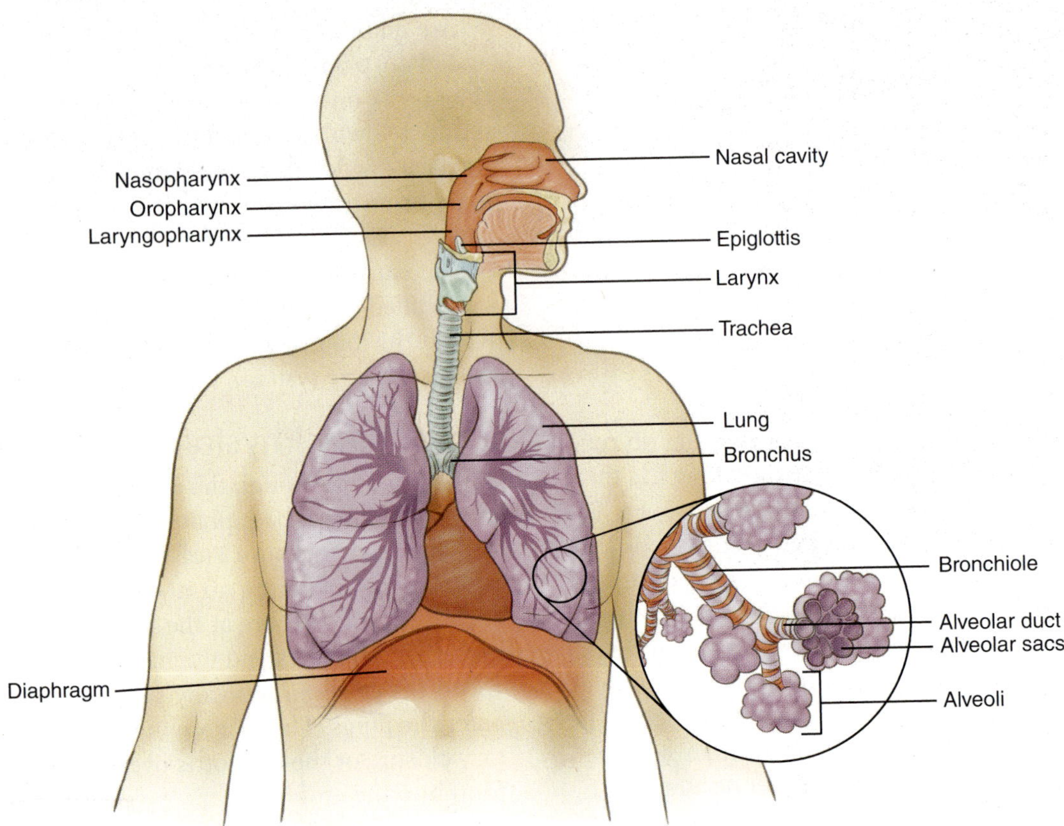

Figure 15-2 ■ Structures of the respiratory system.

When incoming air reaches the alveoli, oxygen and carbon dioxide exchange takes place. These grape-like clusters are surrounded by capillaries, which deposit the carbon dioxide in the lungs and pick up oxygen to carry throughout the body. Their round shape allows for increased surface area for greater exchange capacity. Oxygen-rich blood then travels to the heart, where it is pumped throughout the body. As it circulates, the oxygen is released to the body's tissues, and carbon dioxide by-product is picked up by the bloodstream, and finally excreted by exhalation. The process of breathing is both voluntary and involuntary. That is, we can intentionally alter our breathing, but respiration is most often regulated by the brain stem to steadily continue without conscious thought.

As expiration occurs, the pressure in the lungs drops. When the pressure of the air outside of the body becomes greater than that in the lungs, the *diaphragm*, a thin, dome-like muscle that divides the chest from the abdominal cavity, contracts, pulling the bases of the lung down with it, causing further decreased pressure in the lungs. This results in air being pulled into the lungs, or *inhalation*. When the lungs fill with incoming air, the inside pressure is then greater than the air outside the body and the diaphragm relaxes, allowing the lung bases to rise and air exits the body in *exhalation*. Refer to Figure 15-3 for a diagram that illustrates diaphragmatic movements during inhalation and exhalation.

Meet the **Specialists**

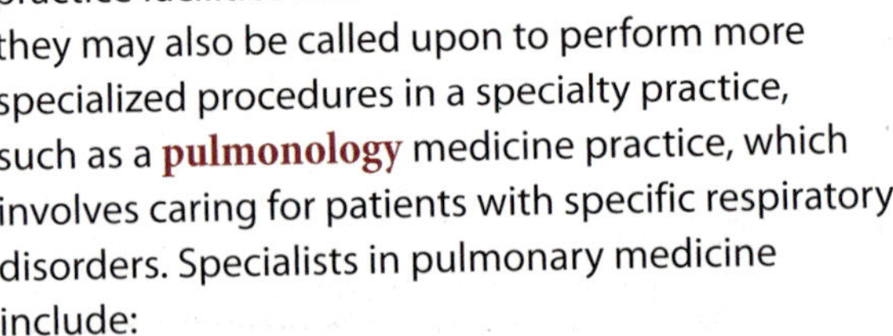

Medical assistants often perform respiratory procedures in family practice facilities but they may also be called upon to perform more specialized procedures in a specialty practice, such as a **pulmonology** medicine practice, which involves caring for patients with specific respiratory disorders. Specialists in pulmonary medicine include:

- **Pulmonologists:** Diagnose and treat problems associated with the lungs and airways
- **Cardiothoracic Surgeons:** Perform surgical procedures on patients with diseases affecting organs of the heart and lungs
- **Respiratory Therapists:** Use equipment and techniques to maintain or improve patients' breathing; administer treatments

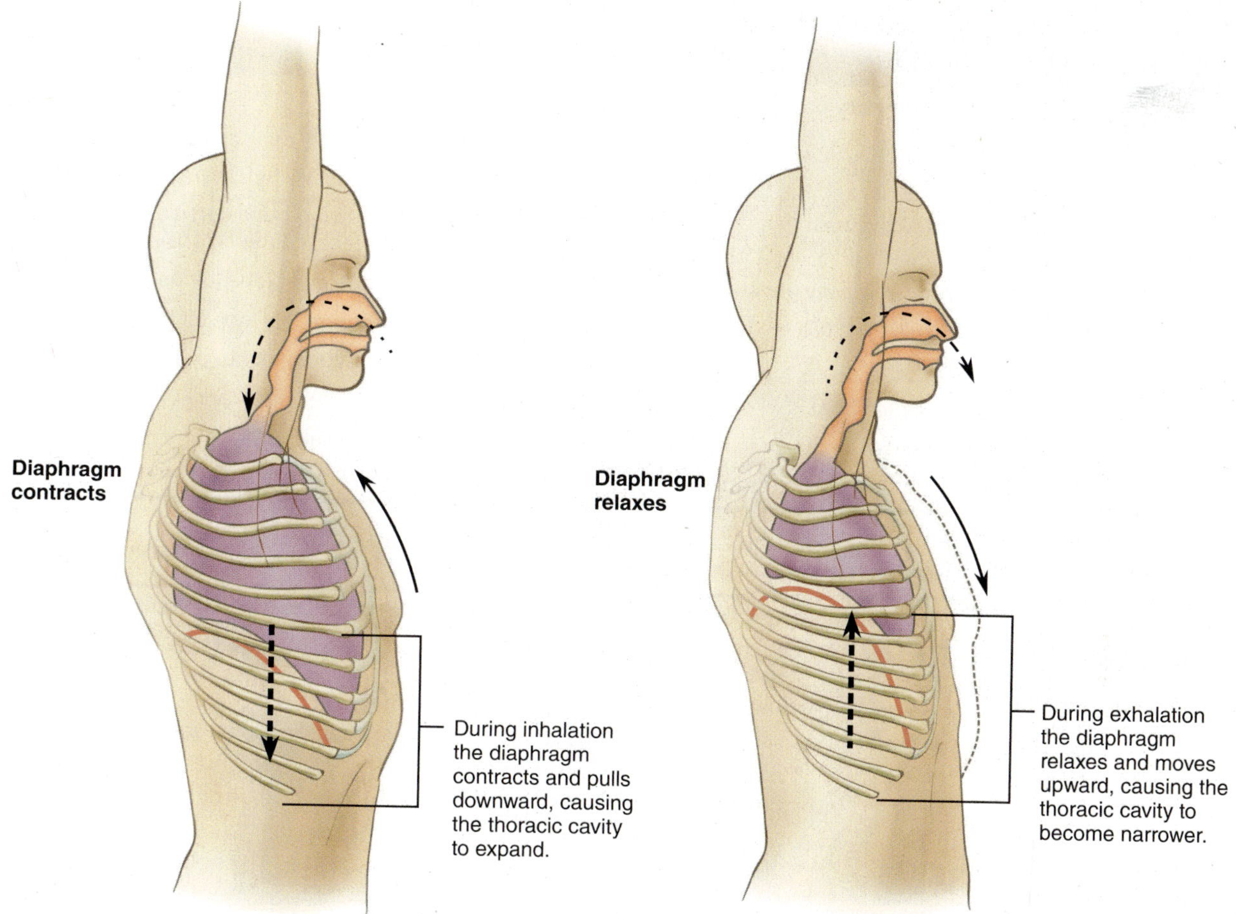
Diaphragm contracts
During inhalation the diaphragm contracts and pulls downward, causing the thoracic cavity to expand.
Diaphragm relaxes
During exhalation the diaphragm relaxes and moves upward, causing the thoracic cavity to become narrower.

Figure 15-3 ■ Movements of the diaphragm and thoracic cavity produce inhalation (left) and exhalation (right).

PULMONARY ABBREVIATION REVIEW

Medical assistants working in pulmonary clinics should be familiar with the abbreviations in Table 15-1.

RESPIRATORY IN-OFFICE SCREENING AND TELEPHONE SCREENING TIPS

Medical assistants may have the responsibility of screening patients prior to provider examination. The depth of screening will be established by office protocol but, in general, medical assistants should be able to ask a series of questions related to the patient's symptoms. Table 15-2 lists types of questions that are typically asked during respiratory screenings and the common procedures that coincide with symptoms.

Important Note: Medical assistants should never perform any procedure unless directed to do so by the provider; however, they can set up various equipment and supplies to help save time in the event that testing is ordered.

COMMON RESPIRATORY DISEASES

There are many forms of pulmonary disease. These include infections that can be caused by viruses, bacteria, or fungi. Another category of disease is obstructive or restrictive disease in which the lungs are not able to properly expand and contract as needed for gas exchange. Abnormal cell growth, such as tumors, can also occur.

Contagious Infections

Contagious infections are those that are transmitted from one person to another. They include those caused by viruses, bacteria, and fungi. The most commonly seen respiratory infection is a viral *upper respiratory*

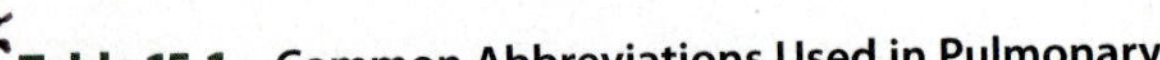

Table 15-1 Common Abbreviations Used in Pulmonary Specialties

Abbreviation	Meaning	Abbreviation	Meaning
BiPAP	Bilevel positive airway pressure	O_2	Oxygen
CA	Cancer	PE	Pulmonary embolus
CO_2	Carbon dioxide	PFT	Pulmonary function testing
COPD	Chronic obstructive pulmonary disease	PPD	Purified protein derivative (skin test to screen for tuberculosis)
CPAP	Continue positive airway pressure	RLL	Right lower lobe (of lung)
CTA(B)	Clear to auscultation (bilaterally)	RML	Right middle lobe (of lung)
CXR	Chest X-ray	RUL	Right upper lobe (of lung)
LLL	Left lower lobe (of lung)	SCLC	Small cell lung cancer
LUL	Left upper lobe (of lung)	TB	Tuberculosis
NHLBI	National Heart Lung Blood Institute	TLC	Total lung capacity

Table 15-2 Patient Screening Instructions for the Respiratory System

Ask the Patient:	• Are you experiencing any shortness of breath, coughing, bringing up phlegm, wheezing, or coughing up blood? • Do you have any history of respiratory disease or frequent infections? • Do you smoke? If so, how many packs per day, and for how many years? • Do you live or work in an environment that makes you vulnerable to certain respiratory conditions or diseases (histoplasmosis, black lung, and so on)?
For Patients Calling on the Telephone	Patient in acute respiratory distress should be encouraged to call the EMS to be on the safe side.
When in the Office:	
Disrobing Instructions	Have patient remove all garments from the waist up and apply provided gown.
Vital Signs	Take patient's temperature, pulse, respiration, blood pressure, and pain/breathing rating
Equipment	Equipment you may need includes nebulizer pulse oximeter, oxygen, and PFT equipment
Possible Procedures	Pulse oximetry, PFT testing, breathing treatments, and oxygen therapy

infection (URI), also known as the common cold. Symptoms include rhinorrhea, nasal and chest congestion, postnasal drip, cough, and fatigue. URIs are usually self-limiting, requiring only comfort care until the virus passes after 3–14 days.

Pneumonia is most commonly a bacterial infection and is treated with antibiotics. Symptoms may include cough, **dyspnea** (difficulty breathing), fever, and fatigue. *Influenza* is a viral illness that spikes in prevalence during fall and winter seasons. It causes fever and body aches, along with sore throat or cough. Immunization exists and vaccines are updated annually for the strains predicted to be most prevalent. Secondary pneumonia is one of the possible complications of influenza.

Tuberculosis

Tuberculosis (TB) is most often considered to be a respiratory infection, though it can manifest in many areas of the body, including lymph nodes, joints, kidneys, spinal meninges, liver, and tissues lining the abdomen. It is caused by *Mycobacterium tuberculosis*, a slow-advancing bacterium. Common symptoms include the following:

- Cough with bloody sputum
- Night sweats
- Tachycardia (rapid heart rate)
- Swelling of lymph nodes in the neck
- Unexplained weight loss

Airborne transmission occurs only if a person has active TB, not latent TB, which cannot be spread but can turn into active TB if not treated. Even though TB can be spread through air and droplets, a single exposure is usually not capable of promoting disease. Repeated exposure to an infected individual, however, increases a person's risk of contracting the disease.

According to the Centers for Disease Control and Prevention (CDC), tuberculosis is responsible for more deaths than any other communicable disease in the world. Approximately one-third of the world's population has some form of TB.

Lung Cancer

Lung cancer occurs when the normal lung cells convert to an abnormal growth pattern. This includes cells that don't function normally and that reproduce at an excessive rate, causing tumors. Alarming data shows that lung cancer kills more people than colon, breast, and prostate cancer combined. It is now the leading cause of cancer death of both genders according to the American Cancer Society (ACS). The ACS estimated 221,000 new cases of lung cancer in 2015, with the number of deaths associated with lung cancer reaching nearly 160,000 annually.

The risk of lung cancer is impacted by many factors, though smoking tobacco is one of the biggest risks. A substance known to cause cancer is known as a **carcinogen**.

Other risk factors include other forms of tobacco use, as well as second hand exposure to tobacco smoke; environmental exposures such as asbestos, radon, uranium, and air pollution; radiation therapy to the lungs; and a diet low in fruits and vegetables.

Health Coach

Smoking Cessation

According to the National Institute on Drug Abuse, tobacco use is the leading preventable cause of disease, disability, and death in the United States. Smoking cessation is difficult due to the addictive nature of the product. In order to be successful, you must make a conscious decision to take charge of your body and to stop letting the nicotine control you. To stay with the program, continually remind yourself of the benefits of quitting, including the following:

- Minimizing your risks for developing lung cancer, heart attack, stroke, and chronic lung disease, as well as many other forms of cancer
- Overall improvement in general health
- No longer putting your family or friends at risk with secondhand smoke
- No more stains on teeth, hands, and fingers
- Avoidance of wrinkles that typically appear as a result of smoking
- No more smoke residue on clothing, hair, furniture, and car upholstery
- An improvement in taste and smell senses
- An overall improvement in the quality of life
- Financial savings

Once you have made the decision to quit, consider the following:

- Join a smoking cessation support group. The American Lung Association offers both educational programs and support groups, with online and telephone components, to assist individuals trying to quit smoking.
- Tell your friends, family, and coworkers so that they can be supportive. They may be more understanding if you are irritable or frustrated.
- Set a date to quit.
- Don't quit during a stressful time.
- Exercise every day.
- Plan a great nutritional program.
- Identify your personal triggers. These include the places, situations, and times that you routinely smoke (e.g., after eating, on break, when in the car, when feeling increased stress). Then develop a plan for an alternative to smoking in each situation (e.g., go for a walk, chew sugarless gum).
- Drink plenty of healthy fluids.
- Plan some fun activity each day.
- Use nicotine replacement such as gums, patches, inhalers, and nasal sprays. These are not as harmful as smoking, if used correctly. They do not have the tars associated with the cigarettes and cigars.
- Consider hypnosis, acupuncture, or other complementary alternative measures.

Emphysema

Emphysema is a form of *chronic obstructive pulmonary disease* (COPD). Asthma can also be considered a form of COPD. Emphysema is most commonly caused by smoking, though other forms of polluted inhalation can also be a risk factor. Progressive damage occurs so that the inner walls of the alveoli weaken and sometimes burst. The grape-like cluster of alveoli then becomes one large air pocket, which is much less effective for gas exchange. The lungs are not able to properly exhale, and air becomes trapped in these damaged areas of the lungs, decreasing the available space for new oxygen to enter.

Patients with emphysema typically have lower oxygen saturation rates, measured through pulse oximetry. Shortness of breath is the most common presenting concern, though typically patients have had the disease for years before diagnosis. Testing to confirm COPD includes chest X-ray, CT scan of the chest, and pulmonary function testing (PFTs).

Treatments are available to help slow the progression of emphysema, but no cure exists. Inhaled medications such as bronchodilators and steroids are often used to decrease inflammation and ease the shortness of breath and cough. Patients with COPD are also at increased risk of pneumothorax (a collapsed lung) and respiratory infections, often requiring antibiotic therapy. Many affected individuals will require supplemental oxygen therapy in later stages of the disease. Figure 15-4 illustrates a patient with emphysema using an oxygen tank in order to breathe.

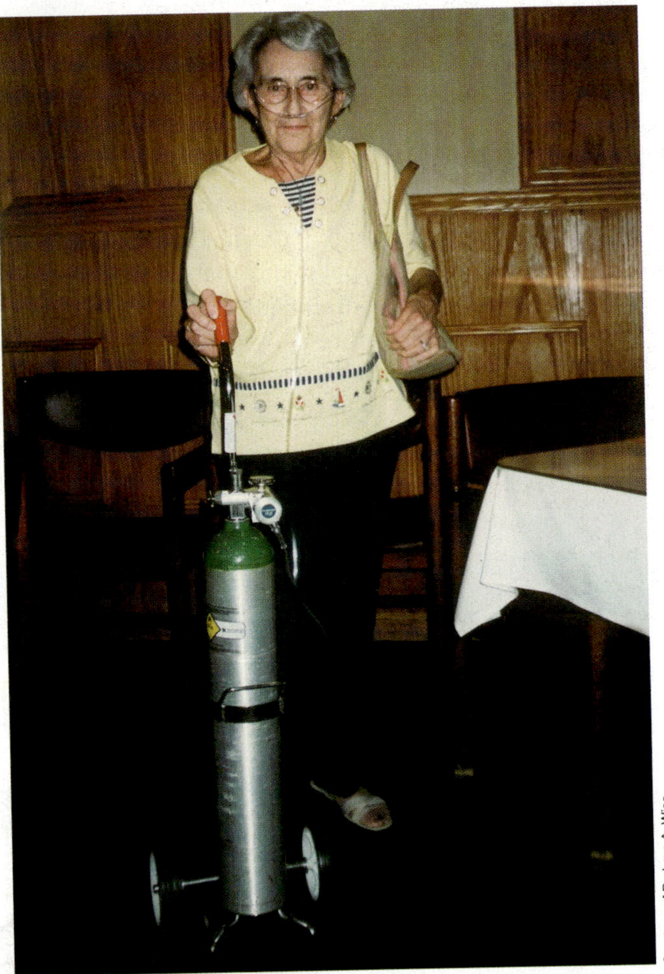

Courtesy of Barbara A. Wise

Figure 15-4 ■ Patients with COPD may need to have portable oxygen when they are away from home.

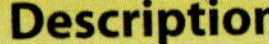

Health Coach

Featured Disease Spotlight: Asthma

Description

Asthma is a very common form of obstructive lung disease. It has two hallmark characteristics: bronchoconstriction and inflammation. Bronchoconstriction occurs when a trigger causes the bronchi and bronchioles to constrict, narrowing the diameter, and making it harder for the same volume of air to pass through. Inflammation of the airways means that the mucosal lining becomes swollen and produces a mucus, further blocking air passage and causing symptoms of chest congestion.

continues

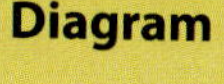

Featured Disease Spotlight: Asthma *continued*

Diagram

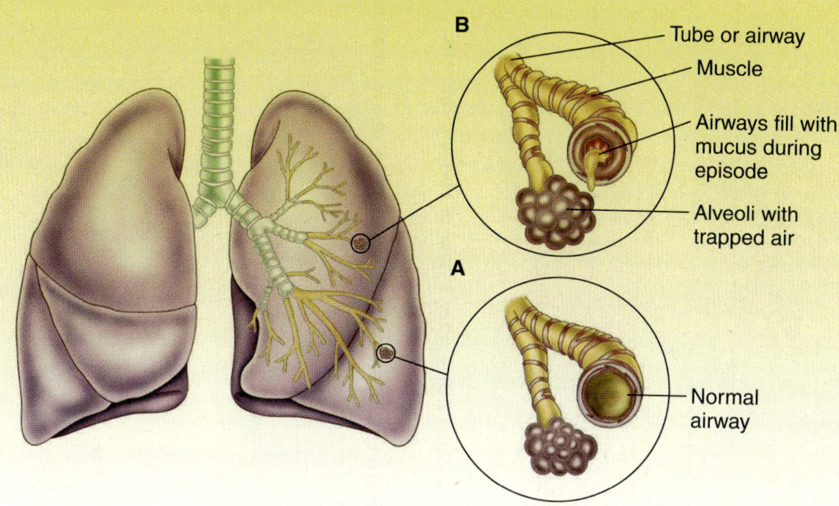

Risk Factors

Family history, exposure to tobacco smoke, and presence of allergies or eczema

Symptoms

Difficulty breathing, chest tightness, wheezing, and cough

Diagnostic Testing

Spirometry (explained later in the chapter)

Peak Flow Meters: Peak flow readings measure how much air can be forcefully blown into a peak flow meter. This helps determine an individual's lung capacity. Physicians and other medical providers use these readings to develop individual treatment plans.

Modifying Factors

Quit smoking. Avoid triggers such as allergens (dust, pollen, and food that triggers allergies); intense exercise (organized sports, recess play, active chores [raking, mowing], going up stairs); infections (any respiratory infection can trigger an asthma attack); and environmental triggers (exhaust fumes, chemicals like bleach/chlorine and tobacco smoke).

Treatment 

To treat asthma appropriately:

1. Identify and avoid triggers.
2. Quit smoking.
3. Develop an Asthma Action Plan (see Figure 15-5) with the help of a health care professional.
4. Monitor symptoms and peak flows and then adjust treatment accordingly.

Bronchodilator therapy, inhaled or oral steroids, and leukotriene modifiers can all be used to treat asthma. These include medications taken by mouth (pills or syrups) and those inhaled (inhalers or nebulizers).

Asthma Action Plan

For: ______ Doctor: ______ Date: ______

Doctor's Phone Number ______ Hospital/Emergency Department Phone Number ______

GREEN ZONE

Doing Well

- No cough, wheeze, chest tightness, or shortness of breath during the day or night
- Can do usual activities

And, if a peak flow meter is used,

Peak flow: more than ______
(80 percent or more of my best peak flow)

My best peak flow is: ______

Take these long-term control medicines each day (include an anti-inflammatory).

Medicine	How much to take	When to take it
Before exercise ❐ ______	❐ 2 or ❐ 4 puffs ______	5 minutes before exercise

YELLOW ZONE

Asthma Is Getting Worse

- Cough, wheeze, chest tightness, or shortness of breath, or
- Waking at night due to asthma, or
- Can do some, but not all, usual activities

-Or-

Peak flow: ______ to ______
(50 to 79 percent of my best peak flow)

First — **Add: quick-relief medicine—and keep taking your GREEN ZONE medicine.**

______ (short-acting beta$_2$-agonist) ❐ 2 or ❐ 4 puffs, every 20 minutes for up to 1 hour
❐ Nebulizer, once

Second — **If your symptoms (and peak flow, if used) return to GREEN ZONE after 1 hour of above treatment:**
❐ Continue monitoring to be sure you stay in the green zone.

-Or-

If your symptoms (and peak flow, if used) do not return to GREEN ZONE after 1 hour of above treatment:
❐ Take: ______ (short-acting beta$_2$-agonist) ❐ 2 or ❐ 4 puffs or ❐ Nebulizer
❐ Add: ______ (oral steroid) mg per day For ______ (3–10) days
❐ Call the doctor ❐ before/ ❐ within ______ hours after taking the oral steroid.

RED ZONE

Medical Alert!

- Very short of breath, or
- Quick-relief medicines have not helped, or
- Cannot do usual activities, or
- Symptoms are same or get worse after 24 hours in Yellow Zone

-Or-

Peak flow: less than ______
(50 percent of my best peak flow)

Take this medicine:

❐ ______ (short-acting beta$_2$-agonist) ❐ 4 or ❐ 6 puffs or ❐ Nebulizer
❐ ______ (oral steroid) mg

Then call your doctor NOW. Go to the hospital or call an ambulance if:
- You are still in the red zone after 15 minutes AND
- You have not reached your doctor.

DANGER SIGNS
- **Trouble walking and talking due to shortness of breath**
- **Lips or fingernails are blue**

- **Take ❐ 4 or ❐ 6 puffs of your quick-relief medicine AND**
- **Go to the hospital or call for an ambulance** ______ (phone) **NOW!**

See the reverse side for things you can do to avoid your asthma triggers.

Courtesy of the Department of Health and Human Services

Figure 15-5 ■ An Asthma Action Plan is individualized to each patient and helps them to manage their asthma.

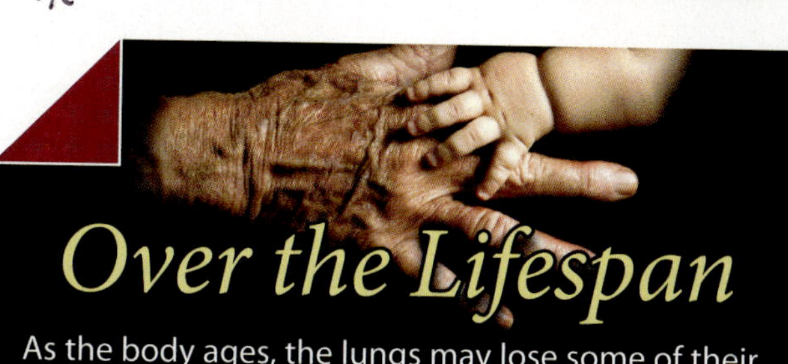

Over the Lifespan

As the body ages, the lungs may lose some of their elasticity, making it more difficult for efficient respiration and gas exchange. Strength and flexibility of the chest also declines. As the lungs become less efficient, the heart often works harder to compensate, resulting in cardiac comorbidities.

FEATURED PULMONARY PROCEDURES

The medical assistant is a valuable team member in the office, able to perform various procedures to study the effectiveness of the lungs or to help diagnose and treat respiratory concerns.

Pulmonary Function Testing

Spirometry, or **pulmonary function testing**, is a noninvasive test that detects the lungs' ability to function. A **spirometer** is the instrument that measures lung function. It can measure how rapidly a patient can move air in and out of the lungs and how much air is moved in and out of the lungs. Pulmonary testing is performed for a variety of different reasons including to detect lung obstructions, to assess lung health prior to surgery [significant reductions in vital capacity (VC) testing can mean that the patient is more prone to respiratory complications following surgery], and to detect how well certain medications are working. The medical assistant is often responsible for performing spirometry testing and for providing the patient with feedback in order to improve performance during testing. Refer to Procedure 15-1 for a complete procedure for performing a spirometry test.

The Importance of Coaching

Coaching can be very effective during spirometry testing (Figure 15-6). Patients will often feel discouraged if they don't perform well during initial testing. The patient, especially when frustrated, might need to be "cheered on" to succeed. The medical assistant might say something like the following to encourage the patient during testing: "Blow, blow, blow! Keep going, you can do it!" This may be necessary in order to achieve the best results possible.

Calibrating the Spirometer

To make certain that the spirometer is working correctly it should be calibrated on any day that testing is scheduled. Spirometry units usually come with a 3-liter calibration syringe that is used to check the unit's performance. Three liters of air is injected into the unit from the 3-liter calibration syringe (Figure 15-7). The results of the calibration should fall within 3% of the 3 liters. A calibration report illustrates whether or not the calibration was successful (Figure 15-8).

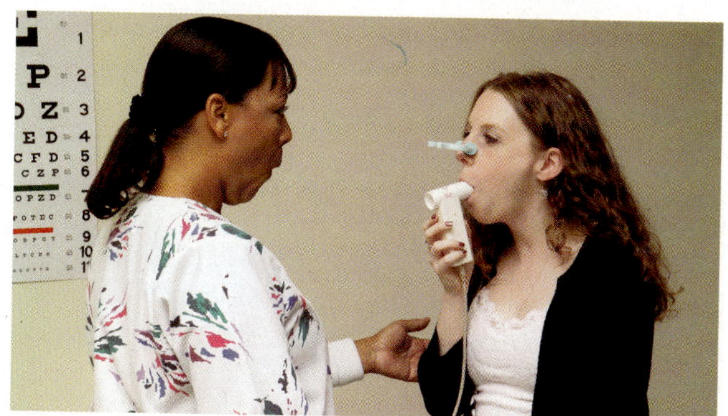

Figure 15-6 ■ The medical assistant coaches the patient during PFT testing.

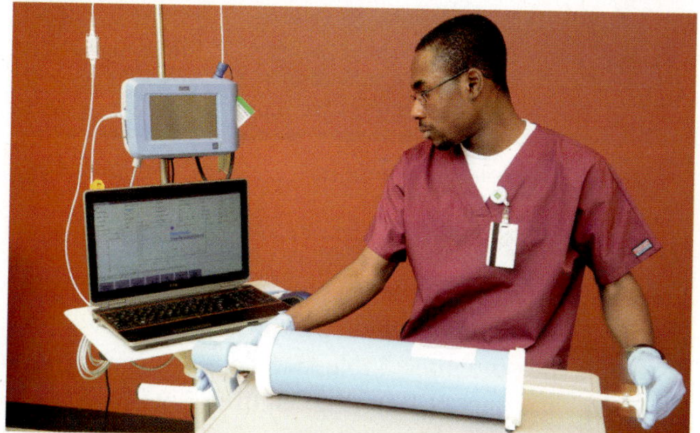

Figure 15-7 ■ Notice how the MA pushes the plunger inward, following the directions on the syringe.

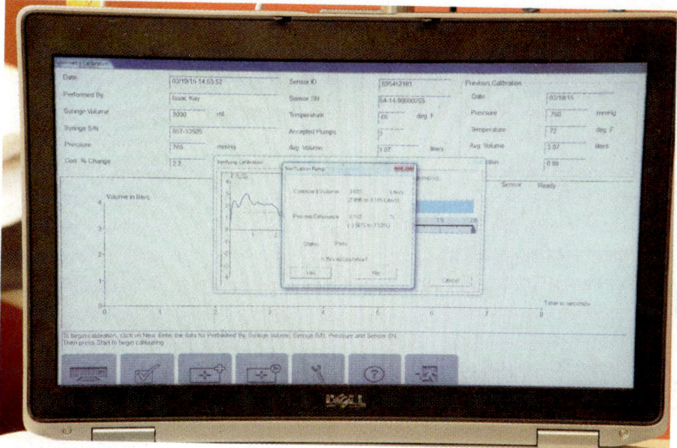

Figure 15-8 ■ This calibration was successful. The medical assistant should refer to the owner's manual when ranges do not fall within the accepted range.

Table 15-3 Definitions of Measurements from Pulmonary Function Tests

Measurement	Definition
Forced expiratory volume after 1 second (FEV1)	The total amount of air forcefully exhaled during the first second of testing. (Patients with healthy lungs should be able to force out 70–75% of the air in their lungs within that first second of testing, emphasizing the need for appropriate education and coaching. Any type of a blockage or restriction may cause the result to drop.)
Forced vital capacity (FVC)	The maximum amount of air forced out of the lungs when the patient exhales as rapidly and forcefully as possible into the tube after taking in a deep inhalation (usually expressed in liters).
Tidal volume (V_t)	The amount of air during inspiration and expiration when breathing normally.
Inspiratory reserve volume (IRV)	The additional amount of air a patient could potentially inhale.
Expiratory reserve volume (ERV)	The additional amount of air a patient could potentially exhale.
Residual volume (RV)	The air that is left in the lungs after the patient forcibly exhales all the air the patient can.
Total lung capacity (TLC)	The amount of air the lungs are able to hold.
Vital capacity (VC)	The maximum amount of air the patient is able to inhale and exhale.
Functional residual capacity (FRC)	The amount of air that is left in the lungs after the patient normally exhales.

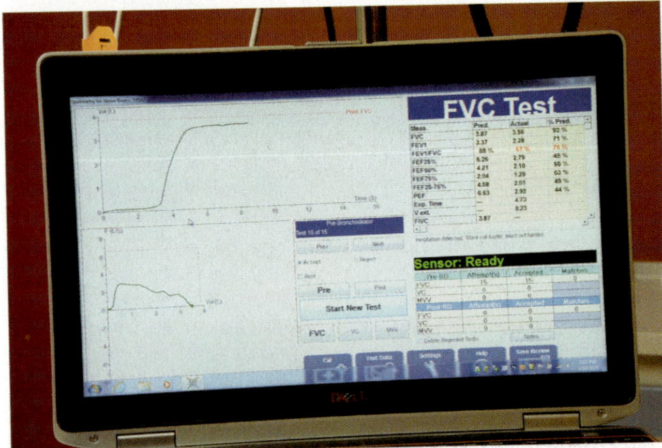

Figure 15-9 ■ A spirometry report.

Understanding the Results

The spirometer will typically graph the results and provide the calculations while the provider reviews and interprets the outcomes. Table 15-3 depicts various measurements used in PFT testing. Figure 15-9 illustrates a PFT report.

Normal Results

Normal results are influenced by several factors, including the patient's age, height, and gender. Results are expressed as a percentage of the predicted lung capacity. There are several online tools for calculating predicted values. Expected outcomes are listed below:

- Normal PFT outcomes: 85% or higher of the predicted value
- Mild disease: 65% to 84% of predicted values
- Moderate disease: 50% to 64% of predicted values
- Severe disease: Less than 50% of predicted values

Another type of pulmonary function test is the exercise challenge test. This test uses spirometry testing prior to and following strenuous activity (using a treadmill or stationary bike). The test correlates any relationship between airflow and activity and assists in diagnosing conditions such as exercise-induced asthma.

Peak Flow Testing

If spirometry proves inconclusive, **peak expiratory flow (PEF)** may be tested with a **peak flow meter** (Figure 15-10). This test is often performed when there are symptoms of asthma but the patient has normal spirometry results. The device for measurement is disposable and inexpensive, enabling the test to be performed at home over a period of two to three weeks. As PEF varies throughout the day, times for testing must be recorded. The test measures the speed of exhalation with the greatest effort.

Peak flow testing is an easy test that can be performed by the patient. A peak flow meter is a small handheld device that measures the fastest speed air can be blown out of the lungs and is a great tool for the patient to monitor lung ailments such as asthma. Refer to Procedure 15-2 for more information.

Significance of a Peak Flow Reading

Peak flow readings are often used to monitor asthma and to help manage treatment. Because everyone has a different lung capacity, everyone has a different "personal best" peak flow reading. The provider will help the patient come up with what is considered a "personal best"

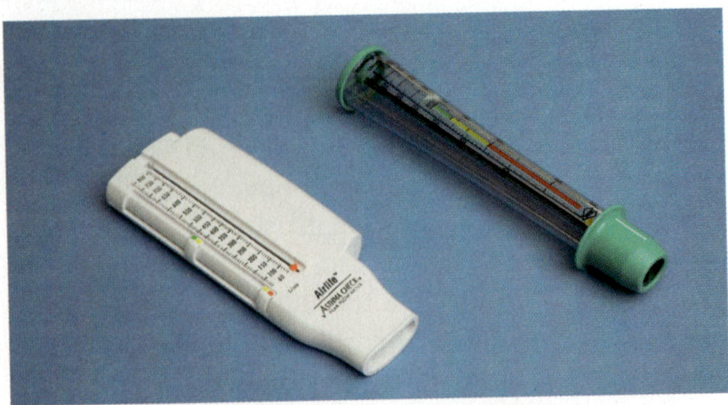

Figure 15-10 ■ Two different peak flow meters.

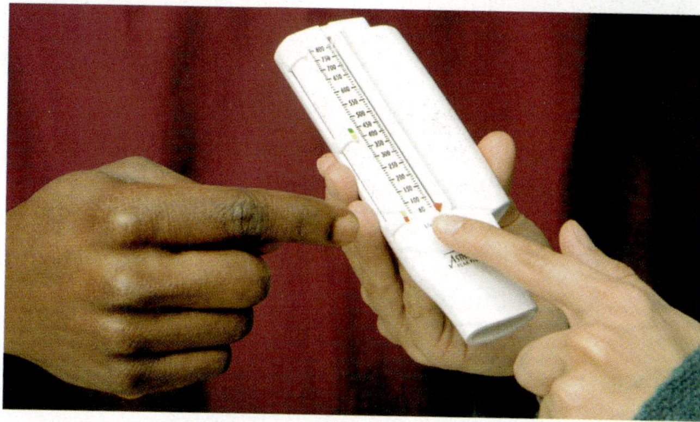

Figure 15-11 ■ The medical assistant shows the patient the red zone.

reading, based on the patient's readings in the office and the patient's personal medical condition. Individualized treatment guidelines can then be set. A common practice now is use of the Asthma Action Plan, which helps patients to easily see if their current readings fall into the green, yellow, or red zone, and adjust their treatment accordingly. This plan is a result of evidence-based guidelines published by the National Institutes for Health. Generally, green zone includes a peak flow rating that is 80% or better of a patient's personal best are well controlled and do not need immediate treatment changes. When an individual's peak flow readings fall into the yellow zone (50–79% of the patient's personal best), a quick relief medication is indicated. Anything below 50% falls into the red zone and means that the patient should immediately seek emergency care. See Figure 15-11 for reference.

Pulse Oximetry Testing

Pulse oximetry is a noninvasive, indirect test that is used to measure pulse rate and oxygen levels in the blood. A pulse oximeter (Figure 15-12) is a device that measures oxygen saturation, abbreviated as SaO_2, in the blood. SpO_2 is a more accurate abbreviation for **oxygen saturation** that is measured through pulse oximetry because the blood sample comes from capillary beds in peripheral circulation, not arterial circulation; however, the abbreviation SaO_2 may be used as well when recording results from this procedure.

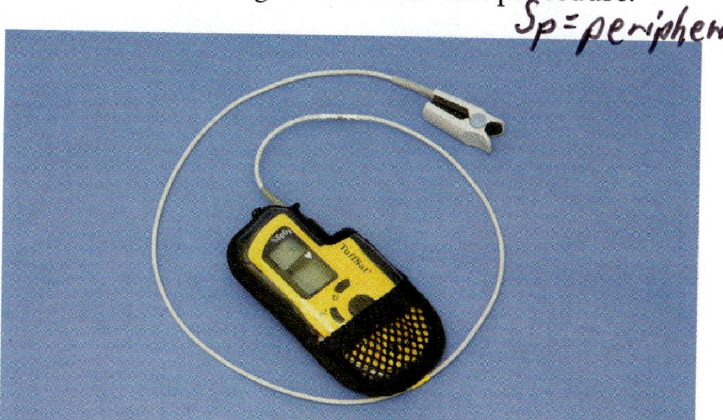

Figure 15-12 ■ A pulse oximeter.

The test is performed by wrapping a small strap around the patient's nail bed on the finger or toe or placing a clip on the bridge of the patient's nose or earlobe. The probe is two-sided. One side of the probe contains a light-emitting diode (LED) that transmits red and infrared red light through the patient's tissues to a photo detector located on the opposite side of the probe. A large portion of the light is absorbed by body tissue but a small amount is able to seep through and is detected by the photo detector. (Refer to Procedure 15-3 for a complete list of steps for performing pulse oximetry.)

Pulse oximetry is not as accurate as arterial blood gases but is very useful in monitoring the patient between arterial blood gases. It is also useful in emergency or outpatient situations when arterial blood gases are not an option. Normal SaO_2 or SpO_2 levels usually fall between 97% and 99%; however, a range of 96–100% is considered normal. *An oxygen saturation percentage of 100% over a prolonged period of time, however, can cause organ toxicity.* Patients are considered **hypoxic** (oxygen level is low) if their SaO_2 drops below 95%. Cyanosis may not set in until the patient's SaO_2 drops below 75%. Pulse oximetry alerts the provider to start oxygen intervention before physiological signs appear, which can decrease complications that arise from hypoxia.

Conditions in Which Pulse Oximetry Is Indicated

Pulse oximetry is indicated in any cardiopulmonary event in which oxygen saturation is a factor. Conditions in which SaO_2 levels may drop include the following:

- Cardiac conditions such as heart attack, congestive heart failure, and coronary artery disease
- Any respiratory disorders such as asthma, pneumonia, or congestive heart failure

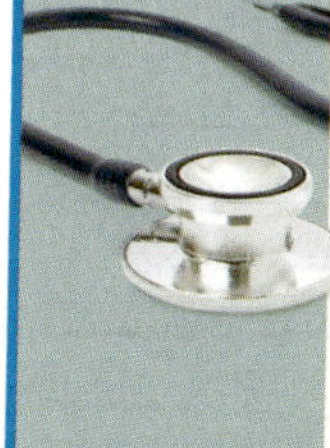

Field Smarts

Complications from hypoxia can start when the patient's SaO_2 level drops below 95%. Severe respiratory failure will most likely occur when arterial saturation of hemoglobin falls between 85% and 90%. This is a life-threatening condition. You should alert the provider when SaO_2 levels fall below acceptable levels and gather the appropriate oxygen equipment and supplies so that you are prepared when the provider gives the order to administer treatment.

Pulse oximetry may also be used to monitor the effectiveness of oxygen therapy and drug therapy as well as to monitor oxygen saturation procedures during surgical procedures. It is quite often used in ambulatory care, especially in urgent care centers. Oxygen saturation is now considered a vital sign.

Medical assistants should do everything possible to ensure accurate readings and should be familiar with readings that indicate immediate intervention.

Variables That Can Affect Oximetry Readings

There are several variables that can interfere with pulse oximetry readings. The medical assistant must do everything possible to ascertain that readings are accurate. An error in oximetry reading can lead to incorrect treatment, which can cause great harm to the patient.

Variables that can affect oximetry readings include:

- Ambient Lighting: If the room contains bright light, either natural or artificial, that shines directly onto the probe, it can interfere with light absorption and produce a false reading. In order to reduce the risk of an inaccurate reading, the medical assistant can turn down or turn off the lights while performing the procedure, or can shield the probe by covering it with a towel or dry wash cloth.
- Callused Digit: A callused digit (finger or toe) can cause an inaccurate reading due to poor perfusion in the area. Try moving the probe to a digit that is not callused or to an earlobe.
- Nail Polish and Nail Overlays: These items can prevent light transmission. Nail polish should be removed from the digit on which the testing is being performed. If the patient has artificial nails, another acceptable location should be selected.
- Patient Movement: Patient movement may cause the electrode to loosen, making it difficult for the probe to pick up a signal. The patient should be instructed to remain still during testing. If patient movement is unavoidable due to uncontrollable tremors or other factors, the probe should be attached to a site that is not affected by movement such as the earlobe or toes.
- Dried Blood, Dirt, or Oil: These items can interfere with light absorption. Make certain that the site is cleansed prior to probe application.
- Applying the Probe on an Extremity with Poor Perfusion: If the patient's digit is cold or there is vasoconstriction in the area, you will not get an accurate reading. Have the patient warm their hands prior to testing or select a site where perfusion is better.

Sputum Collection

The medical assistant will be responsible for obtaining a sputum specimen for a culture or a smear. **Sputum** is a fluid that is produced in the lungs and bronchi. Patients should be told not to use any mouth rinses prior to testing that contain antibacterial agents, as this could interfere with test results. The patient should be encouraged to drink lots of fluids prior to testing to help liquefy the mucus for easier expectoration. Following the test, the medical assistant may want to offer the patient something to drink to rinse out the mouth.

The KOH sputum smear is prepared with potassium hydroxide and may be observed in the office under a microscope. If the office does not have in-house laboratory facilities, it is important for the medical assistant to correctly request a KOH smear if ordered, in place of, or in addition to, a sputum culture.

Miscellaneous Pulmonary Procedures

A variety of testing measures may be instituted to diagnose respiratory disorders. These are performed by a variety of professionals. The type of testing used will be dependent on the patient's symptoms.

Chest X-Ray

Chest X-ray (Figure 15-13) is used for routine screening as well as for diagnostic purposes. It utilizes a very small amount of radiation.

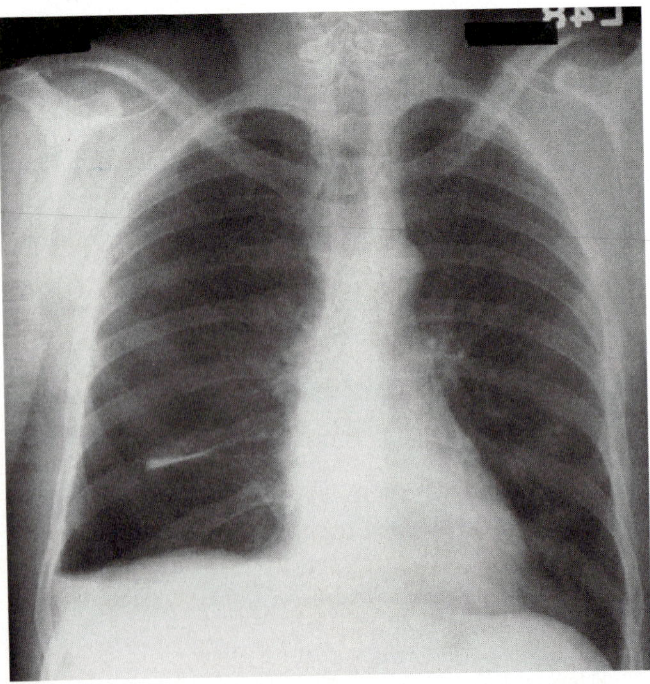

Figure 15-13 ■ A chest X-ray.

Chest CT

The **chest CT** utilizes higher amounts of radiation to provide images of the lungs in cross-sections as the computer rotates completely around the body. Refer to Chapter 29 for a full explanation of a CT scan.

Magnetic Resonance Imaging (MRI)

An MRI uses radio waves and magnets to produce cross-sectional images of the inside of the body. Problems with patients who suffer from claustrophobia must be considered when ordering this type of examination. Refer to Chapter 29 for further information on MRI studies.

Bronchoscopy

During a **bronchoscopy**, a bronchoscope, which is a long flexible tube, is passed through the mouth, down the trachea, and into the bronchi to examine specific structures within the airway. The scope can also be used to remove foreign bodies, identify tumors, obtain culture material, or to obtain tissue biopsies. Biopsies can be performed through the bronchoscope to help in the diagnosis of asthma. The patient is commonly sedated for the procedure and the patient's BP, oxygen saturation levels, and heart are monitored throughout the procedure.

Thoracentesis

A **thoracentesis** is a medical procedure used to withdraw fluids from the pleural space (Figure 15-14). This excess fluid is referred to as a **pleural effusion**. The test is performed by a provider, usually following a chest X-ray indicating excess fluid accumulation. Following injection of an anesthetic agent, a needle is inserted into the lung and the fluid is aspirated by syringe and transferred to a sterile container. The fluid is then analyzed at the laboratory.

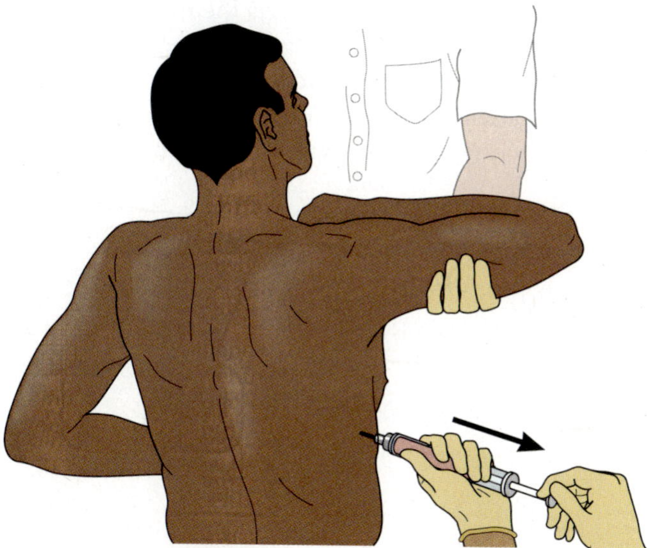

Figure 15-14 ■ Thoracentesis is performed to remove fluid from the pleural cavity.

Sleep Study (Polysomnogram)

The term **sleep apnea** refers to periods of breathing cessation during hours of sleep. While there are three types of sleep apnea (obstructive, central, or mixed), the most common type is obstructive sleep apnea. When a person lies down to sleep, the muscles of the throat and the tongue relax, which can partially block the airway. Major symptoms of this disorder are loud snoring and daytime fatigue and somnolence.

When a patient stops breathing during sleep, it reduces the amount of oxygen in the blood, which, over time, can lead to serious complications such as high blood pressure, heart attack, or stroke.

Sleep apnea is normally diagnosed through a sleep study, which may take place at a sleep center. Electrodes, placed on the patient's scalp and other locations of the body, are hooked up to equipment that records the patient's breathing, snoring, brainwaves, heart rate, leg movements, and eye movements while sleeping. The recording is then evaluated by a sleep specialist and a treatment plan is implemented if sleep apnea is detected. Mild forms of sleep apnea may be treated by instituting a weight loss program for the patient, while moderate to severe cases are treated with a device known as a continuous positive airway pressure (CPAP) machine that keeps the airway open during sleep.

Mantoux Skin Test (PPD Testing)

A **Mantoux skin test** is a common screening test for TB, in which 0.1 ml of tuberculin solution [purified protein derivative (PPD)] is injected intradermally, usually in the forearm, to form a raised wheal (Figure 15-15). The injection site is then examined within 48–72 hours of PPD placement. Development of **induration** (hardening of normally soft tissue) of 5 mm or more (Figure 15-16)

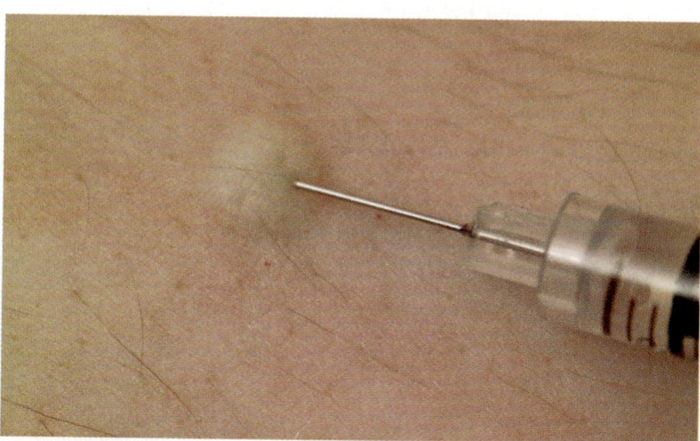

Figure 15-15 ■ A wheal should appear on the surface of the arm following an intradermal injection.

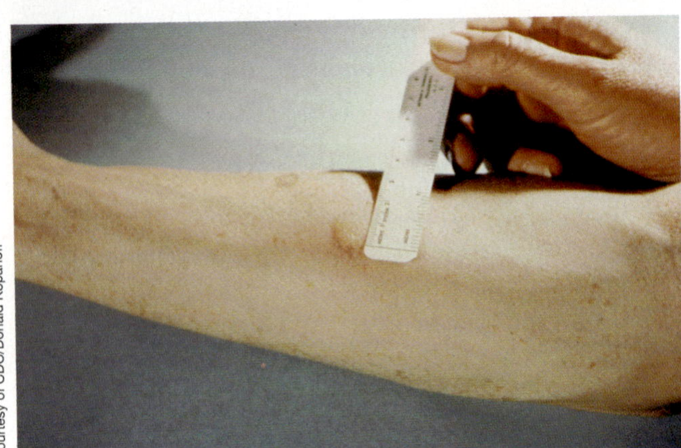
Courtesy of CDC/Donald Kopanoff

Figure 15-16 ■ Measure induration.

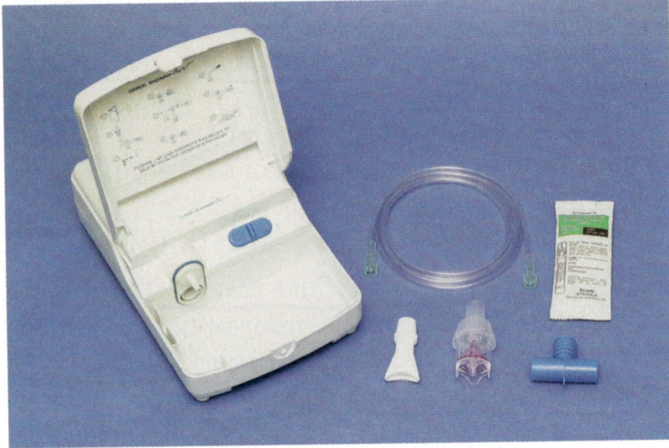

Figure 15-17 ■ A nebulizer is used to administer breathing treatments.

may be considered a positive test, which can indicate TB infection. Erythema alone is *not* measured. Confirmation is done through chest X-ray, sputum collection, or Quantiferon-TB Gold (QFT-G) blood testing.

COMMON PULMONARY TREATMENTS AND MEDICATIONS

There are two forms of inhaled therapy in which medications are delivered directly to the lungs: nebulizers and inhalers.

Nebulizers

Nebulizers (Figure 15-17) are units that change liquid medication into an aerosol mist so that it can be inhaled through a mouthpiece or face mask. Nebulizers are used for the treatment of asthma and other lung conditions. Common types of medications delivered through a nebulizer include anticholinergics, bronchodilators, and corticosteroids.

Nebulizers consists of four major components:

- Compressor: Converts the liquid into a mist and powers the nebulizer
- Nebulizer Tubing: Connects the mouthpiece to the compressor
- Medication Cup: Houses the medication
- Mouthpiece or Face Mask: Delivers the medication into the patient's respiratory system

Nebulizers can be used both in the office and at home. Breathing treatments typically last 15 to 30 minutes. The prescribed medication is properly prepared and poured into the medication cup. The lid is placed and tightened onto the medication cup and connected to the mouthpiece. The underside of the medication cup is connected to the tubing, which is then connected to the compressor. The patient is instructed to place the mouthpiece between the teeth and to purse the lips around the mouthpiece. The patient is encouraged to take in deep breaths lasting two to three seconds throughout the treatment. Once there is no aerosol being produced, the treatment is stopped. Patients should be encouraged to take in deep breaths and cough following the treatment to loosen the secretions. Refer to Procedure 15-5 for a procedure on how to administer a nebulizer treatment.

Inhalers

Inhalers are handheld portable devices that deliver medication directly to the lungs. There are two basic types of inhalers:

- **Metered-Dose Inhalers (MDI)** (Figure 15-18): These inhalers use a chemical propellant to push the medication out of the inhaler. The medication is delivered to the patient's lungs by direct inhalation or by squeezing the canister. Squeezing the top of the canister converts the medication into a fine mist. These inhalers require the patient to squeeze the canister and inhale at the same time. Some patients find this difficult. The dry powder inhalers might be a better choice for those patients.

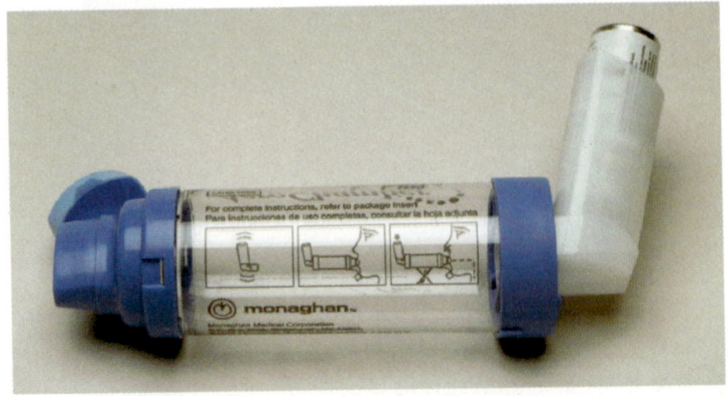

Figure 15-18 ■ An aerosol meter dosed inhaler (MDI).

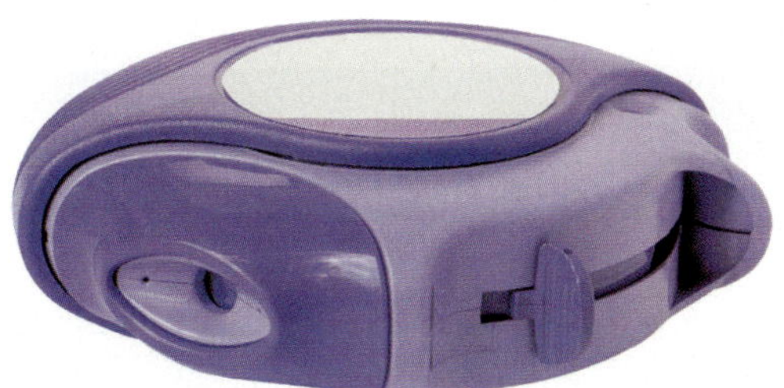

Figure 15-19 ■ A diskus dry powder inhaler. © sumroeng chinnapan /www.Shutterstock.com.

- Dry-Powder Inhalers (Figure 15-19): This type of inhaler does not use a chemical propellant to push the medication out of the inhaler so the patient has to take in rapid inhalations to receive the medication.

Patients who perform in-home nebulizer treatments or who use inhalers should routinely check their peak flow readings. Readings should be performed a minimum of two to three times per week and any time the patient has symptoms. Peak flow measurements should be documented both before and following nebulizer and inhaler treatments.

Oxygen Administration

Oxygen is a colorless, odorless gas that is essential to life. The air that we breathe contains approximately 21% oxygen. Normal oxygen saturation levels range between 96% and 100%; however, a continuous oxygen level saturation of 100% can cause organ toxicity. If oxygen levels drop in the blood, it's difficult for the tissues of the heart to keep pumping. Oxygen therapy is indicated in conditions where the oxygen saturation falls below an acceptable range, usually below 96%.

Even though oxygen is considered a gas, when it is administered to supplement what is normally taken in by atmospheric air, it is considered to be a drug.

The medical assistant may be responsible for gathering the equipment for oxygen therapy and may even be responsible for administering oxygen in some practices; however, the provider or nurse in the practice is usually responsible for the actual administration of oxygen.

Legal Issues to Consider When Administering Oxygen

Because every state has its own guidelines for medication administration, including oxygen delivery, medical assistants should check the law in the state in which they are employed to determine if they are permitted to administer oxygen. Some states are very specific about medication administration, while others are vague. When in doubt, check with the AAMA or AMT for specific guidelines.

Health Coach

Metered-Dose Inhaler (MDI)

Patients should be instructed on how to use a metered-dose inhaler (MDI) using the following steps:

1. Wash your hands very well before starting the procedure. (Bacteria on the hands can be transferred to the mouthpiece or medication cup and delivered into the lungs.)
2. Remove the cap and hold the medication in an upright position. Shake the canister well to properly mix the medication.
3. Open your mouth and hold the canister approximately 1 inch from your mouth. (The gas propellant in the canister can cause the medication to bounce off the throat and into your mouth instead of propelling down toward the lungs.) A spacer, which is a short tube that attaches to the inhaler, may be used to assist with the delivery of the medication. A spacer keeps the medication in the plastic tube for a few seconds following depression so that you have more time to inhale.
4. If not using a spacer, press down on the inhaler one time while breathing in slowly through your mouth. If using a spacer, depress the inhaler and wait a few seconds before inhaling slowly through your mouth.
5. Breathe in slowly for three to five seconds. After breathing in the medication, hold your breath for a total of 10 seconds to allow the medication to reach the lungs.
6. Repeat steps 2 to 6 until the prescribed amount of puffs have been delivered. (You should wait approximately 1 minute between each puff.)
7. Only take the prescribed amount of medication. Taking more medication than prescribed can cause serious side effects. If you start to feel a tingling sensation in your hands and feet or start to feel light-headed, you probably took too much medication and should call the physician right away. If the attack is not relieved by the prescribed number of doses, you should call the EMS.

Table 15-4 Common Pulmonary Medications

Medication Classifications	Description	Medication Examples
Bronchodilators	Drugs that dilate the bronchi and bronchioles. Used in asthma and COPD. There are three main categories: • Beta2-agonists: Short-acting forms are often considered a "rescue inhaler" for acute symptoms; long-acting forms may be part of maintenance therapy. • Anticholinergics: Drugs used in asthma and COPD to block smooth muscle contraction in the airways • Theophylline: Drug used in asthma and COPD to relax bronchial smooth muscle. Considered its own category of bronchodilator.	Short-acting: Ventolin HFA, ProAir HFA, and Proventil HFA Long-acting: Serevent Foradil, and Perforomist Tiotropium (long-acting—inhaled or injected); Atrovent, Apovent, Ipraxa, Aerovent, and Rinatec Theophylline (long-acting—oral or injectable). Usually used in hard to manage cases due to numerous side effects.
Corticosteroids (inhaled)	Anti-inflammatory drugs used daily to keep swelling and mucus production in the airways at bay. Considered a maintenance therapy for asthma and COPD.	Flovent; Pulmicort; Alvesco; Asmanex, Azmax; Beclovent, and Qvar
Corticosteroids (IM, IV, PO)	Anti-inflammatory drugs utilized for more rapid onset of action in acute exacerbations.	Deltasone; Medrol, Depo-Medrol, Solu-Medrol, and Decadron
Combination bronchodilator/ corticosteroid inhalers	Bronchodilators and corticosteroids combined into one medication. Both bronchoconstriction and inflammation are reduced with administration of one medication.	Combivent; Duoneb; Advair; and Symbicort
Leukotriene modifiers	Oral agent used in asthma to relax smooth muscle and decrease inflammation.	Singulair; Accolate
Anti-IgE	Injectable immunological agent that blocks immunoglobulin E, a substance that plays an important role in allergic asthma.	Xolair
Antibiotics	Drugs used to treat bacterial infections such as pneumonia.	**Penicillins:** Amox (amoxicillin) **Cephalosporins:** Keflex; Rocephin **Macrolides:** Z-pack **Tetracyclines:** Vibramycin **Flouroquinolones:** Avelox, Levaquin **TB-specific antibiotics:** Rifadin, Rimactane, Rifamate, and Rifater
Antivirals	Treat some specific viral infections, such as influenza.	Tamiflu and Relenza

Multiple medications exist to treat respiratory disorders, including oral, injectable, and inhaled drugs. Some treatments act rapidly to treat acute symptoms like those of an asthma exacerbation, while others are slow-acting daily agents intended to prevent exacerbations and maintain lung function. Table 15-4 lists many of these classes of medications.

COMMON LAB TESTS THAT COINCIDE WITH RESPIRATORY DISORDERS

Other methods used to diagnose respiratory disease include examination of blood, sputum, and other fluids from the respiratory tract. Often medications are prescribed based on the results of laboratory tests. The medical assistant must be able to obtain these specimens while maintaining the highest level of infection control in order to prevent the spread of communicable disease. Refer to Procedure 15-4 for more information on obtaining a sputum culture.

Although arterial blood gases (ABGs) are usually drawn by a nurse or a respiratory therapist, it is important for the medical assistant to have an understanding in order to provide some patient instruction and preparation for testing. ABGs are ordered and studied for two general reasons:

- To evaluate the health of the respiratory system
- To study the effectiveness of oxygen therapy

ABGs are considered to be a more accurate measurement of oxygen saturation than pulse oximetry. When saturation levels are dangerously low, ABGs should be the preferred testing for oxygen saturation due to the severity of the patient's condition.

Table 15-5 provides some further information on the common lab tests that coincide with respiratory disease.

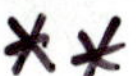

Table 15-5 Common Lab Tests That Coincide with Pulmonary Disorders

Test	Clinical Significance
Sputum culture	Tests for bacteria, blood, or abnormal cells, which can assist in the diagnosis and treatment of various pulmonary disorders.
KOH (a type of sputum smear)	Tests for fungal microorganisms in the respiratory system.
Arterial blood gases (ABGs)	Blood drawn from an artery to measure pH and levels of O_2 and CO_2 in the blood. Used to evaluate the health of the respiratory system and study effectiveness of oxygen therapy.

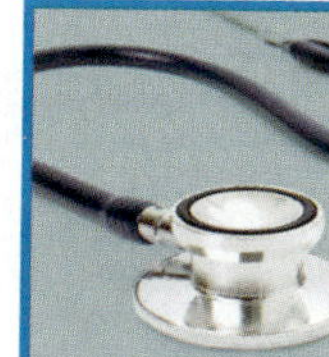

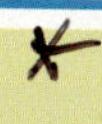

Field Smarts

Patients who have elevated levels of carbon monoxide in the bloodstream may have falsely elevated oxygen saturation levels. Carbon monoxide turns arterial blood bright red, which can trigger the pulse oximeter to display elevated SpO_2 readings. Patients who smoke usually have higher levels of carbon monoxide in the blood due to the presence of carbon monoxide in the cigarettes; therefore, oximetry readings on smokers should be followed up with arterial blood gases when possible. Medical documentation should state the time of the patient's last cigarette, prior to testing. In cases where the patient recently smoked and blood gases are not an option, the provider may want to follow up with SpO_2 readings performed at different time intervals or with continuous monitoring.

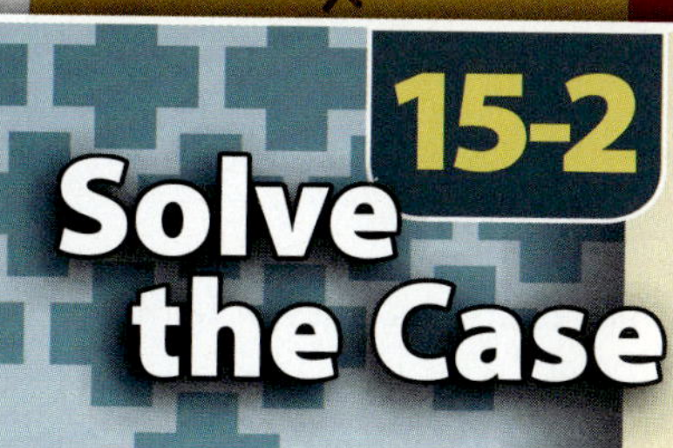

The provider informs Ms. Calhoun that her symptoms suggest an acute asthma exacerbation and orders a nebulizer treatment of albuterol with a repeat pulse oximetry reading 15 minutes after the treatment. Within a few minutes of finishing the treatment, Ms. Calhoun's chest tightness has improved and her O_2 sats are now 98%. Her cough is less persistent, but more productive.

1. **Why would Ms. Calhoun's cough be more productive after the treatment?**
2. **Is Ms. Calhoun's oxygen saturation rate now in a normal range?**
3. **What other tests, if any, do you think the provider may consider ordering for this patient?**
4. **Do you think Ms. Calhoun will be discharged with prescription(s) for new medications/treatments today? Which one(s)?**
5. **Do you think any lifestyle changes would be of benefit to the patient in regards to her current symptoms and diagnosis? Which one(s)?**

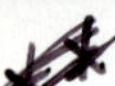

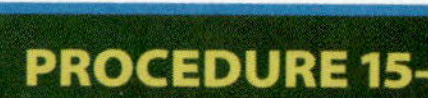

PROCEDURE 15-1

Perform a Spirometry Test

Objective:

To obtain an accurate spirometry reading to evaluate respiratory health and to evaluate medication effectiveness.

Equipment/Supplies:

- Spirometer
- Disposable mouthpiece
- Disposable nose clips
- Disposable tubing
- Spirometer calibration syringe
- Patient's chart/EHR

PROCEDURAL STEPS	DETAILS AND/OR RATIONALE
1. Wash your hands, apply gloves, and gather the equipment.	Washing hands and gloving will help reduce the spread of microorganisms.
2. Calibrate the machine following the manufacturer's instructions.	Calibrating the unit will help to ensure that the machine is working properly.
3. Greet and identify the patient using two identifiers.	Identifying the patient will help to reduce the risk of performing the wrong treatment on the wrong patient.
4. Introduce yourself and ***explain to the patient the rationale for performance of the procedure, showing awareness of the patient's concerns related to the procedure being performed.***	Explaining the procedure helps the patient know what to expect and assists the patient in performing her part of the procedure accurately.
5. Measure the patient's height and weight if not already performed.	This information must be entered into the unit before testing can be performed. (It assists with setting the parameters for expected outcomes.)
6. Have the patient remove constricting clothing, such as belts and sports bras.	Patient comfort will eliminate any constriction that might alter results due to impaired breathing.
7. Position the patient so that the patient is comfortable and safe.	Seating is recommended in case the patient becomes dizzy or faints.
8. Program the unit with the patient's information. Information may include: the patient's name, sex, height, weight, and medication information.	Plugging in this information helps to set the parameters for expected outcome and may transfer data automatically to the electronic health record.
9. Place the nose clip on the patient's nose.	This will prevent air escaping from the nose, which can cause an inaccurate reading.
10. Have the patient inhale as deeply as possible and place the mouthpiece in the mouth. (Some units have the patient take in a deep breath when the tube is in the mouth.) Seal with lips. If the patient has dentures, they are to be left in.	The mouth must be sealed so air does not escape through the lips. This would invalidate the results.

continues

PROCEDURE 15-1 continued

PROCEDURAL STEPS	DETAILS AND/OR RATIONALE
11. Have the patient quickly and forcefully exhale following the prompts on the screen (Figure 15-20). (Press the start button according to manufacturer's instructions.)	It is important to coach the patient during this part of the procedure. For example, "Come on, Mrs. Jones, you can do it, keep it going. Blow … blow … blow."
12. Repeat the test two more times. Record the results from the spirometer and attach the printout to the chart.	Three times shows that the results are reproducible, which is a criterion for accuracy.
13. If ordered, provide medication to the patient.	This test is often used to evaluate the effects of asthma treatments. The test is performed before and after medication for evaluation.
14. Repeat the spirometry procedure, if ordered.	
15. Document or attach the results.	
16. Discard the test products and clean the equipment.	Use recommended precautions with cleaning equipment or discarding in order to prevent contamination.

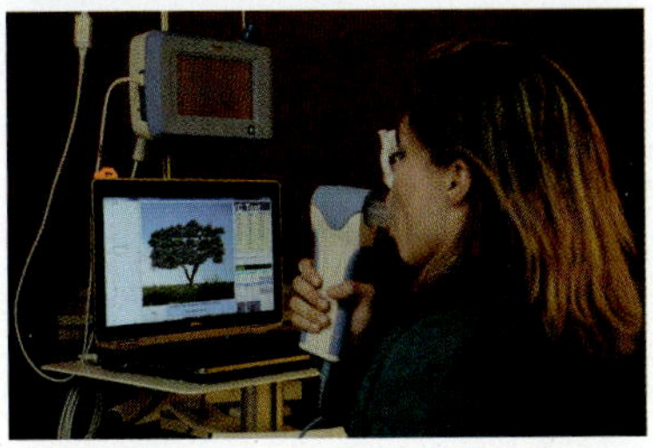

Figure 15-20 ■ Patient seals mouth completely around tube and exhales following the prompts on the screen.

DOCUMENTATION EXAMPLE:

10-14-XX 1430	*Wt. 125 lbs. Ht. 66" T98.8, P 92, R20, BP 142/88: Spirometry testing per Dr. Wong. Dr. Wong ordered inhalation therapy after viewing results: Two puffs of Ventolin administered one minute apart. Spirometry testing repeated. Patient tolerated well. Dr. Wong given the results once again. Results normal. Jacob Green, CMA (AAMA)---------------------------------*

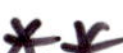

PROCEDURE 15-2

Performing Peak Flow Testing

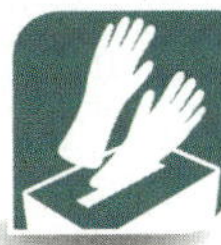

Objective:

To correctly perform peak flow testing, train the patient in home testing, and how to interpret results according to the individualized Asthma Action Plan.

Equipment/Supplies:

- Peak flow meter
- Recording table or graph
- Patient's chart/EHR
- Gloves
- Individualized Asthma Action Plan

continues

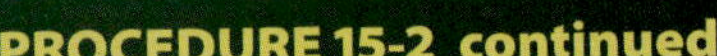

PROCEDURE 15-2 continued

PROCEDURAL STEPS	DETAILS AND/OR RATIONALE
1. Assemble the equipment, including individualized Asthma Action Plan.	Being prepared is a part of professionalism.
2. Identify the patient using two identifiers, introduce yourself, and ***explain the rationale for performance of the procedure, showing awareness of the patient's concerns related to the procedure.***	It is important to always perform the correct procedure on the correct patient.
3. Wash your hands and apply gloves.	Infection control should always be instituted to prevent the spread of microorganisms.
4. Have the patient remove all gum and food from mouth.	This is to avoid any residual food or gum from becoming lodged in the instrument.
5. Start pointer on flow meter at 0.	Starting at 0 is important for an accurate result.
6. Have the patient take in a deep breath.	Filling the lungs fully helps for accuracy.
7. Have the patient place the mouthpiece in mouth behind the teeth, with lips tightly sealed around the tube. Move tongue out of the way.	This enables the air to exit the mouth by the most forceful means.
8. Direct the patient to breathe out as fast and hard as possible (Figure 15-21).	Many patients will not give their full effort without verbal encouragement.
9. Record the results from the gauge; move it back to 0.	Moving the pointer back to 0 each time is important for accuracy.
10. Repeat two more times.	Efforts can be variable.
11. Record the highest reading of the three attempts.	
12. If providing education, give patient peak flow meter, directions and results of personal best reading to take home.	
13. Reference personal best value with their Asthma Action Plan to determine if a change in treatment is indicated at the present time.	It is important for patients to understand how their peak flow reading can help them to better manage their disease.

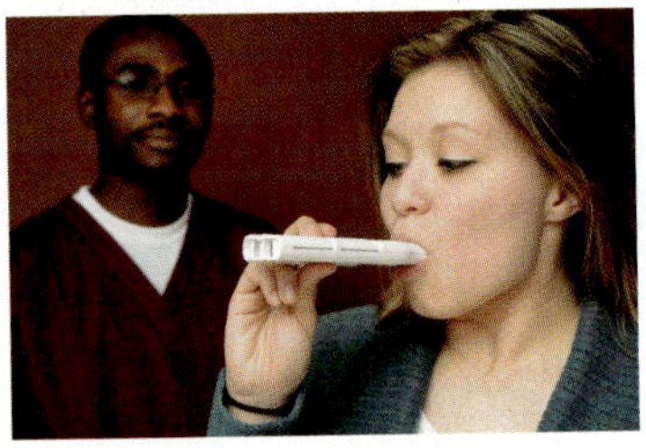

Figure 15-21 ■ The patient is breathing as hard and fast as possible.

DOCUMENTATION EXAMPLE:

10-14-XX 1430	Peak-flow testing practice session per Dr. Joe. Patient performed the test accurately. Patient's highest peak flow reading today was 423. Patient given peak flow meter and instructions to take with her. Asthma Action Plan individualized for patient by Dr. Joe so that patient may know when it is necessary to use her Ventolin inhaler. Kelly Barrett, CMA (AAMA)--

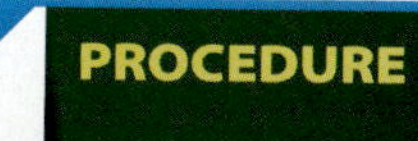

PROCEDURE 15-3

Perform Pulse Oximetry

Objective:

To correctly apply a pulse oximeter to the patient and obtain an accurate reading.

Equipment/Supplies:

- Pulse oximeter unit/finger probe
- Nail polish remover/cotton ball (if indicated)
- Soap/towel
- Patient's chart/EHR

PROCEDURAL STEPS	DETAILS AND/OR RATIONALE
1. Identify the patient using two identifiers, and introduce yourself.	
2. Wash your hands and ***explain to the patient the rationale for performance of the procedure, showing awareness of the patient's concerns related to the procedure being performed.***	Explaining the procedure helps the patient know what to expect and assists the patient in performing her part of the procedure accurately.
3. Have the patient remove nail polish, if necessary, and wash the hands with soap and water. Hands should be rinsed well and dried.	Washing the hands will remove any lotions or grease that could interfere with the results. Nail polish can also interfere with the results.
4. Apply the pulse oximeter probe (Figure 15-22) and observe the perfusion indicator. Observe both the heart rate and the SpO_2 levels.	Make certain that you obtain a proper reading. If the probe is not attached correctly, the unit will not work.
5. Leave the oximeter probe attached to the patient and give the findings to the provider. If the saturation rate is below 95%, notify the provider as soon as possible.	An oxygen saturation below 95% can cause harm to the patient.
6. Continue to monitor as long as the provider wants the patient monitored. (The patient may need to receive oxygen if oxygen is poor.)	If the patient is in respiratory distress, the oximeter probe will remain in place until all symptoms are resolved.
7. Remove the probe once the provider orders the probe to be removed.	
8. Record the results in the chart and assist the patient.	

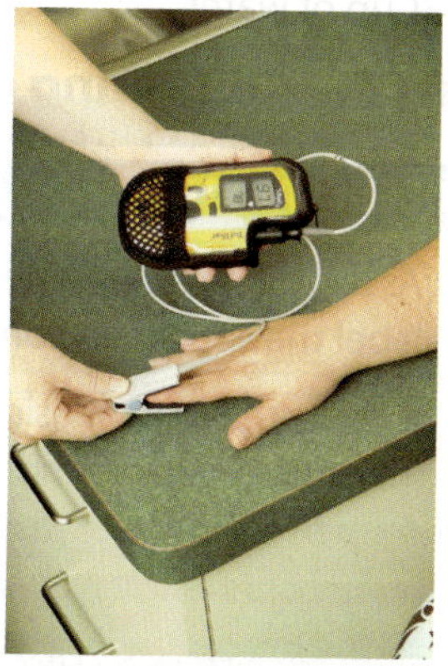

Figure 15-22 ■ The medical assistant places the pulse oximeter probe on the patient's finger.

DOCUMENTATION EXAMPLE:

02-14-XX 1415	Pulse oximetry per Dr. Simon. Patient washed hands prior to application. Hands completely dried. Applied unit to pt.'s right 3rd digit. Pulse rate: 98, SpO_2 96%. Informed provider of results. Ulisha Thompson, CMA (AAMA)--

PROCEDURE 15-5 continued

PROCEDURAL STEPS	DETAILS AND/OR RATIONALE
3. Wash your hands and put on gloves.	This step decreases the spread of microorganisms.
4. Check order (three times) and pour the correct amount of medication and diluent into the medication dispenser. Screw the lid on the dispenser and gently mix the medication (Figure 15-24).	It is important to make certain that you have the correct medication and that it was mixed correctly to ensure the patient is getting the correct dosage of medication.
5. Connect the medication dispenser to the mouthpiece or face mask.	
6. Connect the disposable tubing to the medication dispenser and nebulizer.	
7. Place the patient in a full Fowler's position or upright position.	This is to help the medication disperse correctly.
8. Turn the nebulizer on. When you turn the nebulizer on, you should see a mist.	The mist will show you that the nebulizer is working properly.
9. If using a face mask, place it over the patient's face so that it fits comfortably. If using a mouthpiece, instruct patient to place it in the mouth between the teeth and to purse the lips over the mouthpiece making a seal.	The mouthpiece or face mask has to be applied properly in order for the patient to get the full effect of the medication.
10. Instruct the patient to take in slow deep breaths (Figure 15-25) that last anywhere from two to three seconds.	This helps the medication to disperse throughout the respiratory tract.
11. Continue treatment until the mist disappears.	When the mist disappears it means the medicine has been used up.
12. Turn off the nebulizer and remove and dispose of the mouthpiece or face mask, medicine dispenser, and tubing into the biohazard trash can.	This step stops the spread of microorganisms.
13. Instruct the patient to take in several deep breaths and to try and cough up any secretions that were loosened during the treatment.	Bringing up the secretions will help clear the obstruction.
14. Wash your hands and document the procedure.	
15. Give the patient home care instructions.	Patients will usually need to be instructed on home care instructions to assist them in getting better.

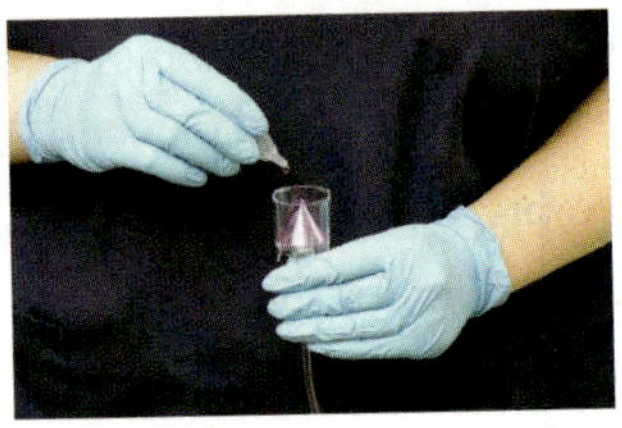

Figure 15-24 ■ The medical assistant pours the medication for the breathing treatment into the medication cup.

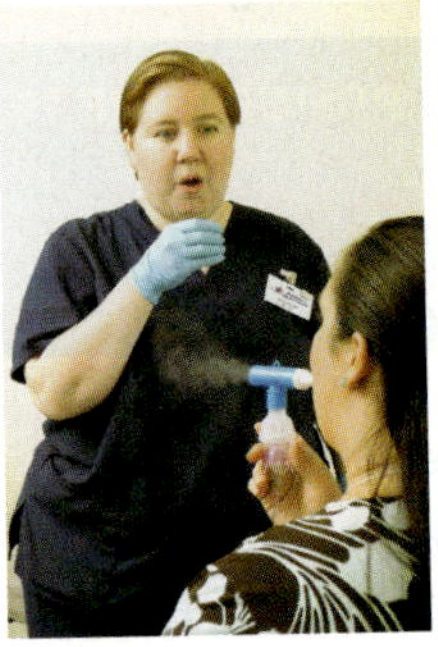

Figure 15-25 ■ The patient is instructed to take in slow deep breaths during the treatment.

PROCEDURE 15-4 continued

Part B—Preparing the Smear

(If the provider orders a smear to be made with the specimen)

PROCEDURAL STEPS	DETAILS AND/OR RATIONALE
1. Wash hands, apply PPE, and label the slide. Smear the sputum on a microscopic slide.	This will be used to observe possible fungal cells in the sputum.
2. Squeeze one drop of potassium hydroxide over the smear and place a cover slip over the smear.	The potassium hydroxide assists with identifying specific types of fungus.
3. Place the slide under the microscope on low power for the provider.	This is done so the provider can identify the microorganism.
4. Clean the area and remove PPE. Throw PPE into appropriate trash or biohazard container.	

DOCUMENTATION EXAMPLE:

1-3-XX 1000	Sputum specimen obtained for a KOH per Dr. Stevens. Substantial amt. blood mixed with sample. Delivered to lab with request. Jessica Hunnicutt, CMA (AAMA)-------------

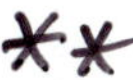

PROCEDURE 15-5
Administer a Nebulizer Treatment

Objective:

To correctly set up the nebulizer unit, select the correct medication, and administer a breathing treatment using a nebulizer.

Equipment/Supplies:

- Nebulizer
- Disposable connecting tubing
- Medication/diluent (if applicable)
- Disposable mouthpiece or face mask
- Disposable medication dispenser
- Patient's chart/EHR

PROCEDURAL STEPS	DETAILS AND/OR RATIONALE
1. Prepare the equipment.	Plugging in the nebulizer before beginning the procedure will save time and confirm that the equipment is working correctly.
2. Identify the patient using two identifiers, introduce yourself, and ***explain to the patient the rationale for performance of the procedure, showing awareness of the patient's concerns related to the procedure being performed.***	It is important to establish that you have the correct patient for safety reasons. Explaining the procedure promotes better compliance.

continues

PROCEDURE 15-5 continued

PROCEDURAL STEPS	DETAILS AND/OR RATIONALE
3. Wash your hands and put on gloves.	This step decreases the spread of microorganisms.
4. Check order (three times) and pour the correct amount of medication and diluent into the medication dispenser. Screw the lid on the dispenser and gently mix the medication (Figure 15-24).	It is important to make certain that you have the correct medication and that it was mixed correctly to ensure the patient is getting the correct dosage of medication.
5. Connect the medication dispenser to the mouthpiece or face mask.	
6. Connect the disposable tubing to the medication dispenser and nebulizer.	
7. Place the patient in a full Fowler's position or upright position.	This is to help the medication disperse correctly.
8. Turn the nebulizer on. When you turn the nebulizer on, you should see a mist.	The mist will show you that the nebulizer is working properly.
9. If using a face mask, place it over the patient's face so that it fits comfortably. If using a mouthpiece, instruct patient to place it in the mouth between the teeth and to purse the lips over the mouthpiece making a seal.	The mouthpiece or face mask has to be applied properly in order for the patient to get the full effect of the medication.
10. Instruct the patient to take in slow deep breaths (Figure 15-25) that last anywhere from two to three seconds.	This helps the medication to disperse throughout the respiratory tract.
11. Continue treatment until the mist disappears.	When the mist disappears it means the medicine has been used up.
12. Turn off the nebulizer and remove and dispose of the mouthpiece or face mask, medicine dispenser, and tubing into the biohazard trash can.	This step stops the spread of microorganisms.
13. Instruct the patient to take in several deep breaths and to try and cough up any secretions that were loosened during the treatment.	Bringing up the secretions will help clear the obstruction.
14. Wash your hands and document the procedure.	
15. Give the patient home care instructions.	Patients will usually need to be instructed on home care instructions to assist them in getting better.

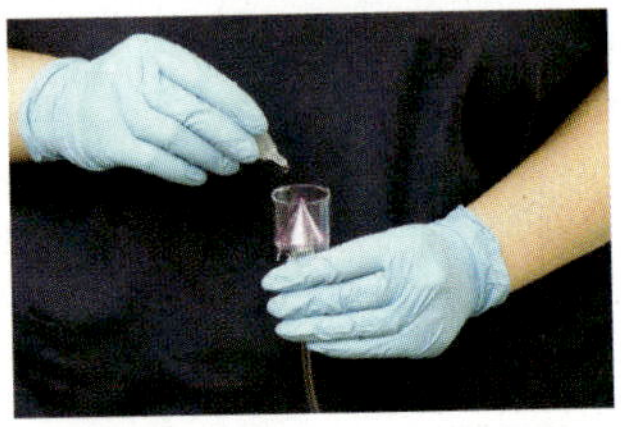

Figure 15-24 ■ The medical assistant pours the medication for the breathing treatment into the medication cup.

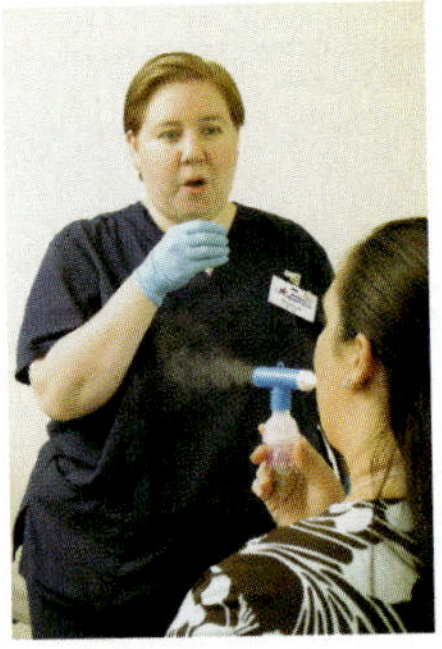

Figure 15-25 ■ The patient is instructed to take in slow deep breaths during the treatment.

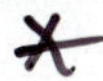

PROCEDURE 15-3

Perform Pulse Oximetry

Objective:

To correctly apply a pulse oximeter to the patient and obtain an accurate reading.

Equipment/Supplies:

- Pulse oximeter unit/finger probe
- Nail polish remover/cotton ball (if indicated)
- Soap/towel
- Patient's chart/EHR

PROCEDURAL STEPS	DETAILS AND/OR RATIONALE
1. Identify the patient using two identifiers, and introduce yourself.	
2. Wash your hands and ***explain to the patient the rationale for performance of the procedure, showing awareness of the patient's concerns related to the procedure being performed.***	Explaining the procedure helps the patient know what to expect and assists the patient in performing her part of the procedure accurately.
3. Have the patient remove nail polish, if necessary, and wash the hands with soap and water. Hands should be rinsed well and dried.	Washing the hands will remove any lotions or grease that could interfere with the results. Nail polish can also interfere with the results.
4. Apply the pulse oximeter probe (Figure 15-22) and observe the perfusion indicator. Observe both the heart rate and the SpO_2 levels.	Make certain that you obtain a proper reading. If the probe is not attached correctly, the unit will not work.
5. Leave the oximeter probe attached to the patient and give the findings to the provider. If the saturation rate is below 95%, notify the provider as soon as possible.	An oxygen saturation below 95% can cause harm to the patient.
6. Continue to monitor as long as the provider wants the patient monitored. (The patient may need to receive oxygen if oxygen is poor.)	If the patient is in respiratory distress, the oximeter probe will remain in place until all symptoms are resolved.
7. Remove the probe once the provider orders the probe to be removed.	
8. Record the results in the chart and assist the patient.	

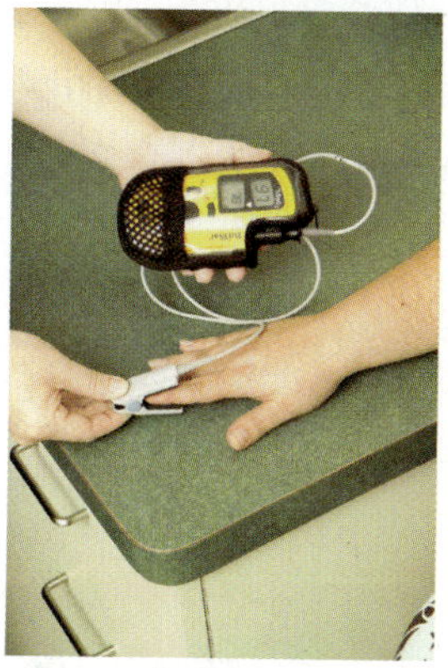

Figure 15-22 ■ The medical assistant places the pulse oximeter probe on the patient's finger.

DOCUMENTATION EXAMPLE:

02-14-XX 1415	Pulse oximetry per Dr. Simon. Patient washed hands prior to application. Hands completely dried. Applied unit to pt.'s right 3rd digit. Pulse rate: 98, SpO_2 96%. Informed provider of results. Ulisha Thompson, CMA (AAMA)--

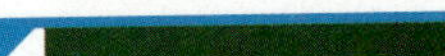

PROCEDURE 15-4

Obtain a Sputum Specimen and Prepare a Smear

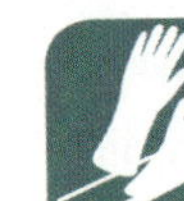

Objective:

To instruct and assist the patient on obtaining a viable sputum specimen that is free of saliva and obtained from deep coughing.

Equipment/Supplies:

- Sterile sputum cup with lid
- Gloves
- Mask
- Waterproof gown
- Goggles
- Cup of water
- Specimen cup with requisition form
- Microscopic slide
- Potassium hydroxide (KOH)
- Patient's chart/EHR

Part A—Obtaining a Sputum Specimen

PROCEDURAL STEPS	DETAILS AND/OR RATIONALE
1. Assemble the equipment and properly label the specimen container.	The patient's name and birth date should be on the cup. Date and time of collection should also be recorded.
2. Identify the patient using two identifiers, introduce yourself, and ***explain the rationale for performance of the procedure, showing awareness of the patient's concerns related to the procedure being performed.***	You want to make certain that you have the correct patient. Explaining the procedure will help the patient in attaining a proper specimen on the first try.
3. Wash your hands and put on all of your PPE.	The patient sometimes will throw up as a result of obtaining the specimen. The PPE is to protect you from splatter.
4. Have the patient rinse out the mouth.	This will get rid of any residual food in the mouth.
5. Carefully remove the lid from the specimen cup and place on the counter without contaminating it.	Contaminating the lid can ruin the test.
6. Instruct the patient to take in three deep breaths and to start forcefully coughing (Figure 15-23A).	Deep coughing will produce a better specimen.
7. Ask patient to expectorate into the center of the specimen container (Figure 15-23B).	This keeps the secretions from running down the sides of the container.
8. Place the lid on the container without contaminating it and tighten it securely. Place the container in a plastic laboratory specimen bag.	Following proper standard precautions helps to reduce disease transmission.
9. Insert the completed lab slip and send to the lab for analysis.	Make sure the lab request name matches the specimen cup for accuracy. Include the appropriate diagnosis codes so that the results will be as expedient as possible.

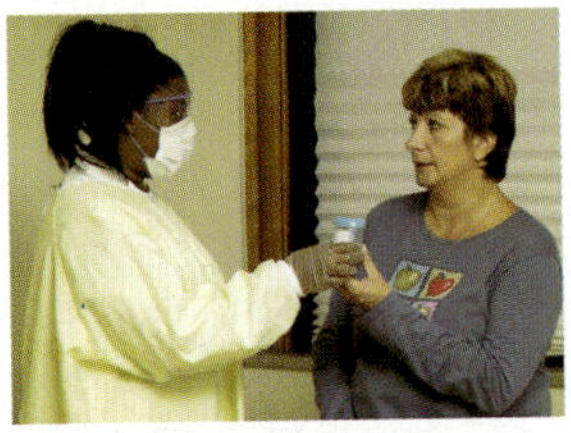

Figure 15-23A ■ The patient is instructed to take three deep breaths before beginning the collection.

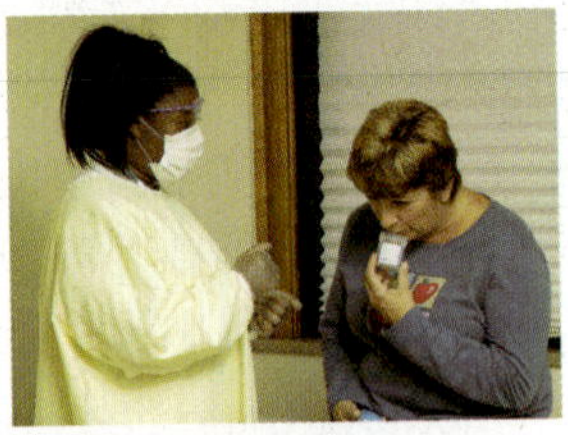

Figure 15-23B ■ The patient should expectorate directly into the cup and avoid contaminating the inner portion of the cup with the mouth or fingers.

continues

DOCUMENTATION EXAMPLE:

12-12-XX 1800	Nebulizer treatment, Albuterol, 2.5 mg per Dr. Jones. Pt. tolerated procedure well. Following treatment patient brought up some mucus secretions that were white and tinged with a bit of green mucus. Pt. reported feeling much better following the treatment. Provider followed up with pt. Jay Craig, RMA (AMT)--

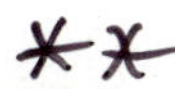

CHAPTER SUMMARY

- The respiratory system consists of the lungs and trachea, mouth, and nose. It has two main functions: to obtain necessary oxygen to fuel the body's cells, and to excrete carbon dioxide waste products from the body.
- Gas exchange takes place in the alveoli. Oxygen from inhaled air enters the bloodstream via tiny capillaries surrounding each alveolus. Carbon dioxide, a waste product of the body, is released from the capillaries into the alveoli and then exhaled.
- There are three primary specialists who diagnose and treat lung disorders: pulmonologists, cardiothoracic surgeons, and respiratory therapists.
- Common diseases of the respiratory system include contagious infections, tuberculosis, lung cancer, emphysema, and asthma.
- Common respiratory procedures include pulmonary function testing, peak flow testing (PFT), and pulse oximetry testing.
- Expected outcomes of pulmonary function testing are as follows: normal PFT outcomes: 85% or higher of the predicted value; mild disease: 65–84% of predicted values; moderate disease: 50–64% of predicted values; severe disease: Less than 50% of the predicted values.
- The Asthma Action Plan is a tool that helps patients self-manage their treatment by using peak flow readings to determine what zone they fall into at the time of testing.
- Respiratory diagnostic tests include radiological examinations such as chest X-ray, CT, and MRI; bronchoscopy; thoracentesis; Mantoux skin test (PPD testing); and sleep apnea studies—overnight study in which electrodes are placed to measure heart rate, respirations, oxygen saturation, and eye movement during sleep.
- Common respiratory treatments need a provider order and include nebulizer treatments, inhalers, and oxygen therapy.
- Common pulmonary medications can be found in Table 15-4, and common pulmonary laboratory tests are found in Table 15-5.
- An important role for medical assistants is to educate patients and to direct them to appropriate resources.

CERTIFICATION REVIEW QUESTIONS

1. Common testing procedures for the diagnosis of tuberculosis include:
   a. Mantoux testing.
   b. vital capacity.
   c. Both of the above
   d. None of the above
2. Which of the following occurs during respiration?
   a. Oxygen enters the body.
   b. Carbon dioxide leaves the body.
   c. Digestion is aided.
   d. Both a and b
3. A procedure that involves looking through a flexible tube to visualize the lungs is called a(n):
   a. colonoscopy.
   b. X-ray.
   c. MRI.
   d. bronchoscopy.
4. Spirometry is used to:
   a. obtain a blood specimen.
   b. help diagnose asthma.
   c. study the effectiveness of the lungs.
   d. Both b and c

5. A treatment in the form of a mist that uses medications to help open up the airways is:
   a. pulse oximetry.
   b. nebulizer.
   c. bronchoscopy.
   d. thoracentesis.
6. According to the Asthma Action Plan, when is a change in asthma treatment first indicated?
   a. When the patient's peak flow changes
   b. When a peak flow reading falls into the red zone
   c. When the patient is experiencing fatigue
   d. When a peak flow reading falls into the yellow zone
7. An available blood test for TB is referred to as:
   a. QFT-G.
   b. PPD.
   c. TB skin.
   d. G-FQT.
8. Which of the following impacts an oxygen saturation level when performing pulse oximetry?
   a. Age of the patient
   b. Nail polish
   c. Temperature of the extremity
   d. Both b and c
9. The most common radiological study to assess the lungs is:
   a. CT.
   b. MRI.
   c. bronchoscopy.
   d. X-ray.
10. Before administering oxygen to a patient, the following is required:
    a. oxygen tank
    b. tubing and delivery system (mask or nasal cannula)
    c. physician order
    d. All of the above

STUDY RESOURCES

Resources to Test and Reinforce Your Knowledge:	
Certification Review Questions	Take this end-of-chapter quiz
Workbook	• Complete the activities for Chapter 15 • Perform the procedures for Chapter 15 using the Competency Checklists
Resources to Promote Critical Thinking:	
***Solve the Case* Activities**	• Consider these case studies and discuss your conclusions
Learning Lab	• Module 15: Respiratory and Circulatory Systems
MindTap	• Complete Chapter 15 readings and activities

REFERENCES

Asthma Action Plan. (2008, July). Retrieved from American Lung Association: http://www.lung.org/lung-disease/asthma/taking-control-of-asthma/AsthmaActionPlan-JUL2008-high-res.pdf

Centers for Disease Control and Prevention. (2014, October). *Trends in Tuberculosis 2012*. Retrieved from Centers for Disease Control and Prevention: http://www.cdc.gov/tb/publications/factsheets/statistics/TBTrends.htm

DrugFacts: Cigarettes and Other Tobacco Products. (2014, September). Retrieved from National Institute on Drug Abuse: http://www.drugabuse.gov/publications/drugfacts/cigarettes-other-tobacco-products

Multidrug-Resistant Tuberculosis. (2014, September). Retrieved from Centers for Disease Control and Prevention: http://www.cdc.gov/tb/publications/factsheets/drtb/mdrtb.htm

National Heart, Lung, and Blood Institute. (n.d.). Retrieved from http://www.nhlbi.nih.gov/health/

Second Hand Smoke. (2014, September). Retrieved from American Cancer Society: http://www.cancer.org/cancer/cancercauses/tobaccocancer/secondhand-smoke

Trends in Tuberculosis. (2014, October). Retrieved from Centers for Disease Control and Prevention: http://www.cdc.gov/tb/publications/factsheets/statistics/TBTrends.htm

What Are the Key Statistics About Lung Cancer? (2014, April 30). Retrieved from American Cancer Society: http://www.cancer.org/cancer/lungcancer-non-smallcell/detailedguide/non-small-cell-lung-cancer-key-statistics

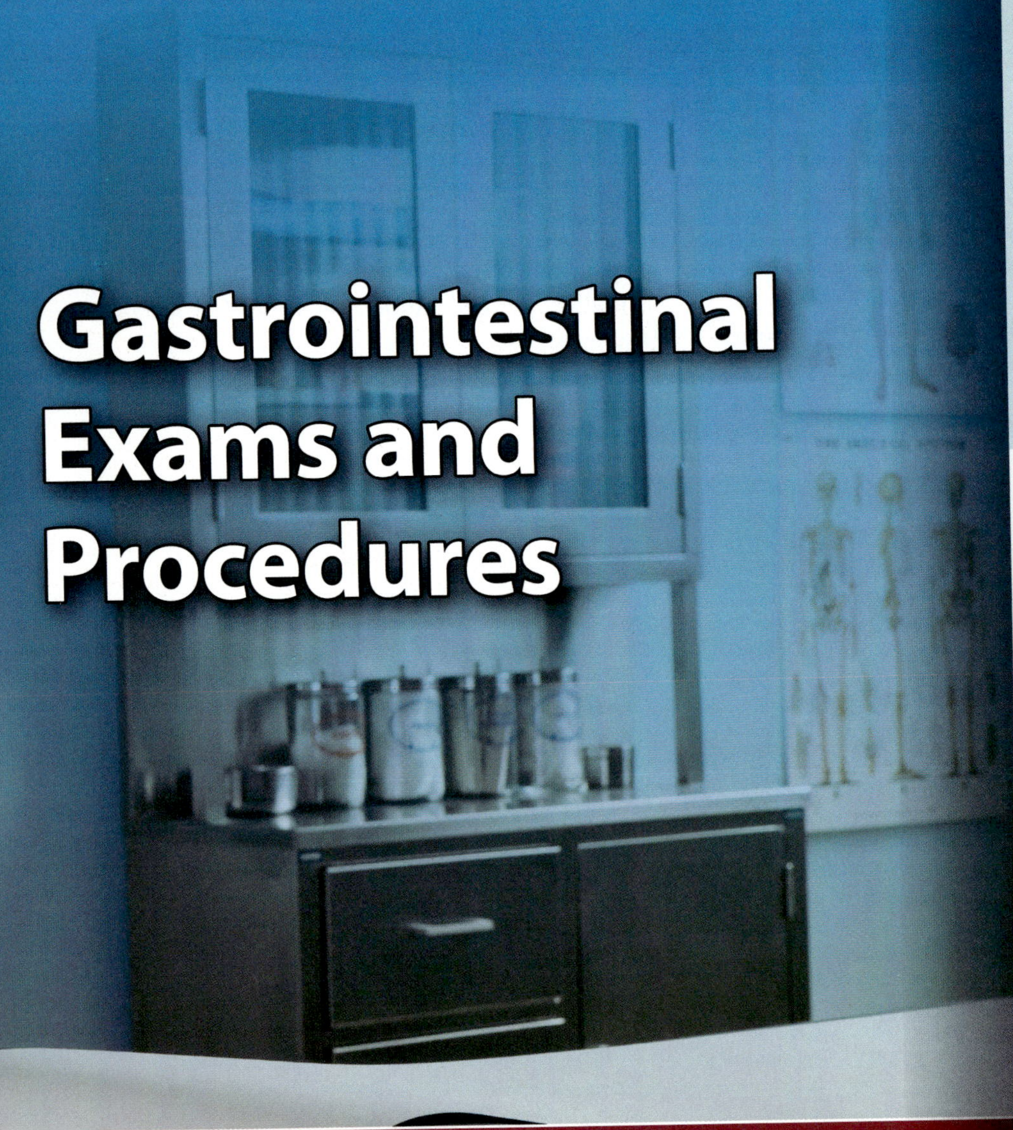

16

Gastrointestinal Exams and Procedures

ESSENTIAL TERMS

anastomosis
anorexia of aging
anoscope
ascites
aspiration pneumonia
colostomy
colonoscopy
constipation
diarrhea
dietitian
endocrinologist
endoscopy
erosion
etiology
fecal occult blood test
fissure
fistula
gastritis
gastroenteritis
gastroenterologist
gastroenterology
gastroesophageal reflux disease (GERD)
hematemesis
hematochezia
hemorrhoids
hepatologist
hiatal hernia
idiopathic
ileostomy
irritable bowel syndrome (IBS)
melena
nonsteroidal anti-inflammatory drug (NSAID)
pancreatitis
peristalsis
polyps
proctologist
proctoscope
rectoscope
sigmoidoscopy
stoma

CHAPTER OUTLINE

Digestive System Snapshot
- Types of Digestion
- Accessory Glands of the Gastrointestinal System

Gastrointestinal Abbreviation Review

Gastrointestinal In-Office and Telephone Screening Tips

Common Gastrointestinal Diseases
- Gastroesophageal Reflux Disease (GERD)
- Ulcerative Colitis and Crohn's Disease
- Cirrhosis
- Colorectal Cancer
- Other Gastrointestinal Conditions

Featured Gastrointestinal Procedures
- Rectal Exams
- Fecal Occult Blood Testing
- Sigmoidoscopy
- Miscellaneous Gastrointestinal Procedures

Common Gastrointestinal Treatments and Medications

Common Lab Tests That Coincide with Gastrointestinal Disorders

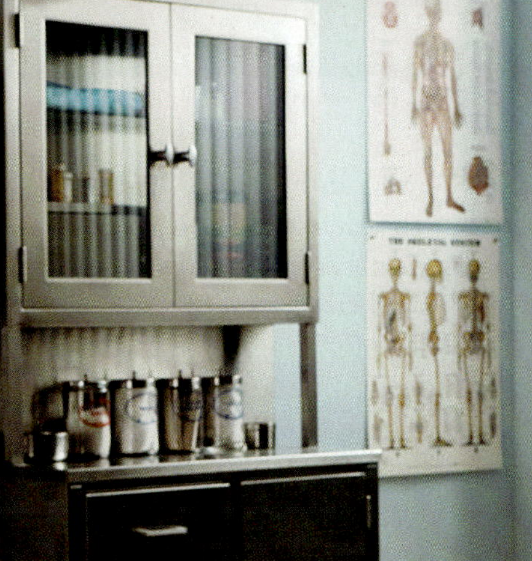

DEVELOPMENTAL OBJECTIVES

After completing this chapter, you should be able to:

1. Correctly spell and define the essential terms.
2. List and provide the anatomical locations of the major structures within the gastrointestinal system.
3. Describe the functions of each structure in the gastrointestinal tract in the process of digestion.
4. List and use common abbreviations associated with the gastrointestinal system.
5. Compile a list of common screening questions that should be asked of patients with gastrointestinal symptoms using established protocols and incorporate critical thinking skills when performing patient assessment.
6. Identify common pathology related to the gastrointestinal system including signs, symptoms, and etiology.
7. Compare structure and function of the gastrointestinal system across the life span.
8. Assist with gastrointestinal procedures, showing awareness of a patient's concerns related to the procedure being performed.
9. Analyze pathology for the gastrointestinal system including diagnostic measures and treatment modalities.
10. Compile a list of common gastrointestinal medication classifications and conclude how each one acts upon body structures to produce a desired effect.
11. Obtain specimens and perform CLIA-waived tests including fecal occult testing.

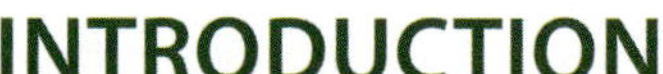

INTRODUCTION

According to the National Digestive Diseases Information Clearinghouse (NDDIC) approximately 60–70 million people suffer from some type of gastrointestinal (GI) disorder, accounting for 48.3 million ambulatory care visits per year.

Disorders of the GI system may have a direct relationship to pathology of other body systems. Often during a routine examination of the patient, complaints of heartburn, abdominal pain, weight fluctuations, or bowel irregularities arise. Laboratory evaluation may indicate dysfunction of organs within or outside of the GI system.

Some tests are noninvasive and can be performed in the office. Testing for occult (hidden) blood in the stool is often assigned to the medical assistant. Various invasive procedures, such as **colonoscopy**, a procedure that examines the colon, are used for diagnosis and treatment, requiring preparation and patient education by the medical assistant. These procedures are performed in a hospital or outpatient facility. Other exams, such as pH monitoring or capsule **endoscopy**, a visual examination of the interior of a body cavity, may be performed within the office setting.

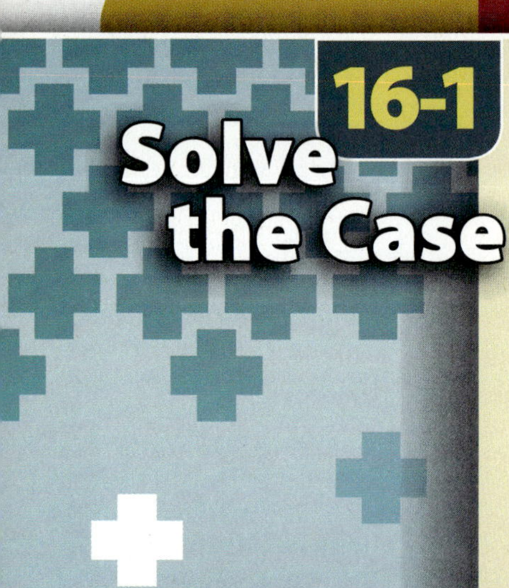

Mr. Reynolds is a 50-year-old man, 5′10″ tall, weighing 280 lb. He has type 2 diabetes and atrial fibrillation and is a heavy smoker. He recently noticed that he has red blood in his stools. Mr. Reynolds complains of abdominal bloating and tenderness. His father died of colon cancer, and now he is worried that he too may have cancer. He is here to have a colonoscopy today. During the history portion of the exam, Mr. Reynolds asks you if you think he has colon cancer. He also asks if his symptoms could be related to anything else.

1. **How should you respond to Mr. Reynolds' question about whether he has colon cancer?**
2. **Do you know of any other diagnoses that may produce similar symptoms?**
3. **What parts of Mr. Reynolds' history increase his risk of colon cancer?**

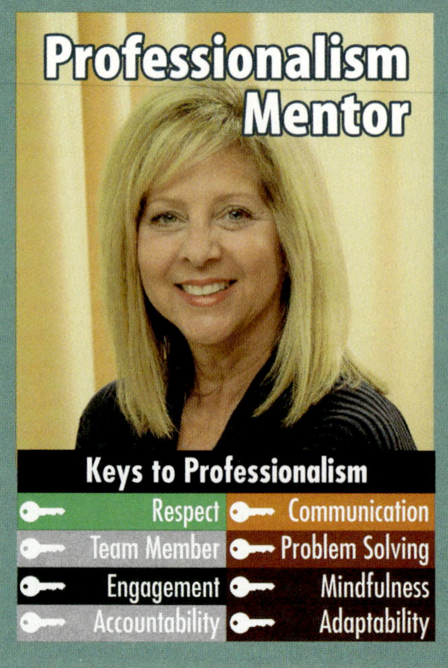

Are you the type of person who can put even the most anxious person at ease? Working in a practice that involves GI procedures requires this skill. Not only can the procedures performed be embarrassing for the patient, but the potential results can make a patient anxious as to what the test may show. Consider the young female who presents to the office with complaints of episodic diarrhea and constipation. Imagine how difficult it is just to talk about it, let alone go through a procedure that is uncomfortable as well as embarrassing. How can you maintain the patient's dignity during an exam that exposes body parts that are considered "private"? Do you acknowledge that the patient may feel uncomfortable and that you understand? All these actions demonstrate clinical empathy toward your patient. Explaining to the patient the importance of the procedure will help the patient trust you and show your concern. You may not realize how much that means to your patient, but it will make even the toughest situation bearable. ■

DIGESTIVE SYSTEM SNAPSHOT

The following are the structures of the digestive system listed in the order in which food and wastes travel:

- Oral cavity
- Esophagus
- Stomach
- Small intestine (consisting of the duodenum, jejunum, and ileum)
- Large intestine (consisting of the sigmoid, ascending, transverse, and descending colon)
- Rectum
- Anus

The digestive system is a long, twisting, hollow tube with an opening at each end (Figure 16-1). The long tube is made of four different layers of tissue including the *mucosa* (innermost layer); *submucosa* (second layer); the *muscularis externa* (third layer); and finally the external layer, the *serosa*, also known as the *visceral peritoneum*, a multilayered membrane that protects and holds the organs in place, within the abdominal cavity. The muscular layer of the GI tract contains both striated and smooth muscle tissue. The striated muscle assists with swallowing and the smooth muscle tissue aids in breaking down food and propelling it through the GI tract, a process referred to as **peristalsis**. Peristalsis is a series of wave-like contractions of the smooth muscles, moving food forward in the digestive tract.

The *peritoneum* is a two-layered membrane: the visceral peritoneum covering the outside of each abdominal organ and the *parietal* layer covering the abdominal cavity. Because of the vastness of this membrane, infection may spread quickly from one organ to another, putting the patient at risk for a widespread infection.

Types of Digestion

The digestive tube has several different names: the *alimentary canal*, the GI tract, and the digestive tract. The major function of the system is digestion by first breaking down food through mechanical and then chemical processes so that nutrients can be absorbed into the bloodstream and utilized by all cells in the body. The final function of the digestive tract is the concentration and elimination of wastes through the act of defecation.

Mechanical digestion is accomplished in the mouth, where food is mechanically broken down into small pieces by the action of the teeth. *Chemical digestion* is initiated in the mouth through the secretion of saliva, which contains

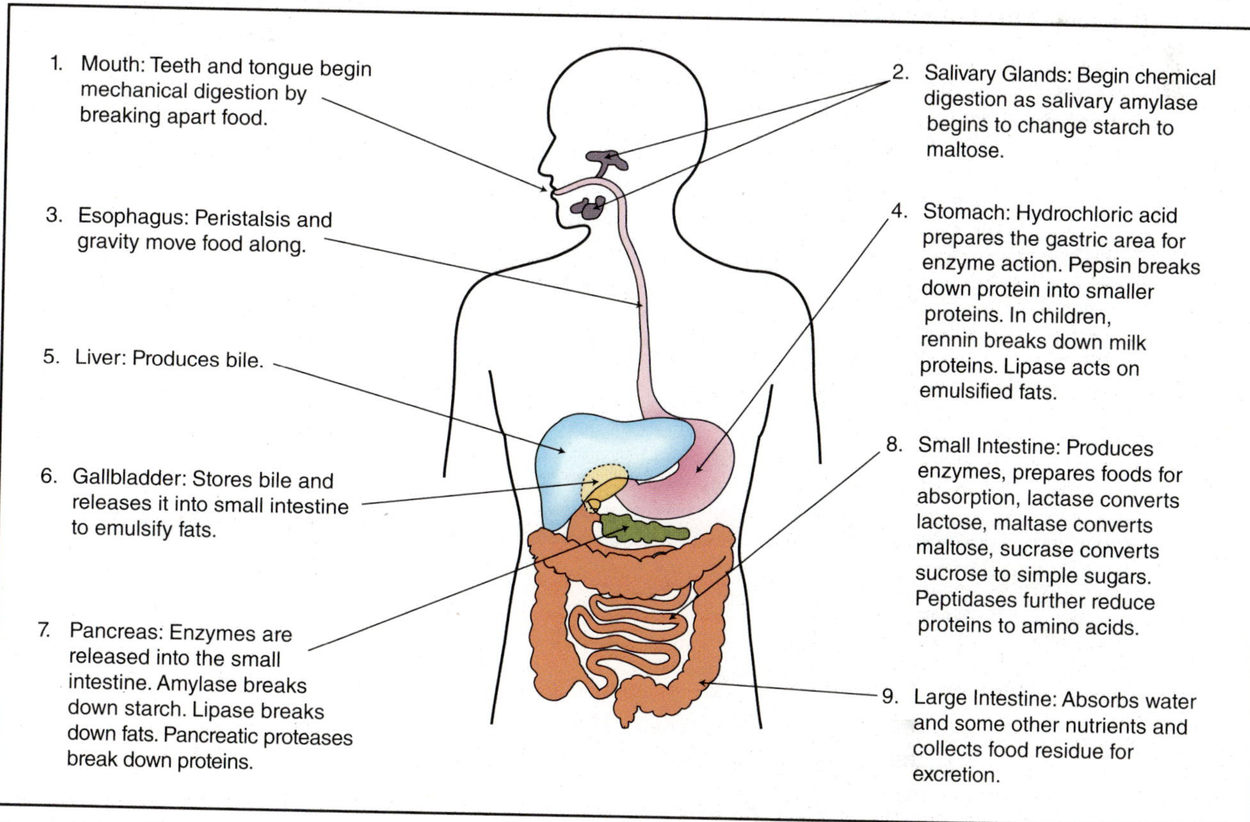

1. Mouth: Teeth and tongue begin mechanical digestion by breaking apart food.
2. Salivary Glands: Begin chemical digestion as salivary amylase begins to change starch to maltose.
3. Esophagus: Peristalsis and gravity move food along.
4. Stomach: Hydrochloric acid prepares the gastric area for enzyme action. Pepsin breaks down protein into smaller proteins. In children, rennin breaks down milk proteins. Lipase acts on emulsified fats.
5. Liver: Produces bile.
6. Gallbladder: Stores bile and releases it into small intestine to emulsify fats.
7. Pancreas: Enzymes are released into the small intestine. Amylase breaks down starch. Lipase breaks down fats. Pancreatic proteases break down proteins.
8. Small Intestine: Produces enzymes, prepares foods for absorption, lactase converts lactose, maltase converts maltose, sucrase converts sucrose to simple sugars. Peptidases further reduce proteins to amino acids.
9. Large Intestine: Absorbs water and some other nutrients and collects food residue for excretion.

Figure 16-1 ■ The digestive system.

Meet the **Specialists**

Specialists are individuals with specific education and training to diagnose and treat GI disorders. GI specialists include the following:

- **Gastroenterologist:** A physician who specializes in the diagnosis and treatment of GI disorders.
- **Hepatologist:** A physician who specializes in the diagnosis and treatment of diseases of the liver, gallbladder, biliary tree, and the pancreas. Hepatology is a subspecialty of gasteroenterology.
- **Proctologist:** A physician specializing in diagnosing and treating diseases of the anus and the rectum.
- **Endocrinologist:** A physician who diagnoses and treats diseases of the endocrine system, which includes the pancreas and the treatment of diabetes.
- **Dietitian:** The above providers often use the services of a dietitian, a professional who counsels patients on the special diets that are required for specific diseases.

The information in this chapter will assist medical assistants who work in GI specialty practices as well as in general practice offices.

a digestive enzyme. Chemical digestion continues in the stomach and the small intestine, which secretes powerful enzymes that turn insoluble food particles into soluble nutrients that can be absorbed into the bloodstream.

Accessory Glands of the Gastrointestinal System

Accessory glands of the digestive tract include the salivary glands, pancreas, liver, and gallbladder. Their function is to secrete chemicals that break down food particles into their primary nutrients. For a full description of the functions of each digestive organ and accessory gland, refer back to Figure 16-1.

GASTROINTESTINAL ABBREVIATION REVIEW

Medical assistants working in GI specialties should be familiar with the medical abbreviations in Table 16-1.

GASTROINTESTINAL IN-OFFICE AND TELEPHONE SCREENING TIPS

Medical assistants are often assigned the responsibility of screening patients over the phone or prior to provider examination in the office. The degree of screening will be established by office protocol, but, in general, medical assistants should be able to ask a series of questions related to the patient's symptoms. Table 16-2 lists the types of questions that are typically asked during a GI screening, indicating the common procedures that coincide with the patient's symptoms.

Important note: Medical assistants should never perform any procedure unless directed to do so by the provider. However, they can anticipate the equipment and supplies required, to help save time in the event that testing is ordered.

Table 16-1 Common Gastrointestinal Abbreviations

Abbreviation	Meaning	Abbreviation	Meaning
ABD	Abdominal	IBD	Inflammatory bowel disease
BM	Bowel movement	IBS	Irritable bowel syndrome
COLO	Colonoscopy	IH	Inguinal hernia
EGD	Esophagogastroduodenoscopy	NG tube	Nasogastric tube
FOBT	Fecal occult blood test	N/V	Nausea and vomiting
GERD	Gastroesophageal reflux (a backward or return flow) disease	PUD	Peptic ulcer disease
GI	Gastrointestinal	TPN	Total parenteral nutrition

Table 16-2 Patient Screening Instructions for the Gastrointestinal System

Ask the Patient:	• Do you have a history of GI disorders? • Have you had any nausea or vomiting, or any change in bowel habits? • Are you experiencing any difficulty in swallowing or any changes in appetite or weight loss? • Are you having any pain? If yes, where is your pain located? Rate your pain on a scale from 0 to 10, with 0 being no pain and 10 being the worst pain you have ever felt.
For Patients Calling on the Telephone	GI pain can range from very mild to severe, which may be a life-threatening event. Patients complaining of severe abdominal pain with a sudden onset should be encouraged to call the EMS. Patients complaining of chronic intermittent abdominal pain can usually be seen in the office (preferably for a same-day appointment). Some patients will confuse chest pain with gastric pain and vice versa. Any symptoms that include prolonged severe diarrhea and vomiting should be considered an emergency, especially in the very young or older adult populations, because of dehydration.
When in the Office:	
Disrobing Instructions	Provide privacy. Check with the provider for clarity, as patients with symptoms above the waist may not disrobe at all or may be directed to disrobe above the waist and to put a gown on so it opens in the back. Patients with rectal bleeding or other anal symptoms should be directed to remove clothing below the waist and draped for modesty.
Vital Signs	Temperature, pulse, respiration, and blood pressure.
Equipment	Anoscope (instrument to examine the anus) or proctoscope (instrument to examine the anus and rectum), lubricant, and 4x4's. Occult blood testing kit and supplies. **Note:** For patient comfort, provide an emesis basin and trash bag if the patient is nauseated or has vomited.
Possible In-Office Procedures	Anoscopy or proctoscopy (if symptoms are related to the rectum or anus), fecal occult blood testing, if applicable.

COMMON GASTROINTESTINAL DISEASES

GI diseases and disorders are quite common, especially as the body ages. Signs and symptoms include nausea, vomiting, stomach cramping, diarrhea, heartburn, loss of appetite, weight loss, indigestion, fatigue, **hematemesis** (vomiting blood), and bright red blood in the feces or black tarry stools. There are several types of GI disorders. In this section, we will focus on some of the more common disorders.

Gastroesophageal Reflux Disease (GERD)

When someone suffers from **gastroesophageal reflux disease (GERD)**, stomach acid backs up (reflux) into the esophagus, due to a defect in the sphincter muscle between the stomach and the esophagus (Figure 16-2). Patients may complain of heartburn or chest pain.

The treatment consists of over-the-counter antacids, prescription medications, diet modifications, and a recommendation to lose weight if applicable. Instruct the patient not to lie flat after a meal and to raise the head of the bed 4" to 6" at night.

Ulcerative Colitis and Crohn's Disease

Crohn's disease and ulcerative colitis are known as inflammatory bowel diseases (IBD).

Colitis is an acute or chronic inflammation of the colon. Symptoms will vary but may include abdominal pain, fatigue, bloody diarrhea, cramping, bloating, and changes in bowel habits.

The treatment is mainly symptomatic and directed at the underlying cause; however, sometimes the condition is **idiopathic**, meaning there is no known cause. Steroids may be used to decrease inflammation, and antibiotics are prescribed when infection is present. Changes in lifestyle are usually recommended, including dietary modifications.

Crohn's disease is an inflammation of any portion of the GI tract, but the terminal ileum is the most common site. Inflammation leads to intestinal thickening, edema, abscesses, and **fistulas**, the abnormal connection between two surfaces. Symptoms depend on the location of the inflammation in the GI tract. Common complaints are cramping, pain, and diarrhea.

Treatment is mainly symptomatic, including the use of steroids to decrease inflammation, antibiotics, and immunosuppressive drugs. Changes in lifestyle are often necessary, including dietary modifications.

Cirrhosis

Cirrhosis is a chronic, progressive inflammatory disease of the liver (Figure 16-3). As liver cells die and are replaced by scar tissue, common complaints include itchy skin, abdominal pain, fatigue, nausea, weight loss,

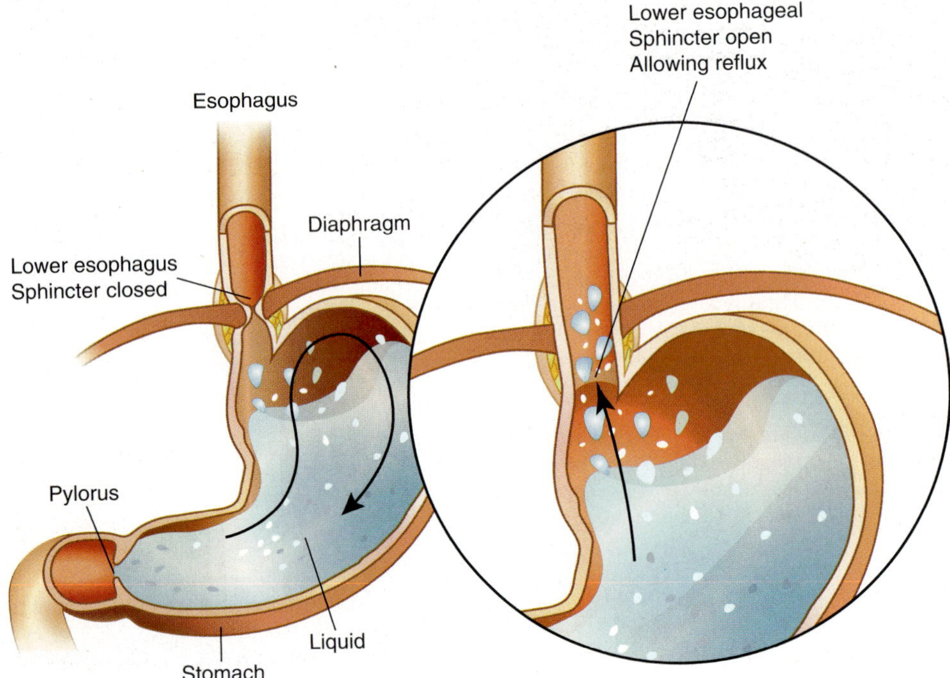

Figure 16-2 ■ In the drawing on the left side, the patient's lower esophageal sphincter is completely closed keeping the acid out of the esophagus, but the drawing on the right side illustrates what occurs when the sphincter doesn't squeeze tightly as in patients with GERD.

and memory loss. As the disease progresses, complications include edema and **ascites**, which is abnormal accumulation of serous fluid in the peritoneal cavity, as well as bruising, bleeding, and jaundice. Treatment cannot cure, but can only delay or reduce complications. Specific treatment depends on the underlying cause, commonly long-term heavy alcohol consumption. Patients with cirrhosis should avoid alcohol consumption and are generally referred to a dietitian for dietary counseling.

Colorectal Cancer

Colorectal cancer accounts for the majority of GI cancers. In the early stages, there may be no symptoms. As the tumor grows, constipation or the complete obstruction of the colon may occur. The treatment of choice is surgical

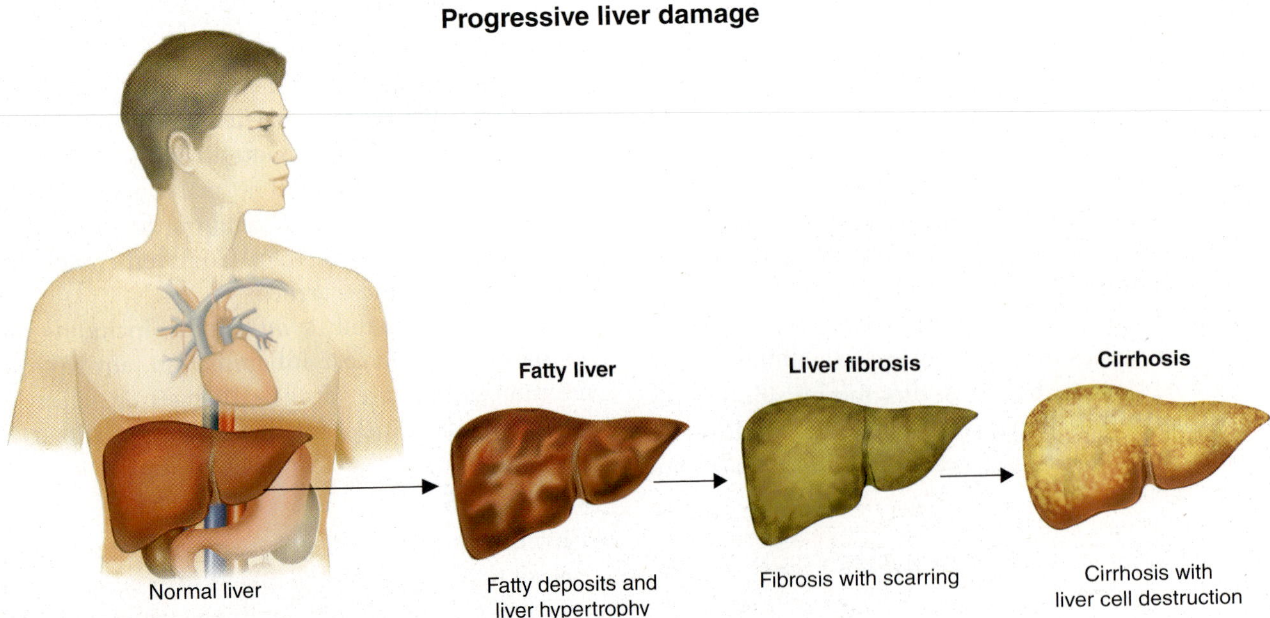

Figure 16-3 ■ Notice how the damage to the liver progresses during each stage of liver disease.

Health Coach

Featured Disease Spotlight: Colorectal Cancer

Description	Colorectal cancer is any cancer that originates in the colon or rectal regions. It accounts for 17% of all cancers diagnosed in the United States and for almost half (47%) of all digestive system cancers. The American Cancer Society estimates that 132,700 cases of colorectal cancers will be diagnosed in 2015. There is a 1 in 20 lifetime risk of developing colorectal cancer. It is one of the most treatable forms of cancer if caught early, yet it is the second leading cause of death in the nation.
Risk Factors	Advancing age; personal or family history of colorectal cancer; ethnicity (Eastern European Jews and African Americans have a higher incidence); a history of intestinal **polyps** (mushroom-like growths from the surface of a mucous membrane); inflammatory bowel disease; inactivity; type 2 diabetes (30% increased risk); smoking (30–40% higher risk); obesity; diet high in red meats and processed meats; and heavy alcohol consumption.
Symptoms	Often symptoms are not present until the tumor grows or metastasizes, which is why cancer screenings are so important. Symptoms may include the following: rectal bleeding, blood in the stools or black tarry stools; cramping, bloating, or abdominal pain; changes in bowel habits such as diarrhea or constipation; unintended weight loss; weakness and fatigue; depression or mood changes; anorexia.
Diagnostic Testing	**Fecal Occult Blood Testing:** Checks for hidden blood in the stool. **Sigmoidoscopy:** A sigmoidoscope is inserted into the sigmoid colon to look for abnormalities. This procedure is limited in that it misses any problems above the sigmoid colon. *Colonoscopy:* A colonoscope is inserted into the colon to look for precancerous polyps and cancerous tumors along the entire length of the colon.
Modifying Factors	Research suggests that a healthy diet may help in the prevention of colorectal cancer. Antioxidants may play a role in the prevention of colorectal and other cancers. They include vitamins A, C, and E; beta-carotene; selenium; and lycopene and can be found in bright-colored fruits and vegetables such as blueberries, carrots, and red cherries. Some of the latest studies show that folic acid, calcium, and vitamin D may help to decrease risks of colon cancers. Cessation of smoking and limiting of alcohol intake also aid in risk reduction.
Treatments	The goal of treatment is to remove the tumor and surrounding tissue to prevent metastasis to other tissues. When a tumor cannot be removed using a colonoscope, a more invasive surgical intervention will be necessary. The goal is to remove the least amount of colon possible. Once a section is removed, it is attached to another segment of the colon, creating an **anastomosis**, the surgical connection between two hollow, or tubular, structures. This allows the stool to exit the body as before. In some cases the colon is too short to connect to lower sections of the colon. A **colostomy** may be necessary. In this procedure, the colon is attached to the abdomen, creating an opening to the outside of the body called a **stoma**. A bag is then worn to collect stool. When a complete colectomy (removal of the entire colon) is performed, the ileum may be used as the site in which a stoma is created. This procedure is referred to as an **ileostomy**. In cases where the tumor has spread to other parts of the body, chemotherapy or radiation may also be necessary.

Table 16-3 Other Common Gastrointestinal Conditions

Condition	Description
Constipation	Constipation is defined as having fewer than three bowel movements in seven days. Occasional constipation is common, but chronic constipation is a problem for some individuals. Treatment depends on the underlying cause. Common causes are a diet too low in fiber, dehydration, and/or physical inactivity. Some diseases also cause constipation, or it may be a side effect of some medications.
Diarrhea	Diarrhea is defined as loose, watery bowel movements. It is normal for individuals to have one or two episodes a year. Remedies for diarrhea may include over-the-counter medications, such as Pepto Bismol, Immodium, and Kaopectate. Patients should drink six (8 oz.) glasses of water each day to replace lost fluids. The most common cause of diarrhea is a virus. Bacterial infections from contaminated food are less common. Other causes include laxative abuse and the side effects of certain medications. More serious cases of diarrhea include the presence of blood and mucus in the stool.
Duodenal ulcer	An **erosion** (the wearing away of a surface) in the duodenum, mainly caused by the bacteria *Helicobacter pylori* and/or hyperacidity, leading to pain. Treated with prescription medications to eradicate *H. pylori* and decrease stomach acidity.
Gastritis	Inflammation of the stomach lining, caused by an irritant (alcohol) or from an infection from a bacteria or a virus, leading to stomach pain. Treated with antacids to decrease stomach acid, diet modifications to decrease irritants, and antibiotics when the infective agent is bacteria.
Gastroenteritis	A self-limiting inflammation of the lining of the stomach and ileum, causing nausea, vomiting, and diarrhea. Typically caused by a virus. Treated with over-the-counter remedies for nausea and vomiting and diarrhea.
Hepatitis (three common types)	• Hepatitis A: Spread by exposure to fecal contaminated water or food. • Hepatitis B: Spread by contact with an infected person's blood or body fluids. • Hepatitis C: Contracted from contaminated needles or from sexual contact.
Hiatal hernia	A hiatal hernia is a protrusion of a portion of the stomach through the thorax due to a weakness in the diaphragm wall.
Irritable bowel syndrome (IBS)	The most common GI disorder in the United States, affecting 30 million people. Causes intermittent abdominal pain, cramping, bloating, and diarrhea and/or constipation. **Etiology** (the cause of disease) is unknown. Treatment focus is stress management and changes in diet and lifestyle.
Pancreatitis	An inflammation of the pancreas, caused by pancreatic enzymes digesting the pancreas itself. Acute pancreatitis can be life-threatening.

intervention to remove the tumor. Refer to the Health Coach Disease Feature to learn more about this disease.

Other Gastrointestinal Conditions

GI specialty practices also see patients with many other conditions. For information on some of these other conditions, refer to Table 16-3.

FEATURED GASTROINTESTINAL PROCEDURES

GI exams in the standard family or general practice office will often consist of an external examination of the abdomen and possible examination of the anus and rectum. The provider may send the patient to a

Over the Lifespan

The 25-foot-long GI tract has a high rate of mucosal cell turnover and is therefore particularly susceptible to age-related disruptions in the growth and replacement of cells. Changes in GI physiology play a role in the following: **anorexia of aging** (the loss of appetite for food in the later years of life), **aspiration pneumonia** (inhaling a foreign substance into the upper respiratory tract, resulting in inflammation of the lung), drop in blood pressure after eating, and bowel incontinence. As a person ages, the stomach takes much longer to empty and the protective lining thins. **Nonsteroidal anti-inflammatory drugs (NSAIDs)** decrease the protective mucous lining in the GI tract and can increase the likelihood of gastritis and ulcers.

Other age-related changes include the small intestine being less efficient in absorbing Vitamin D, B_{12}, and calcium. The large intestine also loses wall strength, leading to the development of diverticulosis. Peristalsis through the intestine slows, resulting in constipation. Finally, there is an increased incidence of colon polyps and colon cancer as one ages.

hospital or X-ray facility for further testing or refer the patient to a GI specialist.

Rectal Exams

The provider will typically perform an exam of the rectum when the patient complains of rectal bleeding or pain. The provider will palpate the anus and rectum for any tenderness, nodules, or other irregularities. The medical assistant should prepare the following equipment and supplies for the exam: **anoscope**, (Figure 16-4) an instrument to examine the anus, **rectoscope**, an instrument to examine the rectum, or **proctoscope**, an instrument to examine both the anus and rectum (refer to Figure 16-5 for a sketch showing the length of these scopes); occult blood testing supplies (to test for hidden blood in the stool); lubricant; gloves; and tissues.

Typical positions used during rectal exams include the following:

- Sims' position or left lateral position
- **Lithotomy** position (to examine the pelvis and lower abdomen)
- A standing position with the patient bent over the exam table

Patients should not be positioned until just prior to the examination and should be draped for modesty and comfort. The room should be well lit and at a comfortable temperature. A fecal specimen obtained during the examination is tested to see if any blood is present. Often, patients are unaware that they have blood in their stool because it is not visible.

Blood in the stool that is not visible is referred to as fecal occult blood. Blood in the stool can indicate different pathological conditions, including **hemorrhoids**, swollen blood vessels both inside and outside the anus that stretch under pressure and bleed. **Fissures** are cracks in the anal skin usually caused by hard bowel movements, causing bleeding. Blood in the stool may also indicate ulcers or cancers in the GI tract. Typically bright red blood in the stool indicates bleeding in the colon or hemorrhoids. Dark black stool indicates bleeding from the upper GI tract.

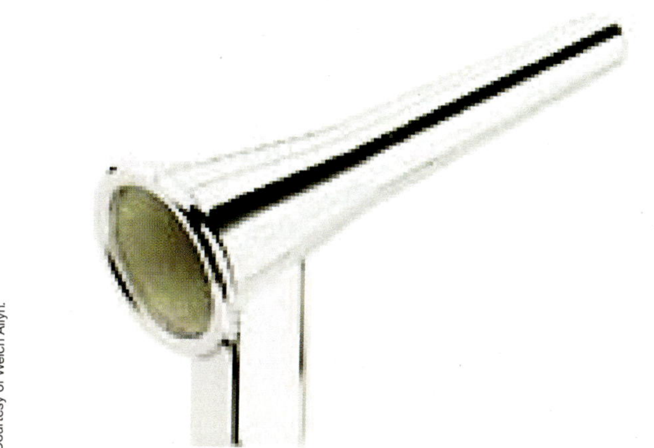

Courtesy of Welch Allyn.

Figure 16-4 ■ A disposable anoscope.

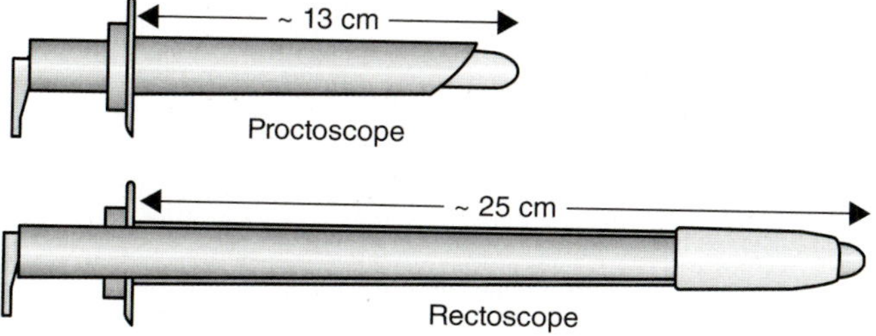

Figure 16-5 ■ Notice how the scopes get longer the deeper it has to be inserted into the rectum.

Proper Collection Technique for a Stool Sample

Patients may be requested to gather additional fecal specimens at their home. Stool samples are required for various types of testing, including the following:

- Stool Culture: A test that looks for various types of bacteria or other microorganisms.
- *Clostridium difficile* or "C-Diff" Testing: Done when a patient suffers from explosive diarrhea that is often the side effect of antibiotic therapy.
- Ova and Parasite (O&P) Testing: Testing to identify intestinal parasites and their eggs or cysts in patients with symptoms of GI infection.

The medical assistant is often responsible for providing the patient with instructions for proper stool collection at home. The patient must have a thorough understanding of special dietary requirements, how to collect the sample, and the specific instructions for sending the specimens back. Patients may feel embarrassed or awkward when discussing the stool collection process because it seems dirty or unpleasant. It is therefore important to make the patient feel at ease during the education session, but the medical assistant must stress the importance of the ordered tests and suggest the use of disposable gloves. Collection and preservation instructions should be given in writing and reviewed with the patient prior to leaving the office.

Every stool test begins with stool collection. Patients should be given a toilet collection hat (Figure 16-6) along with a specimen container. The medical assistant should explain how to place the hat under the toilet seat and how to transfer parts of the stool from the collection hat to the specimen container. Patients should be instructed that nothing other than stool should be collected in the hat and that they should

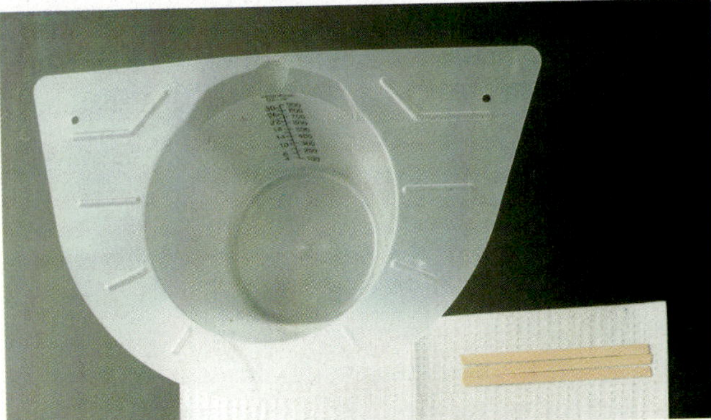

Figure 16-6 ■ The toilet hat fits right underneath the seat of the toilet for easy retrieval of stool samples.

urinate in the commode before setting up the collection hat. Patients should remove the hat immediately following collection and avoid wiping until the hat has been removed. Using a collection spoon or tongue depressor, patients should remove small scoops of stool from different sections of the stool, especially sections that appear darker or contain blood. For a full procedure on stool collection, refer to Procedure 16-1.

Fecal Occult Blood Testing

Blood in the stool can occur from a number of different conditions, including hemorrhoids, polyps, fissures, diverticulitis, ulcers, and colorectal cancer. The term **melena** refers to stool that is black and tarry and is often the result of blood entering the stool from the upper GI tract (stomach and small intestines). This condition is common in patients with peptic ulcers. The black color is caused by the hemoglobin in the blood being altered by digestive chemicals and intestinal bacteria.

There are a number of test kits that check for blood in the stool. The medical assistant will provide dietary and collection instructions for the patient. The patient will collect the specimen and apply it to the test cards in the privacy of his or her own home (Figure 16-7)

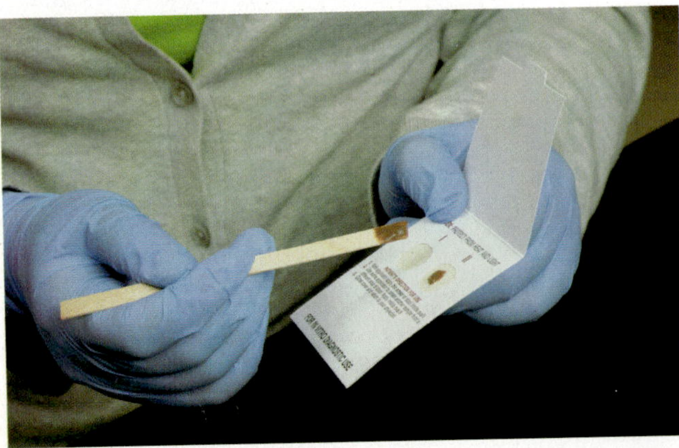

Figure 16-7 ■ The patient places the specimen in the window that reads, "patient sample" in the privacy of her home.

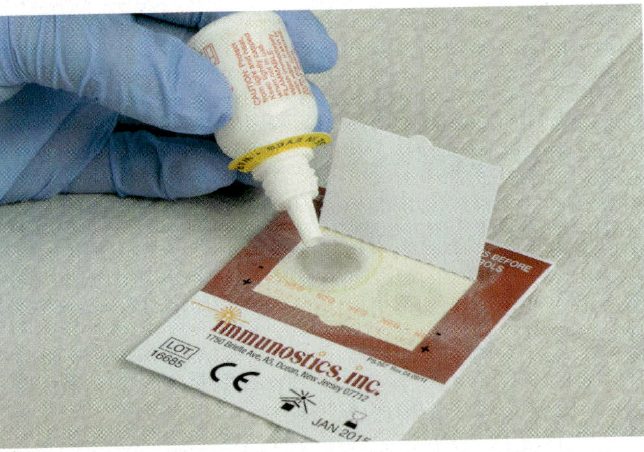

Figure 16-8 ■ Once the card is sent back to the office the medical assistant opens the opposite side of the window and places the reagent over the correct area.

and send it back to the office to be tested. The medical assistant will test the specimen for blood by applying reagent to the opposite side of the card from where the specimen was applied (Figure 16-8).

Quality Control Measures

In order to ensure accurate results, quality control measures should be instituted throughout the process. Test kits should be stored according to the manufacturer's instructions as the reagents used during testing as well as the reagent impregnated on the filter paper are highly sensitive to both light and temperature changes. The developer is first applied to the sample and interpreted before the developer is added to control monitoring areas of the slide (Figure 16-9). This helps to prevent false-positive and false-negative results because of migration of the controls into the testing areas of the slides. Refer to Procedure 16-2 for a full procedure on testing for occult blood in the stool.

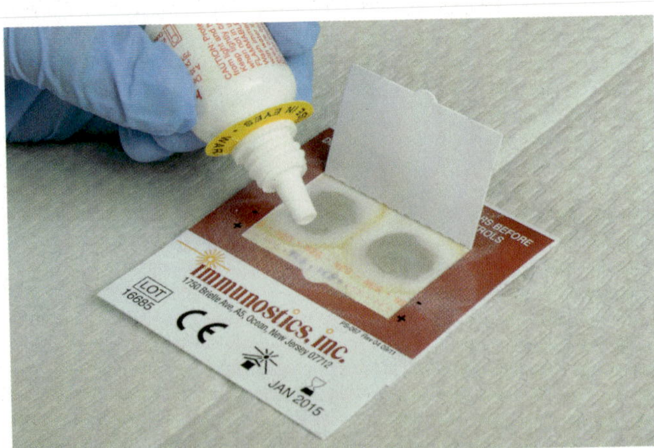

Figure 16-9 ■ The medical assistant then places a drop of control over the control area. Placing a drop of reagent over the area prior to testing could have caused the blue color to bleed into the sample region creating a false positive result.

Health Coach

Instructions for Fecal Occult Blood Testing

When providing patients with fecal occult blood testing supplies, it is important to include both verbal and written instructions, including the following:

- Avoid taking NSAIDs such as ibuprofen or naproxen and aspirin for seven days prior to and during testing.
- Avoid taking more than 250 mg per day of vitamin C for three days prior to testing.
- Avoid red meat, raw vegetables, and raw fruits. No rectal suppositories for at least three days prior to testing. Examples of what may be eaten include well-cooked pork, poultry, fish, cooked vegetables, and fruit.
- For sanitary purposes, complete the blanks on the front of the test cards prior to testing.
- Select samples from three different days and follow the collection instructions supplied with the test kit.

Hematochezia is the term used when bleeding originates in the lower GI tract (colon, rectum, and anus) and is generally associated with bright red blood, but hematochezia can also occur in the case of high-volume upper GI bleeds. Often tumors or lesions bleed minute amounts in their early stages before symptoms are present. This is why occult blood testing should be performed annually in high-risk populations such as patients 50 years of age and older.

Sigmoidoscopy

A sigmoidoscopy is an examination of the lower colon or sigmoid colon. In this test, a flexible tube called a sigmoidoscope (Figure 16-10) is used to examine the sigmoid colon. This test is convenient because it can be performed in a provider's office, does not require the use of anesthesia, has less preparation, and less chance of intestinal tearing than a colonoscopy procedure. This screening test helps to detect colorectal cancer in its early stages but may miss cancers that occur in more distant sections of the colon. Colonoscopy is able to view the full length of the colon and is therefore a better screening test for colorectal cancer than sigmoidoscopy.

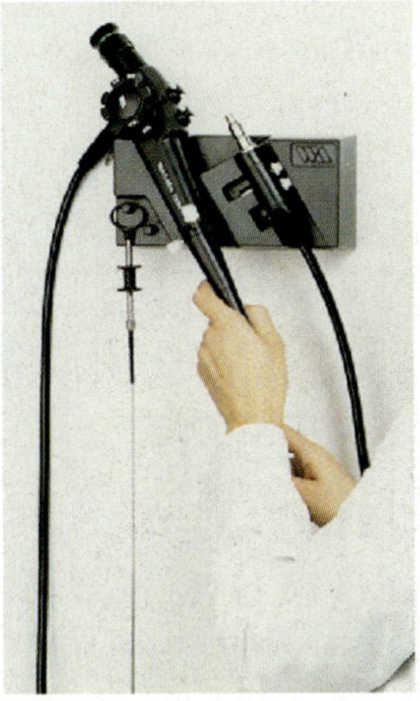

Figure 16-10 ■ A picture of a flexible sigmoidoscope.

Due to the convenience of sigmoidoscopy, some patients prefer this method over colonoscopy. Medical assistants are often responsible for educating patients on how to prepare for the test, setting up the test, and providing home care instructions following the test. Cleaning and disinfecting the sigmoidoscope is also a task that is performed by the medical assistant. Refer to Procedure 16-3 for a complete procedure on assisting the provider with a sigmoidoscopy.

Preparing for a Sigmoidoscopy

The patient will need to clean out his colon prior to examination so that the doctor can view the entire sigmoid section of the colon. This is known as a partial bowel prep because the patient is clearing out the lower third of the colon.

The patient is directed not to eat the day before the exam. Drinks may be limited to clear liquids such as plain water, broth, clear carbonated beverages, tea, and coffee without milk or cream. Then nothing should be taken by mouth after midnight prior to the procedure.

Patients should take a laxative the night before the exam and possibly the morning of the exam. Patients are directed to refer to the specific instructions provided by the provider.

Patients taking aspirin or NSAIDs will need to stop these medications two days before the procedure is to be performed. Other prescription medicines will need to be adjusted according to the provider's orders.

Table 16-4 Miscellaneous Gastrointestinal Tests and Procedures

Procedure	Description
Cologuard	A stool-based colorectal screening test, to detect DNA mutations in shed cells, which may indicate the presence of colon cancer.
Capsule endoscopy	A video camera is placed inside a capsule that the patient swallows. As the capsule tumbles through the small intestine, video images are recorded and analyzed via a computer. This is useful in diagnosing Crohn's disease, ulcers, and colon cancer.
24-hour pH monitoring	A probe is placed through the patient's nose down to the distal esophagus and left in place for 24 hours. The probe is attached to a small recorder and continuous pH values are obtained. This is useful in diagnosing acid reflux (GERD) and stomach ulcers.
Hydrogen breath test	The patient ingests a standard dose of lactose, followed by the measurement of exhaled hydrogen. An increase in the hydrogen exhalation by 20 ppm (parts per million) indicates lactose intolerance.
Procedures Requiring Patient Sedation:	
Esophagogastroduodenoscopy (EGD) (AKA Upper Endoscopy)	The esophagus, stomach, and first portion of the small intestine (duodenum) are examined with a scope.
Endoscopic retrograde cholangiopancreatography (ERCP)	A scope is placed near the opening of the common bile duct and the pancreatic duct followed by the use of catheters to access the appropriate duct. Incisions can be made through the scope and stones may be extracted.
Enteroscopy	A long scope called an enteroscope is used to examine the distal duodenum and jejunum.
Endoscopic ultrasound (EUS)	A scope with an ultrasound device at the tip allows examination of either the upper or the lower GI tract. Sound waves create visual images for diagnosis.

Table 16-5 Recommended Intervals for GI Tests

Test	Interval
Fecal occult blood	Every year, when applicable.
Flexible sigmoidoscopy	Every five years, with fecal occult blood every three years, when applicable.
Double contrast barium enema	Every five years, when applicable.
CT colonography (virtual colonoscopy)	Every five years, when applicable.
Colonoscopy	Every 10 years, following the initial screening procedure. Those with strong risk factors should evaluate the recall frequency with their gastroenterologist. Those with a history of polyps should repeat the procedure every one to six years.

Miscellaneous Gastrointestinal Procedures

Certain diagnostic procedures are specific to the field of **gastroenterology** or general surgery. Many of these procedures require special patient preparation, which must be carefully followed. Preparation for most GI procedures includes some form of fasting. It is important to follow the protocol for patient preparation that is mandated by the facility where the procedure will be performed. Fully explain all preparation instructions to patients and give them a printed copy of the instructions to take home. In general, any examination of the colon will require dietary restrictions and include procedures to cleanse the bowel through the use of laxatives.

Any examination of the upper GI tract may involve only fasting. Table 16-4 lists some of the diagnostic procedures that are particular to the field of gastroenterology. Table 16-5 lists recommended intervals for some of the most common GI tests.

COMMON GASTROINTESTINAL TREATMENTS AND MEDICATIONS

Many of the medications used to treat GI conditions are over-the-counter medications that treat constipation, diarrhea, and excess stomach acid while other prescription drugs treat specific GI diseases. Table 16-6 features some of the most common GI medications.

COMMON LAB TESTS THAT COINCIDE WITH GASTROINTESTINAL DISORDERS

Several lab tests can be performed to evaluate specific GI disorders. Table 16-7 features some of the common lab tests that coincide with GI disorders.

Health Coach

Preparing for a Colonoscopy

During a colonoscopy, a colonoscope (a flexible lighted viewing scope with a camera) will be inserted into the patient's rectum. The scope will be attached to a video display so that the provider can view the lining of the colon. The physician will view the colon for any polyps, tumors, or other abnormalities. If the provider does find any abnormalities such as a polyp, it will be removed and sent to a pathologist for examination.

Upon arrival at the center, the nurse will take the patient's vital signs, take a short medical history, and put an IV in the patient's arm. An anesthesiologist will put medication into the IV to sedate the patient during the procedure. Most patients do not recall the procedure upon waking up. Due to medications used, the procedure requires that the patient have a driver to take him home following the procedure.

Instructions Given to Patients before Colonoscopy:

Days before Procedure	Instructions
7 days	No iron supplements. Includes multivitamins with iron.
5 days	Stop aspirin and all NSAIDs.
3–7 days	Stop blood thinners/anticoagulants. Specific number of days defined by GI specialist.
3 days	Diet: No nuts, popcorn, raw fruits, raw vegetables, salad, corn, seeds, or Metamucil. Cooked foods are okay.
1 day	Diet: No milk products. Only clear liquids, such as jello, tea, coffee, broths, and sodas. No red or purple dyes in Jello or drinks.
1 day	Start prescription laxative preparation. Drink 8 oz. fluids every hour, to replace lost fluids.
Procedure day	Take morning meds with a sip of water. No insulin or pills for diabetes.
	Nothing to drink within three hours of appointment

Table 16-6 Common Gastrointestinal Medications

Medication Classifications	Description	Medication Examples
Laxatives	Medications used to promote passage of stool	Biscodoyl, Milk of Magnesia, Senna, Dulcolax, Benefiber, Miralax, Metamucil, Citrucel, castor oil, Peri-colase, glycerine suppositories
Antacids	Medications to decrease stomach acid	Pepcid Complete, Prilosec, Protonix, Zantac
Antidiarrheal	Medications to decrease/stop diarrhea	Dificid to treat C-Diff, Imodium, Pepto Bismol, Kaopectate
Antiemetics	To reduce/stop nausea and vomiting	Compazine, Benadryl, Dramamine, Zyprexa, Zofran
Medications for IBS	Medications to relax the colon and increase fluid secretion in small intestine	Lotronex, Amitiza
Medications for GERD	Decreases stomach acidity and eradicates *H. pylori*	Aciphex, Nexium
Medications for ulcerative colitis	Decreases inflammation in the colon	Asacol
Medications for intra-abdominal infections	Antibiotics to kill bacteria that cause infections	Cipro, Flagyl, Rocephin, Dificid

Table 16-7 Common Lab Tests That Coincide with Gastrointestinal Disorders

Test	Clinical Significance
Comprehensive GI function panel	Measures inflammatory, digestive, and immune markers, to detect abnormal GI function
Complete blood count	Detects abnormalities in the total blood profile, such as a low hematocrit, which could indicate blood loss
Protein, bilirubin, alkaline, phosphatase, gamma-globulin	Tests liver function

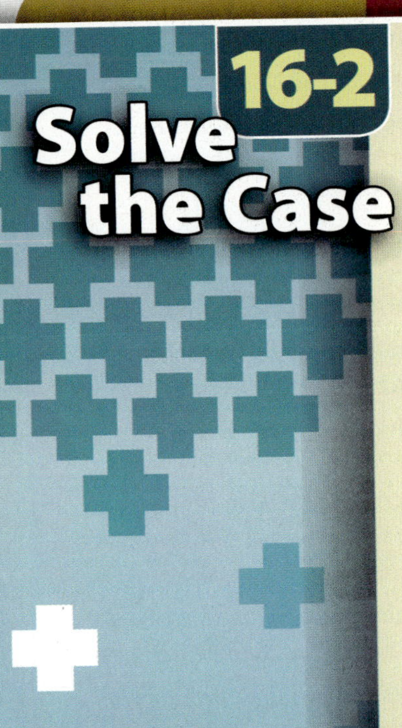

Mr. Reynolds has returned to the office and is pacing anxiously awaiting the results of his colonoscopy.

Assessment Information: The report of the colonoscopy states that 10 polyps were removed. The pathology report reveals that two were positive for cancer.

Today's Vital Signs: BP 160/100, T 98.8 °F, P 84 and slightly irregular, R 18. The provider reviewed the results of the colonoscopy with the patient and told Mr. Reynolds that at least a portion of the colon would have to be surgically removed. Mr. Reynolds is worried that he may need to have a colostomy, as his father did. He is visibly upset.

Provider's Plan: Refer to surgeon for evaluation. Follow-up referral to the oncologist.

1. **What may be the cause of the elevated blood pressure reading?**
2. **What is the purpose of a referral to the oncologist?**
3. **Based on other parts of Mr. Reynold's medical history, found in the first Solve the Case, what other specialists may need to see Mr. Reynolds prior to surgery?**

PROCEDURE 16-1

Instruct the Patient on How to Collect a Fecal Specimen

Fecal specimens are collected for tests that can detect occult (hidden) blood, ova and parasites (O & P), and *Clostridium difficile*. The reliability of these tests depends on patient preparation and the directions for specimen collection being carefully followed. It is important to be aware of the patient's concerns as they relate to this procedure.

Objective:

To instruct a patient on the correct way to collect and preserve a fecal specimen.

Equipment/Supplies:

- Laboratory request form
- Specimen container with a lid and label
- Collection container or hat
- Tongue depressors
- Printed instructions
- Patient chart/EHR

continues

PROCEDURE 16-1 continued

PROCEDURAL STEPS	DETAILS AND/OR RATIONALE
1. Assemble all the equipment, complete lab requisition form, and adhere label with patient's information on specimen container.	Assembling the equipment ahead of time eliminates interruptions in the teaching process.
2. Identify the patient using two identifiers and identify yourself.	Using two identifiers confirms that you have the correct patient.
3. Explain the provider's orders and ***rationale for ordering the procedure to the patient, showing awareness of the patient's concerns related to the procedure being performed.***	Explaining the orders will help the patient to comprehend the instructions.
4. Instruct patient to write the date and time of collection on the affixed label prior to collection.	Completing the label prior to collection will reduce the handling of the container following collection. (Less chance of contamination.)
5. Instruct the patient to fully empty the bladder before the collection procedure starts. Stress the importance of not contaminating the specimen with urine, toilet tissue, or any other foreign material.	This will keep urine and toilet paper from mixing with the stool and contaminating the specimen.
6. Instruct the patient to lift the toilet seat and place the toilet hat in the bowl, following manufacturer's instructions.	The hat can be used for both urine and stool collection. The patient needs to have the hat turned in the proper direction so that the sample is fully contained.
7. Instruct the patient to use the tongue depressors or collection spoons to collect a small portion (approximately three to four tablespoons) of the next bowel movement from different sections of the stool and to place it in the specimen container.	The specimen may not contain the products you are looking for throughout the specimen so it is important to obtain samples from different regions of the stool to improve chances of finding bacteria, ova, and parasite or blood during testing.
8. Instruct the patient to place the lid tightly onto the specimen container and to return the specimen to the office or laboratory within two hours of collection. If the specimen is to be tested for O & P, it must not be refrigerated.	Refrigeration decreases bacterial growth in the specimen and may kill parasites.
9. Provide the patient with a copy of the printed instructions.	Printed instructions will help the patient to remember the proper steps for collecting the specimen.
10. Document the procedure in the patient record.	

DOCUMENTATION EXAMPLE:

10-10-XX 10:30 a.m.	Instructed pt. on proper method of collecting a fecal sample per Dr. Leonard's orders. Provided pt. with printed instructions. Kate Lilly, RMA (AMT)----------------------------------

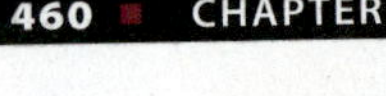

PROCEDURE 16-2

Perform a Fecal Occult Blood Test

Objective:

To instruct a patient how to properly prepare for fecal occult blood testing; how to collect the sample for testing; and how to accurately perform the testing once the sample has been collected.

Equipment/Supplies:

- Gloves
- Collection Container/Hat
- Test cards, spatulas, and developer
- Return envelope or biohazard bag
- Patient chart/EHR
- Home care instruction form

PROCEDURAL STEPS	DETAILS AND/OR RATIONALE
1. Assemble the supplies.	Having all the supplies ready saves time. *Note:* An expired test kit can result in an inaccurate result.
2. Identify the patient using two identifiers and identify yourself.	Using two identifiers will ensure that you have the correct patient.
3. ***Explain to the patient the rationale for performance of the procedure, showing awareness of the patient's concerns related to the procedure.***	Adequate preparation and careful collection of the specimen by the patient assures accurate results.
4. Explain special dietary instructions for the patient to follow prior to collecting the specimen, ***showing awareness of the patient's concerns regarding a dietary change***. Start collection with the first bowel movement following three days of dietary restriction. Patients on NSAIDs or Aspirin should restrict these medications for seven days prior to testing.	Dietary Instructions Include the Following: Avoid red and processed meats and liver. No turnips, broccoli, cauliflower, or melons. Avoid aspirin, iron supplements, and large doses of vitamin C for seven days before the test. Do not start test during or three days after menses, or if bleeding from hemorrhoids. Consume a high-fiber diet and drink liquids to promote bowel movements.
5. Explain how to properly collect a stool sample following the directions in Procedure 16-1.	Allowing the stool to fall into the toilet water or mixing the stool with urine or toilet paper contaminates the specimen.
6. Explain how to properly label the cards prior to collection.	To label the cards prior to testing will prevent the patient from contaminating their hands following the procedure.

continues

PROCEDURE 16-2 continued

PROCEDURAL STEPS	DETAILS AND/OR RATIONALE
7. Explain instructions for collecting the samples (Figure 16-11), and the number of samples the patient is to collect. Most guaiac test slides have two windows for each slide (A&B) The patient is to obtain a tiny section of stool using the provided spatula or spoon from one part of the stool and to spread a thin film of the stool in window A and to repeat the procedure using a different section of the stool for window B. Instruct the patient to close the front flap of the collection slide.	The patient must understand how to properly collect the samples to ensure test accuracy. Instruct the patient to store test slides at room temperature and to protect from exposure to heat, sun, and fluorescent light.
8. Instruct the patient to repeat steps 5–7 for the second and third day of testing, using the remaining two cards.	
9. Review the instructions for sending the samples back to the office. These specimens are usually mailed back in a foil lined envelope and must arrive for testing within 14 days of collection.	

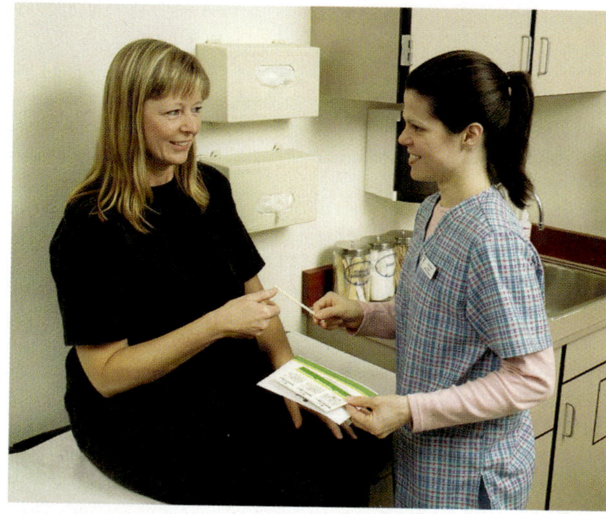

Figure 16-11 ■ The medical assistant explains the procedure to the patient.

TESTING PROCEDURE	
10. When the completed test cards arrive in the office, wash your hands, gather supplies (developer), and apply gloves before testing begins. Check the expiration date on the developer.	Standard precautions must be practiced when completing tests on all human samples. Using expired developer can produce inaccurate results.
11. Correctly follow the developing instructions (Figure 16-12), including performing a control on each test following testing and interpretation of each sample. A blue color indicates a positive result for the presence of blood.	The instructions must be followed exactly and correct timing is crucial for accurate results. Performing controls ensures that the testing cards and developer are working correctly.
12. Properly dispose of the test cards in a trash receptacle or by following institutional guidelines.	Fecal contents are not considered medical wastes and can be thrown into the regular trash.
13. Remove gloves and wash your hands.	To reduce the risk of contamination.
14. Document the procedure and the results in the patient record.	Accurate charting is essential to ensure proper patient care.

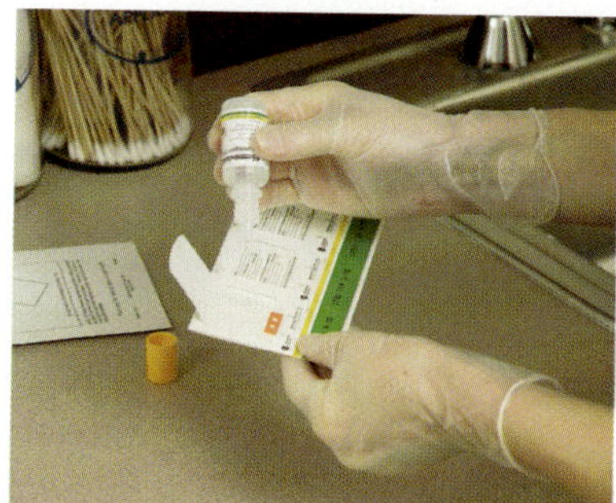

Figure 16-12 ■ The medical assistant places the developing solution on the slides over the appropriate regions.

DOCUMENTATION EXAMPLES:

12-13-XX 9:45 a.m.	Hemawipe testing instructions per Dr. Jones. Pt. supplied with testing cards and spatulas to obtain three test samples at home. Verbal and written preparation and collection instructions given. Pt. expressed understanding of procedure and will return test cards to the office. Judith Jones, CMA (AAMA)--------------------------------

12-20-XX 10:30 a.m.	Hemoccult test cards received in office today. Test completed. Results: negative (–) for all three specimens. Judith Jones, CMA (AAMA) --------------------------------

PROCEDURE 16-3

Assist with a Flexible Sigmoidoscopy

Objective:

To ensure that the equipment is set up and properly functioning, prepare the patient for the examination, providing assistance to the provider and support to the patient during the procedure, and sterilizing the equipment after the procedure.

Equipment/Supplies:

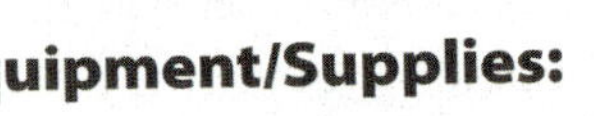

- Disposable gloves
- Sterile specimen container
- Flexible sigmoidoscope
- Lubricant
- Biopsy forceps
- Light source
- Tissue
- Gown and drape
- Patient chart/EHR
- Pen

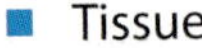

PROCEDURAL STEPS	DETAILS AND/OR RATIONALE
1. Wash hands and apply gloves.	Hand washing is the principal method of preventing the spread of infection.
2. Assemble the equipment. Ensure that all is in acceptable working condition.	Having all equipment and supplies ready will save time.
3. Identify the patient using two identifiers and identify yourself. ***Explain to the patient the rationale for performance of the procedure, showing awareness of the patient's concerns related to the procedure.*** Label the sterile specimen container with all pertinent patient information.	Identifying the patient provides assurance that the procedure and examination performed is on the correct patient. Explaining the procedure increases patient compliance and comfort during the procedure.
4. Ask the patient to use the restroom to empty the bladder and bowel.	Emptying the bladder and bowel will allow for a more comfortable procedure.
5. Supply the patient with a gown, instructing the patient to disrobe below the waist and place the gown with the opening in the back. Provide a drape for added privacy.	This provides the most privacy possible during a sigmoidoscopy.

continues

PROCEDURE 16-3 continued

PROCEDURAL STEPS	DETAILS AND/OR RATIONALE
6. ***Demonstrating empathy***, reassure the patient that the exam should only last a few minutes.	
7. Assist the patient into the Sims' position and instruct the patient to breathe deeply through the mouth to relax the abdominal muscles.	This is the position of choice for the procedure. The draping technique allows for only a minimal portion of the drape to be moved for the procedure. This provides the most privacy.
8. Provide the physician with suitable disposable gloves. When gloved, provide lubrication to the first digit for rectal examination.	Lubrication makes insertion easier.
9. Lubricate the end of the flexible scope.	Lubrication makes insertion of the scope into the anus easier.
10. ***Incorporate critical thinking skills when performing patient care***, and be prepared for any requests by the provider. Assist with suctioning during the procedure and give support to the patient.	
11. Hand biopsy forceps to the provider, if requested. Be certain the specimen container is maintained in a functional position. Place the biopsy specimen into the sterile container.	The specimen is placed in a sterile container to maintain the integrity of the specimen.
12. Following completion of the procedure, provide tissue to the patient to remove any excess lubrication from the anal region.	
13. Assist the patient into a sitting position and instruct the patient to remain sitting while you assess the patient's status, ***incorporating critical thinking skills when performing patient assessment***.	The patient may become dizzy if allowed to stand up too soon.
14. Once the patient is stable, assist with dressing, if requested, ***while demonstrating the principles of self-boundaries***.	
15. Prepare the specimen for transport to the laboratory. Be certain lab requests are filled out in their entirety.	An incomplete lab requisition could delay testing.
16. Clean the equipment and examination room. Follow the manufacturer's instructions for cleaning the scope.	Each scope is different and each manufacturer has its own set of cleaning and maintenance instructions.
17. Document the exam and procedure in the patient record.	

DOCUMENTATION EXAMPLES:

11-14-XX 10:30 a.m.	Assisted physician with flex sig, Biopsy obtained and sent to lab. Pt. tolerated well, f/u appt. given. Instructed pt. to contact office with any c/o discomfort. Diet reviewed as requested by physician. Dispensed 4 Sample packs of Nexium (20 mg) per Dr. Davis. Malcolm Jones, RMA (AMT)--

CHAPTER SUMMARY

- Gastrointestinal diseases are common in the population. Around 60–70 million people suffer from some type of GI disorder. Complaints include heartburn, abdominal pain, weight fluctuations, and bowel irregularities. Testing, both noninvasive and invasive, may be required to diagnose and treat these conditions.
- The two major functions of the GI tract are digestion (both mechanical and chemical) and the elimination of food waste products. The order in which food travels through the GI tract is oral cavity, esophagus, stomach, small intestine (duodenum, jejunum, ileum), large intestine (ascending, transverse, descending, and sigmoid), rectum, and anus.
- Accessory glands of the digestive tract include the salivary glands, pancreas, liver, and gall bladder. The salivary glands secrete saliva and sodium bicarbonate. The pancreas secretes digestive juices and sodium bicarbonate. The liver secretes bile through the gallbladder for the digestion of fats.
- GI specialists include the gastroenterologist, hepatologist, proctologist, endocrinologist, and dietitian.
- Common GI diseases include GERD, the reflux of stomach acid into the esophagus; colitis, an acute or chronic inflammation of the colon; cirrhosis, a chronic, progressive inflammatory disease of the liver; and colorectal cancer, which is cancer of the colon, rectum, or both.
- Colorectal cancer is the second leading cause of death in the United States. It comprises 17% of all cancer diagnoses and 47% of all digestive system cancers. The average person has a 1 in 20 lifetime risk of developing colorectal cancer. Risk factors for the development of colorectal cancer include advancing age, a personal or family history of colorectal cancer, history of intestinal polyps or inflammatory bowel disease, obesity, type 2 diabetes, inactivity, a diet high in red and processed meats, and heavy alcohol consumption. Symptoms of colorectal cancer may include blood in the stool, cramping and abdominal pain, unintended weight loss, and weakness and fatigue. However, some may have colorectal cancer and have no symptoms.
- Other common GI diseases include Crohn's disease, a chronic inflammation of the ileum; duodenal ulcer, erosion of the duodenum mainly caused by the bacteria *H. pylori*; gastroenteritis, a self-limiting inflammation of the lining of the stomach and ileum; gastritis, the inflammation of the stomach lining; hepatitis (A, B, C), an inflammation and destruction of liver cells; hiatal hernia, herniation of a portion of the stomach through the diaphragm; pancreatitis, pancreatic enzymes digest the pancreas itself.
- Elimination problems from the GI tract are the most common of all GI conditions, including diarrhea (watery, loose stools) and constipation (less than three bowel movements in seven days).
- The aging of the GI tract can cause anorexia of aging; dysphagia and aspiration pneumonia; postprandial hypotension; slowed peristalsis and constipation; fecal incontinence; an increased incidence of gastric ulcers and gastric bleeding; decreased absorption of vitamin D, B_{12}, and calcium; increased incidence of diverticulosis, colon polyps, and colon cancer.
- Common GI procedures include instructing the patient how to collect and preserve a fecal specimen, performing a fecal occult blood test, and assisting with a flexible sigmoidoscopy.
- Procedures that can be carried out in the provider office, hospital, or outpatient facility include rectal and anal exam, pH monitoring, capsule endoscopy, sigmoidoscopy, testing stool sample for occult blood and ova and parasites, colonoscopy, esophagogastroduodenoscopy (EGD), endoscopic retrograde cholangiopancreatography (ERCP), enteroscopy, endoscopic ultrasound, and upper GI series (barium swallow).

- Exams for rectal or anal symptoms may require a fecal occult blood test kit and two instruments: an anoscope and/or a proctoscope.
- Typical patient positions for a rectal exam include Sims' (left lateral), lithotomy, and a standing position bent over a table.
- A limitation of a sigmoidoscopy is that it can only visualize the sigmoid colon. However, colonoscopy can visualize the entire length of the colon.
- Patient preparations for colonoscopy include no iron for one week prior to the exam; discontinuing NSAIDs five days before the exam; stopping blood thinners three to seven days before the exam; no uncooked fruits, vegetables, or meats, including popcorn, nuts, seeds, and Metamucil for three days. The day prior to the exam, no milk products and only clear liquids. No purple or red dyes in foods or fluids. Nothing to drink three hours prior to the exam. Patient should take morning meds with a sip of water, but no insulin or pills for diabetics.
- When the colon is surgically resected, there are three possible outcomes: anastomosis at the site of the resection, the surgical creation of a colostomy, or the surgical creation of an ileostomy.
- Common medication for the GI tract treats constipation, excess stomach acid, diarrhea, GERD, ulcerative colitis, and intra-abdominal infections.
- Common tests that coincide with GI disorders include abdominal ultrasound, CT abdominal scan, complete blood count (CBC), and blood tests for liver function, including protein, bilirubin, alkaline phosphatase, and gamma-globulin.
- Common blood and GI lab tests are ordered to detect abnormal blood chemistry, occult blood in the stool, measure hydrochloric acid (HCl) levels in the stomach, and detect bacteria as well as the presence of ova and parasites.
- Fecal testing includes occult blood, stool culture, *Clostridium difficile* (C-Diff), and testing for ova and parasites.
- Patient instructions prior to occult blood testing include not ingesting NSAIDs seven days prior to the exam; avoiding raw meats, raw vegetables, and raw fruits; taking no more than 250 mg of vitamin C for three days prior to the exam; and not using rectal suppositories for three days prior to the exam.
- Recommended intervals for GI tests include a fecal occult blood test every year; every five years a flexible sigmoidoscopy, double contrast barium enema, and CT colonography. A colonoscopy should be done a minimum of every 10 years following the initial screening, but every one to six years when there is a history of polyps.

CERTIFICATION REVIEW QUESTIONS

1. A reason for performing a fecal occult blood test is to:
   a. detect abnormal organisms in the stool.
   b. screen for hepatitis.
   c. evaluate the digestion of food elements.
   d. test for any bleeding in the GI tract.

2. Examination of the entire colon with a flexible lighted video scope is referred to as:
   a. sigmoidoscopy.
   b. colonoscopy.
   c. capsule endoscopy.
   d. cholangiogram.

3. Prior to occult blood studies, patients should be advised to avoid which of the following?
   a. Red meat
   b. NSAIDs
   c. Raw vegetables
   d. All of the above

4. Patients calling the office and complaining of severe abdominal pain should be advised to do which of the following?
   a. Take an NSAID for pain.
   b. Make an appointment to see the practitioner.
   c. Apply heat to the abdomen.
   d. Call EMS.

5. The treatment of GERD includes all of the following, except:
   a. weight reduction.
   b. prescription medications.
   c. modifying the type of foods in the current diet.
   d. decreasing the amount of liquids in the diet.

6. Risk factors for the development of colorectal cancer include all of the following, except:
   a. personal or family history of polyps.
   b. high-fiber diet.
   c. obesity.
   d. type 2 diabetes.

7. All of the following is true regarding stool colors, except:
   a. bright red blood may indicate upper GI tract bleeding.
   b. brown stools may have occult blood.
   c. black stools indicate bleeding in the upper GI tract.
   d. brown stools may include both ova and parasites.

8. NSAIDs are drugs that do the following, except:
   a. increase bleeding tendencies.
   b. decrease inflammation.
   c. increase muscle function.
   d. decrease pain.

9. The main cause of duodenal ulcers is:
   a. NSAIDs.
   b. bacterial infection.
   c. high-stress environments.
   d. *H. pylori.*

10. Patients should avoid all but which of the following before and during stool collection for fecal occult blood testing?
   a. Red meats
   b. Food high in fiber
   c. Raw vegetables
   d. NSAIDs
   e. Dairy Products

STUDY RESOURCES

Resources to Test and Reinforce Your Knowledge:	
Certification Review Questions	Take this end-of-chapter quiz
Workbook	• Complete the activities for Chapter 16 • Perform the procedures for Chapter 16 using the Competency Checklists
Resources to Promote Critical Thinking:	
***Solve the Case* Activities**	• Consider these case studies and discuss your conclusions
Learning Lab	• Module 17: Immune and Digestive Systems
MindTap	• Complete Chapter 16 readings and activities, including medical terminology and patient navigation study tools.

REFERENCES

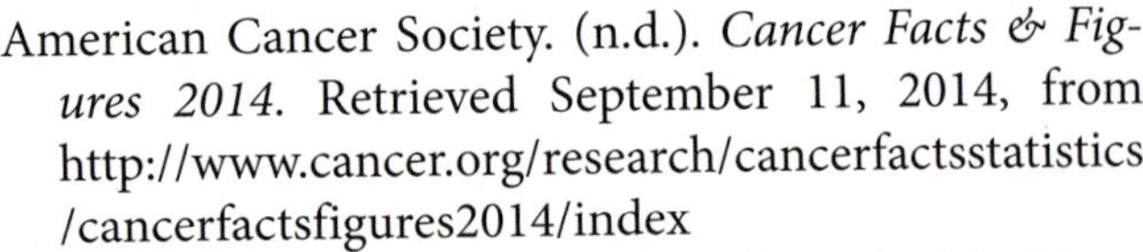

American Cancer Society. (n.d.). *Cancer Facts & Figures 2014*. Retrieved September 11, 2014, from http://www.cancer.org/research/cancerfactsstatistics/cancerfactsfigures2014/index

American College of Gastroenterology. (n.d.). *Digestive health statistics*. Retrieved October 8, 2014, from http://gi.org/media/digestive-health-statistics-niddk

American Society for Gastrointestinal Endoscopy. (n.d.). *Understanding EUS (endoscopic ultrasonography*. Retrieved September 11, 2014, from http://www.asge.org/patients/patients.aspx?id=380

Crohn's & Colitis Foundation of America. (n.d.). *What are Crohn's & colitis?* Retrieved October 13, 2014, from http://www.ccfa.org/what-are-crohns-and-colitis/

Laboratory Tests of Gastrointestinal Disease. (2010, April 27). Retrieved September 11, 2014, from http://ucsdlabmed.wikidot.com/chapter-5

Mayo Clinic (n.d.) *Diseases and conditions: Constipation*. Retrieved September 30, 2014, from www.mayoclinic.org/diseases-conditions/constipation/basics/resk-factors/con-20032773

Mayo Clinic (n.d.) *Diseases and conditions: Irritable bowel syndrome*. Retrieved October 13, 2014, http://www.mayoclinic.org/diseases-conditions/irritable-bowel-syndrome/basics/definition/con-20024578

Testing for Food Allergies: Fatigue Panel. (2012, July 11). Retrieved October 13, 2014, from http://ibstreatmentcenter.com/2012/07/testing-food-allergies-fatigue-panel.html

The Basics of Diarrhea. (n.d.) Retrieved September 13, 2014, from www.webmd.com/digestive-disorders/digestive-diseases-diarrhea

The Clinical Significance of Gastrointestinal Changes with Aging. (2008, September 11). Retrieved October 2, 2014, from http://www.ncbi.nlm.nih.gov/pubmed/18685464

U.S. Food and Drug Administration. (2014, November 23). Press announcements. Retrieved October 8, 2014, from http://www.fda.gov/newsevents/newsroom/PressAnnouncements/default.htm

Weight-control Information Network. (2014, January 24). *Bariatric surgery for severe obesity*. Retrieved September 15, 2014, from http://www.win.niddk.nih.gov/publications/gastric.htm

17

Women's Health Issues: Obstetrics and Gynecology

CHAPTER OUTLINE

Female Reproductive System Snapshot
- Ovaries
- Fallopian Tubes
- Uterus
- Vagina
- The Menstrual Cycle
- Menopause

Obstetric and Gynecologic Abbreviation Review

Gynecologic In-Office and Telephone Screening Tips

Common Obstetric and Gynecologic Diseases
- Vulvodynia
- Vaginitis
- Uterine Fibroids
- Breast Cancer
- Other Common Obstetric and Gynecologic Diseases

Featured Gynecologic Procedures
- Gynecological Exam
- Medical Assistant's Responsibility During a Pap and Pelvic Exam
- Pelvic Exam for Women Who Have Vaginal Symptoms
- Mammography
- Miscellaneous Gynecologic Procedures

Common Gynecologic Treatments and Medications

Common Lab Tests That Coincide with Women's Health Issues

Featured Obstetric Procedures
- The Initial or First Prenatal Exam
- Return Prenatal Visits
- Miscellaneous Prenatal Diagnostic Tests and Procedures

Common Obstetric Treatments

Common Lab Tests That Coincide with Pregnancy

Labor and Delivery

Postnatal or Postpartum Period
- Six-Week Postpartum Visit

ESSENTIAL TERMS

abnormal uterine bleeding (AUB)
abortion
amenorrhea
amniocentesis
atypical
Braxton-Hicks contractions
cesarean section (C-section)
colposcopy
cytologic
cytology
dilation
dysmenorrhea
eclampsia
ectopic
effacement
gestation
gravida
infertility specialist
lochia
meconium
menarche
menopause
menses
menstruation
midwife (midwives)
miscarriage
OB-GYN
para
parturition
perimenopause
postpartum
preeclampsia
prenatal
puerperium
sexually transmitted disease (STD)
sexually transmitted infections (STIs)
toxemia
trimester

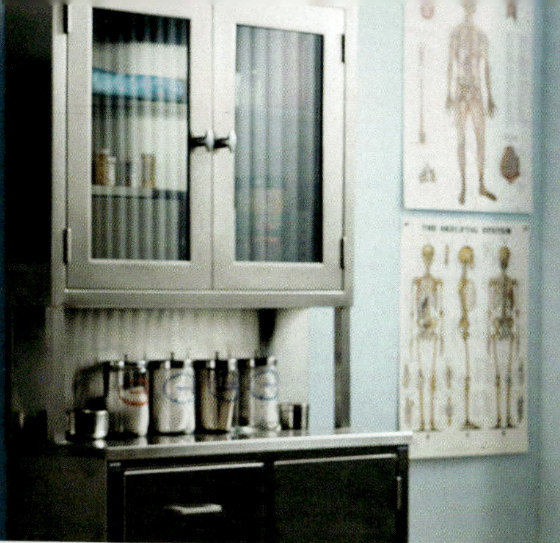

DEVELOPMENTAL OBJECTIVES

After completing this chapter, you should be able to:

1. Correctly spell and define the essential terms.
2. List and provide the anatomical locations of the major structures within the female reproductive system and describe their functions.
3. List and use abbreviations associated with the female reproductive system.
4. Compile a list of common screening questions that should be asked of patients regarding the female reproductive system using established protocols and incorporate critical thinking skills when performing patient assessment.
5. Identify common pathology related to the female reproductive system including signs, symptoms, and etiology.
6. Compare structure and function of the female reproductive system across the life span.
7. Analyze pathology for the female reproductive system including diagnostic measures and treatment modalities.
8. Compile a list of common female reproductive system medication classifications and conclude how each one acts upon body structures to produce a desired effect.
9. List and describe different methods of contraception.
10. List the parts of a thorough gynecologic (GYN) exam and describe the role of the medical assistant during each exam.
11. Explain the importance of breast self-examinations (BSE) and regular mammography for females over 40.
12. Discuss the pros and cons of hormone replacement therapy (HRT) during menopause.
13. List and explain each part of the initial prenatal exam and what occurs in each subsequent exam.
14. List and describe the rationale for each of the prenatal lab tests performed throughout pregnancy.
15. List the stages of labor and explain the importance of the postpartum exam.

INTRODUCTION

The field of obstetrics and gynecology (OB-GYN) has many facets. Tracking a patient through the prenatal period can be very exciting. Watching the joy on an expectant mother's face when you confirm her deepest desire is priceless; but the field of OB-GYN has its downsides as well. Due to financial constraints or a lack of support from loved ones, some patients are saddened by the news that they are expecting a baby. Some expectant mothers end up losing their babies or learn that their unborn baby has a congenital or hereditary defect that cannot be corrected through surgical intervention or medical treatment. Some expectant mothers become so ill during their pregnancy that they must choose to risk premature delivery to save themselves and, possibly, their child.

The gynecological side of OB-GYN involves regular screening exams by the provider and a myriad of opportunities to educate patients about disease prevention and management. The medical assistant is often the health care professional responsible for providing the patient with educational materials and teaching the patient how to perform breast self-exams.

This chapter will help prepare you to work in an OB-GYN practice and will assist you in learning common instruments and tray setups used in the specialty. Additionally, this chapter will prepare you to assist the provider with common OB-GYN procedures and provide you with tips for educating your patients.

FEMALE REPRODUCTIVE SYSTEM SNAPSHOT

The female reproductive system consists of a vagina, cervix, uterus, fallopian tubes, and ovaries (Figure 17-1). The major functions of the female reproductive system are sexual and procreative.

Ovaries

The *ovaries* are inside of the body and are referred to as the gonads. The ovaries mature eggs (ova) and are the primary site of female hormone production. Ovarian activity is determined by the amount of hormones in the body including luteinizing hormone (LH), follicle-stimulating hormone (FSH), estrogen, progesterone, and even testosterone.

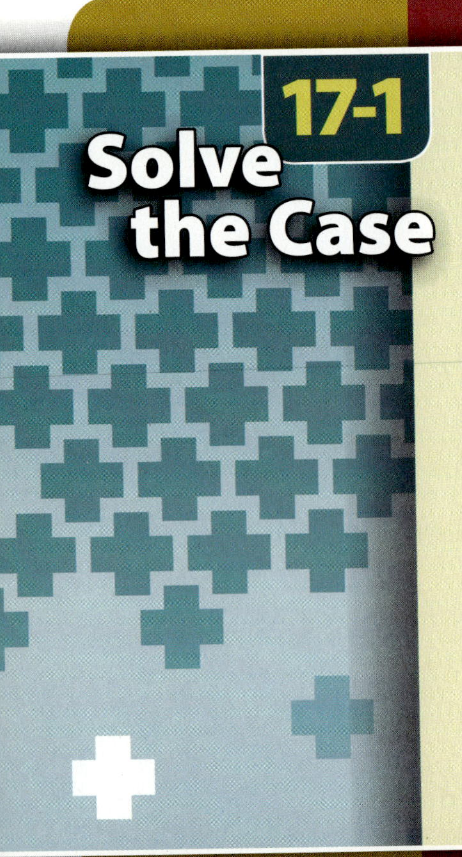

Danielle Rosman, a 26-year-old female is being seen in the office today for her yearly GYN exam with Dr. Ayerick. Your responsibility is to set up the equipment, obtain needed information from the patient, and instruct the patient to empty her bladder. When the patient is prepared, you enter the room with the provider for the exam. The provider performs a pelvic exam and Pap smear and collects the specimen and places it in the ThinPrep solution. When the exam is completed, you notice that the lid on the ThinPrep container is on crooked. You reach over to reposition the lid, and the lid separates from the container, causing the contents to spill on the floor. The patient just finished checking out but has not left the office yet. Given the situation and your current level of knowledge, what should you do? Consider the following questions.

1. **Will the test need to be repeated?**
2. **Would it be best to stop the patient before she leaves the office or call her on the telephone for a new appointment?**
3. **If you do stop the patient, should you tell her what happened before you tell the provider?**
4. **How should you approach the provider to advise of the situation?**
5. **Reviewing the steps taken to resolve, how could this incident have been prevented?**

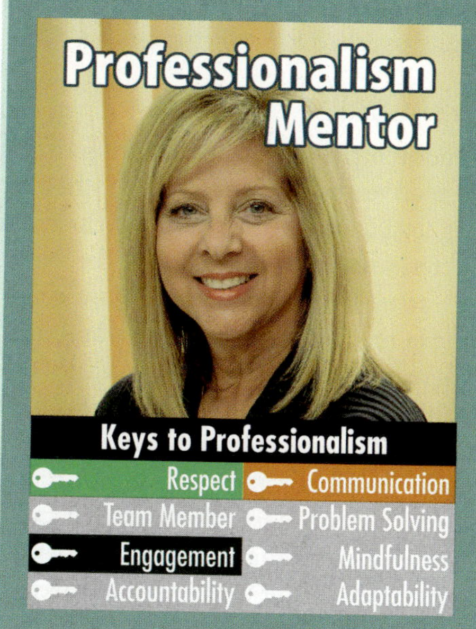

Occasionally, I will place a student medical assistant in an OB/GYN practice for their externship. Some medical assistants worry that working in an OB/GYN office will be too routine for them. While many of the patient appointments are for routine examinations, most patients don't consider these visits to be routine at all. Women in all stages of life will come to the OB/GYN practice and most will feel some level of apprehension or uneasiness. In one room there may be a new mother-to-be and in the next room a woman experiencing abnormal test results. As the medical assistant for both patients, you need to be both knowledgeable about the procedures being performed and respectful of both patients' feelings, however different they may be. In your journal, write down some of the conditions and procedures you may see while working with the OB/GYN patient. Try to imagine how they may be feeling so that when you interact with them, your actions will demonstrate your professionalism. ■

Without the ovarian production of estrogen, puberty would not lead to the menstrual cycle or female fertility. The interplay and cyclic nature of hormones is essential to fertility. Fertility involves multiple factors that include the release of an ovum every month to the fallopian tubes.

Fallopian Tubes

The *fallopian tubes* and uterus are structurally derived from embryonic ureter material called the *müllerian ducts*. The fallopian tubes are attached to the uterus and reach to the ovaries with finger-like fimbriae that capture the ovum. The ovum is guided through the fallopian tubes by small projections called cilia inside the tubes. Additionally, the fallopian tubes are the location where sperm and egg merge into a single cell (zygote). The transport of the zygote to the uterus is essential to a successful pregnancy.

Uterus

The uterus (refer to Figure 17-1) is composed of a *myometrium* (muscle) and *endometrium* (vascular tissue). The *endometrium* is the lining that allows the zygote to attach and feed nutrients from the mother's blood supply through

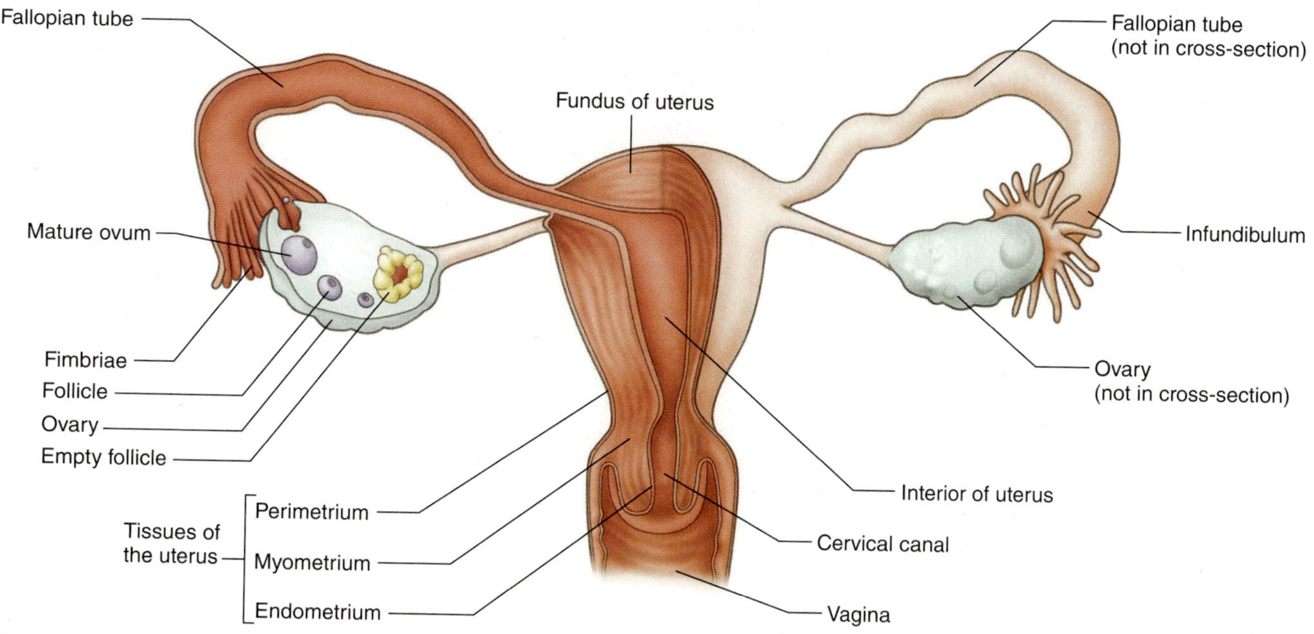

Figure 17-1 ■ The female reproductive system.

diffusion and, later, the placenta. When pregnancy fails to occur, the body sloughs this endometrial lining monthly and is referred to as menstruation, menses, or a period.

The myometrium of the uterus is a muscle that leads to cramps and contractions. This muscle facilitates the delivery of the baby, decrease of blood flow to the placenta after birth, the delivery of the placenta, and then reduction of bleeding in the postpartum period. The uterus and vagina are connected by the cervix.

Vagina

The *vagina* is a structure that allows for sexual intercourse. The *vulva* and labial folds form the entrance and the *cervix* connects the vagina to the uterus. Structures of the *vulva* (external genitalia) include the *clitoris* (organ of arousal), urethral orifice (opening to the urethra), and the labia minora (inner vaginal folds) and majora (outer vaginal folds) (Figure 17-2). Two tiny glands referred to as *Bartholins glands* are under the skin and usually not visible. They secrete a lubricant which moistens the vulva. The vagina is lined by *rugae* (ribbed regions) and by *mucosa* (a mucous producing thin lining), which allows for lubrication and cleanliness. The cervix is of particular importance in that it is the opening that allows menstrual flow, receives sperm during sexual intercourse, and allows the passage of the newborn during delivery. Tissue obtained from the cervical region during a Pap smear is usually checked for cell changes.

The Menstrual Cycle

Each month, the endometrial lining (inner lining of the uterus) prepares to receive and nourish a zygote (the first set of cells following fertilization). If fertilization does not occur, the lining deteriorates and flows out of the body, a process known as **menses** or **menstruation**. A woman's first menstrual cycle is referred to as **menarche** and usually occurs somewhere between the ages of 11 and 15, but this varies among different ethnicities and the girl can be as young as 9 years old. The monthly cycle continues for approximately 35 years until complete cessation occurs, a process referred to as **menopause.** A menstrual cycle begins with the first day of woman's menstrual period and lasts until the first day of the next monthly period. The average menstrual cycle is right around 28 days but may range anywhere from 21 to 35 days depending on the individual. The average length of the bleeding portion of the cycle can last anywhere from three to eight days. Terms related to menstrual flow include the following:

- **Amenorrhea:** Absence of menstrual flow, either primary (never had a menses) or secondary (stops due to an event such as pregnancy or menopause).
- **Dysmenorrhea:** Difficult or painful menstruation

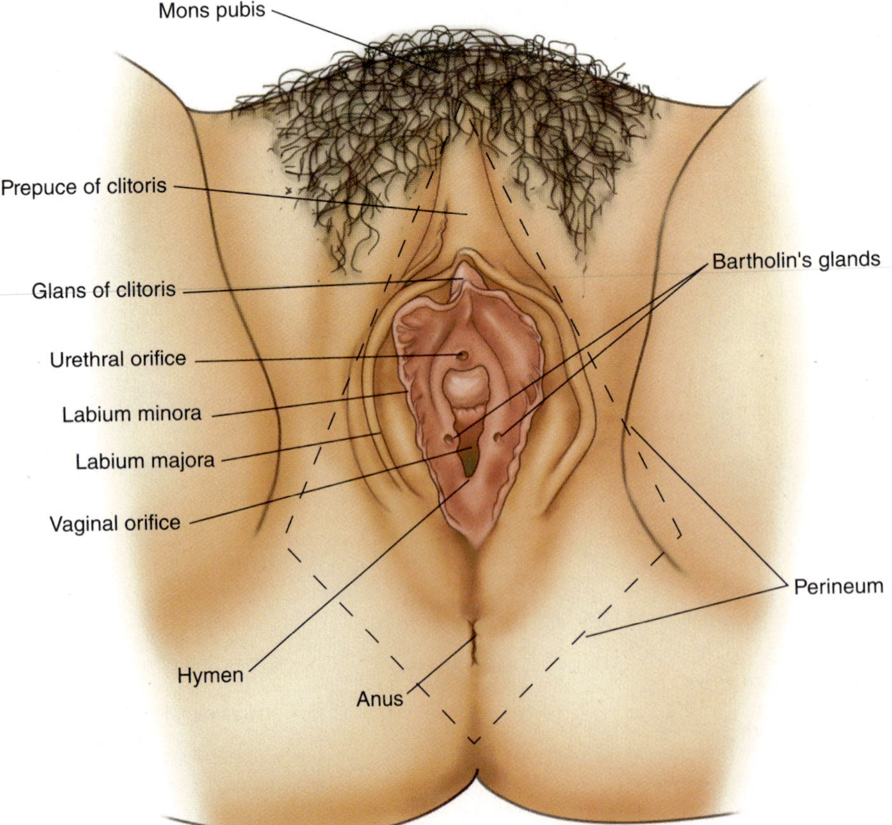

Figure 17-2 ■ Female external genitalia.

- **Abnormal Uterine Bleeding (AUB)**: AUB has replaced the terms *menorrhagia* (excessive menses) and *metorrhagia* (abnormal timing or bleeding between periods).

The menstrual cycle is controlled by hormonal activity within the body. As a woman ages, hormone activity diminishes, stimulating both physiological and psychological changes within the woman. Figure 17-3 illustrates the hormonal and physical changes that occur throughout the menstrual cycle.

Menopause

Menopause, defined earlier as cessation of menses, occurs around the age of 52, but can occur any time after the age of 40. Women can be thrown into "premature" or "induced menopause" as a result of a complete

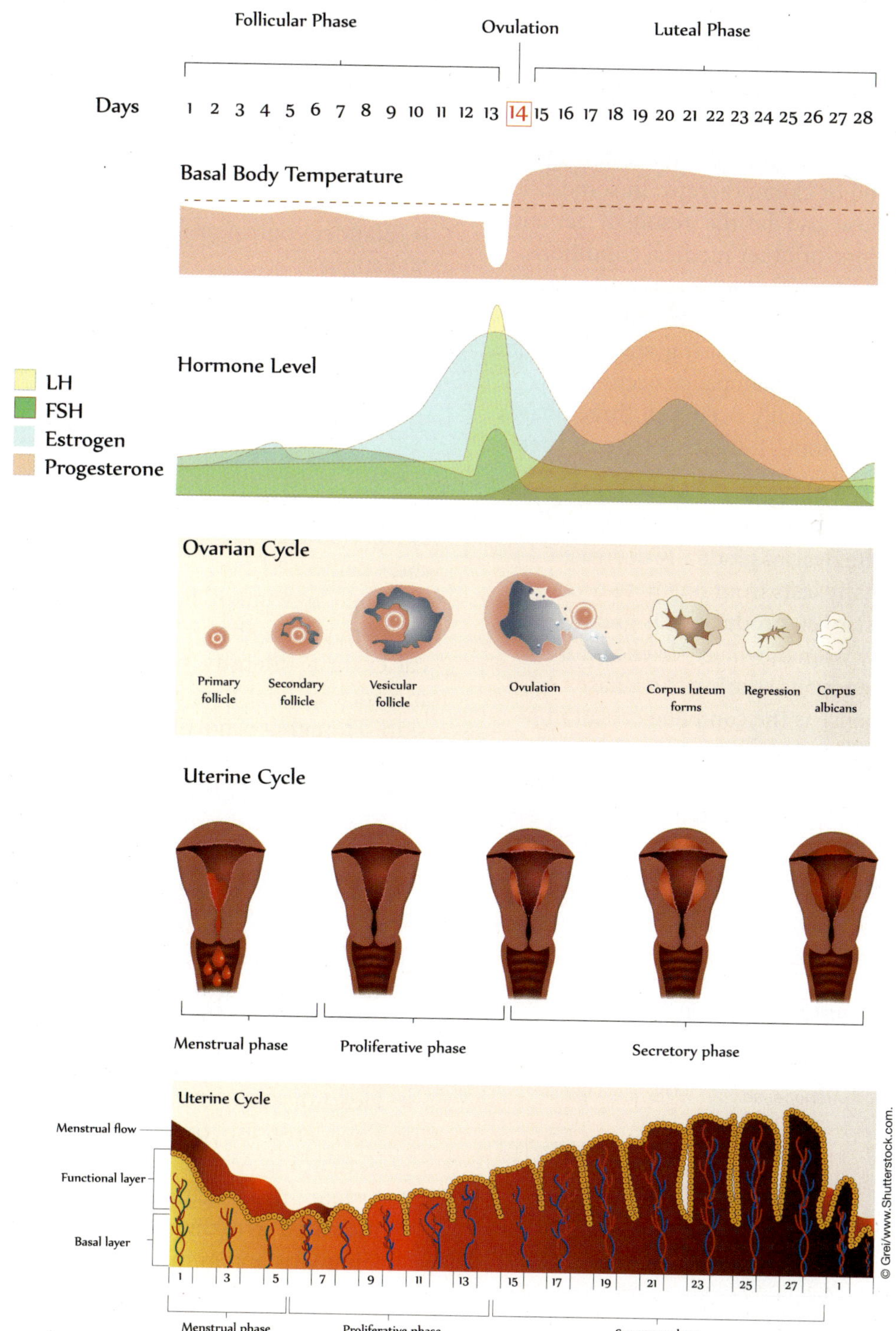

Figure 17-3 ■ A graphic example of the menstrual cycle.

CRITICAL THINKING CHALLENGE

Refer to Figure 17-3 and answer the following questions:

1. **What day of the menstrual cycle are women most likely to ovulate?**
2. **Which hormones are at their highest level during ovulation?**
3. **What vital sign is a good indicator that ovulation is near?**

hysterectomy or certain treatments that can damage the ovaries, like radiation or chemotherapy. In some cases, premature menopause can be the result of genetics, autoimmune disorders, or other medical conditions.

The ovaries are responsible for storing and releasing eggs and for the production of estrogen and progesterone. When the ovaries stop releasing eggs, hormone production decreases, and menopause occurs.

Natural menopause usually occurs in three phases. Figure 17-4 lists symptoms for each phase of menopause and the time intervals for each phase.

- Phase 1: **Perimenopause** begins when estrogen production by the ovaries gradually decreases. This stage normally lasts from one to two years, at which time estrogen production is greatly decreased. Many women will experience the symptoms of menopause during this phase.
- Phase 2: Menopause is the complete cessation of menstrual flow. The ovaries have now stopped producing almost all estrogen and have stopped releasing eggs. A diagnosis of menopause is determined after a female has not had a period for 12 months.

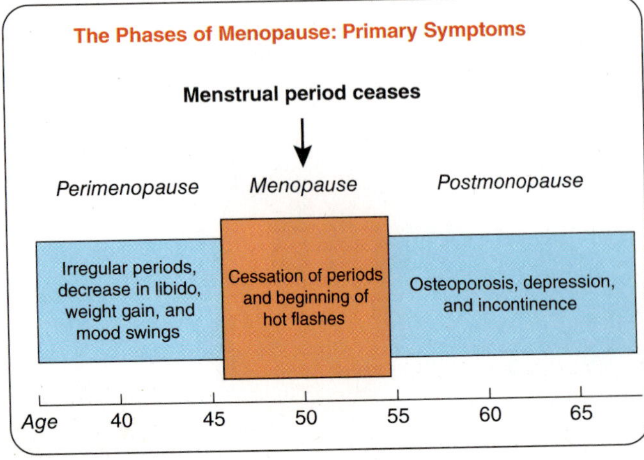

Figure 17-4 ■ The phases of menopause.

- Phase 3: Postmenopause is the phase that includes all years after menopause. Usually, menopausal symptoms will stop, but other health risks such as osteoporosis and cardiovascular disease related to loss of estrogen will continue to increase with natural aging.

Symptoms of Menopause

The most common complaint of women during menopause is "hot flashes." The body experiences a sudden warmness that can range from mild to extremely hot, the skin can become red, and heavy perspiration often occurs. Other symptoms include:

- Headaches
- Joint and muscle pain
- Vaginal dryness
- Bladder control problems
- Fatigue
- Mood swings
- Insomnia
- Decrease in concentration
- Depression
- Irritability

Most symptoms are nothing more than a nuisance and only a small percentage of women experience symptoms that are uncomfortable enough to hinder their daily activities.

When a woman begins to experience symptoms of menopause, the provider will usually do a physical exam to identify signs of decreased estrogen that includes vaginal dryness and thin or fragile mucosal skin. Though it is not always necessary, blood tests may be ordered to confirm decreased estrogen production. The level of follicle-stimulating hormone (FSH) rises as the ovaries have decreased estrogen production.

Long-Term Health Issues Linked to Menopause

The following health problems can be directly linked to the decrease in estrogen that occurs with the onset of menopause. These health issues include:

- Poor bowel and bladder function
- Heart disease
- Poor brain function with an increased risk of developing Alzheimer's disease
- Osteoporosis (brittle bone disease)
- Increased wrinkling of the skin due to poor elasticity
- Gingivitis and gum recession
- Loss of muscle tone and power
- Vision problems, such as cataracts or macular degeneration

Several treatment options exist to combat the health problems associated with menopause. The provider and patient should work together to determine the best course of treatment.

Hormone Replacement Therapy

Hormone replacement therapy (HRT) used to be common among perimenopausal and postmenopausal women. Women were placed on hormones to help alleviate hot flashes and sleep problems and to help protect them from diseases such as colon cancer, osteoporosis, and heart disease. The latest studies now conclude that HRT may be linked to breast cancer, blood clots, dementia (in a small number of women), and cardiovascular disease. The Food and Drug Administration (FDA) has changed their guidelines and recommendations for the use of this type of treatment and now recommends that HRT only be used:

- To treat or prevent osteoporosis in those women at high risk of developing the disorder. The risks of taking HRT must be weighed against the possible side effects.
- Short-term use to relieve perimenopausal symptoms. Again, women must decide if the benefits of using HRT outweigh the risks.
- Alternatives to HRT for hot flashes include certain selective serotonin reuptake inhibitors (SSRIs), serotonin norepinephrine reuptake inhibitors (SNRIs), and gabapentin.

Health Coach

Hormone Replacement Therapy Alternatives

Patients should be made aware of alternative treatment methods to HRT. There are many herbal remedies on the market as well as transdermal creams and patches that claim to relieve menopausal symptoms. Some medical providers specialize in homeopathic medicine and design specially formulated creams and herbal supplements for individuals looking for alternatives to HRT. There are even compounding pharmacies that specialize in designing these unique formulas and "bio-identical" preparations. Just because a medication is termed as "natural" or "homeopathic" doesn't mean that it is without risks especially since there are no regulatory bodies that ensure purity or efficacy. Some natural remedies may also contain trace amounts of estrogen and may pose slight risks for the patients that use them. In the case of bio-identical products, studies suggest inferior results when compared to conventional HRT. Whatever the case, patients should be educated about the benefits and risks of all treatments so that they can make informed decisions that are right for their bodies.

Meet the **Specialists**

Specialists who treat women's health: obstetrics and gynecology include the following:

- **OB-GYN**: A provider who specializes in diagnosing and treating diseases of the female reproductive system and breasts, and caring for a woman while she is pregnant. The "OB" portion of the term is the abbreviation that is used for obstetrics and is the branch of medicine that involves caring for a woman while she is pregnant. Some physicians, especially those close to retirement age, may cease to care for obstetric patients and will only practice the gynecology side of OB-GYN medicine.
- **Infertility Specialist:** A provider who specializes in assisting patients who are experiencing problems with conception or carrying pregnancies to term delivery.
- **Midwife:** Both Certified Nurse Midwives (CNM) and Certified Professional Midwives (CPM) have specialty training in the care of the pregnant female as well as labor, delivery, and the postpartum period. Both are accredited through the same process, but CNM's are registered nurses prior to their midwifery training. Midwives can work in the hospital and some will offer home labor management to those who don't want to deliver in the hospital setting.

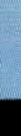
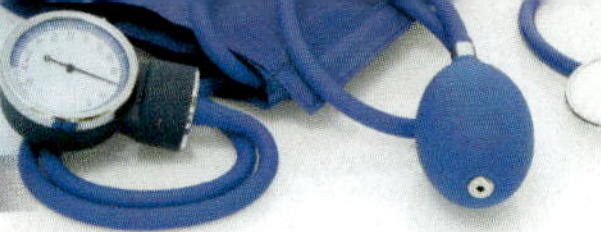

Table 17-1 Common OB-GYN Abbreviations

Abbreviation	Meaning	Abbreviation	Meaning
Cx Bx	Cervical biopsy	PCO	Polycystic ovarian disease
C/S	Cesarean section	PMS	Premenstrual syndrome
D&C	Dilation and curettage of the uterus	Q	Quickening
EAB	Elective abortion	STD	Sexually transmitted disease
EDC	Estimated day of confinement (delivery due date)	STI	Sexually transmitted infection
EGA	Estimated gestational age	SAB	Spontaneous abortion
FHT	Fetal heart tones	SUI	Stress urinary incontinence
IUFD/FDIU	Intrauterine fetal demise/fetal death in utero	TAH	Total abdominal hysterectomy
LMP	Last menstrual period	TVH	Total vaginal hysterectomy
OCT	Oxytocin challenge test	TL	Tubal ligation
PID	Pelvic inflammatory disease	U/S	Ultrasound

OBSTETRIC AND GYNECOLOGIC ABBREVIATION REVIEW

Medical assistants working in obstetrics and gynecology should be familiar with the abbreviations listed in Table 17-1.

GYNECOLOGIC IN-OFFICE AND TELEPHONE SCREENING TIPS

Medical assistants may have the responsibility of screening patients prior to provider examination or over the telephone. The depth of screening will be established by office protocol, but in general, medical assistants should be able to ask a series of questions related to the patient's symptoms. Table 17-2 lists types of questions that are typically asked during a GYN screening and lists common procedures that coincide with symptoms.

Important note: Medical assistants should never perform any procedure unless directed to do so by the provider; however, they can set up various equipment and supplies to help save time in the event that testing is ordered.

COMMON OBSTETRIC AND GYNECOLOGIC DISEASES

There are many conditions that affect women's health. In this section we will describe some of the most common conditions that affect women, and in particular obstetrics and gynecology.

Vulvodynia

Vulvar pain, burning, stinging, irritation, or rawness, is common and difficult to treat due to the extensive differential diagnosis. Treatment is often aimed at the root cause such as inadequate stimulation or lubrication prior to sexual intercourse through a variety of modalities that includes hygiene, medications, lubrications, biofeedback, pelvic physiotherapy, sexual counseling, and occasionally surgery. One of the diagnoses that causes significant vulvodynia (pain in the vulvar area) is herpes simplex virus, which causes painful ulcerations of mucosal and surrounding tissues.

Vaginitis

Irritation of the vaginal region usually related to local irritant, infection, or inflammation often associated with vaginal discharge. Yeast infections, contact dermatitis, bacterial vaginosis, and urinary tract infections are common, but any woman with sexual contact should be evaluated for sexually transmitted infections (STIs).

Uterine Fibroids

A benign myometrial tumor can lead to severe cramping and uterine bleeding. It is one of the most common reasons females have hysterectomies, but smaller fibroids can be removed by ablation (procedure that destroys the uterine lining), surgical removal of just the fibroids, and embolization (blocking blood vessels that provide blood to the fibroids). These tumors can be quite large and numerous and can be identified by ultrasonography.

Table 17-2 Patient Screening and Instructions for Patients with Breast Concerns, Urogenital Concerns, or Pregnancy Concerns

Breast Screenings	
Ask the Patient:	■ Are you experiencing any pain, fever, tenderness, lumps, swelling, nipple drainage, odor, change in the size, or any dimpling? ■ Is there a familial history of breast disease?
For Patients Calling on the Telephone	Patients calling with any of the symptoms above should usually be seen for an appointment.
When in the Office:	
Disrobing Instructions	Remove all clothing from the waist up.
Vital Signs	Blood pressure, temperature, pulse, respiratory rate, and pain
Equipment	Drape or disposable gown
Possible Procedures	In office: Skin scrapings Out of office: Breast ultrasound, mammogram, or breast biopsy
Urogenital Symptoms	
Ask the Patient:	Are you experiencing any vaginal pain, discharge, unusual odor, pain during intercourse, any urinary symptoms, abdominal or lower back pain, or fever?
For Patients Calling on the Telephone	Patients with vaginal or urinary symptoms should usually be seen as soon as possible to avoid migration of bacteria to other structures.
When in the Office:	
Disrobing Instructions	If the patient exhibits vaginal symptoms, disrobe from the waist down.
Vital Signs	Blood pressure, temperature, pulse, respiratory rate, and pain
Equipment	Pelvic tray with cultures, if applicable
Possible Procedures	Pelvic exam, Pap smear, HPV co-testing, sexually transmitted infection (STI) polymerase chain reaction (PCR), swab (to check for diseases like chlamydia, gonorrhea, and herpes), urinalysis (if the patient complains of urinary symptoms)
Pregnant Patients	
Ask the Patient:	■ What is your expected date of delivery? ■ Are you experiencing any swelling in extremities, any vaginal discharge or discomfort, vaginal bleeding, fetal movement, any headaches, dizziness, or vision problems, any nausea or vomiting?
For Patients Calling on the Telephone	Amniotic leak concerns or vaginal bleeding should be evaluated immediately.
When in the Office:	
Disrobing Instructions	*First visit:* Completely disrobe *Subsequent visits until week 36:* Abdominal exam with Doppler for fetal heart rate *Weeks 36 and beyond:* Disrobe below waist for Group B Streptococcus (GBS) testing and possibly a cervical exam
Vital Signs	Blood pressure, temperature, pulse, respiratory rate, and pain
Equipment	Fetal doppler, ultrasound gel, ultrasound equipment (if applicable), tape measure, urine dipsticks, pelvic tray and cultures, and (first visit only) blood drawing equipment
Possible procedures	Urinalysis, ultrasonography (if applicable), blood draws (when applicable), Leopold maneuvers (to check position of baby), doptones (fetal heart rate), and pelvic and cervical exam

Breast Cancer

A diagnosis of breast cancer is devastating to women and their families. According to the American Cancer Society, more than 232,000 women were diagnosed with breast cancer in 2014 alone in the United States. About 40,000 women will die each year from breast cancer. Refer to the Health Coach Disease Feature to learn more about this disease.

Other Common Obstetric and Gynecologic Diseases

Other Cancers

There are several other cancers that affect female patients including cervical, ovarian, uterine, and endometrial cancers (Table 17-3). Providers screen for cervical cancer based on the American Society for

Health Coach

Featured Disease Spotlight: Breast Cancer

Description	Abnormal breast cells that can grow and spread throughout the body.
Diagram	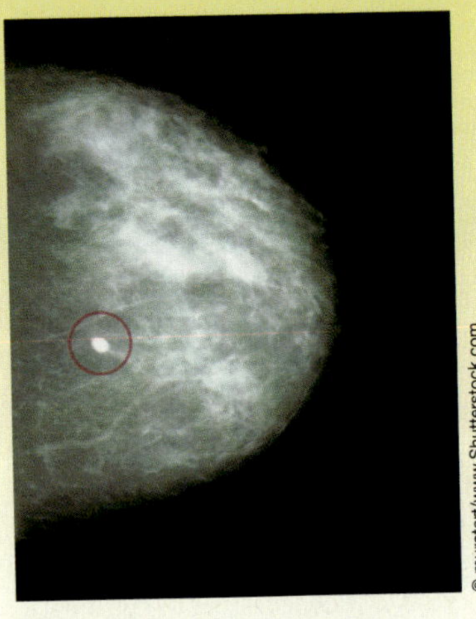 © muratart/www.Shutterstock.com. **Figure 17-5** ■ Breast cancer detected on mammography.
Risk Factors	Age, sex (female), genetics (BRCA1 and BRCA2), family history, ethnicity (Caucasian), dense breast tissue, smoking, alcohol consumption, unopposed estrogen (an imbalance of estrogen and progesterone due to obesity, hormone therapy and so on), radiation exposure, no prior pregnancies by 30 years of age, menarche (first period) younger than 12 years of age, menopause after 55 years of age, sedentary lifestyle, and chemical exposures. BRCA1 and BRCA2 are human genes that produce tumor suppressor proteins that help repair damaged DNA. If the BRCA genes mutate, a women's risk for developing breast or ovarian cancer, or both, is greatly increased.
Symptoms	Nipple discharge, lump, armpit swelling, breast tenderness, abnormal skin findings (color, texture, contour), skin flattening or dimpling.
Diagnostic Testing	Mammogram, ultrasound, fine-needle biopsy
Modifying Factors (if applicable)	Smoking cessation, diet, hormone therapy, weight control
Treatment	Lumpectomy, mastectomy, bilateral mastectomy, chemotherapy, radiation, lymph node dissection

Colposcopy and Cervical Pathology (ASCCP) screening and management guidelines. Pap smears screening begins at 21 years of age and continues every three years for patients based on the 2013 guidelines. Ovarian and uterine cancers are not screened for due to low benefit and the scarcity of disease in the absence of symptoms. However, symptoms such as abdominal fullness, pain, and abnormal uterine bleeding may lead to further evaluation of these diseases. Patients over the age of 40–45 years old with abnormal uterine bleeding may be offered an endometrial biopsy to evaluate for signs of endometrial cancer.

Table 17-3 Female Cancers

Age Group	Cancer Screening Testing Recommendations Related to the Female Reproductive System
20–29	*Breast Cancer Testing:* Clinical breast exam every three years. If there is a family history of breast cancer, clinical breast exams should be conducted more often. Check with the provider to determine when mammograms should be started. *Cervical Cancer Testing:* Ages 21–29 all women should have a Pap test every three years. Human papillomavirus (HPV) tests should not be used unless a Pap test is abnormal. If patient is in a high risk group for cervical cancer, testing should be performed more often.
30–39	*Breast Cancer Testing:* Same as 20–29 age group *Cervical Cancer Testing:* Starting at age 30, patients at average risk should have a Pap smear and HPV test every five years or a Pap test only every three years. High-risk groups should be tested more often. No testing is necessary for patients who have had hysterectomies that include removal of the uterus and cervix not related to cervical cancer.
40–49	*Breast Cancer Testing:* Clinical breast exam and mammogram every year. *Cervical Cancer Testing:* Same as 30–39 group
50–65	*Breast Cancer Testing:* Same as 40–49 group *Cervical Cancer Testing:* Same as 30–39 group
65 plus	*Breast Cancer Testing:* Same as 40–49 group *Cervical Cancer Screening:* No testing is necessary if patient has had normal results during previous 10 years.

Health Coach

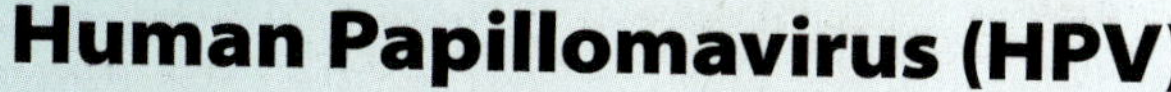

Human Papillomavirus (HPV)

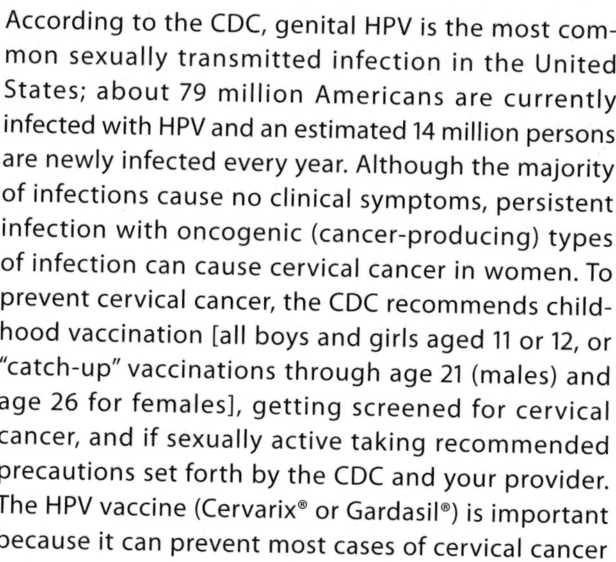

According to the CDC, genital HPV is the most common sexually transmitted infection in the United States; about 79 million Americans are currently infected with HPV and an estimated 14 million persons are newly infected every year. Although the majority of infections cause no clinical symptoms, persistent infection with oncogenic (cancer-producing) types of infection can cause cervical cancer in women. To prevent cervical cancer, the CDC recommends childhood vaccination [all boys and girls aged 11 or 12, or "catch-up" vaccinations through age 21 (males) and age 26 for females], getting screened for cervical cancer, and if sexually active taking recommended precautions set forth by the CDC and your provider. The HPV vaccine (Cervarix® or Gardasil®) is important because it can prevent most cases of cervical cancer in females if it is given before a person is exposed to the virus. Cervarix® is one of the two vaccines on the market and is given to females only. Gardasil® is given to both male and female patients. The vaccine is given in a series of separate shots. The series has had a great success, and the number of women with HPV infection is expected to plummet over the next several years. Patients should be warned, however, that the vaccine does not protect them from all forms of HPV. Though there is still some concern regarding the efficacy of the HPV vaccinations in preventing cervical cancer risk, several well-conducted studies have shown reductions in cervical cancer rates. For patients who choose not to vaccinate, avoiding smoking should be highly encouraged as smoking decreases the clearance of HPV at the level of the cervix.

Sexually Transmitted Infections

Sexually transmitted diseases (STDs), also sometimes referred to as **sexually transmitted infections (STIs)**, continue to be a problem despite all of the education available on the topic. STDs and STIs are defined as infections that are transmitted through sexual contact, such as chlamydia, gonorrhea, and syphilis. Not all STIs turn into an STD, however all STDs start with an STI. STDs affect all age groups, including seniors. The Centers for Disease Control and Prevention (CDC) estimates that 20 million new STIs occur every year in the United States, and half of those infections affect young people aged 15–24. STIs can lead to severe reproductive health complications. In 2012 it was estimated that the costs to diagnose and treat STIs runs almost $16 billion annually. While anyone can become infected with an STI, certain groups, including gay and bisexual men, and young people, are at greatest risk according to the CDC.

Table 17-4 Sexually Transmitted Infections (STIs)

STI	Symptoms	Treatment
Chlamydia (bacterial infection)	Vaginal discharge, burning sensation or pain with urination. Maybe none.	Azithromycin or doxycycline, but erythromycin and levofloxacin are also used
Gonorrhea (bacterial infection)	Women are usually asymptomatic, but may develop inflammation with a greenish discharge	Ceftriaxone or cefixime with co-treatment for chlamydia
Genital herpes (viral infection)	Fluid-filled vesicles on the genitalia that erupt and become painful ulcers	No cure; treatment with antiviral medication can help prevent outbreaks
Syphilis (bacterial infection)	Vary according to stage of the disease: during the first stage, a painless lesion called a chancre appears; in the second stage, an infectious rash on hands and feet appears; in the third stage, no symptoms are seen until nerve or organ damage is present	Benzathin penicillin G

Of course, all groups are at risk for contracting STIs. The medical assistant is usually responsible for delivering patient education in this area. The CDC website has links to many brochures and fact sheets regarding this topic. Log on to the CDC website and search the topic "Sexually Transmitted Diseases (STDs)." Some brief information regarding STIs can be found in Table 17-4.

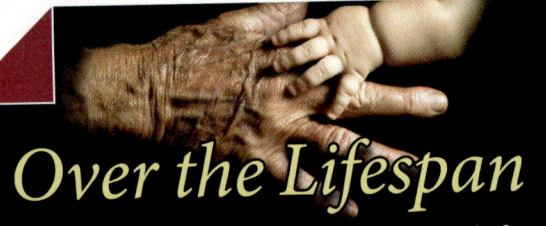

Over the Lifespan

Adult women have a monthly cycle comprised of proliferative (development) and secretory phases. In the proliferative phase (also known as the follicular phase), estrogen is the predominant circulating hormone. Estrogen causes the proliferation of the endometrium in preparation for ovulation, fertilization, and implantation. Midcycle is pronounced by the peak secretion of follicle-stimulating hormone, estrogen in response, and then ovulation (the release of the egg). In the secretory phase, progesterone is the predominant circulating hormone. Progesterone causes the thickened endometrium to become porous and leaky, ready to receive the fertilized egg. This cycle is repeated monthly for the entirety of a woman's fertile years.

While a woman is fertile, mucous membranes within the vagina are pliable and moist. When the menstrual cycle begins to fail or become irregular around 40 to 50 years of age, menopause begins. The mucous membranes begin to dry. Additionally, the structures around the vagina become less supported and can lead to cystoceles (herniation of the urinary bladder into the vagina) and bladder incontinence issues. Vaginal bleeding after menopause is abnormal and warrants evaluation. In menopause, estrogen levels are very low but follicle-stimulating hormones are elevated.

FEATURED GYNECOLOGIC PROCEDURES

Medical assistants often have the responsibility of assisting the provider during examination or procedures, setting up outside procedures (procedures not performed in the office), and educating patients in the proper preparation of specific procedures. This section will focus on procedures routinely performed by medical assistants, within their scope of practice.

Gynecological Exam

The gynecological (GYN) exam consists of a breast exam, abdominal and pelvic exam, and a Pap test. The Pap test, which derived its name from the developer of the test (Dr. George Papanicolaou), is performed to detect early signs of cervical cancer. The GYN exam may also include a wet mount, hanging drop, KOH wet prep, or STI testing if the patient is complaining of vaginal symptoms (Chapter 27 discusses these three tests in detail). It is recommended that women have an annual GYN exam when they become sexually active or by the time they reach age 20. This exam may be included as part of a complete physical exam or may be performed separately.

The GYN exam is not only useful for early detection of cervical cancer, but also breast cancer and other potential health risks related to the female reproductive system. While the order in which steps are performed may differ, the following is a listing of the steps that take place during a GYN exam:

1. Complete and thorough breast exam
2. External pelvic and vaginal exam
3. Collection of tissue for Pap smear and possible cultures when indicated
4. Bimanual pelvic/abdominal exam
5. Rectal–vaginal exam

All of these exams are explained in greater detail later in this chapter. The provider may conduct a pelvic exam without performing a Pap test. This is common when the patient comes in complaining of gynecological symptoms.

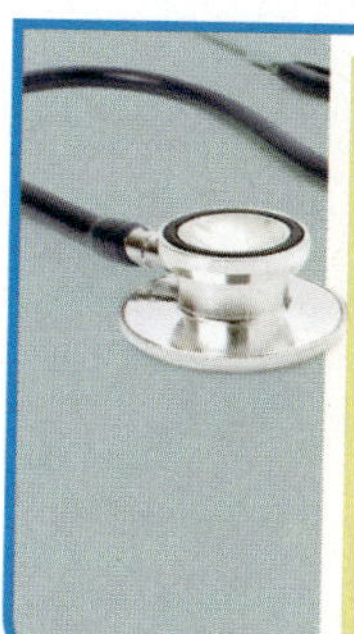

Field Smarts

It is highly recommended that male providers have a female assistant present whenever performing breast or genital exams. This will help to alleviate false accusations and reduce lawsuits that are unjust.

If the patient is a new patient, a complete GYN and medical history should be obtained prior to beginning the exam. If the patient is an established patient, the history should be reviewed and amended as necessary. The patient can complete the history herself or the medical assistant may obtain the information by interview. Pertinent information to be included in a complete GYN history includes the following:

- Age at onset of menstrual cycle
- **Gravida** (how many pregnancies?), **para** (how many live births?), and abortions (specify how many and whether they were spontaneous or elective); the para portion is often reported in the TPAL (Term delivery, preterm delivery, abortions, and currently living) format. G2T1P1A0L1 would be two pregnancies, one term birth, one preterm birth, no abortions, and one living child.
- Date of last menstrual period (LMP)
- Regularity and duration of cycles
- Date of last Pap
- Any history of abnormal Pap or biopsies
- Contraception method used
- HRT information
- Date of last mammogram for women over 40 or who are at high risk
- Types and dates of GYN surgeries
- Sexual activity and history (up to the provider)
- Signs or symptoms of GYN disorders including vaginal discharge or painful intercourse

Breast Exam

The American Cancer Society recommends that all females 20 years of age and older be educated on breast self-examinations (BSEs) and that females aged 20 to 39 also have a clinical exam of the breast every three years, with yearly clinical breast exams recommended for patients over 40 years old.

The provider usually begins the clinical breast exam with the patient in a sitting position. A visual inspection of each breast is performed noting any redness, puckering, or dimpling of the skin. The patient is then instructed to lie back and place both hands behind or over her head. The provider then palpates both breasts and armpits for any lump or thickening. The patient will also be asked if she is performing BSEs. Written instructions should be provided, in case the patient has questions about the procedure once she leaves the office. Figure 17-6 illustrates the proper technique for performing three methods of BSE, Figure 17-7 shows a breast self-examination model, and Procedure 17-1 lists the proper steps for instructing a patient on the correct way to perform BSE.

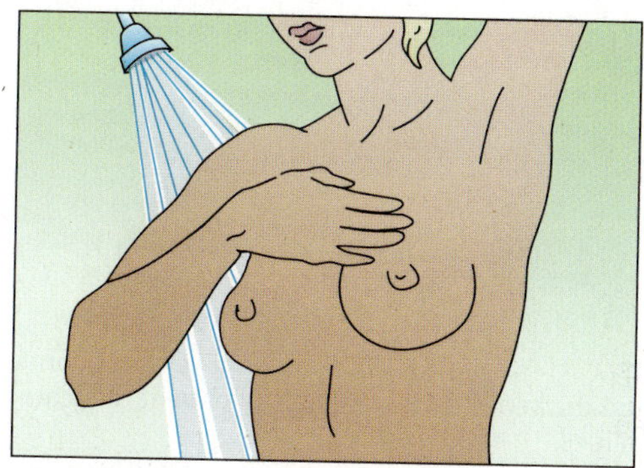

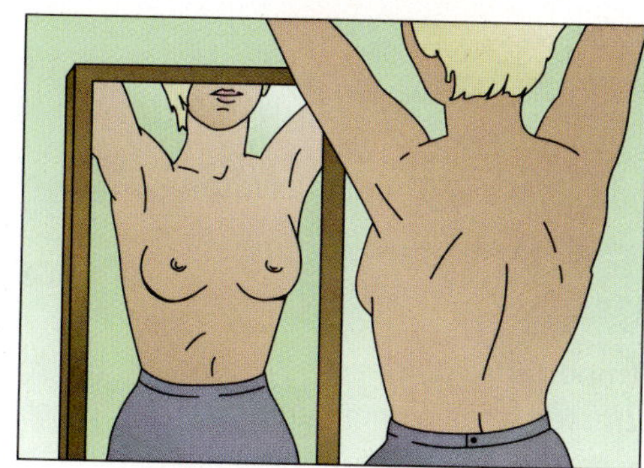

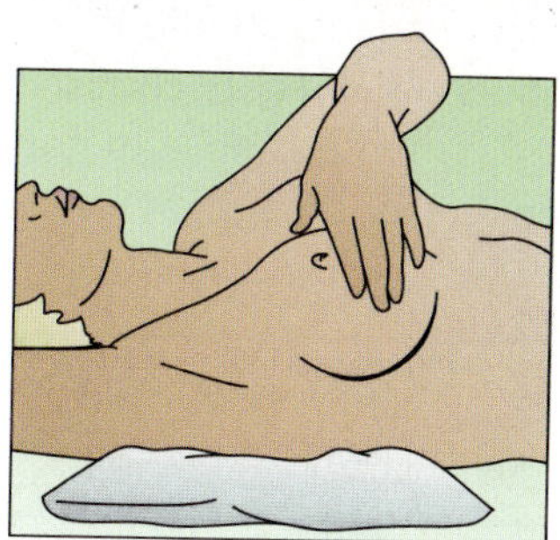

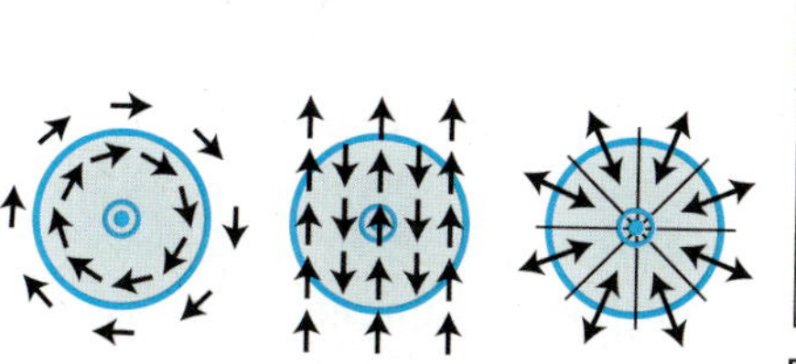

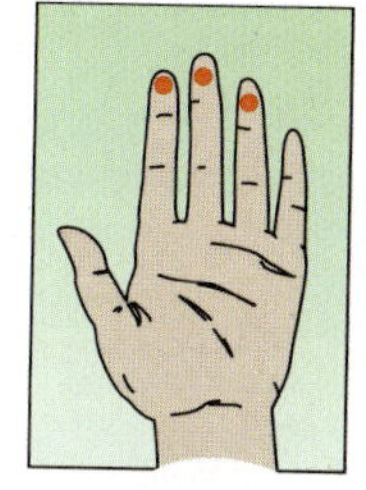

Figure 17-6 ■ Three methods of BSE should be performed monthly, using the pads of the first three fingers: in the shower, in front of a mirror, and while lying down. Refer to Procedure 17-1 for details.

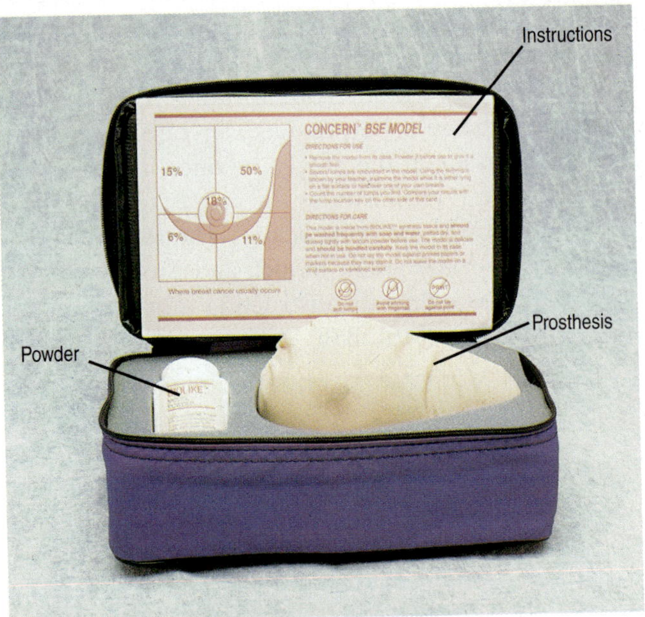

Figure 17-7 ■ The breast self-examination model contains lumps and thickenings for training the patient to locate and feel abnormalities.

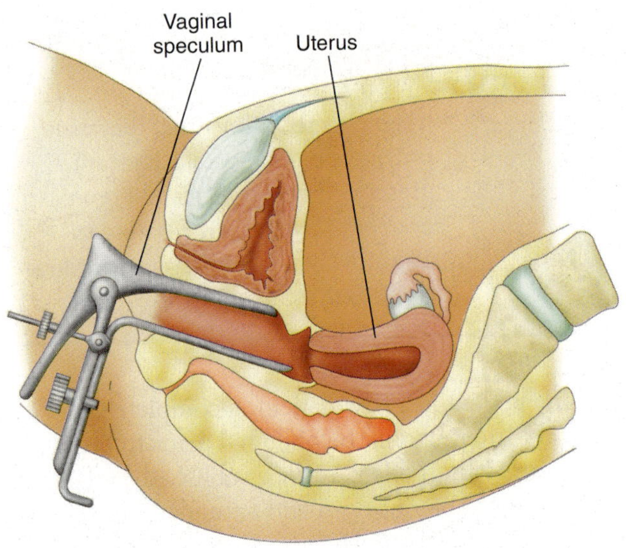

Figure 17-8 ■ A vaginal speculum is inserted to observe the vagina and cervix and to obtain a sample for the Pap test.

Health Coach

Breast Self-Exam

The importance of breast self-examination (BSE) must be stressed to all women above age 20. Breast cancer does not occur just in older women, but in younger women as well. Patients should be comfortable with their own bodies, and if they choose, be able to conduct a BSE. If patients choose to conduct BSE, they should be looking for changes as well as signs of breast cancer.

Signs to look for include the following:

- A prominent lump or nodule
- Bloody, brown, or serous discharge from the nipple
- Dimpling
- Nipple retraction
- Skin discoloration

The patient should become familiar with her breasts and report any changes to her provider immediately.

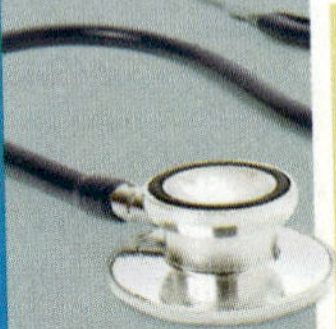

Field Smarts

Speculums are available in different sizes and are either disposable plastic or reusable metal. A metal speculum should be warmed before insertion for patient comfort. Holding the metal speculum under warm running water for several seconds should accomplish this and will also provide some lubrication.

Pelvic Exam

The provider will conduct a pelvic exam that consists of several components. First, a visual inspection of the external genitalia is conducted. Next, the cervix and vagina are visually examined by the use of a sterile speculum exam. Figure 17-8 illustrates proper speculum insertion.

Collection of Tissue for Pap Smear

If a Pap test is to be performed, cells from the cervix are obtained for **cytologic** evaluation (the examination of material for the purposes of cytology). **Cytology** is a branch of science dealing with the configuration, structure, and

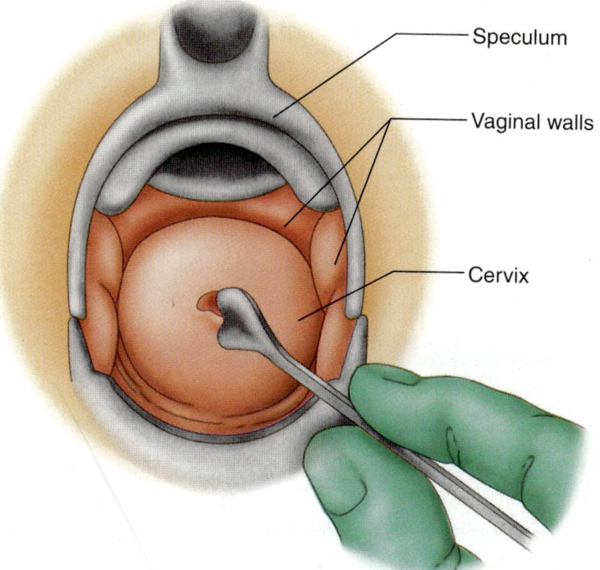

Figure 17-9 ■ The cervix is scraped with a spatula to obtain cells for a Pap test.

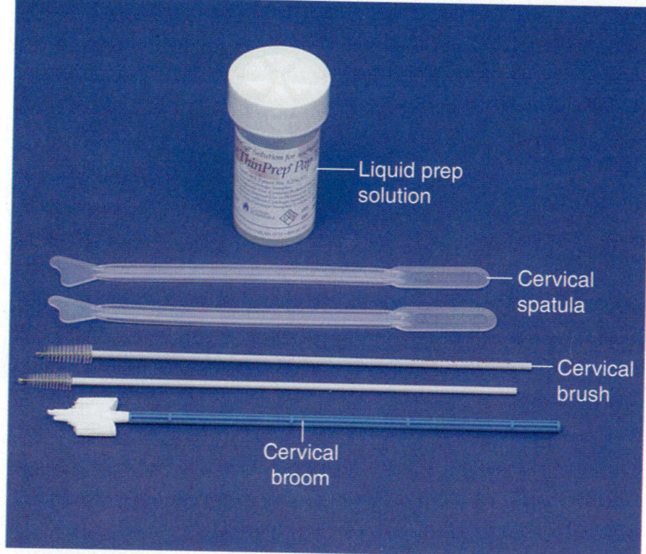

Figure 17-10 ■ A spatula and brush, or just a broom, may be used to collect cells when obtaining a specimen for the liquid prep method.

functions of cells, and also refers to a laboratory department that performs microscopic examination of cells, such as Pap tests. The Pap test, mentioned earlier, can detect cervical cancer in the early stages and can also detect any **atypical** cells or inflammation that may be present. Cells are collected from the cervix and endocervical canal by scraping the area (Figure 17-9) with a cervical spatula and brush or just a cervical broom (Figure 17-10).

Once the specimen is collected, the medical assistant will prepare the slides to be sent to the laboratory for evaluation. The slides must be properly labeled and must be accompanied by a cytology lab requisition (Figure 17-11) containing all pertinent information. Slides must be labeled with the proper patient identification, and the source of the specimen labeled as (V) for vaginal, (C) for cervical, or (E) for endocervical.

Health Coach

Preparing for a Pap Test

To provide the laboratory with the best possible specimen for cytologic evaluation, the patient must be properly prepared. The patient must adhere to the following preparation guidelines.

- Do not douche prior to the test. Douching washes away many of the cells and the specimen produces fewer cells for evaluation.
- Do not insert vaginal medications or spermicide for two days prior to the test. Both change the pH of the vagina, making the specimen invalid.
- Abstain from sexual intercourse for two days prior to the test. Intercourse can produce inflammation that can make the cells look abnormal.

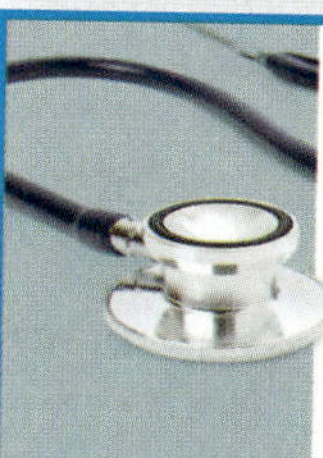

Field Smarts

It is important to remember that a Pap test detects cervical cancer and some other benign conditions of the cervix and vagina. Women who have had partial hysterectomies are still at risk of cervical cancer and should continue to have Pap smears. The Pap test does not, however, provide any information about the status of the endometrium inside the uterus. An endometrial biopsy must be performed in order to evaluate the lining of the uterus for abnormalities or endometrial cancer.

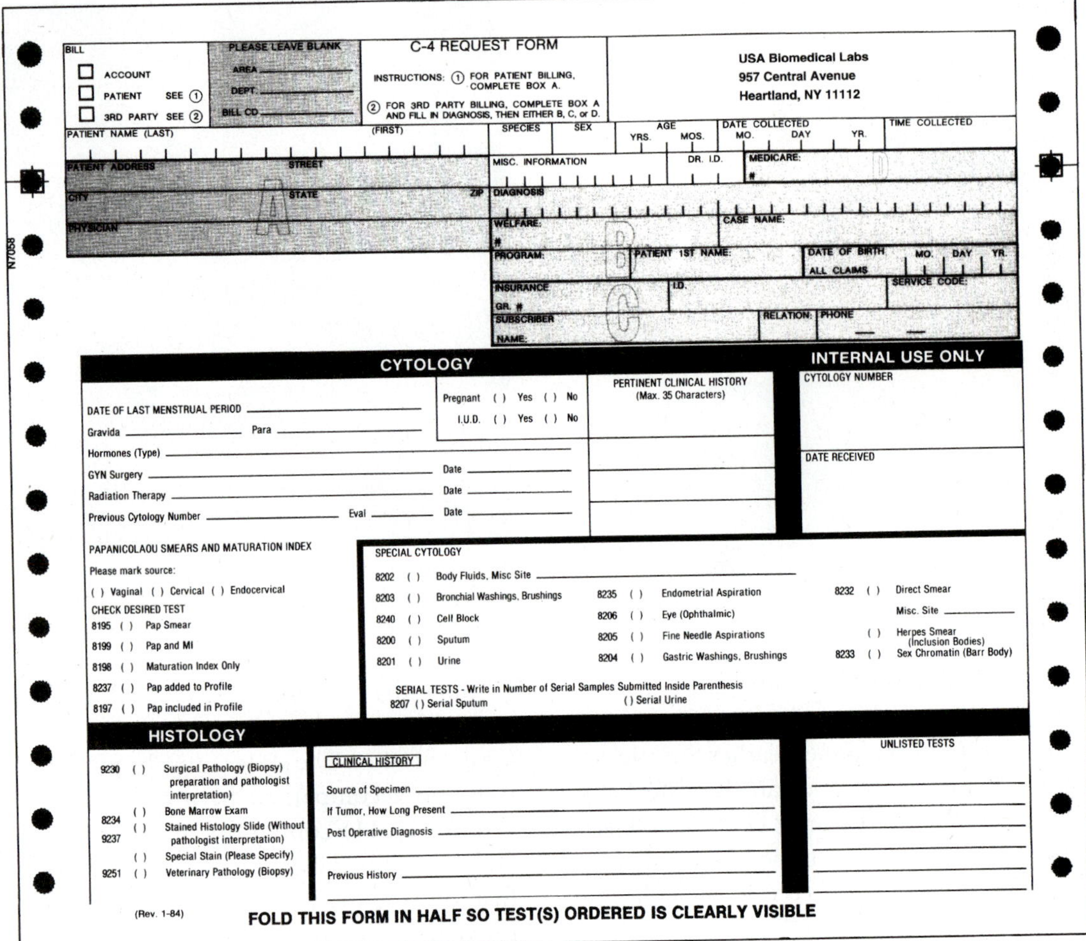

BILL
☐ ACCOUNT
☐ PATIENT SEE ①
☐ 3RD PARTY SEE ②

PLEASE LEAVE BLANK
AREA
DEPT.
BILL CD

C-4 REQUEST FORM
INSTRUCTIONS: ① FOR PATIENT BILLING, COMPLETE BOX A.
② FOR 3RD PARTY BILLING, COMPLETE BOX A AND FILL IN DIAGNOSIS, THEN EITHER B, C, or D.

USA Biomedical Labs
957 Central Avenue
Heartland, NY 11112

PATIENT NAME (LAST) | (FIRST) | SPECIES | SEX | AGE YRS. MOS. | DATE COLLECTED MO. DAY YR. | TIME COLLECTED

PATIENT ADDRESS | STREET | MISC. INFORMATION | DR. I.D. | MEDICARE: #
CITY | STATE | ZIP | DIAGNOSIS
PHYSICIAN | WELFARE: # | CASE NAME:
PROGRAM: | PATIENT 1ST NAME: | DATE OF BIRTH MO. DAY YR. | ALL CLAIMS
INSURANCE | I.D. | SERVICE CODE:
GR. #
SUBSCRIBER NAME: | RELATION: | PHONE

N7058

CYTOLOGY

DATE OF LAST MENSTRUAL PERIOD ______
Gravida ______ Para ______
Pregnant ( ) Yes ( ) No
I.U.D. ( ) Yes ( ) No
Hormones (Type) ______
GYN Surgery ______ Date ______
Radiation Therapy ______ Date ______
Previous Cytology Number ______ Eval ______ Date ______

PERTINENT CLINICAL HISTORY (Max. 35 Characters)

INTERNAL USE ONLY
CYTOLOGY NUMBER
DATE RECEIVED

PAPANICOLAOU SMEARS AND MATURATION INDEX
Please mark source:
( ) Vaginal ( ) Cervical ( ) Endocervical
CHECK DESIRED TEST
8195 ( ) Pap Smear
8199 ( ) Pap and MI
8198 ( ) Maturation Index Only
8237 ( ) Pap added to Profile
8197 ( ) Pap included in Profile

SPECIAL CYTOLOGY
8202 ( ) Body Fluids, Misc Site ______
8203 ( ) Bronchial Washings, Brushings
8240 ( ) Cell Block
8200 ( ) Sputum
8201 ( ) Urine
8235 ( ) Endometrial Aspiration
8206 ( ) Eye (Ophthalmic)
8205 ( ) Fine Needle Aspirations
8204 ( ) Gastric Washings, Brushings
8232 ( ) Direct Smear
Misc. Site ______
( ) Herpes Smear (Inclusion Bodies)
8233 ( ) Sex Chromatin (Barr Body)

SERIAL TESTS - Write in Number of Serial Samples Submitted Inside Parenthesis
8207 ( ) Serial Sputum ( ) Serial Urine

HISTOLOGY

9230 ( ) Surgical Pathology (Biopsy) preparation and pathologist interpretation)
8234 ( ) Bone Marrow Exam
9237 ( ) Stained Histology Slide (Without pathologist interpretation)
( ) Special Stain (Please Specify)
9251 ( ) Veterinary Pathology (Biopsy)

CLINICAL HISTORY
Source of Specimen ______
If Tumor, How Long Present ______
Post Operative Diagnosis ______
Previous History ______

UNLISTED TESTS

(Rev. 1-84)

FOLD THIS FORM IN HALF SO TEST(S) ORDERED IS CLEARLY VISIBLE

Figure 17-11 ■ A lab request form for a cytology examination.

One of two methods may be used to collect and preserve cells for a Pap test:

1. Conventional/Direct Method: Cells are collected and spread onto a slide that is placed into a jar with a liquid fixative, or the slide may be sprayed with a fixative and placed in a protective slide holder to be sent to the lab. (The fixative should be applied immediately after the cells are placed on the slide. Allowing the cells to dry on the slide can cause inaccurate readings.)
2. Liquid Prep Method: A specimen is collected and the collection device is agitated in a vial of liquid preservative to remove the cells. The vial is sent to the laboratory where slides are prepared, fixed, and stained. The liquid prep method has certain advantages over the direct method (see Table 17-5).

ViraPap

ViraPap® is another testing method that can be performed on the same specimen as the ThinPrep. This test detects the presence of human papillomavirus (HPV), which has been found to increase a woman's risk of developing cervical cancer.

Table 17-5 Direct versus ThinPrep Pap Method

Direct Method	Liquid Prep Method
Only a small portion of cells is smeared on the slide; 80% of the cells remain on the collection device.	Almost 100% of the specimen is rinsed from the collection device, providing the laboratory with a complete specimen for evaluation.
Cells can be unevenly distributed, and the slide may be contaminated with debris such as mucus and blood cells, making it difficult to evaluate.	The preparation process eliminates debris and evenly distributes a thin layer of cells on the slide.
Detects only cervical cancer	The same specimen may be used to detect chlamydia, human papillomavirus (HPV), and gonorrhea.

Interpreting Pap Test Results

The National Cancer Institute (NCI) developed a system for grading Pap tests that provides detailed information about the results. This system of reporting Pap results is known as the Bethesda system (TBS) and is divided into three parts. Any patient with an abnormal Pap will receive further testing.

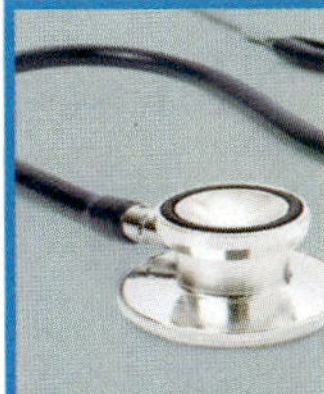

Field Smarts

The U.S. Food and Drug Administration (FDA) recently approved the first FDA-approved HPV DNA test for women 25 and older known as the cobas HPV test. The cobas HPV test can be used alone to help the health care provider assess the need for a woman to undergo additional diagnostic testing for cervical cancer as well as provide information about the patient's risk for developing cervical cancer in the future. Although medical guidelines have not been changed, it has been speculated that this may replace traditional testing in the future.

For more information on the Bethesda system, visit the National Institute of Health website at www.nih.gov and search for "Bethesda System."

Bimanual Pelvic Exam

Following the collection of the sample for the Pap test, the provider will remove the speculum to perform the bimanual exam. The provider lubricates the index and middle fingers of a gloved hand and gently inserts them into the vagina and presses on the abdomen with the other hand, to palpate the internal pelvic organs (uterus and ovaries). The organs are palpated for abnormalities such as lumps or areas of tenderness. If any abnormalities are detected, further testing is indicated.

Rectal Vaginal Exam

The rectal exam may or may not be performed. The provider will insert one finger in the rectum or one finger in the rectum and vagina simultaneously. Tone and position of the pelvic organs are assessed along with detecting the presence of any rectal abnormalities, such as masses, hemorrhoids, fistulas, and fissures. Some providers may also obtain a small fecal sample for occult blood testing.

Medical Assistant's Responsibility During a Pap and Pelvic Exam

The medical assistant is usually responsible for setting up the room and patient prior to the pelvic exam. After obtaining a complete GYN history, the medical assistant will prep the patient by instructing her to empty her bladder and giving her proper disrobing instructions. The patient should be instructed to sit on the exam table until the provider enters the room to begin the exam. Sitting on the table is more comfortable than being placed in the lithotomy position for a prolonged period of time.

Another responsibility of the medical assistant will be preparing the liquid prep solution or Pap slides to be sent to the laboratory. A cytology request form must accompany the specimen to the laboratory. After the exam is completed, the medical assistant will clean the exam room and prepare it for the next patient. Procedure 17-2 lists the steps involved in assisting with a GYN exam.

The medical assistant should obtain the patient's weight and perform a set of vital signs either prior to or following the GYN history. Patients around the age of menopause and following menopause should also be measured to see if there is a decline in height due to a loss of bone density.

EHR Application

Many EHR software programs have templates designed for specialty exams. Templates allow the user to just point to the usual questions asked during a GYN screening, and click on responses given to those questions. This cuts down on the amount of documentation that has to be entered and saves time for all parties involved.

Setting up the Equipment

The medical assistant usually begins by setting up the Pap tray and related supplies and placing all other necessary equipment in a convenient location. Table 17-6 lists the equipment and supplies that are necessary to complete a GYN exam and Figure 17-12 illustrates the tray set up with the equipment used during the exam. The pelvic tray should be placed at the appropriate height for the provider.

Labeling any Cultures or Vials

Labeling of cultures and samples requires specific information. Information that is mandatory for all studies include site of collection, name of patient, date of birth, sex, medical record number, ordering facility, ordering provider name, the lab ordered, designation of fasting

Table 17-6 Pap Tray Setup (When Using a Liquid Prep)
Refer to Figure 17-12 for a photo of the tray items.

On the Tray	Off to the Side
(a) Vaginal speculum (may be metal or plastic); light source if applicable	Patient gown and drape
(b) Liquid prep solution (ThinPrep® or SurePath®)	Tissues
(c) Endocervical brush or broom	Gooseneck lamp
(d) Lubricant	Biohazard container
(e) Two pairs of gloves (one pair for the provider and one pair for the medical assistant)	Cytology requisition form
(f) STI PCR swabs, if needed	
(g) Fecal occult test supplies for women over the age of 40	

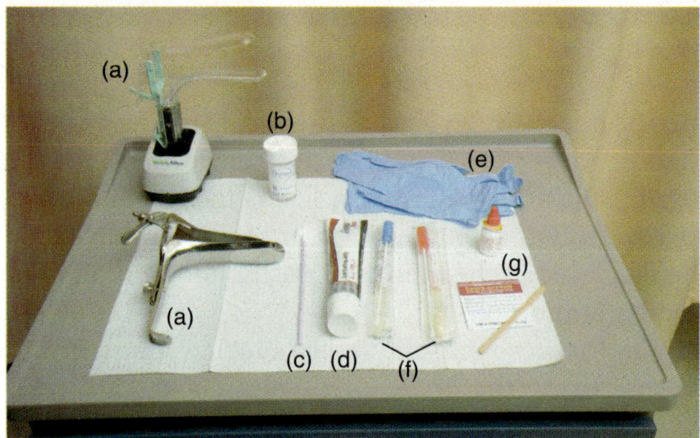

Figure 17-12 ■ A tray set up for a pelvic exam and Pap test when using a liquid prep solution. (Refer to Table 17-6 for a description of each item.)

or nonfasting, and an attached order form. Occasionally additional information is necessary such as height and weight.

Completing the Lab Requisition Forms

Medical assistants will often be required to fill out lab requisition forms. Besides the information required for a given lab test, insurance information, patient demographic and contact information, and specific diagnostic codes are often required. The use of electronic health records has significantly decreased the number of paper requisitions, but specialized testing still often require lab requisition forms.

Rooming the Patient

The medical assistant is often the face of the clinic. Interactions should be a personal, professional, courteous encounter that welcomes the patient to divulge information as if they were a close friend. Patients should feel comfortable allowing the medical assistant to take their vital signs, obtain their weight, update their medical history, and obtain details of the sexual and gynecologic history. The patients will often be requested to empty their bladder prior to the exam as well as disrobe to allow a full physical exam. Patients who present for vaginal or uterine symptoms often only need to disrobe from the waist down, but occasionally patients must fully disrobe. Patients should be provided with disposable gowns, opened to the back, to ensure that the patient maintains as much privacy and modesty as possible throughout their exam. The assistant should leave the room to allow the patient to prepare while they await their provider.

Assisting Provider with Breast Exam and the Actual Pap Smear Procedure

Preparation prior to the provider entering the room is often helpful as specific complaints prompt specific exams. Complaints regarding the urogenital tract often require speculum, culture, swabs, and a bimanual exam. Visits for cervical cancer screening require a patient to undress from the waist down, have a speculum exam, and have cervical cell sampling for Pap smear. Patients should be prepared for a thorough external and internal exam with encouragement to be as calm as possible but to feel free to voice any discomfort. Preparation of the speculum, a light source, lubrication, gloves, and sampling materials are often necessary for this procedure. Complaints regarding the chest and breast region often prompt a breast exam. Breast exams require the drapes to open to the front. The breast exam is a visual and tactile exam which usually requires gloves and a good light source.

Patient Education

Following a wellness visit, there are several topics which may be discussed. Besides education on avoiding tobacco products, encouraging diet and exercise regimens, and the importance of stress management on overall health, there are specific topics that are purely related to female health; education on cervical cancer screening, breast cancer screening, sexual health, STI prevention, birth control options, self-exams, and preparation for childbearing.

Pelvic Exam for Women Who Have Vaginal Symptoms

When a woman recognizes a change in her vaginal secretions, pattern, odor, or sensation, they should be encouraged to come in for a full pelvic evaluation. Generally the exam will include a sterile speculum exam, swabs for chlamydia and gonorrhea, swabs for microscopic evaluation, and bimanual exam. If a sexually transmitted infection is possible, blood tests may be necessary.

STI Cultures

Gonorrhea and chlamydia remain the most common sexually transmitted diseases, but other infections including syphilis, herpes simplex virus, human papillomavirus, HIV, and Hepatitis B and C can coexist. STI PCR sampling or collection supplies should be available in the event the provider wants to test the patient for any of the condition listed above.

KOH/Wet Prep/Wet Mount

Supplies for the wet prep (wet mount) and KOH prep include a pipette, cotton-tipped swabs, small test tube, and microscope slide with coverslip, saline, and KOH (potassium hydroxide) solution. The KOH/wet mount is a clinic procedure with the purpose to determine the cause of vaginitis in women. This test for fungal infections in the vagina is used to identify *Candida albicans* (yeast), bacterial vaginosis, and trichomoniasis, which usually require treatment.

Mammography

Mammography is an X-ray of the breast tissue used as a screening method for the early detection of breast cancer. During a mammogram, each breast is compressed between two plates to flatten the tissue, making visualization easier. A view of each breast is taken from top to bottom and side to side.

The American Cancer Society (ACS) guidelines recommend that all females aged 40 and over should have a yearly mammogram and clinical breast exam. Those females with a strong family history should begin mammography at a younger age. Although mammography is not "foolproof," numerous studies have clearly shown that getting a mammogram and a breast exam reduces the risk of dying from breast cancer (ACS). Early detection of a tumor leads to improved chances of successful treatment and better outcomes. There are conflicting guidelines on the use of mammography. Many physicians follow the the United States Preventive Services Task Force (USPSTF) guidelines, which recommend a mammogram every two years for patients 50–74 years old.

Miscellaneous Gynecologic Procedures

When potential problems are discovered by the patient or their provider, further diagnostic testing may be necessary to arrive at a diagnosis and to determine the best course of treatment. Table 17-7 lists some of the common diagnostic tests and procedures.

Table 17-7 Gynecologic Diagnostic Tests and Procedures

Procedure Name	Description	Rationale
Amplified DNA probe	Rapid test kit for the detection of chlamydia and gonorrhea. Swab or dirty urine sampling.	Screening test for men and women. Performed on all pregnant females.
Biopsies: Breast	Open surgical removal of the lump or a needle biopsy in which a small incision is made and a vacuum-needle is inserted and the specimen is obtained	Performed after a clinical exam, mammography, or when an ultrasound reveals a suspicious mass of any kind
Cervical biopsy	Tissue samples are taken using a colposcope and biopsy forceps	Usually performed after abnormal Pap results to detect the presence of malignant cells
Endometrial biopsy	Removal of endometrial tissue for microscopic evaluation	Abnormal bleeding Infertility
Colposcopy	Visualization of the vaginal and cervical tissue with a colposcope (an instrument to examine the vagina)	Abnormal Pap results based on the ASCCP management guidelines
Cryosurgery	Cervix is frozen using liquid nitrogen	Cervicitis Cervical erosion
Dilation and curettage (D & C)	Cervix is dilated and some of the endometrial lining is scraped off	Evaluation of tissue due to excessive bleeding. Removal of remaining tissue after a miscarriage.
Loop electrosurgical excision procedure (LEEP)	Removal of abnormal tissue from the cervix using thin wire loop electrodes	High-grade cervical dysplasia or cancer
Ultrasonography	Harmless sound waves are bounced off internal structures, which produce images of the uterus, ovaries, and the fetus	To detect abnormalities of the ovaries and uterus. Also used to diagnose tubal or ectopic pregnancies, fibroids, and ovarian cysts.

COMMON GYNECOLOGIC TREATMENTS AND MEDICATIONS

There are a variety of treatments in the form of procedures and medications that treat women's health issues. Some treatments were already discussed in the Health Coach features throughout the chapter. Others can be found in Table 17-8.

There are also several medications used in the treatment of women's health issues. Table 17-9 features some of the most common medications.

Table 17-8 Common Gynecologic Treatments

Treatment Name	Description	Rationale
Doppler Fetal Heart Tones (Doptones)	The use of a Doppler to hear the fetal heartbeat at every prenatal visit	To ensure a viable fetus as well as note any arrhythmias
Endometrial ablation	Use of electricity or hot water to destroy (ablate) the endometrial tissue	Used for excessive bleeding and benign overgrowth of the endometrium
Essure	Use of a metal coil and ultrasound heat to scar the fallopian tube	Contraceptive process that prevents the ova from being fertilized, like tubal ligation without abdominal surgery
Hysterectomy bilateral salpingo-oopherectomy	Removal of the uterus and both fallopian tubes	This procedure removes the source of bleeding as well as the hormone producing organs to limit cancer and anemia
Hysterosalpingogram	Use of a hysteroscope (an instrument to examine the uterus) to visualize fluid flow in the fallopian tubes and uterus	This procedure identifies any blockages or abnormalities in the fallopian tubes
Tubal ligation	Removal or disruption of the fallopian tubes	Contraceptive process that prevents the ova from being fertilized
Ultrasonography	Use of harmless sound waves to identify the fetus and fetal structures	Allows for identification of organs, sex of the fetus, and proper development

Table 17-9 Common Gynecologic Medications

Medication Classifications	Description	Medication Examples
Antibiotics	Used to treat sexually transmitted disease/infections	Ceftriaxone, Penicillin, Doxycycline, Azithromycin, Flagyl
Antiestrogen	Used to prevent the effects of estrogen on estrogen-receptive tissues or tumors	Tamoxifen
Antifungals	Used to treat yeast infections	Miconazole, Fluconazole
Estrogen-containing contraceptives	The estrogen and progesterone mimic the natural cycle while preventing ovulation	Ortho Tricyclen, Ortho Evra, Nuva Ring, Yaz
Intrauterine devices	Prevent fertilization and implantation; contraceptives. Paragard is copper and causes local inflammation; Skyla and Mirena secrete progesterone and thin the endometrium to prevent implantation and bleeding.	Skyla, Mirena, Paragard
Ovulation agents	Promotes the development and release of an ovum	Clomid
Progesterone-only contraceptives	Progesterone mimics pregnancy and prevents ovulation	Depo-Provera, Mini-pill, Nexplanon

COMMON LAB TESTS THAT COINCIDE WITH WOMEN'S HEALTH ISSUES

Several lab tests can be performed to evaluate specific issues relating to women's health. Table 17-10 features some of the common lab tests that coincide with women's health issues.

FEATURED OBSTETRIC PROCEDURES

Obstetrics (OB) is the medical specialty that provides care and treatment to the pregnant female. Obstetrical care is provided during pregnancy (prenatal), labor and delivery, and the **postpartum** period, also known as the **puerperium** period. A full-term pregnancy is

Table 17-10 Common Lab Tests That Coincide with Women's Health Issues

Test	Clinical Significance
Estradiol (estrogen level)	Ensures that there is estrogen available. Low-levels suggest ovarian failure or suppression.
Follicle-stimulating hormone (FSH) (hormone secreted when there is inadequate estrogen available)	If this level is high and remains high, a lack of estrogen production is likely
Glucola (use of 50-, 75-, or 100-gram glucose solution and measurement of fasting, one-, two-, and three-hour glucose levels)	Identifies abnormal response to glucose. Used to diagnose gestational diabetes.
Hemoglobin A1C (percent of hemoglobin molecules that are glycosylated)	This is a test used to help diagnose diabetes, but can also show signs of insulin resistance
Human chorionic gonadotropin (hCG) (hormone produced with placental implantation)	A test that checks for pregnancy
Prolactin (produced in the pituitary gland of the brain, promotes lactation)	In high enough levels, this hormone prevents ovulation
Testosterone	Ensures that there is low-circulating "male" hormone
Thyroid-stimulating hormone (produced in response to low thyroid levels, limited by high thyroid levels)	Both hyper- and hypothyroidism can interfere with ovulation

Table 17-11 Schedule of Exams

Initial exam: approximately 6 to 12 weeks gestation
Every four weeks until 34 weeks gestation
Every two weeks from 34 to 38 weeks gestation
Every week from 38 weeks gestation to delivery
Six weeks after delivery

considered to be from 37 to 42 weeks **gestation** and is divided into three **trimesters** at approximately three months each. Adhering to a regular schedule of prenatal visits is important in order to follow the progression of the pregnancy and to monitor the health of both the mother and fetus. Early detection of potential problems can prevent serious complications for the mother and baby. Table 17-11 lists the recommended schedule for prenatal and postpartum visits.

Due to a wide variety of in-home pregnancy tests, a woman can now confirm a pregnancy almost immediately upon implantation. Prenatal care can begin sooner, due to early confirmation, and new mothers can begin preparing much earlier than ever before for their baby's arrival. It is vital for expectant mothers to adhere to the schedule of prenatal visits, as recommended by the provider.

The Initial or First Prenatal Exam

The first **prenatal** exam (see Procedure 17-3) is usually scheduled after a woman obtains a positive pregnancy test result at home or after she has missed a second menstrual cycle. Confirmation of the pregnancy and a thorough history and physical will be completed during the first office visit. Baselines will also be established to be used as future reference points. The provider will be looking for any potential disorders that could have an adverse effect on the mother or child. Early detection of potential problems can alert the provider to possible complications that may occur during the pregnancy and birth process.

Sufficient time should be allotted to complete the initial prenatal exam. A larger block of time will be needed to obtain the history, complete the physical exam, and provide the patient with important information regarding her pregnancy.

Parts of the initial exam include the following:

- Complete Medical History, Including Menstrual and Prenatal History: A thorough database can assist the provider in identifying high-risk patients. Any problems related to previous pregnancies and deliveries should also be noted including **miscarriages** and **abortions**.
- Physical exam, which includes a breast, abdominal, pelvic, and vaginal exam
- Patient education
- Laboratory tests

The patient's menstrual history is also reviewed to determine onset, regularity, length of cycle, and amount of flow. Any past gynecological problems can also be reviewed. It should also be noted if the patient became pregnant while on birth control.

Estimated Date of Confinement

Once the pregnancy is confirmed, the mother is anxious to determine the expected delivery date (EDD) or estimated date of confinement (EDC). Although there are no perfect methods for determining an exact date of delivery, a formula known as *Nagele's rule* is considered to be fairly accurate:

Nagele's Rule:

First day of LMP + 7 days – 3 months + 1 year

Example:

January 11, 2016 + 7 days = January 18, 2016

January 18, 2016 – 3 months = October 18, 2015

October 18, 2015 + 1 year = October 18, 2016 (EDD)

A pregnancy wheel or gestational calculator, such as the one pictured in Figure 17-13, may also be used.

Patient Preparation

After completing the prenatal record, the medical assistant will obtain the patient's height, weight, and vitals and then ask the patient to empty her bladder into a sterile urine cup for urinalysis and culture. While the patient is voiding, the medical assistant can set up the exam room with any equipment needed by the provider, and place a gown and drape on the exam table for the patient. The medical assistant should give thorough disrobing instructions and should instruct the patient to sit on the exam table until the provider enters the room to begin the exam.

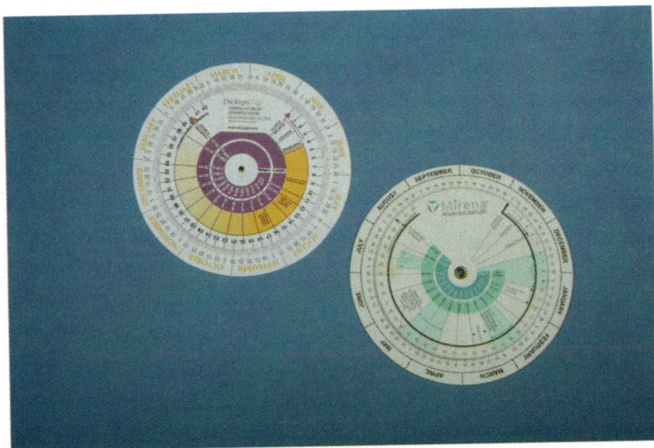

Figure 17-13 ■ An example of a gestational wheel for calculating the estimated delivery date of the fetus.

Parts of the Initial Prenatal Exam

Components that are generally included in the first prenatal exam are listed in Table 17-12 along with the rationale for each component.

Following completion of the exam, the patient should be encouraged to ask any questions before leaving the office. They should also be instructed to report any signs or symptoms of possible problems immediately. Table 17-13 lists signs and symptoms that could be cause for concern.

CRITICAL THINKING CHALLENGE

A patient in her fourth month of pregnancy phones the office to say she is experiencing fever, chills, frequent urination, and vaginal discharge.

1. How soon should the patient be seen?
2. What should you instruct the patient to bring with her to the office?

Table 17-12 Segments of the First Prenatal Exam

Segment	Conducted By	Rationale
Complete medical and prenatal history	Provider or medical assistant	Reference base
Vital signs: TPR and BP	Medical assistant	Reference point for return prenatal visits
Weight	Medical assistant	Beginning weight must be measured for a baseline
General physical exam	Provider	Determines the woman's overall general health
Breast exam	Provider	Examine the breasts to determine if there are any potential problems and to check for breast changes that are normally present during pregnancy
Abdominal exam with fundal height measurement and fetal heart tones, if applicable	Provider	Detection of any abnormalities, such as lumps or swelling that are not part of normal fetal development
Pelvic exam including cultures for chlamydia and gonorrhea	Provider	Detection of any abnormalities that could complicate the pregnancy or delivery. Screen for STDs. Estimation of gestational age.
Rectal–vaginal exam	Provider	Detection of any abnormalities in the rectum and to estimate vaginal strength (rarely performed)
Pelvic measurement	Provider	Determination of the size and shape of the pelvis for the purpose of delivery

Table 17-13 Signs and Symptoms of Possible Pregnancy-Related Problems

Potential Problem	Sign/Symptom
Preeclampsia/toxemia	Edema, headache, rapid weight gain, increased blood pressure, visual disturbances
Hyperemesis gravidum (could result in dehydration)	Severe nausea and vomiting
Possibility of a miscarriage, placenta previa, placenta abruptio	Abdominal pain, bleeding, discharge
Possible infection	Fever, chills, decreased urine output, frequent or painful urination, vaginal discharge
Preterm labor	Cramping, pelvic pressure, low-back pain, regular contractions

Note: Descriptions of the medical terms used in this table can be found in Table 17-9.

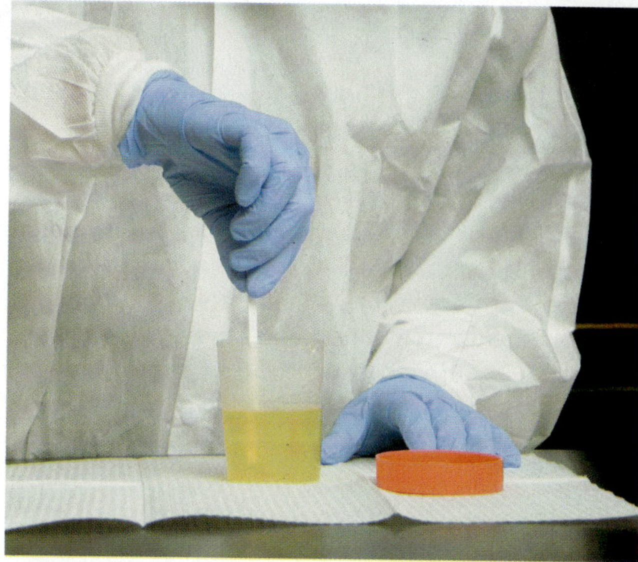

Figure 17-14 ■ A medical assistant usually tests the urine for glucose and protein; however, here a physician performs the test.

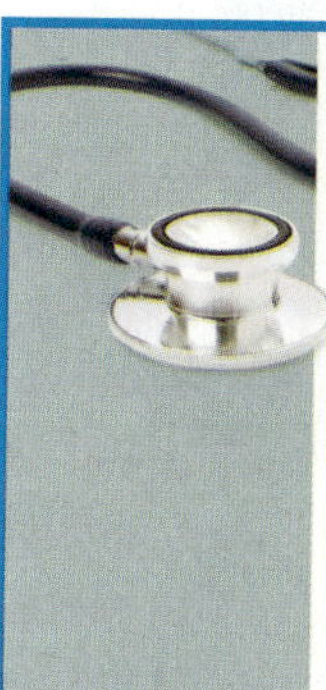

Field Smarts

Providers often request that pregnant patients be placed on their left side when their blood pressure reading is elevated. This positional change helps to reduce blood pressure. The blood pressure is monitored throughout the visit to see if there are any changes.

Return Prenatal Visits

Once the initial visit is completed and the prenatal database has been established, the patient is seen at regular intervals until the baby is delivered. The schedule for return visits may differ somewhat from one provider to the next, but will usually be as stated in Table 17-14.

During subsequent OB-GYN visits, the medical assistant will be responsible for weighing the patient and obtaining a blood pressure reading as well as any tests requested by the provider. A urine sample may be collected and tested for a urinary tract infection as well as glucosuria and proteinuria (Figure 17-14), which may be signs of diabetes and preeclampsia.

The medical assistant will then obtain information from the patient about any problems since their last visit. Questions posed to the patient should include the following:

- Any vaginal bleeding? If so, list amount, any clots or tissue passed, or any cramping.
- Any fluid leakage?
- Any unusual vaginal discharge?
- Any headaches, dizziness, or vision problems?
- Any unusual swelling?
- Any nausea or vomiting?

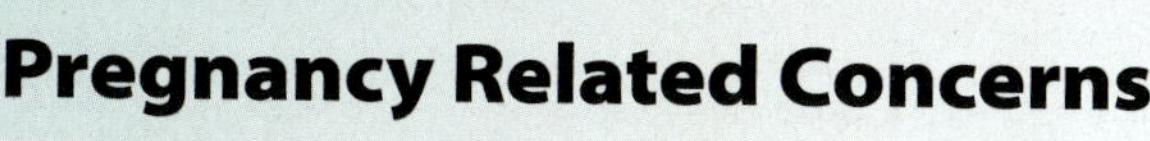

Health Coach

Pregnancy Related Concerns

Patients should be educated regarding facts related to alcohol, tobacco, and recreational drug use during pregnancy. Patients must be warned of the complications that can occur when these products are used. Smoking can cause low birth weight and premature births. Using alcohol and other drugs can cause birth defects like fetal alcohol syndrome (FAS). Children with FAS often have distinctive facial features including a small head and eyes, a wide flat nasal bridge, and a small jaw. They may also experience abnormalities in growth and central nervous system (CNS) malfunctions, along with mental retardation.

Health Coach

Preeclampsia (Toxemia)

Preeclampsia (also known as toxemia) is a dangerous complication that can develop during pregnancy. The patient often presents with elevated blood pressure and protein in the urine. Some studies have shown a direct relationship between a lack of protein and other nutrients in the diet and the development of metabolic toxemia. Therefore, proper nutrition may play an important role in preventing toxemia. Patients should be encouraged to take in a minimum of 75 to 100 grams of protein a day along with other essential vitamins and minerals. Water should be increased to help keep the kidneys functioning.

The stage of pregnancy will determine which exam techniques and tests are conducted during standard OB visits. Once the medical assistant has finished recording pertinent screening information, the provider will perform the following tasks.

Fundal Height

As the uterus increases in size, fundal measurements are taken by using a tape measure and measuring from the top of the pubic bone to the top of the uterus. This is recorded in centimeters and is usually within 1–3 cm of the gestational age of the fetus in weeks, so a fundal height of 22 cm would be normal for a patient who is 24 weeks pregnant. Fundal height measurements help the provider to determine duration of pregnancy and may also help to detect abnormalities that should be further evaluated. The first measurement, obtained at the initial prenatal visit, serves as a baseline for comparison of future measurements. Figure 17-15 shows the physician obtaining a fundal height measurement.

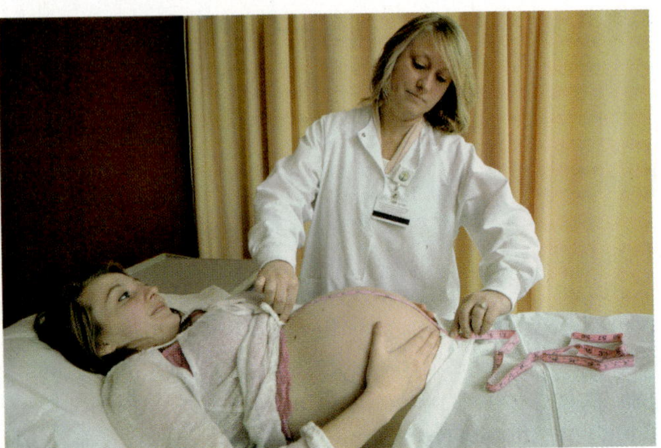

Figure 17-15 ■ The fundal height measurement is obtained.

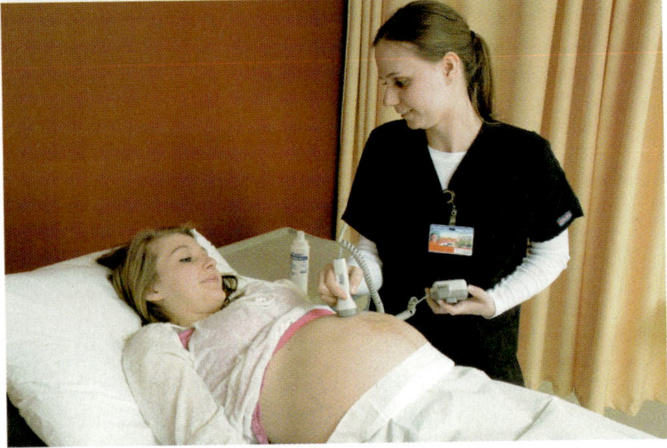

Figure 17-16 ■ Fetal heart tones are measured using a handheld Doppler for detecting fetal heart tones.

Monitoring Fetal Heart Tones

Somewhere between 10 and 12 weeks gestation, the fetal heart tones can be heard with a fetal pulse detector (Figure 17-16) through the mother's abdominal wall. Normal fetal heart rate is 120 to 160 BPM. A slow or rapid rate could be an indication of fetal distress and requires further investigation.

Vaginal/Internal Exam

A vaginal or internal exam may be performed at any time during the pregnancy, but is typically performed two to three weeks prior to delivery. The obstetrician will assess cervical dilation and **effacement** (thinning of the cervix). To facilitate fetal delivery, the cervix must be completely effaced and dilated to 10 cm.

Miscellaneous Prenatal Diagnostic Tests and Procedures

Additional tests or procedures may be performed at specific intervals during the prenatal period to detect possible genetic abnormalities. Table 17-14 lists specialized prenatal diagnostic tests.

Table 17-14 Prenatal Diagnostic Tests

Test	Description	When Performed	Possible Indications
Alpha-fetoprotein (AFP)	Test is performed to detect neural tube defects.	15 to 18 weeks gestation Patient permission required	Decreased levels indicate an increased risk of Down syndrome. Increased levels may indicate an increased risk of spina bifida or anencephaly.
Amniocentesis	Amniotic fluid is aspirated and tested for chromosomal abnormalities.	Positive screening test (Quad or integrated screen; CF screen) Family history of genetic disorders	Congenital abnormalities Fetal lung capacity
Chorionic villi sampling (CVS)	Sample of tissue that surrounds the fetus is suctioned.	8 to 10 weeks gestation	Thalassemia Sickle cell anemia Tay-Sachs
Fetal heart rate monitoring	*Nonstress test:* monitors changes in the baby's heart rate during fetal movement *Contraction stress test*: monitors changes in the baby's heart rate when mild uterine contractions are stimulated	Later in pregnancy after viability	Detects placental function Performed on patients with: Gestational diabetes Increased fetal movement or growth Decreased amniotic fluid Hypertension
Glucose challenge	Screening test for gestational diabetes	24 to 28 weeks gestation; earlier if obese prior to pregnancy	A positive result will require a longer glucose tolerance test to determine if gestational diabetes is present.
Ultrasound	High-frequency sound waves produce an image of the fetus.	Performed at different intervals throughout pregnancy	Detects: Ectopic pregnancies Abnormal bleeding Fetal growth Gender determination Multiple fetuses Placental position

Ultrasound

Since ultrasound uses sound waves, not X-rays, it is safe to administer during pregnancy and will pose no threat to either the mother or fetus. An ultrasound exam allows the provider to obtain a multitude of information about the pregnancy and the fetus and can detect problems such as **ectopic** (tubal) pregnancy. The ultrasound can be performed at any time during pregnancy, but is typically performed at:

12 weeks to:
- Detect fetal heart beat
- Confirm gestational age

18 to 20 weeks to:
- Detect multiple fetuses
- Examine the brain, spinal cord, internal organs, and extremities
- Check the position of the placenta
- Perform a measurement of fetal growth, size, and weight
- Detect any congenital abnormalities present

34 to 37 weeks to:
- Measure fetal growth, size, and weight
- Determine fetal position
- Determine position of placenta

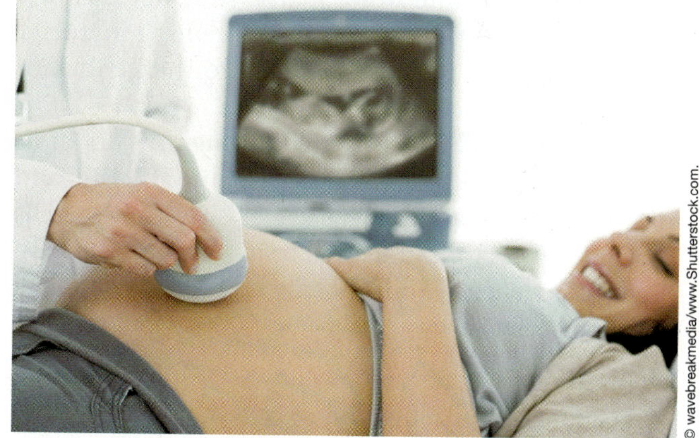

Figure 17-17 ■ A technician performs a prenatal abdominal ultrasound.

Ultrasounds can be performed abdominally or intravaginally (Figure 17-17). An ultrasound study is also performed during an amniocentesis to guide the needle (to prevent injury to the fetus), to detect any abnormalities present, and to confirm a suspected intrauterine death.

Amniocentesis

An **amniocentesis** is a prenatal procedure performed to detect certain genetic abnormalities, metabolic

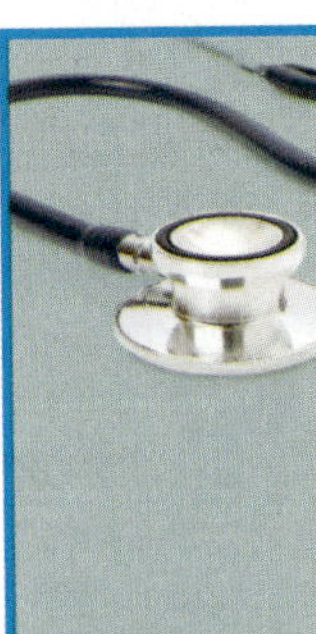

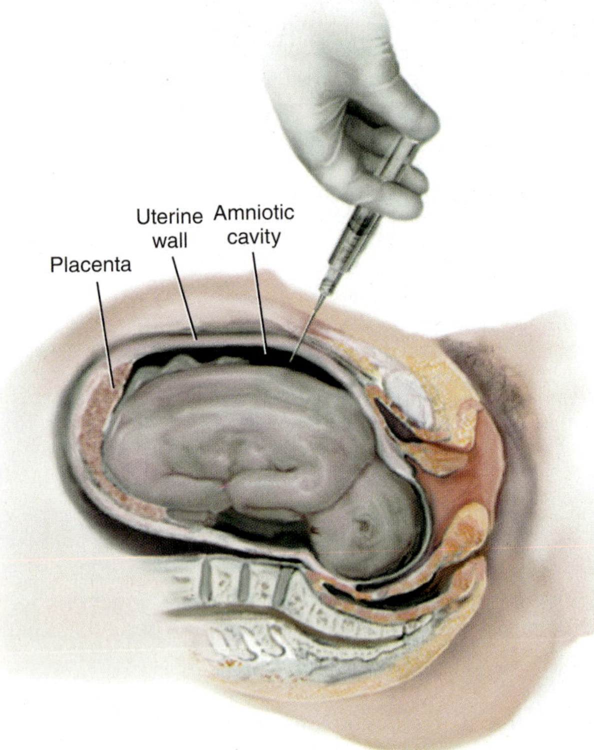

Figure 17-18 ■ Amniocentesis is performed to withdraw amniotic fluid for analysis.

disorders, and chromosomal disorders such as Down syndrome and other neural tube defects. It is sometimes performed to evaluate the lung maturity of the fetus and can also determine the gender of the fetus.

A long thin needle is inserted through the abdominal wall into the amniotic sac (Figure 17-18), and amniotic fluid is withdrawn for analysis. While there is a low risk of complications as a result of amniocentesis, slight risks do exist. Some potential problems that may occur are as follows:

- Bleeding
- Leaking of amniotic fluid
- Infection
- Miscarriage

COMMON OBSTETRIC TREATMENTS

Many complications can arise during pregnancy, labor, and delivery. Table 17-15 lists some of the possible complications that can occur, along with their corresponding treatments.

Field Smarts

Because an amniocentesis is not risk-free, it is usually performed only under certain conditions. Amniocentesis is often recommended under the following conditions:

- The mother is 35 or older
- The mother already had a child with a genetic disorder or neural tube defect
- The mother's blood work is abnormal
- One parent has a known chromosomal abnormality
- One parent is a known carrier of a metabolic disorder

COMMON LAB TESTS THAT COINCIDE WITH PREGNANCY

Certain laboratory tests are performed as part of the initial prenatal exam. Conditions may exist that could pose a danger to the mother and the fetus. Cytology, blood, and urine specimens are collected. Table 17-16 lists the traditional prenatal lab tests.

LABOR AND DELIVERY

Labor or **parturition** begins when the uterus begins to contract and ends with the delivery of the baby.

As delivery nears, decreased levels of progesterone signal the uterus to produce prostaglandin and to begin contracting. Prostaglandin causes the pituitary to release oxytocin, a hormone that produces strong uterine contractions. Occasionally, **Braxton-Hicks contractions** or false labor can be mistaken for true labor. Braxton-Hicks are intermittent and painless contractions occurring every 10 to 20 minutes. Braxton-Hicks do not occur in all pregnancies.

If spontaneous rupture of the fetal membrane has not occurred, the provider may rupture the amniotic sac by puncturing it with an instrument. The rupture of the membrane may decrease the mother's time in labor.

Labor occurs in three stages:

- Stage I (Dilation): Once labor begins, dilation and effacement of the cervix must occur for the fetus to be delivered. The cervix must dilate or expand to an opening of 10 cm and must be completely effaced or thinned out to facilitate delivery.

Table 17-15 Complications of Pregnancy and Corresponding Treatments

Complication	Description/Symptoms	Treatment
Eclampsia	Same symptoms as preeclampsia along with: Grand mal seizures Coma	Immediate seizure management Induction of labor Cesarean section (C-section)
Gestational diabetes	Mild form of diabetes that begins in the second or third trimester of pregnancy and resolves when the pregnancy ends.	Diet Medications
Hyperemsis gravidarum	Excessive vomiting Severe nausea Severe fatigue Severe dehydration Anorexia Possible starvation	IV fluids Mild sedation
Miscarriage/ abortion	Pregnancy ends before the fetus is viable. Six types of miscarriage/abortion: *Spontaneous*: also known as miscarriage; cause unknown *Threatened*: uterine bleeding, but no dilation or contractions *Inevitable*: uterine bleeding with cervical dilation *Elective*: fetus and placenta are evacuated from the mother's uterus; performed due to a threat to the mother's health or by maternal request *Incomplete*: partial expulsion of fetus and placenta *Complete*: expulsion of all fetal and placental tissue *Missed*: fetus must be removed after intrauterine death	If bleeding occurs following any of the types of miscarriage or abortion, a D&C is usually performed.
Placenta abruptio	Placenta abruptly or prematurely detaches from the uterus. Maternal symptoms: Severe pain Tight abdomen Extreme uterine tenderness Absence of fetal heart tones Profuse bleeding Shock	Varies with type and extent of abruption Supportive treatment Surgical intervention if abruption is moderate to severe
Placenta previa	Placenta implants low in the uterus and partially or completely blocks the cervical opening. Maternal symptoms: Painless vaginal bleeding	Prevention or control of postpartum hemorrhage Prevention of sepsis Treatment for anemia
Preeclampsia/toxemia	Condition that causes: Increased blood pressure Proteinuria	Bed rest High protein diet Antihypertensives Mild sedative Magnesium sulfate

- Stage II (Expulsion): The cervix is completely dilated and effaced and birth occurs. During the birth process, the mother is instructed to "bear down" once the baby has crowned, that is, the top of head is visible. Strong uterine contractions and pushing by the mother move the baby's head through the vaginal opening. Once the head is out, the baby should turn sideways so the shoulders can pass. When the baby has been delivered, its nose and mouth are wiped or suctioned to remove mucus and it begins to cry. Crying inflates and clears the baby's lungs. The umbilical cord is then clamped and severed.
- Stage III (Placental): The placenta, which nourishes and oxygenates the fetus during pregnancy, is expelled after a few more contractions. The uterus should continue to gently contract to close off blood vessels and control postpartum bleeding.
- Observation of certain signs during labor may indicate complications. Signs include the following:
  - Sudden increase or decrease in maternal blood pressure
  - Heavy vaginal bleeding
  - Headache or visual disturbances

Table 17-16 Traditional Prenatal Lab Tests

Test	Clinical Significance
ABO and Rh Blood Types	To determine ABO and Rh compatibility of mother and fetus
Blood glucose/Oral Glucose Challenge Test (OGCT)	To screen for gestational diabetes
CBC	To detect anemia or a possible asymptomatic infection
Complete urinalysis (cultures should be performed)	To screen for a UTI, hypertension, diabetes mellitus, renal disease
Group B strep screen	To detect the presence of group B strep in the vagina or rectum. If present, it could produce life-threatening infections in the infant.
Hepatitis B and C	To screen for hepatitis B and C in the mother
HIV	To detect the presence of the HIV virus or antibodies against it
Renal function tests	To determine proper renal function and to detect the presence of renal disease
Rubella titer	To detect levels of antibodies to the rubella virus. If the mother is not immune, contracting the disease during pregnancy could cause serious birth defects. Mothers with no immunity are given an immunization within six weeks of delivery.
Smear from cervix, rectum, or vagina	To screen for chlamydia, gonorrhea, and HPV
Sterile speculum exam with Pap	To screen for any cervical abnormalities or vaginal infections (such as herpes simplex virus)
Trichomonas/Candida screen (if unusual vaginal discharge is present)	To rule out trichomoniasis and candidiasis
Varicella titer	To detect varicella virus (chicken pox) antibodies. Same rationale as the rubella titer.
VDRL and RPR	To detect syphilis

- Increased fetal activity
- **Meconium** (earliest stools of the newborn) in the vaginal discharge

- If the fetus cannot be delivered through the vagina, it may be necessary to perform a **cesarean section (C-section)**. The physician makes a surgical incision through the abdominal wall and into the uterus to remove the fetus and placenta. The incision can be made either transversely (across the abdomen) or vertically (up and down). The rationales for performing C-sections include the following:
    - Small pelvic size
    - Breech position (the fetus is not head first)
    - Ineffective contractions
    - Fetal distress
    - Maternal distress

POSTNATAL OR POSTPARTUM PERIOD

Upon delivery of the fetus, the postnatal or postpartum period begins. This period, also referred to as puerperium, lasts from four to six weeks. During the postpartum period, the body and its systems are returning to their prepregnant state. Definite changes occur during this period. The uterus returns to a normal size (involution) and any tissue injuries that occurred during the birth process are healing.

A vaginal discharge called **lochia,** which consists of white blood cells, mucus, bacteria, and tissue occurs in different stages following delivery:

- Lochia rubra: Bright red discharge for the first three days postpartum
- Lochia serosa: Pink or brownish discharge occurring on about day four postpartum
- Lochia alba: Decreased amount of a yellowish-white discharge that usually stops at approximately three weeks postpartum, but sometimes lasts for up to six weeks

Menstrual flow usually resumes after two months in a nonnursing mother and after three to six months in a nursing mother.

Six-Week Postpartum Visit

Six weeks after delivery, the patient is seen in the office for her postpartum visit. The provider will examine the patient and evaluate her overall health to determine whether there are any problems that were created by the birth process.

The medical assistant will conduct the first part of the postpartum exam by measuring the patient's weight and obtaining her temperature, pulse, and respiratory rate (TPR) and blood pressure (BP). The provider will then assess the patient's general appearance and will also perform a breast and pelvic exam. A Pap is

Health Coach

Following Delivery

Following delivery, the mother should be instructed to avoid certain activities such as heavy lifting. She should also get lots of rest and engage in a well-balanced diet. The mother should also report any of the following: an increase in the amount of discharge, cessation of discharge within the first two weeks following delivery, discharge with a foul odor, a yellowish-white discharge that changes to red. The mother should be cautioned to report any feelings of depression, as this could be an indication of postpartum depression.

usually not performed at this time due to the presence of abnormal cells expelled by the cervix and vagina as part of the normal healing process.

Blood work may be performed to detect possible anemia due to blood loss during and following delivery. A rubella immunization is also given if it was determined that the mother did not have antibodies to the rubella virus.

The postpartum visit is an excellent time to stress the importance of breast self-examination and yearly checkups by the provider. Different forms of contraception may also be discussed.

Health Coach

Postpartum Depression

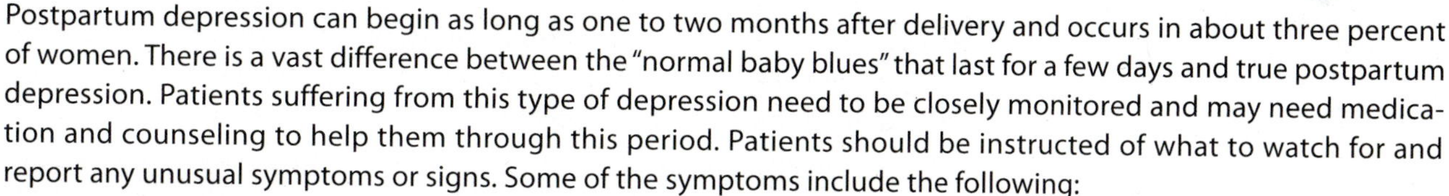

Postpartum depression can begin as long as one to two months after delivery and occurs in about three percent of women. There is a vast difference between the "normal baby blues" that last for a few days and true postpartum depression. Patients suffering from this type of depression need to be closely monitored and may need medication and counseling to help them through this period. Patients should be instructed of what to watch for and report any unusual symptoms or signs. Some of the symptoms include the following:

- Uncontrollable crying
- Despondency
- Feelings of hopelessness
- Unable to care for the infant
- Mood swings
- Extreme anxiety when it comes to the infant
- Guilty feelings about not loving the infant
- Irritability
- Fatigue
- Thoughts of abandoning or hurting the baby

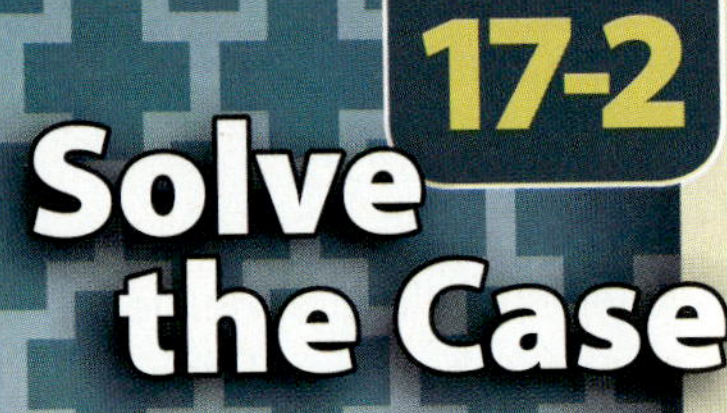

Review the following notes from Ms. Rosman's visit with Dr. Ayerick.

Patient Symptoms. Patient here for annual physical exam and Pap smear. Patient complains of "lumpy breasts" and unable to perform BSE, otherwise no GYN complaints.

Current Medications include: Birth control pill Yaz® (drospirenone/ethinyl estradiol), Vitamin D, Calcium Citrate, and prenatal multivitamin.

Today's ***Vital Signs*** include a BP of 122/68, a pulse rate of 66, and a respiration of 20. Patient's height is 5′ 4″ and weight is 132 pounds.

Assessment Information: Patient's vital signs are within normal limits. Review of lab work, all within normal limits. Sexually active with one partner. Performed second Pap smear, using ThinPrep (first test contaminated). Completed manual breast exam, result negative. Patient has not received the HPV vaccination series, discussed benefits.

Provider's Plan includes referral for screening mammogram, administer Gardasil® dose 1 of 3 today for HPV. Set up return visit for subsequent Gardasil® dose 2 of 3 in 30–60 days, and dose 3 of 3 six months from today. Provide patient education for BSE and HPV vaccine. If results of Pap smear are negative, patient to return in three years for repeat Pap. Schedule patient for annual physical exam in one year.

1. **Based on the patient's symptoms and the provider's diagnoses, what concerns will you address with the patient after the visit?**
2. **Why did the provider recommend the HPV vaccine today?**
3. **Where would you be able to locate the education materials requested per the provider's plan?**
4. **Go to the Internet and look up educational materials for the prescribed medication and vaccine. Role play with a classmate discharging the patient and going over educational materials.**

PROCEDURE 17-1

Instruct the Patient in Breast Self-Examination

Objective:

To instruct a patient in the proper procedure for performing monthly breast self-exam.

Equipment/Supplies:

- Pamphlet/shower hanger on BSE
- Breast model
- Patient's chart/EHR

continues

PROCEDURE 17-1 continued

PROCEDURAL STEPS	DETAILS AND/OR RATIONALE
1. Greet the patient, identify yourself, and ***explain the rationale for the performance*** of BSE, ***showing awareness of a patient's concerns related to the procedure being performed***.	Explaining the importance of performing monthly BSEs will result in better patient compliance.
2. Give the patient a brochure, such as the ones shown in Figure 17-19, and begin explaining the proper procedure for performing BSE. Explain to the patient that the breasts should be examined in the shower, in front of a mirror, and while lying down (see Figure 17-6).	Written instructions and pictures can help to explain the procedure more clearly. Examining the breasts in three different positions is the most thorough method for detecting abnormalities.
3. Instruct the patient to examine the breasts at the same time each month, preferably a few days to a week following menstrual period.	Normal changes of the breast tissue due to hormonal fluctuations during the cycle could be mistaken for an abnormality.
4. While the patient is in the shower, instruct her to cover the right breast with soapy lather and place the right arm over the head. Gently glide the fingers over the entire breast and axilla feeling for any lumps or thickening. Repeat the procedure with the left breast.	Fingers can glide smoothly over the skin while in the shower, making detection of any abnormalities easier.
5. When the patient has finished showering, she should stand before a mirror and look for: ■ Puckering or dimpling of the skin ■ Redness or a change in skin texture ■ Nipple retraction ■ Any change in size or shape The exam should be repeated first with the hands raised over the head and then with the hands on the hips, while pressing down.	A tumor may pull the skin inward, creating dimpling or puckering of the skin or retraction of the nipple. Raising the arms over the head changes the position of the breasts and pressing down flexes the chest muscles.
6. Instruct the patient to gently squeeze each nipple and look for any discharge.	A bloody discharge is usually the only reason for concern, but any discharge should be reported to the provider.
7. Instruct the patient to lie down and place a small pillow under her right shoulder and to raise her right arm over her head.	This position helps to evenly distribute the breast tissue.
8. Instruct the patient to use the pads of the first three fingers and, using firm pressure and a circular motion, examine the entire breast, including the nipple and the underarm area (Figure 17-20). Repeat the entire process with the left breast.	Each area of the breast needs to be examined along with the underarm area.

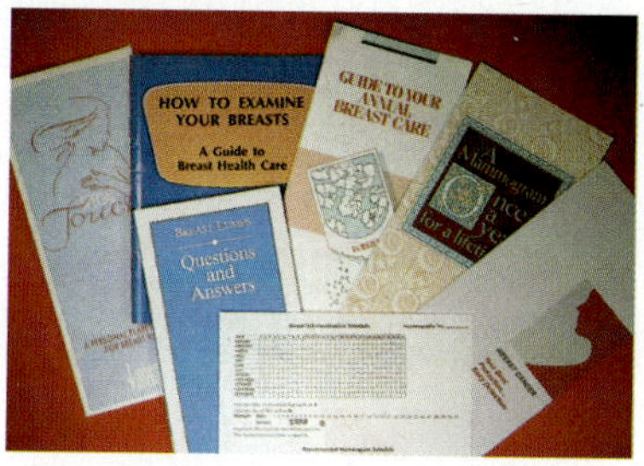

Figure 17-19 ■ Samples of BSE pamphlets for home use.

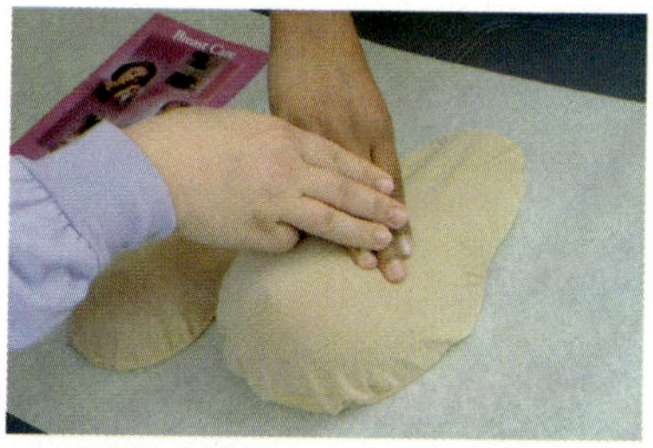

Figure 17-20 ■ A medical assistant instructs the patient on how to perform a BSE using a breast model.

continues

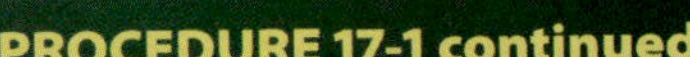

PROCEDURE 17-1 continued

PROCEDURAL STEPS	DETAILS AND/OR RATIONALE
9. Answer any questions and instruct the patient to repeat the instructions and perform an exam on the breast model. Instruct the patient to report any changes immediately.	Early detection is the key.
10. Document the education session in the patient's chart.	All education sessions must be documented.

DOCUMENTATION EXAMPLE:

10-18-XX 1030	Instructed pt. on proper BSE. Pt. performed BSE on breast model and successfully stated where lumps were located. Pt. given BSE pamphlet and encouraged to call with any additional questions. Joni Leonard, RMA (AMT)--

PROCEDURE 17-2
Assist with a GYN Exam and Pap Test

Objective:

To prepare all necessary equipment and assist the provider with a routine GYN exam including a Pap test.

Equipment/Supplies:

- Exam gloves, two or three pairs
- Patient gown and drape
- Vaginal speculum
- Lubricant
- Light source
- Tissues
- Biohazard specimen bag
- Lab requisition
- Patient's chart/EHR

Conventional/Direct Method:

- Glass slides
- Fixative/specimen jar
- Cervical spatula
- Endocervical brush
- Slide holder

ThinPrep Method:

- ThinPrep vial
- Cervical spatula
- Endocervical brush
- Endocervical broom (when using broom for collection)

PROCEDURAL STEPS	DETAILS AND/OR RATIONALE
1. Wash your hands and set up all needed equipment. Warm the speculum.	All equipment should be readily available to prevent any delays during the exam.

continues

PROCEDURE 17-2 continued

PROCEDURAL STEPS	DETAILS AND/OR RATIONALE
2. Label the specimens. *Direct method:* Label slides with the patient's name, the date, and source (V) = vaginal, (C) = cervical, or (E) = endocervical. *ThinPrep method:* Label the specimen container with the patient's name, date, and ID number (from lab request form).	Labeling specimens before collection reduces slide mix-ups.
3. Identify the patient using at least two identifiers, identify yourself, and instruct the patient to empty her bladder and collect the urine specimen.	An empty bladder makes examination easier and the specimen is often used for a urinalysis.
4. Obtain the patient's blood pressure and weight and update her medical and GYN history.	Updated information may alert the provider to potential health problems.
5. ***Explain the rationale for performance of the procedure*** to the patient and instruct her to undress completely and to put the gown on so that it opens correctly (check provider preference), ***showing awareness of the patient's concerns related to the procedure being performed***.	Patients are often more comfortable if they know what to expect.
6. Instruct the patient to sit on the exam table until the provider enters the room.	Placing the patient in the lithotomy position for a prolonged period can be uncomfortable.
7. After the provider enters, assist the patient into the supine position and drape for the breast exam.	
8. Assist the patient into the lithotomy position and drape for privacy.	Patients often have difficulty getting into the lithotomy position on their own.
9. Hand the warmed vaginal speculum to the provider.	Warming the speculum provides patient comfort.
10. Adjust the light source for easy visualization.	
11. Hand the spatula and brush to the provider when using the direct method, and the broom when using the ThinPrep method.	Each method has different collecting supplies.

continues

PROCEDURE 17-2 continued

PROCEDURAL STEPS	DETAILS AND/OR RATIONALE
12. Apply PPE (gloves) and: *Direct method:* Hold the slides so the provider can apply the collected cells to the slides. Immediately spray the slides with fixative from a distance of six inches. Allow the slides to dry for 10 minutes before placing in a holder. *ThinPrep method (broom method):* Hold the opened vial so the provider can place the broom in the vial (Figure 17-21). Agitate the broom in the solution until all of the specimen has been suspended in the liquid. Dispose of the broom in a biohazard container.	Prevents the cells from drying on the slide, which distorts their appearance.
13. Squeeze the lubricant on the provider's gloved fingers for the bimanual and rectal exam.	Makes insertion of the fingers easier and more comfortable for the patient.
14. After the provider completes the exam, assist the patient into a sitting position and give her tissues for cleansing the vaginal and rectal area.	Some patients may feel dizzy and unsteady after lying down.
15. Properly dispose of biohazardous wastes and other used supplies and soak the stainless steel speculum in a solution. Sanitize and sterilize the speculum per office protocol.	
16. Instruct the patient to get dressed.	
17. Prepare the specimen and lab requisition for transport (see Figure 17-22).	
18. Remove gloves and wash your hands.	
19. Document the procedure in the patient's chart.	

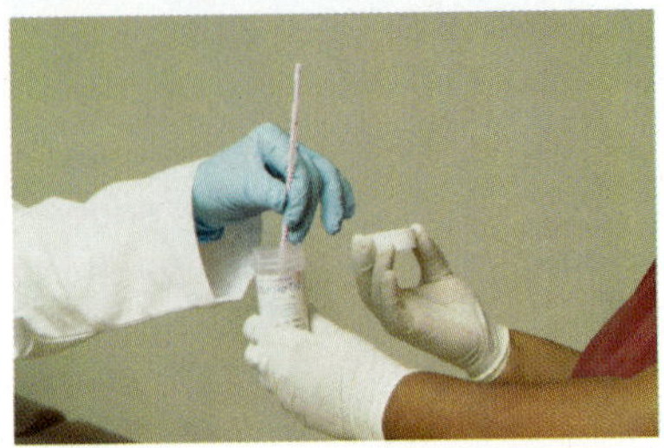

Figure 17-21 ■ A medical assistant holds the vial for the provider as the provider places the broom into the solution.

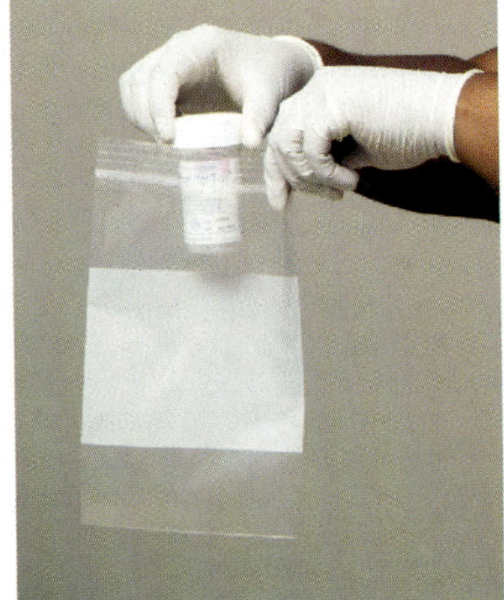

Figure 17-22 ■ A medical assistant prepares the specimen for transport to the lab.

DOCUMENTATION EXAMPLE:

9-18-XX 1030	Pt. here for annual Pap & pelvic. Last Pap, 10-18-XX (normal), G3T2P1A0L3, LMP 09-1-XX, BC Ortho Evra, GYN surg. None, Sex part. (1), no breast concerns or changes, "performs monthly BSE." Latania Carter, CMA (AAMA)--

PROCEDURE 17-3

Assist with the Prenatal Exam

Objective:

To assist the provider with prenatal exams to monitor the progression of a pregnancy.

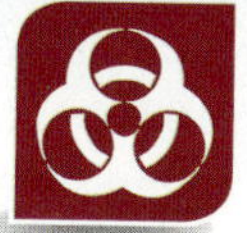

Equipment/Supplies:

- Scale
- Sphygmomanometer
- Stethoscope
- Tape measure
- Patient gown
- Urine specimen cup
- Urine reagent strips
- Doppler fetoscope with coupling agent
- Biohazard waste container
- Patient's chart/EHR

PROCEDURAL STEPS	DETAILS AND/OR RATIONALE
1. Wash your hands and set up the equipment.	Hands must be washed before and after each patient contact.
2. Identify the patient using two identifiers and instruct the patient to collect a urine specimen. Dip the urine for protein and glucose.	Initial visit: A pregnancy test may be repeated at this visit. Return visits: Urine is tested for protein and glucose, which screens for preeclampsia and gestational diabetes.
3. Obtain the patient's weight and blood pressure. Both measurements are obtained at each prenatal visit.	The patient's weight and blood pressure are monitored throughout the pregnancy to assess maternal nutrition and fetal growth and to alert the provider of the possible development of complications.
4. *Initial visit:* ***Showing awareness of the patient's concerns related to the procedure being performed***, have the patient disrobe completely and put on a gown. Assist the provider in conducting a thorough exam including a breast exam and pelvic exam.	A thorough exam is needed in the initial visit.
Return visits: The fundal height is measured and the fetal heart tones are assessed. Assist the provider by supplying a tape measure for the fundal height measurement and a fetal monitor and gel to listen to the fetal heart tones. (After the initial visit, an internal exam will not be performed again until approximately 36 weeks gestation, and thereafter.)	Measuring the fundal height assists the provider in determining fetal growth
5. After completion of the exam, assist the patient into a sitting position and have her remain there for a few minutes.	A sudden drop in blood pressure can occur when rising from a supine position.
6. Provide the patient with educational materials.	Providing the patient with education promotes patient and baby health.

continues

PROCEDURE 17-3 continued

PROCEDURAL STEPS	DETAILS AND/OR RATIONALE
7. Apply gloves, clean the exam room, properly dispose of used supplies, and disinfect or sterilize equipment.	These precautions reduce the risks of cross-contamination.
8. Wash hands and document the visit in patient's chart.	Careful records must be kept throughout the prenatal and postpartum period.

DOCUMENTATION EXAMPLE:

10-18-XX 0900	Return prenatal visit, pt. is at 25 wks. gestation, BP 120/70, weight 156 lb., pt. reports no problems or concerns, urine negative for glucose and protein. Megan Speck, CMA (AAMA)--

CHAPTER SUMMARY

- The system snapshot provides an overview of the female reproductive system including ovaries, fallopian tubes, uterus, vagina, and the menstrual cycle and menopause.
- Specialists who treat diseases and disorders of the female reproductive system include the OB-GYN, a provider who specializes in diagnosing and treating diseases of the female reproductive system and breasts, and caring for a woman while she is pregnant; the infertility specialist, who specializes in assisting patients who are experiencing problems with conception or carrying pregnancies to term delivery; and the midwife, someone who has specialty training in the care of the pregnant female as well as labor, delivery, and the postpartum period.
- You have been introduced to abbreviations related to the female reproductive system.
- Medical assistants may have the responsibility of screening patients prior to provider examination or over the telephone. The depth of screening will be established by office protocol, but in general, medical assistants should be able to ask a series of questions related to the patient's symptoms.
- Common GYN diseases of the female reproductive system include vulvodynia, vaginitis, uterine fibroids, and breast, uterine, and ovarian cancers.
- The medical assistant will room the patient and assist providers in procedures such as the gynecological exam, breast exam, pelvic exam, setting up the equipment, assisting with the collection and labeling of cultures, completing lab requisition forms, and providing patient education.
- For women who have vaginal symptoms, the medical assistant will assist the provider with obtaining STI cultures, and the KOH/Wet prep.
- Medical assistants should never perform any procedure unless directed to do so by the provider; however, they can set up various equipment and supplies to help save time in the event that testing is ordered.
- Medical assistants can often be instrumental in helping patients reduce their risks of GYN infections and diseases with proper education.
- Providing for patient's modesty and explaining what to expect will help to alleviate anxiety.
- Obstetrics (OB) is the medical specialty that provides care and treatment to the pregnant female. Obstetrical care is provided during pregnancy (prenatal), labor and delivery, and the postpartum period, also known as the puerperium period.
- Prenatal care begins earlier than ever and prepares new mothers for their baby's arrival. It is vital for expectant mothers to adhere to the schedule of prenatal visits, as recommended by the provider.

The first prenatal exam is usually scheduled after a woman obtains a positive pregnancy test result at home or after she has missed a second menstrual cycle.

- Many complications can arise during pregnancy, labor, and delivery, including miscarriage/abortion, hyperemis gravidarum, gestational diabetes, preeclampsia/toxemia, eclampsia, placenta previa, and placenta abruptio.
- Labor or parturition commences when the uterus begins to contract and ends with the delivery of the baby.
- Upon delivery of the fetus, the postnatal or postpartum period begins. This period, also referred to as puerperium, lasts from four to six weeks. During the postpartum period, the body and its systems are returning to their prepregnant state.
- The medical assistant is a key member of the obstetric staff and has many responsibilities.
- Demonstrating professionalism, being an active listener, and performing accurate testing will assist the provider in keeping mother and baby healthy and safe.

CERTIFICATION REVIEW QUESTIONS

1. Another term for labor is:
   a. parity.
   b. puerperium.
   c. parturition.
   d. postpartum.
2. Which of the following tests should be performed to diagnose endometrial cancer?
   a. Pap
   b. Biopsy
   c. Maturation index
   d. Hormone level
3. Which instrument is used to view dysplastic cells of the cervix?
   a. Laproscope
   b. Hysteroscope
   c. Colposcope
   d. Uteroscope
4. Braxton-Hicks contractions are also known as:
   a. preterm labor.
   b. false labor.
   c. early labor.
   d. true labor.
5. Pregnancy is divided into three trimesters and lasts approximately how long?
   a. 40 weeks
   b. 36 weeks
   c. 10 months
   d. 35 weeks
6. What can an AFP test detect?
   a. Neural tube defects
   b. Intrauterine death
   c. Cystic fibrosis
   d. Gender of the fetus
7. Ovulation occurs on approximately day ___ of the menstrual cycle.
   a. 12
   b. 10
   c. 21
   d. 14
8. Natural menopause occurs at what age?
   a. After age 40
   b. After age 35
   c. 55
   d. 52
9. Which condition produces symptoms such as irritability, vaginal dryness, and mood swings?
   a. Postpartum depression
   b. Early-stage cervical cancer
   c. Menopause
   d. End-stage breast cancer
10. Freezing of atypical cells on the cervix is known as:
    a. LEEP.
    b. cryosurgery.
    c. electrosurgery.
    d. nitrosurgery.

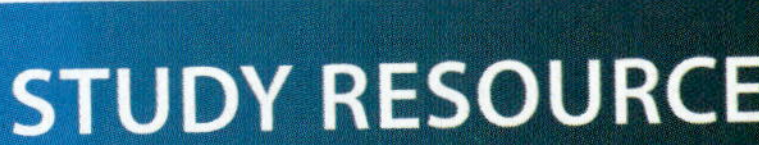

STUDY RESOURCES

Resources to Test and Reinforce Your Knowledge:	
Certification Review Questions	Take this end-of-chapter quiz
Workbook	• Complete the activities for Chapter 17 • Perform the procedures for Chapter 17 using the Competency Checklists
Resources to Promote Critical Thinking:	
***Solve the Case* Activities**	• Consider these case studies and discuss your conclusions
Learning Lab	• Module 17: Urinary, Endocrine, and Reproductive Systems
MindTap	• Complete Chapter 17 readings and activities

REFERENCES

American Cancer Society (n.d.). Breast cancer overview. Retrieved November 23, 2014, from American Cancer Society (Sept 2014). Mammograms. Retrieved November 25, 2014 from http://www.cancer.org/cancer/breastcancer/moreinformation/breastcancerearlydetection/breast-cancer-early-detection-acs-recs-mammograms

American Cancer Society (n.d.). Why Get Screened? Retrieved November 25, 2014, from http://www.cancer.org/healthy/toolsandcalculators/remind-me

American Society for Colposcopy and Cervical Pathology (ASCCP)

Centers for Disease Control and Prevention (CDC) (2012).CDC Fact Sheet: Reported STDs in the United States. 2012 National Data for Chlamydia, Gonorrhea, and Syphilis. Retrieved November 25, 2014, from http://www.cdc.gov/nchhstp/newsroom/docs/std-trends-508.pdf

Centers for Disease Control and Prevention (CDC) (2013). Vaccine Information Statement (VIS). HPV. Retrieved November 25, 2014, from http://www.cdc.gov/vaccines/hcp/vis/vis-statements/hpv-cervarix.html

Centers for Disease Control and Prevention (CDC) (2013). Vaccine Information Statement (VIS). HPV. Retrieved November 25, 2014, from http://www.cdc.gov/vaccines/hcp/vis/vis-statements/hpv-gardasil.html

Johns Hopkins Medicine National Cancer Institute (n.d.). BRCA 1 and BRCA2: Cancer Risk and Genetic Testing. Retrieved January 27, 2015, from http://www.cancer.gov/cancertopics/factsheet/Risk/BRCA

U.S. Department of Health and Human Services (May 2011). Centers for Disease Control and Prevention. Vaccine Information Statement. HPV Vaccine Cervarix® (Human Papillomavirus) What You Need to Know. Retrieved November 25, 2014, from http://www.cdc.gov/vaccines/hcp/vis/vis-statements/hpv-cervarix.pdf

U.S. Department of Health and Human Services (May 2013). Centers for Disease Control and Prevention. Vaccine Information Statement. HPV Vaccine Gardasil® (Human Papillomavirus) What You Need to Know. Retrieved November 25, 2014, from http://www.cdc.gov/vaccines/hcp/vis/vis-statements/hpv-gardasil.pdf

U.S. Food and Drug Administration (2014, April). FDA approves first human papillomavirus test for primary cervical cancer screening. Retrieved June 14, 2015, from http://www.fda.gov/NewsEvents/Newsroom/PressAnnouncements/ucm394773.htm

18

Urology and Male Reproductive Exams and Procedures

CHAPTER OUTLINE

Urological and Male Reproductive System Snapshot
- The Urinary System
- The Male Reproductive System

Urological Abbreviation Review

Urinary System In-Office and Telephone Screening Tips

Male Reproductive System In-Office and Telephone Screening Tips

Common Urological Diseases and Conditions
- Urinary Tract Infection (UTI)
- Overactive Bladder (OAB)
- Renal Calculi (Kidney Stones)
- Erectile Dysfunction (ED)
- Benign Prostatic Hypertrophy (BPH)
- Testicular Cancer

Provider Examination

Featured Urological Procedures
- Urinary Catheterization
- Diagnostic Testing
- Intravenous Pyelogram (IVP)
- Percutaneous Suprapubic Bladder Aspiration
- Transrectal Ultrasound (TRUS)
- Vasography

Common Surgical Procedures for Male Reproductive Organs
- Vasectomy
- Transurethral Resection of the Prostate (TURP)
- Circumcision

Common Urological Treatments and Medications
- Kidney Stone Treatments
- Urethral Dilatation
- Dialysis
- Kidney Transplant
- Common Urological Medications

Common Lab Tests That Coincide with Urological Disorders

ESSENTIAL TERMS

anuria
benign prostatic hyperplasia (BPH)
catheterization
circumcision
cystitis
cystoscopy
dialysis
digital rectal exam (DRE)
dilatation
dysuria
erectile dysfunction (ED)
extracorporeal
extracorporeal shock wave lithotripsy (ESWL)
Foley catheter
hemodialysis
hernia
hypertrophy
intravenous pyelogram (IVP)
lithotripsy
nephrologist
nocturia
oliguria
polyuria
prophylactic
prostatitis
pyelonephritis
retroperitoneal
testosterone
testicular self-examination (TSE)
transrectal ultrasound (TRUS)
transurethral resection of the prostate (TURP)
urethritis
urologist
urology
vasectomy
vasography

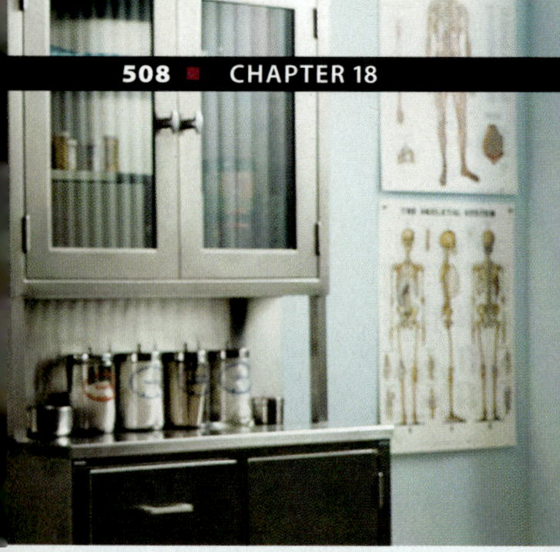

DEVELOPMENTAL OBJECTIVES

After completing this chapter, you should be able to:

1. Correctly spell and define the essential terms.
2. List and provide the anatomical locations of the major structures within the urinary and male reproductive systems.
3. Describe the normal functions of the urinary and male reproductive systems.
4. List and describe providers who specialize in treating diseases and disorders of the urinary tract, kidney, and the male reproductive system.
5. List and use common abbreviations associated with the urinary and male reproductive systems.
6. Compile a list of common screening questions that should be asked of patients with urinary or male reproductive disorder symptoms using established protocols and incorporate critical thinking skills when performing patient assessment.
7. Identify common pathology related to the urinary and male reproductive systems including signs, symptoms, and etiology.
8. Compare the structure and function of the urinary and male reproductive systems across the life span.
9. List and describe steps for performing a testicular self-examination (TSE).
10. Analyze pathology for the urinary and male reproductive systems including diagnostic measures and treatment modalities.
11. Compile a list of common urological medication classifications and conclude how each one acts upon body structures to produce a desired effect.

INTRODUCTION

The promotion of health in the field of **urology** requires an understanding of the structure, physiology, and diseases of the urinary system and the male reproductive system. A complete physical exam includes an assessment of these areas, often with the assistance of the medical assistant.

Common urological issues for both women and men include bladder control, urinary tract infections, kidney stones, and chronic kidney disease, leading to end-stage renal failure. Common issues for men include erectile dysfunction and cancer of the prostate and testicles.

The primary role of the medical assistant is to provide the patient with instructions to prepare for an exam and ordered procedures, as well as to offer emotional support during testing and provide the patient with educational information following the procedure. The medical assistant may also perform urinary catheterizations after instruction by the provider and supervised practice. Both male and female catheterization techniques require an accomplished level of skill.

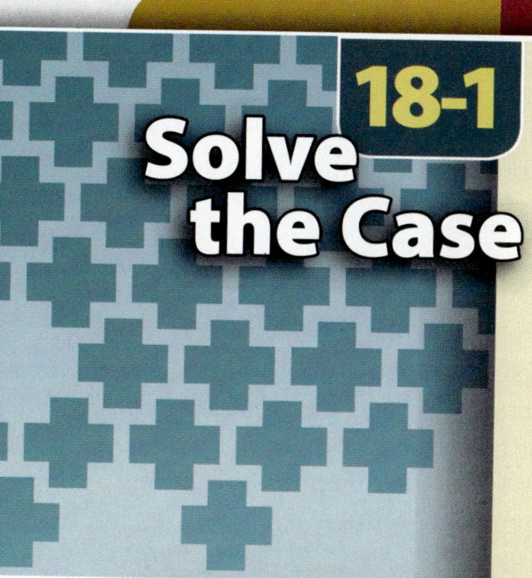

Mr. Taylor is a 58-year-old male who complains of difficulty urinating. He states that when he tries to expel his urine, he is only able to urinate a few drops; however, when he doesn't want to urinate he sometimes experiences urinary urgency and uncontrollable dribbling. Mr. Taylor states that he now has to wear "Depend" and that it is quite embarrassing. He also has some other concerns that he only wants to discuss with the provider. His vital signs are unremarkable, and he does not have a fever. Overall, he has been in good health and has no known medical ailments.

1. **How hard do you think it was for Mr. Taylor to reveal his current symptoms?**
2. **Should you press Mr. Taylor into telling you about his other concerns?**
3. **Is there anything you can say or do to make Mr. Taylor feel more at ease?**

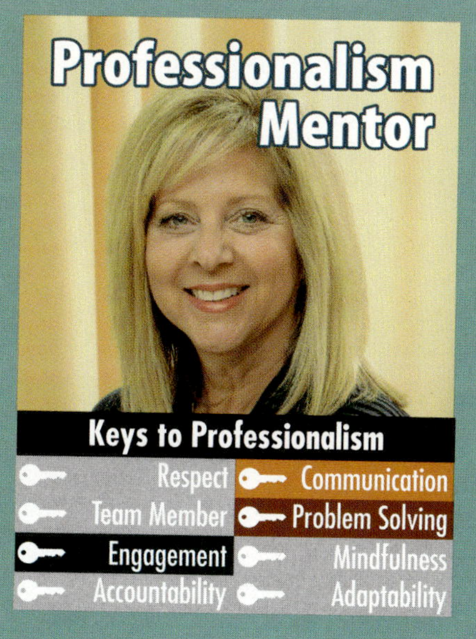

I had the opportunity to shadow a new medical assistant grad at a busy internal medicine practice. He was feeling overwhelmed by the acuity of the patients that the practice serves. He stated that he didn't realize how devastating some diseases can be. He wasn't sure how to handle patients who are too embarrassed to discuss sensitive health topics. We discussed the importance of putting the patient at ease and encouraging the patient to be open and honest from the start. We also discussed how being professional and demonstrating a compassionate attitude can help to alleviate some of the uneasiness patients feel when discussing private matters. In your journal, discuss ways you can help to alleviate some of the uneasiness associated with sensitive health questioning. ■

UROLOGICAL AND MALE REPRODUCTIVE SYSTEM SNAPSHOT

The urinary system is responsible for the filtration of blood and the excretion of nitrogenous wastes, salts, and water. Other excretory organs include the lungs, skin, and intestines. Substances excreted by these other organs include the following:

- Lungs: Elimination of carbon dioxide and water vapor
- Skin: Elimination of dissolved salts
- Intestines: Removal of solid wastes and water.

The kidneys are also responsible for acid–base balance, the maintenance of blood pressure, and the production of erythropoietin, a hormone responsible for the stimulation of red blood cells.

The male reproductive system is responsible for *spermatogenesis* (production of sperm) and producing male hormones in the body.

The Urinary System

The urinary system (Figure 18-1) consists of the kidneys, ureters, bladder, and urethra.

The *kidneys* are bean shaped and reside against the posterior wall of the upper abdominal cavity. They are referred to as **retroperitoneal** because they are behind the peritoneum. Each kidney is made up of more than a million *nephrons*, which are responsible for the filtration of blood and the removal of wastes.

The two *ureters* are long tubes extending from each kidney and are responsible for the transportation of urine from the kidneys to the bladder. *The urinary bladder* is the structure that stores the urine until it is expelled and is capable of stretching to accommodate large volumes of urine. The urge to urinate typically occurs when the bladder contains around 200 milliliters of urine; however, an average size adult can hold up to 500 milliliters of urine, if necessary.

The *urethra* is the tube that leads from the bladder to the outside of the body. The female urethra is around 1.5 inches in length and the male urethra is about 8 inches. Because the female urethra is so much shorter than the male urethra, microbes have a shorter distance to travel to get to the bladder, making urinary tract infections more common in females than in males.

The *urinary meatus* is the opening through which urine is released.

The Male Reproductive System

Male reproductive anatomical structures include the testes, scrotum, vas deferens, prostate, urethra, Cowper's gland also known as the bulbourethral gland, and penis (Figure 18-2). Table 18-1 lists the functions of each the major structures of the male reproductive system.

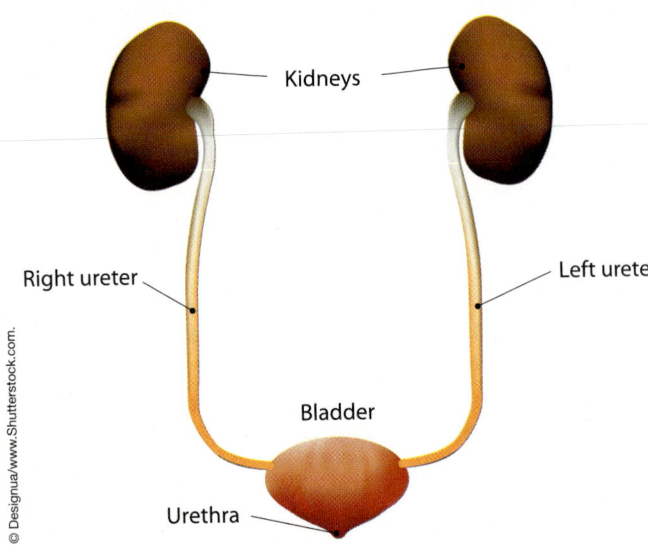

Figure 18-1 ■ Structures of the urinary system.

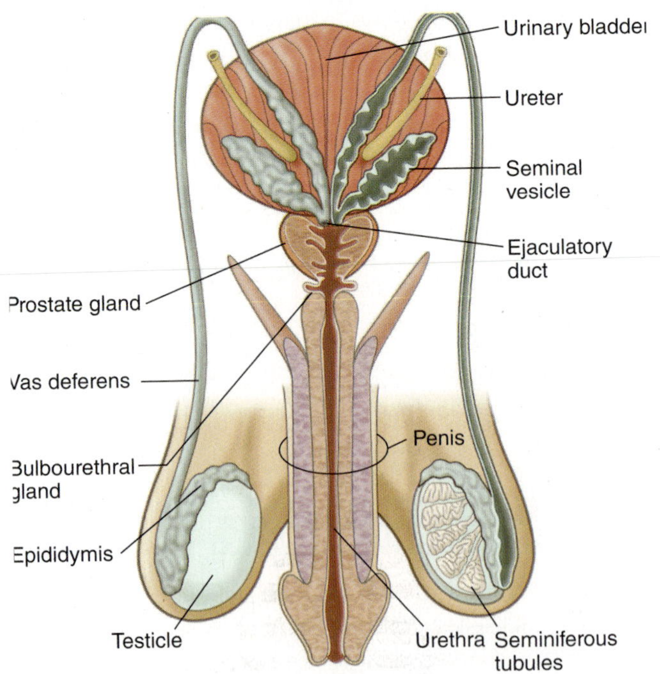

Figure 18-2 ■ Structures of the male reproductive system.

Table 18-1 Structures of the Male Reproductive System

Structure	Description
Testis (singular)/Testes (plural)	The *testes* are responsible for the production of the male gamete, spermatozoa, and the production of testosterone. Each testis contains twisted convoluted tubules referred to as the *seminiferous tubules* in which the sperm is made. These tubules will eventually unite to form the *epididymis*, which connects the testes to the vas deferens. The sperm continues to develop and is stored here until needed. **Testosterone** is a natural steroid in the body and is found in males and in lesser amounts in females. Testosterone is responsible for the secondary sex characteristics such as the development of a deeper voice, muscle mass, facial hair, and the development of male genitalia during puberty. Testosterone also increases sex drive in both males and females.
Scrotum	The *scrotum* is one of two external structures of the male reproductive system. This is the external sac that encases each testis.
Vas deferens	The *vas deferens* is a continuation of the epididymis. Each duct runs up through the inguinal canal and down and around the side of the urinary bladder. Eventually the vas deferens joins the *ejaculatory duct* and descends through the prostate gland where it joins the urethra.
Seminal vesicles	The *seminal vesicles* are two tiny glands located behind the prostate. These glands add a large volume of liquid to the ejaculate, which aids in nourishing the sperm.
Prostate gland	The *prostate gland* is around the size of a walnut and located in front of the rectum between the bladder and the penis. The urethra extends down through the center of the prostate before entering the penis. The prostate contracts during ejaculation releasing a fluid, which also helps to nourish the sperm and aids in the expulsion of semen outside the body.
Urethra	The *urethra* is the structure that carries the sperm and seminal fluid to the urethral meatus during ejaculation. Also transports urine.
Bulbourethral gland or Cowper's glands	The two *Cowper's glands* are located on each side of the urethra below the prostate gland. These glands secrete a fluid upon sexual arousal, which aids in lubrication during sexual intercourse and in making the semen less acidic.
Penis	The *penis* is the second external structure of the male reproductive system. Upon sexual stimulation, the brain sends chemical messages to the penile vessels, causing them to relax. This allows blood to flow freely into the penis where it gets trapped. The high pressure in chambers of the penis causes it to expand, resulting in an erection. The skin around the tip of the penis called the *prepuce* can be removed through circumcision.

Meet the **Specialists**

The primary care provider often treats minor infections and conditions involving the urinary tract and male reproductive system. When conditions are more complex, the patient may be referred to the following specialists:

- **Urologist:** A physician who specializes in treating diseases and disorders of the urinary tract and male reproductive systems
- **Nephrologist:** A physician specializing in the treatment of diseases and disorders of the kidneys

UROLOGICAL ABBREVIATION REVIEW

Medical assistants working in urological specialties should be familiar with the abbreviations listed in Table 18-2.

Common terms that are often used to describe urine flow are listed in Table 18-3.

When screening the patient's complaint, use the common terms provided by the patient. Only use the technical terms when in the presence of the provider.

Table 18-2 Common Abbreviations Used in Urological Practices

Abbreviation	Meaning	Abbreviation	Meaning
BPH	**Benign prostatic hypertrophy**	PSA	Prostate specific antigen
CC	Circumcision	PD	Peritoneal dialysis
ED	Erectile dysfunction	RCC	Renal cell carcinoma
ESWL	**Extracorporeal shock wave lithotripsy**	TUIP	Transurethral incision of the prostate
GN	Glomerulonephritis	TUNA	Transurethral needle ablation of the prostate
HD	Hemodialysis	TURB	Transurethral resection of the bladder
IVP	Intravenous pyelogram	TURP	Transurethral resection of the prostate
KUB	Kidney, ureter, bladder	UA	Urinalysis
LUTS	Lower urinary tract symptoms	URS	Ureterorenoscopy

Table 18-3 Terms Used to Describe Urine or Urine Flow

Term	Meaning
Anuria	No urine is being formed by the kidneys
Dysuria	Difficult or painful urination
Incontinence	An inability to retain urine
Nocturia	The need to urinate frequently at the time of sleep
Oliguria	Scanty urination
Polyuria	Excessively large amounts of urine
Urgency	An immediate need to urinate

URINARY SYSTEM IN-OFFICE AND TELEPHONE SCREENING TIPS

Medical assistants may have the responsibility of screening patients prior to provider examination or over the phone. The depth of screening will be established by office protocol. Table 18-4 lists types of questions that are typically asked during urinary screenings and common actions that should be offered when screening over the phone. The table also

Table 18-4 Patient Screening Instructions for the Urinary System

Ask the Patient	• Are you experiencing any pain upon urination; increase in urination; need to urinate at night; immediate need to urinate; weak or unsteady stream; inability to completely empty your bladder; a loss in force of your urine stream; changes in urine volume; bedwetting; lower abdominal or lower back pain; fever; vaginal or penile symptoms? • Do you have any history of urinary disease?
For Patients Calling on the Telephone	Any time the patient complains of urinary symptoms, he or she should be offered an appointment as soon as possible.
When in the Office:	
Disrobing Instructions	Patients typically do not need to disrobe for urinary symptoms unless genital symptoms are also present. In that case patients should be instructed to disrobe from waist down and given a drape for modesty.
Vital Signs	Blood pressure and temperature
Possible Equipment	Equipment you will need includes clean-catch urine container, urinary dipsticks, microscopic supplies, and culture supplies for urinary symptoms. When urogenital symptoms are present, set up a pelvic tray for females and genital swabs and PCR collection kit for both females and males.
Possible Procedures	*Females*: A pelvic exam if vaginal symptoms are present. *Males*: An exam of the penis, if penile symptoms are present. *For both males and females*: Catheterization, if the patient is unable to void or when a sterile specimen is absolutely necessary; UA and culture, if urinary symptoms are present; urethral dilatation, if the patient has urethral constriction.

lists common procedures that may be ordered when the patient comes into the office.

Important Note: Medical assistants should never perform any procedure unless directed to do so by the provider; however, they can set up related equipment and supplies to help save time in the event that testing is ordered.

MALE REPRODUCTIVE SYSTEM IN-OFFICE AND TELEPHONE SCREENING TIPS

Table 18-5 lists types of questions that are typically asked during male reproductive system screenings and lists common actions that should be offered when screening over the phone. The table also lists common procedures that may be ordered when the patient comes into the office.

COMMON UROLOGICAL DISEASES AND CONDITIONS

There are many conditions that affect the urinary and male reproductive systems. In this section, we will describe some of the most common conditions.

Urinary Tract Infection (UTI)

A urinary tract infection (UTI) can occur anywhere along the urinary tract from the kidneys to the urethra.

- **Pyelonephritis** is an infection of the renal pelvis and kidney
- **Cystitis** is an infection in the bladder
- **Urethritis** is an infection in the urethra
- **Prostatitis** is an infection in the prostate

UTIs occur mainly in women and the infective agent is typically *Escherichia coli* from the gastrointestinal tract. The symptoms of a UTI include a strong, persistent urge to urinate with a burning sensation during urination. Other signs of a UTI include blood in the urine or cloudy urine that is foul-smelling. Women often complain of pain in the pelvis and men complain of pain in the rectal area.

Overactive Bladder (OAB)

Overactive bladder (OAB) is not a disease, but the term used for troubling urinary symptoms. OAB is a problem with the bladder-storage function. Thirty-three million Americans have OAB, representing 30% of all men and 40% of all women. OAB results in a sudden urge to urinate that can be difficult to stop, causing incontinence. Although it is common among older adults, it is not considered to be a normal part of aging.

OAB causes the bladder muscles to start to involuntarily contract, even when the urine volume is low in the bladder, leading to the intense urge to urinate. Certain neurological conditions such as Parkinson's, multiple sclerosis, and strokes can also cause bladder muscle contractions.

Testing for OAB includes postvoiding residual urine volume, urine flow rate, and measurement of bladder pressures. Treatment choices include behavioral management techniques; medications such as Detrol and Vesicare; neuromodulation therapy, which delivers electrical impulses to the nerves, changing how those nerves work; as well as Botox injections into the bladder muscle to keep the bladder from contracting so frequently.

Table 18-5 Patient Screening Instructions for the Male Reproductive System

Ask the Patient	• If experiencing any urinary symptoms, ask questions in Table 18-4. • Are you experiencing penile discharge, itching, or odor; swelling in or around the testicle area? • Are you sexually active? • Are you experiencing any problems holding an erection or any pain during intercourse? • Are you performing testicular self-examinations? If so, how often?
For Patients Calling on the Telephone	Patients experiencing any signs of infection should be seen as soon as possible.
When in the Office:	
Disrobing Instructions	Have the patient disrobe from the waist down and provide a drape for modesty.
Vital Signs	Blood pressure and temperature
Equipment	Clean-catch urine container; genital swabs and PCR collection kit, if indicated.
Possible Procedures	Complete urinalysis (for urinary symptoms), culture and sensitivity (for urinary symptoms), STI cultures (for penile symptoms)

Health Coach

Guidelines for Prevention of Bladder Infections

Some general guidelines for prevention of cystitis (bladder infection) include the following:

- Drink plenty of fluids. Cranberry juice keeps the pH of the urine acidic, which is an unsuitable environment for bacterial growth.
- Urinate when needed and urinate completely.
- Cotton underwear is useful as it does not trap excessive moisture that would promote bacterial growth.
- Use good hygiene skills. For women, go from front to back when wiping to prevent fecal contamination of the urethra.
- Urinate after intercourse.
- If using a diaphragm for birth control, remove it when not in use.
- If chronic UTIs occur, a **prophylactic** (preventive) antibiotic may be ordered by the provider to reduce the risk of infection.

Renal Calculi (Kidney Stones)

Renal calculi are small, hard deposits that form inside the kidney pelvis. The stones are made of mineral and acid salts, but most commonly are composed of calcium. The size of the calculi range from tiny to a staghorn (a calculi that fills the kidney pelvis).

When the stone starts to pass down the ureter, there may be a sudden, severe pain that radiates into the abdomen, flank, or groin. This pain is often intermittent and recurs with the natural peristalsis or gentle contractions of the ureter. If the stone cannot pass down the ureter, surgical intervention may be necessary.

Risk factors for the development of renal calculi include the following, being male, increasing age (over 40), dehydration, obesity, and some digestive diseases.

Erectile Dysfunction (ED)

Erectile dysfunction (ED), also called impotence, is defined as the inability to keep an erection long enough to complete intercourse. Because of the sensitivity of the issues involved with ED, the medical assistant must show empathy and demonstrate a professional demeanor when discussing ED concerns with the patient.

Sexual arousal in the male is a very complex process that involves the brain, emotions, and hormones as well as nerves and blood vessels. ED can develop if there are any problems in any of these areas. Typically, the cause of ED is physical, such as heart disease, hypertension, diabetes, obesity, or low testosterone. Some prescription medications, alcoholism, depression, injuries, or surgeries affecting the pelvic area or spinal cord can also contribute to ED symptoms.

Tests for ED include blood tests, urine tests, ultrasound, overnight erection test, and a psychological exam. Medications can be prescribed to enhance the effects of nitric oxide, the neurotransmitter that stimulates an erection. Medications include sildenafil (Viagra), tadalafil (Cialis), or vardenafil (Levitra/Staxyn). However, these drugs are contraindicated for those taking nitrate drugs (nitroglycerine) or certain anticoagulants, or those with certain conditions such as stroke, uncontrolled diabetes, hypertension, or hypotension.

Devices such as penis pumps can be used by the patient, or penile implants can be surgically inserted into the penis. Surgery can also be performed on blood vessels when indicated.

Benign Prostatic Hypertrophy (BPH)

Benign prostatic hypertrophy (BPH) means a benign (noncancerous) **hypertrophy** (enlargement) of the prostate, which typically occurs in males around the age of 45, with its incidence increasing with age. Risk factors include family history, lack of physical exercise, obesity, erectile dysfunction, and type 2 diabetes. This condition often causes the patient to have problems emptying his bladder. The patient may also experience urinary urgency (the immediate need to urinate) and dribbling. Medications may be beneficial; however, some patients need surgical intervention to correct the problem.

Testicular Self-Examination

Testicular self-examination should be performed once a month after a warm bath or shower. The heat will relax the scrotum, making it easier to find abnormalities. (A) Stand in front of the mirror. Look for swelling on the skin of the scrotum. (B) Examine each testicle with both hands. Position your index and middle fingers under the testicle with the thumbs on top. Gently roll the testicle between your thumbs and fingers. (Having one testicle larger than the other is normal.) (C) Find the epididymis (the soft, tubelike structure and the back of the testicle). Do not mistake the epididymis for an abnormal lump. (D) If you find a lump, notify your doctor right away. Most lumps are found on the sides of the testicle, but some are located on the front. Testicular cancer is highly curable when detected early and treated promptly.

(A) (B)

Epididymis
Testicle
(C)

Vas deferens
Epididymis
Nodule
(D)

Figure 18-3 ■ Instructions for TSE.

Testicular Cancer

Although rare, testicular cancer can occur at any age, even in infants. Early detection of testicular cancer involves knowing the signs of cancer and understanding the methods for performing **testicular self-examination (TSE)**. Over 50% of testicular cancers occur in males between the ages of 20 and 34. Symptoms may include any of the following: hard lumps or nodules in the testicle region, scrotal swelling or pain or enlarged breasts caused by hormonal activity from the tumor. The medical assistant may be called upon to provide educational materials for performing TSE. Figure 18-3 is an example of a TSE instruction card. It is important to stress the necessity for regular monthly self-examination. Any abnormalities should be reported immediately for further evaluation.

PROVIDER EXAMINATION

Before the provider examines the patient, the medical assistant should ask the patient's chief complaint and take vital signs. Initial interactions and questions during the screening process must always communicate at the level of the patient's ability to understand as well as ensure patient confidentiality, which will create an environment for open and honest communication.

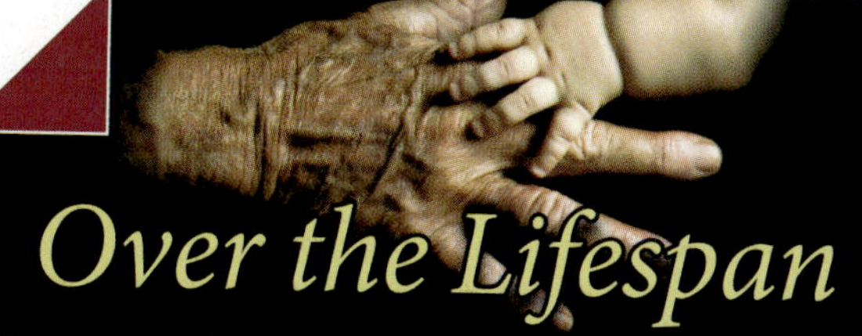

Over the Lifespan

Urological ailments typically start around the age of 45 with their incidence increasing over time. Muscular changes affect bladder control and also produce changes in the reproductive system. There is a decrease in kidney tissue and the number of filtering units. Blood vessels supplying the kidneys become narrowed by atherosclerosis, resulting in slower filtering of the blood. Medications can also affect the ability of the kidneys to function normally.

The bladder walls become less elastic as bladder muscles weaken. Impingement or blockage of the urethra can occur in men with BPH. Women can experience bladder and/or uterine prolapse from weakened pelvic muscles.

The changes in the male reproductive system with age can cause a decrease in the testicle tissues or mass, decreased rate of sperm and testosterone production, erectile dysfunction, decreased libido, and an increase in the size of the prostrate, causing a slowing in urination and ejaculation.

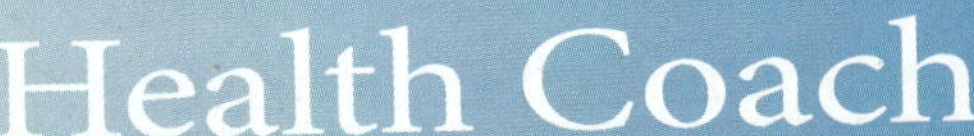

Health Coach

Featured Disease Spotlight: Prostate Cancer

Description	Prostate cancer is a malignancy of the prostate gland and is common in males over the age of 65. According to the National Cancer Institute, the incidence of prostate cancer in the United States was an estimated 220,800 new cases in 2015, representing 13% of all cancers. The five-year survival rate is 98.9%, with a lifetime risk of developing prostate cancer at 14%. Prostate cancer is slow-growing and highly curable when detected early. Current recommendations discourage routine screening for prostate cancer.
Diagram	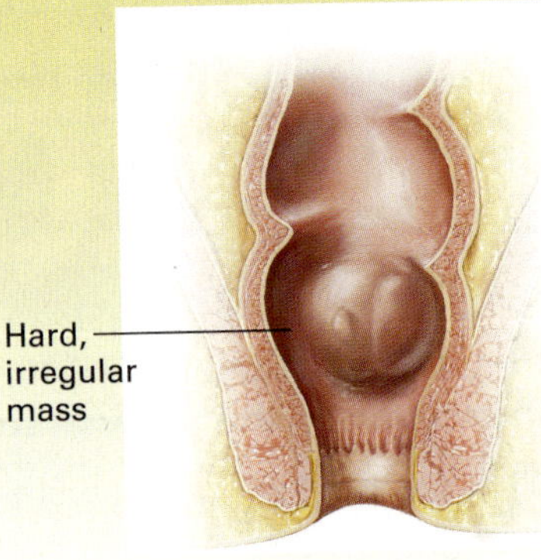 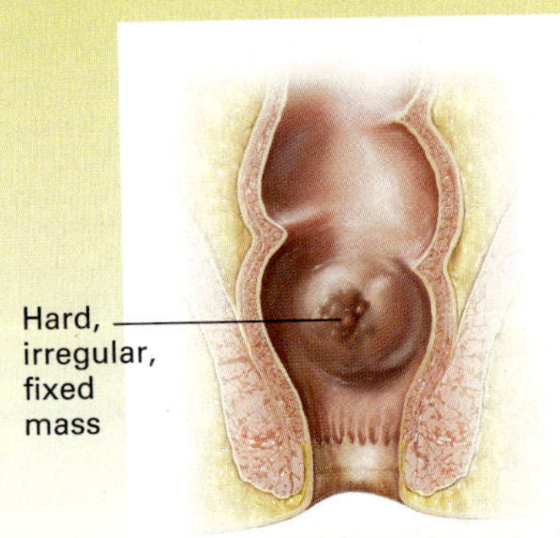
Risk Factors	Certain risk factors for the development of prostate cancer are unknown, but it appears that advancing age, family history, race (African-Americans are more prone to prostate cancer than Caucasians), and a high-fat diet are associated with the development of prostate cancer.
Symptoms	While cancer of the prostate does not usually cause symptoms in the early stages, the first sign the patient may notice is problems with urination. Other symptoms may include difficulty starting the urine stream; weaker than normal stream; not being able to urinate at all; frequency; retention; nocturia; dysuria; hematuria; pain deep in the lower back, abdomen, hips, or pelvis.
Diagnostic Testing	Prostate cancer may be suspected following a physical exam. If so, the provider will order a blood test to measure prostate-specific antigen (PSA), which usually increases in patients with this type of cancer. However, the only definitive diagnosis of prostate cancer is made through a biopsy.
Modifying Factors	There are many factors that decrease the risk of prostate cancer, including drinking six or more cups of coffee daily, avoiding tobacco, avoiding obesity and diabetes, regular exercise, and nonsteroidal anti-inflammatory drug (NSAID) and aspirin use. Though multivitamins don't seem to influence the incidence of prostate cancer, zinc, folic acid, selenium, vitamin E, dairy sources of vitamin D, and calcium increase the risk of prostate cancer. Prostatitis, agent orange, insecticides, bisphenol A (BPA), UV light exposure, and radiation exposure also increase the rate of prostate cancer.
Treatment	Treatment involves surgery and/or radiation to remove or destroy the cancer, which unfortunately can leave the patient impotent.

Inspection by the provider during the physical exam may involve visual examination of the external genitalia of the patient. Lesions, drainage, rashes, and inflammatory signs should be noted.

When examining a male, the provider will carefully look at the skin of the penis, the prepuce or foreskin, and the glans. Normally there should be no discharge noted through the urethral meatus. If there is a discharge, this can be examined on a slide under a microscope, or cultured for evaluation. The medical assistant may be assigned preparation of the slide or culture.

In addition to the penis, the scrotum should be inspected by the provider, to include the skin, the posterior surface, and any swelling or excessive veins in the area. Bulges might also be noted, which could indicate a hernia, either inguinal or femoral. **Hernias** are the protrusion of a body part though a surrounding area into a body cavity, creating the bulge. Figure 18-4 illustrates an inguinal type with a portion of the intestine protruding into the scrotal sac.

The provider may conclude the exam with a **digital rectal exam (DRE)**.

The tray setup for a DRE includes 4 × 4s, water-soluble lubricant, and possible occult blood test supplies under special conditions. During this part of the exam, the provider will insert a gloved finger into the rectum and feel the prostrate for enlargement, lumps, or any other abnormalities. Patients may be especially anxious regarding this part of the exam asking several questions prior to the exam. Reassure patients who are particularly nervous.

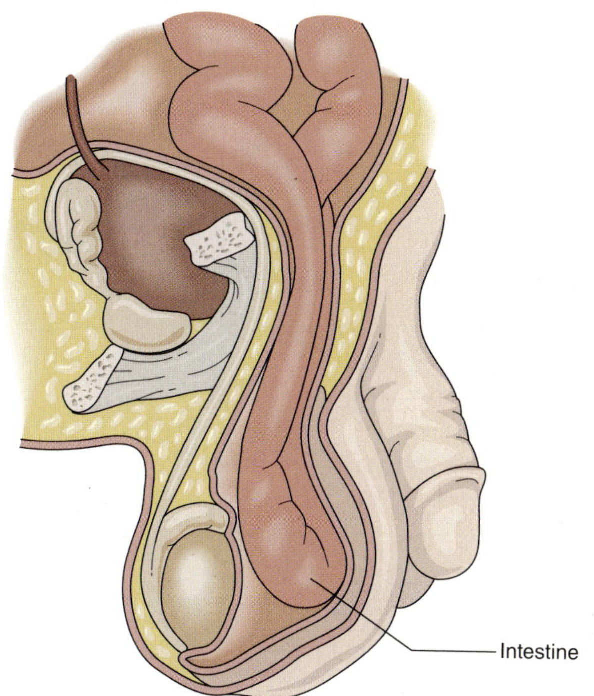

Figure 18-4 ■ An inguinal hernia.

FEATURED UROLOGICAL PROCEDURES

Medical assistants often have the responsibility of performing procedures, setting up outside procedures (procedures not performed in the office), and educating patients in the proper preparation of specific procedures. There are a variety of tests that are performed to help in the diagnosis of urological conditions. This section will focus on procedures routinely performed by medical assistants.

Urinary Catheterization

Some laboratory analyses require a sterile urine specimen, which may be obtained by **catheterization**. This process involves the insertion of a sterile tube directly into the bladder through the urethra using a strict sterile technique. The medical assistant may assist the provider or may actually perform the procedure themselves. (*Note*: Check state laws for any restrictions on medical assistants performing catheterization.)

Two common types of catheters are used to perform catheterizations, *straight catheters* and *Foley catheters* (Figure 18-5). Straight catheters are used for obtaining a single specimen and then discarded. They may also be utilized by the urologist for conditions, such as paralysis, that might cause urinary retention in the bladder.

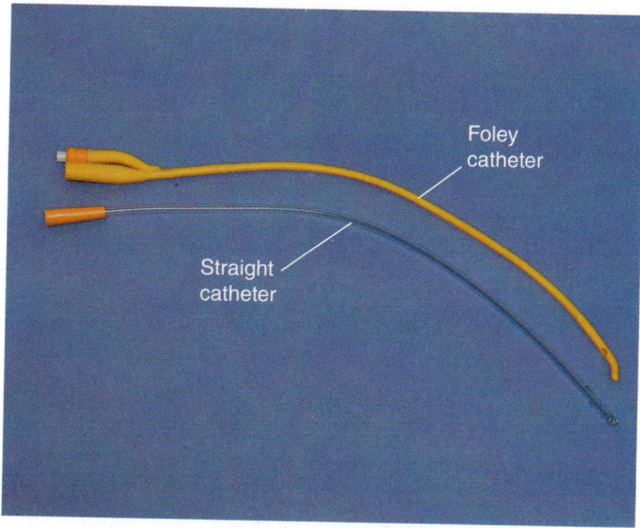

Figure 18-5 ■ Types of catheters: straight and Foley.

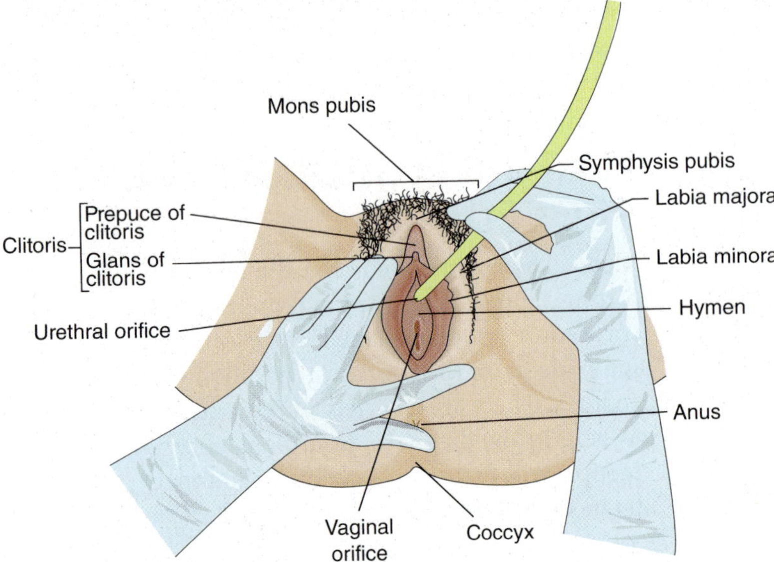

Figure 18-6a ■ The medical assistant inserts the catheter tube through the urinary meatus on a female.

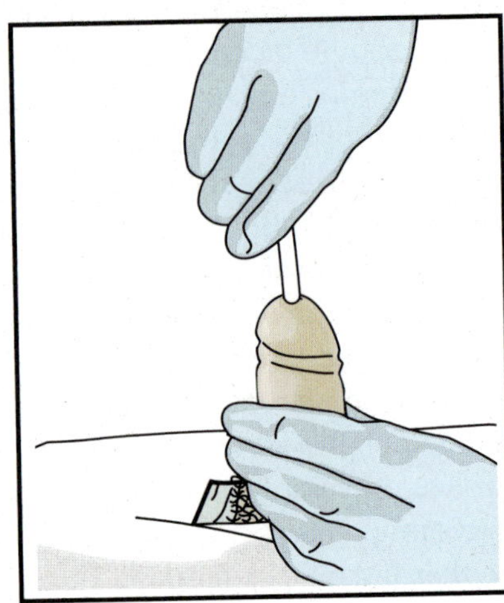

Figure 18-6b ■ The medical assistant inserts the catheter tube through the urinary meatus on a male.

Foley catheters have a balloon that inflates to keep the catheter in place in the bladder for an extended period of time. These catheters are also used short-term for patients during and following surgery.

Removing urine via a straight catheter will help eliminate bladder distention and discomfort. The catheter tubing is inserted through the urinary meatus, into the urethra, and finally into the bladder (see Procedure 25-4). Refer to Figures 18-6a (female) and 18-6b (male) for illustrations of a catheter being inserted into a patient's urinary meatus. Inserting a catheter is often a delicate and embarrassing procedure for an adult. Remember to provide privacy along with emotional support.

As a medical assistant, you are often responsible for calling the patient with the test results or making results available in the patient portal. This may prompt questions from the patient. Never give out more information than what was approved by the provider. Questions or requests for additional information should be documented and routed to the provider for clarification.

Diagnostic Testing

A variety of diagnostic tests may be ordered to evaluate the health of the urinary system. Medical assistants must be able to explain the tests ordered and to instruct the patient in the preparation for these tests. This information decreases patient anxiety and ensures a high-level of patient compliance.

Cystoscopy

Following the initial patient assessment, inspection, palpation, and laboratory analysis, the provider may want to inspect the interior of the urethra and bladder. This can be accomplished by a test called **cystoscopy** (Figure 18-7). This procedure involves the insertion of a thin scope with a light into the urethra, which is then directed into the bladder. The physician can visualize and examine the pathway for any abnormal pathology that could include tumors, stones, infection, and bleeding.

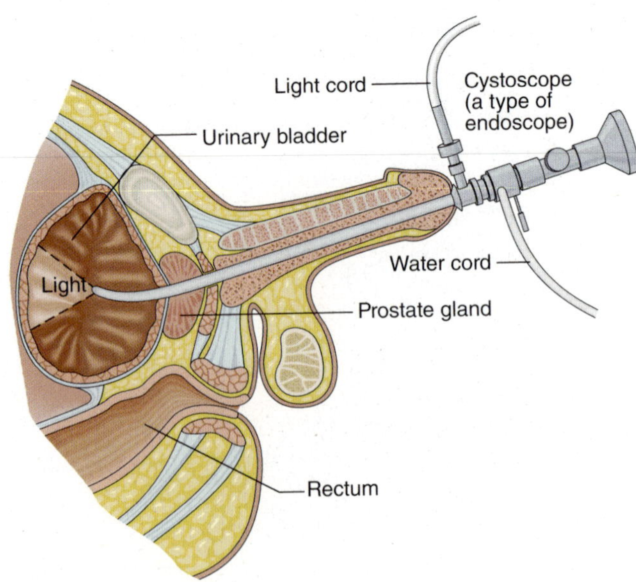

Figure 18-7 ■ A cystoscope is inserted through the urethra into the bladder.

When giving a patient information about a cystoscopy, first ask the following questions:

- Are there any allergies, including those to anesthetic agents? (Local, spinal, or general anesthesia may be used.)
- Are there any bleeding problems or are any anticoagulant medications being taken?

Reinforce any directions given by the provider. Depending on the type of anesthesia, clarify that the patient understands directions for food and drink restrictions prior to the procedure. Local anesthesia may not be affected by intake, while general anesthesia requires that the patient be NPO (nothing by mouth) for at least eight hours prior to the test.

Prophylactic antibiotics may be prescribed before the procedure to prevent urinary tract infections. Ensure that the patient understands the importance of taking the antibiotics as prescribed both before and following the procedure. After the procedure, provide the patient with the following postprocedure instructions:

- A urinary tract infection may occur, indicated by pain or burning with urination, urgency, frequency, dribbling, foul-smelling urine, or pain in lower abdomen. Any signs or symptoms of a UTI, as well as a fever, need to be reported immediately.
- A pinkish tint to the urine following the procedure is normal and should persist only for a few days.
- Increasing fluid consumption after cystoscopy is important and may help prevent complications.

Intravenous Pyelogram (IVP)

An **intravenous pyelogram (IVP)** is an X-ray examination of kidney, ureters, and bladder urethra by injecting a contrast dye. Allergies to iodine may be a contraindication for the use of this injectable contrast dye, but shellfish is likely not. The reasons for ordering an IVP include blood in the urine, flank pain, a tumor in the urinary tract, to determine the location of a kidney stone, or to evaluate an injury to the urinary tract. The patient must be NPO 8–12 hours prior to the procedure.

Before the procedure ask if there are any allergies to iodine or seafood. For female patients, ask if the woman is pregnant or has an intrauterine device (IUD) in place. If breast feeding, the patient must plan to use formula for two days following the procedure.

Weakness, nausea, or lightheadedness may normally occur shortly after the test. Encourage the patient to drink plenty of fluids after the test to flush out the contrast dye from the body.

Percutaneous Suprapubic Bladder Aspiration

This procedure is sometimes performed on small children to obtain a sterile specimen when a UTI is suspected. The medical assistant should assist with maintaining a sterile environment while providing patient and parental support. Refer to Chapter 10 for preparing and maintaining a sterile environment.

At times, a Foley or straight catheter cannot be inserted through the urethra, and yet, entry into the bladder is necessary. After the medical assistant prepares the suprapubic region for a sterile procedure, the provider inserts a 22 to 23 gauge, 3½ inch needle (spinal needle) above the pubic symphysis into the urinary bladder (a smaller size needle would be used for infants and small children). Urine can then be withdrawn into the 20 mL syringe. This technique is illustrated in Figure 18-8. Indications for this procedure may include the following:

- Insertion of medication directly into the bladder
- Obtaining a sterile urine specimen
- Relief of urinary retention

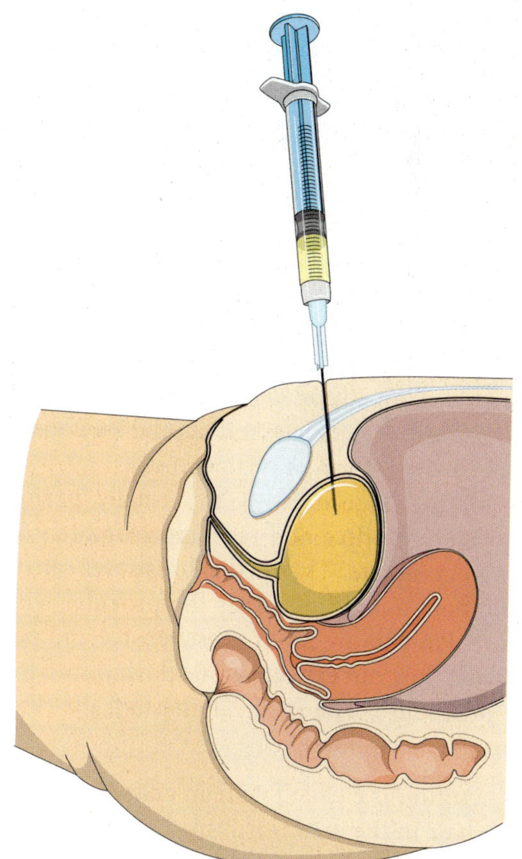

Figure 18-8 ■ Suprapubic aspiration.

Transrectal Ultrasound (TRUS)

Transrectal ultrasound (TRUS) uses reflected sound waves to produce pictures of internal body parts. During TRUS, an ultrasound probe is inserted into the rectum to produce images to examine the prostrate in men suspected to have BPH (enlargement of the prostate). The procedure is often used after the prostate has already been determined to be enlarged. When the PSA level is high, a biopsy may be required, and the TRUS guides the location of the needle for the biopsy. Other indications for ordering a TRUS are to:

- Estimate prostate size
- Evaluate lumps that are detected with a physical exam
- Evaluate the vas deferens
- Evaluate the seminal vesicles
- Evaluate the ejaculatory duct

Vasography

A **vasography** is a radiological procedure that is used to evaluate the patency (openness) of the vas deferens and ejaculatory ducts. A contrast material is injected into the vas deferens and radiographs are taken as the dye flows through the ducts.

COMMON SURGICAL PROCEDURES FOR MALE REPRODUCTIVE ORGANS

The common procedures performed on structures within the male reproductive tract include vasectomy, the TURP procedure, and circumcision.

Vasectomy

Vasectomy is a surgical procedure in which the vas deferens is cut, clamped, or sealed to prevent the sperm from entering the ejaculate and should be considered to be a permanent form of birth control.

Vasectomies (Figure 18-9) are usually performed in the provider's office and take approximately 20–30 minutes to complete. The medical assistant sets up all the equipment and often assists the provider with the procedure. Patients are often apprehensive and need to be told what they can expect before, during, and following the procedure. The medical assistant may explain the procedure as follows:

- The scrotum is cleaned with an antiseptic and pubic hair in the area is trimmed if necessary.
- The patient is given an oral or intravenous (IV) medication to relax and relieve anxiety.
- A local anesthetic is injected into the surgical area.

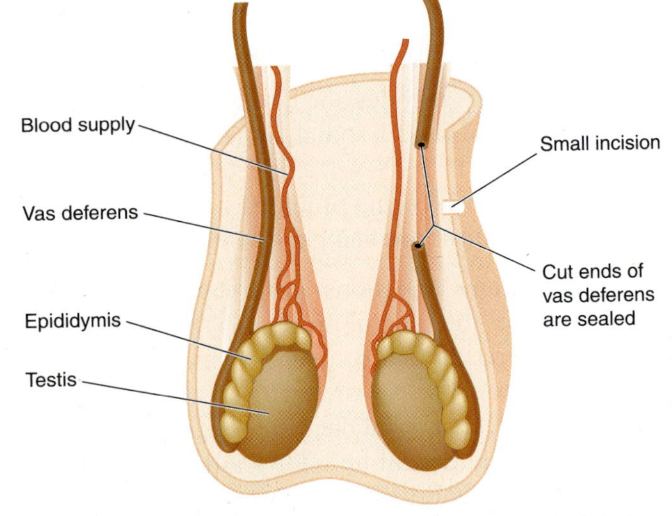

Figure 18-9 ■ The vas deferens is separated and sealed during a vasectomy.

- One to two small incisions are made in the scrotum and the vas deferens are identified, isolated, cut, and then sutured or sealed by electrocautery.
- The vas deferens is placed back inside the scrotum and the skin may be closed with dissolvable sutures.

Other less invasive methods of performing vasectomies that differ from the traditional method include the no-scalpel method and the Vasclip implant, although there is some controversy about the use of these procedures.

The No-Scalpel Method

This method uses a small clamp instead of a scalpel. The clamp is poked through the skin to retrieve the vas deferens. The vas is then cut and replaced, and the site is sealed. This method takes approximately 10 minutes and the time required to heal is less than with the traditional vasectomy.

Vasclip Implant

In this method, the vas deferens is not cut, sutured, or cauterized. Instead, it is locked closed with the Vasclip device. There appears to be less pain with this method, but some studies have indicated that it may not be as effective as other methods.

Transurethral Resection of the Prostate (TURP)

The **transurethral resection of the prostate (TURP)** is a procedure performed on males who have BPH. In this procedure, the surgeon cuts away overgrown tissue of the prostate to facilitate urination (Figure 18-10). This may be performed as an inpatient or outpatient procedure.

Health Coach

Vasectomy Post-Op Instructions

Whatever vasectomy procedure is used, patients must strictly adhere to the following vasectomy post-op instructions to prevent complications from developing or impregnating their partners:

- Lie on your back and apply ice packs to the area for the remainder of the day.
- Expect some swelling and minor pain for several days.
- Return to work in one to two days, depending on your job duties.
- Avoid heavy lifting until healed, usually two weeks.
- You may resume sexual activity, but must use contraception until the sperm count reaches zero, around 12 weeks post-op, to avoid pregnancy.

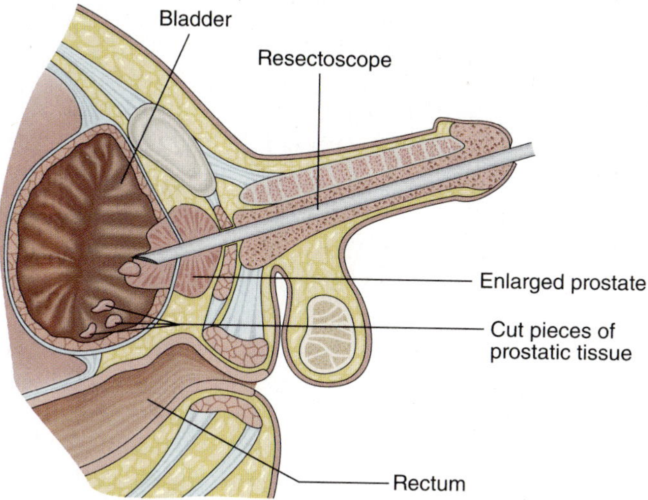

Figure 18-10 ■ An illustration of what occurs during a TURP procedure.

Circumcision

Circumcision is a procedure in which the prepuce or foreskin of the penis is cut away. It is usually performed within one to two days following birth, but may also be performed in the office up to two weeks of age. The medical assistant may be responsible for setting up the circumcision tray, obtaining the anesthetic, and restraining the infant by placing him on a papoose board. Males who were not circumcised as infants may decide to have this procedure performed later in life for physiological or religious reasons.

COMMON UROLOGICAL TREATMENTS AND MEDICATIONS

There are a variety of treatments in the form of procedures and medications that treat disorders and diseases involving the urinary tract and kidneys.

Kidney Stone Treatments

Kidney stone treatments include extracorporeal shockwave lithotripsy (ESWL), ureteroscopy and laser lithrotripsy, and percutaneous nephrolithotomy (PCNL).

Extracorporeal Shockwave Lithotripsy

ESWL is used for small to medium stones. **Extracorporeal** (outside the body) shockwaves produce pressure waves that pass through the body to the kidney stone, crushing the stone in a process called **lithotripsy** into small pieces, which can then be passed down the ureter and into the bladder, and then removed from the bladder through urination.

Ureteroscopy and Laser Lithrotripsy

This treatment is accomplished by passing a scope through the urinary opening into the bladder and up into the ureter/kidney pelvis, using the laser to break up the stones.

Percutaneous Nephrolithotomy

This procedure is used for very large/complex stones. The surgeon makes a channel directly into the drainage system of the kidney, through a small incision in the back, in order to break up and remove the stones.

Urethral Dilatation

Dilatation is a procedure in which the urethra is dilated with graduated dilators to treat a urethral stricture. A urinary stricture often causes excruciating pain upon urination and may also be the source of repeated infections due to urine reflux caused by the narrowing of the urethra. This procedure should be performed using strict sterile technique.

Dialysis

There are more patients suffering from end-stage renal disease as longevity increases and aging changes occur in the kidney. Damage can also occur due to complications from diseases, such as diabetes or autoimmune diseases. With end-stage renal disease (85–90% kidney function is lost) patients must resort to dialysis to sustain life. **Dialysis** removes wastes, extra water, and salts as it balances the levels of potassium, sodium, and bicarbonate and helps to control blood pressure. There are two main types of dialysis: hemodialysis and peritoneal dialysis.

Hemodialysis

During **hemodialysis**, the patient is connected to a machine (Figure 18-11) by tubes that are attached to the patient's blood vessels. Blood is slowly pumped through a filter or a dialyzer where waste products and extra fluid are removed before the blood is returned back to the body. One session lasts about four hours and must be performed one to three times a week at a dialysis center.

In order to be attached to a dialysis machine, a surgically created port for the blood to flow into and out of the body is required. There are three types of hemodialysis access:

- *Venous Catheter/Port*: This type of access is usually only used temporarily. A tube is placed in one of the veins of the neck, chest, or groin. The port can easily become clogged and can be a site for the development of infection.
- *Fistula*: This type of access is created by connecting an artery and a vein in the lower arm. The fistula does not clot as easily as the venous catheter and is considered to be the most durable dialysis access

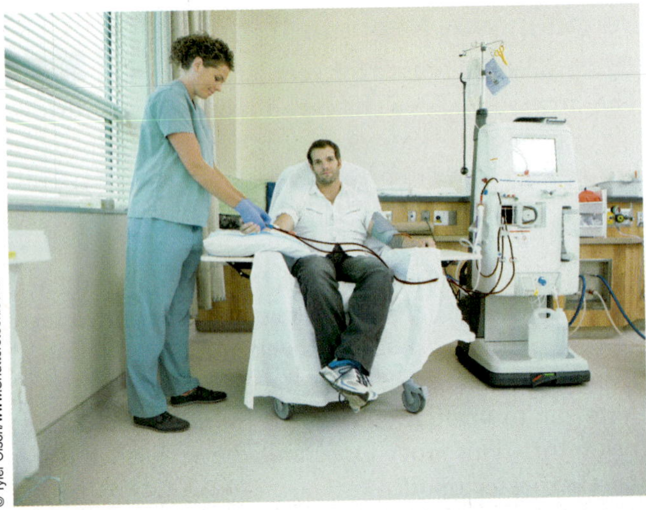

Figure 18-11 ■ A dialysis machine filters waste products from the blood of patients whose kidneys have failed.

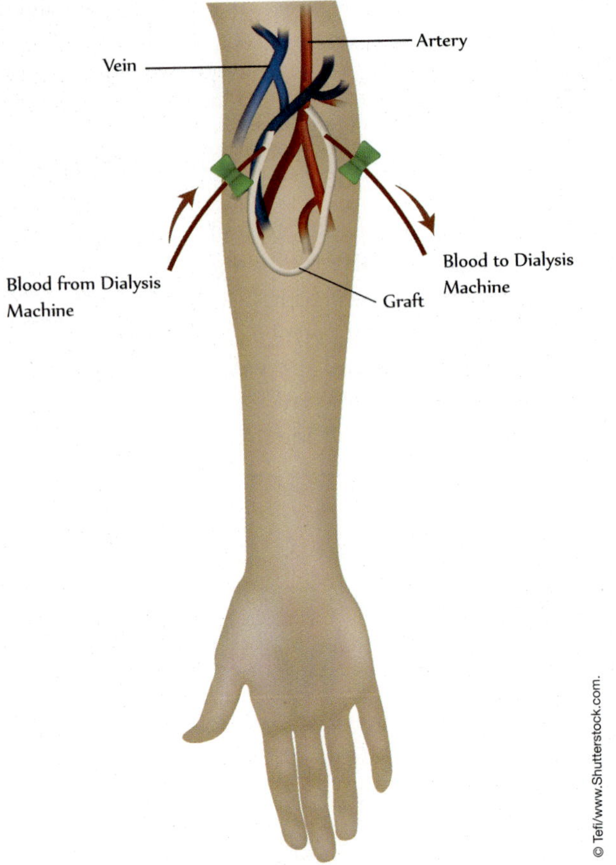

Figure 18-12 ■ An example of a graft that can be used for dialysis.

- *Graft*: This type of access is created by implanting a tube under the skin of the arm, which serves as an artificial vein. Grafts also have problems with clotting and infection and need to be replaced frequently (Figure 18-12).

Peritoneal Dialysis

This process includes three steps:

1. The fluid enters the body through a tube into the peritoneal cavity in the abdomen (Figure 18-13).
2. Wastes and extra fluids are filtered across the semipermeable peritoneal membrane into the dialysis fluid.
3. The dialysis fluid is then drained out of the body after several hours and new dialysis fluid is instilled.

There are two types of peritoneal dialysis: continuous ambulatory peritoneal dialysis (CAPD) and continuous cycling peritoneal dialysis (CCPD). Patients may choose the one that best fits their lifestyle.

In CAPD, dialysis fluid is instilled into the peritoneal cavity in the abdomen and remains anywhere from four to five hours before it is drained. Fresh dialysis fluid is

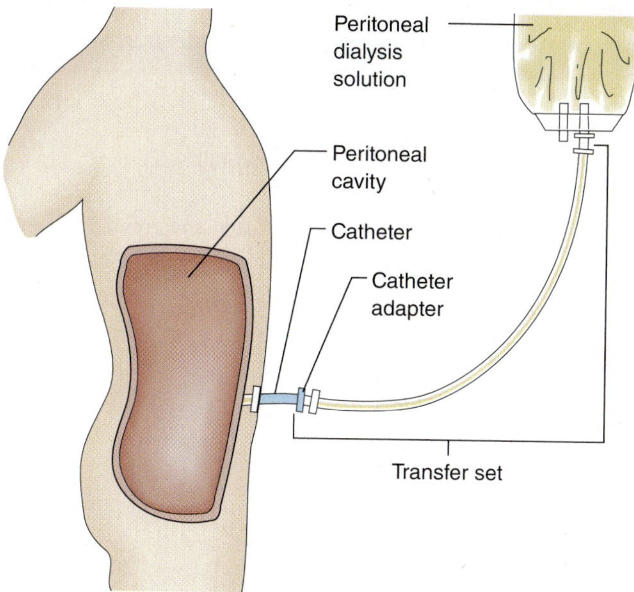

Figure 18-13 ■ The tube is inserted into the patient's peritoneal cavity.

then instilled. The patient will perform the exchange four times a day and no machines are involved. This is the most common type of peritoneal dialysis used.

The CCPD requires a machine that fills and drains the dialysate fluid from the abdomen. This method takes 10–12 hours to complete and is usually performed in the patient's home, at night while sleeping.

When working with dialysis patients, symptoms such as headache, weight gain, edema, thirst, and confusion are important to note. Patients exhibiting any of these symptoms should be evaluated immediately (usually in the emergency room [ER]) for electrolyte abnormalities.

Cost of Dialysis

These treatments are expensive, but 80% of the cost of dialysis is paid for patients with Medicare. Private health insurance and state Medicaid also help with some of these expenses. In addition, there are also Safety Net Grants programs through The American Kidney Foundation, The Kidney and Urology Foundation, The National Kidney Foundation, and the United Way.

Kidney Transplant

Many patients find dialysis to be a difficult process to maintain long-term and request a kidney transplant. However, there are established criteria that are used to determine acceptable candidates. The provider will explain the risks and protocols with the patient.

Transplantation involves removing a diseased or damaged kidney and surgically replacing it with a donor kidney, either from a living or deceased donor. Much preparation and instruction is involved, both before and after the transplant surgery. Criteria to be designated as a recipient include the following:

- End-stage renal disease must be determined and a decision that no other methods would correct the kidney failure other than transplantation.
- The patient must not have an active infection anywhere in the body.
- The patient should not have another comorbidity life-shortening condition such as cancer or lung disease.
- Age may be a consideration.

Postoperatively, the patient will be on immunosuppressant therapy to prevent rejection of the kidney transplant. These medications will have to be taken indefinitely. The risk associated with these drugs is that with suppression of the immune system, infections are more likely.

Common Urological Medications

There are also several medications used in the treatment of urinary and male reproductive system disorders. Table 18-6 features some of the most common medications used.

COMMON LAB TESTS THAT COINCIDE WITH UROLOGICAL DISORDERS

Laboratory tests are important in the evaluation of urological health. Blood tests and urine tests may provide indications that pathology is present. A complete analysis of the urine involves physical, chemical, and microscopic examination. In order to obtain accurate results, the medical assistant must ask the patient to collect a clean-catch urine specimen. A clean-catch specimen means that the patient has cleaned the vaginal or penile openings to rid the area of sloughing cells and microorganisms that may contaminate the urine sample. The medical assistant must give clear instructions so that the patient understands how to properly collect the sample. Chapter 25 includes a procedure for obtaining a clean-catch urine sample and includes procedures for performing a urinalysis.

Table 18-7 features some of the common lab tests that coincide with urological disorders.

Table 18-6 Common Urological Medications

Medication Classifications	Description	Medication Examples
Analgesic	Drugs used to treat pain, burning, and discomfort associated with UTIs	Pyridium
Androgen	Drugs used in hormone replacement	Androderm (testosterone topical), Depo-Testerone, Testoderm
Antibacterial	Drugs used to treat bacterial infections	Bactrim, Septra, Cipro, Levaquin, Macrobid, Trimpex
Anticholinergic	Drugs used to treat bladder cramps and spasms	Cystospaz, Levbid
Anticholinergic *Antibacterial* *Analgesic*	Drugs used to treat painful and irritating symptoms of the urinary tract	Prosed/DS, Urised
Antieurnetic	Drugs used to treat bed wetting	Elavil, Tofranil
Anti-inflammatory	Drugs used to treat interstitial cystitis	Elmiron
Antineoplastic	Drugs used to decrease testosterone levels in the treatment of cancer	Eligard, Trelstar
Antispasmodic	Drugs used to decrease bladder spasms and frequent urge to urinate	Detrol, Ditropan, Enablex, Vesicare
BPH agents	Drugs used to increase urine flow past the enlarged prostate	Avodart, Flomax, Hytrin, Proscar, Uroxatral
Erectile dysfunction	Drugs used to help produce an erection	Cialis, Levitra, Viagra
Urinary alkalinizing agent	Drugs used for reduction of some acid in urine to decrease crystal formation	Urocit-K

Table 18-7 Common Lab Tests That Coincide with Urological Disorders

Test	Clinical Significance
General lab tests [blood, urea, nitrogen (BUN); creatinine; uric acid; and blood protein levels]	These tests are used to evaluate renal function. If any of these tests results are outside normal limits, further diagnostic testing may be indicated.
Semen analysis	Measures sperm count and motility for infertility studies
Hormone levels	Detects infertility and glandular conditions
Prostate-specific antigen (PSA)	Test that measures the level of PSA in a man's blood

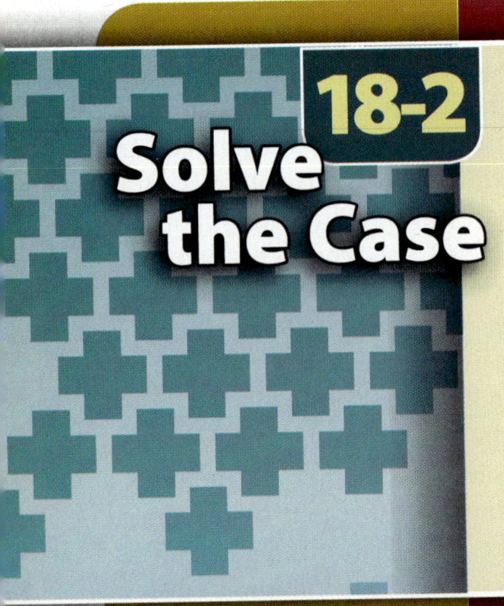

At the end of the visit, Dr. Dorado asks you to draw blood on Mr. Taylor for a PSA level and basic metabolic panel. He would also like for Mr. Taylor to have educational handouts for BPH and ED and prescriptions for Flomax (0.4 mg/daily) and Levitra (10 mg prn [or as needed]).

1. **What are BPH and ED? Describe common symptoms for each condition.**
2. **Levitra is the prescription for which of Mr. Taylor's conditions? How about Flomax?**
3. **What procedure may be necessary if the medication doesn't help to solve Mr. Taylor's BPH?**
4. **Role play with a classmate, one playing the MA and the other playing the patient, to practice going over these conditions.**

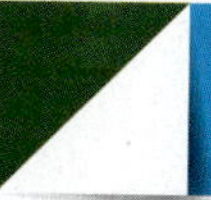

CHAPTER SUMMARY

- The urinary system consists of the kidneys, ureter, bladder, and urethra. The kidneys filter waste products and excess water out of the blood, producing urine that is then stored in the bladder until urination.
- The male anatomical structures include the vas deferens, epididymis, testes, scrotum, urethra, and penis.
- Provider specialists in the field of urology include the urologist and the nephrologist.
- A variety of terms are used to describe urine flow: anuria, oliguria, polyuria, nocturia, urgency, incontinence, and dysuria.
- Urinary tract infections (UTI) include pyelonephritis, cystitis, and urethritis. The symptoms of a UTI include a strong persistent urge to urinate with a burning sensation on urination.
- Overactive bladder (OAB) is not a disease, but a term for troubling urinary symptoms. Although OAB is common in older adults, it is not considered a normal part of aging.
- Renal calculi are small, hard deposits that form inside the kidney pelvis.
- Erectile dysfunction (ED) is also called impotence. The causes for ED are typically physical, such as heart disease, hypertension, diabetes, obesity, or low testosterone.
- Benign prostatic hypertrophy (BPH) is the enlargement of the cells of the prostate.
- Prostate cancer is common in men over the age of 45, with a lifetime risk of 14% for developing the disease. The first sign of prostate cancer may be problems with urination.
- Over the life span, changes occur in both urinary and male reproductive structures.
- Early detection of testicular cancer requires testicular self-examination (TSE).
- Urinary catheterization requires the use of sterile technique, using either a Foley catheter or a straight catheter. Urinary catheterization is a sterile procedure and specific procedural steps must be followed exactly.
- A cystoscopy allows the inspection of the interior of the urethra and bladder.
- Allergies to iodine may contraindicate the use of the contrast dye used for an IVP, but shellfish may not.
- Percutaneous suprapubic bladder aspiration is a technique to obtain a sterile urine specimen.
- Transrectal ultrasound (TRUS) is a procedure to examine an enlarged prostate.
- Vasography is a procedure to examine the patency of the vas deferens and the ejaculatory ducts.
- Vasectomies can be performed using one of three procedures: The surgical cutting of the vas deferens; the no-scalpel method; and the Vasclip implant. A vasectomy is considered to be a permanent form of birth control.
- Transuretheral resection of the prostate (TURP) is used to reduce the size of the prostate in order to facilitate urination.
- Circumcision is usually performed one to two days after birth, but it can also be performed on older infants and adults.
- Treatments for kidney stones include extracorporeal shockwave lithotripsy, ureteroscopy with laser lithrotripsy, and percutaneous neprolithotomy.
- Urethral dilatation treats strictures of the urethra.
- There are two types of dialysis: peritoneal dialysis and hemodialysis. There are two types of peritoneal dialysis: continuous ambulatory peritoneal dialysis (CAPD) and continuous cycling peritoneal dialysis (CCPD).
- Kidney transplants are considered for those with end-stage renal disease and when no method other than transplantation would correct the kidney failure.

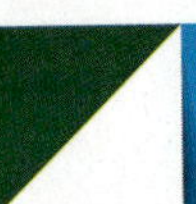

CERTIFICATION REVIEW QUESTIONS

1. The ureter is:
   a. a single tube from the bladder to the urinary meatus.
   b. a renal filtering unit.
   c. a tube from each kidney to the bladder.
   d. the lower portion of the renal pelvis.
2. The normal functioning urinary system includes:
   a. kidneys.
   b. ureter.
   c. bladder.
   d. All of the above
3. Dysuria means which of the following?
   a. Frequency in urination
   b. Blood in the urine
   c. Urgent need to urinate
   d. Painful urination
4. The recommended screening questions for the male reproductive system does not include which of the following:
   a. Are you experiencing any pain upon urination?
   b. Are you bedwetting?
   c. Are you experiencing lower abdominal or lower back pain?
   d. Do you use birth control?
5. Overactive bladder is caused by:
   a. drinking too many fluids.
   b. the aging process.
   c. bladder hypertrophy.
   d. involuntary muscle contractions.
6. Which urological change is not associated with changes over the life span?
   a. Bladder prolapse
   b. Blood vessels supplying the kidneys become narrowed by atherosclerosis
   c. BPH
   d. Overactive bladder
7. The preparation for a cystoscopy does not include:
   a. asking the patient about gluten allergies.
   b. asking the patient about any bleeding problems.
   c. asking if the patient has been NPO.
   d. asking if the patient has taken an antibiotic.
8. Common medication classifications in urology do not include:
   a. androgens.
   b. antieurnetics.
   c. alkalinizing agents.
   d. antispasmodics.
9. Which of the following is a criterion that is not used in designating a kidney transplant recipient?
   a. Age
   b. The absence of infection
   c. An intact immune system
   d. Any life-shortening comorbidities
10. The three types of hemodialysis access are:
    a. CAPD, venous catheter port, and fistula.
    b. fistula, graft, and IV.
    c. CCPD, fistula, and graft.
    d. venous catheter port, fistula, and graft.

STUDY RESOURCES

Resources to Test and Reinforce Your Knowledge:	
Certification Review Questions	Take this end-of-chapter quiz
Workbook	• Complete the activities for Chapter 18
Resources to Promote Critical Thinking:	
***Solve the Case* Activities**	• Consider these case studies and discuss your conclusions
Learning Lab	• Module 18: Urinary, Endocrine and Reproductive Systems
MindTap	• Complete Chapter 18 readings and activities

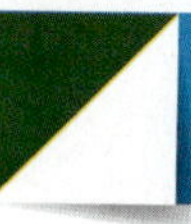

REFERENCES

Manski, D. (2014, November 26). *Medical Abbreviations*. Retrieved December 30, 2014, from http://www.urology-textbook.com/medical-abbreviations.html

Mayo Clinic. (2015, February 4). *Diseases and Conditions: Erectile Dysfunction*. Retrieved March 11, 2015, from http://www.mayoclinic.org/diseases-conditions/erectile-dysfunction/basics/definition/con-20034244

Mayo Clinic. (2015, February 26). *Diseases and Conditions: Kidney Stones*. Retrieved March 11, 2015, from http://www.mayoclinic.org/diseases-conditions/kidney-stones/basics/definition/con-20024829

Mayo Clinic. (2012, August 29). *Diseases and Conditions: Urinary Tract Infection (UTI)*. Retrieved December 30, 2014, from http://www.mayoclinic.org/diseases-conditions/urinary-tract-infection/basics/definition/con-20037892

MedlinePlus. (2012, November 10). *Aging Changes in the Kidneys and Bladder*. Retrieved December 30, 2014, from http://www.nlm.nih.gov/medlineplus/ency/article/004010.htm

Northwest Suburban Urology Associates, S.C. (n.d.). *Urology and Male Infertility*. Retrieved March 11, 2015, from http://www.nsua.com/urology-medications.shtml

U.S. Department of Health and Human Services. (2014, August 6). *National Kidney and Urologic Diseases Information Clearinghouse (NKUDIC)*. Retrieved December 30, 2014, from http://kidney.niddk.nih.gov/clinicaltrials/clinicaltrials.aspx

Washington University School of Medicine in St. Louis. (n.d.). *Surgery for Kidney Stones*. Retrieved December 30, 2014, from http://urology.wustl.edu/en/Patient-Care/Kidney-Stones/Surgery-for-Kidney-Stones

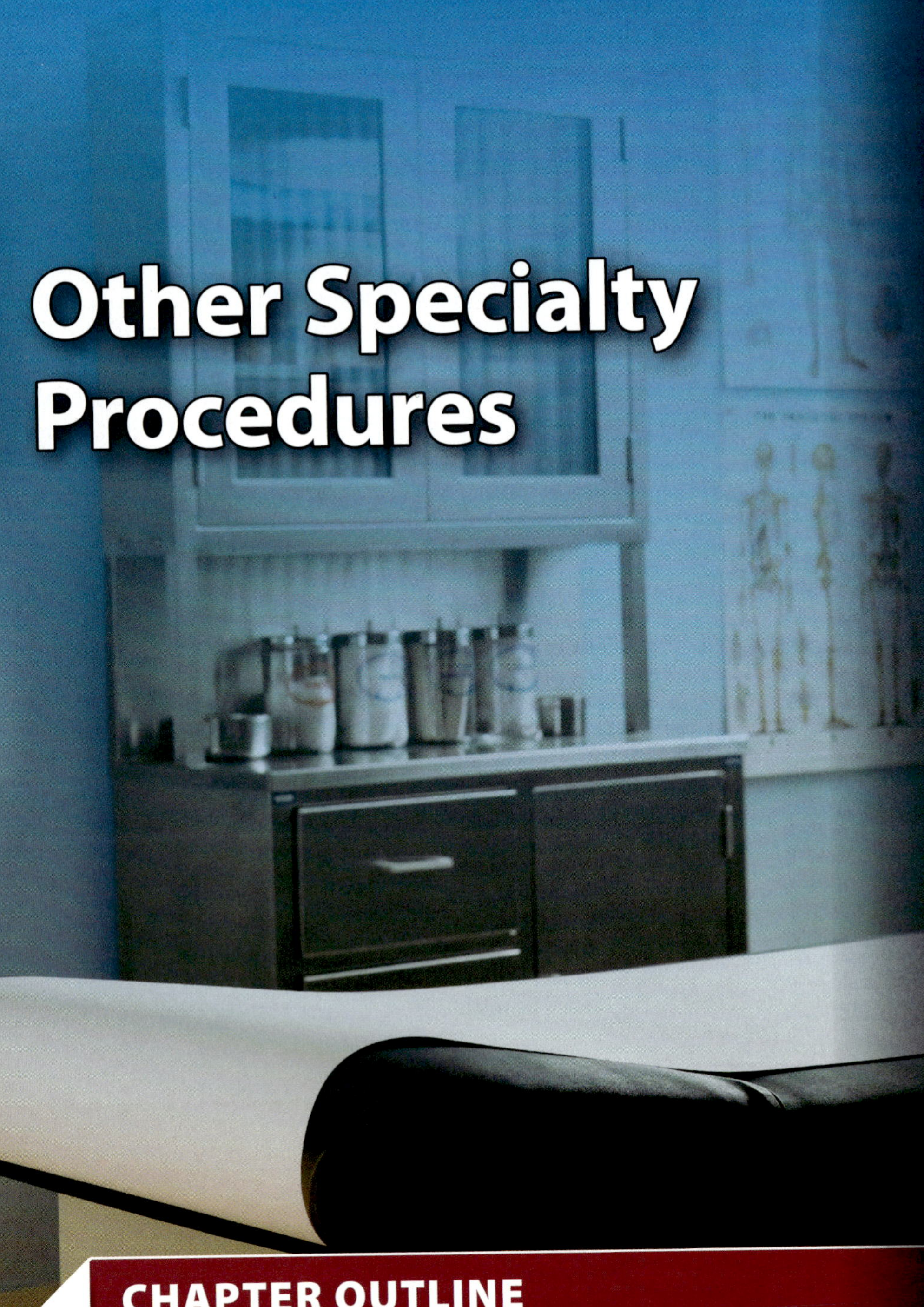

19

Other Specialty Procedures

ESSENTIAL TERMS

acupressure
acupuncture
acupuncturist
allergen
allergist
alternative therapy
anaphylaxis
angioedema
antigen
aroma therapy
art and/or music therapy
Ayurveda
biofeedback
chelation
chiropractor
complementary and alternative medicine (CAM)
contact dermatitis
cosmetic dermatologist
dentist
dermatologist
doctor of osteopathy
epidermis
epinephrine
faith and prayer
homeopathy
hypnosis
immunotherapy
integrative health care
kinesiology
light therapy
Mantoux test
massage therapy
massage therapist
melanocytes
mindfulness meditation
multiple allergosorbent test system (MAST)
naturopathic medicine
ophthalmologist
optometrist

continues

CHAPTER OUTLINE

Allergy Specialty
- Types and Causes of Allergies
- Common Allergy Diagnostic Tests
- Allergy Treatments

Anti-aging Procedures
- Anti-aging Treatments
- The Role of the Medical Assistant in Assisting with Anti-aging Procedures

Complementary and Alternative Medicine (CAM)
- Description and Purpose of CAM
- Provider Concerns
- Types of CAM

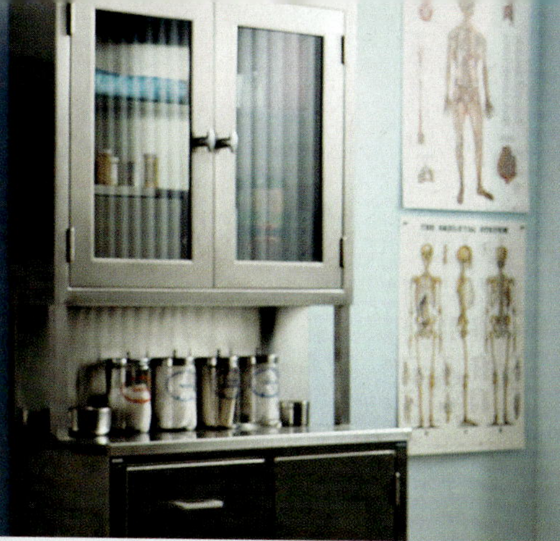

orthomolecular medicine
osteopathic manipulative therapy (OMT)
otorhinolaryngologist
pain management specialist
placebo effect
plastic surgeon
progressive muscle relaxation
radioallergosorbent test (RAST)
subcutaneous
traditional Chinese medicine
urticaria
wheal
yoga

DEVELOPMENTAL OBJECTIVES

After completing this chapter, you should be able to:

1. Correctly spell and define the essential terms.
2. Identify and describe health care specialists who treat allergies, anti-aging, and perform complementary and alternative medicine (CAM).
3. Identify the types and causes of allergies.
4. Describe allergy treatments.
5. Identify, discuss, and perform common allergy diagnostic tests and procedures.
6. Perform allergy testing.
7. Explain anti-aging procedures and treatments.
8. Explain the role and responsibilities of the medical assistant in administering allergy shots and assisting with anti-aging procedures.
9. Describe the injection routes that are used for testing and receiving allergy injections.
10. List and describe the purpose and types of CAM.
11. Instruct and prepare a patient for a procedure or treatment.

INTRODUCTION

There are many specialty areas and procedures that do not fit into the body systems featured in this text. The purpose of this chapter is to introduce readers to a few specialty areas that are really growing and expanding in today's health care community.

Two of the most common health problems include asthma and allergic diseases. It is estimated that approximately 50 million Americans have asthma, hay fever, or other allergy-related conditions (according to the American College of Allergy, Asthma, and Immunology [ACAAI]). Some allergies are mild and may not need any treatment; however, some allergies can interfere with day-to-day activities and may even be life-threatening. It is important to know when it is time to see a specialist.

Thanks to medical advancements and technology, people are living longer than ever in today's modern society. Antiaging medicine is biotechnology coupled with advanced clinical preventive medicine. There are a variety of treatments and techniques used by medical professionals to combat the aging appearance.

Complementary and alternative medicine (CAM) refers to a broad set of health care practices that are not part of that country's own tradition and are not integrated into the dominant health care system. **Integrative health care** is a growing trend where providers and health care systems are integrating various practices into treatment and health promotion.

ALLERGY SPECIALTY

Allergies exist in many different forms and cause a variety of symptoms that range from minor to severe. Allergy (sometimes called hypersensitivity) is a reaction by the immune system. People who have allergies can often be sensitive to more than one thing. The body's defense mechanism (immune system) normally fights germs. In most allergic reactions, the body is responding to a "false alarm." A variety of tests are used to diagnose allergies, and treatments include medications, allergy shots, and avoiding the substance that causes the reaction.

Types and Causes of Allergies

Allergies exist in many forms and the effects of an allergy can vary from person to person. For example, according to the Centers for Disease Control and Prevention (CDC) more than 50 million Americans suffer from some type of allergy and 4–6 percent of children and 4 percent of adults suffer from food allergies alone.

Hypersensitivity Reactions

There are four types of hypersensitivity reactions that vary in response time (immediate to delayed) and severity (irritation to life-threatening anaphylaxis).

Type I hypersensitivity is an immediate reaction to a known allergen (medications, foods, or proteins). The reaction is IgE (immunoglobulin E)-mediated and

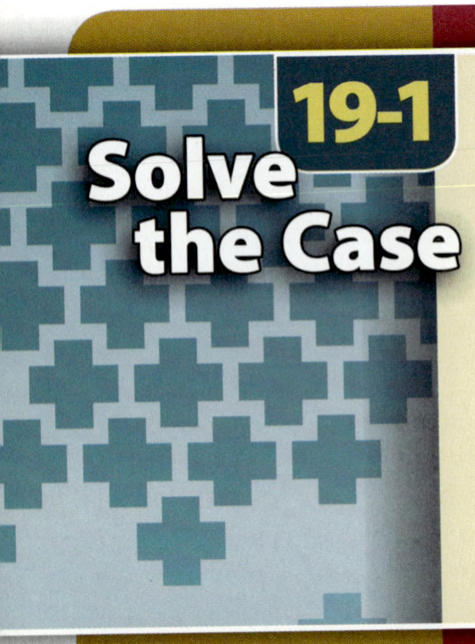

Patient Jonae Williamson, a 36-year-old female, comes to the office today to see Dr. Angela Lim, D.O. who specializes in osteopathic manipulative therapy (OMT). Jonae has been complaining of recurring headaches over the past 6 weeks and has questions about the type of treatment available to provide relief of her symptoms. Your responsibility is to interview the patient, document the chief complaint, record current medications, and prepare the patient for her visit with Dr. Lim. Dr. Lim's schedule is extremely full today. Given your current level of knowledge, consider the following questions.

1. **What information would you obtain from the patient?**
2. **The patient asks you the difference between an M.D. and D.O. How would you respond?**
3. **How would you prepare the patient for the provider's examination?**

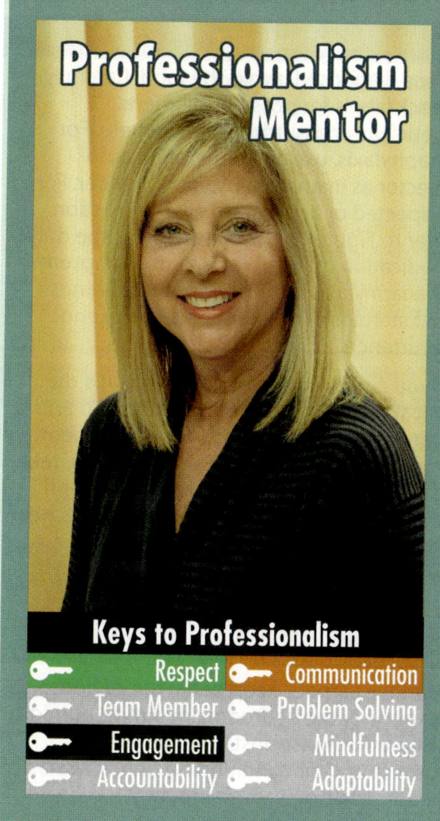

A young man who played collegiate baseball came to the physician's office looking for some relief for the constant neck pain he had been having. He had been given lots of pain meds which left him groggy and tired, not a good combination to have when catching 90 mph fastballs. Upon rooming the patient, the MA looked up from his note taking and asked him what kind of treatment he was seeking? The young baseball player said he would like to try some alternative treatments he had been reading about, that involved manipulation to help get his cervical spine in better alignment. What I saw next impressed me. The MA nodded and without missing a beat, wrote this information in the notes and nodded in agreement saying "that would be much better than all the pain meds." This level of understanding and compassion cannot be taught. The MA recognized a frustrated young man and voiced his empathy by stating that he really understood. That comment was sincere and the patient knew it. Being open-minded when a patient suggests something that might not be a main stream option is an important key to success. Years from now, certain alternative treatments may be the norm. To be successful, we always need to consider the patients ideas and suggestions and work together as a team. In your journal, write how the keys listed in this feature apply to this scenario. Would you have added any other keys? Why? ■

causes a release of histamine, which causes symptoms such as rhinitis, allergic asthma, conjunctivitis, nausea, and abdominal upset. Serious reactions include **urticaria** (also known as hives), **angioedema** (swelling under the skin), and anaphylaxis leading to respiratory compromise and possibly death.

Type II hypersensitivity is referred to as a cytotoxic hypersensitivity where antibodies bind to antigens on the cell surface to respond to foreign tissues and proteins. An example is ABO incompatibility where a patient that receives mismatched red blood cells reacts through a complement cascade resulting in cellular destruction.

Type III hypersensitivity is the result of the accumulation of antigen–antibody complexes that overwhelm the immune system and leads to excess inflammation. Examples of this type of reaction include Henoch–Schönlein purpura (a disorder that causes inflammation and bleeding in the small blood vessels in the skin [purple spots], joint pain, gastrointestinal problems), and vasculitis (inflammation of blood vessels). These types of reactions are delayed and have variable severity depending on the therapy received.

Type IV hypersensitivity is referred to as delayed type hypersensitivity because it can take several days to develop. This reaction is cell-mediated. The most common example of this is contact dermatitis to poison ivy, metals, and the **Mantoux test** (tuberculin skin test).

An overview of the types, triggers, symptoms, and treatments for some of the most common allergies are outlined in Table 19-1.

For more information on allergies, visit the websites for the American College of Allergy, Asthma, and Immunology (www.acaai.org), Centers for Disease Control and Prevention (www.cdc.gov), and Asthma and Allergy Foundation of America (www.aafa.org).

Identifying Anaphylaxis

Anaphylaxis is a serious allergic reaction with excessive release of histamine, which compromises the pulmonary and circulatory systems, and can lead to death if not properly treated. Histamine release causes itching, hives, and swelling initially, followed by respiratory symptoms which include wheezing, coughing, postnasal drip, and eventually respiratory distress. As vasodilation progresses and swelling worsens, the volume of fluid in the circulatory system decreases and patients exhibit signs of shock starting with tachycardia (rapid heart beat) and ending in hypoperfusion (lack of blood flow to vital organs). The combination of respiratory and circulatory compromise can lead to death if not identified and treated early.

Meet the **Specialists**

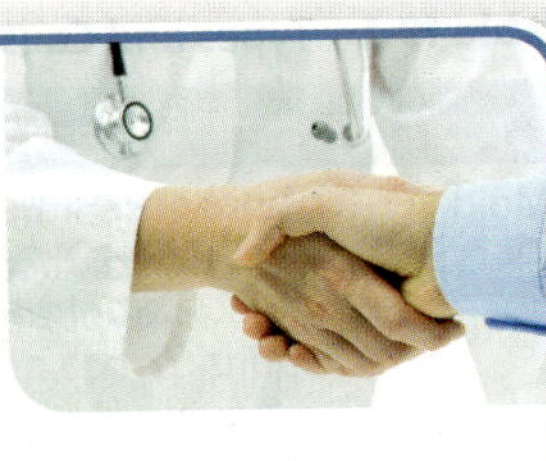

Specialists who treat allergies include the following:

- **Allergist**: An allergist is a provider who is specially trained to diagnose, treat, and manage allergies, including specialty training to identify factors that trigger allergies or asthma.
- Ear, Nose, and Throat (ENT) (**Otorhinolaryngologist**): A provider who specializes in assisting patients who are experiencing sinus problems, including those associated with allergies.
- **Dermatologist**: A provider who specializes in assisting patients with itchy skin associated with allergies.
- **Ophthalmologist** and **Optometrist** (Eye Doctor): A provider who specializes in eye disease, including eyes that itch or burn from allergies.

Common Allergy Diagnostic Tests

In order to diagnose an allergy, specific tests will be performed (see Procedure 19-1). A variety of treatments are available to treat symptoms that vary from minor to severe.

Skin Prick Tests

In the skin prick or scratch test (Figure 19-2), a tiny drop of the possible allergen is pricked or scratched into the skin. This is sometimes called a percutaneous test, and is the most common type of skin test.

Intradermal Test

The intradermal test is often performed if the scratch test is negative or unclear and shows whether someone is allergic to things such as insect stings and penicillin. Intradermal test sites are performed at spaced intervals on the forearm or scapular area. If the initial test is negative, it is often repeated with a stronger solution.

Skin Patch Test

The patch test determines if you have contact dermatitis. A small amount of the possible allergen is placed on the skin, covered with a bandage, and checked for reactions after 48 hours (Figure 19-4a and 19-4b). A rash develops if the test is positive for the allergen.

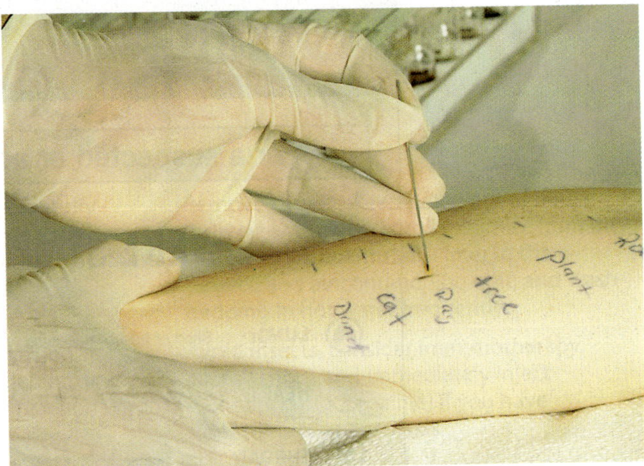

Figure 19-2 ■ A person receiving a skin prick test.

Patient Preparation for Skin Scratch Testing

The skin is prepared with alcohol and allowed to air dry. The skin, usually on the forearm or back, is marked with a pen to illustrate where each drop of

Health Coach

Intradermal Injections

A fine-gauge needle (usually 26 G and $\frac{3}{8}$ to $\frac{5}{8}$ inches long) is used to perform an intradermal test. The antigen is introduced into the dermal layer of the skin in minute dosages of 0.01 to 0.02 mL by sterile technique. The area will appear as a small blister from the fluid raising the skin known as a **wheal**. The reaction period is up to 30 minutes, and the interpretation of the results is the same as in the scratch tests. Some antigens such as fungi and bacteria produce delayed reactions 24–48 hours after administration. The provider will interpret the size of the wheal after the designated time period (Figure 19-3). Wheals are measured in centimeters by using a tape measure or by comparison.

Table 19-1 Types and Causes of Allergies *(continued)*

Type of Allergy	Triggers	Symptoms	Management/Treatment
Mold	Breathing in or coming in contact with mold spores. Type I hypersensitivity.	Sneezing; runny or stuffy nose; itchy throat or inside of ears; hives; swollen eyelids and itchy eyes; and coughing, wheezing, and trouble breathing.	Avoid or limit contact with mold, take action to prevent or get rid of mold, take medication to relieve symptoms.
Sinus	Any allergen such as mold, dust or pollen. Left untreated, sinusitis may lead to bacterial infections. Type I hypersensitivity.	Postnasal drip, discolored nasal discharge (greenish in color) headache or facial pain, fever, coughing, nasal congestion, and bad breath. Many symptoms of a bad cold are often mistaken for sinusitis.	Avoid or limit contact with allergen. Most recent studies suggest that a nasal topical steroid is equivalent to treatment with antibiotics (drugs that kill the germs causing the infection).

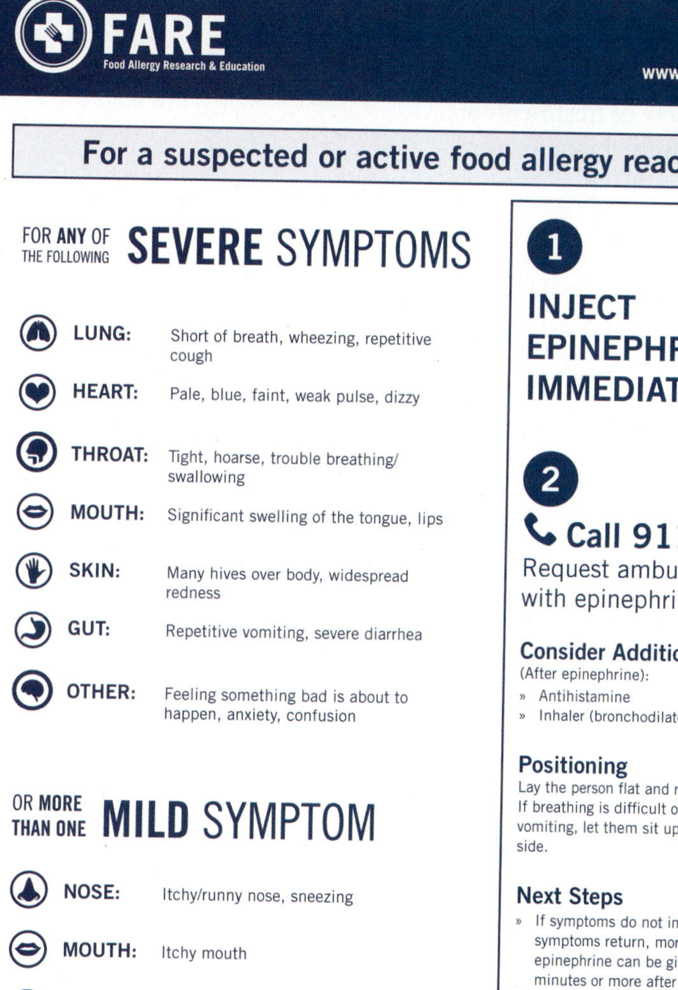

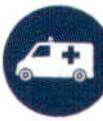

Figure 19-1 ■ FARE Allergy Symptoms.

Meet the **Specialists**

Specialists who treat allergies include the following:

- **Allergist**: An allergist is a provider who is specially trained to diagnose, treat, and manage allergies, including specialty training to identify factors that trigger allergies or asthma.
- Ear, Nose, and Throat (ENT) (**Otorhinolaryngologist**): A provider who specializes in assisting patients who are experiencing sinus problems, including those associated with allergies.
- **Dermatologist**: A provider who specializes in assisting patients with itchy skin associated with allergies.
- **Ophthalmologist** and **Optometrist** (Eye Doctor): A provider who specializes in eye disease, including eyes that itch or burn from allergies.

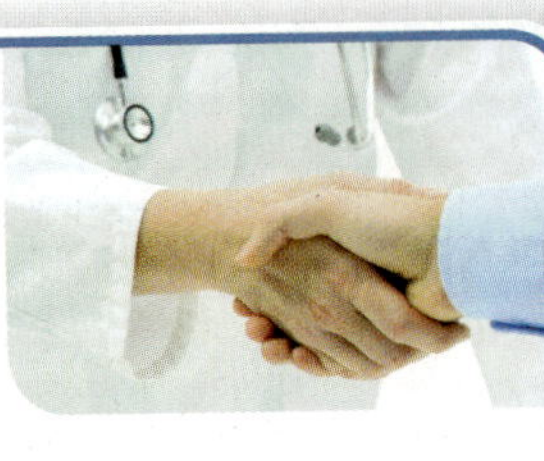

Common Allergy Diagnostic Tests

In order to diagnose an allergy, specific tests will be performed (see Procedure 19-1). A variety of treatments are available to treat symptoms that vary from minor to severe.

Skin Prick Tests

In the skin prick or scratch test (Figure 19-2), a tiny drop of the possible allergen is pricked or scratched into the skin. This is sometimes called a percutaneous test, and is the most common type of skin test.

Intradermal Test

The intradermal test is often performed if the scratch test is negative or unclear and shows whether someone is allergic to things such as insect stings and penicillin. Intradermal test sites are performed at spaced intervals on the forearm or scapular area. If the initial test is negative, it is often repeated with a stronger solution.

Skin Patch Test

The patch test determines if you have contact dermatitis. A small amount of the possible allergen is placed on the skin, covered with a bandage, and checked for reactions after 48 hours (Figure 19-4a and 19-4b). A rash develops if the test is positive for the allergen.

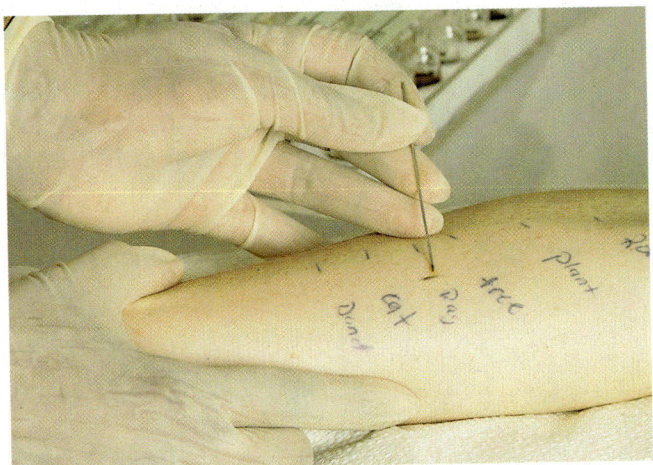

Figure 19-2 ■ A person receiving a skin prick test.

Patient Preparation for Skin Scratch Testing

The skin is prepared with alcohol and allowed to air dry. The skin, usually on the forearm or back, is marked with a pen to illustrate where each drop of

Health Coach

Intradermal Injections

A fine-gauge needle (usually 26 G and ⅜ to ⅝ inches long) is used to perform an intradermal test. The antigen is introduced into the dermal layer of the skin in minute dosages of 0.01 to 0.02 mL by sterile technique. The area will appear as a small blister from the fluid raising the skin known as a **wheal**. The reaction period is up to 30 minutes, and the interpretation of the results is the same as in the scratch tests. Some antigens such as fungi and bacteria produce delayed reactions 24–48 hours after administration. The provider will interpret the size of the wheal after the designated time period (Figure 19-3). Wheals are measured in centimeters by using a tape measure or by comparison.

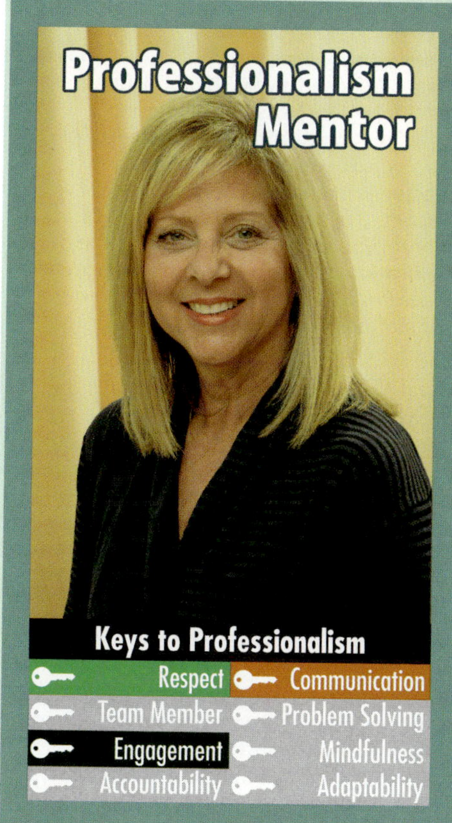

A young man who played collegiate baseball came to the physician's office looking for some relief for the constant neck pain he had been having. He had been given lots of pain meds which left him groggy and tired, not a good combination to have when catching 90 mph fastballs. Upon rooming the patient, the MA looked up from his note taking and asked him what kind of treatment he was seeking? The young baseball player said he would like to try some alternative treatments he had been reading about, that involved manipulation to help get his cervical spine in better alignment. What I saw next impressed me. The MA nodded and without missing a beat, wrote this information in the notes and nodded in agreement saying "that would be much better than all the pain meds." This level of understanding and compassion cannot be taught. The MA recognized a frustrated young man and voiced his empathy by stating that he really understood. That comment was sincere and the patient knew it. Being open-minded when a patient suggests something that might not be a main stream option is an important key to success. Years from now, certain alternative treatments may be the norm. To be successful, we always need to consider the patients ideas and suggestions and work together as a team. In your journal, write how the keys listed in this feature apply to this scenario. Would you have added any other keys? Why? ■

causes a release of histamine, which causes symptoms such as rhinitis, allergic asthma, conjunctivitis, nausea, and abdominal upset. Serious reactions include **urticaria** (also known as hives), **angioedema** (swelling under the skin), and anaphylaxis leading to respiratory compromise and possibly death.

Type II hypersensitivity is referred to as a cytotoxic hypersensitivity where antibodies bind to antigens on the cell surface to respond to foreign tissues and proteins. An example is ABO incompatibility where a patient that receives mismatched red blood cells reacts through a complement cascade resulting in cellular destruction.

Type III hypersensitivity is the result of the accumulation of antigen–antibody complexes that overwhelm the immune system and leads to excess inflammation. Examples of this type of reaction include Henoch–Schönlein purpura (a disorder that causes inflammation and bleeding in the small blood vessels in the skin [purple spots], joint pain, gastrointestinal problems), and vasculitis (inflammation of blood vessels). These types of reactions are delayed and have variable severity depending on the therapy received.

Type IV hypersensitivity is referred to as delayed type hypersensitivity because it can take several days to develop. This reaction is cell-mediated. The most common example of this is contact dermatitis to poison ivy, metals, and the **Mantoux test** (tuberculin skin test).

An overview of the types, triggers, symptoms, and treatments for some of the most common allergies are outlined in Table 19-1.

For more information on allergies, visit the websites for the American College of Allergy, Asthma, and Immunology (www.acaai.org), Centers for Disease Control and Prevention (www.cdc.gov), and Asthma and Allergy Foundation of America (www.aafa.org).

Identifying Anaphylaxis

Anaphylaxis is a serious allergic reaction with excessive release of histamine, which compromises the pulmonary and circulatory systems, and can lead to death if not properly treated. Histamine release causes itching, hives, and swelling initially, followed by respiratory symptoms which include wheezing, coughing, postnasal drip, and eventually respiratory distress. As vasodilation progresses and swelling worsens, the volume of fluid in the circulatory system decreases and patients exhibit signs of shock starting with tachycardia (rapid heart beat) and ending in hypoperfusion (lack of blood flow to vital organs). The combination of respiratory and circulatory compromise can lead to death if not identified and treated early.

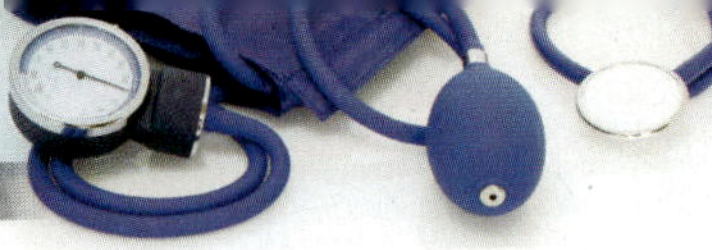

Table 19-1 Types and Causes of Allergies

Type of Allergy	Triggers	Symptoms	Management/Treatment
Food	Eight food types account for about 90% of all reactions. They include eggs, milk, peanuts, tree nuts, fish, shellfish, wheat, and soy (Type I hypersensitivity).	Mild to severe, with the most severe reaction being **anaphylaxis** (an acute allergic reaction to an **antigen** to which the body has become hypersensitive). An antigen is a toxin or other foreign substance that induces an immune system response.	Once diagnosed, avoid the food. Carefully check labels for possible allergens. Dieticians and nutritionists can help. For anaphylaxis, use an epinephrine auto-injector as instructed by your provider. For suspected or active food allergy reaction refer to Figure 19-1. **Epinephrine** is the only medication that can reverse the symptoms of anaphylaxis, but use of antihistamines and steroids can lessen the severity and recurrence.
Skin	Rashes can be caused by plants (poison ivy for example), food, medication, or illness. **Contact dermatitis** (a reaction that appears when the skin comes in contact with an irritant or an allergen) symptoms usually occur within 10 days from the first time a person comes in contact with the irritant (Type IV hypersensitivity).	Contact dermatitis symptoms range from mild to severe and may include redness and swelling, itching, bumps or blisters, rash, warm or hot to the touch, and cracking or peeling of the skin.	If you suffer from contact dermatitis do not scratch the rash; wash with soap and water, apply medicated lotion, ointment, or cream (may require a prescription), take an antihistamine, and call the allergist if rash is large, doesn't stop itching, or is near your eyes.
Dust	Dust mites, cockroaches, mold, pollen, pet hair, fur, or feathers. This can be nonallergic or Type I hypersensitivity.	Sneezing; runny or stuffy nose; red, itchy, or teary eyes; wheezing, coughing, shortness of breath; itching	Remove carpets, keep pet(s) out of house (especially the bedroom), minimize humidity within the house, install a filter in the furnace and air conditioning unit, and wash bedding in hot water frequently.
Insect sting	Stings from bees, wasps, hornets, yellow jacket, red or black fire ant. Type I hypersensitivity.	Pain, redness, swelling, flushing, hives, itching, and the most severe reaction of anaphylaxis.	Avoid insects, consider immunotherapy, allergy shots, and immediately inject epinephrine (adrenaline) if you have symptoms of anaphylaxis.
Pet	Pet (animals). Type I hypersensitivity.	Sneezing, runny or stuffy nose, nasal congestion (which may cause face pain), coughing, wheezing, skin rash or hives.	Avoid or limit exposure to cats and dogs, use nasal spray, antihistamines, consider immunotherapy (allergy shots).
Eye	Outdoor allergens (pollen), indoor allergens (pet dander, dust mites, and mold), irritants (smoke from cigarettes, perfume, exhaust). **Allergen** is defined as a substance that causes an allergic reaction. Type I hypersensitivity.	Itching, redness, burning, and clear, watery discharge.	Avoid triggers and modify home and behaviors (e.g., keep windows closed, wash hands after petting animal), use over-the-counter medications (artificial tears, antihistamines), seek an allergist, including prescription medications.
Drug	Penicillin and related antibiotics, sulfa drugs, anticonvulsants, nonsteroidal anti-inflammatory drugs (NSAIDs), and chemotherapy drugs. Type I or IV hypersensitivity.	Skin rash or hives, itching, wheezing or shortness of breath, swelling, and in the most serious form, anaphylaxis.	Make sure all medical providers are aware of the allergy and symptoms, ask about related drugs to avoid, ask for alternative drugs, wear an emergency medical alert bracelet, avoid triggers, take antihistamines to control some of the symptoms, and seek immediate care and treatment for multiple symptoms or anaphylaxis.
Latex	A medical or dental procedure conducted by health care workers wearing natural latex gloves; blowing up a rubber balloon. Type I or IV hypersensitivity.	Hives, itching, stuffy or runny nose; asthma symptoms, and in the most severe cases, anaphylaxis.	Avoidance of latex products, wear a medical alert identification, and carry an epinephrine auto-injector for emergency use.

allergen extract will be applied. You can also use alcohol to remove the ink after the test is completed. A positive control (histamine) and negative control (glycerin or saline) are usually applied initially to make certain the patient's results will be accurate. If the patient doesn't respond to the positive control he or she may not respond to the allergy extract and the testing will be invalid. These results are also used for comparison in interpreting the results. A sterile needle or lancet tears the surface of the skin in a scratch

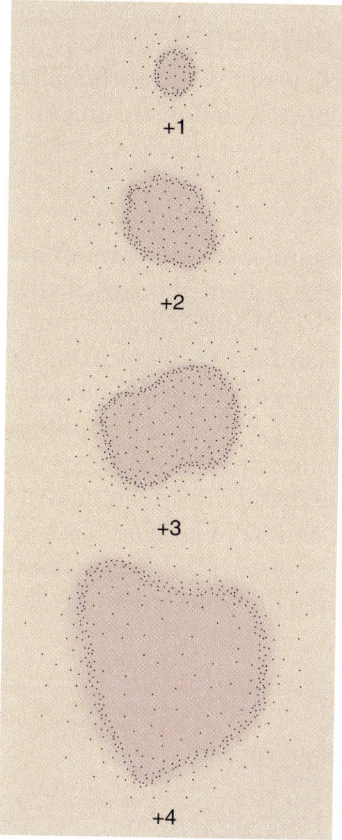

Figure 19-3 ■ Sizes of wheals from +1 to +4 in reaction to scratch test of allergens.

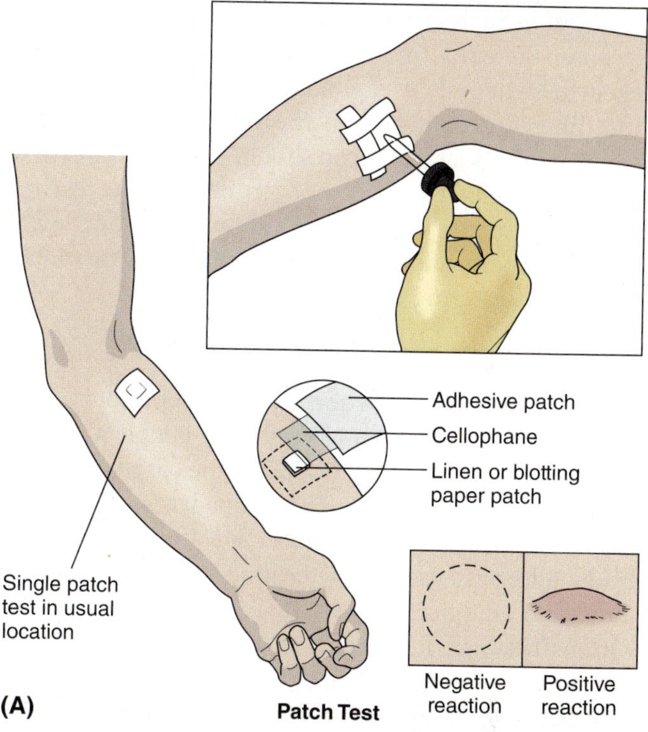

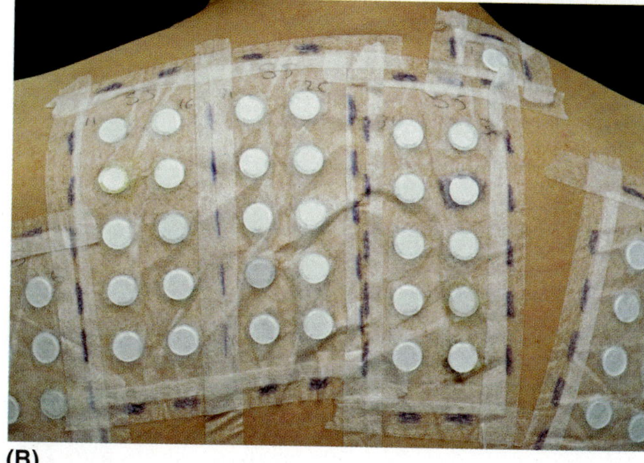

Figure 19-4 ■ (a) Patch test being applied. Tell the patient to keep the patch clean, dry, and covered until the provider reads the results. (b) Skin allergy patch test on back.

Health Coach

Allergy Testing

Prior to administering allergy testing, advise the patient to discontinue allergy medications, antihistamines, and tricyclic antidepressants such as Pamelor and Tofranil which can interfere with testing. Failure to stop these medications will result in inaccurate test results. Using professional behavior and showing awareness of the patient's concerns, explain the rationale for performing the procedure. Advise the patient that there is some discomfort when administering either the scratch test or the intradermal test, but that it will not last long. Instruct the patient to inform you of any itching, redness, or swelling at the site of injection. Advise the patient to avoid scratching the area to allow for accurate interpretation following the prescribed timing of the test(s).

of about 1/8 inch or less to allow a drop of the antigen to enter the epidermis. Some test materials are packaged in sealed glass capillary tubes. The contents of the tubes are shaken onto the skin after the tube is snapped. Only a small drop should be used, otherwise antigens might run together, rendering the test results inaccurate. The scratches should be from 1½ to 2 inches apart, allowing possible reactions to spread without interfering with each other.

Blood Tests

Blood samples are taken and sent to a laboratory where the lab adds the allergen to the blood sample and then measures the amount of antibodies the blood produces to attack the allergen(s). The **radioallergosorbent test (RAST)** is a blood test to detect specific IgE antibodies to allergens used to determine the substance(s) a patient is allergic to. The RAST is used when medications that can interfere with test results cannot (or should not) be discontinued, the patient suffers severe skin condition(s), or has a high sensitivity to allergens that could result in serious side effects. The **multiple allergosorbent test system (MAST)** is a method for measuring total and allergen-specific IgE levels.

Oral Food Challenges (OFC)

If a definitive allergy diagnosis is still unclear after performing the skin and blood tests, the allergist may suggest an oral food challenge (OFC). The OFC is a highly accurate diagnostic test for food allergies and should only be performed by an experienced allergist in a facility where appropriate medications and equipment are available. During the food challenge, the provider feeds the suspect food in measured doses (starting with very small amounts) and observes the patient for a reaction. Gradually larger doses are given, again while the provider observes for possible reaction. If a reaction is seen, the challenge is stopped. If no symptoms are observed during the challenge, the food allergy can be ruled out.

Allergy Treatments

There are a variety of treatments for allergy symptoms. Some of the most common treatments are discussed below.

Allergy Shots

Subcutaneous (under the skin) immunotherapy treatment is when a patient receives increasingly higher doses of an injected allergen over time and gradually becomes less sensitive to it by changing the antibody response from IgE to IgG production. **Immunotherapy** is the prevention or treatment of disease that stimulates the immune response. Allergy shots are proven to be an effective method for relief of symptoms caused by grass, tree, and weed pollens. Shots are also used to treat symptoms of allergic reaction to dust mites, cat dander, certain molds, and insect stings.

Health Coach

Allergy shots (Immunotherapy)

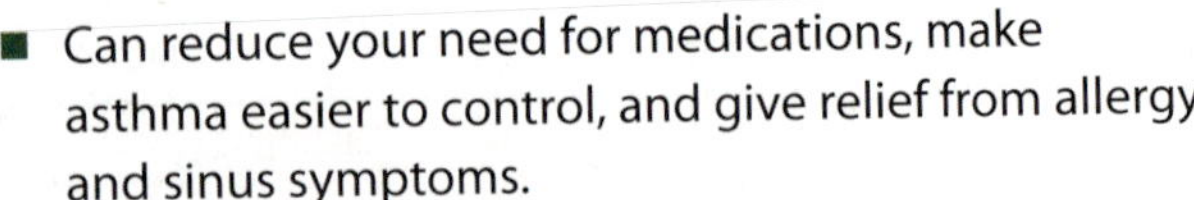

- Can reduce your need for medications, make asthma easier to control, and give relief from allergy and sinus symptoms.
- Do not contain medications. Allergy injections contain the natural protein extracts of these allergens.
- Can reduce or eliminate your allergic reactions to future exposures by making your immune system more tolerant of the allergens.
- Reactions to shots are mostly localized and appear as redness and swelling at the injection site, typically occurring within a couple of hours of the injection, and clears up within a few hours. Rarely, a more serious systemic reaction can occur that includes swelling of the throat, wheezing, and dizziness. Very rarely this can be life-threatening.
- Due to possible reactions, injections must be given in the presence of a qualified medical provider and the patient must wait in the office for 30 minutes following the injection, so any reaction can be safely treated.

For more information on allergy shots (immunotherapy), visit the website www.allergypartners.com.

(Source: Allergy Partners of Richmond)

The Medical Assistant's Responsibilities in Administering Allergy Shots

Because medication delegation laws vary from one state to another, you must refer to the particular laws set forth in the state where you work and the policies set forth by your provider and practice. If a medical assistant is authorized to administer allergy shots, he or she would follow safety and privacy protocols, including but not limited to the following:

- Ensuring a licensed physician is available at the facility at the time the allergy shot is given and for 30 minutes after
- Confirming that a patient is not taking a beta-blocker medication prior to receiving the allergy shot. This is because emergency drugs used to treat an allergic reaction may not be as effective if the patient is taking beta-blockers.
- Rotating injection sites each visit
- Asking the patient to remain in the office for up to 30 minutes after injection to be observed for any adverse reactions
- Having the equipment and medications available to treat anaphylaxis
- Documenting required safety checks, including peak flows measured before and 30 minutes after allergy shots for patients with asthma, the concentrations and dose of each allergy shot, and any reactions occurring after
- Immediately reporting any reactions to the provider

ANTI-AGING PROCEDURES

People are living longer than ever in today's modern society thanks to the advancement of medicine, drugs, and lifestyle changes. In 1970 the average life expectancy was 70.8 years, and by 2020 the U.S. Census Bureau projects that will increase to 79.5 years. People are searching for ways to live longer, healthier, and more active lives. Anti-aging medicine is a medical specialty concerned with detecting, preventing, and treating aging-related disease, as well as promoting research into methods to delay and optimize the human aging process. It is biotechnology coupled with advanced clinical preventive medicine.

Anti-aging Treatments

There are a variety of treatments and techniques used by medical professionals to combat the aging appearance.

Microdermabrasion

Microdermabrasion is a noninvasive procedure that gently exfoliates the skin by spraying tiny crystals onto the skin and gently removing the outer layer of skin. Microdermabrasion performed by a medical professional (versus the type of treatment you would perform with a home kit) goes a bit deeper into the skin but is safe for all skin colors. This procedure can provide a more youthful look without downtime by diminishing a dull complexion, uneven skin tone, age or dark spots, and melisma (patches of brown discoloration).

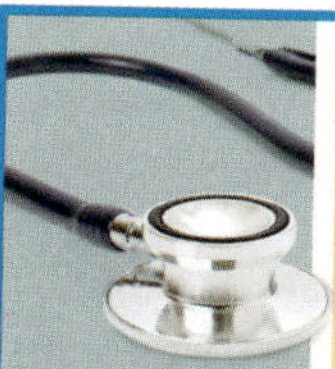

Field Smarts

Reducing the Possibility of a Local or Systemic Reaction when Administering Allergy Shots

To decrease local reactions when administering allergy shots, the medical assistant should do the following:

1. Remove the needle that was used to draw up the injection and replace it with a brand new needle before administering the injection. This prevents allergy serum from getting on the skin when administering the injection.
2. Using a 90-degree angle rather than a 45-degree angle to reduce the potential for back flow of allergy serum onto the skin when there is an adequate amount of adipose tissue to do so.

Always, ask the patient the following questions prior to administration:

1. Did you have any reactions following your last injection? (If yes, ask patient to describe reaction.)
2. Are you currently ill?
3. Is there a possibility you are pregnant (females only)?

If patient answered yes to any of the questions above, check with provider before administering the injection. Also, if the patient is behind on shots, follow office protocol for reducing the dosage.

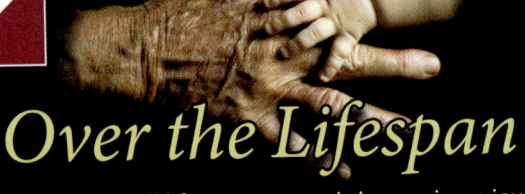

Over the Lifespan

While the overall life expectancy is increasing, views on aging are also changing. Where disease and disability were once considered inevitable, many older adults can be healthy and active well into their advancing years, and want to retain a youthful look as long as possible. Skin changes are one of the most visible signs of aging. With aging, the **epidermis** (outer skin layer) thins, and the number of **melanocytes** (pigment-containing cells) decreases. Changes in the connective tissue reduce the skin's strength and elasticity. Blood vessels become more fragile, leading to bruising and bleeding under the skin. To slow down or reverse some of the aging signs seen with the skin, patients resort to anti-aging treatments such as microdermabrasion, topical retinoids, skin-tightening procedures, skin fillers, and Fraxel Restore. Some of the best ways to preserve the skin is by not smoking, avoiding direct sun exposure (using sunblock), and reducing stress, obesity, and other related diseases.

Meet the Specialists

Specialists who specialize in anti-aging procedures include the following:

- **Dermatologist:** A provider who specializes in diagnosing and treating diseases concerned with the skin and its structure, hair, nails, and mucous membranes.
- **Cosmetic Dermatologist:** In addition to those conditions treated by a dermatologist, treatments that fall into the category of cosmetic dermatology include surgery to diminish acne scars, injecting fillers and botulinum toxins (Botox) to give an aging face a more youthful appearance, chemical peels, and laser surgery to diminish or remove small veins, age spots, and wrinkles.
- **Plastic surgeon:** A surgical specialist who deals with the repair, reconstruction, or replacement of physical defects of form or function involving the skin, musculoskeletal system, craniomaxillofacial structures, extremities, breast and trunk, and external genitalia.
- **Dentist:** A provider who diagnoses and treats the teeth, oral cavity, and associated structures, and treats related diseases including prevention and the restoration of defective and missing tissue (e.g., cosmetic dentistry). Many dentists are now providing anti-aging procedures including Botox and fillers, such as Juvaderm.

Chemical Peels

Unlike microdermabrasion, a chemical peel (also called chemexfoliation and derma peeling) often requires downtime. A chemical solution is applied to the skin that causes exfoliation and eventual peel off. New, regenerated skin is usually smoother and less wrinkled, and is often more sensitive to the sun.

Laser/Light Therapy

Laser/light therapy is a noninvasive procedure that uses light energy to repair and regenerate damaged skin. Effects of this treatment may not be seen until several weeks after the procedure.

Laser Resurfacing

Laser resurfacing is a procedure that improves the appearance of skin or minor flaws by using a laser to remove layers of skin. Two of the most common types of resurfacing lasers are carbon dioxide (CO_2) and erbium. Because the procedure can be painful, medication is often given to help the patient relax and to relieve pain. For small treatment areas a topical anesthetic is used to numb the area, and for larger areas, a nerve block or conscious sedation may be used.

Fraxel Restore

Another noninvasive laser therapy that is said to help reverse the visible signs of aging is known as Fraxel

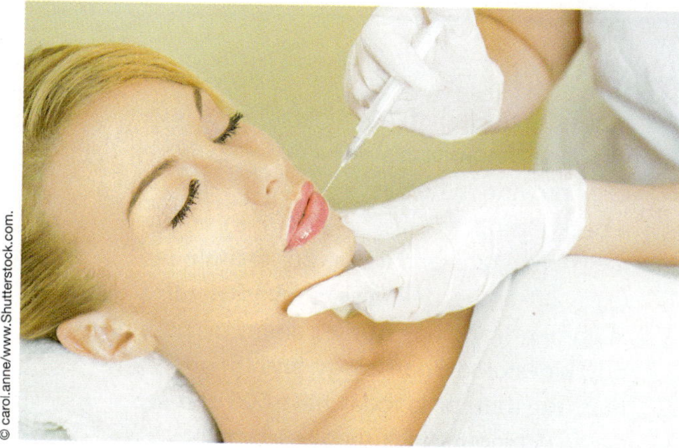
© carol.anne/www.Shutterstock.com.

Figure 19-5 ■ A cosmetic dermatologist injecting dermal filler to give patient a more youthful appearance.

Restore. Fraxel Restore generates tiny microscopic wounds in the dermal layer of the skin, stimulating the body's own healing process and collagen production. This gives the skin a more youthful appearance. Treatments are between 15 and 45 minutes and require one to five treatments to obtain the best results.

Dermal Fillers

There are a number of well-known dermal fillers such as Juvaderm, Restylane, Belotero, and Voluma. Each contains some form of hyaluronic acid. Other fillers include Radiesse (a calcium hydroxyapatite filler) and Sculpra, which contains L-poly(lactic acid). Fillers are used to plump lips, raise depressed scars, and level wrinkled skin temporarily (Figure 19-5).

Botox

Botox (various forms of botulinum toxin) injections are used to temporarily paralyze muscle activity, most noted to reduce the appearance of some facial wrinkles. Newer products on the market include the brands Dysport, Myobloc, and Zeomin.

Retin-A (Tretinoin)

Retin-A is a form of Vitamin A that helps the skin renew itself. Retin-A has been widely used to treat acne, but also helps improve the skin's appearance and minimize fine wrinkles.

The Role of the Medical Assistant in Assisting with Anti-aging Procedures

The medical assistant should be well educated about all procedures offered in the office.

The role of the medical assistant will vary from one practice to another, but may include the following:

- Placing numbing gel on the patient prior to the procedure
- Setting up the room and the patient prior to the procedure
- Assisting the provider during procedures
- Providing education following the procedure

Many of these procedures can be very painful. The medical assistant should be supportive throughout the procedure and alert the provider when the patient's discomfort appears to be heightened.

COMPLEMENTARY AND ALTERNATIVE MEDICINE (CAM)

As Americans strive to meet today's personal health care needs, there is an ever-increasing reliance on complementary, alternative, or integrative medicine. Complementary and alternative medicine (CAM) refers to a broad set of health care practices that are not part of that country's own tradition and are not integrated into the dominant health care system. As many as 40 percent of Americans use health care approaches outside of Western or conventional medicine. The National Center for Complementary and Integrative Health defines complementary medicine as using a nonmainstream approach together with conventional medicine. Using alternative medicine refers to using a nonmainstream approach in place of conventional medicine. **Integrative health care** is a growing trend where providers and health care systems are integrating various practices into treatment and health promotion.

Description and Purpose of CAM

CAM includes a variety of services that are not considered standard of care but may have some evidence of effectiveness. While acupuncture and osteopathic manipulative therapy (OMT) have evidence for efficacy in the treatment of certain ailments and are readily adopted as adjunctive therapies in Western medicine, other CAM therapies do not have significant evidence and are viewed with skepticism.

Provider Concerns

Using a method other than conventional medicine is sometimes referred to as **alternative therapy**. Some providers are hesitant about this type of medicine as often there is no scientific evidence or validation by research that it is or can be therapeutic. While some people have claimed cures from alternative and other

Meet the Specialists

Specialists who perform complementary and alternative medicine include the following:

- **Doctor of Osteopathy (D.O.)**: Both D.O.s and M.D.s are fully qualified physicians licensed to prescribe medication and perform surgery. Osteopathic medicine is a parallel branch of American medicine with a distinct philosophy and approach to patient care, practicing a "whole person" approach. D.O.s focus on preventive health care and have received extra training in the musculoskeletal system. A D.O. incorporates osteopathic manipulative treatment into his or her practice, using their hands to diagnose illness and injury and to encourage the body's natural tendency toward good health.
- **Chiropractor**: Providers who practice a drug-free, hands-on health care approach that focuses on the musculoskeletal and nervous systems. The most common procedure performed is "spinal manipulation," also referred to as "chiropractic adjustment." The purpose of chiropractic manipulation is to restore joint mobility.

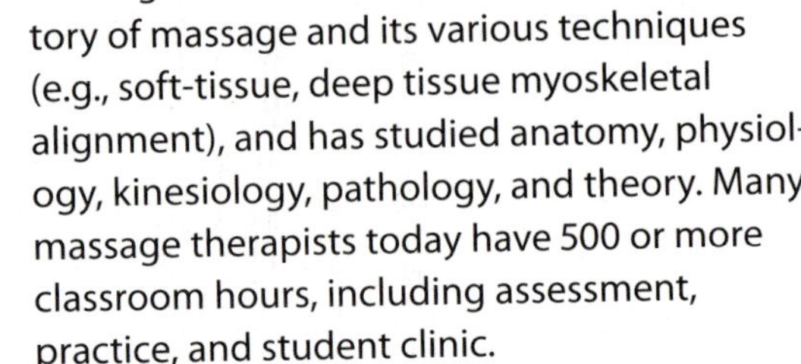

- **Massage therapist**: A massage therapist is a CAM provider who has a background and history of massage and its various techniques (e.g., soft-tissue, deep tissue myoskeletal alignment), and has studied anatomy, physiology, kinesiology, pathology, and theory. Many massage therapists today have 500 or more classroom hours, including assessment, practice, and student clinic.
- **Acupuncturist**: A provider who inserts very thin needles through a patient's skin in varying depths at specific points on the body. Licensure varies from state to state. Log on to www.nccaom.org to learn more about acupuncture.
- **Pain management specialist**: A medical doctor (M.D.) or doctor of osteopathy (D.O.) who has specialized training in managing pain. Many pain management specialists also have specialty training as an anesthesiologist.

remedies, the placebo effect or spontaneous healing cannot be ruled out. A **placebo effect** refers to the fact that some people respond favorably to a known ineffective treatment because they believe it is working. This occurs in about 30–40 percent of patients.

Types of CAM

CAM encompasses a variety of techniques and therapies. Combined with traditional medicine, use of CAM has greatly increased in recent years and has proven to improve the physical and mental health of those receiving such services. In 2012, the National Center for Health Statistics published the 10 most common complementary health approaches among adults (Figure 19-6).

Whole Medical Systems

The National Center for Complementary and Integrative Health (NCCAM) groups CAM practices into four domains (see Figure 19-7). Whole medical systems cut across all four domains.

Treatments can be focused on one of the four types of CAM therapy (biologically-based practices, mind–body medicine, energy medicine, or manipulation and body-based practices) or can take on a more specific approach to medicine. Homeopathy, naturopathic medicine, and traditional Chinese medicine are models which are unique.

- **Homeopathy**: A 200-year-old system of medicine based on the Law of Similars: If a dose of a substance can cause a symptom, that same substance in minuscule amounts can cure the symptom. It is a highly controversial form of medicine and lacks scientific evidence of efficacy.
- **Naturopathic Medicine**: A combination of traditional practices and health care popular in nineteenth-century Europe, naturopathy utilizes diet, herbs, homeopathy, therapeutic massage, exercise, and lifestyle counseling to influence health.
- **Traditional Chinese medicine**: An ancient Chinese approach to health care utilizing mind–body practices, acupuncture, tai chi, moxibustion, herbs, qi gong, and tui na (Chinese therapeutic massage).

Energy Therapies

There are of two types of energy therapies:

1. Biofield therapies intended to affect energy fields that supposedly surround and penetrate the human body.
2. Bioelectromagnetic-based therapy, which involves the unconventional use of electromagnetic fields.

Energy therapies can include applied **kinesiology** (the study of the principles of mechanics and anatomy in relation to human movement), color therapy, magnet

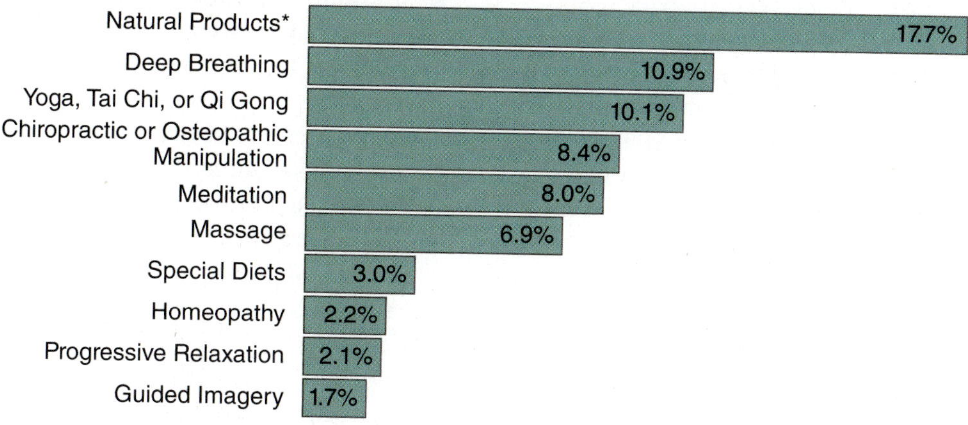

Figure 19-6 ■ 10 Most common complementary health approaches among adults—2012.

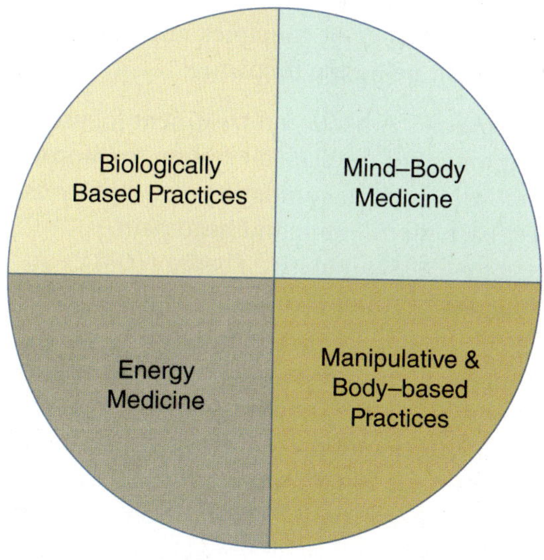

Figure 19-7 ■ The Four Domains of Whole Medical Systems for CAM Practices.

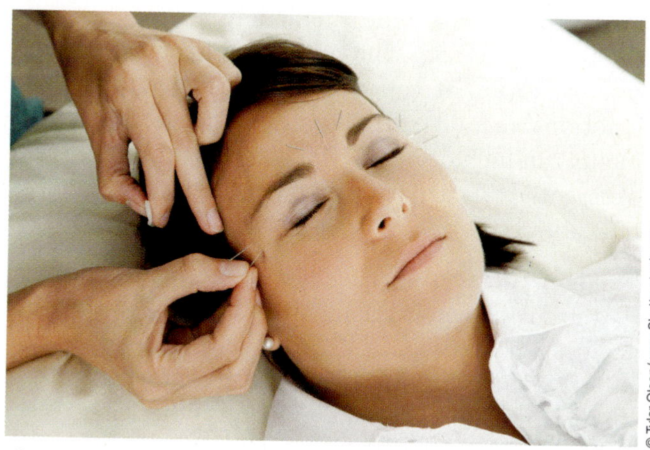

Figure 19-8 ■ A patient receives acupuncture on her face.

therapy, polarity therapy, Qi Gong, Reiki, yoga, therapeutic touch, and acupuncture. **Acupuncture** is a form of traditional Chinese medicine with at least 2,500 years of practice. It is widely practiced in the United States for pain relief. Thin needles are placed at specific points along 14 energy pathways or meridians (Figure 19-8) to release the flow of the body's vital energy ("chi"). The needles can be electrified with low voltage to stimulate the meridians. **Acupressure**, also a method used to stimulate acupoints, uses a firm pressure to massage the acupoints.

Biologically-Based Therapies

Biologically-based therapies are treatments that use substances found in nature, such as herbs, foods, and vitamins. Other therapies include the following:

- **Chelation**: Therapy used to remove excess or toxic metals or minerals from the body using a chemical substance to bind molecules, such as metal or minerals, and hold them tightly so they can be removed from the body.
- **Diet**: The use of specialized diet regimens to treat a myriad of diseases ranging from cardiovascular

disease to cancer. Diets can include widely studied regimens such as the Mediterranean diet, but can also include Ornish, low-fat vegetarian, or other personalized regimens.

- **Herbs and Nutritional Supplements:** The most common CAM therapy utilized by patients. Currently there is no regulatory body reviewing safety or contents of supplements, but the FDA is beginning this process. Herbal medicines often have precursors to refined pharmaceutical products and have some efficacy.
- **Orthomolecular Medicine**: The administration of vitamins, minerals, amino acids, hormones, and metabolic intermediates for the prevention and treatment of disease.

Mind–Body Medicine (MBM)

The NCCAOM defines mind–body medicine as a field that "uses a variety of techniques designed to enhance the mind's capacity to affect bodily function and symptom." Standard treatment approaches include meditation, prayer, and creative outlets. Mind–body medicine focuses on the interactions among the brain, the rest of the body, the mind, and behavior. Behavioral factors that can directly affect health include emotions; mental, social, and spiritual factors. Treatments can include **aroma therapy**, the use of the scent of essential oils to have a therapeutic response such as relaxation.

- **Light Therapy**: Viewing light at specific times of the day to encourage the natural circadian rhythm in the patient.
- **Art and/or Music Therapy**: Use of art forms to express thoughts and emotions otherwise repressed.
- **Biofeedback**: A therapy used to enable a person to learn to control otherwise involuntary bodily functions, usually with the help of electronic equipment.
- **Hypnosis**: The induction of a deeply relaxed state to facilitate or suggest wellness for conditions such as tobacco use, anxiety, headache, pain, depression, and irritable bowel.
- **Mindfulness Meditation**: An adaptation from prayer that focuses on mindfulness of ones thoughts, feelings, and sensations.
- **Ayurveda**: The traditional medicine of India that emphasizes reestablishing balance in the body through diet, lifestyle, exercise, cleansing of the body, and on the health of the mind, body, and spirit.
- **Progressive Muscle Relaxation**: The active process of relaxing bodily tension in a way to reach significant relaxation. Useful for anxiety and insomnia.
- **Faith and Prayer**: Both faith and prayer have been shown to improve the resiliency of the individual likely through the belief of a higher power and purpose.
- **Yoga**: The practice of combining postures, breathing, meditation, and relaxation provides relief of stress as well as cardiovascular conditioning.

Manipulative and Body-Based Therapies

Massage and other body-based therapies are known to be healing. These techniques are based on the manipulation and/or movement of one or more body parts. There are a number of therapies and techniques, the most common being the following:

- **Chiropractic**: A hands-on treatment focused on realignment of the skeletal system to improve function. These manipulations are mainly used to treat back, neck, joint, and head pain.
- **Osteopathic Manipulative Therapy (OMT)**: A hands-on treatment where D.O.s use their knowledge of physiology and their hands to examine the back and other parts of the body such as joints, tendons, ligaments, and muscles, for pain and restrictions of motion that representing an injury, impaired function, or underlying disease process (American Osteopathic Association).
- **Massage Therapy**: Use of pressure on muscles and soft tissues to relieve tension and pain. There are many types of massage techniques.

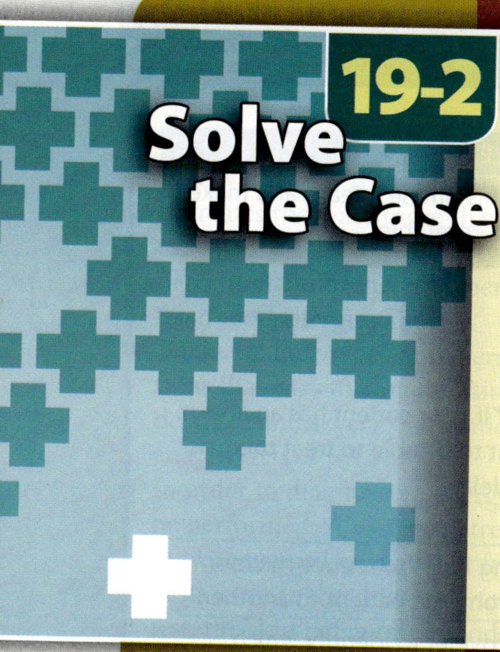

Dr. Lim has been running more than 30 minutes behind schedule. Given your current level of knowledge, consider the following questions.

1. **What steps should you take to keep Ms. Williamson informed?**
2. **What information should you provide to Ms. Williamson regarding OMT?**

Dr. Lim has now completed her exam and treatment of Ms. Williamson. Dr. Lim performed OMT to relieve her neck and headache symptoms. In addition, she wants to see Ms. Williamson again in one week, and then every two weeks after that for six weeks total. Dr. Lim would also like Ms. Williamson to consider acupuncture as an additional form of treatment and has recommended to Ms. Williamson that if her headaches are not relieved with OMT that she would like to refer her to Dr. Sachdeva, a well-respected neurologist.

3. **After the treatment by Dr. Lim, what steps should you take before Ms. Williamson leaves the office?**

PROCEDURE 19-1

Perform Allergy Testing

Objective:

Identify allergens that the patient reacts toward.

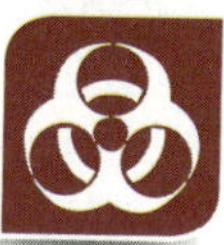

Equipment/Supplies:

- Personal protective equipment (PPE)
- Histamine control
- Purified allergen
- Alcohol swabs
- Individual skin prick device
- EpiPen
- Antihistamine
- Glycerin or saline control
- Patient's chart/EHR

PROCEDURAL STEPS	DETAILS AND/OR RATIONALE
1. Review provider's order and gather all supplies.	It is important to make certain you are performing the correct testing or the test will need to be repeated.
2. Identify yourself and identify the patient using at least two identifiers.	Performing allergy testing on the wrong patient can cause problems for the patient and practice.
3. Ask the patient if she held her allergy medications for the prescribed amount of days before the appointment.	Medications such as antihistamines, antidepressants (nortriptyline and desipramine), cimetidine, ranitidine, and omlizumab (Xolair) will make the test invalid by suppressing the reaction. Having patients bring their medications allows for medication reconciliation as well as to have a supply if the patient has a reaction during the test.

continues

3. The most common example of Type _____ hypersensitivity is contact dermatitis to poison ivy, metals, and the Mantoux test (tuberculin skin test).
   a. I
   b. II
   c. III
   d. IV
4. A serious allergic reaction with excessive release of histamine, which compromises the pulmonary and circulatory systems and can lead to death if not properly treated is known as:
   a. Type III hypersensitivity.
   b. anaphylaxis.
   c. Mantoux test.
   d. None of the above
5. A provider who specializes in assisting patients who are experiencing sinus problems, including those associated with allergies, is known as:
   a. an otolaryngologist.
   b. ear, nose, and throat (ENT) specialist
   c. an allergist.
   d. both a. and b.
6. A hands-on treatment where the provider uses their knowledge of physiology and their hands to examine the back and other parts of the body such as joints, tendons, ligaments, and muscles is known as:
   a. chiropractic.
   b. osteopathic manipulative therapy.
   c. massage therapy.
   d. Alexander technique.
7. A noninvasive procedure that gently exfoliates the skin by spraying tiny crystals onto the skin and gently removing the outer layer of skin is known as:
   a. microdermabrasion.
   b. a chemical peel.
   c. chemexfoliation.
   d. laser resurfacing.
8. To reduce the possibility of a local or systemic reaction when administering allergy shots, the medical assistant should ask which of the following questions of the patient?
   a. Did you have any reactions to your last injection?
   b. Are you currently ill?
   c. Is there a possibility you are pregnant (females only)?
   d. All of the above.
9. Which of the following statements accurately represents whether it is important to know if a patient is currently taking a beta-blocker before administering an allergy shot.
   a. No. There are no known reactions to a beta-blocker when receiving allergy shots.
   b. Yes, because emergency drugs used to treat an allergic reaction may not be as effective if the patient is taking beta-blockers.
   c. Yes, because beta-blockers can cause an allergic reaction.
   d. No. Beta-blockers can improve the results of allergy shots.
10. A 200-year-old system of medicine based on the Law of Similars is known as:
   a. naturopathic medicine
   b. osteopathic medicine.
   c. traditional Chinese medicine.
   d. homeopathy.

STUDY RESOURCES

Resources to Test and Reinforce Your Knowledge:	
Certification Review Questions	Take this end-of-chapter quiz
Workbook	• Complete the activities for Chapter 19 • Perform the procedure for Chapter 19 using the Competency Checklist
Resources to Promote Critical Thinking:	
***Solve the Case* Activities**	• Consider these case studies and discuss your conclusions
MindTap	• Complete Chapter 19 readings and activities

CHAPTER SUMMARY

- Allergies exist in many forms and the effects of an allergy can vary from person to person. The CDC estimates there are more than 50 million Americans that suffer from some type of allergy, and 4–6 percent of children, and 4 percent of adults suffer from food allergies alone.
- There are four types of hypersensitivity reactions that vary in response time (immediate to delayed) and severity (irritation to life-threatening anaphylaxis).
- In order to diagnose an allergy, specific tests will be performed. A variety of treatments are available to treat symptoms that vary from minor to severe. Tests include the skin prick test, the intradermal test, the skin patch test, blood tests, and the oral food challenge (OFC).
- There are a variety of treatments for allergy symptoms. Some of the most common treatments are subcutaneous allergen-specific immunotherapy/immunomodulation (allergy shots).
- There are a variety of treatments and techniques used by medical professionals to combat the aging appearance, including microdermabrasion, chemical peels, laser/light therapy, laser resurfacing, Fraxel Restore, dermal fillers, Botox, and Retin-A.
- The medical assistant should be well educated about all procedures offered in the office. The role of the medical assistant will vary from one practice to another, and may include placing numbing gel on the patient prior to the procedure, setting up the room and the patient prior to the procedure, assisting the provider during procedures, providing education following the procedure, being supportive throughout the procedure, and alert the provider when the patient's discomfort appears to be heightened.
- Complementary and alternative medicine (CAM) refers to a broad set of health care practices that are not part of that country's own tradition and are not integrated into the dominant health care system. As many as 40 percent of Americans use health care approaches outside of Western or conventional medicine.
- CAM includes a myriad of services that are not considered standard of care but may have evidence, anecdotal experience, or mixed results of efficacy. While acupuncture and OMT have evidence for efficacy in the treatment of certain ailments and readily adopted as adjunctive therapies in Western medicine, other CAM therapies do not have significant evidence and are viewed with skepticism.
- Some providers are hesitant about this type of medicine (CAM) as often there is no scientific evidence or validation by research that they are or can be therapeutic. While some people have claimed cures from alternative and other remedies, the placebo effect or spontaneous healing cannot be ruled out.
- The most common CAM approaches are outlined in Figure 19-6.
- The NCCAOM groups CAM practices into four domains (see Figure 19-7) in which there is often overlap. Whole medical systems cut across all domains. Treatments can be focused on one of the four types of CAM therapy (biologically-based practices, mind–body medicine, energy medicine, or manipulation and body-based practices) or can take on a more specific approach to medicine. Homeopathy, naturopathic medicine, and traditional Chinese medicine are models that are unique.

CERTIFICATION REVIEW QUESTIONS

1. A growing trend where providers and health care systems are integrating various practices into treatment and health promotion is known as:
   a. complementary and alternative medicine.
   b. integrative health care.
   c. complementary and integrative medicine.
   d. alternative and integrative medicine.

2. Type _____ hypersensitivity is an immediate reaction to a known allergen (medications, foods, or proteins).
   a. I
   b. II
   c. III
   d. IV

3. The most common example of Type _____ hypersensitivity is contact dermatitis to poison ivy, metals, and the Mantoux test (tuberculin skin test).
   a. I
   b. II
   c. III
   d. IV

4. A serious allergic reaction with excessive release of histamine, which compromises the pulmonary and circulatory systems and can lead to death if not properly treated is known as:
   a. Type III hypersensitivity.
   b. anaphylaxis.
   c. Mantoux test.
   d. None of the above

5. A provider who specializes in assisting patients who are experiencing sinus problems, including those associated with allergies, is known as:
   a. an otolaryngologist.
   b. ear, nose, and throat (ENT) specialist
   c. an allergist.
   d. both a. and b.

6. A hands-on treatment where the provider uses their knowledge of physiology and their hands to examine the back and other parts of the body such as joints, tendons, ligaments, and muscles is known as:
   a. chiropractic.
   b. osteopathic manipulative therapy.
   c. massage therapy.
   d. Alexander technique.

7. A noninvasive procedure that gently exfoliates the skin by spraying tiny crystals onto the skin and gently removing the outer layer of skin is known as:
   a. microdermabrasion.
   b. a chemical peel.
   c. chemexfoliation.
   d. laser resurfacing.

8. To reduce the possibility of a local or systemic reaction when administering allergy shots, the medical assistant should ask which of the following questions of the patient?
   a. Did you have any reactions to your last injection?
   b. Are you currently ill?
   c. Is there a possibility you are pregnant (females only)?
   d. All of the above.

9. Which of the following statements accurately represents whether it is important to know if a patient is currently taking a beta-blocker before administering an allergy shot.
   a. No. There are no known reactions to a beta-blocker when receiving allergy shots.
   b. Yes, because emergency drugs used to treat an allergic reaction may not be as effective if the patient is taking beta-blockers.
   c. Yes, because beta-blockers can cause an allergic reaction.
   d. No. Beta-blockers can improve the results of allergy shots.

10. A 200-year-old system of medicine based on the Law of Similars is known as:
   a. naturopathic medicine
   b. osteopathic medicine.
   c. traditional Chinese medicine.
   d. homeopathy.

STUDY RESOURCES

Resources to Test and Reinforce Your Knowledge:	
Certification Review Questions	Take this end-of-chapter quiz
Workbook	• Complete the activities for Chapter 19 • Perform the procedure for Chapter 19 using the Competency Checklist
Resources to Promote Critical Thinking:	
***Solve the Case* Activities**	• Consider these case studies and discuss your conclusions
MindTap	• Complete Chapter 19 readings and activities

19-2 Solve the Case

Dr. Lim has been running more than 30 minutes behind schedule. Given your current level of knowledge, consider the following questions.

1. **What steps should you take to keep Ms. Williamson informed?**
2. **What information should you provide to Ms. Williamson regarding OMT?**

Dr. Lim has now completed her exam and treatment of Ms. Williamson. Dr. Lim performed OMT to relieve her neck and headache symptoms. In addition, she wants to see Ms. Williamson again in one week, and then every two weeks after that for six weeks total. Dr. Lim would also like Ms. Williamson to consider acupuncture as an additional form of treatment and has recommended to Ms. Williamson that if her headaches are not relieved with OMT that she would like to refer her to Dr. Sachdeva, a well-respected neurologist.

3. **After the treatment by Dr. Lim, what steps should you take before Ms. Williamson leaves the office?**

PROCEDURE 19-1

Perform Allergy Testing

Objective:

Identify allergens that the patient reacts toward.

Equipment/Supplies:

- Personal protective equipment (PPE)
- Histamine control
- Purified allergen
- Alcohol swabs
- Individual skin prick device
- EpiPen
- Antihistamine
- Glycerin or saline control
- Patient's chart/EHR

PROCEDURAL STEPS	DETAILS AND/OR RATIONALE
1. Review provider's order and gather all supplies.	It is important to make certain you are performing the correct testing or the test will need to be repeated.
2. Identify yourself and identify the patient using at least two identifiers.	Performing allergy testing on the wrong patient can cause problems for the patient and practice.
3. Ask the patient if she held her allergy medications for the prescribed amount of days before the appointment.	Medications such as antihistamines, antidepressants (nortriptyline and desipramine), cimetidine, ranitidine, and omlizumab (Xolair) will make the test invalid by suppressing the reaction. Having patients bring their medications allows for medication reconciliation as well as to have a supply if the patient has a reaction during the test.

continues

PROCEDURE 19-1 continued

PROCEDURAL STEPS	DETAILS AND/OR RATIONALE
4. ***Demonstrating professional behavior, explain to the patient the rationale for performance of the procedure, showing awareness of the patient's concerns related to the procedure being performed.*** Counsel the patient that positive reactions will likely itch, but they must not scratch.	Scratching will cause local histamine release and make the results of the test uninterpretable.
5. ***Incorporating critical thinking skills when performing patient care***, ensure that you have all emergency medications as well as standard supplies for the procedure.	"Luck favors the prepared." If your patient has an anaphylactic reaction, it is best to be able to treat them as soon as possible without delay.
6. Wash hands and apply gloves.	Washing hands and gloving helps to reduce microorganisms that are carried from one patient to another.
7. Mark out a grid on the forearms or back according to your standard operating procedure (SOP). Ensure that the controls are marked appropriately.	This allows you and the provider to identify which allergens are positive or negative.
8. Clean the skin with an alcohol pad prior to skin prick or scratch.	Removes other allergens that are on the skin.
9. Dip the tip of the individual skin prick device into the purified allergen or appropriate controls based on the grid map and allow 15 minutes for full reaction.	Each grid square represents one allergen. After 15 minutes, any reaction will be assessed and compared to the histamine and control saline controls. If the patient reacts to saline or if they don't react to histamine, the test is not interpretable.
10. Identify and measure areas of induration as well as noting the erythema for each grid square.	This will allow the provider to interpret positive and negative results.
11. Remove gloves and wash hands.	
12. Provide patient with self-care instructions such as use of antihistamines, topical steroids, and washing site with soap and water.	These are ways to minimize the itch and discomfort following the procedure.
13. There will likely be a skin test report form that needs to be completed. This is a rather lengthy process and may be completed by the provider or medical assistant.	
14. Document the procedure in the patient's chart.	

DOCUMENTATION EXAMPLE:

10/12/XX 1300	Prepped skin and performed skin prick tests per Dr. Dorado. Doctor examined and measured the test sites at the appropriate time intervals. Results are in the results section of the chart. No complications during or following procedure. Patient given home care instructions. S. Burtilli, CCMA---

REFERENCES

Acupressure.com (n.d.). What Is Acupressure? Retrieved April 4, 2015, from http://www.acupressure.com/

Allergy Partners of Richmond (n.d.). Allergy Shots (Immunotherapy). Retrieved April 19, 2015, from http://www.allergypartners.com/richmond/SitePages/AllergyShots.aspx

American Academy of Dermatology (n.d.). Microdermabrasion. Retrieved April 4, 2015, from https://www.aad.org/dermatology-a-to-z/diseases-and-treatments/m-p/microdermabrasion

American Chiropractic Association (n.d.). What Is Chiropractic? Retrieved April 5, 2015, from http://www.acatoday.org/level2_css.cfm?T1ID=13&T2ID=61

American College of Allergy, Asthma & Immunology (n.d.). When to See an Allergist. Retrieved April 3, 2015, from http://acaai.org/allergies/treatment/when-to-see-allergist

American Osteopathic Association (n.d.). Osteopathic Medicine and Your Health. Retrieved April 5, 2015, from http://www.osteopathic.org/osteopathic-health/about-your-health/health-conditions-library/general-health/Pages/back-pain.aspx

American Society for Dermatologic Surgery (n.d.). Dermal Fillers. Retrieved April 4, 2015, from https://www.asds.net/Dermal-Fillers-Info/

American Society for Dermatologic Surgery (n.d.). Laser Resurfacing. Retrieved April 4, 2015, from https://www.asds.net/LaserResurfacingInformation.aspx

Anonymous (n.d.). Alternative Therapies and Treatments. Retrieved April 4, 2015 from http://altmedicine.about.com/od/treatmentsremedies/u/treatments.htm

Asthma and Allergy Foundation of America (AAFA) (n.d.). Allergy Overview. Retrieved April 4, 2015, from http://www.aafa.org/display.cfm?id=9&cont=80

Asthma and Allergy Foundation of America (AAFA) (n.d.). Immunotherapy. Retrieved April 4, 2015, from http://www.aafa.org/display.cfm?id=9&sub=21&cont=303

Barnes, M., Bloom, B., Nahin, R. (2008, December). CDC National Health Statistics Report #12. Complementary and Alternative Medicine. Use among Adults and Children; United States, 2007.

Blesi, M. (2017). *Medical Assisting: Administrative & Clinical Competencies* (8th ed.). Clifton Park, NY: Cengage Learning.

Clark, T., Black, L., Stussman, B., Barnes, P., Nahin, R. (2015). Trends in the Use of Complementary Health Approaches among Adults. United States, 2002–2012. National health statistics reports; no 79. Hyattsville, MD: National Center for Health Statistics 2015.

Dallas Allergy Immunology (n.d.). Physician's Consent to Administer Allergy Shots. Retrieved April 4, 2015, from http://www.dallasallergy.net/wp-content/uploads/2013/10/I.T.-Outside-Facility-Consent.2011.pdf

Food Allergy Research & Education (n.d.). About Food Allergies. Retrieved April 4, 2015, from http://www.foodallergy.org/about-food-allergies

Fraxel (n.d.). Fraxel and You. Retrieved April 4, 2015, from http://www.fraxel.com/fraxel-and-you

Johns Hopkins Asthma & Allergy Center (n.d.). Patient Information Letter: Xolair (omalizumad). Retrieved April 4, 2015, from http://www.hopkinsmedicine.org/allergy/new/Xolairptinfoversion2C.pdf

Mayo Clinic (n.d.). Botox Injections. Retrieved April 4, 2015, from http://www.mayoclinic.org/tests-procedures/botox/basics/definition/prc-20009036

Merriam-Webster Dictionary (n.d.). Define Kinesiology. Retrieved April 4, 2015, from http://www.merriam-webster.com/dictionary/kinesiology

National Center for Complementary and Integrative Health (n.d.). Complementary, Alternative, or Integrated Health: What's in a Name? Retrieved April 4, 2015, from https://nccih.nih.gov/health/whatiscam

National Certification Commission for Acupuncture and Oriental Medicine (n.d.). State Licensure Requirements. Retrieved April 5, 2015, from http://www.nccaom.org/regulatory-affairs/state-licensure-map

National Institute of Allergy and Infectious Diseases (n.d.). Pollen allergy. Retrieved April 4, 2015, from http://www.niaid.nih.gov/topics/allergicDiseases/Documents/PollenAllergyFactSheet.pdf

National Institutes of Health (n.d.). Allergy. Retrieved April 4, 2015, from http://www.nlm.nih.gov/medlineplus/allergy.html

Olivas, Evelyn, CMT (2015). Massage Therapist Definition.

Ownby D. R. and Bailey J. (1986 Jan). Comparison of MAST with Radioallergosorbent and Skin Tests for Diagnosis of Allergy in Children. Retrieved April 19, 2015, from http://www.ncbi.nlm.nih.gov/pubmed/3510527

U.S. Department of Health & Human Services (n.d.). NIH: Mind–Body Medicine Practices in Complementary and Alternative Medicine. Retrieved April 4, 2015, from http://report.nih.gov/nihfactsheets/viewfactsheet.aspx?csid=102

WebMD (n.d.). Retin—A Topical. Retrieved April 4, 2015, from http://www.webmd.com/drugs/2/drug-1192/retin-a-topical/details

Wheeler M. D. PhD, Claire (2010 June). What Is Mind–Body Medicine? *Psychology Today*. Retrieved April 4, 2015, from https://www.psychologytoday.com/blog/head-toe-happiness/201006/what-is-mind-body-medicine

Wong, Cathy ND (2015, January). What Is Ayurveda? Retrieved April 4, 2015, from http://altmedicine.about.com/cs/2/a/AyurvedaDef.htm

Wong, Cathy ND (2014, December). What Is Chelation? Retrieved April 4, 2015, from http://altmedicine.about.com/od/treatmentsfromatod/a/chelation.htm

20

Diet and Nutrition

CHAPTER OUTLINE

The Digestive Process

Nutritional Abbreviations Review

Nutrients

- Fiber, Electrolytes, and Metabolism
- Functions of Vitamins and Minerals in the Body

Nutrition through the Life Cycle

- Infancy (The First Year of Life)
- Childhood (Ages 1 to 10)
- Adolescence (Ages 10 to 19)
- Adult (Age 20+)
- Seniors

Planning a Healthy Diet

- Reading Food Labels
- Health Benefits of the Food Groups
- Nutritional Guidelines

Educating Patients about Good Nutrition

Exercise for Weight Maintenance

Nutrition Screening and Assessment

Obesity

- Health Effects of Obesity

Weight Loss Diets

Bariatric Surgery

Special Diets

Eating Disorders

- Anorexia Nervosa
- Bulimia Nervosa
- Compulsive Overeating
- Night Eating Syndrome

Foodborne Illnesses

ESSENTIAL TERMS

bariatrics
binge
BMI (body mass index)
bulimia nervosa
Campylobacter
carbohydrates
DASH (Dietary Approaches to Stop Hypertension)
dietetic technician
dietitian
E. coli
electrolyte
fiber
gastroenterologist
gluten
glycemic index (GI)
insulin
lactose
kcalorie
malabsorption syndrome
metabolic syndrome
metabolism
minerals
nutrient
nutrition
nutritionist
norovirus
obesity
proteins
Salmonella
supplements
transfats
vegan
vegetarian
vitamins

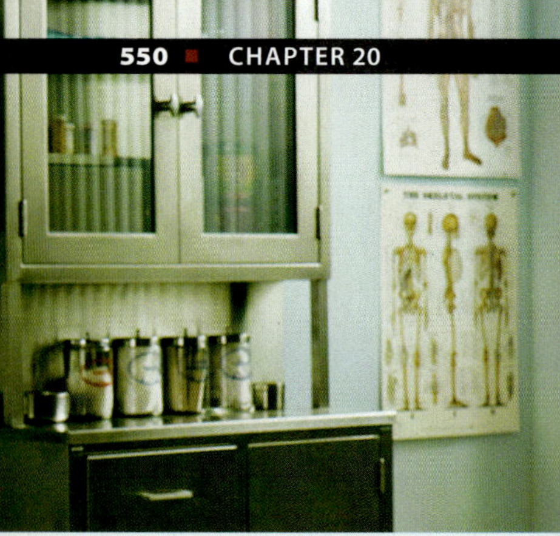

DEVELOPMENTAL OBJECTIVES

After completing this chapter, you should be able to:

1. Correctly spell and define the essential terms.
2. Describe the following eight nutrients: carbohydrates, fats, proteins, minerals, vitamins, fiber, water, and electrolytes.
3. Define the function of dietary supplements.
4. List and define the different parts of a food label.
5. Explain the importance of diet and nutrition as it relates to the development of health issues.
6. List five different food groups in the ChooseMyPlate food plan with examples of foods in each group.
7. Show awareness of the patient's concerns regarding dietary changes.
8. Develop a meal plan utilizing the basic principles of nutrition.
9. Discuss the role of exercise in a healthy lifestyle.
10. Identify the special dietary needs for weight control, diabetes, cardiovascular disease, hypertension, cancer, lactose sensitivity, gluten-free, and food allergies.
11. Identify categories of patients who require special diets or diet modifications.
12. Instruct a patient according to the patient's special dietary needs, applying the nutrition guidelines.
13. Name and define one foodborne illness.

INTRODUCTION

The food choices you make each day may or may not benefit you on that day. However, when the same choices are repeated over the years, the rewards as well as the consequences are significant. A lack of knowledge about **nutrition**, the process by which organisms take in and utilize food materials, and carelessness about food choices can contribute to the development of many chronic diseases.

Both adults and children throughout the world have become increasingly more overweight, and obesity has now reached epidemic proportions. Statistics gathered by the Food Research and Action Center show that approximately 69% of adults in the United States are overweight and 34.9% are obese. Approximately 32% of children are overweight and 17% are classified as obese. These obesity rates have doubled since the 1970s. Nutrition not only plays a big role in a person's weight, but in overall health as well. Inappropriate food choices and eating habits may contribute to the development of conditions such as type 2 diabetes, heart disease, and colon cancer. Health care professionals therefore have a responsibility to teach patients the fundamentals of nutrition.

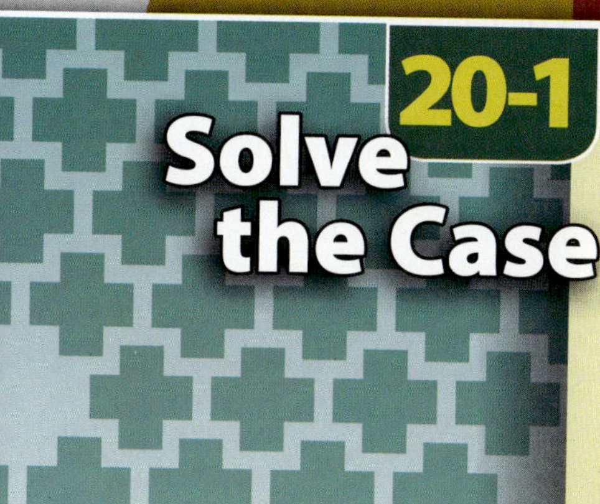

Jane Winters is a 20-year-old college student who is 5'4" tall and weighs 160 pounds. Compared to the standardized height and weight chart, she is 20 pounds overweight. She wants to know the basics of nutrition so that she can make better food choices and also lose weight.

1. **Based on your current level of understanding, what are some short and long term ramifications of obesity?**
2. **Why would it be valuable to have her keep a food diary for a week?**
3. **Where can Jane find additional information about nutrition?**

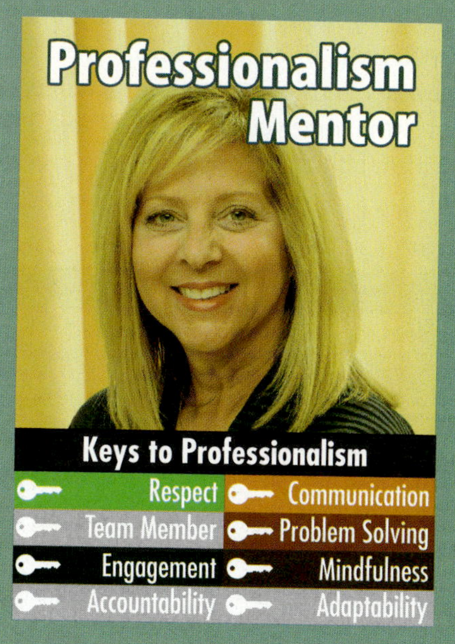

If you are like me, going to the doctor and being asked to stand on the scale to get weighed will make you sigh in resignation. Consider this the perfect time to ask the patient if he partakes in an exercise program or has any questions about his dietary needs. Some patients want to lose weight while others wish they could have more energy, and still others wish they could gain some weight. The key to success when discussing this part of the patient's lifestyle is being *tactful*. How can you collect information without sounding "preachy"? You demonstrate professionalism when you possess a nonjudgmental *attitude*. What are some phrases that you can use when reviewing diet and nutrition with your patients that won't make them feel like you are judging them? In your journal, jot down some ideas on what phrases you would use when speaking to your patient. ■

THE DIGESTIVE PROCESS

Many structures are involved in the process of digestion. Table 20-1 summarizes the role of each structure. Refer to Chapter 16 for an in-depth review of the digestive system.

Table 20-1 Structures Involved in the Digestive Process

Digestive Structure	Role in the Digestive Process
Oral cavity	Teeth mechanically grind food into smaller particles. Saliva is secreted to start the process of digesting carbohydrates.
Stomach	Digestive enzymes break down fats, proteins, and carbohydrates into their basic components, which can then be absorbed and used by the body.
Small intestine	Secretes digestive juices to further break down food components and absorbs these components into the blood stream.
Large intestine	Reabsorbs water from food wastes.
Anus	Site for evacuation of wastes from the large intestine.
Accessory organs of digestion:	Pancreas, liver, and gallbladder secrete substances that break down food into their components.
Pancreas	In addition to producing **insulin** (a hormone secreted by the beta cells of the pancreatic islet in response to high-levels of glucose in the blood stream), the pancreas produces digestive juices and sodium bicarbonate to neutralize the acidity of food leaving the stomach.
Liver	Manufactures bile, necessary for the digestion of fats.
Gallbladder	Stores and concentrates bile from the liver, when not needed in the digestion of fats.

Meet the Specialists

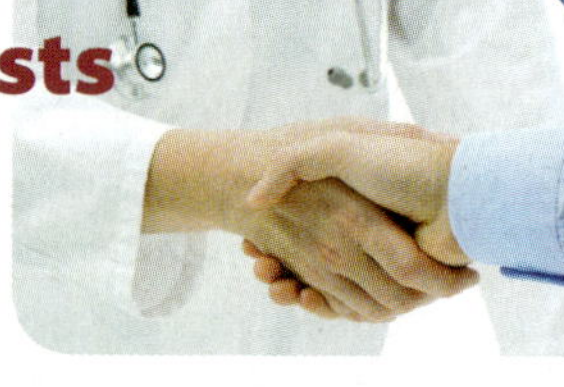

Professionals who diagnose and treat digestive and nutritional disorders include the following:

- **Gastroenterologist:** A physician who specializes in the diagnosis and treatment of diseases and disorders of the stomach and intestines.
- Registered **Dietitians** and **Nutritionists:** All registered dietitians are nutritionists, but not all nutritionists are registered dietitians. The credentials "RDN" indicate a registered dietitian nutritionist, with a bachelor's degree and the completion of an extensive internship program. Employment specialty areas include clinical/medical and community settings as well as teaching and management positions.
- **Dietetic Technician:** DTR indicates dietetic technician registered. DTRs have a two-year associate degree with training in food and nutrition. They are employed in health care and food service settings.

NUTRITION ABBREVIATIONS REVIEW

Some abbreviations are unique to dietetics and others are the same abbreviations in other practice areas that have different meanings in this setting. For instance, GI can mean gastrointestinal or glycemic index. Table 20-2 lists common nutrition abbreviations.

Table 20-2 Common Nutrition Abbreviations

Abbreviation	Meaning	Abbreviation	Meaning
A, D, E, K	Fat-soluble vitamins	GI	Glycemic index
AI	Adequate intake	kcal	Kilocalorie
CA	Calcium	meg	One-thousandths of a gram equivalent
CHO	Carbohydrate	mcg	Microgram
BMI	Body mass index	mg	Milligram
DRI	Dietary reference intake	mEq	Milliequivalent
EAR	Estimated average requirement	MVI	Multivitamin
Fe	Iron	Na	Sodium
FBS	Fasting blood sugar	RDA	Recommended dietary allowance
FTT	Failure to thrive	REE	Resting energy expenditure
		UL	Tolerable upper limit

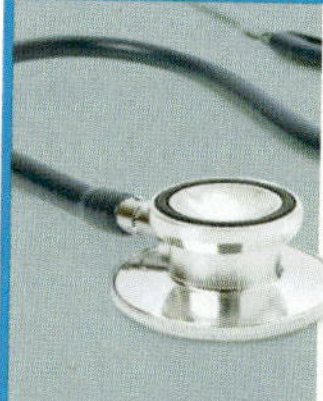

Field Smarts

Some important dietary reference standards to know include reference information found on most food labels. Refer to the following:

- Recommended Dietary Allowance (RDA): The amount of a nutrient that will meet the requirements of 97.5% of healthy individuals.
- Dietary Reference Intake (DRI): The levels of nutrients needed for dietary consumption. (The DRI replaced the RDA in 1989, but both are still in use.)
- Estimated Average Requirements (EAR): The intake of a nutrient that will meet the requirements of 50% of all healthy individuals.

NUTRIENTS

A **nutrient** is a substance, usually from foods, that is necessary for normal functioning of the body and for good health. Six nutrients are necessary for cellular functioning throughout the body: water, proteins, carbohydrates, fats/lipids, vitamins, and minerals.

1. Water: Water makes up 65% of the total body weight and is contained in all body tissues. Water transports substances throughout the body and is involved in all biochemical reactions. It serves as a lubricant both for joints and for the digestive tract. Through the evaporation of sweat, water helps control body temperature.
2. Proteins: **Proteins** are large molecules composed of one or more chains of amino acids. They are required for the structure, function, and regulation of the body's cells, tissues, and organs. Proteins are important in the growth and repair of all tissues. They also regulate the rate of chemical reactions. When glucose is unavailable, protein can be used as a source of energy.
3. Carbohydrates: **Carbohydrates** are the main source of energy for the body when converted to glucose. When consumed in excess, they are converted into fat and stored in the adipose tissues.
4. Fats/Lipids: Fats/lipids are the primary stored source of energy for the body and are a component in all cell membranes.
5. Vitamins: **Vitamins** are organic substances in foods that are essential in minute quantities for normal growth and the maintenance of good health.
6. Minerals: **Minerals** are chemicals contained in foods, and necessary for normal growth and tissue maintenance.

Fiber, Electrolytes, and Metabolism

In addition to nutrients, the following are essential for the proper functioning of the body.

- **Fiber** is that part of plant foods that is not digested. Fiber is found in whole grains, vegetables, and fruits. It is essential for the normal functioning of the GI system.
- **Electrolytes** are mineral salts dissolved in water that carry an electrical current. Electrolytes with a positive electrical charge are sodium (Na^+), potassium (K^+), calcium (Ca^{2+}), and magnesium (Mg^{2+}). Electrolytes with a negative charge are chloride (Cl^-), bicarbonate (HCO_3^-), phosphate (HPO_4^{2-}), sulfate ($SO4^{2-}$), organic acids (lactate and pyruvate), and proteins. The cells in the body

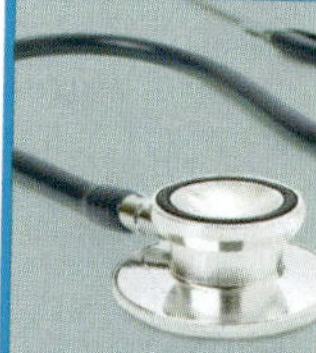

Field Smarts

All foods are made up of proteins, carbohydrates (simple and complex), and fats.

In addition, vitamins are organic substances found in both plants and animals. Vitamins are necessary for normal growth and development. There are two types of vitamins: *fat-soluble*, which includes A, D, E, and K, and *water-soluble*, which includes the B complex and C vitamins. Minerals are inorganic elements that are essential for normal body function including elements such as sodium, potassium, and magnesium.

Supplements are products containing a dietary ingredient intended to add further nutritional value to the diet, such as vitamins, minerals, herbs, and over-the-counter medications. These can interact with some prescription medications, so always get a complete list of these supplements from the patient when obtaining a medication history.

Table 20-3 The Major Minerals

Mineral	Function in the Body
Calcium (Ca)	Calcium plus vitamin D and adequate weight-bearing physical activity builds strong bones. Is involved in muscle and nerve function, blood pressure, and blood clotting.
Chloride (Cl)	Maintains fluid and electrolyte balance. Required for normal digestion as a component of hydrochloric acid in the stomach.
Iron (Fe)	The essential component of hemoglobin in the red blood cells, transferring oxygen from the lungs to the tissues.
Magnesium (Mg)	Regulates protein synthesis, muscle and nerve function, blood glucose control, and blood pressure.
Phosphorus	Makes up 1% of total body weight and is present in every cell of the body. Primary function is formation of bones and teeth. Also works with B vitamins for kidney function, muscle contraction, normal heartbeat, and nerve conduction.
Potassium (K)	A mineral important in body functions to build muscle, control the electrical activity in the heart, and to break down carbohydrates for use in the body.
Sodium (Na)	The primary regulator of extracellular fluid volume. Essential for nerve conduction and muscle contraction.
Sulfate	Contained within proteins. A component of insulin.

are involved in the direct movement of the major minerals to control the movement of water into and out of the cells.

- **Metabolism** includes all of the processes involved in the body's use of nutrients. In those processes, energy contained within different foods is released, measured by the amount of heat generated, and called **kcalories** or kilocalories.

Function of Vitamins and Minerals in the Body

Table 20-3 describes the major minerals and their function in the body.

Table 20-4 describes the major vitamins and their function in the body.

Table 20-4 The Major Vitamins

Vitamin	Function in the Body
A	A fat-soluble vitamin involved in immune function, vision, reproduction, and cellular communication. Plays a critical role in the maintenance of heart, lungs, kidneys, and other organs.
B (folate)	A coenzyme involved in the synthesis of DNA, RNA, and amino acids.
C	Necessary for repair and growth of tissues. An antioxidant that blocks some free radicals (molecules with unpaired electrons making them unstable and more prone to forming disease).
D	A fat-soluble vitamin stored in the body's fatty tissues. Vitamin D + phosphate helps the body absorb calcium.
E	A group of fat-soluble compounds with antioxidant activities. Vitamin E protects the cells from the damaging effects of the free radicals.
K	Makes proteins for healthy bones and tissues and the proteins for blood clotting.

NUTRITION THROUGH THE LIFE CYCLE

Malnutrition can be defined as too little, too much, or an imbalance of energy or nutrients. There are two types of nutritional deficiencies: primary and secondary. Primary is the inadequate consumption of the nutrient. A secondary deficiency is the result of decreased absorption, accelerated utilization, or increased excretion. These nutritional requirements increase and decrease throughout the life span, from infancy through old age.

Infancy (The First Year of Life)

Infants grow rapidly and their energy requirements (calories) are high at 100 kcalories per kilogram of weight, compared to adult requirements of fewer than 40 kcalories per kilogram according to the Centers for Disease Control and Prevention (CDC). The nutrient most essential for this rapid growth is protein, for building body tissues. A healthy infant doubles its birth weight in three months and triples it by the first birthday.

Childhood (Ages 1 to 10)

Appetites decrease consistent with the slowing rate of growth. Standardized growth charts show a gain of an average of 2–3 inches of height and 5–6 pounds per year to adolescence.

Adolescence (Ages 10 to 19)

Adolescence is a period of intense growth when energy and nutrient needs increase dramatically. For the first time, individuals are making more of their own decisions for the foods that they consume and their participation in physical activities. Dietary Guidelines for Americans recommend that adolescents should have 60 minutes or more of physical activity daily, with encouragement to spend no more than one to two hours watching television, playing electronic games, or sitting at the computer for recreation.

Adult (Age 20+)

Promoting health and slowing aging motivates adults to pay attention to their diets and to exercise. Six lifestyle behaviors appear to have the greatest influence on people's health and their physiological age:

- Eating well-balanced meals that are rich in fruits, vegetables, whole grains, poultry, fish, and low-fat milk products
- Regular physical activity
- Not smoking
- No alcohol, or use only in moderation
- Maintaining a healthy body weight
- Adequate sleep

Individuals who follow the above guidelines live longer and have fewer disabilities as they age. Physical activity appears to be the most influential in preventing or slowing the many changes associated with aging. Many physical limitations in aging occur because of inactivity, not as a consequence of advancing age.

Seniors

A balanced nutritional intake with sufficient protein at each meal and regular physical activity can help maintain muscle mass and strength, minimizing the changes in body composition associated with aging. Falls common in the elderly are less likely when muscle strength and flexibility are maintained.

PLANNING A HEALTHY DIET

When planning a healthy diet, remember that no individual foods are "good" or "bad." The first step in making good food decisions is learning how to read and interpret food labels. Be aware that there are 4 calories per gram in carbohydrates and proteins, compared to fats at 9 calories per gram.

Reading Food Labels

Food labels such as the one in Figure 20-1 list all the information required by law on each product. The U.S. Food and Drug Administration recommends that individuals pay close attention to the following sections of a food label:

- Serving size and calories per serving—many people think that a serving size is the whole container and calories for the whole container are the same as a single serving. This is usually not the case.
- Limited nutrients are listed, including total and saturated fats, cholesterol, and sodium.
- The number of carbohydrates, fiber, sugars, and proteins in the product.
- Net carbohydrates can be calculated by subtracting fiber grams from total carbohydrates grams.
- List of nutrients, which include vitamins.
- Footnotes, which list the Percent Daily Value of key nutrients.

For more information on reading food labels, visit the FDA website (www.fda.gov).

Health Benefits of the Food Groups

A balanced combination of foods provides all the nutrients necessary for a diet to be considered "healthy." The health benefits from including various food groups in the daily diet include a reduction in the risk of developing coronary artery disease, stroke, type 2 diabetes, and osteoporosis. Table 20-5 lists the different food groups and some of the health benefits of consuming foods from each group.

Nutritional Guidelines

"ChooseMyPlate" from the Department of Agriculture details the latest nutritional guidelines to use in planning a healthy diet (Figure 20-2). One of the major challenges in putting these guidelines into practice is accepting the portion sizes that are defined by the United States Department of Agriculture (USDA). Restaurants and fast food chain servings have morphed portions into supersize, and Americans have lost sight of the meaning of "normal" portions. Figure 20-3 demonstrates what is referred to as "portion distortion."

Daily Food Plan

The ChooseMyPlate website offers a daily food plan worksheet called My Plan (Figure 20-4). The My Plan worksheet provides specific tips on what an individual should eat daily, based on a specific calorie allowance. The default allowance is 2,000 calories, but this can be adjusted for a more individualized plan. To calculate your own daily required

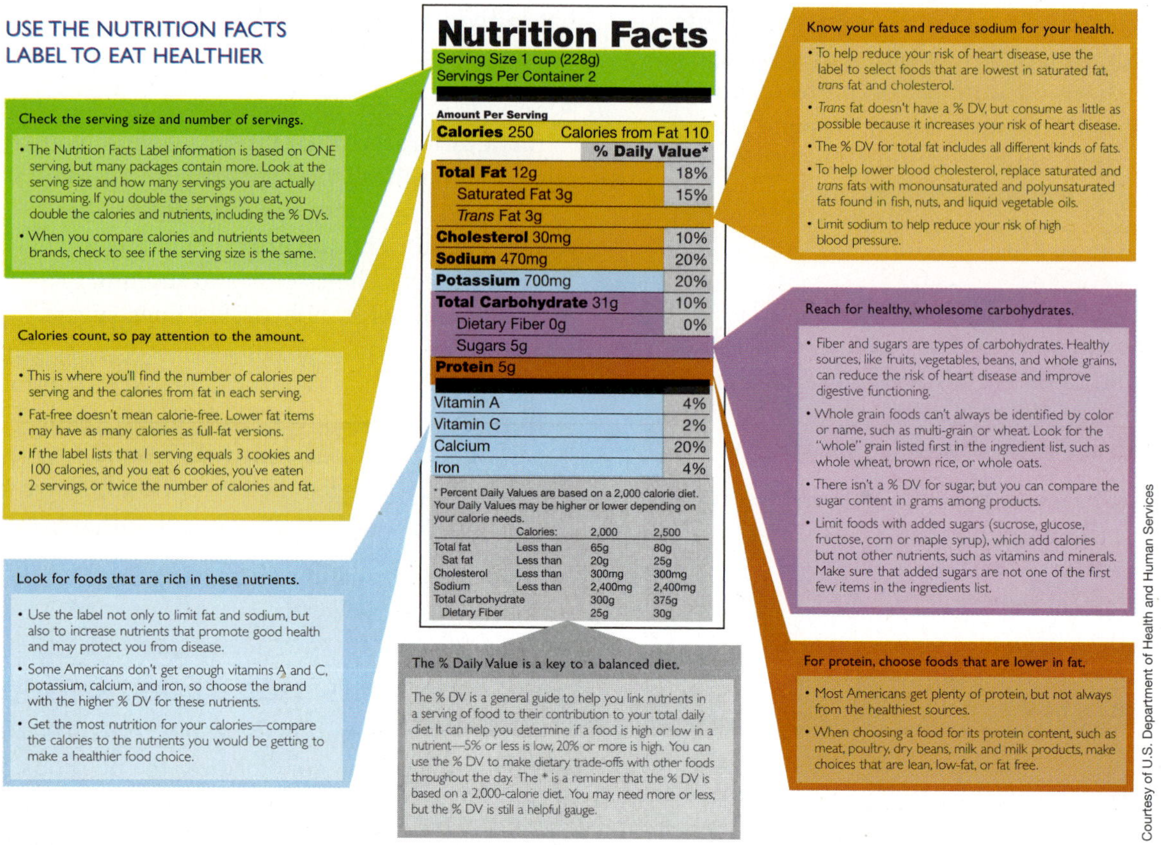

USE THE NUTRITION FACTS LABEL TO EAT HEALTHIER

Check the serving size and number of servings.

- The Nutrition Facts Label information is based on ONE serving, but many packages contain more. Look at the serving size and how many servings you are actually consuming. If you double the servings you eat, you double the calories and nutrients, including the % DVs.
- When you compare calories and nutrients between brands, check to see if the serving size is the same.

Calories count, so pay attention to the amount.

- This is where you'll find the number of calories per serving and the calories from fat in each serving.
- Fat-free doesn't mean calorie-free. Lower fat items may have as many calories as full-fat versions.
- If the label lists that 1 serving equals 3 cookies and 100 calories, and you eat 6 cookies, you've eaten 2 servings, or twice the number of calories and fat.

Look for foods that are rich in these nutrients.

- Use the label not only to limit fat and sodium, but also to increase nutrients that promote good health and may protect you from disease.
- Some Americans don't get enough vitamins A and C, potassium, calcium, and iron, so choose the brand with the higher % DV for these nutrients.
- Get the most nutrition for your calories—compare the calories to the nutrients you would be getting to make a healthier food choice.

Nutrition Facts

Serving Size 1 cup (228g)
Servings Per Container 2

Amount Per Serving

Calories 250	Calories from Fat 110
	% Daily Value*
Total Fat 12g	18%
Saturated Fat 3g	15%
Trans Fat 3g	
Cholesterol 30mg	10%
Sodium 470mg	20%
Potassium 700mg	20%
Total Carbohydrate 31g	10%
Dietary Fiber 0g	0%
Sugars 5g	
Protein 5g	
Vitamin A	4%
Vitamin C	2%
Calcium	20%
Iron	4%

* Percent Daily Values are based on a 2,000 calorie diet. Your Daily Values may be higher or lower depending on your calorie needs.

	Calories:	2,000	2,500
Total fat	Less than	65g	80g
Sat fat	Less than	20g	25g
Cholesterol	Less than	300mg	300mg
Sodium	Less than	2,400mg	2,400mg
Total Carbohydrate		300g	375g
Dietary Fiber		25g	30g

The % Daily Value is a key to a balanced diet.

The % DV is a general guide to help you link nutrients in a serving of food to their contribution to your total daily diet. It can help you determine if a food is high or low in a nutrient—5% or less is low, 20% or more is high. You can use the % DV to make dietary trade-offs with other foods throughout the day. The * is a reminder that the % DV is based on a 2,000-calorie diet. You may need more or less, but the % DV is still a helpful gauge.

Know your fats and reduce sodium for your health.

- To help reduce your risk of heart disease, use the label to select foods that are lowest in saturated fat, *trans* fat and cholesterol.
- *Trans* fat doesn't have a % DV, but consume as little as possible because it increases your risk of heart disease.
- The % DV for total fat includes all different kinds of fats.
- To help lower blood cholesterol, replace saturated and *trans* fats with monounsaturated and polyunsaturated fats found in fish, nuts, and liquid vegetable oils.
- Limit sodium to help reduce your risk of high blood pressure.

Reach for healthy, wholesome carbohydrates.

- Fiber and sugars are types of carbohydrates. Healthy sources, like fruits, vegetables, beans, and whole grains, can reduce the risk of heart disease and improve digestive functioning.
- Whole grain foods can't always be identified by color or name, such as multi-grain or wheat. Look for the "whole" grain listed first in the ingredient list, such as whole wheat, brown rice, or whole oats.
- There isn't a % DV for sugar, but you can compare the sugar content in grams among products.
- Limit foods with added sugars (sucrose, glucose, fructose, corn or maple syrup), which add calories but not other nutrients, such as vitamins and minerals. Make sure that added sugars are not one of the first few items in the ingredients list.

For protein, choose foods that are lower in fat.

- Most Americans get plenty of protein, but not always from the healthiest sources.
- When choosing a food for its protein content, such as meat, poultry, dry beans, milk and milk products, make choices that are lean, low-fat, or fat free.

Courtesy of U.S. Department of Health and Human Services

Figure 20-1 ■ Use the nutrition facts label to eat healthier.

Table 20-5 Health Benefits of the Food Groups

Food Group	Description and Health Benefits
Grains (any food made from wheat, rice, oats, cornmeal, barley, or another cereal grain)	Grains provide nutrients for a healthy body, including fiber, which decreases cholesterol and helps reduce constipation. Grains are divided into two subgroups: whole grains and refined grains. Whole grains contain the whole grain kernel. Refined grains have been milled, removing the bran, germ, and dietary fiber; iron; and many B vitamins. Most refined grains are "enriched," meaning certain vitamins and iron are added back after processing. Vitamins and minerals found in grains include folate, iron, and magnesium. **Tip:** Make at least half of your grains, whole grains.
Fruits and vegetables	Fruits provide nutrients vital for health and the maintenance of the body, including fiber to keep you regular and antioxidants to ward off disease. Vegetables are divided into five subgroups, based upon their nutrient content: dark green, starchy, red and orange, beans and peas, and other. Vitamins and minerals found in fruits and vegetables include fiber, potassium, vitamin A, vitamin B (folic acid), and vitamin C. **Tip:** Make half of your plate fruits and vegetables.
Dairy products	Vitamins and minerals found in milk and dairy products include calcium, potassium, phosphorus, and vitamin D. This food group helps with building bone and teeth and maintaining bone mass. **Tip:** Choose fat-free or low-fat milk products.
Protein foods (meats, poultry, eggs, beans and peas, processed soy products, nuts, and seeds)	Protein is necessary to build bones, muscles, cartilage, skin, and blood. Proteins supply energy, assist in tissue repair, and help to keep immune system functioning properly. Processed meats such as ham, sausage, hot dogs, and deli meats have added sodium and should be restricted. Vitamins and minerals found in meats and beans include B vitamins, vitamin E, magnesium, omega-e fatty acids, and iron. **Tip:** Choose unsalted nuts and seeds to keep sodium intake low. **Tip:** Choose lean or low-fat meats and poultry. Limit processed and deli meats to limit sodium.

Table 20-5 Health Benefits of the Food Groups (*continued*)

Food Group	Description and Health Benefits
Oils (Fats that are liquid at room temperature. Oils come from many different plants and from fish. **Transfats** are unhealthy substances made through the hydrogenation of oils, turning liquids into fats that are solid at room temperature.)	Oils are not a food group, but they provide essential nutrients. Foods that contain mainly oil include mayonnaise, some salad dressings, and soft margarine. Check the nutrition label to find margarines with 0 grams of transfat. Polyunsaturated fats containing essential fatty acids are necessary for normal cell function throughout the body. Fats are required in the body to process the fat-soluble vitamins: A, D, E, and K.

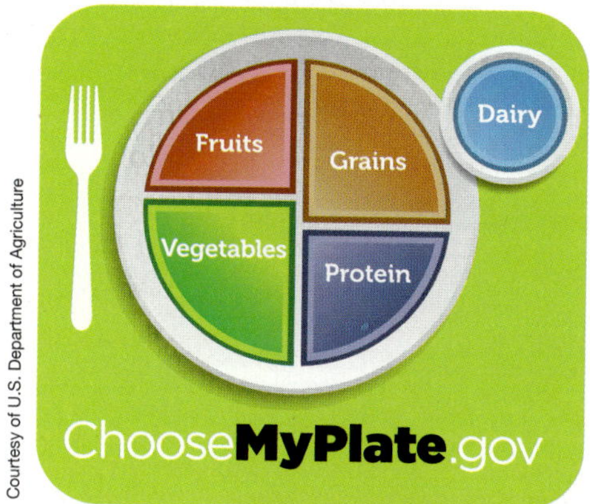

Courtesy of U.S. Department of Agriculture

Figure 20-2 ■ MyPlate, the icon for the USDA Daily Food Plan.

calories and specific food plan, visit www.choosemyplate.gov and calculate your Daily Food Plan (Figure 20-5).

In Table 20-6, notice the change in the daily amounts for each food group as the calories change from 2,000 calories per day to 1,200 calories per day. The challenge in accomplishing weight loss is cutting calories modestly to avoid a fasting state, remembering that a "safe" rate of weight loss is 1 to 2 pounds per week. Fasting causes the body to conserve energy by increasing the break down of stored fats, resulting in ketones (compounds that are formed from the incomplete breakdown of fats when glucose is not available in the cells), which affect the brain by decreasing appetite, slowing the rate of metabolism, and further decreasing the rate of weight loss.

After determining the food plan, a tool to use in following the plan is a Daily Food Plan worksheet (see Figure 20-6). See step-by-step Procedures 20-1 and 20-2 for the details on developing a meal plan and instructing a patient.

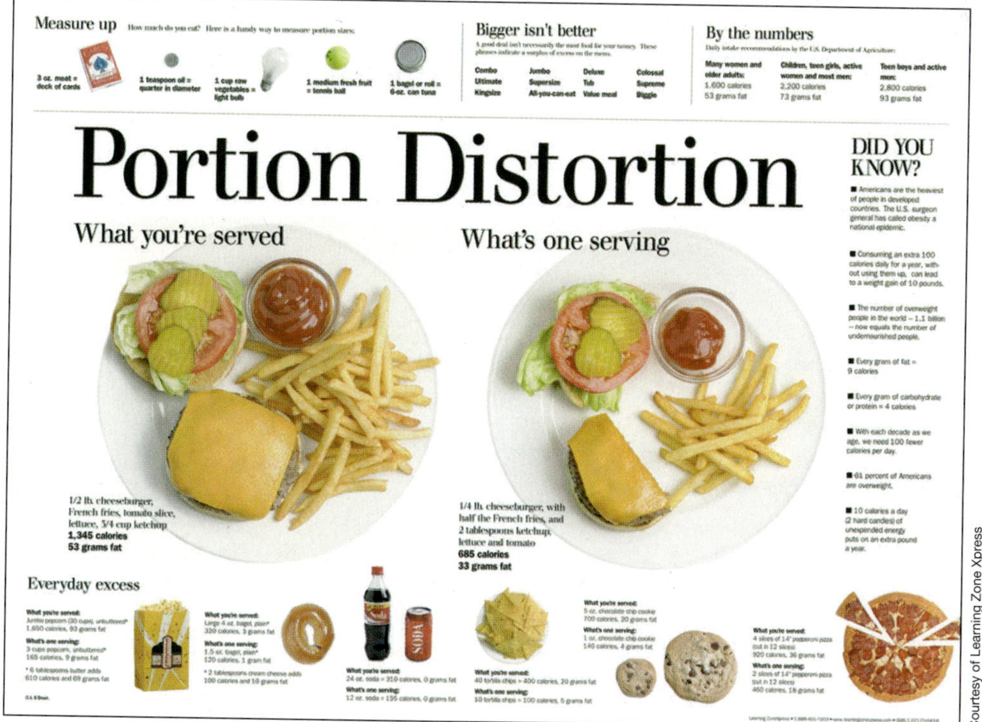
Measure up
3 oz. meat = deck of cards
1 teaspoon oil = quarter in diameter
1 cup raw vegetables = light bulb
1 medium fresh fruit = tennis ball
1 bagel or roll = 6-oz. can tuna
Bigger isn't better
Combo
Ultimate
Kingsize
Jumbo
Supersize
All-you-can-eat
Deluxe
Tub
Value meal
Colossal
Supreme
Biggie
By the numbers
Many women and older adults: 1,600 calories 53 grams fat
Children, teen girls, active women and most men: 2,200 calories 73 grams fat
Teen boys and active men: 2,800 calories 93 grams fat
Portion Distortion
What you're served
What's one serving
1/2 lb. cheeseburger, French fries, tomato slice, lettuce, 3/4 cup ketchup
1,345 calories
53 grams fat
1/4 lb. cheeseburger, with half the French fries, and 2 tablespoons ketchup, lettuce and tomato
685 calories
33 grams fat
DID YOU KNOW?
■ Americans are the heaviest of people in developed countries. The U.S. surgeon general has called obesity a national epidemic.
■ Consuming an extra 100 calories daily for a year, without using them up, can lead to a weight gain of 10 pounds.
■ The number of overweight people in the world – 1.1 billion – now equals the number of undernourished people.
■ Every gram of fat = 9 calories
■ Every gram of carbohydrate or protein = 4 calories
■ With each decade as we age, we need 100 fewer calories per day.
■ 61 percent of Americans are overweight.
■ 10 calories a day (2 hard candies) of unexpended energy puts on an extra pound a year.
Everyday excess
What you're served:
What's one serving:
What you're served: 24 oz. soda = 310 calories, 0 grams fat
What's one serving: 12 oz. soda = 155 calories, 0 grams fat
SODA

Courtesy of Learning Zone Xpress

Figure 20-3 ■ Portion distortion. The amount of food Americans actually eat vs. what is considered a single serving.

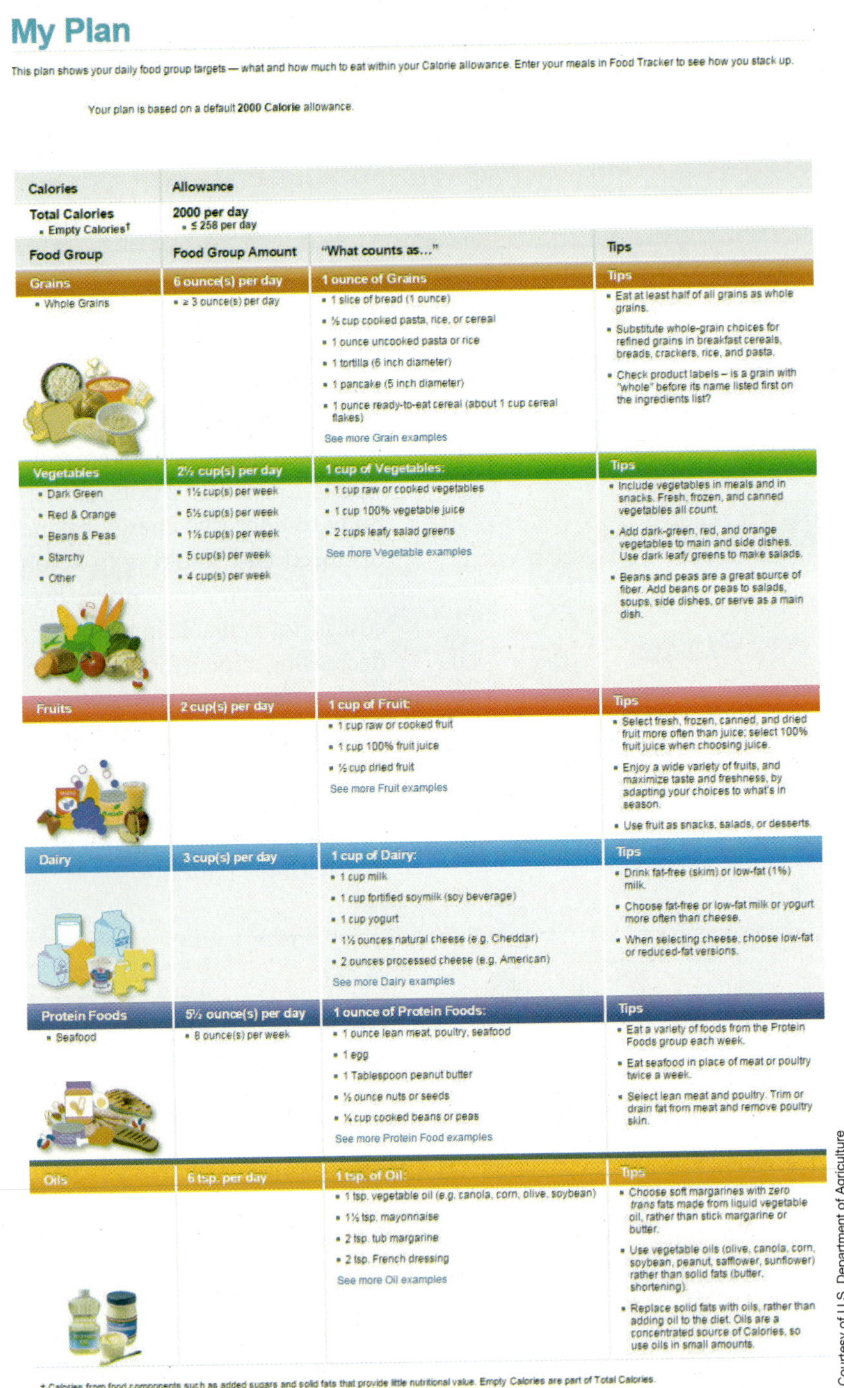

Today	Physical Activity Target		Daily Calorie Limit	
12/30/14	Week of 12/28/14 to 01/03/15		Allowance	2000
	Target	AT LEAST 150 minutes per week	Eaten	0
	Actual	0 minutes	Remaining	2000

Daily Food Group Targets More Info>

	Grains	Vegetables	Fruits	Dairy	Protein Foods
Target	6 oz.	2½ cup(s)	2 cup(s)	3 cup(s)	5½ oz.
Eaten	0 oz.	0 cup(s)	0 cup(s)	0 cup(s)	0 oz.
Status	-	-	-	-	-

My Plan

This plan shows your daily food group targets — what and how much to eat within your Calorie allowance. Enter your meals in Food Tracker to see how you stack up.

Your plan is based on a default **2000 Calorie** allowance.

Calories	Allowance		
Total Calories • Empty Calories†	2000 per day • ≤ 258 per day		
Food Group	**Food Group Amount**	**"What counts as..."**	**Tips**
Grains • Whole Grains	**6 ounce(s) per day** • ≥ 3 ounce(s) per day	**1 ounce of Grains** • 1 slice of bread (1 ounce) • ½ cup cooked pasta, rice, or cereal • 1 ounce uncooked pasta or rice • 1 tortilla (6 inch diameter) • 1 pancake (5 inch diameter) • 1 ounce ready-to-eat cereal (about 1 cup cereal flakes) See more Grain examples	**Tips** • Eat at least half of all grains as whole grains. • Substitute whole-grain choices for refined grains in breakfast cereals, breads, crackers, rice, and pasta. • Check product labels – is a grain with "whole" before its name listed first on the ingredients list?
Vegetables • Dark Green • Red & Orange • Beans & Peas • Starchy • Other	**2½ cup(s) per day** • 1½ cup(s) per week • 5½ cup(s) per week • 1½ cup(s) per week • 5 cup(s) per week • 4 cup(s) per week	**1 cup of Vegetables:** • 1 cup raw or cooked vegetables • 1 cup 100% vegetable juice • 2 cups leafy salad greens See more Vegetable examples	**Tips** • Include vegetables in meals and in snacks. Fresh, frozen, and canned vegetables all count. • Add dark-green, red, and orange vegetables to main and side dishes. Use dark leafy greens to make salads. • Beans and peas are a great source of fiber. Add beans or peas to salads, soups, side dishes, or serve as a main dish.
Fruits	**2 cup(s) per day**	**1 cup of Fruit:** • 1 cup raw or cooked fruit • 1 cup 100% fruit juice • ½ cup dried fruit See more Fruit examples	**Tips** • Select fresh, frozen, canned, and dried fruit more often than juice; select 100% fruit juice when choosing juice. • Enjoy a wide variety of fruits, and maximize taste and freshness, by adapting your choices to what's in season. • Use fruit as snacks, salads, or desserts.
Dairy	**3 cup(s) per day**	**1 cup of Dairy:** • 1 cup milk • 1 cup fortified soymilk (soy beverage) • 1 cup yogurt • 1½ ounces natural cheese (e.g. Cheddar) • 2 ounces processed cheese (e.g. American) See more Dairy examples	**Tips** • Drink fat-free (skim) or low-fat (1%) milk. • Choose fat-free or low-fat milk or yogurt more often than cheese. • When selecting cheese, choose low-fat or reduced-fat versions.
Protein Foods • Seafood	**5½ ounce(s) per day** • 8 ounce(s) per week	**1 ounce of Protein Foods:** • 1 ounce lean meat, poultry, seafood • 1 egg • 1 Tablespoon peanut butter • ½ ounce nuts or seeds • ¼ cup cooked beans or peas See more Protein Food examples	**Tips** • Eat a variety of foods from the Protein Foods group each week. • Eat seafood in place of meat or poultry twice a week. • Select lean meat and poultry. Trim or drain fat from meat and remove poultry skin.
Oils	**6 tsp. per day**	**1 tsp. of Oil:** • 1 tsp. vegetable oil (e.g. canola, corn, olive, soybean) • 1½ tsp. mayonnaise • 2 tsp. tub margarine • 2 tsp. French dressing See more Oil examples	**Tips** • Choose soft margarines with zero *trans* fats made from liquid vegetable oil, rather than stick margarine or butter. • Use vegetable oils (olive, canola, corn, soybean, peanut, safflower, sunflower) rather than solid fats (butter, shortening). • Replace solid fats with oils, rather than adding oil to the diet. Oils are a concentrated source of Calories, so use oils in small amounts.

† Calories from food components such as added sugars and solid fats that provide little nutritional value. Empty Calories are part of Total Calories.

Courtesy of U.S. Department of Agriculture

Figure 20-4 ■ My Plan Worksheet.

Estimating Portion Sizes

Food scales and measuring cups are not always available when estimating the amounts of foods that are defined for daily consumption on a food plan. It is useful to be able to estimate the amount per serving using hand symbols (see Figure 20-7).

EDUCATING PATIENTS ABOUT GOOD NUTRITION

Patient's food and exercise diaries provide important information about the patient's nutritional intake. Patients are asked to record everything they eat for a

Daily Food Plan

Want to know the amount of each food group you need daily? Enter your information below to find out and receive a customized Daily Food Plan.

NOTE: Daily Food Plans are designed for the general public ages 2 and over; they are not therapeutic diets. Those with a specific health condition should consult with a health care provider for a dietary plan that is right for them. More tailored Daily Food Plans are available for preschoolers (2-5y) and women who are pregnant or breastfeeding.

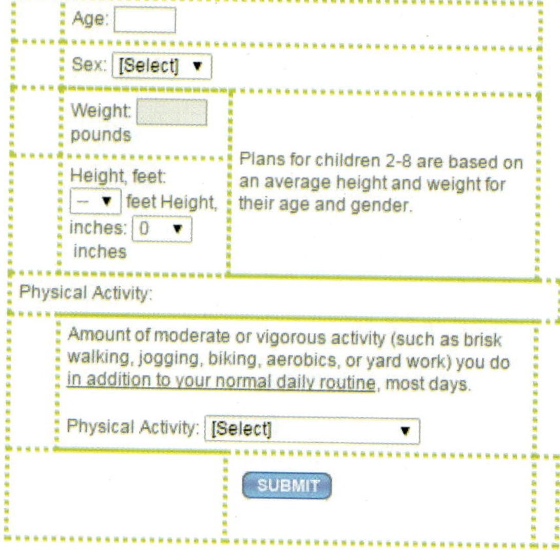

Age:
Sex: [Select]
Weight: pounds
Height, feet: -- feet Height, inches: 0 inches
Plans for children 2-8 are based on an average height and weight for their age and gender.
Physical Activity:
Amount of moderate or vigorous activity (such as brisk walking, jogging, biking, aerobics, or yard work) you do in addition to your normal daily routine, most days.
Physical Activity: [Select]
SUBMIT

Courtesy of U.S. Department of Agriculture

Figure 20-5 ■ Daily Food Plan calculator.

Table 20-6 Daily Amounts for Each Food Group Based on Calorie Intake

Food Group	2,000 Calories	1,600 Calories	1,400 Calories	1,200 Calories
Fruit	2 cups	1½ cups	1½ cups	1 cup
Vegetables	2½ cups	2 cups	1½ cups	1½ cups
Grains	6 ounces	5 ounces	5 ounces	4 ounces
Protein	5½ ounces	5 ounces	4 ounces	3 ounces
Dairy	3 cups	3 cups	2½ cups	2½ cups
Oils	6 teaspoons	5 teaspoons	4 teaspoons	4 teaspoons

prescribed number of days. The provider then reviews the diary and checks to see if the patient is consuming an adequate number of calories and getting all of the nutrients that are necessary for normal functioning of the body and for good health. Primary nutrients are carbohydrates, fats, proteins, vitamins, and minerals. The provider will calculate the Daily Food Plan, including the amount of daily exercise, consistent with predetermined goals, such as weight loss management, disease management, or overall health maintenance. After instituting a plan of action, the food and exercise diary should be reviewed periodically for feedback on progress made toward reaching the goal. To make good food choices the patient must be able to read and understand food labels (see Figure 20-1).

Providers who do not feel qualified to counsel patients about their diet may share some general dietary information, but will then send the patient to a licensed dietician or nutritionist for specific dietary instructions.

It is often the medical assistant's duty to make an appointment for the patient with a dietician. Preauthorization by the patient's insurance company is normally required for dietitian services to be covered. The medical assistant may be responsible for any or all of the following:

- Providing general information about good food choices with the use of brochures, educational handouts, and so on.
- Teaching patients how to use the "ChooseMyPlate" website.
- Obtaining a preauthorization from the insurance company to see a dietician.
- Sending the pertinent records to both the insurance company and dietician.
- Scheduling the appointment with the dietician.

My Daily Food Plan Worksheet

Check how you did today and set a goal to aim for tomorrow

Write in Your Food Choices for Today	Food Group	Tip	Based on a 1400 Calorie pattern. Your Goals Are:	Match Your Food Choices with Each Food Group	Estimate Your Total
______	GRAINS	Make at least half your grains whole grains	**5 ounce equivalents** (1 ounce equivalent is about 1 slice bread; 1 ounce ready-to-eat cereal; or ½ cup cooked rice, pasta, or cereal)	______	______ ounce equivalents
______	VEGETABLES	Aim for variety every day; pick vegetables from several subgroups: Dark green, red & orange, beans & peas, starchy, and other veggies	**1½ cups** (1 cup is 1 cup raw or cooked vegetables, 2 cups leafy salad greens, or 1 cup100% vegetable juice)	______	______ cups
______	FRUITS	Select fresh, frozen, canned, and dried fruit more often than juice	**1½ cups** (1 cup is 1 cup raw or cooked fruit, ½ cup dried fruit, or 1 cup 100% fruit juice)	______	______ cups
______	DAIRY	Include fat-free and low-fat dairy foods every day	**2½ cups** (1 cup is 1 cup milk, yogurt, or fortified soy beverage; 1½ ounces natural cheese; or 2 ounces processed cheese)	______	______ cups
______	PROTEIN FOODS	Aim for variety—choose seafood, lean meat & poultry, beans, peas, nuts, and seeds each week	**4 ounce equivalents** (1 ounce equivalent is 1 ounce lean meat, poultry, or seafood; 1 egg; 1 Tbsp peanut butter; ¼ cup cooked beans or peas; or ½ ounce nuts or seeds)	______	______ ounce equivalents
______	PHYSICAL ACTIVITY	Be active every day. Choose activities that you like and fit into your life.	Be physically active for at least **60 minutes** each day.	Some foods and drinks, such as sodas, cakes, cookies, donuts, ice cream, and candy, are high in fats and sugars. Limit your intake of these.	______ minutes

How did you do today? ☐ Great ☐ So-So ☐ Not so Great

My food goal for tomorrow is: ______________________

My activity goal for tomorrow is: ______________________

Courtesy of U.S. Department of Agriculture

Figure 20-6 ■ My Daily Food Plan Worksheet.

EXERCISE FOR WEIGHT MAINTENANCE

With obesity now defined by the American Medical Association (AMA) as a disease, there is increased public awareness of the importance of physical activity requirements, combined with a healthy Daily Food Plan. Some studies suggest that as many as 60% of American adults do not participate in enough physical activity, and 25% are physically inactive.

As people become more sedentary, there is an associated increase in weight gain. Before partaking in any increased level of activity or beginning a new exercise program, one should check with his primary physician for any restrictions. Some important guidelines and recommendations for physical activity include the following:

- Adults should attempt to engage in at least 30 minutes of moderate activity (over normal daily activity) each day. A longer duration would be even more beneficial.
- Prevention of weight gain may require 60 minutes of activity per day, depending on the level of daily calorie consumption.
- Weight loss may require 60 to 90 minutes of moderate activity on most days.
- Alter the workout plan to prevent boredom.
- Include cardiovascular conditioning by increasing the heart rate during exercise. To calculate the maximum exercising heart rate for healthy individuals, subtract the individual's age from 220.
- Include stretching before and after exercise to maintain or improve flexibility.
- Incorporate resistance exercises to improve strength and endurance.
- Children and adolescents should participate in at least 60 minutes of physical activity every day.
- Pregnant women, when cleared for exercise by their physician, should engage in 30 minutes of activity on most days. The activities should be designed to avoid falls or any sudden impact to the abdominal region.
- Older adults should exercise as tolerated. Exercise may slow the functional declines associated with aging.

Adjusting the requirements for caloric intake and exercise can be assessed by using BMI and waist circumference measurements. BMI is discussed in Chapter 11.

Serving-Size Comparison Chart

FOOD	SYMBOL	COMPARISON	SERVING SIZE
Milk & Milk Products			
Cheese (string cheese)		Pointer finger	1½ ounces
Milk and yogurt (glass of milk)		One fist	1 cup
Vegetables			
Cooked carrots		One fist	1 cup
Salad (bowl of salad)		Two fists	2 cups
Fruits			
Apple		One fist	1 medium
Canned peaches		One fist	1 cup
Grains, Breads & Cereals			
Dry cereal (bowl of cereal)		One fist	1 cup
Noodles, rice, oatmeal (bowl of noodles)		Handful	½ cup
Slice of whole wheat bread		Flat hand	1 slice
Meat, Beans & Nuts			
Chicken, beef, fish, pork (chicken breast)		Palm	3 ounces
Peanut butter (spoon of peanut butter)		Thumb	1 tablespoon

Figure 20-7 ■ Estimating portion sizes, using common household items.

Table 20-7 Information Used for a Nutritional Assessment

Information	Rationale
Past medical and surgical history	To discover any conditions that could interfere with intake of foods or the assimilation of nutrients.
Family health history	There is a genetic tendency for some major conditions, such as heart disease, to run in families.
Current symptoms	Symptoms can point to conditions suggesting dietary or digestive problems.
Medications and supplements	Some medications and supplements can interfere with the assimilation of nutrients in the body.
Lifestyle	Physical activity level, the use of alcohol, and smoking all impact nutritional status.
Weight history	Previous and current weights are compared to reference charts specific for sex, age, and height.
Digestive history	To reveal food intolerances and allergies.
Diet intake	To determine adequacy of the diet through the analysis of nutritional intake, compared to the dietary reference intake (DRI).
Dietary goals	To determine what the patient wants to accomplish through dietary and lifestyle changes.
Physical exam	The hair, fingernails, skin, and tongue can provide clues that may be indicative of poor nutrition.
Laboratory tests	Blood and urine sample components are compared to normal values, to detect deficiencies or excesses.

NUTRITION SCREENING AND ASSESSMENT

To conduct a nutritional assessment for a patient, the dietitian uses information gathering tools. Findings are then interpreted to create a comprehensive view of the patient's nutritional status. Table 20-7 describes the information used by a dietitian to provide a nutritional assessment.

OBESITY

Bariatrics is a branch of medicine concerned with the prevention and control of obesity and associated diseases. A simple definition of **obesity** is having too much body fat for the height, gender, and age of the individual. Another definition of obesity is severe overweight with a BMI equal to or greater than the 95th percentile. Calculation of the **BMI (body mass index)** can determine the degree of obesity. You can determine your BMI using the formulas below:

$$\text{BMI} = \frac{(\text{Weight in pounds} \times 703)}{\text{Height in inches}^2}$$

$$\text{BMI} = \frac{(\text{Weight in kilograms})}{\text{Height in meters}^2}$$

Most EHRs will automatically generate the BMI after entering the height and weight. There are also BMI calculators that can be purchased to make the process easier. Table 20-8 lists weight classifications by BMI.

Table 20-8 Weight Classifications by BMI

BMI	Classification
<18.5	Underweight
18.5–24.99	Normal weight
25.0–29.99	Overweight
30.0–34.99	Class I obesity
35.0–39.99	Class II obesity
>40.00	Class III obesity

Being overweight or obese is the result of a daily calorie intake that is higher than the body requires and exercise that is insufficient to offset the higher number of calories consumed. Although genetic inheritance and endocrine disorders can contribute to weight gain, their contribution to the development of obesity is minimal. In 2013, the American Medical Association classified obesity as a disease.

Health Effects of Obesity

Childhood obesity is now at epidemic proportions worldwide. The Food Research and Action Center (FRAC) states that in the United States, 31.8% of children are overweight or obese, with 16.9% obese, defined as a BMI ≥ 95th percentile. Obesity among children is a public health concern, as many continue the inappropriate eating patterns into adulthood, maintaining the obesity and placing them at high risk for negative effects on their health, such as diabetes, heart disease, cancer, and osteoarthritis. Heart disease and cancer are now the leading causes of death in the United States and worldwide.

Obesity is known to decrease life expectancy. FRAC reports that in the United States, 68.5% of adults are overweight or obese, with 34.9% obese, defined as a BMI ≥ 30. The average life expectancy in the United States in 2011 was 76 years for men and 81 years for women. Compared to 36 countries in the Organization for Economic Cooperation and Development (OECD) the United States ranks only 26th in longevity, yet it spends the most of all countries on health care [17.7% of the national gross domestic product (GDP)].

Metabolic Syndrome

Metabolic syndrome is a combination of medical disorders, primarily caused by obesity, including high blood pressure, high blood sugar levels, abnormal cholesterol levels, and the accumulation of body fat around the waist. Any one condition increases the risk of serious disease, but more than one increases that risk further. Metabolic syndrome is linked to insulin resistance.

Insulin Resistance

Increases in body fat alter the body's response to insulin, causing the body to no longer use insulin effectively. Glucose then rises in the bloodstream, instead of being used in the cells for energy. This condition leads to pre-diabetes and type 2 diabetes.

WEIGHT LOSS DIETS

With 68% of adults classified as overweight or obese, Americans are obsessed with weight loss diets, yet very few lose weight and fewer still maintain that weight loss. There are many commercial weight loss diets that make money for the promoters, yet most are not nutritionally sound. Unfortunately, most diets are not eating plans, which can be continued indefinitely for the weight loss to be maintained. For example, eliminating an entire food group, such as carbohydrates, is simply not sustainable over the long term.

When individuals start a weight loss diet, their expectations for the rate of weight loss are typically unrealistic, compared to the accepted safe weight loss rate of 0.5 to 2 pounds per week, or 10% of body weight in 6 months. When unrealistic expectations are not met, many dieters give up and return to their previous eating patterns.

Examples of sound eating plans that can be maintained are the Mediterranean diet and an eating plan called **DASH (Dietary Approaches to Stop Hypertension)**.

DASH emphasizes vegetables, fruits, and fat-free dairy and includes whole grains, poultry, fish, seeds, and beans. Sodium is limited, as are sweets, high-sugar beverages, and red meats. DASH is low in saturated fats, but rich in magnesium, potassium, and protein.

Counting calories will always be a basic requirement in any weight loss program, but being aware of the glycemic index of various foods is also useful.

The **glycemic index (GI)** measures how quickly carbohydrate foods raise the blood glucose level. The highest value is for plain sugar and the lowest for complex carbohydrates such as nonstarchy vegetables and fruits. To be avoided are what are referred to as "empty calories" from solid fats and/or sugars, which have few or no nutrients, as in high-sugar beverages. To offset the empty calories in a 20 oz. sugary drink would require 5 miles of walking. Of greater importance is the clear link between the high consumption of sugar and poor health, including increased rates of obesity, type 2 diabetes, and tooth decay.

But regardless of the GI value, portion sizes are still relevant for managing blood glucose. Using the GI may be useful, but the first step must be some type of carbohydrate or calorie counting, or both.

BARIATRIC SURGERY

Surgery may be considered for those who have failed weight loss and exercise programs and remain obese. All surgical procedures restrict food intake, which promotes weight loss and decreases the risk of type 2 diabetes.

The American College of Physicians defines surgical candidates as those with a BMI greater than 40 or those with a BMI of 35–40, who also have a serious health condition linked to obesity such as diabetes, heart disease, or severe sleep apnea.

Surgical procedures for reducing the size of the stomach include a gastric band, resection of the stomach, or resection/rerouting the small intestine into a small pouch (bypass surgery).

Complications following surgery are not infrequent, both during the hospital stay and after discharge, including the need for repeated surgery, gallbladder disease, and GI **malabsorption syndrome** (the inability of the GI tract to absorb some nutrients).

Unfortunately there is no sure method, including surgery, to produce and maintain weight loss. Those who succeed after bariatric surgery are those who are totally committed to changing eating habits and agree to follow-up medical care for the rest of their lives.

SPECIAL DIETS

Special diets are either a reflection of how individuals choose to eat or a necessity due to food intolerances, weight gains, or medical conditions. Table 20-9 lists different types of special diets, including those followed by **vegetarians**, individuals who do not eat fish, fowl, or animal flesh, but may include dairy and eggs.

Table 20-9 Types of Special Diets

Special Diet	Diet Modification
Lacto vegetarian	No beef, chicken, fish, or eggs. Includes dairy products.
Lacto-ovo vegetarian	No beef, chicken, or fish. Includes eggs and dairy products.
Vegan	No animal or animal by-products including beef, chicken, fish, eggs, dairy, or any other products that come from animals.
Gluten-free	Excludes gluten, which causes inflammation of the small intestine in some individuals. **Gluten** is a protein found in grains such as wheat, rye, triticale (a cross between wheat and rye), and barley.
Food allergies	Excludes foods that cause an allergic reaction. Nearly all allergens are proteins such as eggs, fish, milk, nuts from trees, peanuts, shellfish (shrimp, crabs, mussels), soy, and wheat.
Lactose sensitivity or intolerance	The consumption of **lactose**, a protein found in milk products, is reduced but not eliminated.

Table 20-10 Medical Conditions Requiring a Diet Modification

Medical Condition	Diet Modification
Cardiovascular	Sodium (Na) is restricted to lower blood pressure or to reduce fluid retention. Saturated fats are restricted.
Hypertension	Sodium (Na) is restricted to lower blood volume and blood pressure.
Cancer	High-calorie and high-protein diet
Diabetes	Carbohydrate levels are based on metabolic needs and the type of insulin that is being used. High fiber, minimally processed foods, including complex carbohydrates. Reduction in saturated fats.
GERD	Limit foods that increase gastric acid secretion or irritate the esophagus.
Malabsorption (the result of conditions such as celiac disease, lactose intolerance, gastrointestinal surgeries, and genetic diseases)	Testing to identify nutrients that are insufficient and then providing supplements that may include folate, iron, vitamins B_{12} and D, as well as calcium. If necessary, these nutrients may be administered intravenously.
Acute intestinal disturbances	Low-fiber or liquid diet

Table 20-10 lists medical conditions that require a diet modification.

EATING DISORDERS

Radical changes in eating patterns or eating behaviors are characteristic of an eating disorder. It is not unusual that the person with this type of disorder is an overachieving female. Such factors as high stress levels from unreasonable work and personal responsibilities and an unrealistic body image, are thought to influence overachieving women to develop eating disorders. Eating disorders have been linked to psychological and physical causes. Therefore, both areas must be addressed for treatment. Failure to resolve the disorder will prove hazardous to the patient's health, and can be fatal. Due to the high incidence of eating disorders in adolescents, discussions of anorexia and bulimia are included in Chapter 21. Classifications of eating disorders follow.

Anorexia Nervosa

Anorexia nervosa is characterized by a drastic reduction of food intake in an effort to minimize body weight. The individual perceives any weight gain negatively. This disorder is primarily seen in adolescents, but can also occur in adulthood. Medical and psychological support is essential in the treatment of this disorder.

Bulimia Nervosa

Bulimia nervosa involves a dangerous pattern of eating or binging followed by purging. The purge may be by vomiting, using laxatives, diuretics, or diet pills, or by excessive exercise. Any method to rid the body of the excess food intake may be attempted.

Compulsive Overeating

Compulsive overeating is characterized by excessive **binge** eating when huge amounts of foods are consumed. This eating behavior is used in an attempt to relieve stress or depression, but in turn, causes them to increase.

Night Eating Syndrome

This disorder occurs when patients are awakened by hunger throughout the night. Binging occurs during the late hours, causing the person to not be hungry in the morning hours.

FOODBORNE ILLNESSES

According to the most recent CDC estimates (2011), one out of every six persons in the United States will be sickened by a foodborne illness each year. As many as 128,000 will be hospitalized and 3,000 will die. There are more than 250 different foodborne diseases that are caused by bacteria, viruses, and parasites, which can contaminate foods.

Common symptoms of a foodborne illness are nausea, vomiting, and abdominal cramps with diarrhea. Table 20-11 describes several different foodborne illnesses.

Protection from foodborne illnesses require simple, basic precautions when preparing and cooking foods. See Table 20-12 for more information.

Table 20-11 Foodborne Illnesses

Foodborne Illness	% U.S. Incidence	Description
Salmonella	35%	A bacteria that is present in the intestines of birds, reptiles, and mammals. It is transmitted through feces, either through direct contact with animals or by eating contaminated raw or undercooked meats, eggs or unpasteurized milk, and cheese products.
Norovirus	26%	A virus that spreads from an infected person to another through contaminated food preparation surfaces, contaminated food, and water.
Campylobacter	15%	The most common cause of diarrhea worldwide. The bacteria are present in the intestines of healthy birds. Most raw poultry is contaminated.
E. coli	4%	Six different types of *E. coli* bacteria cause diarrhea, transmitted through contaminated foods that have not been cooked properly. The illness develops two to eight days after swallowing the organism. Most recover within seven days. However, a type of kidney failure can occur at any age, but is most common in children under the age of five and the elderly.

Table 20-12 Protection against *E. coli* and Other Foodborne Illness

1. Those at higher risk of foodborne illness are pregnant women, newborns, children, older adults, and those with weakened immune systems.
2. Good handwashing is very important. See www.cdc.gov/handwashing for more information on proper handwashing techniques.
3. Cook meats thoroughly to an internal temperature of 160 degrees or more.
4. In food preparation areas, thoroughly wash hands, counters, cutting boards, and utensils after they come into contact with raw meats.
5. Avoid raw milk, unpasteurized dairy products, as well as unpasteurized juices, including fresh apple cider.

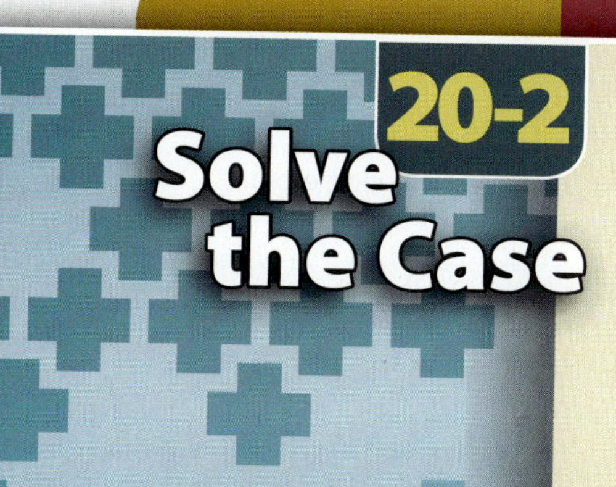

Miss Winters has returned to the clinic three months after her initial visit, for a routine checkup. She has lost 5 pounds and does not know why she has not lost more weight.

1. **What is considered a normal weight loss per week?**
2. **What questions would you ask her, to try to understand why she did not lose more weight?**
3. **How many calories should she consume, at 5'4" and 155 pounds, for a "safe" weight loss?**

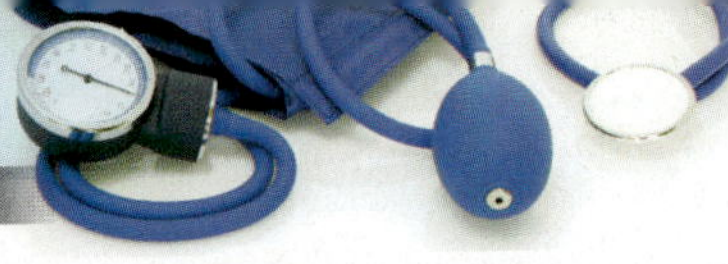

PROCEDURE 20-1

Develop a 2,000-Calorie Meal Plan Utilizing Basic Principles of Nutrition

Objective:

To develop a 2,000-calorie daily meal plan, applying DRI information for a nutritionally balanced diet.

Equipment and Supplies:

- Patient's chart/EHR
- Height and weight reference chart
- My Daily Food Plan
- My Daily Food Plan Worksheet

PROCEDURAL STEPS	DETAILS AND/OR RATIONALE
1. Read the patient's chart and note the patient's height and weight. Review the list of diagnoses and note those requiring dietary modifications. Review the patient's usual daily physical activity.	In order to develop a meal plan you must know the patient's diagnosed medical conditions and understand why diet planning is appropriate. Comparing the patient's height and weight to the height/weight chart will help you conclude if the patient is under-, over-, or normal weight. Anticipate any special modifications that might be necessary. Know that to balance a 2,000-calorie diet, 150 minutes per week of physical activity is required.
2. Review the Daily Food Plan for 2,000 calories/day.	Recommended daily allowances for a 2,000/day diet are: 6 oz. grains—at least half are whole grains 2½ cups vegetables—include dark green and red/orange, plus beans and peas, starchy, and other vegetables 2 cups fruit—plan a variety of whole/cut up fruits more often than fruit juices. 3 cups dairy—fat-free or low-fat milk; yogurt and cheese that is fat-free or low fat 5½ ounces protein—seafood twice a week; include beans, peas, nuts, and seeds; keep meat and poultry portions small and lean. 6 teaspoons oil Sodium at less than 2,300 mg/day
3. Apply the food plan to the Daily Food Plan Worksheet.	Practice applying the food plan principles to the worksheet, before working with the patient.

PROCEDURE 20-2

Instruct a Patient According to the Patient's Special Dietary Needs

Objective:

To review and develop a daily food plan with the patient, including nutrition labels and portion sizes.

Equipment/Supplies:

- Patient chart/EHR
- My Daily Food Plan (two copies) from www.choosemyplate.gov
- My Daily Food Plan Worksheet (two copies) from www.choosemyplate.gov
- Review and print "Use the Nutrition Facts Label to Eat Healthier"; see Figure 20-1
- Additional reference information at www.fda.gov/nutritionandhealth (for) "Understanding and Using the Nutrition Facts Label"
- Estimating portion sizes (two copies); see Figure 20-7

PROCEDURAL STEPS	DETAILS AND/OR RATIONALE
1. Prepare for patient instruction by writing a list of talking points. Assemble teaching materials, including print copies for the patient to take home.	Preparation and organization make the sharing of information more effective. Reference materials at home reinforce teaching.
2. Introduce yourself to the patient. Instruct the patient what educational materials she should review and ask if she has any questions	Know that sharing information about behaviors around foods can be embarrassing. Be sensitive to feelings, both verbal and nonverbal.
3. Ask the patient about her dietary goals and her realistic commitment to changing her diet, ***showing awareness of the patient's concerns regarding a dietary change***.	Determine if the patient wants only information or if she is also committed to making dietary and lifestyle changes.
4. Review and discuss the Daily Food Plan (Figure 20-8).	Hand the patient My Daily Food Plan and review each of the five food categories.
5. Complete the Food Plan worksheet with the patient.	Applying new information to a worksheet checks understanding of the patient's dietary goals.
6. Review how to read and use the nutrition facts label with the patient	Understanding the information on food labels helps consumers make better food choices.
7. Teach the patient how to estimate portion sizes (Figure 20-9).	Knowing how to estimate portion sizes recommended in the Daily Food Plan will ensure that diet nutrient intake is adequate and not over or under the recommended levels.

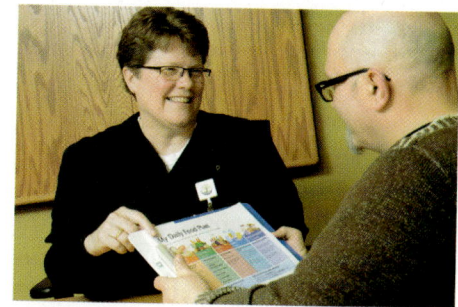

Figure 20-8 ■ The medical assistant reviews the daily food plan with the patient.

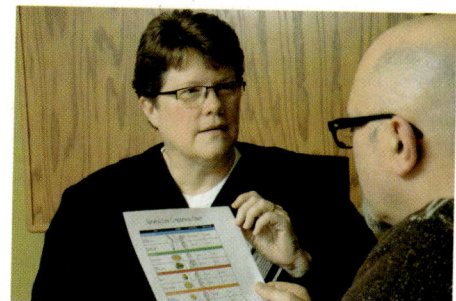

Figure 20-9 ■ The medical assistant shows the patient how to estimate portion sizes.

continues

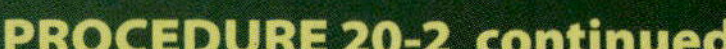

PROCEDURE 20-2 continued

PROCEDURAL STEPS	DETAILS AND/OR RATIONALE
8. Review the amount of time the patient spends in physical activity each day.	Share the general recommendation that to balance food and physical activity to maintain weight, on a 2,000/day calorie diet, 150 minutes of physical activity each week is recommended.
9. Provide the website address for more information on ChooseMyPlate food plans.	Information can be found at the USDA website: www.choosemyplate.gov
10. Document the patient education provided in the patient's chart.	

CHAPTER SUMMARY

- All foods are made up of proteins, carbohydrates, fats, and fiber. Vitamins are either fat-soluble (vitamins A, D, E, K) or water-soluble vitamins. Minerals are inorganic elements (e.g., sodium, potassium, and magnesium) that are essential for normal body functioning.
- It is important to know and understand the nutrients and their primary function in the body: calcium; potassium; phosphorus; magnesium; iron; and vitamins A, B, C, D, E, and K.
- Individuals must be able to read and interpret food labels in order to make good food choices.
- Vegetables are divided into five subgroups: dark green, starchy, red and orange, beans and peas, and other. Half the daily diet should be fruits and vegetables.
- Appropriate protein choices are fat-free or low-fat dairy products, lean or low-fat meats and poultry, and a limited amount of processed and deli meats, to restrict sodium.
- Inappropriate food choices and eating habits may contribute to the development of type 2 diabetes, but nutritionally sound food plans can be calculated using the USDA ChooseMyPlate.
- Nutrition procedures to calculate a meal plan and to then teach the patient require assessment information and specific reference documents.
- As people become more sedentary, there is increased weight gain. It is recommended that adults should engage in at least 30 minutes of moderate physical activity each day.
- Obesity for adults and children has reached epidemic proportions worldwide. The degree of obesity is defined by the calculated BMI (body mass index).
- Metabolic syndrome is a combination of medical disorders, primarily caused by obesity, high blood pressure, high blood sugar levels, abnormal cholesterol, and the accumulation of fat around the waist.
- There are two types of diabetes: type 1 and type 2. Diabetes is diagnosed when the blood glucose is higher than normal limits.
- The glycemic index measures how quickly carbohydrate foods raise the blood glucose levels.
- Bariatric surgery restricts food intake in order to promote weight loss and to decrease the risk of type 2 diabetes.
- There are three types of vegetarian diets: lacto-ovo, lacto, and vegan.
- Gluten is a protein found in grains such as wheat, barley, and rye. In some individuals gluten causes inflammation of the small intestine.
- Diet modifications are necessary for common food allergies such as eggs, fish, milk, nuts, peanuts, and shellfish. Medical conditions also often require modification of the diet.
- There are four emotional eating disorders: anorexia nervosa, bulimia nervosa, compulsive overeating, and night eating syndrome. Any treatment must address both physical and psychological factors.
- Foodborne illnesses include *E. coli*, *Salmonella*, norovirus, and *Campylobacter*.

CERTIFICATION REVIEW QUESTIONS

1. Nutrients that provide energy are:
   a. fats and vitamins.
   b. minerals, fats, and water.
   c. fiber, fats, and vitamins.
   d. carbohydrates, fats, and proteins.
2. Weight control success requires:
   a. decreasing proteins and restricting carbohydrates.
   b. drinking water and taking dietary supplements.
   c. reducing calorie intake and increasing physical activity.
   d. avoiding all fats.
3. Eating disorders are:
   a. only psychological.
   b. psychological and physical.
   c. only physical.
   d. drug-induced.
4. Diets can influence the development of all of the following diseases, except:
   a. Cancer
   B. Strokes
   c. Type 1 diabetes
   d. Cardiovascular disease
5. Diet modifications for those with cardiovascular disease include:
   a. increased carbohydrates.
   b. decreased proteins.
   c. decreased fats and salt.
   d. decreased salt.
6. Meal planning includes:
   a. knowing the calorie content of foods.
   b. using the five food groups to plan meals.
   c. eliminating fats.
   d. providing adequate proteins.
7. The foods listed in each of the five food groups in the ChooseMyPlate food plan are similar in:
   a. fiber.
   b. vitamins.
   c. calories.
   d. carbohydrates.
8. Food labels list ingredients:
   a. in alphabetical order.
   b. by weight in descending order.
   c. by the manufacturer's preference.
   d. according to nutrient density.
9. The role of exercise in a healthy lifestyle is to:
   a. decrease sodium.
   b. increase calories burned.
   c. increase balance.
   d. decrease food cravings.
10. Foodborne illnesses do not include:
    a. *E. coli.*
    b. *Clostridium difficile.*
    c. *Salmonella.*
    d. norovirus.

STUDY RESOURCES

Resources to Test and Reinforce Your Knowledge:	
Certification Review Questions	Take this end-of-chapter quiz
Workbook	• Complete the activities for Chapter 20 • Perform the procedures for Chapter 20 using the Competency Checklists
Resources to Promote Critical Thinking:	
***Solve the Case* Activities**	• Consider these case studies and discuss your conclusions
Learning Lab	• Module 27: Rehabilitation and Healthy Living
MindTap	• Complete Chapter 20 readings and activities

REFERENCES

Allison, D. B. et al. (1999, October). Annual deaths attributable to obesity in the United States. *JAMA, 282*(16), 1530–1538.

American Diabetes Association. (n.d.) *Understanding carbohydrates.* Retrieved from http://www.diabetes.org/food-and-fitness/food/what-can-i-eat/understanding-carbohydrates/

Anderson, A. I. et al. (2011). Dietary patterns and survival of older adults. *Journal of the American Dietetic Association, 111.*

Caballero, B. (2007). The global epidemic of obesity: An overview. *Epidemiologic Reviews, 29.*

Centers for Disease Control and Prevention. (2014, May 20). E. coli *infection and food safety.* Retrieved from http://www.cdc.gov/Features/ecoliinfection/

Centers for Disease Control and Prevention. (2014, September 10). *Overweight and obesity.* Retrieved from www.cdc.gov/obesity

Ford, E. S. et al. (2011). Low-risk lifestyle behaviors and all-cause mortality: Findings from the National Health and Nutrition Examination Survey III Mortality Study. *American Journal of Public Health, 101.*

The Huffington Post. (2013, November 21). U.S. life expectancy ranks 26th in the world, OECD report shows. Retrieved from http://www.huffingtonpost.com/2013/11/21/us-life-expectancy-oecd_n_4317367.html

Koopman, R. and vanLoon, L.J. (2009). Aging, exercise and muscle protein Metabolism. *Journal of Applied Physiology.*

The Mayo Clinic. (2014, August 22). *Metabolic syndrome.* Retrieved from www.mayoclinic.org/diseases-conditions/metabolicsyndrome/basics/definition/con-20027243

Medline Plus. (2014, August 9). *Malabsorption syndromes.* Retrieved from www.nih.gov/medlineplus/malabsorptionsyndromes.html

MyNetDiary. (n.d.). *Measuring and estimating portion size.* Retrieved from http://www.mynetdiary.com/estimating-portions-for-food-diary.html

National Heart, Lung, and Blood Institute. (2014, June 6). *What is the DASH eating plan?* Retrieved from http://www.nhlbi.nih.gov/health/health-topics/topics/dash/

National Institutes of Health, Office of Dietary Supplements. (n.d.). *Dietary supplement fact sheets.* Retrieved from https://owl.english.purdue.edu/owl/resource/560/10/

Ogden, C. L. et al. (2011–2012). Prevalence of childhood and adult obesity in the United States. *Journal of the American Medical Association, 311*(8), 806–814.

Pollack, A. (2013, June 18). AMA recognizes obesity as a disease. *The New York Times.*

Rolfes, S. R., Pinna, K., and Whitney, E. (2015). *Understanding normal and clinical nutrition* (10th ed.). Boston, MA: Cengage Learning.

U.S. Department of Health and Human Services. (2014, September 10). National Diabetes Information Clearinghouse. Retrieved from http://diabetes.niddk.nih.gov/dm/pubs/insulinresistance/

United States Department of Agriculture. (n.d.). ChooseMyPlate. Retrieved from http://www.choosemyplate.gov/

Weight-Control Information Network. (2011, June). *Bariatric surgery for severe obesity.* Retrieved from www.win.niddk.nih.gov/publications/gastric.htm

21

Evaluation and Care of the Pediatric Patient

CHAPTER OUTLINE

Pediatric Age Classifications

Age-Appropriate Communication

Infant/Toddler Measurements

- Height/Length
- Weight
- Circumferences
- Pediatric Vital Signs

Pediatric Development

- Motor Development
- Sensory Development
- Language Development

Visual and Hearing Screenings

- Visual
- Auditory

Immunizations

- Schedules
- Controversies

Pediatric Injections

- Reducing Pain During Immunizations
- Intranasal Route for Giving Immunizations

Newborn Screenings

Circumcision

Adolescent Care

- Height and Weight
- Puberty
- Sports and Athletics

Behavioral and Mental Health Issues

- Depression
- Eating Disorders
- Abuse
- Suicide

ESSENTIAL TERMS

adolescent
anorexia nervosa
bulimia nervosa
child
circumcision
familial stature
head circumference
hypothyroidism
galactosemia
immunizations
infant
language development
macrocephaly
microcephaly
milestones
motor development
neonate
newborn
pediatric
pediatrician
percentiles
phenylketonuria (PKU)
puberty
reflexes
secondary sex characteristics
sensory development
sudden infant death syndrome (SIDS)
toddler
vaccinations

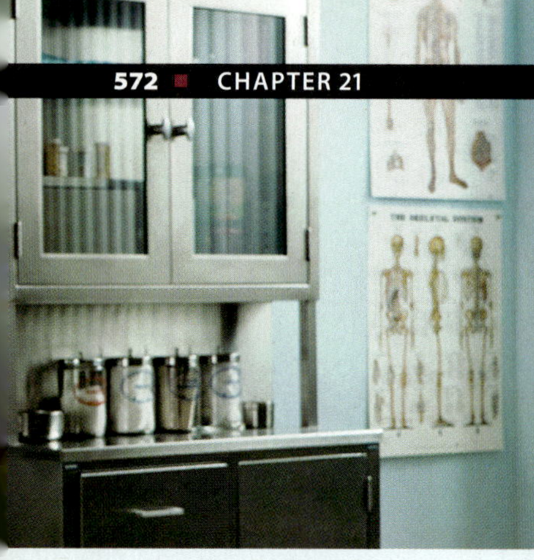

DEVELOPMENTAL OBJECTIVES

After completing this chapter, you should be able to:

1. Correctly spell and define the essential terms.
2. Discuss the different age groups of patients within the practice of pediatrics.
3. Compare and contrast the different methods used when communicating with toddlers, adolescents, and parents.
4. Explain the need for precise documentation when recording height, weight, and circumference measurements.
5. Explain the normal pulse respiratory rates, and blood pressure for all age groups within the pediatric population.
6. List and describe three types of blood screening tests for newborns.
7. Discuss the development of motor, sensory, and language milestones throughout the growth of the pediatric patient.
8. List and explain six common reflexes tested in the newborn.
9. Explain the methods used to determine if a child is hearing impaired.
10. List the childhood immunization guidelines and the ages at which each immunization is administered.
11. Debate controversies over childhood vaccinations.
12. Describe the different signs and changes during puberty, including secondary sex characteristics.
13. Provide patient education guidelines regarding baby safety and sudden infant death syndrome (SIDS).
14. Discuss social issues that are affecting our youth's health of today.

INTRODUCTION

A **pediatric** practice presents special challenges in education due to the diversity of the patient population. The office setting might include any patient from a newborn to a young adult. In addition, there are often various caregivers involved in the patient's care, which can create multiple levels of health and education needs.

The medical assistant must be knowledgeable in all areas of pediatric wellness and must also be able to deal with the unique health challenges presented by this patient population.

Character traits necessary to work in pediatrics include patience, honesty, and a love for children. Communication skills and the needs of the patient will often fluctuate at each unique developmental level. As the pediatric patient ages, ethical issues along with degrees of confidentiality become increasingly relevant. Social issues and concerns become a growing part of the pediatric patient's development; therefore, it is important for all health care workers to be current in societal issues, pressures, and expectations.

Apprehension and anxiety are often associated with areas of growth and development, as children

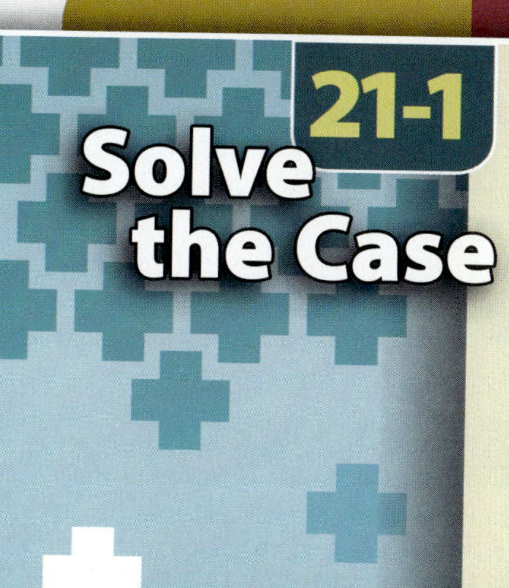

Mrs. Parsons brings her daughter, Gabby, in for her six-month well-baby check today. Mrs. Parsons is a new mom and a bit apprehensive about her child hitting all the normal gross and fine motor development milestones on time. She is also concerned about whether or not to continue having her daughter immunized. She states that she has been reading some materials that link certain physiological defects to particular immunizations.

1. **What can you say to Mrs. Parsons about her daughter hitting all of the normal gross and fine motor development milestones on time?**
2. **What can you say to Mrs. Parsons regarding her concerns on whether or not to have her daughter immunized going forward?**
3. **Should you share this information with the provider? Why or why not?**

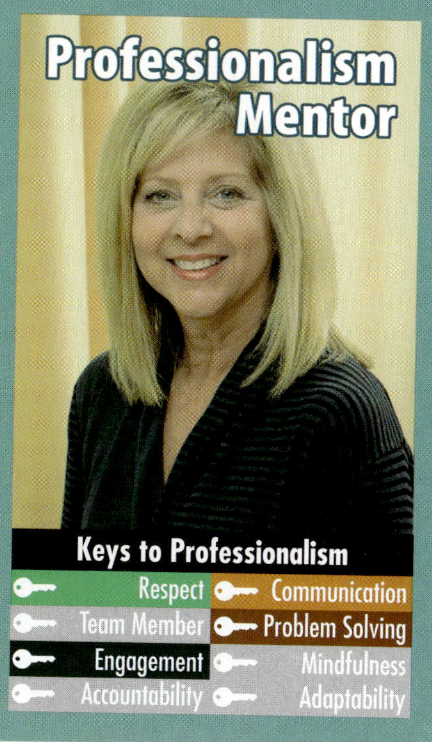

Working with the pediatric patient is probably one of the toughest yet most rewarding services a medical assistant can provide. I recently had the opportunity to visit one of our pediatric clinics and witnessed first-hand the compassion of the staff caring for a young toddler. He was by nature a sweet boy but challenging nonetheless when it came time for his yearly vaccinations and was visibly afraid. The medical assistant in the office was fairly new but she greeted the little boy and his mother with a big smile. His mother seemed on the edge herself, probably worried about the staff and how they would react to her son's aversion to needles. The medical assistant spoke softly to the mom and told her everything would be "okay." Her voice and demeanor exhibited patience and empathy, two important keys to success when caring for pediatric children, especially those having a painful procedure. I can't in all honesty say it was an easy task giving that little boy his injection, but the medical assistant did her best to provide the tenderness that mother and child needed. As they were leaving the clinic, the medical assistant handed the little boy his "sticker" and gave him a big hug and in return he smiled at her. How about you? Do you have what it takes to work in a pediatric office? In your journal, express why you would or wouldn't be a fit for a pediatric office. ■

unfortunately do not come with an instructional manual. Patient and family empathy must be developed. Educational support may be a large portion of the medical assistant's role in the pediatric practice.

PEDIATRIC AGE CLASSIFICATIONS

When thinking of the patients of a **pediatrician**, you might envision small babies in diapers. However, this is only a portion of the pediatric population. Many practices consider pediatrics to cover care from newborn through 18 years of age. The classification terms used for the various age ranges are as follows:

- **Newborn**: Usually refers to the initial period following birth
- **Neonate**: The first month of life
- **Infant**: The first year of life
- **Toddler**: Begins late in the first year of life and continues into the preschool years
- **Child**: Often correlates with school attendance and can be broken down into early childhood and middle childhood
- **Adolescent** or teenager: Related to the onset of **puberty** (age at which reproduction is possible) and development of secondary sex characteristics

Some pediatricians may also address care of the unborn. Others provide continued health care over the age of 18, if special needs are identified.

Some practices may define the levels of age based on school age, using terminology such as preschool development and school-aged development. Still other groups might classify patients into categories like infancy, early childhood, middle childhood, and adolescence. An understanding of these terms and how they may coexist is important in communication, patient education, and documentation.

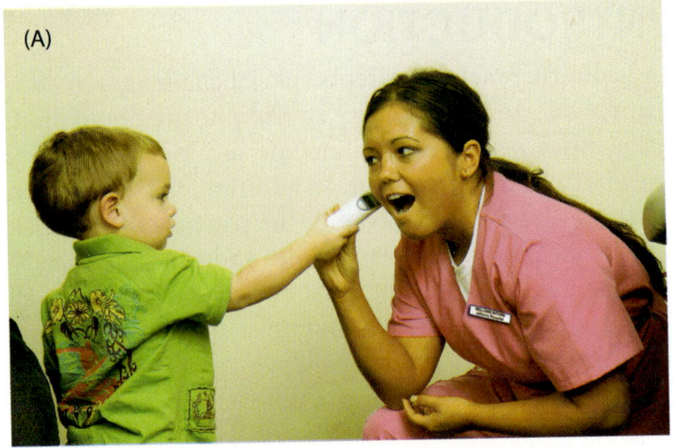

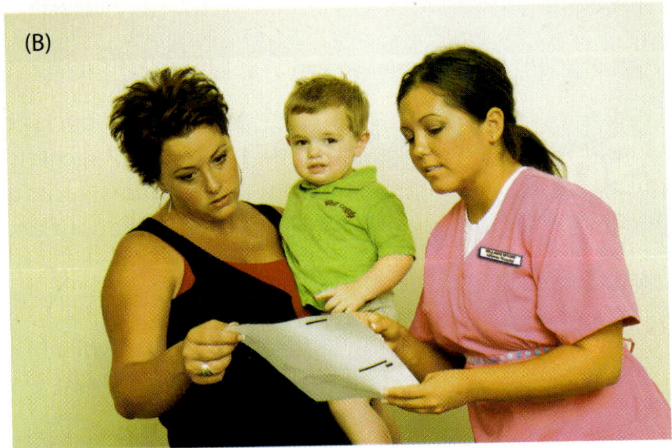

Figure 21-1 ■ (a) The medical assistant communicates with the toddler by getting down to his level and allowing him to examine the equipment. (b) The medical assistant adopts a more professional demeanor when communicating with the patient's mother.

AGE-APPROPRIATE COMMUNICATION

Age- and education-appropriate communication is important in developing a relationship with the patient and the patient's family; especially in the field of pediatrics. Figure 21-1 illustrates the differences in the way the medical assistant communicates with the patient and the way she communicates with the patient's mother.

Speaking down to or over the head of an individual often creates barriers that hinder high standards of care, which may decrease patient compliance. Remember when conversing with a parent or adult caregiver of a young child that it is important to speak to the adult's level of understanding. Remain professional and use correct but understandable terminology. Address parents by name and not "mommy" or "daddy." The medical assistant must remember that he is no longer speaking to the infant or young child.

Communication with small children often involves nonverbal interactions. Language may not yet be developed; therefore, expressions and motions must be considered. Often spoken language from the caregiver will conflict with the nonverbal communication from the infant. The health care worker must be aware of these possible contradictions. Squeals may be interpreted as pain or pleasure. A single word or sound may have multiple meanings. Caregivers are often the only interpreters available.

When speaking with older children or adolescents, a communication barrier may exist. Current terms and expressions might be used by the patient that the medical assistant finds unfamiliar. Never assume a meaning or an intention. Always attempt to clarify what the

CRITICAL THINKING CHALLENGE

While gathering patient history information, Ben, a 16-year-old patient, begins to use profanities that make you feel uncomfortable. He is watching you intently, while smirking. He also explains that his mom hates it when he uses "cuss" words, but that she is mean and just doesn't understand.

1. How should you respond to Ben?
2. What are Ben's intentions?
3. Should you say something to the provider or to Ben's parents?

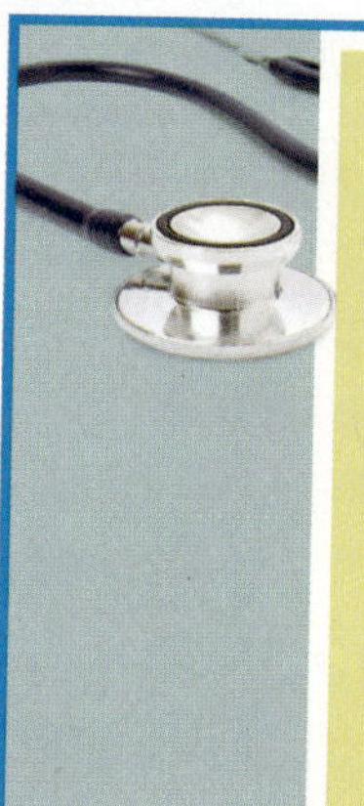

Field Smarts

If a child is in the 10th percentile for the child's height, it means that based on averages, the child is shorter than 90 percent of other children in the same age range. If a child is in the 90th percentile for the child's height, it means that based on averages, only 10 percent of children in the same age range are taller than the patient being measured.

patient is communicating. Consider that the patient may be attempting to test your reaction to words and phrases. Do you show disapproval, embarrassment, or acceptance?

Communication, if appropriate, can be a major tool for successful evaluations and examinations. It can assist in providing quality health care while increasing patient and parent compliance.

INFANT/TODDLER MEASUREMENTS

Infants and toddlers proceed through a rapid period of growth and change. Accurate and consistent measurements are necessary to evaluate normal and abnormal growth patterns. Trends are often tracked to identify any potential health care problems. Early detection is the key to prompt intervention. The medical assistant must be proficient in obtaining these measurements for evaluation. Sometimes, the behavior of young infants and toddlers can be unpredictable. For this reason, the medical assistant must be creative and flexible. Encourage parental assistance instead of interference while being tolerant and empathetic. Use of distraction methods is an effective technique in this age group.

Height/Length

Height/length and weight measurements in the young child can be an indicator of potential health problems. The medical assistant must be proficient in obtaining these measurements for all levels of pediatric patients. Members of the pediatric team must perform procedures similarly to ensure consistency and accuracy.

Accurate documentation on approved records and charts is necessary to enable the health provider to assess growth patterns. The National Center for Health Statistics provides charts for height, weight, and head circumference. Figure 21-2 illustrates various growth charts, based on gender and age.

These charts use **percentiles**, which compare the child's measurements with an average range of growth for children in the United States. Many factors might come into play when assessing the measurement, including but not limited to, **familial stature**, gestational age at birth, and chronic disease. Refer to Figure 21-3 for an example of a growth chart that has been plotted.

When measuring the length of an infant, it is often helpful to have a second set of hands, possibly those of the parent or guardian. Children younger than two years of age are measured in a supine position with the body fully extended.

When using a caliper (an instrument used to measure the distance between two points), the top of the infant's head is placed against the stationary head board of the caliper and the bottom of the foot is placed against the sliding foot board (Figure 21-4). Refer to Procedure 21-1 for detailed instructions on obtaining a height measurement. An alternative method is using a tape measure. The infant is placed in a supine position on the exam table with its legs fully extended. A tape measure is then placed along the side of the infant's body and the measurement is recorded. A pencil mark is quickly made on the table paper at the top of the head and the bottom of the heel. The infant is then removed from the exam table and the distance between the two marks is measured to determine the length of the infant. It is important to measure in a straight line for accuracy.

Children who are older than two years of age can be measured while standing on an upright scale. Remove the patient's shoes and have the patient stand erect. Bring the slide bar down so that it is flat against the patient's

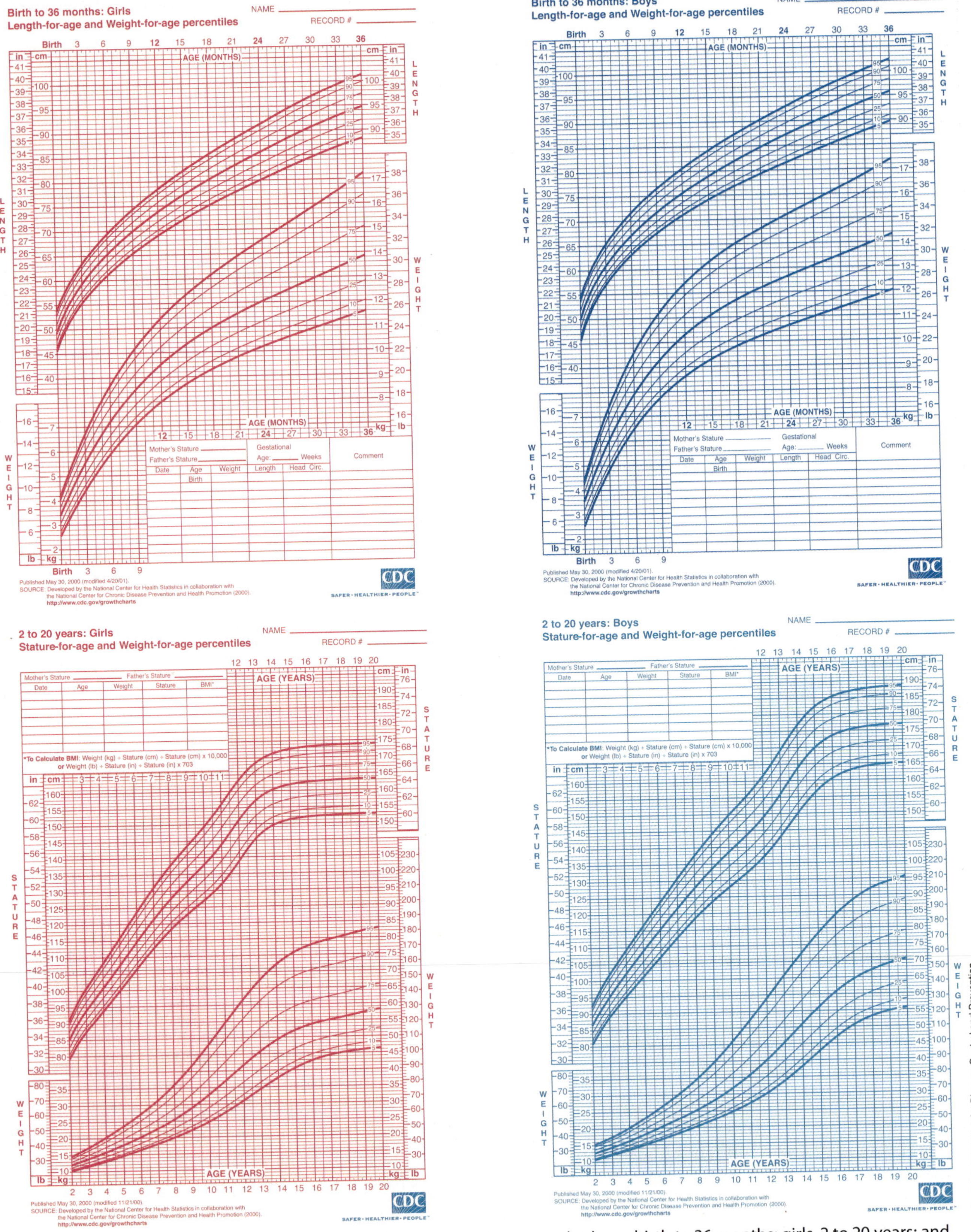

Figure 21-2 ■ Height and weight growth charts for girls, birth to 36 months; boys, birth to 36 months; girls, 2 to 20 years; and boys, 2 to 20 years.

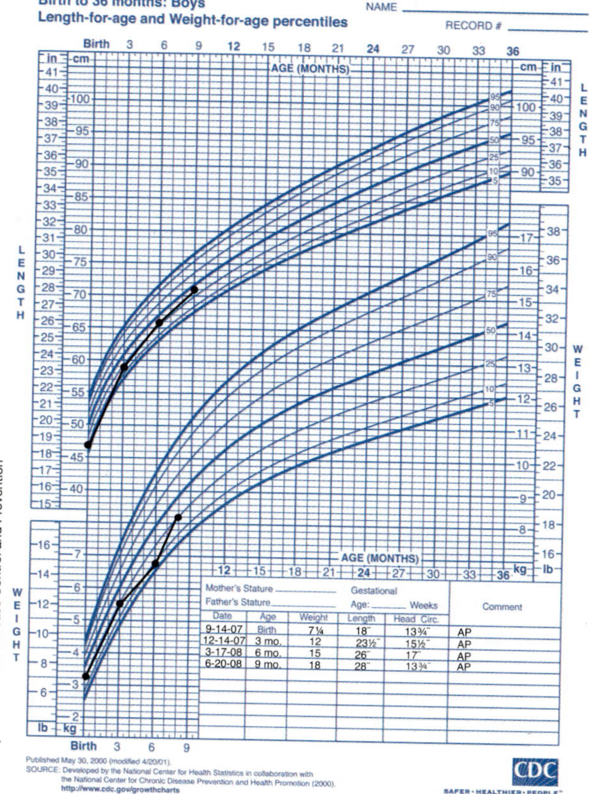

Figure 21-3 ■ A growth chart with patient information plotted and documented.

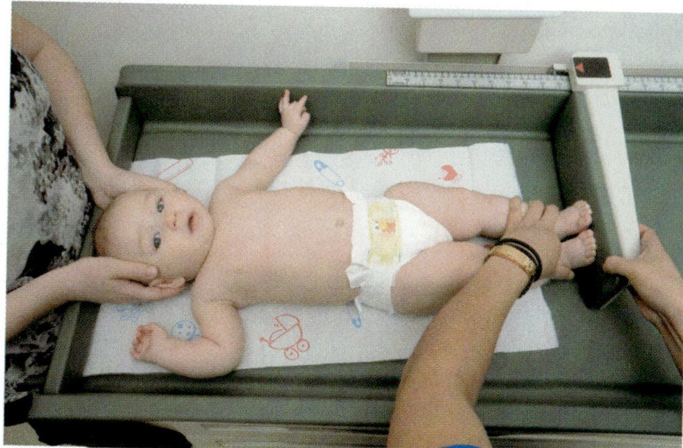

Figure 21-4 ■ Recumbent length measurement using a table scale.

head at a 90 degree angle. The child should look straight ahead and stand still during the measurement, which is sometimes very challenging for younger children.

Weight

Weight measurements provide another means for evaluating the pediatric patient's growth and development. As with height, accurate measurement and documentation on a standardized growth chart is an important skill for the medical assistant. Young infants are weighed directly on an infant scale or table scale (Figure 21-5). Ideally, they should be weighed without clothing or only in a fresh diaper. Remember, any paper, diaper, or clothing also has mass; therefore, these items need to be weighed individually and subtracted from the total weight, if left on during the measurement.

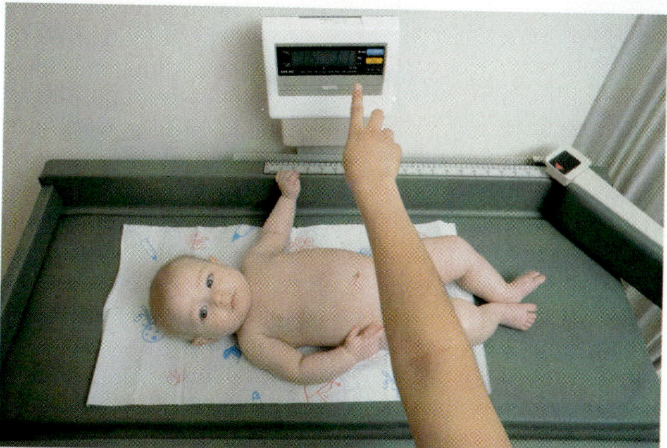

Figure 21-5 ■ Example of a baby being weighed using an infant table scale.

As children get older, screening techniques must be tailored to the comfort level of the child. Young children can often be weighed in their clothing, using a standing scale. As they move into school age, a gown can be worn for overall comfort and accurate evaluation. The weights of the gowns and underwear do not need to be determined for the older child because a fluctuation of ounces in these children would not be nearly as significant as they would be for an infant. The use of consistent equipment is important.

Circumferences

Accurate head circumferences record the growth of the cranium and the brain. Abnormally large or small head sizes must be monitored closely. **Macrocephaly**, an abnormally large head, may indicate a pathologic disorder. This is often indicated if the head circumference measurement is larger than the 97th percentile. Again, familial or genetic trends also need to be considered before jumping to conclusions. **Microcephaly**, an abnormally small head, may also indicate an abnormal condition, such as a genetic disorder.

When measuring the head circumference, it is important to consistently measure the same area of the head. Place the tape measure just above the eyebrows making sure that it fits snuggly and lies over the occipital protuberance and the supraorbital prominence (Figure 21-6). The circumference can be documented in either inches or centimeters according to office protocol.

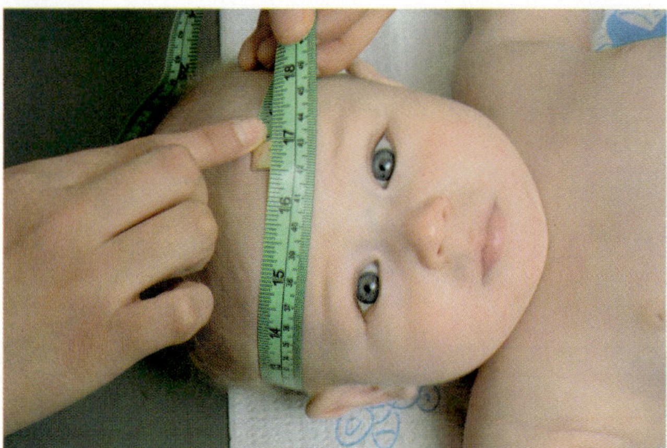

Figure 21-6 ■ The correct area for measuring head circumference.

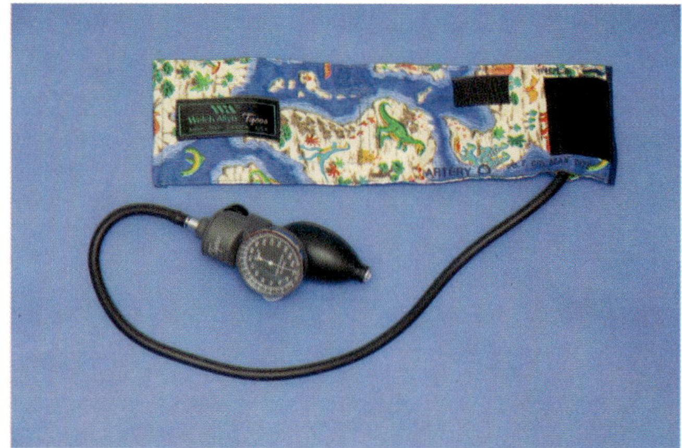

Figure 21-7 ■ A brightly colored pediatric blood pressure cuff.

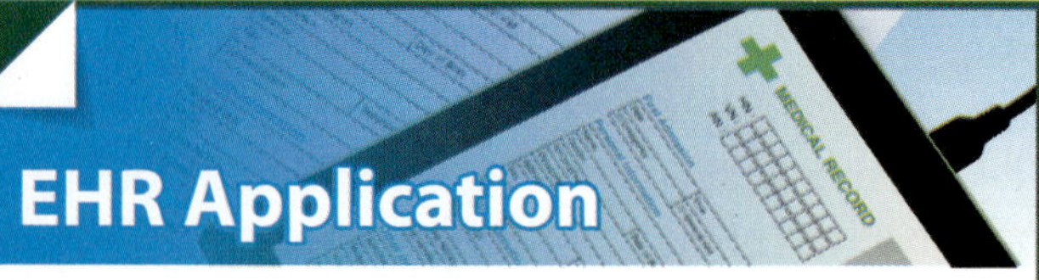

EHR Application

Many EHR software programs include graphing features. To graph growth percentiles on an electronic growth chart, you just click on the appropriate tab and enter the measurements within the requested field; the computer automatically graphs the measurements onto the electronic growth chart. Electronic results are usually more accurate because you don't have to rely on the naked eye to trace where the horizontal line matches up with the vertical line.

Abdominal circumference may be ordered to evaluate a problem with one of the abdominal organs or abnormal swelling of the abdomen. If the health care provider requests an abdominal circumference, identify the umbilicus when documenting results.

Pediatric Vital Signs

Obtaining vital signs on the pediatric patient may be a bit challenging at times. Blood pressures are usually not obtained until the age of two. The size of the blood pressure cuff must be proportionate to the size of the patient. Cuffs come in various sizes to match the stages of child development. A child cuff is normally used on smaller children; however, a larger child may require the use of an adult cuff, just as a petite adult might require the use of a pediatric cuff. Size is important in the accuracy of blood pressure measurement.

New or unfamiliar equipment is often traumatic for a young child. Many pediatric offices purchase equipment that is appealing to children. Pediatric cuffs are supplied in a variety of different colors and with different characters and scenes on the outside of the cuff (Figure 21-7). Allow the child to safely touch and test the sphygmomanometer and stethoscope (Figure 21-8). Demonstration of the procedure on the parent or older sibling often helps relieve anxiety. Another comforting method is to allow the young child to perform the procedure on a doll or stuffed animal. Of course, this should always be supervised for safety. Role playing and games often make evaluation tests more tolerable, even for the medical assistant.

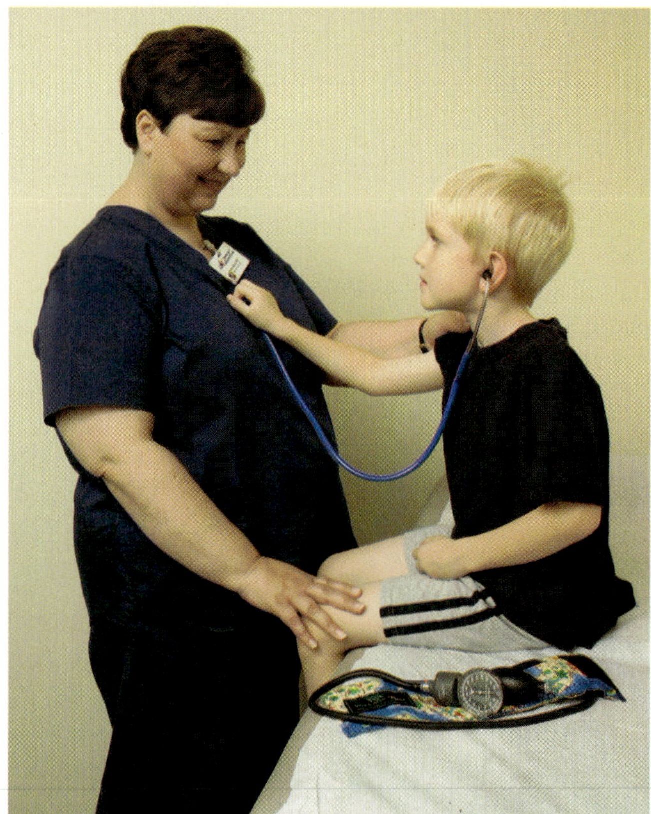

Figure 21-8 ■ The child listens to the medical assistant's heart before she listens to his heart.

The pulse rate in a child varies with age and growth. Most average pulse rates refer to a resting pulse. The primary locations for measuring pulse in infants and young children are different than the locations used for measuring pulse in the adult. The radial artery is normally used to check pulse rate on older children and adults but the radial artery is not very prominent in infants and small children. The femoral or brachial arteries (Figure 21-9) are the arteries of choice for pulse rate in infants and young children.

The most accurate method for obtaining heart rate is through auscultation (listening to the heart with a stethoscope). As the child ages and develops, the radial pulse becomes easier to obtain.

Respirations in the infant and toddler can be measured along with the pulse. The rates will vary, depending on the level of activity or illness. Remember that a fever can elevate the respiratory and pulse rate. Refer to Table 21-1 for normal ranges of pulse and respiratory rates as well as blood pressure in pediatrics.

Obtaining an accurate body temperature is another skill that is essential for the medical assistant. Fevers are quite common in pediatric patients and often their fevers have higher peaks than fevers that are typically seen in adult patients. There are several methods that can be used to obtain a body temperature reading on a pediatric patient.

In children and adolescents, auditory canal or aural readings are quick and relatively comfortable, which encourages patient compliance. Infants younger than two months of age are best evaluated with a temporal thermometer (refer to Chapter 11 for a further discussion of temporal temperatures). If it is necessary to obtain a rectal temperature reading, it must be completed with extreme caution, as it is moderately invasive. Refer to Procedure 21-2 for a detailed instruction and rationale for obtaining body temperature readings in the pediatric patient.

Pediatric measurements and vital signs are key evaluation tools for identification of any potential disorders.

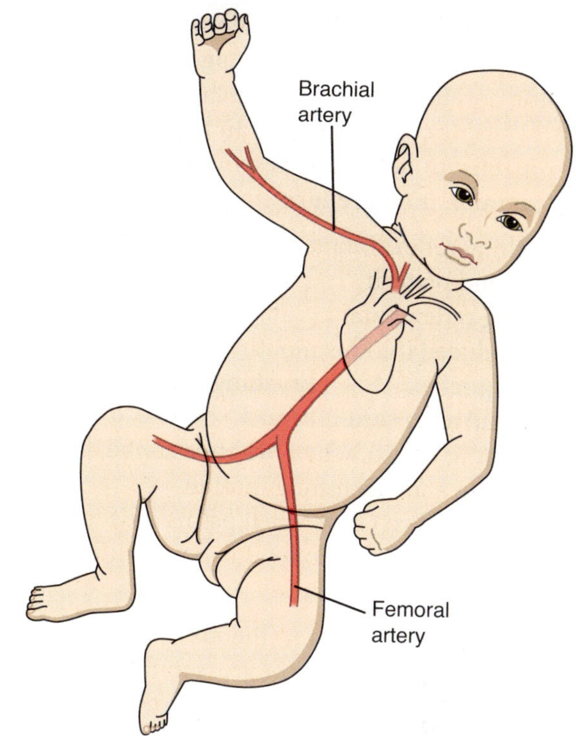

Figure 21-9 ■ The pulse is taken in the brachial or femoral artery in an infant.

PEDIATRIC DEVELOPMENT

In addition to physical measurements used to evaluate pediatric progress, other areas of growth and development include **motor**, **sensory**, and **language development**. Different ages have normal **milestones**, which indicate acceptable growth and development patterns; however, keep in mind that all children develop at their own pace and just because a child doesn't reach a specific milestone at the age listed doesn't mean there is a problem. The provider will use many tools to assess a child's progress.

Motor Development

Motor skills provide visible and exciting changes in the growth of the child. These are usually celebrated developments that are documented by parents and compared for generations. **Motor development** allows the

Table 21-1 Average Heart Rates, Respiratory Rates, and Blood Pressures in Pediatrics

Age	Average Heart Rate Beats per Minute (BPM)	Average Respiratory Rate	BP (Systolic)	BP (Diastolic)
Newborn to 3 months	80–160	30–60/min	<60–70 mmHg	—
3 months to 2 years	75–160	30–60/min	<70–74 mmHg	—
2 to 3 years	60–140	24–40/min	84–113 mmHg	39–69 mmHg
2–10 years	60–140	18–30/min	84–123 mmHg	39–82 mmHg
10 and above	60–100	12–16/min	100–139 mmHg	59–89 mmHg

child to develop more independence, which encourages sensory, cognitive, and language growth.

Motor development usually includes three areas of growth: **reflexes**, gross motor, and fine motor skills. Reflexes refer to automatic responses to any stimulation. Common infant reflexes are listed below:

- Breathing reflex: Infant displays a normal breathing depth and pattern
- Sucking reflex: Infant is able to suck when a nipple is introduced into his mouth
- Rooting reflex: When brushing the cheek, the infant turns toward it to suck
- Swimming reflex: When held horizontal, begins stretching and swimming motion
- Grasping reflex: Grips when palms are touched
- Moro reflex: Startles to loud banging and other environmental stimuli

These reflexes are seen in the normal newborn and lead to voluntary responses or gross motor skills. Gross motor skills include motions such as rolling, scooting, crawling, and walking.

Just as gross motor skills involve the development of large muscles groups, fine motor skills develop by utilizing smaller movements. These include motions such as touching, grabbing, poking, pulling, and pinching. Gross and fine motor skills often develop during the same time periods, usually complementing each other's growth. Refer to Table 21-2 for a general timetable for normal gross and fine motor development.

Sensory Development

During motor development, sensory, perceptual, and cognitive growth is also progressing. Vision and hearing are improving along with depth perception and motion assessment. All of these **sensory developments** continue to promote further motor development. Any single area that exhibits impairments will affect the growth in other areas of development. For example, if vision is impaired, some fine motor skills may be slow to develop and a lack of depth perception can inhibit gross motor skills.

Visual development involves increasing distances in sight as the brain matures. This maturation allows for better focus and increased tracking of objects as the child grows. Color perception also develops with normal growth.

Hearing improves in normal sensory development as the child matures. Varying pitches and frequencies can be differentiated. Notice how babies listen to cooing or baby talk from others. A positive response occurs with higher pitched baby jargon. As they grow and develop, deeper noises also attract interest. The ability to locate sounds also occurs as the child develops. Initially, infants have a difficult time identifying the direction of a noise or voice. As they develop, they are better able to locate the noise.

Language Development

From infancy forward, the child begins with noises that elicit a response. This progresses to words, phrases, and finally sentences. Normal language milestones help identify intellectual development. The timing may differ due to educational and environmental circumstances, but it appears that universal trends occur in language development. Refer to Table 21-3 for normal developmental trends in language.

Table 21-2 Normal Gross and Fine Motor Developmental Milestones

Patient's Age (Months)	Gross Motor Development	Fine Motor Development
Newborn to 1 month		The hands are in fists and the hands and legs are pulled inward and upward to the body
2	Lifts the head when on stomach	
3	Rolls over; sits when propped	Touches an object
6	Sits without support	Grabs an object and holds
8	Stands with support	Transfers an object between hands
9	Walks while holding on	Attempts to catch thrown objects
9–10	Stands alone	Uses thumb with forefinger to grasp
12–15	Walks alone	
17	Walks on stairs with help	
20	Kicks a ball	

Table 21-3 Language Development in the Pediatric Patient

Patient's Age (Months)	Language Development Trends
Newborn	Reflexive: cries, expressions
2	Coos, cries, laughs
3–6	Squeals, trills, uses vowel sounds
6–10	Babbles, repeats sounds
10–12	Understands simple words and commands
13–18	Speaks first true words and number of words begins to increase rapidly
20	Starts putting words together into very short sentences
24	Puts longer sentences together

Disclaimer: The above ages are merely guidelines and not exact. Because of the differences from one child to the next, one may perform tasks at a certain age while another will not. This does not necessarily indicate a cause for alarm.

VISUAL AND HEARING SCREENINGS

Sight and hearing screenings are also conducted at different age intervals throughout a child's development. Periodic screenings can alert the provider to potential problems that can be treated or corrected.

Visual

Pediatric visual screenings and examinations begin in infancy. Charts used to conduct pediatric visual screenings are discussed in Chapter 13.

Prior to early school age, visual milestones are evaluated. These include blinking, fixation on objects, coordination of eye movements, and reaching for objects. The medical assistant can help the health provider evaluate these milestones. Shaking eye movements and wandering eyes might also be observed and documented.

As the child matures, more standard eye exams can be utilized to test visual acuity. Pediatric visual screenings are performed utilizing an age appropriate chart, refer back to Chapter 13, Procedure 13-1, which lists the steps involved.

Auditory

Screening for hearing in the newborn and infant begins immediately at birth. Newborn hearing exams are mandated to be completed prior to discharge from the birth hospital in many states. Communication with parents or caregivers may enlighten the health care provider to signs of a hearing deficit. Clues include responses to loud noises, facial expressions, and turning the head toward noises.

IMMUNIZATIONS

In an effort to prevent the spread of identified communicable diseases, a series of **immunizations** (or **vaccinations**) has been recommended by the Centers for Disease Control and Prevention, American Academy of Pediatrics, American Academy of Family Practitioners, and the World Health Organization.

Schedules

Pediatric schedules include the suggested age of the patient along with the specific immunizations (IMZ) for the country in which the patient lives. The Centers for Disease Control and Prevention (CDC) provides guidelines for immunizations. The medical assistant is often responsible for administration of the vaccination, either orally, topically, or by injection. In addition, the medical assistant will be involved in providing the necessary patient education related to the risks and side effects of each individual vaccine. For a detailed description of the childhood immunization schedule along with concise descriptions of each vaccine, refer to Figure 21-10.

Controversies

Even as the infant mortality rate has improved due to the increased provision of vaccinations throughout the world, health concerns and patient rights topics have created additional controversy. Risks versus benefits associated with vaccines need to be understood by the medical assistant along with the parents/patient. In the United States, immunizations are voluntary.

Refer parents to appropriate website to enable them to make educated decisions regarding their children. The World Health Organization's website, www.WHO.int, discusses suggested schedules along with vaccine safety. The Global Advisory Committee in Vaccine Safety (GACVS) is also a useful resource. When discussing these choices, do not belittle personal preferences such as religious beliefs. The CDC provides vaccine information statements that are given to the patient and caregiver prior to vaccination. An educated choice by the parents is the desired outcome along with respecting patient rights.

Documentation of the vaccine must be thorough. Figure 21-11 is a screen shot from Harris CareTracker illustrating the information that needs to be entered when documenting an immunization. The information should automatically populate in the immunization log section of the EHR after entering the pertinent information (Figure 21-12). Caregivers should sign a consent form for every immunization given and should receive a vaccination information statement (VIS) (Figure 21-13).

Figure 1. Recommended immunization schedule for persons aged 0 through 18 years—United States, 2015.
(FOR THOSE WHO FALL BEHIND OR START LATE, SEE THE CATCH-UP SCHEDULE [FIGURE 2]).

These recommendations must be read with the footnotes that follow. For those who fall behind or start late, provide catch-up vaccination at the earliest opportunity as indicated by the green bars in Figure 1. To determine minimum intervals between doses, see the catch-up schedule (Figure 2). School entry and adolescent vaccine age groups are shaded.

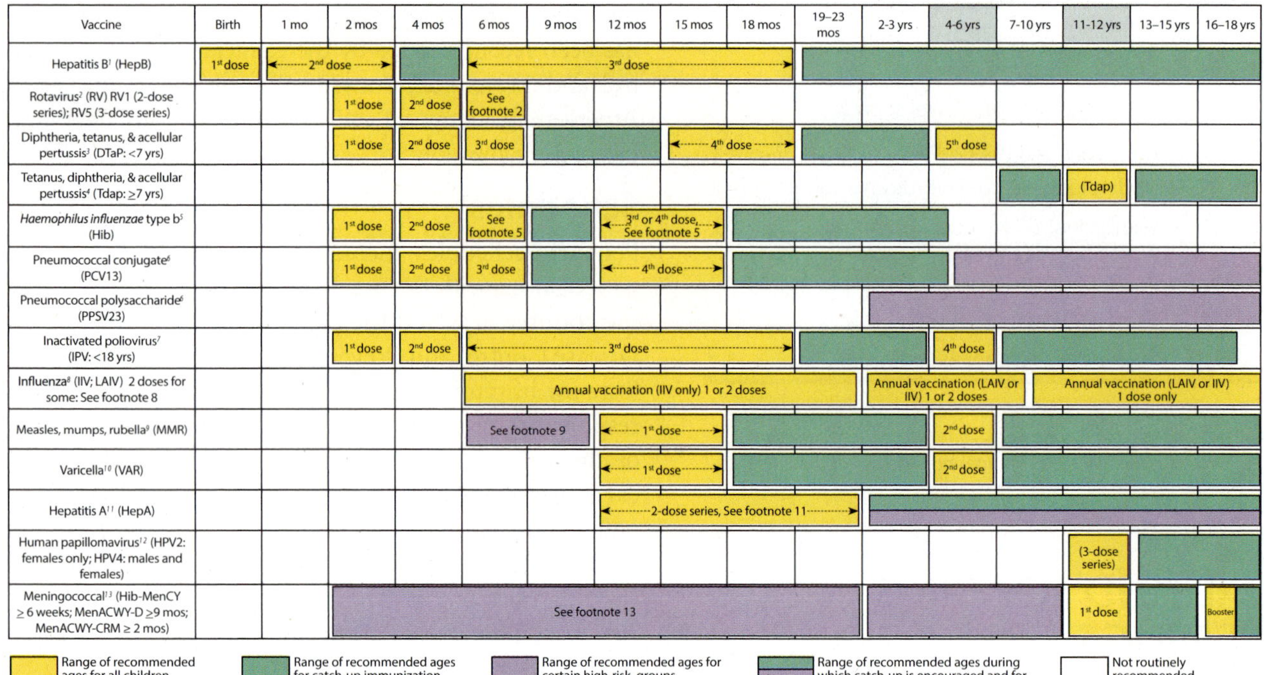

Vaccine	Birth	1 mo	2 mos	4 mos	6 mos	9 mos	12 mos	15 mos	18 mos	19–23 mos	2-3 yrs	4-6 yrs	7-10 yrs	11-12 yrs	13–15 yrs	16–18 yrs
Hepatitis B[1] (HepB)	1st dose	←2nd dose→			←3rd dose→											
Rotavirus[2] (RV) RV1 (2-dose series); RV5 (3-dose series)			1st dose	2nd dose	See footnote 2											
Diphtheria, tetanus, & acellular pertussis[3] (DTaP: <7 yrs)			1st dose	2nd dose	3rd dose			←4th dose→				5th dose				
Tetanus, diphtheria, & acellular pertussis[4] (Tdap: ≥7 yrs)														(Tdap)		
Haemophilus influenzae type b[5] (Hib)			1st dose	2nd dose	See footnote 5		←3rd or 4th dose, See footnote 5→									
Pneumococcal conjugate[6] (PCV13)			1st dose	2nd dose	3rd dose		←4th dose→									
Pneumococcal polysaccharide[6] (PPSV23)																
Inactivated poliovirus[7] (IPV: <18 yrs)			1st dose	2nd dose	←3rd dose→							4th dose				
Influenza[8] (IIV; LAIV) 2 doses for some: See footnote 8					Annual vaccination (IIV only) 1 or 2 doses						Annual vaccination (LAIV or IIV) 1 or 2 doses		Annual vaccination (LAIV or IIV) 1 dose only			
Measles, mumps, rubella[9] (MMR)					See footnote 9		←1st dose→					2nd dose				
Varicella[10] (VAR)							←1st dose→					2nd dose				
Hepatitis A[11] (HepA)							←2-dose series, See footnote 11→									
Human papillomavirus[12] (HPV2: females only; HPV4: males and females)														(3-dose series)		
Meningococcal[13] (Hib-MenCY ≥ 6 weeks; MenACWY-D ≥9 mos; MenACWY-CRM ≥ 2 mos)			See footnote 13											1st dose		Booster

Range of recommended ages for all children | Range of recommended ages for catch-up immunization | Range of recommended ages for certain high-risk groups | Range of recommended ages during which catch-up is encouraged and for certain high-risk groups | Not routinely recommended

This schedule includes recommendations in effect as of January 1, 2015. Any dose not administered at the recommended age should be administered at a subsequent visit, when indicated and feasible. The use of a combination vaccine generally is preferred over separate injections of its equivalent component vaccines. Vaccination providers should consult the relevant Advisory Committee on Immunization Practices (ACIP) statement for detailed recommendations, available online at http://www.cdc.gov/vaccines/hcp/acip-recs/index.html. Clinically significant adverse events that follow vaccination should be reported to the Vaccine Adverse Event Reporting System (VAERS) online (http://www.vaers.hhs.gov) or by telephone (800-822-7967). Suspected cases of vaccine-preventable diseases should be reported to the state or local health department. Additional information, including precautions and contraindications for vaccination, is available from CDC online (http://www.cdc.gov/vaccines/recs/vac-admin/contraindications.htm) or by telephone (800-CDC-INFO [800-232-4636]).

This schedule is approved by the Advisory Committee on Immunization Practices (http//www.cdc.gov/vaccines/acip), the American Academy of Pediatrics (http://www.aap.org), the American Academy of Family Physicians (http://www.aafp.org), and the American College of Obstetricians and Gynecologists (http://www.acog.org).

NOTE: The above recommendations must be read along with the footnotes of this schedule.

Figure 21-10 ■ The recommended immunization schedule for infants to adolescents.

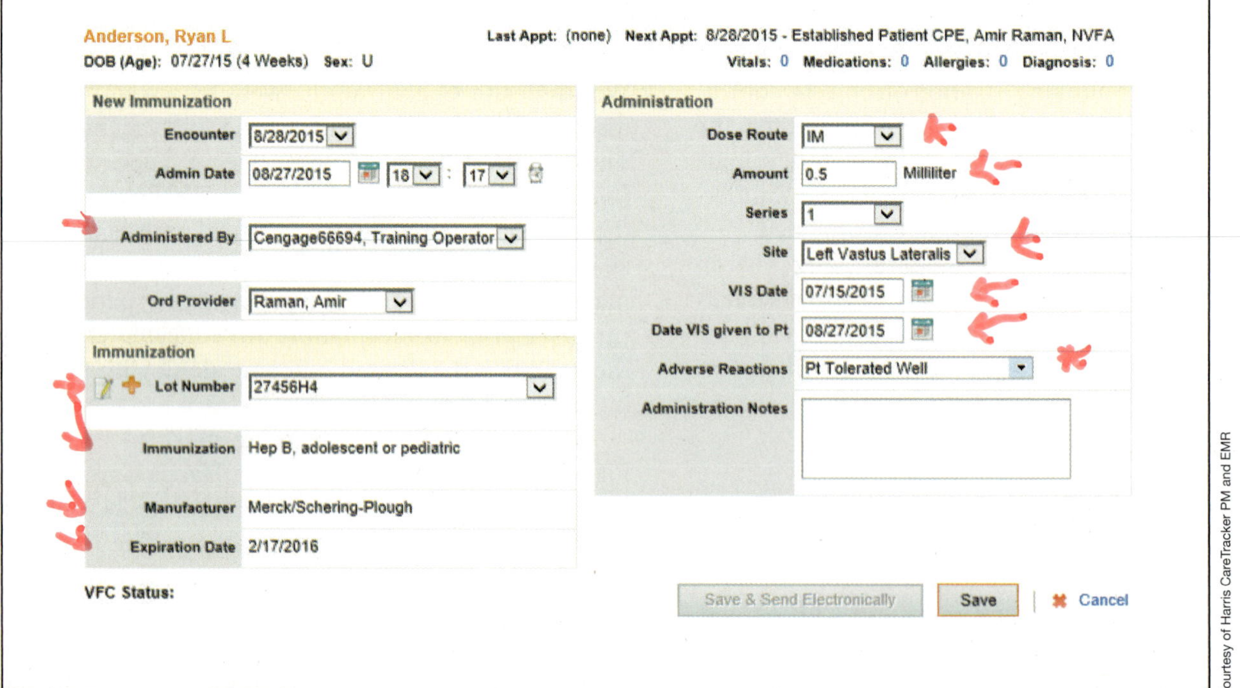

Anderson, Ryan L
DOB (Age): 07/27/15 (4 Weeks) Sex: U
Last Appt: (none) Next Appt: 8/28/2015 - Established Patient CPE, Amir Raman, NVFA
Vitals: 0 Medications: 0 Allergies: 0 Diagnosis: 0

New Immunization
Encounter: 8/28/2015
Admin Date: 08/27/2015 18 : 17
Administered By: Cengage66694, Training Operator
Ord Provider: Raman, Amir

Immunization
Lot Number: 27456H4
Immunization: Hep B, adolescent or pediatric
Manufacturer: Merck/Schering-Plough
Expiration Date: 2/17/2016

Administration
Dose Route: IM
Amount: 0.5 Milliliter
Series: 1
Site: Left Vastus Lateralis
VIS Date: 07/15/2015
Date VIS given to Pt: 08/27/2015
Adverse Reactions: Pt Tolerated Well
Administration Notes:

VFC Status:

Save & Send Electronically | Save | Cancel

Figure 21-11 ■ An example of an infant immunization entry screen from Harris CareTracker. Notice all of the information that needs to be entered when documenting an immunization.

Anderson, Ryan L
Chart #326525
DOB 07/27/15 (1 mos/0 wks)
Sex Unknown

PCP N/A Insurance N/A
Next Appt 08/28/15 Established Patient CPE

Info Viewer Prog Rx Order OrdSet Immu Attach Recalls Letters MsgCntr Edu Refer E&M Visit

Chart Summary
Problem List
Medications
Allergies
Immunizations
Vital Signs
Progress Notes

All | Last Encounter | Past 6 months | Past Year | Immunization Schedules: Adult | Child

Send to Registry

Add Past/Refused Immunization

Immunizations

Immunization	CPT	Date	Admin Provider	Series	Amount	Refused
Hep B, adolescent or pediatric	90744	08/27/15	Cengage88694, Training Operator	1	0.5 Milliliter	No

Courtesy of Harris CareTracker PM and EMR

Figure 21-12 ■ Example of an immunization log in the patient's EHR.

VACCINE INFORMATION STATEMENT

Hib Vaccine

(*Haemophilus Influenzae* Type b)

What You Need to Know

Many Vaccine Information Statements are available in Spanish and other languages. See www.immunize.org/vis

Hojas de información sobre vacunas están disponibles en español y en muchos otros idiomas. Visite www.immunize.org/vis

1 Why get vaccinated?

Haemophilus influenzae type b (Hib) disease is a serious disease caused by bacteria. It usually affects children under 5 years old. It can also affect adults with certain medical conditions.

Your child can get Hib disease by being around other children or adults who may have the bacteria and not know it. The germs spread from person to person. If the germs stay in the child's nose and throat, the child probably will not get sick. But sometimes the germs spread into the lungs or the bloodstream, and then Hib can cause serious problems. This is called invasive Hib disease.

Before Hib vaccine, Hib disease was the leading cause of bacterial meningitis among children under 5 years old in the United States. Meningitis is an infection of the lining of the brain and spinal cord. It can lead to brain damage and deafness. Hib disease can also cause:

- pneumonia
- severe swelling in the throat, making it hard to breathe
- infections of the blood, joints, bones, and covering of the heart
- death

Before Hib vaccine, about 20,000 children in the United States under 5 years old got Hib disease each year, and about 3% - 6% of them died.

Hib vaccine can prevent Hib disease. Since use of Hib vaccine began, the number of cases of invasive Hib disease has decreased by more than 99%. Many more children would get Hib disease if we stopped vaccinating.

2 Hib vaccine

Several different brands of Hib vaccine are available. Your child will receive either 3 or 4 doses, depending on which vaccine is used.

Doses of Hib vaccine are usually recommended at these ages:

- First Dose: 2 months of age
- Second Dose: 4 months of age
- Third Dose: 6 months of age (if needed, depending on brand of vaccine)
- Final/Booster Dose: 12–15 months of age

Hib vaccine may be given at the same time as other vaccines.

Hib vaccine may be given as part of a combination vaccine. Combination vaccines are made when two or more types of vaccine are combined together into a single shot, so that one vaccination can protect against more than one disease.

Children over 5 years old and adults usually do not need Hib vaccine. But it may be recommended for older children or adults with asplenia or sickle cell disease, before surgery to remove the spleen, or following a bone marrow transplant. It may also be recommended for people 5 to 18 years old with HIV. Ask your doctor for details.

Your doctor or the person giving you the vaccine can give you more information.

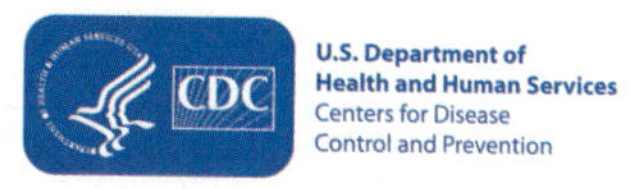

Courtesy of U.S. Department of Health and Human Services, Centers for Disease Control and Prevention

Figure 21-13 ■ Example of a vaccination immunization statement. Notice the date on the VIS form.

3 Some people should not get this vaccine

Hib vaccine should not be given to infants younger than 6 weeks of age.

A person who has ever had a life-threatening allergic reaction after a previous dose of Hib vaccine, OR has a severe allergy to any part of this vaccine, should not get Hib vaccine. *Tell the person giving the vaccine about any severe allergies.*

People who are mildly ill can get Hib vaccine. People who are moderately or severely ill should probably wait until they recover. Talk to your healthcare provider if the person getting the vaccine isn't feeling well on the day the shot is scheduled.

4 Risks of a vaccine reaction

With any medicine, including vaccines, there is a chance of side effects. These are usually mild and go away on their own. Serious reactions are also possible but are rare.

Most people who get Hib vaccine do not have any problems with it.

Mild Problems following Hib vaccine:

- redness, warmth, or swelling where the shot was given
- fever

These problems are uncommon. If they occur, they usually begin soon after the shot and last 2 or 3 days.

Problems that could happen after any vaccine:
Any medication can cause a severe allergic reaction. Such reactions from a vaccine are very rare, estimated at fewer than 1 in a million doses, and would happen within a few minutes to a few hours after the vaccination.

As with any medicine, there is a very remote chance of a vaccine causing a serious injury or death.

Older children, adolescents, and adults might also experience these problems after any vaccine:

- People sometimes faint after a medical procedure, including vaccination. Sitting or lying down for about 15 minutes can help prevent fainting, and injuries caused by a fall. Tell your doctor if you feel dizzy, or have vision changes or ringing in the ears.
- Some people get severe pain in the shoulder and have difficulty moving the arm where a shot was given. This happens very rarely.

The safety of vaccines is always being monitored. For more information, visit: **www.cdc.gov/vaccinesafety/**

5 What if there is a serious reaction?

What should I look for?

- Look for anything that concerns you, such as signs of a **severe allergic reaction**, very high fever, or unusual behavior.

  Signs of a severe allergic reaction can include hives, swelling of the face and throat, difficulty breathing, a fast heartbeat, dizziness, and weakness. These would usually start a few minutes to a few hours after the vaccination.

What should I do?

- If you think it is a severe allergic reaction or other emergency that can't wait, call 9-1-1 or get the person to the nearest hospital. Otherwise, call your doctor.
- Afterward, the reaction should be reported to the Vaccine Adverse Event Reporting System (VAERS). Your doctor might file this report, or you can do it yourself through the VAERS web site at **www.vaers.hhs.gov**, or by calling **1-800-822-7967**.

VAERS does not give medical advice.

6 The National Vaccine Injury Compensation Program

The National Vaccine Injury Compensation Program (VICP) is a federal program that was created to compensate people who may have been injured by certain vaccines.

Persons who believe they may have been injured by a vaccine can learn about the program and about filing a claim by calling **1-800-338-2382** or visiting the VICP website at **www.hrsa.gov/vaccinecompensation**. There is a time limit to file a claim for compensation.

7 How can I learn more?

- Ask your doctor. He or she can give you the vaccine package insert or suggest other sources of information.
- Call your local or state health department.
- Contact the Centers for Disease Control and Prevention (CDC):
  - Call **1-800-232-4636** (**1-800-CDC-INFO**) or
  - Visit CDC's website at **www.cdc.gov/vaccines**

Vaccine Information Statement
Hib Vaccine

4/02/2015

42 U.S.C. § 300aa-26

Office Use Only

Figure 21-13 ■ *(Continued)*

PEDIATRIC INJECTIONS

This chapter only covers the procedure for administering a pediatric injection. It does not cover preparing the medication or the seven rights associated with medication administration. Please refer to Chapter 32 for this information.

The medical assistant is often responsible for performing pediatric injections. Proper skills need to be developed for the comfort and safety of the patient. Undue trauma, either physical or emotional, needs to be minimized. Assistance from the parent or caregiver may be necessary.

Most pediatric injections are administered intramuscularly. The location of an intramuscular injection is usually the vastus lateralis muscle of the thigh in infants and very small children. The type of medication or vaccine administered will dictate the location of the injection. The age and size of the patient also helps to determine the most effective injection site. Table 21-4 compares the various sites.

An important part of the medical assistant's responsibility is to calm the patient both before and after the injection. Children are often alarmed about receiving an injection and every effort should be made to calm their fears so they are not apprehensive about receiving injections in the future. The medical assistant can be instrumental in achieving this goal.

Reducing Pain During Immunizations

- Most texts, including this one, teach that the skin should be held taut when administering intramuscular injections; however, grasping the skin by pinching up on the muscle and surrounding subcutaneous tissue may be used to help reduce discomfort during the injection. If this method is used, the needle should be slightly longer to ensure it reaches the muscle.
- Order of injections: Pain often increases with each new injection. When administering multiple immunizations, the more painful immunizations such as the MMR, PCV13, or HPV vaccines should be given last to decrease the amount of pain associated with the injection.

Table 21-4 **Intramuscular Injection Sites in the Pediatric Patient**

Injection Site	Maximum Amount	Age/Needle Size	Technique
Deltoid	1 mL	Not typically used until the child is three years of age or older. Provider preference will be the rule. Size of the needle: 5/8 to 1 inch (16 to 25 mm)	The deltoid is held taut. The needle is inserted into the muscle at a 90° angle.
Gluteal (Ventrogluteal) Iliac crest Anterior superior iliac spine Greater trochanter of femur	2 mL	Age two and older. Size of the needle: 1 to 1¼ inch (25 to 31 mm)	Place the child on one side or the other with the hip facing upward. The muscle is held taut and the needle is inserted into the muscle at a 90° angle.
Vastus lateralis	4 mL	Seven months and older. Length of the needle: Birth to 1 mo: 5/8" (16 mm) 1 mo/1 yr: 1" (25 mm) 1 to 18 yr: 1 to 1¼" (25 to 31 mm)	The infant is placed on the back, often in the lap of the caregiver. The parent can stabilize the patient. The muscle is held taut while also stabilizing the patient's leg. The injection is given at a 90° angle.

- Changes in Advisory Committee's Immunization Practices (ACIP) recommendations: The ACIP no longer recommends slow administration of immunizations or the practice of aspiration during injection procedures. Studies reveal that there have been no reported adverse effects for either one of these practices and that the patient tolerated the immunizations much better without aspiration and when pushing the medication in quickly.
- Using tactile stimulation (the rubbing or stroking of skin) near the injection site, both prior to and during the injection, may decrease pain associated with the procedure.

For more information, access the CDC website at www.cdc.gov and search "Vaccines."

As the child matures and can understand procedural explanations, honesty is important. Never promise the child, "This won't hurt." This will instill distrust for future injections, even to the point of hysteria. Provide an explanation of the minimal discomfort that might occur. Parent comfort may also be necessary. Parent involvement needs to be evaluated to ensure a positive encounter. Some parents may elicit a calming environment, while others may cause more anxiety for the patient. Once again the goal is to avoid future fears, making the provision of quality health care a realistic possibility. Refer to Procedure 21-4 for instructions on how to perform a pediatric injection.

Chapter 8 has several tips for communicating with pediatric patients and provides helpful hints for performing invasive procedures on children.

Intranasal Route for Giving Immunizations

Another method used for immunization administration in pediatric patients is the intranasal route. Intranasal means "pertaining to within the nasal cavity." There is only one vaccine given via this route, which is the live attenuated influenza vaccine (LAIV, Flumist). The vaccine is in a sprayer device divided into two equal parts (one for each nostril). The patient should be seated, sitting erect with the head tilted back. The medical assistant should place one hand behind the patient's head while placing the tip of the sprayer into one of the patient's nostrils with the other hand. The dose divider tip is removed and the procedure is repeated in the opposite nostril.

NEWBORN SCREENINGS

A complete evaluation of the newborn involves analysis of the blood to identify any potential diseases that may be treated early for better outcomes. Screening tests can be initiated in the hospital, but may occur up to seven days later. States have varying requirements as to what is included in the infant blood screenings. Capillary blood is collected from the infant's heal (Procedure 21-3) and may be tested for a variety of conditions or diseases. Newborn screening saves thousands of babies each year from disability and premature death. Screening requirements will vary by state policy. The following are examples of some of the screening tests required for newborns in different states:

- **Phenylketonuria (PKU)**: PKU is a congenital familial disease. Patients with this disorder are deficient in the enzyme phenylalanine hydroxylase, making them unable to metabolize or break down the amino acid phenylalanine. This causes increased levels of phenylalanine in the blood, which can cause mental retardation, seizures, and muscular difficulties. Since phenylalanine is present in milk, the test for PKU is attempted 24 hours after the ingestion of milk, either from the breast or formula. The evaluation will demonstrate whether or not phenylalanine has been metabolized. Most states require this blood test within the first several days of life. If not obtained, a urine test can be evaluated after six weeks of age. Prompt diagnosis is essential for a favorable prognosis so that a diet that restricts phenylalanine (often seen in meat and dairy products) can be quickly implemented. A procedure for collecting a sample for PKU testing can be found in Procedure 21-3.
- **Hypothyroidism**: The decreased function of the thyroid gland affects the metabolism of the infant. A thyroid panel assists the provider in making a diagnosis.
- **Galactosemia**: This condition is characterized by the inability to metabolize galactose and is the result of an absence of one of two enzymes that are needed to convert galactose into glucose.

Other blood tests may also be ordered depending on the state. Check your state's guidelines for additional testing.

CIRCUMCISION

Circumcision, or removal of foreskin of the penis, is commonly performed on newborn infants while they are still in the hospital after birth. However, due to unforeseen circumstances, the procedure is sometimes performed in the office. The decision to have a child circumcised is a family decision and not a medical decision in the majority of children. The medical assistant must remain unbiased, empathetic, and supportive during the decision process.

Health Coach

Suddent Infant Death Syndrome (SIDS)

Sudden infant death syndrome (SIDS) is the second leading cause of death of infants in the United States. It is often related to nighttime apnea (stoppage of breathing for approximately 20 seconds). SIDS is the death of an infant, usually under one year of age, with no known cause. If a cause is identified, it is not SIDS. Apnea combined with bradycardia (slow pulse) is a precursor of SIDS, which usually occurs from the second to the fourth month, but not exclusively. Pathological changes may be related to the respiratory, cardiovascular, or nervous system. Discussing measures such as limiting smoking during pregnancy and after birth, reducing low birth rates, and placing sleeping infants on their backs has reduced the number of SIDS deaths. If a family loses a child to SIDS, reinforce that there is no known cause of SIDS. It cannot be predicted and fault cannot be placed on the caregiver if an infant dies of SIDS.

Health Coach

Childhood Obesity

Childhood obesity is becoming a serious problem in today's society. Many factors contribute to this problem, including genetics. Most families are dual employed leaving children to prepare their own nutritionally challenged meals. Some parents are so fatigued after a long day that fast food is often the meal of choice. Many households have televisions and computers that have become the primary focus instead of some type of physical activity. Obesity leads to many disorders as the child grows, including diabetes, heart disease, orthopedic injuries, and respiratory disorders. Proper nutrition and exercise need to be addressed early in a child's development to prevent obesity from occurring.

Some community health centers now have kitchens to teach mom and children how to prepare nutritious meals. Getting everyone involved helps assists with overall compliance.

ADOLESCENT CARE

The period of adolescence begins at the onset of puberty. This is when the secondary sex characteristics emerge. This is also the time frame when youths attempt to display more independence. Exploration into various avenues, such as drugs, tobacco, alcohol, and other substances that alter the mind, can occur. Body images are questioned. The challenges of daily life expand.

Communication during this period of development is crucial. The patient may wish to discuss issues with health care providers in private. Since the patient is a minor, this often poses ethical and legal concerns. Adolescents may also attempt to challenge health care workers and providers by trying to intimidate or shut down verbally. It is important to remain nonjudgmental, while exhibiting empathy and compassion in a professional manner.

Height and Weight

Height and weight can present significant concerns for the adolescent. Obesity is prevalent in today's American society. Various forms of media attempt to set standards that are not necessarily realistic, healthy, or achievable. Always use sensitivity when discussing "normal" heights and weights.

Height and weight chart figures vary, depending upon the company and the purpose for which it was developed. They do not often account for growth periods, muscle mass, levels of exercise, and health conditions such as diabetes and should only be used as a guideline, not as exact scientific information.

A more recently used tool for evaluation is the body mass index (BMI). This method incorporates body fat into standardized height and weight measurements. The relationship of body fat to size is a valuable assessment for health. Further discussion of BMI can be found in Chapter 11.

Puberty

As the pediatric patient grows and develops, sexual changes begin to develop and reproduction becomes a possibility. With girls, breast buds become apparent, pubic hair begins to grow, and the first menstrual cycle may occur. There is often a height and weight growth spurt before the secondary sex characteristics. During this time, estrogen and progesterone hormones are increasing. All of these changes combined can easily create emotional fluctuations. The exact age of this development may vary, but generally follows a standard pattern. Questions of sexuality and independence arise. Self-image becomes very important.

Boys will have an increase in the production of testosterone during puberty. Their testes, scrotum, and penis will enlarge, while pubic hair will begin growing. Adolescent boys may experience a height and weight growth spurt after the onset of secondary sex characteristics. The widening of shoulders also becomes apparent. Facial hair and lowering of the voice may create embarrassment and discomfort regarding self-image. Boys may also go through a brief period of time where their voice is similar to an adult female (such as their mother), which the adolescent may find embarrassing.

The onset of puberty varies between different cultures. Certain cultures and nations proceed through these changes at different rates. This might be attributed to health, sanitation, and nutrition. Certain medications may cause variances. As health care workers, it is important to remember that individuals differ in development. Normal is not necessarily synonymous with average. **Secondary sex characteristics** are the changes seen as girls and boys develop differently. Breasts, hips, and voice are examples. These are sexual features that are not necessarily related to reproduction. An adolescent male growing a beard may indicate puberty, but this is not directly related to reproduction.

Sports and Athletics

High school creates a competitive environment, not only academically, but athletically. Examination of pediatric patients involved in athletic programs must include both physical and emotional components, and most schools are now requiring annual physicals prior to participation. Injuries are often a consequence of playing sports. Refer to Chapter 33 for information on concussions and other types of injuries.

CRITICAL THINKING CHALLENGE

Scott, a 15-year-old patient, arrives in the office with his father. His father wants to be involved in the examination because he suspects that Scott might be sexually active. Scott is willing to talk to the provider and you, but only if his father leaves the room. When alone, he asks that his father not be told anything. He proceeds to discuss his sexual preferences.

1. **How should you handle this situation?**
2. **Should you inform his father about the information you received?**
3. **Is this a legal or an ethical situation?**

BEHAVIORAL AND MENTAL HEALTH ISSUES

Some problems such as depression, eating disorders, abuse, and suicide are thought to be primarily adult issues, but they can also occur in the pediatric patient. The health care provider must be aware of the signs and symptoms in order to arrive at a diagnosis for these problems.

Depression

Often a hidden disorder, the diagnosis of depression may be overlooked, and yet, this may begin in the very young child. Temporary sadness must be differentiated from depression. A diagnosis of depression is often difficult because of the different developmental changes experienced throughout the pediatric time frame. The cues may be confusing to the parent. For example, irritability may be related to hormonal changes or to depression.

Signs that could indicate depression are as follows:

- Increased physical complaints that cannot be directly related to any syndrome or illness
- Decreased performance in school or activities
- Increased periods of crying or complaining
- Increased boredom
- Dangerous behavior
- Isolation from peers and family
- Substance abuse
- Wanting to run away
- Increased fear of failure
- Feelings of hopelessness

Identification of depression is important for prompt treatment. Many evaluation tests are available such as the Beck Depression Inventory (BDI). An evaluation of the family history is also important as depressive conditions can be inherited. Girls are also more likely to develop depression than boys, but depression in boys is more difficult to diagnose. Other areas to consider as risk factors include the following:

- Loss of family member
- Loss of pet
- Breakup of relationship
- Confusion about sexual orientation
- Illness
- Abuse

Depression must be identified as it can progress down dangerous avenues, which might include eating disorders or suicide. Be particularly aware of abuse, both physical and psychological, from family, friends, or schoolmates.

Eating Disorders

Common eating disorders seen during the pediatric years are **anorexia nervosa** and **bulimia nervosa**. Primarily seen in the adolescent years, these conditions require both medical and psychological support. Self-image is a major concern for youths. Peer pressure and media input often encourage appearances that are unobtainable with healthy eating patterns. Refer to Chapter 20 for a more thorough discussion on eating disorders.

Abuse

Health care providers are mandated to report any suspected abuse of a pediatric patient. Determination of abuse might be revealed during the physical examination portion of the exam; however, the medical assistant may detect concerns by incorporating active listening during the screening portion of the exam. During the pediatric examination, the provider will observe for signs of bruising, lacerations, scarring, and tenderness. Remember, however, children have accidents and some bruising is normal. Medical assistants should listen for clues during the patient screening phase that may indicate physical or emotional abuse, and discuss with the provider any concerns they may have. Keep in mind the safety for all involved including the patient, family, and health providers. It is not the responsibility of the medical assistant to confront any potential abuses.

Suicide

An alarming statistic is that suicide is the third leading cause of death in 10- to 20-year-old patients. Because of this, all health care providers, including the medical assistant, must take any suicide threat seriously. It is a complete myth that anyone who talks about suicide will usually not complete the act.

CRITICAL THINKING CHALLENGE

When preparing to obtain a two-year-old's height and weight, you notice some round scars on the back of the leg, the shoulder, and one of the hands. The scars resemble cigarette burns and you are concerned about child abuse.

1. How should you handle this situation?

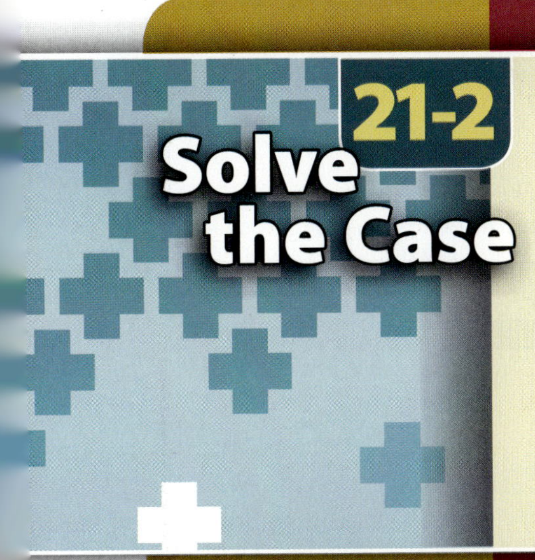

The pediatrician finishes his exam of Gabby and is pleased with her progress. He orders all of the immunizations for a normal six-month-old. Mrs. Parsons is still concerned about having her daughter immunized even though the doctor reassured her that the statistics are much more favorable for immunizing than not immunizing.

1. **Look up the usual immunizations for a six-month-old using the chart provided in this chapter or look it up on the CDC's website. Write down all the immunizations Gabby should receive today.**
2. **List the routes of administration and state where you will administer each immunization.**
3. **Once again, how will you deal with Mrs. Parson's concerns since she already discussed them with the provider?**

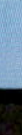

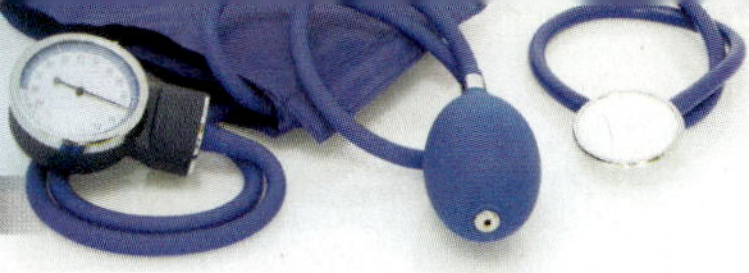

PROCEDURE 21-1

Obtain the Height/Length and Weight of an Infant

Objective:

To obtain accurate measurements of the height and weight of an infant and correctly plot them on a growth chart.

Equipment/Supplies:

- Exam gloves
- Exam table paper
- A measuring device/caliper
- Infant scale, balanced
- Length and weight percentiles flow sheet
- Pen
- Patient's chart/EHR

PROCEDURAL STEPS	DETAILS AND/OR RATIONALE
1. Wash your hands and assemble the equipment.	Handwashing is the principle method of preventing the spread of infection. Having all of the equipment ready prior to handling the infant ensures more efficient use of time with the child.
2. Identify the patient using two identifiers, and identify yourself. Ask the parent to remove the child's clothing, except for the child's diaper.	This allows for a more complete examination. The parent assisting will comfort the infant and allow you to measure the infant.
3. Place the infant face up on the paper on the exam table with the top of the infant's head flush with the top measuring bar of the caliper.	In this position, eye contact can be made with the infant.
4. Stretch the infant's legs to their full length and place the sole of the foot flush with the bottom measuring bar of the caliper. Use caution when extending the joints, ***incorporating critical thinking when performing patient assessment***. Do not pull on the neck or legs. Be gentle. Have the parent support the head and neck, if needed (Figure 21-14).	Be prepared to work rapidly but accurately. Babies do not lie still for very long.
5. Document your results immediately on the patient record and the growth chart.	Immediately documenting the results prevents errors.

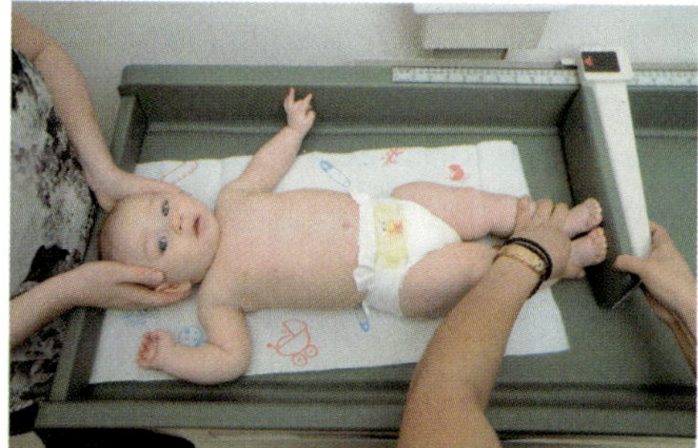

Figure 21-14 ■ Mother holds the infant's head against the top of the table and the medical assistant flattens out the legs and pushes the feet against the foot board.

continues

PROCEDURE 21-1 continued

PROCEDURAL STEPS	DETAILS AND/OR RATIONALE
6. After completing measurement of length, place the infant on the infant scale, lined exam paper, or towel. The scale should be balanced to zero prior to the exam.	Paper or a towel provides a cleaner, warmer environment.
7. Have the parent comfort and support the infant. Make sure that the parent does not exert additional weight.	This will decrease squirming, which will make reading the scale easier.
8. Obtain a reading (Figure 21-15). Remove the infant from the scale. Remove the diaper from the infant. Place the diaper on the scale and weigh.	The weight of the diaper and paper alone will allow you to calculate the weight of the infant. Another option is to weigh the infant without a diaper.
9. Calculate the infant's weight. Remember: total weight – diaper = infant weight.	Avoid math errors.
10. Document your results immediately on the patient record and growth chart.	Accurate documentation is the only method for tracking growth and development trends.

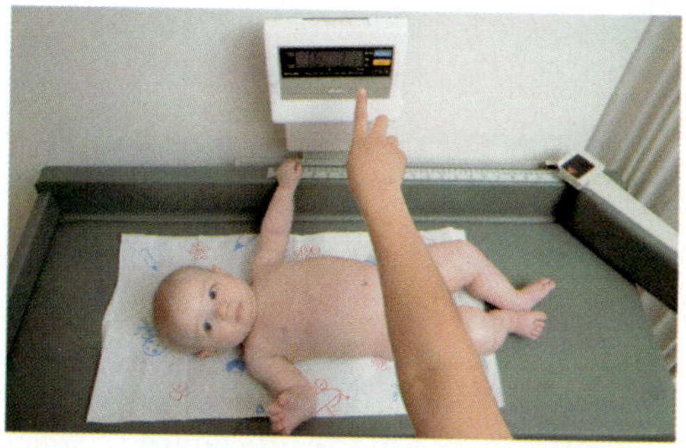

Figure 21-15 ■ The medical assistant obtains the reading when the infant is completely still.

DOCUMENTATION EXAMPLE:

7-02-XX 11.30	Pt. here for five month well baby exam. Length: 22', Weight: 19 lb. Parent assisted with measurements. Tara Smith, RMA (AMT) --

PROCEDURE 21-2

Obtain the Temperature of an Infant or Young Child

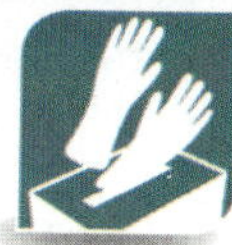

Objective:

To obtain an accurate body temperature reading on an infant by performing a rectal, aural, or temporal temperature.

Equipment and Supplies:

- Electronic rectal thermometer and probe cover, tympanic thermometer and probe cover, or temporal thermometer
- Lubricant
- Tissues
- Gloves
- Watch or clock
- Patient's chart/EHR

continues

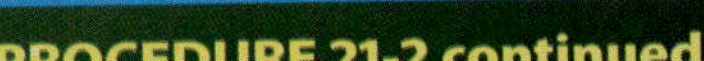

PROCEDURE 21-2 continued

PROCEDURAL STEPS	DETAILS AND/OR RATIONALE
1. Wash your hands and assemble all the equipment. Put on gloves.	Handwashing is the principle method of preventing the spread of infection. Having all of the equipment ready prior to handling of the infant ensures more efficient use of time with the child.
2. Identify the patient using two identifiers, and identify yourself.	Performing any procedure on the wrong patient can cause problems for the patient and using an incorrect chart can cause administrative problems.
3. ***Explain the rationale for performance of the procedure, showing awareness of the patient's and parent's concerns related to the procedure being performed.*** Have the parent remove the infant's clothing.	This will be more comforting to the infant. This will also provide quality time for you to interact with the parent.
Rectal temperature:	
4. Place the infant on the abdomen in your lap, or the infant may be placed in a supine position (Figure 21-16).	These positions provide the most comfort for the patient and the most control for the medical assistant.
5. Apply a clean probe cover and lubricant to the rectal thermometer.	The probe cover protects the thermometer from contamination. The lubricant allows for easiest insertion into the rectum.
6. Gently insert the thermometer into the infant's rectum approximately one inch. Hold it securely. Leave the thermometer in place until the signal that indicates the reading is complete.	Gentle insertion prevents damage to the rectal area. Holding the thermometer securely will prevent it from being drawn into the colon.
7. Remove the thermometer. Remove the sheath and discard it in the biohazard container.	
8. Observe the reading, disinfect the probe with alcohol, and place the probe into its storage slot on the unit.	Proper storage of the probe will prevent damage.
9. Remove excess lubricant from the anal area of the infant. Discard the tissue appropriately.	

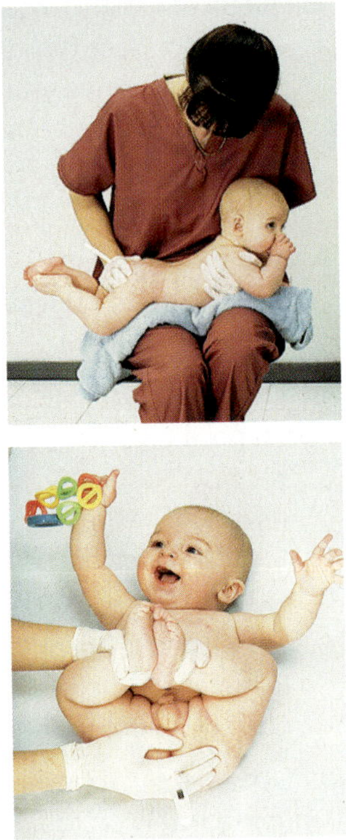

Figure 21-16 ■ Different methods used to take rectal temperatures on an infant. Remember that this route shouldn't be used unless specified by provider.

continues

PROCEDURE 21-2 continued

PROCEDURAL STEPS	DETAILS AND/OR RATIONALE
Aural temperature:	
10. Place the probe cover on the thermometer.	Covering the probe eliminates cross-contamination.
11. Insert the thermometer gently into the ear canal and press the activation button. For best placement and most accurate results, pull gently down and backward on children under the age of three (Figure 21-17) and up and back on children three and over.	Gently pulling the ear lobe down and back in children below the age of three and up and back in children over the age of three helps to properly position the canal for a more accurate reading.
12. After the signal sounds indicating that the reading is complete, remove the thermometer and note the reading.	
13. Discard the probe cover in the appropriate container.	
Temporal temperature:	
14. Clean the thermometer with an alcohol swab and check to be sure the thermometer is in working order.	Cleaning the thermometer between patients helps to prevent cross-contamination.
15. Check the forehead for any moisture and begin with the probe at the midline of the forehead. Keeping the probe flush with the skin, press and hold the scan button and slowly glide the thermometer across the forehead to the location of the temporal artery (Figure 21-18).	Holding the probe flush with skin will ensure an accurate reading.
16. Remove gloves, if worn, and accurately record the information on the patient's record indicating the method performed.	The method must always be recorded. Otherwise, it will be assumed it was by the oral method.

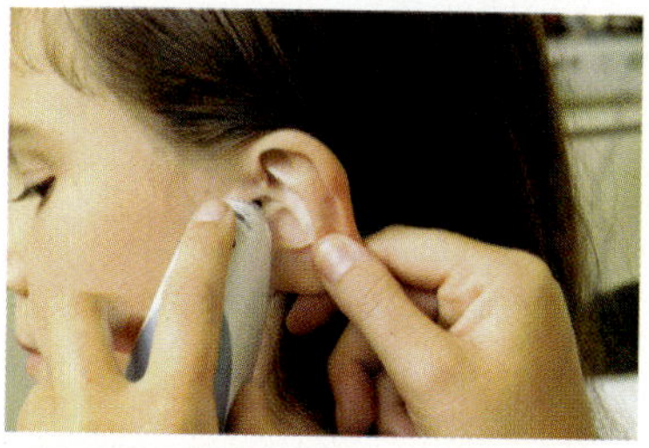

Figure 21-17 ■ Pull down and back when straightening the ear canal on a child.

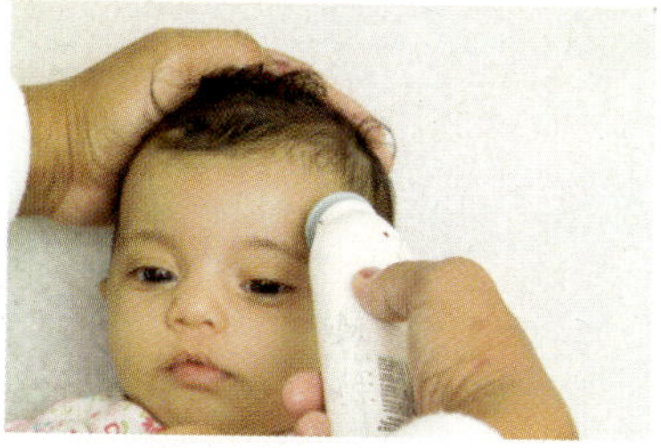

Figure 21-18 ■ Glide the temporal thermometer across the infant's forehead to the side of the forehead where the temporal artery is located.

DOCUMENTATION EXAMPLES:

6-02-XX 0920	T- 102.4° (Rectal). Pt. tolerated procedure well. Shamika Thomas, CMA (AAMA)------------
5-7-XX 1000	T- 99.2° (Aural). Sara Moore, RMA (AMT)---

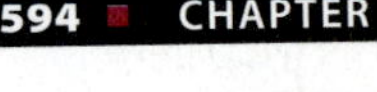

PROCEDURE 21-3

Perform a PKU on a Newborn

Objective:

To obtain a blood sample from a newborn and correctly apply the sample to the test card for evaluation of PKU.

Equipment/Supplies:

- Personal protective equipment (PPE)
- Antiseptic wipe
- Sterile gauze or 2 × 2
- Lancet (sterile)
- Gloves
- Newborn Examination Test Card with envelope
- Sharps container
- Small adhesive bandage
- Pen
- Patient's chart/EHR

PROCEDURAL STEPS	DETAILS AND/OR RATIONALE
1. Wash your hands and assemble the equipment. Complete all required information in the patient section of the test card (Figure 21-19).	Proper handwashing is the single most effective way to prevent the spread of contaminants. Having the equipment ready and the card completely filled out makes the procedure run smoothly. This is important when dealing with infants.

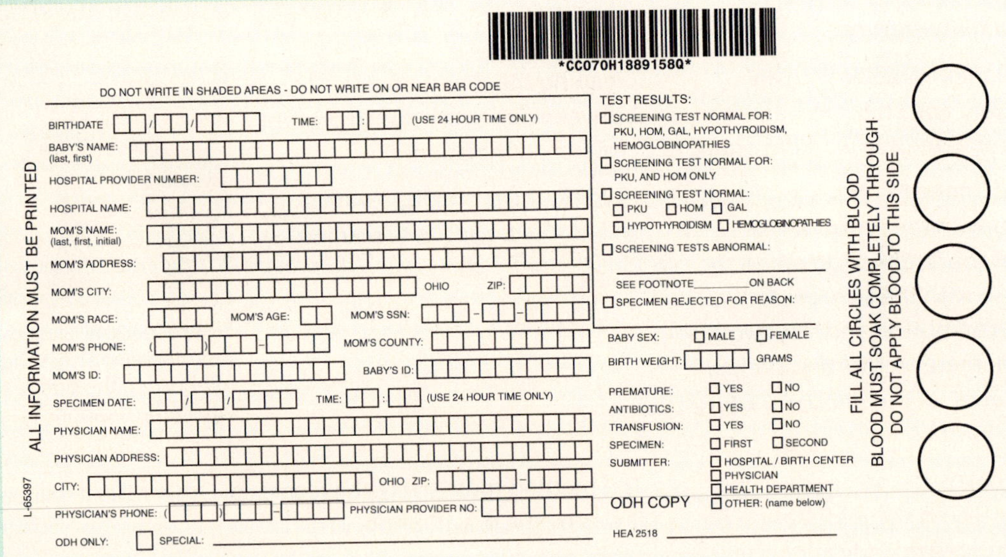

CC070H1889158Q

DO NOT WRITE IN SHADED AREAS - DO NOT WRITE ON OR NEAR BAR CODE

ALL INFORMATION MUST BE PRINTED

BIRTHDATE / / TIME: : (USE 24 HOUR TIME ONLY)
BABY'S NAME: (last, first)
HOSPITAL PROVIDER NUMBER:
HOSPITAL NAME:
MOM'S NAME: (last, first, initial)
MOM'S ADDRESS:
MOM'S CITY: OHIO ZIP:
MOM'S RACE: MOM'S AGE: MOM'S SSN: - -
MOM'S PHONE: ( ) - MOM'S COUNTY:
MOM'S ID: BABY'S ID:
SPECIMEN DATE: / / TIME: : (USE 24 HOUR TIME ONLY)
PHYSICIAN NAME:
PHYSICIAN ADDRESS:
CITY: OHIO ZIP: -
PHYSICIAN'S PHONE: ( ) - PHYSICIAN PROVIDER NO:
ODH ONLY: SPECIAL:

L-65397

TEST RESULTS:
☐ SCREENING TEST NORMAL FOR: PKU, HOM, GAL, HYPOTHYROIDISM, HEMOGLOBINOPATHIES
☐ SCREENING TEST NORMAL FOR: PKU, AND HOM ONLY
☐ SCREENING TEST NORMAL: ☐ PKU ☐ HOM ☐ GAL ☐ HYPOTHYROIDISM ☐ HEMOGLOBINOPATHIES
☐ SCREENING TESTS ABNORMAL:
SEE FOOTNOTE ______ ON BACK
☐ SPECIMEN REJECTED FOR REASON:

BABY SEX: ☐ MALE ☐ FEMALE
BIRTH WEIGHT: GRAMS
PREMATURE: ☐ YES ☐ NO
ANTIBIOTICS: ☐ YES ☐ NO
TRANSFUSION: ☐ YES ☐ NO
SPECIMEN: ☐ FIRST ☐ SECOND
SUBMITTER: ☐ HOSPITAL / BIRTH CENTER ☐ PHYSICIAN ☐ HEALTH DEPARTMENT ☐ OTHER: (name below)

ODH COPY

HEA 2518

FILL ALL CIRCLES WITH BLOOD
BLOOD MUST SOAK COMPLETELY THROUGH
DO NOT APPLY BLOOD TO THIS SIDE

Figure 21-19 ■ A PKU test card.

PROCEDURAL STEPS	DETAILS AND/OR RATIONALE
2. Identify the patient using two identifiers, and identify yourself.	Performing any procedure on the wrong patient can cause problems for the patient and using an incorrect chart can cause administrative problems.
3. ***Explain the rationale for performance of the procedure to the parent or caregiver, showing awareness of the parent's concerns related to the procedure being performed.*** Put on gloves.	Explaining the procedure will provide comfort to the parent. Gloving provides safety to the medical assistant when coming in contact with body fluids such as blood.

continues

PROCEDURE 21-3 continued

PROCEDURAL STEPS	DETAILS AND/OR RATIONALE
4. Expose the infant's heel and locate the position on the heel used to obtain blood. Warm with compresses for approximately five minutes.	Select the location that provides the best access for a successful blood specimen. Warming the area increases the blood flow to the capillaries in the heel.
5. Cleanse the area with the antiseptic wipe. Allow to dry.	This prevents contamination of the sample. Do not touch the clean site. If touched, the area will need to be cleaned again.
6. Securely grasp the foot to be punctured. Using the lancet, quickly puncture the heal perpendicular to the line on the sole of the foot (Figure 21-20). Discard the lancet in the sharps container.	Securing the foot prevents excessive motion that could cause trauma during puncture. Discarding the lancet immediately prevents puncture to self or other health professionals.
7. Gently wipe the first drop of blood away with sterile gauze and discard in the biohazards container.	The first drop of blood contains excess tissue fluid along with alcohol from the antiseptic wipe, which could produce inaccurate results.
8. Gently squeeze the heel, expressing large drops of blood. The test card is placed, as per directions, on the puncture site.	Gently squeeze to expel only blood products. Excessive pressure will dilute the sample with tissue fluid.
9. Fill each circle on the test card with blood, obtained directly from the puncture site. All circles must be saturated for accurate results (Figure 21-21). Place the card aside for drying.	Providing an adequate sample allows for a more accurate evaluation.
10. Cover the puncture site with gauze and apply pressure. Maintain pressure until the bleeding has stopped.	This will assist in controlling bleeding.
11. Cover the site with a small adhesive bandage.	This will absorb any additional blood expelled during the remainder of the exam. It is also comforting to the caregiver.
12. Discard all materials in the appropriate container. Remove gloves and wash hands.	Discarding all materials in the appropriate container and handwashing will prevent the spread of any possible contaminants.
13. Document the results of the procedure in the patient record.	Every procedure must be documented in the patient record.
14. After the card is completely dry (approximately two hours), place the card in an envelope to transport to lab.	The card must be dried for best results.

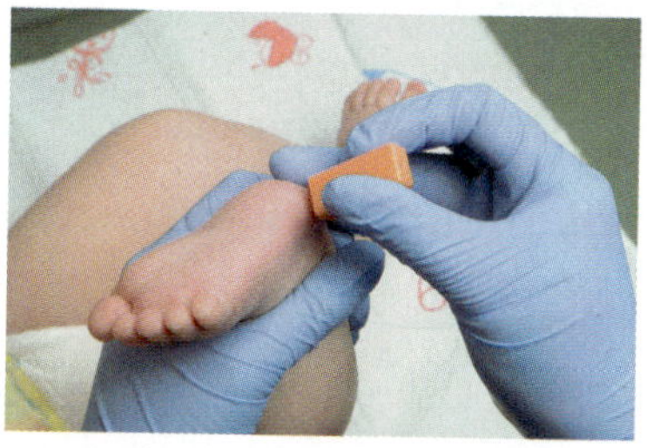

Figure 21-20 ■ The medical assistant goes into the bottom side of the infant's heel to obtain a blood sample.

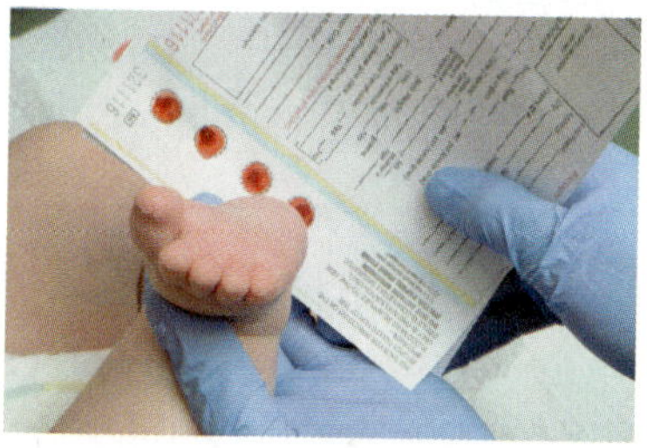

Figure 21-21 ■ Circles must be properly filled for accurate results.

DOCUMENTATION EXAMPLE:

10-6-XX 1500	PKU screening per Dr. Heinz. Blood specimen obtained from medial L heel. Bleeding stopped without difficulty. Pt. comforted easily. All circles on screening card completely covered and mailed to XYZ lab at 2:30 p.m. Justin Danick, RMA (AMT) --------------------------------

PROCEDURE 21-4

Perform a Pediatric Injection

Objective:

To properly administer a medication into the vastus lateralis muscle of a pediatric patient.

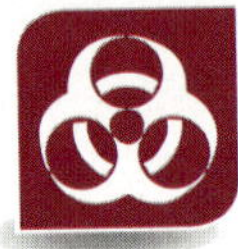

Equipment/Supplies

- Appropriate sized needle and syringe unit
- Antiseptic wipe
- 2 × 2 gauze sponges
- Adhesive bandage
- Medication tray
- Sharps container
- Disposable gloves
- Patient's chart/EHR

PROCEDURAL STEPS	DETAILS AND/OR RATIONALE
1. Wash your hands, assemble the equipment, and prepare the medication.	Handwashing is the number one defense against disease transmission. The medication should be prepared before beginning the procedure.
2. Identify the patient using two identifiers, identify yourself, and ***explain the rationale for performance of the procedure, showing awareness of the patient's and parent's concerns related to the procedure being performed.***	Giving a medication to the wrong patient can result in serious consequences to the patient.
3. Rewash your hands and put on gloves.	Hands become soiled again once you touch any surfaces such as doorknobs, countertops, or the chart. Gloves should be worn when there is a possibility of contact with blood.
4. Select and locate the proper site for the injection.	The medication must be placed in the muscle for proper absorption.
5. Cleanse the site with an antiseptic and allow to completely air dry.	Allowing the alcohol to dry completely will be more comfortable for the patient.
6. Remove the needle cap and properly position the hand on the injection site.	
7. Pull the skin taut and insert the needle at a 90° (Figure 21-22).	The medication needs to be delivered into the muscle.
8. Swiftly inject the medication into the muscle.	Injecting the medication quickly helps to decrease the amount of pain associated with the injection.

Figure 21-22 ■ The medical assistant goes in at a 90 degree angle for an infant injection.

continues

PROCEDURE 21-4 continued

PROCEDURAL STEPS	DETAILS AND/OR RATIONALE
9. Remove the needle quickly at the same angle as insertion.	Removing the needle in this fashion prevents injury to the surrounding tissue.
10. Place a gauze sponge over the injection site and gently massage.	Massaging the site speeds absorption of the medication and soothes the area.
11. Engage the safety device on the needle and dispose of the entire unit in the sharps container.	Safety devices are designed to prevent needle stick injuries.
12. Apply an adhesive bandage to the site.	If there is any bleeding after the injection, the blood will be absorbed by the bandage.
13. Remove the gloves and wash your hands.	
14. Document the procedure in the patient's chart.	

DOCUMENTATION EXAMPLE:

10-05-XX 1100	DTaP Inj, R. vastus lateralis, IM, per Dr. Leonard. Manufacturer: Squibb, Lot # M98760, exp. date 12-05-XX. Kaley Karnes, CMA (AAMA) --

CHAPTER SUMMARY

- The medical assistant must be knowledgeable in all areas of pediatric wellness and must also be able to deal with the unique health challenges presented by this patient population.
- Pediatric classifications include the following: Newborn (initial period following birth); neonate (the first month of life); infant (first year of life); toddler (begins late in the first year of life and continues into the preschool years); child (often correlates with school attendance and can be broken down into early and middle childhood); and adolescent (related to the onset of puberty)
- Adaptations in communication are often necessary when working with small children.
- Accurate and consistent measurements are necessary to evaluate normal and abnormal growth patterns in infants and toddlers.
- Growth charts compare the child's measurements with an average range of growth for children in the United States.
- Children under the age of two are often measured in a supine position. Children over the age of two can be measured in a standing position.
- Infants should be weighed either without clothing or in a plain diaper. The diaper should then be weighed separately and subtracted from the infant's weight.
- A head circumference is performed to help detect micro- or macrocephaly.
- Abdominal circumference may be ordered to evaluate a problem with one of the abdominal organs or abnormal swelling of the abdomen.
- The younger the child, the faster the heart and respiration rate. Blood pressure will be lower in younger populations. Pulse is often performed through auscultation in infants and small children.
- Motor skills provide visible and exciting changes in the growth of the child. These are usually celebrated developments that are documented by parents and compared for generations.
- Motor development usually includes three areas of growth: reflexes, gross motor, and fine motor skills. Reflexes refer to automatic responses to any stimulation.

- During motor development, sensory, perceptual, and cognitive growth is also progressing. Vision and hearing are improving along with depth perception and motion assessment.
- Children should stay on track with all immunizations. Charts or tables can be found at the CDC website.
- The most common site used for pediatric injections is the vastus lateralis.
- Three newborn screening blood tests performed in all 50 states include: PKU, hypothyroidism, and galactosemia.
- Circumcision is the removal of the foreskin from the penis and is often performed following birth at the hospital.
- SIDS is the second leading cause of death in infants in the United States.
- Some problems such as depression, eating disorders, abuse, and suicide are thought to be primarily adult issues, but they can also occur in the pediatric patient.
- Health care providers are mandated to report any suspected abuse of a pediatric patient.

CERTIFICATION REVIEW QUESTIONS

1. At six months, a toddler can:
   a. string two to three words together.
   b. only listen with no response.
   c. complete sentences.
   d. babble, squeal, and produce other noises.
2. Common reflexes seen in the infant include all of the following except:
   a. rooting reflex.
   b. sucking reflex.
   c. skipping reflex.
   d. swimming reflex.
3. A required newborn screening test is:
   a. pneumonia.
   b. PKU.
   c. scoliosis.
   d. allergies.
4. Childhood obesity can be attributed to:
   a. fast food.
   b. televisions and computers that have become the primary focus instead of physical activity.
   c. genetics.
   d. All of the above.
5. What pediatric classification is considered the first month of life?
   a. Newborn
   b. Neonate
   c. Toddler
   d. Young baby
6. You take a toddler's blood pressure and it is 82/34. This would be considered:
   a. normal.
   b. high.
   c. low.
   d. hypertensive.
7. You take a respiration rate on a newborn and it is 58 breaths per minute. This would be considered:
   a. normal.
   b. high.
   c. low.
   d. bradypnea.
8. Billy comes in for his three-month check-up. You need to take his weight. What should you do with his diaper and T-shirt?
   a. Remove the diaper and the T-shirt
   b. Leave on the diaper and the T-shirt
   c. Remove the diaper but leave on the T-shirt
   d. Remove the T-shirt but leave on the diaper
9. Eight-year-old Lucy comes in today for a well-child check. How should she be weighed?
   a. With her clothes and shoes on
   b. Remove her outer clothing but keep on undergarments
   c. With her clothes on but shoes off
   d. None of the above
10. Four-month-old Noah needs immunizations today. Which immunizations shouldn't he receive?
    a. RV
    b. Varicella
    c. Hib
    d. PCV

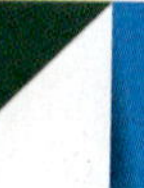

STUDY RESOURCES

Resources to Test and Reinforce Your Knowledge:	
Certification Review Questions	Take this end-of-chapter quiz
Workbook	• Complete the activities for Chapter 21 • Perform the procedures for Chapter 21 using the Competency Checklists
Resources to Promote Critical Thinking:	
***Solve the Case* Activities**	• Consider these case studies and discuss your conclusions
Learning Lab	• Module 21: Clinical Procedures
MindTap	• Complete Chapter 21 readings and activities

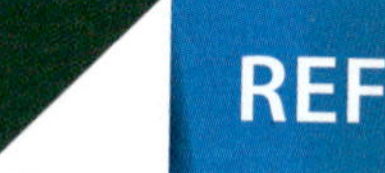

REFERENCES

ExitCare, LLC. *Intramuscular Injections, How and Where to Give*. Baylor Scott & White Health. March 11, 2013. Web. July 12, 2015.

22

Orthopedics, Rehabilitation, and Physical Therapy

CHAPTER OUTLINE

Musculoskeletal System Snapshot

Musculoskeletal Abbreviation Review

Musculoskeletal In-Office and Telephone Screening Tips

Common Orthopedic Conditions

- Strain
- Sprain
- Dislocation
- Fracture
- Osteoporosis
- Other Orthopedic Conditions

Featured Orthopedic Procedures

- Assisting with the Orthopedic Exam
- Application of Immobilization Devices
- Ambulatory Assistive Devices
- Common Exams Using Diagnostic Imaging

Common Orthopedic Treatments

- Surgical Procedures
- Rehabilitation
- Arthritis Treatments
- Exercises

Common Orthopedic Medications

Common Diagnostic Tests That Coincide with Orthopedic Disorders

ESSENTIAL TERMS

allograft
ambulation
anterior cruciate ligament (ACL)
arthritis
arthroscopy
assistive device
atrophy
autograft
bisphosphonates
bursitis
calcitonin
carpal tunnel syndrome
cartilage
cast
chiropractor
Colles (fracture)
comminuted (fracture)
compression (fracture)
cryotherapy
debridement
dislocation
fracture
greenstick (fracture)
heat therapy
kyphosis
massage
modalites
neurologist
occupational therapist (OT)
orthopedist
osteoporosis
physiatrist
physical therapist (PT)
physical therapy
plantar fasciitis
podiatrist
prosthesis
range of motion (ROM)
reduction
rehabilitation
scoliosis
splint

continues

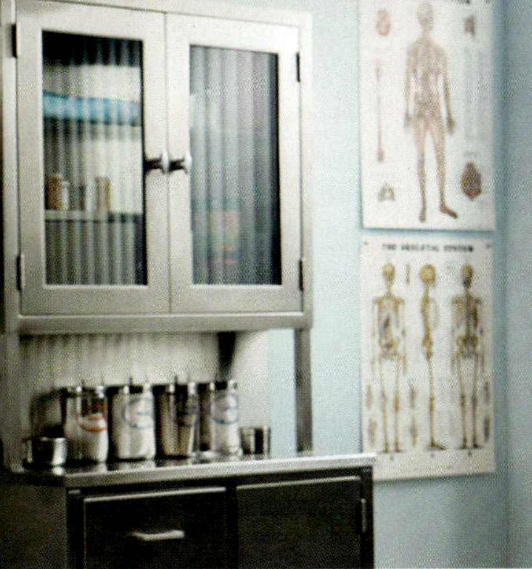

sprain
strain
thermotherapy
ultrasound
vasodilation
viscosupplementation

DEVELOPMENTAL OBJECTIVES

After completing this chapter, you should be able to:

1. Correctly spell and define the essential terms.
2. List and provide the anatomical location of the major structures within the musculoskeletal system.
3. Describe the normal functions of the musculoskeletal system.
4. List and use common abbreviations associated with the musculoskeletal system.
5. Compile a list of common screening questions that should be asked of patients with musculoskeletal symptoms, using established protocols and incorporate critical thinking skills when performing a patient assessment.
6. Identify common pathology related to the musculoskeletal system, including signs, symptoms, and etiologies.
7. Compare the structure and function of the musculoskeletal system across the life span.
8. Analyze pathology for the musculoskeletal system, including diagnostic measures and treatment modalities.
9. Explain the difference between physical therapy and occupational therapy.
10. Describe the different types of hot and cold modalities.
11. List the different types of therapeutic exercises.
12. Compile a list of common musculoskeletal medication classifications and conclude how each one acts upon the body structures to produce the desired effect.
13. Apply a commercial splint to the patient's limb
14. Provide education for the use of canes, crutches, and walkers.
15. Properly apply therapeutic modalities for heat and cold application.
16. Properly transfer a patient from wheelchair to exam table and from exam table to wheelchair.

INTRODUCTION

Orthopedics is the branch of medicine that deals with injuries and disorders of the musculoskeletal system and the following structures: bones, muscles, joints, tendons, and ligaments. Goals for treatment in this specialty are centered on restoring the function of the affected area and improving the patient's quality of life.

The orthopedic team typically includes a host of specialists who all work together to provide the patient with individualized comprehensive care for the best outcome possible. Medical assistants working in orthopedic offices will have a variety of responsibilities including screening patients, assisting the provider, and applying various treatments, as well as educating patients.

MUSCULOSKELETAL SYSTEM SNAPSHOT

The human adult skeletal system consists of 206 bones and has five primary functions: (1) to provide support; (2) to protect the internal organs; (3) to serve as an anchor for muscles that enable movement; (4) to provide storage for minerals; and (5) to provide a site for blood cell formation.

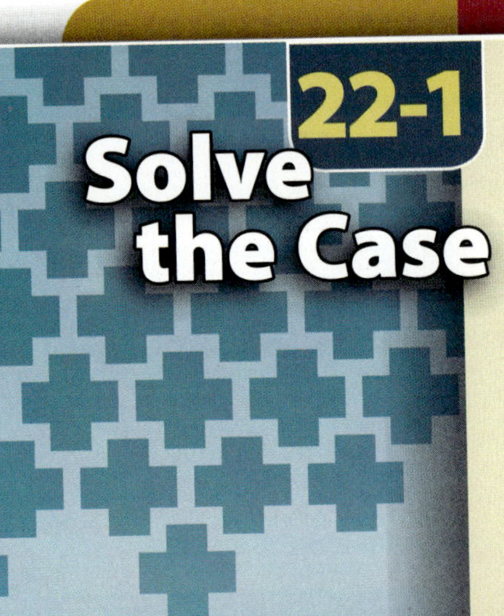

Mr. Conklin is a 70-year-old man who reports falling down five steps in his home. He is sitting on the exam table holding his left forearm with his right hand. There is bruising from the elbow to the wrist. He is very frustrated and concerned that his arm is broken. Mr. Conklin is a farmer who lives on his own and even though he sold several acres of land, he still has 60 acres that he farms all by himself.

1. **Do you think Mr. Conklin's arm may be broken? If so, what symptoms point to a possible fracture?**
2. **What do you speculate may be going through Mr. Conklin's mind as he waits for the provider?**
3. **Is there anything you can do to make Mr. Conklin feel more comfortable as he waits for the provider?**

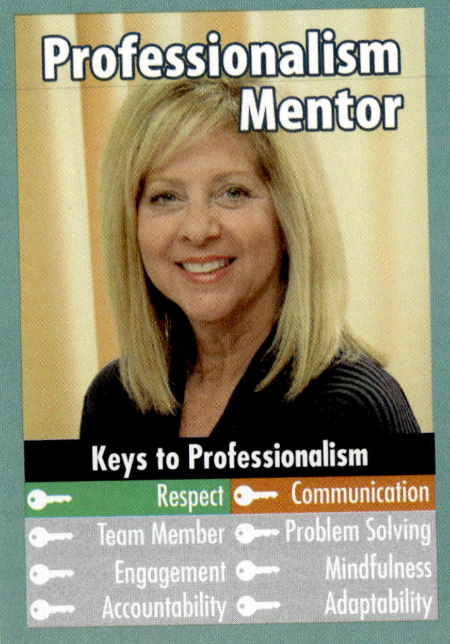

Imagine this: you are all set to go on a vacation and you break an arm, twist a knee, or hurt your back. Has this ever happened to you? If you work in an orthopedic practice you will see all kinds of accidents happen to people at the most inopportune times. Navigating a complex treatment plan many times includes casting or bracing, or possibly surgery followed by physical therapy. It can be long and frustrating for a patient trying to get back to everyday life. How can you help? Being organized and helping your patient get organized with all their appointments may be one place you can start. Demonstrate compassion, and help the patient deal with the stress of this new event in their lives. Be honest: sometimes the patient will have months of physical therapy ahead of them. It doesn't help to underplay a situation but it will help if you are encouraging. The orthopedic practice is a very rewarding place to work. Many times you get to see patients working toward regaining their mobility and independence. In your journal, describe how the keys listed in this feature apply to this scenario. ■

The largest bone in the body is the femur and the smallest bones are the three auditory bones in the ear, commonly referred to as: the hammer, anvil, and stirrup. The skeleton has two major divisions—the axial skeleton and the appendicular skeleton (Figure 22-1). The axial skeleton consists of 80 bones: the skull, spinal column, ribs, sternum, and hyoid bones. The appendicular skeleton consists of 126 bones: shoulder girdles, arms, wrists, hands, and the lower extremities: hip, legs, ankles, and feet.

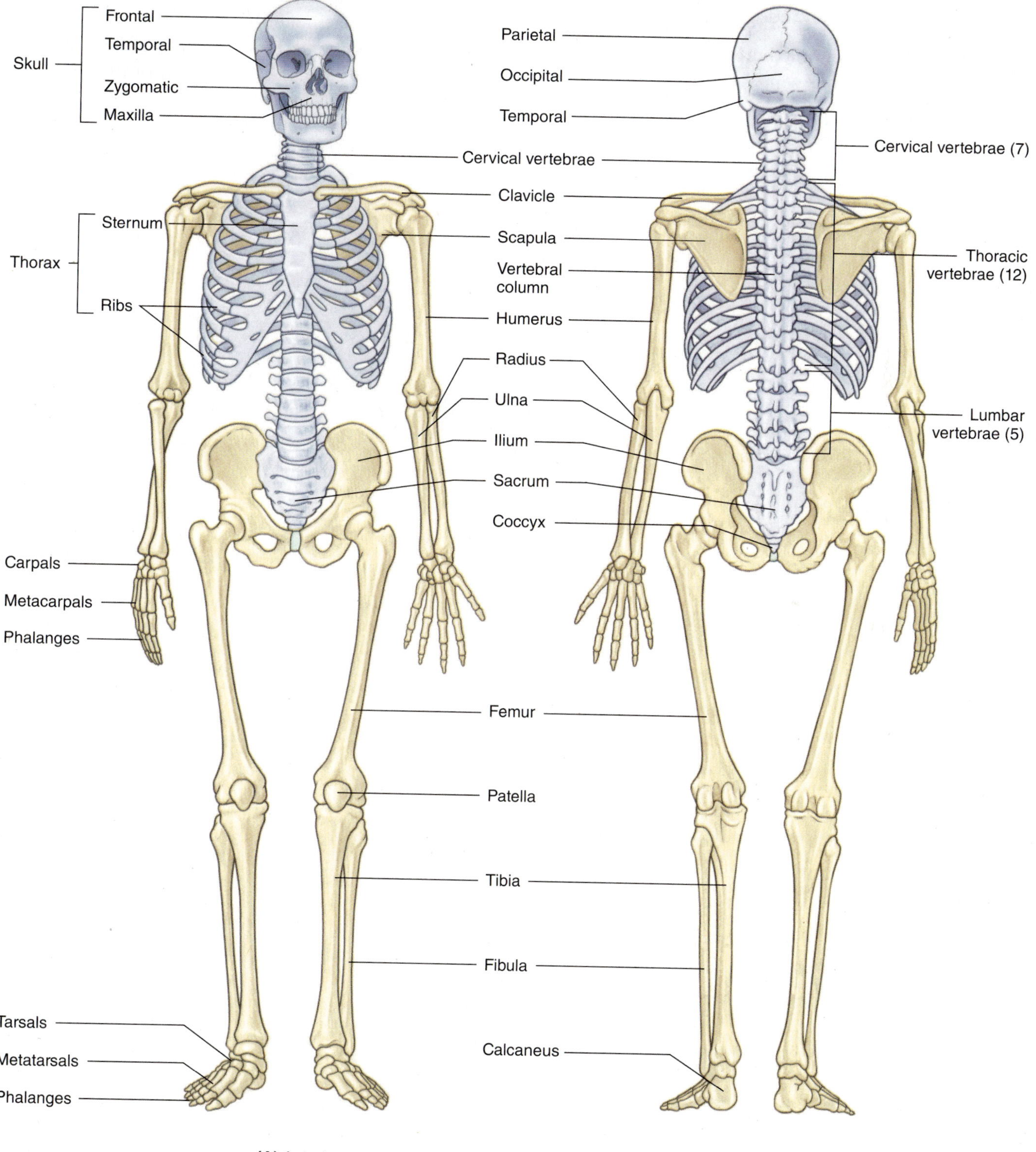

Figure 22-1 ■ The axial skeleton (blue) and the appendicular skeleton (bone color).

The vertebrae consists of five sections which include the following:

- Cervical (includes 7 bones)
- Thoracic (includes 12 bones)
- Lumbar (includes 5 bones)
- Sacral (includes 5 fused bones)
- Coccyx or tailbone (includes 4 fused bones)

The bones reach their maximum density around the age of 30. After that the window for building strong bones closes. See the osteoporosis health coach box to learn more about the physiological aspects of bone health. Medical assistants who take X-rays need to be very familiar with the bones to ensure proper placement of the X-ray tube.

The muscles of the body (Figures 22-2 and 22-3), attached to the skeleton, enable movement, give the body shape and facilitate the maintenance of posture. There are over 650 muscles in the body and three types of muscle tissue: skeletal, smooth, and cardiac. Skeletal

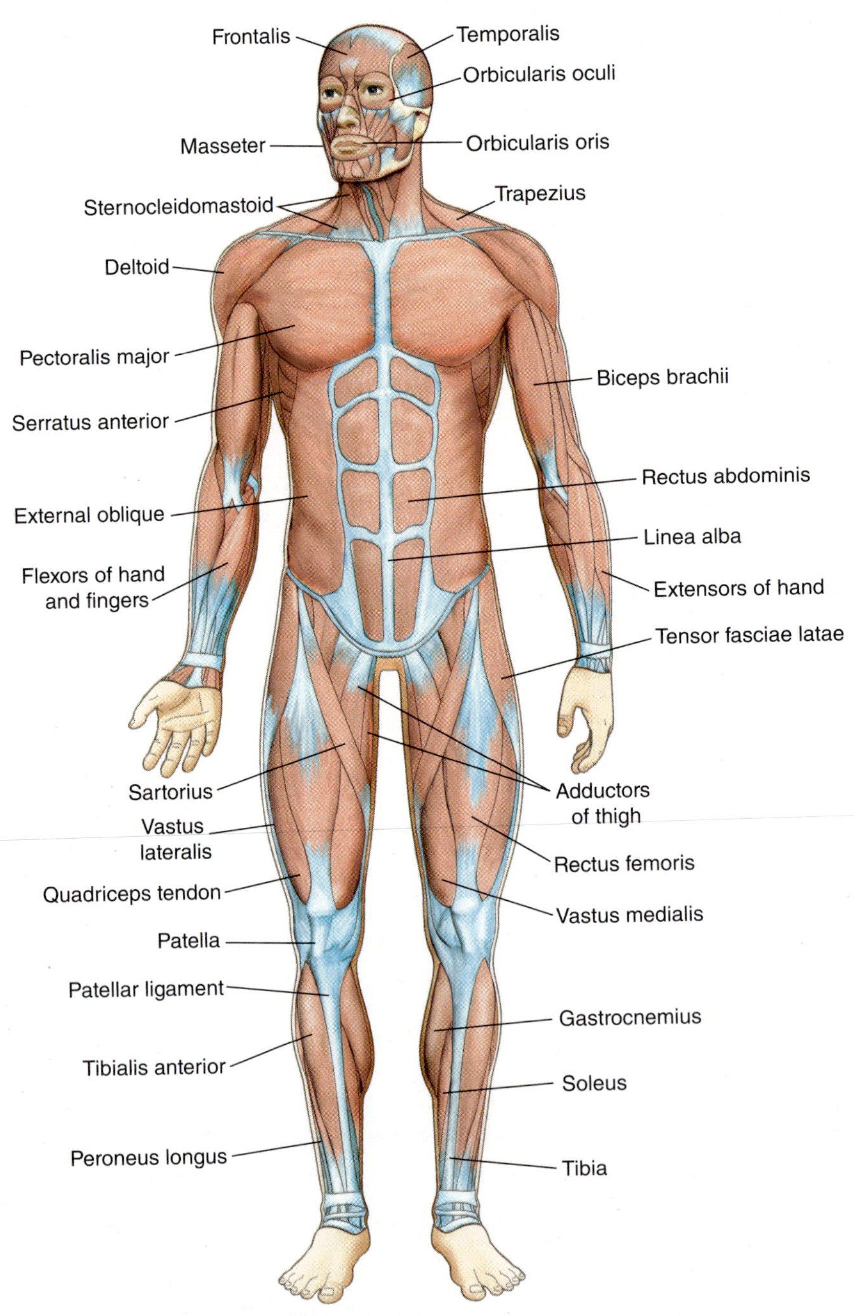

Figure 22-2 ■ Principal skeletal muscles of the body—anterior view.

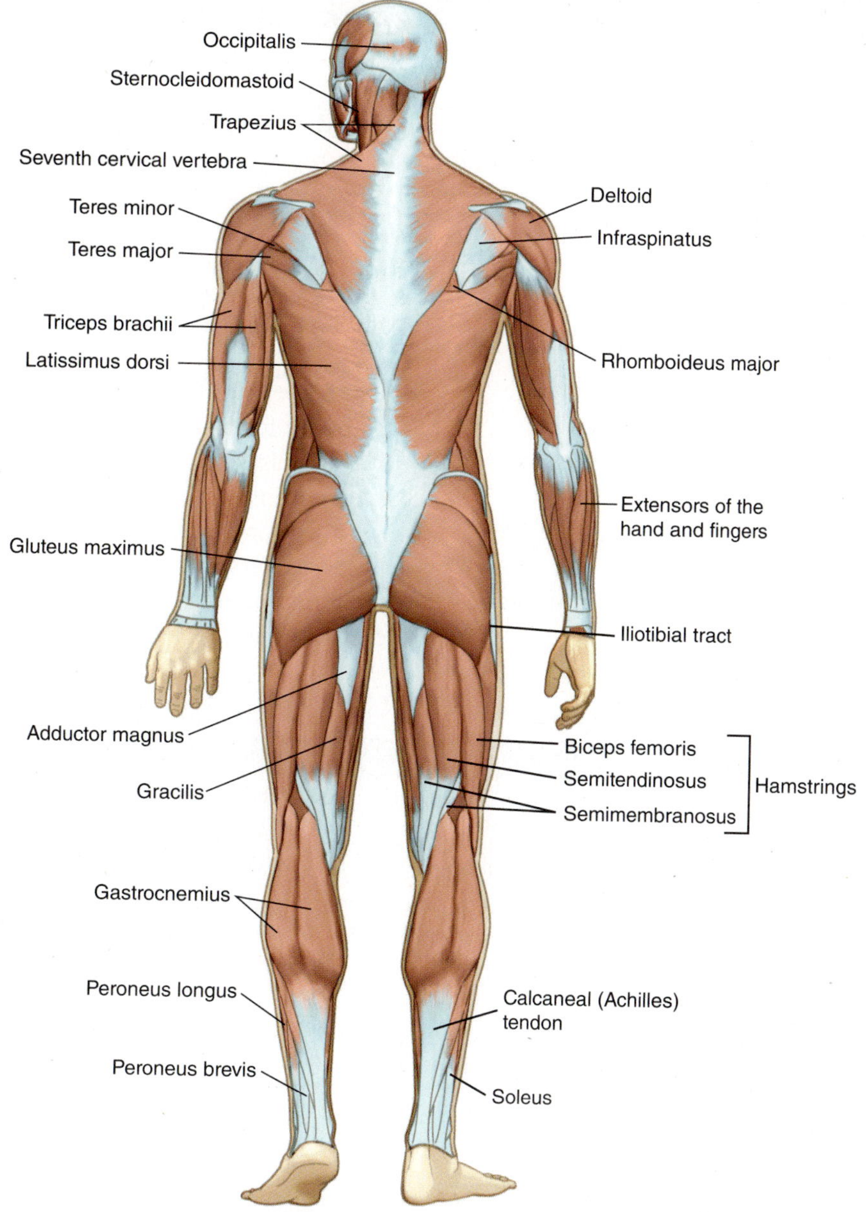

Figure 22-3 ■ Principal skeletal muscles of the body—posterior view.

Meet the **Specialists**

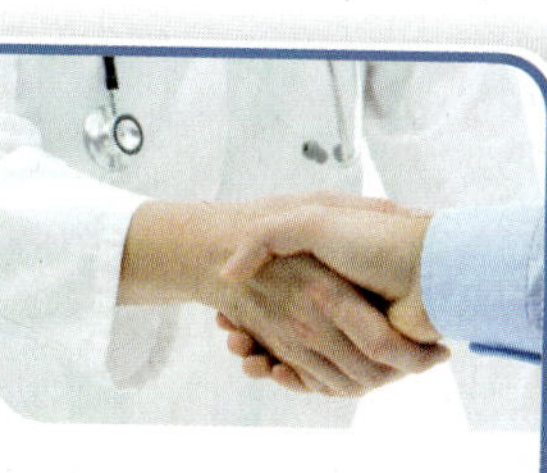

An **orthopedist** is a medical doctor who treats diseases and disorders of the bones and muscles and often performs orthopedic surgeries. This specialist treats acute conditions such as trauma caused by injuries and chronic conditions such as **arthritis**, the inflammation of a joint or multiple joints with pain, swelling, stiffness, or deformity.

An orthopedist's work often overlaps that of the plastic surgeon, pediatrician, **chiropractor** (a doctor of chiropractic who uses manipulation techniques to treat disorders of the spine), or **podiatrist** (a doctor specializing in the diagnosis and treatment of foot conditions). Some orthopedists specialize in treating particular conditions including spinal deformities such as **scoliosis** (abnormal lateral curvature of the spine) and **kyphosis** (abnormal forward curvature of the spine), congenital foot disorder, sports injuries, growth plate fractures, joint dysfunction, and the management of complex fractures. Orthopedists often work in conjunction with other specialists and members of the health care team to provide the patient with the best care possible. Table 22-1 lists specialists who work in conjunction with an orthopedist.

muscles are striated or striped and attached to bone tissue. This tissue is considered voluntary. Smooth muscle can be found in the layers of particular organs and within the blood vessels. Cardiac muscle is only found in the heart and is the layer of tissue that allows the heart to contract. Both smooth and cardiac muscle tissue is considered nonvoluntary. Muscles also contribute to the maintenance of body temperature through the generation of heat.

Other supporting structures of the musculoskeletal system include the following:

- *Tendons*. Dense, fibrous connective tissue that attaches the muscles to the bones of the skeleton.
- *Ligaments*. Fibrous connective tissue that attach and connect one bone to another, such as the bones in the fingers.
- *Joints*. Formed where bones are connected to each other by ligaments.

MUSCULOSKELETAL ABBREVIATION REVIEW

Medical assistants working in musculoskeletal specialties should be familiar with the abbreviations listed in Table 22-2.

MUSCULOSKELETAL IN-OFFICE AND TELEPHONE SCREENING TIPS

The bones form the framework for the entire body and serve as points of attachment for muscles, tendons, ligaments, and other connective tissue. There are a multitude of diseases, disorders, and injuries that can affect this system.

Medical assistants may have the responsibility of screening patients prior to provider examination. The depth of screening will be established by office protocol,

Table 22-1 Specialists Who Work with the Orthopedist

Specialist	Description/Treatment Duties
Neurologist	A physician who specializes in the diagnosis and treatment of diseases of the nervous system, including the brain, spinal cord, and nerves
Neurosurgeon	A physician who specializes in performing surgery on structures of the nervous system
Physiatrist	A physical medicine doctor who diagnoses and treats neuromuscular and bone diseases and injuries and works closely with physical therapists
Physical therapist (PT)	A specialist who helps to restore function, improve mobility, and decrease pain to an area that has been damaged by injury or disease
Occupational therapist (OT)	A medical professional who is responsible for assisting patients with basic motor function, reasoning, and activities of daily living (ADLs)

Table 22-2 Common Musculoskeletal Abbreviations

Abbreviation	Meaning	Abbreviation	Meaning
AK	Above the knee	MUSC	Muscles
BDT	Bone density testing	MSP	Muscle spasm
BJM	Bones, joints, and muscles	OA	Osteoarthritis
BK	Below the knee	ORIF	Open reduction internal fixation
BMD	Bone mineral density	RA	Rheumatoid arthritis
CTS	**Carpal tunnel syndrome**	RLE	Right lower extremity
DJD	Degenerative joint disease	RUE	Right upper extremity
EMG	Electromyogram	SKM	Skeletal muscle
EMS	Electrical muscle stimulation	SM	Smooth muscle
FX	Fracture	TBMM	Total body muscle mass
HNP	Herniated nucleus pulposus	THA	Total hip arthroplasty
LAT	Latissimus dorsi	THR	Total hip replacement
LLE	Left lower extremity	TKA	Total knee arthroplasty
LUE	Left upper extremity	TKR	Total knee replacement
MFT	Muscle function test		

Table 22-3 Patient Screening and Instructions for the Musculoskeletal System

Ask the Patient:	• *Injury:* Are you experiencing any pain or swelling in the affected area, skin discoloration, loss of feeling, or tingling? Can you describe the injury? • *General:* Are you experiencing any joint pain, swelling, stiffness, or weakness? Do you have any history of musculoskeletal disorders?
For Patients Calling on the Telephone	If a patient has an injury that includes extensive swelling, pain, loss of feeling, or tingling, he or she should be seen the same day, if at all possible.
When in the Office:	
Disrobing Instructions	Expose affected areas but provide privacy
Vital Signs	Blood pressure, pulse, respirations, and temperature
Equipment	Casting materials or splints for possible fracture, wrapping materials for possible strain or sprain
Possible Procedures	X-rays of the affected areas, casting, splinting, or wrapping procedures

but in general, medical assistants should be able to ask a series of questions related to the patient's symptoms. Table 22-3 lists types of questions that are typically asked when patients complain of musculoskeletal symptoms and common procedures that coincide with symptoms.

Important note: Medical assistants should never perform any procedure unless directed to do so by the provider; however, they can set up various equipment and supplies to help save time in the event that testing is ordered.

COMMON ORTHOPEDIC CONDITIONS

There are many conditions that affect the musculoskeletal system. In this section, we will describe some of the most common conditions.

Strain

A **strain** is an injury to a muscle or tendon caused by excessive use or overexertion; and it is not considered to be as serious as a sprain. Patients with a suspected strain injury should be examined by a provider to determine the extent of the injury. A strain causes pain upon movement and is usually treated by rest and heat. Occasionally the physician will prescribe a muscle relaxant.

Sprain

A **sprain** is a more serious injury than a strain. It involves trauma to ligaments and may also involve injury to the tendons and muscles. A sprain may cause swelling and bruising of the affected area, and should be treated with rest and the application of ice, with compression and elevation.

Patients must properly care for a strain or sprain in order for the injury to heal correctly. Recommended home care includes the following:

- RICE (rest, ice, compression, elevation)
- Immobilization
- Anti-inflammatory medications
- Analgesics
- Massage

Proper home care will speed up the recovery process and help to return the injured part to its normal function.

Dislocation

Dislocation is a temporary displacement of a bone from its usual position in the joint. A dislocation must be returned to its proper position to prevent further injury and damage. Indications of a possible dislocation may include the following:

- Pain and tenderness
- Obvious deformity of the joint
- Swelling
- Discoloration
- Loss of function

After a dislocation has been reduced, a **splint**, a stiff device used to support and immobilize a part of the body that has been injured or fractured, may be used to immobilize the joint to allow for healing. Surgery to correct a dislocation is being performed much more often today, especially in athletes, for once a dislocation occurs, the affected area is much more susceptible to further injury.

Fracture

A **fracture** or break in a bone can be caused by a pathological condition, injury, or trauma. The main objective of the orthopedist is to realign the bones that are broken to their original position, a process that is known as **reduction**. This process promotes healing, decreases pain and deformity, and helps the patient regain the use of the injured body part. Unexpected complications such as infection, fat embolisms, or blood clots may arise from fractures. An embolism or a clot can circulate to the lungs, which can be fatal.

Featured Disease Spotlight: Osteoporosis *continued*

Symptoms	Early warning signs may include a gradual loss of height, back pain, stooped posture, and a dowager's hump. However, later in the disease process, patients may incur fractures. Common fracture sites include the spine, hips, and wrists.
Diagnostic Testing	DEXA (dual X-ray absorptiometry) scan measures bone density to determine fracture risks in the spine, hip, or entire body; bone densitometry (measures density of bone quickly); qualitative computed tomography (QCT); ultrasound; and blood test markers that check bone metabolism and the degree of disease progression.
Modifying Factors	You can decrease risks of this disease or slow its progress and complications by living an active lifestyle in early life (preteen and teenage years when bone mass is developing), incorporating a diet rich in calcium and vitamin D, not smoking (or participating in a smoking cessation program), and limiting alcohol use. A good exercise program (particularly weight bearing) and stretching regimen throughout your entire life will assist in limiting ramifications from this disease.
Treatments	Supplements of calcium and other nutrients, weight-bearing exercises, estrogen and bisphosphonate drugs such as Fosamax and Boniva.

Other Orthopedic Conditions

Orthopedic specialty practices also see patients with many other conditions, including arthritis. For information on some of these other conditions, refer to Table 22-5.

Arthritis

Arthritis is an inflammatory process that affects one or more joints. Over 50 million people are affected by arthritis. There are different types of arthritis but the two most common are osteoarthritis and rheumatoid arthritis.

Osteoarthritis is the most common form of arthritis and is a progressive degenerative disease. In this form of arthritis, the cartilage breaks down, causing the bones to rub against each other. This results in pain and loss of mobility. Risk factors may include obesity, increasing age, genetics, and previous injuries to the joints. Joint soreness and stiffness in the knees, hips, and lower back following inactivity are all symptoms of this form of arthritis; however, other structures may also be affected including the fingers, toes, ankle, and neck. Anti-inflammatory drugs and physical therapy may help to manage the symptoms of the disease.

Table 22-5 Other Common Orthopedic Conditions

Condition	Description
ACL injuries	The ACL connects the shinbone (tibia) to the thighbone (femur). A severe twist of the knee can tear the ACL and cause the knee to give out. There are an estimated 100,000 ACL surgical repairs each year in the United States.
Bursitis	The bursa functions as a cushion between the bones and the overlying soft tissues. When there is inflammation of the bursa, there is pain at the outside of the joint whenever the tendon moves over the bursa. This condition is usually treated with anti-inflammatory agents.
Carpal tunnel syndrome	This syndrome is caused by the compression of the median nerve, located at the base of the palm. Common symptoms are numbness and tingling in the hand, with clumsiness in handling objects. Surgical intervention relieves the compression on the median nerve.
Plantar fasciitis	This condition is one of the most common causes for heel pain. Inflammation is caused by too much tension on the fascia, as a result of obesity, arthritis, diabetes, or poorly fitting shoes. This condition is usually treated with anti-inflammatory agents.

may be serious enough that realignment and immobilization are not enough to ensure proper healing. Often, the orthopedist must perform surgery and place screws, wires, pins, and plates to repair and realign the damaged bones. In some instances, the pins and wires can be removed once the healing process has taken place.

Osteoporosis

Osteoporosis is a disease resulting in weak and brittle bone, occurring primarily in females. Refer to the Health Coach Disease Feature to learn more about this disease.

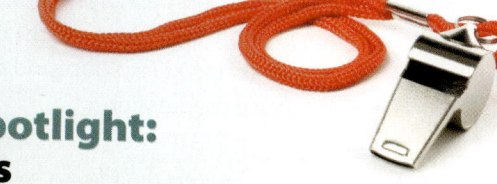

Health Coach

Featured Disease Spotlight: Osteoporosis

Description

Osteoporosis is a condition in which the bones become porous and brittle. Women have a greater risk of acquiring the disease due to denser bone mass and the role estrogen plays in the disease; however, males may also develop osteoporosis. After age 30, calcium deposition into the bone is greatly diminished while more calcium is withdrawn from the bones to maintain normal blood clotting, and cardiac and nervous system functioning. This means that you are withdrawing more calcium from the bank than you are putting into the bank. This demineralization process results in weak and brittle bones. Even a mild physical stress, such as coughing, can result in a fracture in patients with osteoporosis.

Diagram

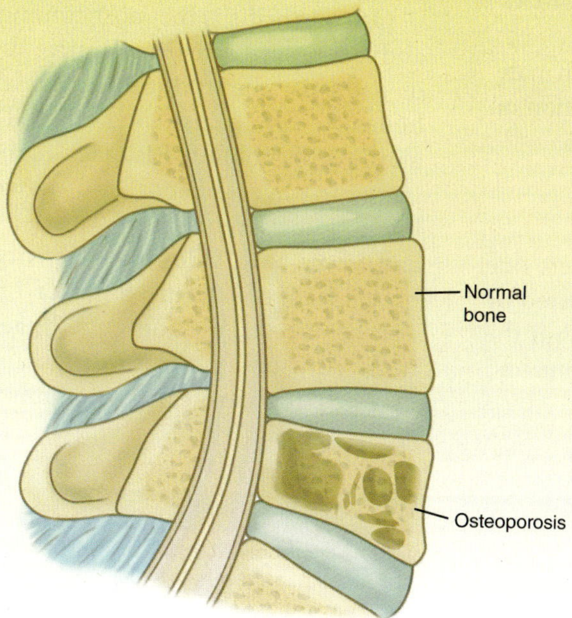

Risk Factors

Gender (females are more prone than males); Early menopause (before age 45. This is because estrogen levels drop following menopause. Estrogen assists with the absorption and utilization of calcium. The drop in estrogen accelerates osteoporosis in females.); thin, small body frame; family history; increasing age; inadequate intake of calcium; long-term corticosteroid use; sedentary lifestyle; smoking; and excessive alcohol consumption all contribute to osteoporosis.

continues

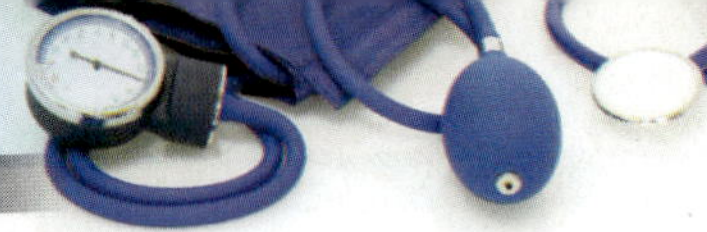

Featured Disease Spotlight: Osteoporosis *continued*

Symptoms	Early warning signs may include a gradual loss of height, back pain, stooped posture, and a dowager's hump. However, later in the disease process, patients may incur fractures. Common fracture sites include the spine, hips, and wrists.
Diagnostic Testing	DEXA (dual X-ray absorptiometry) scan measures bone density to determine fracture risks in the spine, hip, or entire body; bone densitometry (measures density of bone quickly); qualitative computed tomography (QCT); ultrasound; and blood test markers that check bone metabolism and the degree of disease progression.
Modifying Factors	You can decrease risks of this disease or slow its progress and complications by living an active lifestyle in early life (preteen and teenage years when bone mass is developing), incorporating a diet rich in calcium and vitamin D, not smoking (or participating in a smoking cessation program), and limiting alcohol use. A good exercise program (particularly weight bearing) and stretching regimen throughout your entire life will assist in limiting ramifications from this disease.
Treatments	Supplements of calcium and other nutrients, weight-bearing exercises, estrogen and bisphosphonate drugs such as Fosamax and Boniva.

Other Orthopedic Conditions

Orthopedic specialty practices also see patients with many other conditions, including arthritis. For information on some of these other conditions, refer to Table 22-5.

Arthritis

Arthritis is an inflammatory process that affects one or more joints. Over 50 million people are affected by arthritis. There are different types of arthritis but the two most common are osteoarthritis and rheumatoid arthritis.

Osteoarthritis is the most common form of arthritis and is a progressive degenerative disease. In this form of arthritis, the cartilage breaks down, causing the bones to rub against each other. This results in pain and loss of mobility. Risk factors may include obesity, increasing age, genetics, and previous injuries to the joints. Joint soreness and stiffness in the knees, hips, and lower back following inactivity are all symptoms of this form of arthritis; however, other structures may also be affected including the fingers, toes, ankle, and neck. Anti-inflammatory drugs and physical therapy may help to manage the symptoms of the disease.

Table 22-5 Other Common Orthopedic Conditions

Condition	Description
ACL injuries	The ACL connects the shinbone (tibia) to the thighbone (femur). A severe twist of the knee can tear the ACL and cause the knee to give out. There are an estimated 100,000 ACL surgical repairs each year in the United States.
Bursitis	The bursa functions as a cushion between the bones and the overlying soft tissues. When there is inflammation of the bursa, there is pain at the outside of the joint whenever the tendon moves over the bursa. This condition is usually treated with anti-inflammatory agents.
Carpal tunnel syndrome	This syndrome is caused by the compression of the median nerve, located at the base of the palm. Common symptoms are numbness and tingling in the hand, with clumsiness in handling objects. Surgical intervention relieves the compression on the median nerve.
Plantar fasciitis	This condition is one of the most common causes for heel pain. Inflammation is caused by too much tension on the fascia, as a result of obesity, arthritis, diabetes, or poorly fitting shoes. This condition is usually treated with anti-inflammatory agents.

Table 22-3 Patient Screening and Instructions for the Musculoskeletal System

Ask the Patient:	• *Injury:* Are you experiencing any pain or swelling in the affected area, skin discoloration, loss of feeling, or tingling? Can you describe the injury? • *General:* Are you experiencing any joint pain, swelling, stiffness, or weakness? Do you have any history of musculoskeletal disorders?
For Patients Calling on the Telephone	If a patient has an injury that includes extensive swelling, pain, loss of feeling, or tingling, he or she should be seen the same day, if at all possible.
When in the Office:	
Disrobing Instructions	Expose affected areas but provide privacy
Vital Signs	Blood pressure, pulse, respirations, and temperature
Equipment	Casting materials or splints for possible fracture, wrapping materials for possible strain or sprain
Possible Procedures	X-rays of the affected areas, casting, splinting, or wrapping procedures

but in general, medical assistants should be able to ask a series of questions related to the patient's symptoms. Table 22-3 lists types of questions that are typically asked when patients complain of musculoskeletal symptoms and common procedures that coincide with symptoms.

Important note: Medical assistants should never perform any procedure unless directed to do so by the provider; however, they can set up various equipment and supplies to help save time in the event that testing is ordered.

COMMON ORTHOPEDIC CONDITIONS

There are many conditions that affect the musculoskeletal system. In this section, we will describe some of the most common conditions.

Strain

A **strain** is an injury to a muscle or tendon caused by excessive use or overexertion; and it is not considered to be as serious as a sprain. Patients with a suspected strain injury should be examined by a provider to determine the extent of the injury. A strain causes pain upon movement and is usually treated by rest and heat. Occasionally the physician will prescribe a muscle relaxant.

Sprain

A **sprain** is a more serious injury than a strain. It involves trauma to ligaments and may also involve injury to the tendons and muscles. A sprain may cause swelling and bruising of the affected area, and should be treated with rest and the application of ice, with compression and elevation.

Patients must properly care for a strain or sprain in order for the injury to heal correctly. Recommended home care includes the following:

- RICE (rest, ice, compression, elevation)
- Immobilization
- Anti-inflammatory medications
- Analgesics
- Massage

Proper home care will speed up the recovery process and help to return the injured part to its normal function.

Dislocation

Dislocation is a temporary displacement of a bone from its usual position in the joint. A dislocation must be returned to its proper position to prevent further injury and damage. Indications of a possible dislocation may include the following:

- Pain and tenderness
- Obvious deformity of the joint
- Swelling
- Discoloration
- Loss of function

After a dislocation has been reduced, a **splint**, a stiff device used to support and immobilize a part of the body that has been injured or fractured, may be used to immobilize the joint to allow for healing. Surgery to correct a dislocation is being performed much more often today, especially in athletes, for once a dislocation occurs, the affected area is much more susceptible to further injury.

Fracture

A **fracture** or break in a bone can be caused by a pathological condition, injury, or trauma. The main objective of the orthopedist is to realign the bones that are broken to their original position, a process that is known as **reduction**. This process promotes healing, decreases pain and deformity, and helps the patient regain the use of the injured body part. Unexpected complications such as infection, fat embolisms, or blood clots may arise from fractures. An embolism or a clot can circulate to the lungs, which can be fatal.

Fractures are classified as simple or closed, or compound or open. In a closed or simple fracture, the bone is broken, but does not penetrate the skin. In an open or compound fracture, the broken bone protrudes through the skin, resulting in an open wound. When the bone penetrates the skin, there is also the danger of severing a vein or an artery, which may cause a life-threatening hemorrhage.

Fractures are treated differently from strains, sprains, or dislocations. Fractures must be reduced as soon as possible, which involves placing the broken bone fragments back into their original position. Two types of reductions may be used:

- Closed reduction: The bone is realigned or "set" without making an incision into the skin.
- Open reduction: An incision is made into the skin to realign the bones. The orthopedist will sometimes use screws, rods, and plates to hold the bones in place.

Table 22-4 lists information on the different types of fractures, and Figure 22-4 illustrates the various types of fractures.

Once a fracture has been reduced, a cast or other immobilization device is applied to the affected body part. Splints or casts support and protect the broken bone during the healing process. Fractures and other injuries

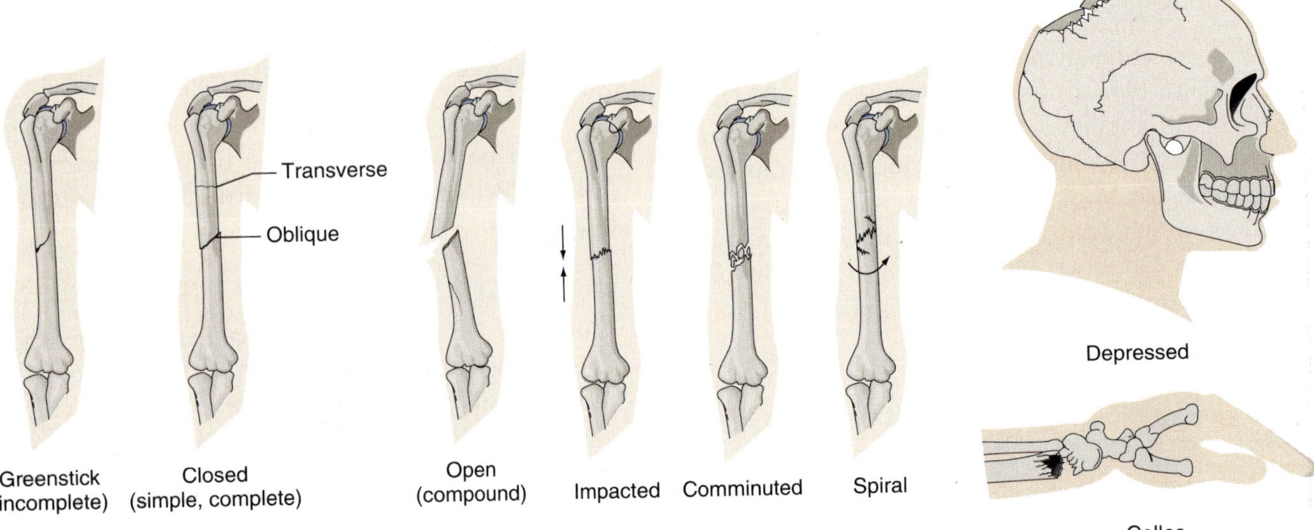

Figure 22-4 ■ Examples of different types of fractures.

Table 22-4 Types of Fractures

Type of Fracture	Description
Complete	The bone is completely broken into two or more pieces.
Incomplete	The bone is partially broken.
Complicated	The bone is broken and surrounding tissue is also damaged.
Greenstick	The bone is partially bent and partially broken (often seen in children).
Compression	A piece of the broken bone is driven inward. Sometimes seen in skull fractures.
Hairline	A crack in the bone that can be seen on an X-ray. The bone ends are perfectly aligned and the break does not go all the way through the bone.
Impacted	A break in which one bone fragment is wedged into the other bone fragment.
Pathological	A fracture due to a disease condition such as osteoporosis.
Pott's	A fracture that occurs at the distal end of the tibia or fibula just above the ankle.
Spiral	A fracture that occurs as a result of twisting the bone. The fracture spirals around a long bone.
Stress	A fine hairline fracture that occurs as a result of repetitive traumas due to running, aerobics, or marching. Difficult to diagnose by X-ray.
Colles	A fracture of the distal end of the radius bone in the wrist.
Comminuted	The bone is broken or splintered into fragments.
Transverse	The bone is fractured at a right angle to the axis of the bone.
Oblique	A diagonal fracture of a bone.

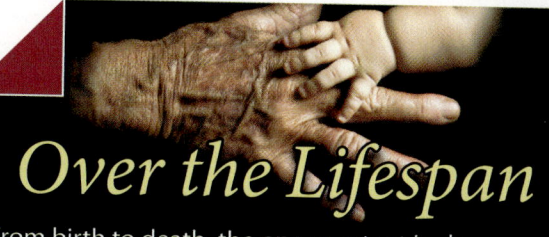

Over the Lifespan

From birth to death, the one constant is change. Around the age of 40, bone mass starts to decrease and muscle loss begins as fiber tissues replace muscle tissue. With aging, joints stiffen as cartilage and connective tissue changes cause the joints to be less mobile. Shrinkage of the intervertebral cartilage results in a decrease in height. The loss of **cartilage**, the connective tissue located between the articular surfaces of the bones, joints, and vertebrae, which act as a shock absorber, in both the hips and knees causes diminished mobility. Muscles gradually show a degree of **atrophy** (shrinkage due to inadequate nutrition to the muscle) as ligaments, tendons, and joints harden, causing increased rigidity and decreased flexibility.

Common problems for the musculoskeletal system over time include the development of osteoporosis, fractures, osteoarthritis, gait changes, and loss of balance. All these may be slowed or prevented with regular exercise. Often the difficulties associated with aging reflect not the advanced age but a lack of physical exercise.

Rheumatoid arthritis is an autoimmune disease in which the body's immune system attacks its own joints and organs such as the heart. This form of arthritis occurs most commonly between the ages of 30 and 60. Symptoms may include joint pain, erythema (redness of the skin), and warmth over the skin of the joint. Symptoms are often bilateral, meaning on both sides. Good nutrition and staying physically active will help to keep joints flexible; however, patients often need medications to help manage symptoms.

FEATURED ORTHOPEDIC PROCEDURES

There are a variety of procedures performed in orthopedic offices. Procedures will vary by the type of orthopedic practice (sports medicine verses general orthopedics) and the skills of the personnel working in the practice. This section will focus on skills that medical assistants may be capable of performing or procedures or exams that medical assistants may assist with.

Assisting with the Orthopedic Exam

In the orthopedist's office, the medical assistant's main duty is assisting with the general exam. Other duties may include ordering X-rays and other diagnostic tests, assisting with casting or cast removal, administering treatment modalities, and patient education regarding home therapies, cast care, and the use of assistive devices such as a cane, crutches, walker, or wheelchair. The medical assistant may also be asked to drape, position, or help support the patient during an exam.

Application of Immobilization Devices

Immobilization devices are used in the treatment of fractures. Once a fracture has been identified and reduced, an immobilization device is applied to the affected body part in order to protect the broken bone during the healing process. There are a variety of immobilization devices that can be used.

Splint

A splint is a stiff device used to support and immobilize a part of the body that has been injured or fractured. A splint typically consists of an inflexible material, like plastic, fiberglass, or metal and may come with Velcro straps (Figure 22-5) to hold it in place. Orthopedists can also make a custom splint of plaster or fiberglass for a better fit. Temporary splints may be used before a cast is applied to allow for swelling. Once the swelling has decreased, a cast can then be applied.

Procedure for Splinting

Procedures used for splinting will vary according to the materials that are available. Many first aid kits come complete with commercial splints. These splints are usually very easy to apply and come with a set of detailed instructions. If a commercial splint is not available, items such as magazines, books, pieces of wood, and pillows may be used temporarily. Also, items to secure the splint such as string, strips of sheet material, or roller gauze will be needed. Sometimes a triangular bandage and gauze can be used to splint a limb when no splints are available.

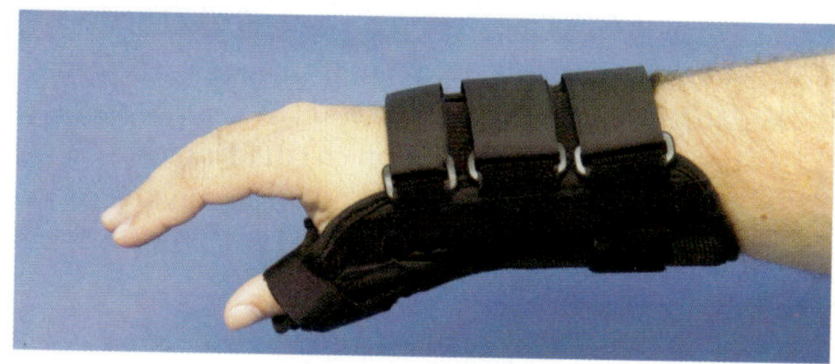

Figure 22-5 ■ A wrist splint with Velcro fasteners.

Refer to Procedure 22-1 for a complete procedure on applying a professional splint.

Application of Casts

Once the swelling has diminished from a fracture, the patient will come back to have a cast applied. The role of the medical assistant may include the following:

- Setting up the required supplies
- Assisting the provider as directed
- Educating the patient on proper care of the cast
- Alerting the patient to signs of complications that should be reported to the provider immediately

Cast

A **cast** is composed of a hard plaster or fiberglass layer (Figure 22-6) placed over a soft cotton layer. The cast usually extends to the joints above and below the fracture site. Half casts are sometimes used to allow for swelling; however, they offer less support than a full cast.

Plaster is cheaper and shapes better, but fiberglass is lightweight, durable, air permeable, and waterproof. Casting materials (Figure 22-7) usually come in rolls that are dipped in water and then applied over a layer of cotton or synthetic padding. The material is smoothed and shaped during application so it will hold the bone in the correct position after it hardens. The casting material will heat as it hardens, so patients should be warned so they know what to expect. Extra padding may be used to diminish the heating sensation.

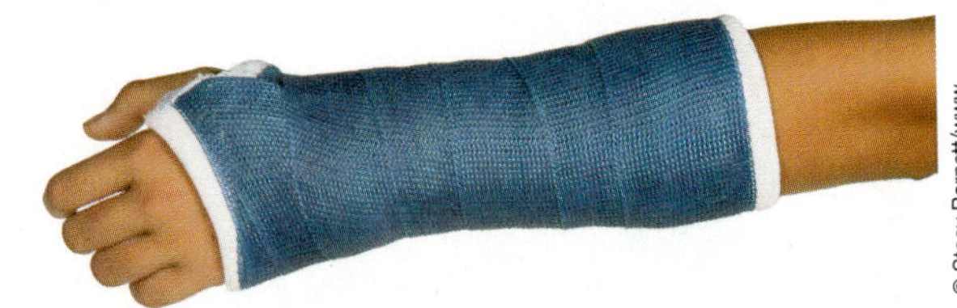

Figure 22-6 ■ An example of a fiberglass cast.

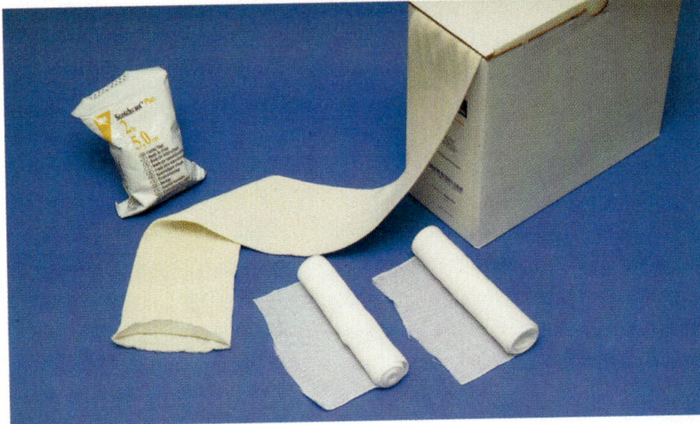

Figure 22-7 ■ Various casting materials.

Cast Removal

Patients often follow up for a cast removal 6 to 10 weeks following its application. Equipment necessary for cast removal includes the following:

- Electric cast cutter
- Cast spreader
- Bandage scissors
- Materials for washing the limb post cast removal
- Supportive bandages and appliances

Health Coach

Guidelines for Cast Care

The following guidelines will help to ensure proper healing of the fractured bone and improve the longevity of the cast:

- Allow the cast material to dry completely.
- The casted extremity should be elevated to reduce swelling (swelling during the first 48 to 72 hours may cause pressure and tightness).
- Move toes or fingers often and check for a color or temperature change, which could indicate restricted blood flow in the tissues below the cast.
- Apply an ice bag over the area of the break so that it wraps around the cast.
- Keep the cast dry. (Some manufacturers of fiberglass materials state that patients may bathe and swim while wearing a cast.)
- Cover the cast with a protective waterproof covering, such as a plastic bag, when bathing.
- Do not pull on the padding inside the cast.
- Do not stick objects inside the cast.
- Do not trim the edges of the cast.
- Report the following symptoms to the provider immediately:
  - Increased pain, numbness, or tingling
  - Excessive swelling
  - Cold fingers or toes or loss of movement (could indicate that the cast is too tight)
  - Burning or stinging (could also indicate that the cast is too tight)

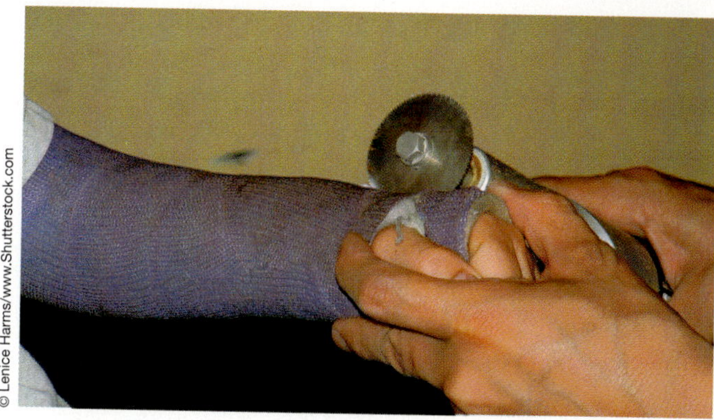

Figure 22-8 ■ A cast being removed using an electric cast cutter.

The medical assistant will gather all of the supplies for the provider and explain the procedure to the patient. Patients may be fearful of the look and sound of the electric cast cutter, which is an electronic saw with a circular blade (Figure 22-8). The patients can listen to music with headsets to help drown out the sound from the saw.

The blade oscillates or vibrates against hard surfaces, thus it doesn't typically cut tissue. To prevent injury, many providers place a plastic skin protector between the skin and the saw to avoid any burns or other injuries to the patient's skin.

Traction

Traction can also be used to immobilize a body part by attaching a weight to pull or draw the bones into proper alignment.

Ambulatory Assistive Devices

The term **ambulation** means the ability to walk or move about freely. Following an injury, surgery, or prolonged illness, it may be necessary for a patient to use an assistive device in order to ambulate, including a cane, crutches, walker, or wheelchair. It may be the responsibility of the medical assistant to instruct the patient in the use of these devices.

The specific type of assistive device prescribed by the provider will depend upon the amount of support needed by the patient. The age of the patient and the amount of muscle strength will also be considered before deciding on the proper device.

When transferring or assisting patients with assistive devices, a gait belt should be placed around the patient's trunk to support the patient and prevent falls.

Canes

A cane will usually be prescribed for the patient who needs slight support on one side of the body. Canes are generally used long term, especially for patients with a weakness on one side of the body due to a stroke or those with poor balance. Canes are usually made of wood or metal and have either a curved or T-shaped handle (Figure 22-9). The basic types of canes include the following:

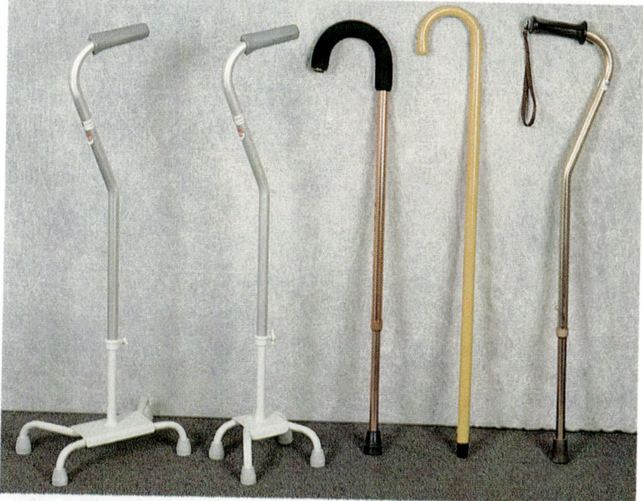

Figure 22-9 ■ Various types of canes that work with the patient's mobility level.

- Standard: Used for patients needing little support
- Tripod: Three-legged base, which provides greater stability than a standard cane
- Quad: Rests on four legs and also provides a greater amount of support and stability than other types of canes

Both the tripod and quad canes are adjustable, have T-shaped handles, and can stand alone, which allows the patient to use both arms when standing from a sitting position.

Canes must be the correct height in order to provide optimum support for the patient. When the patient stands tall and places the hand on the handle of the cane it should be even with the top of the hipbone, and the elbow should be flexed at a 20°–30° angle. The patient should not lean on the cane, but use it as a support for better ambulation and balance. The cane is held in the hand on the strong side of the body.

The medical assistant may be asked to instruct the patient on the proper use of a cane or to reinforce the instructions given by the provider. Refer to Procedure 22-2 for instructions on the use of a cane.

Crutches

Crutches are usually used when weight bearing on the foot or leg is prohibited. Patients recovering from a sprain or fracture and those with certain diseases or congenital deformities may be required to use crutches in order to ambulate.

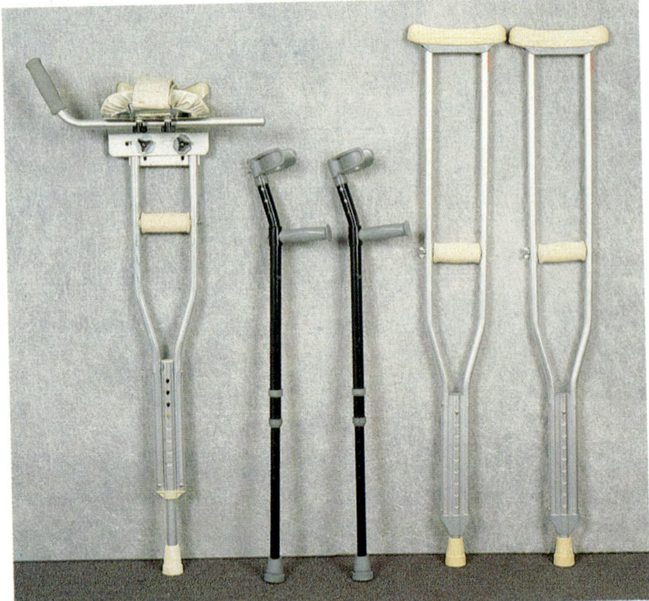

Figure 22-10 ■ A platform crutch, forearm/Lofstrand crutches, axillary crutches.

Crutches are made from wood or aluminum with rubber tips to prevent slippage on the floor. Three types of crutches are shown in Figure 22-10: platform, forearm, and axillary crutches.

Axillary crutches, usually used during healing of a lower extremity, have a shoulder rest and a handgrip and extend from the floor to just beneath the armpit. Figure 22-11a shows a patient using axillary crutches. The forearm or Lofstrand/Canadian crutch extends from the ground to the forearm. A plastic or metal cuff is attached to the crutch, which wraps around the patient's forearm. With this type of crutch, the weight is borne on the handgrip, which is protected by rubber. This crutch type requires greater strength and coordination and is usually used long term by patients with cerebral palsy or paraplegia (Figure 22-11b).

Platform crutches are designed for use by patients who cannot bear weight on their hands or wrists or who have difficulty gripping the handles. A platform with a handgrip is attached to the top of the crutch and is designed so that the patient bears weight on the entire forearm (Figure 22-11c).

Measuring for Axillary Crutches

Axillary crutches must be properly fitted to each individual patient. Improperly fitting crutches can cause nerve damage and injuries to the axilla and palms of the hands.

Crutches that are too long can create pressure in the armpits and force the patient's shoulders forward, which can cause back strain and make walking difficult. Crutches that are too short cause the patient to bend forward when walking, which causes poor balance.

To determine the correct crutch height, the patient should be instructed to stand erect. The crutch tips should be placed two inches in front of and four to six inches to the side of each foot. Adjust the crutch length so that the axillary bar is two to three finger widths below the axilla (Figure 22-12). The handgrips should be adjusted so that the elbows are bent at an angle of approximately 20°–30°.

Crutch Gaits

Generally, there are five crutch gaits used: two-point, three-point, four-point, swing-to, and swing-through.

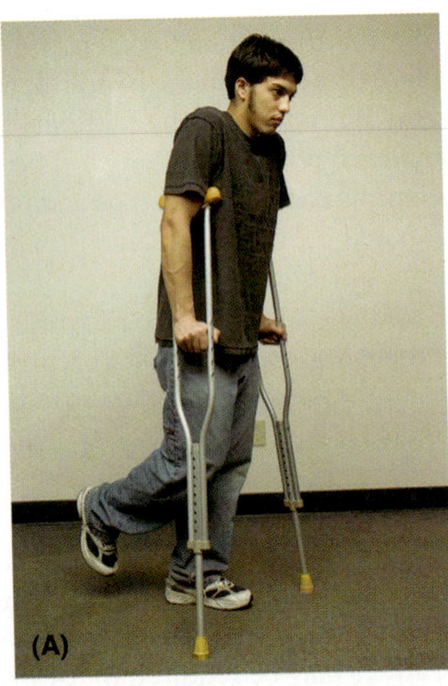

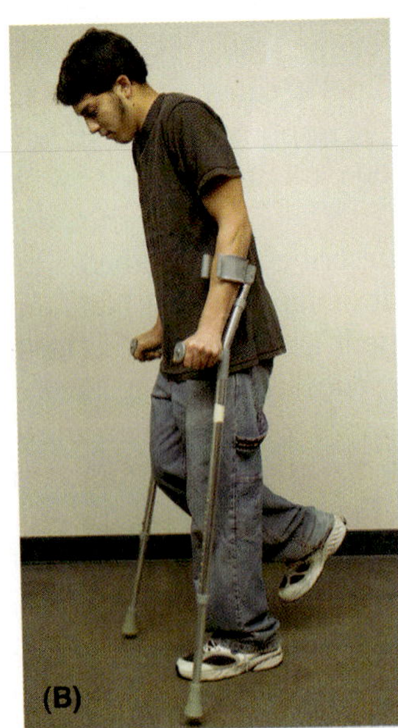

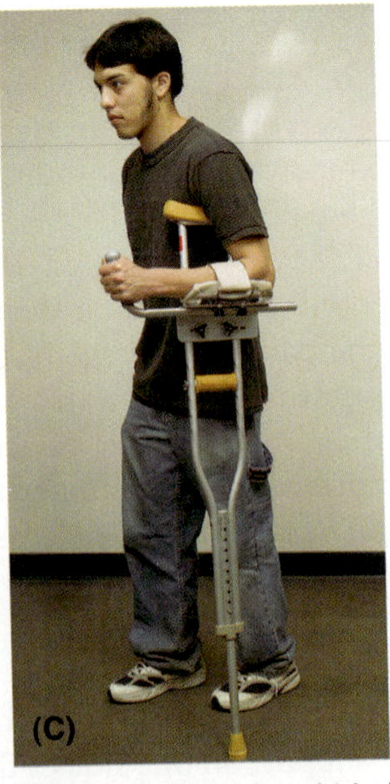

Figure 22-11 ■ A patient demonstrating the use of different types of crutches: (a) axillary, (b) forearm/Lofstrand, and (c) platform.

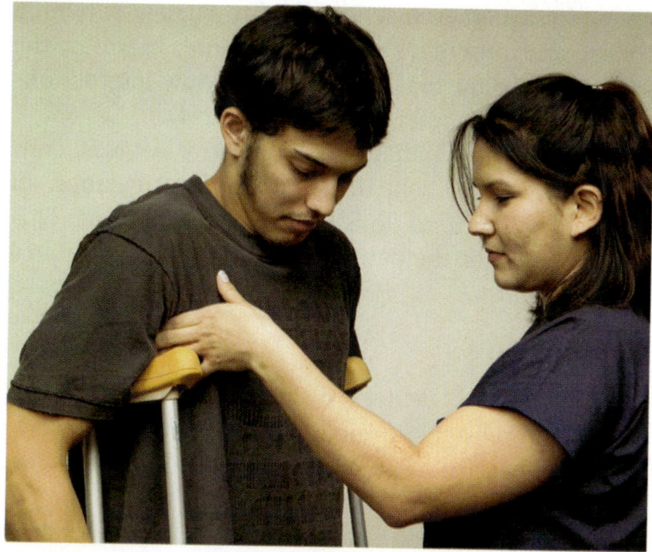

Figure 22-12 ■ Correctly measure the patient for axillary crutches by adjusting them so that the crutches are two or three finger widths below the patient's armpits.

The gait used depends on the amount of weight bearing allowed and the patient's physical condition. Table 22-6 lists an explanation of the different gaits. When describing a gait, the term "point" refers to when the patient's foot or the crutch touches the ground. Figure 22-13 illustrates the two-point, three-point, and four-point crutch gaits.

Caution patients to bear their weight on the hands and not on the armpits. Bearing weight on the axilla can cause permanent nerve damage, as well as soreness, which can cause muscle weakness in the hands, wrists, and forearms.

Helping the patient use the crutches will require a knowledge of the various crutch gaits to first demonstrate the gait and then supervise the patient.

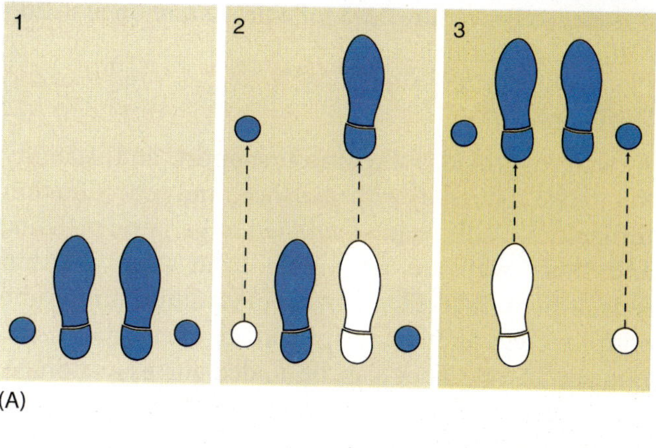

(A)

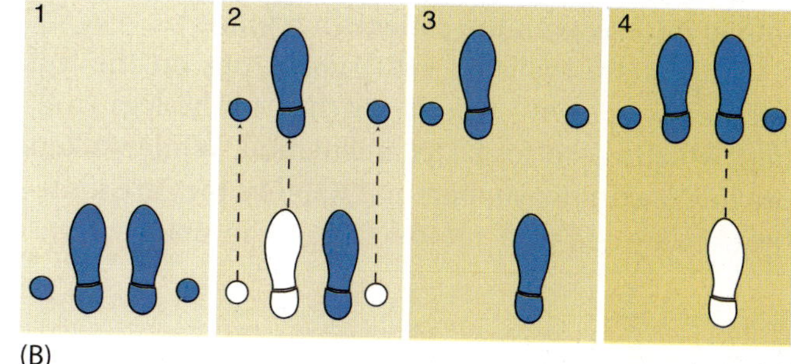

(B)

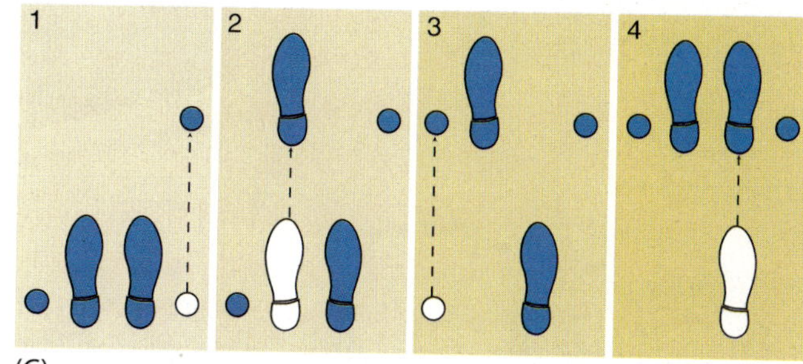

(C)

Figure 22-13 ■ Examples of crutch gaits: (a) two-point, (b) three-point, and (c) four-point.

Table 22-6 Crutch Gaits

Gait	Description	Uses
Four-point	Basic and slow gait, which allows the patient to bear weight on both the legs. Provides three points of support at all times; very stable and safe.	Patients with muscle weakness in the legs, poor balance or coordination, and degenerative diseases.
Three-point	The patient must support the weight on only one leg. Both the crutches and the weak leg are moved forward at the same time. The weight is then transferred to the crutches and the strong leg is moved forward.	Amputees without prostheses; patients with lower extremity trauma, fractures, and sprains; and patients recovering from surgery.
Two-point	Two points support the body at the same time. More advanced gait, used after mastery of the four-point gait.	Partial weight bearing on both legs in patients with good muscle coordination.
Swing-to	The crutches are moved forward simultaneously and the weight is transferred forward. Both feet are then moved forward together, ending even with the crutches.	Patients suffering from paralysis or severe disabilities of the lower extremities; patients wearing leg braces.
Swing-through	The crutches are moved forward simultaneously while transferring the weight forward. Both feet are then moved forward together, ending slightly in front of the crutches.	Same as swing-to.

Refer to Procedure 22-3 for a procedure on assisting patients with crutches.

Walkers

A walker provides the most support and stability for those patients with balance and coordination difficulties. Walkers are often used by geriatric patients, and those who are recovering from knee and hip replacement. Walkers are made of an aluminum frame with four legs and handgrips and are open on one side (Figure 22-14). They can be folded for easy storage. The height of the walker may be adjusted by having the patient stand on a level surface. The top of the walker should be level with the patient's hip joint.

Walkers are available with rubber tips on the legs (stationary) or with wheels attached to the legs (rolling), which allows for faster ambulation. While walkers provide maximum support and stability, they are sometimes bulky and difficult to maneuver in small areas.

A physical therapist usually fits the patient for a walker and provides training in its use; however, the medical assistant may be asked to review instructions with the patient (refer to Procedure 22-4).

When helping patients with assistive devices, consider using a gait belt. If the patient loses balance, all that you will have to do is lift up on the gait belt. This helps to prevent the patient from sustaining an injury due to a fall.

Wheelchairs

Wheelchairs are devices that enable a patient who would otherwise be immobile to move about. Wheelchairs can be manual or large motorized models. Figure 22-15 illustrates the parts of a manual wheelchair.

Medical assistants must familiarize themselves with the parts of the wheelchair prior to working with patients. Know how to lock the wheels, how to remove and apply the foot pedals, and how to collapse

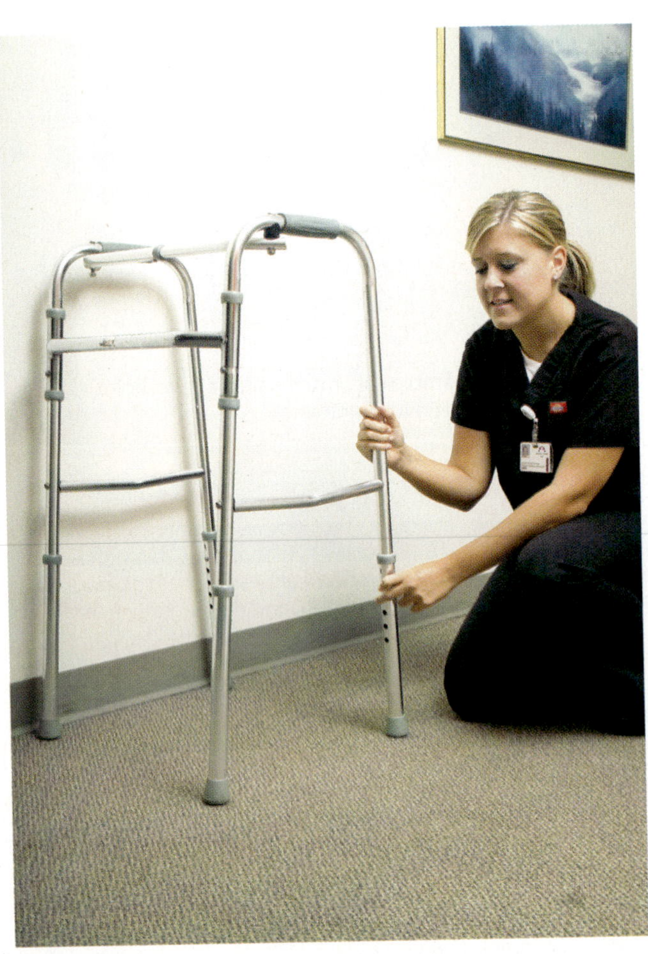

Figure 22-14 ■ A stationary walker.

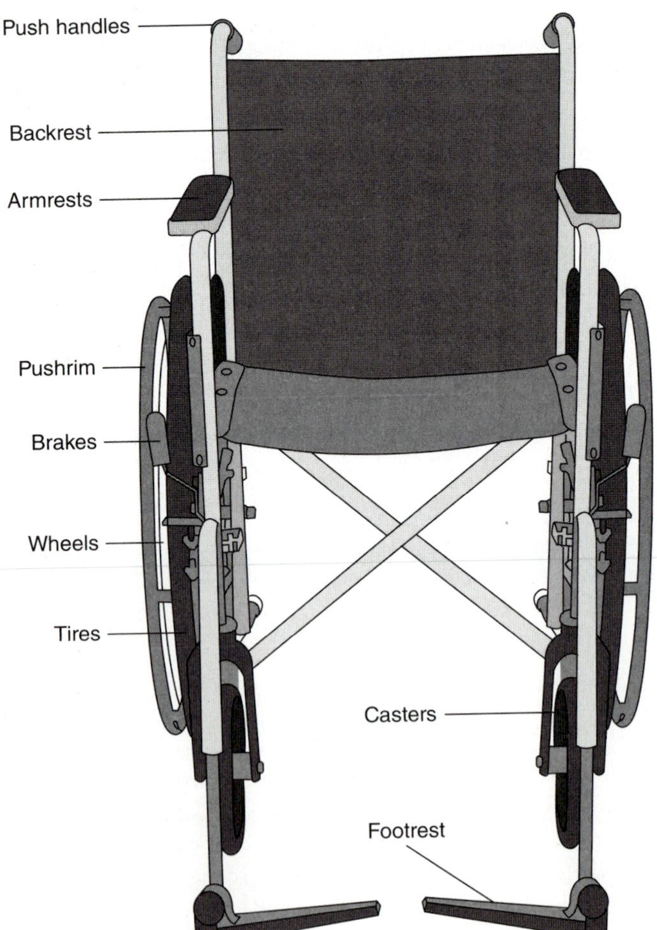

Figure 22-15 ■ The parts of a wheelchair. (Knowing the parts of the wheelchair will assist you in wheelchair transfers.)

the wheelchair just in case you have to park it out of the way during an X-ray or examination. Always use a gait belt for wheelchair transfers and remember to bend your knees, not your back, when lifting patients to avoid injuring yourself. For a complete procedure in transferring a patient from the wheelchair to the exam table, refer to Procedure 22-5.

Common Exams Using Diagnostic Imaging

Table 22-7 lists common exams using diagnostic imaging that are used in the evaluation and diagnosis of orthopedic conditions and diseases.

COMMON ORTHOPEDIC TREATMENTS

There are a variety of treatments in the form of procedures and medications that treat orthopedic conditions. Some orthopedic treatments were already featured in the Health Coach Disease Feature earlier in the chapter. Others can be found in the following section.

Surgical Procedures

Advances in medical science have given the orthopedist the skills, tools, and materials to not only repair badly broken bones, but to reconstruct and even replace damaged parts of the skeleton. Hands can now be reconstructed, the spinal vertebrae can be fused together, and whole joints can be replaced.

Minimally invasive surgeries using an arthroscope vs. standard, open surgical techniques, have revolutionized orthopedic surgery. Such techniques result in less postoperative swelling, less postoperative pain, a decreased risk of complications, and a more rapid recovery time than with open surgical techniques. Almost all arthroscopic procedures can be performed in an outpatient setting.

Total joint replacement surgery for knees, hips, shoulders, and ankles are now possible for patients with injuries, deformities, or severe arthritic conditions. Knees, hips, and shoulders can also be surgically restored by removing certain damaged parts of the joint and substituting a plastic or metal device called a **prosthesis** (artificial joint). Patients may be considered candidates for partial or total joint replacement if they have

- limited function and mobility affecting work, recreation, and activities of daily living (ADLs);
- pain that has not been relieved by medications, physical therapy, using a cane, or restricting activity;
- significant joint stiffness;
- X-rays revealing advanced arthritis or other issues; and
- pain that has not been relieved through **arthroscopy** (the visualization of a joint and joint capsule through a lighted instrument for treatment).

The four most common orthopedic surgeries are the following:

1. Total joint (knee, hip, and ankle) replacement
2. Total shoulder replacement
3. Spine surgery
4. **Anterior cruciate ligament (ACL)** repair. The ACL is the major stabilizing ligament of the knee.

Other common orthopedic procedures include the surgical treatment of hand dysfunctions such as carpal tunnel syndrome, foot deformities, and systemic diseases, such as gout, osteoarthritis, and osteomyelitis, including neoplasms (cancer).

Table 22-7 Common Exams Using Diagnostic Imaging

Exam	Description	Uses
CT scan	X-rays that produce cross-sectional views of different areas of the body	To diagnose a variety of diseases and conditions of the bones and muscles
MRI	Uses magnetic waves to produce images of the inside of the body	To visualize any bone, joint, or muscle in the body
Bone scan	Visualizes the distribution of an IV-injected radioactive isotope that collects in the bones and joints	To detect and evaluate areas of arthritis, increases and decreases in bone metabolism, and cancerous metastases
Arthrography	Dye is injected into a joint and X-rays are taken	To view ligaments, tendons, cartilage, and the joint capsule
Discography	Dye is injected into one or more intervertebral discs and a CT scan is performed	Evaluation of discs to determine the cause of pain or the presence of a disorder
X-rays	Permanent film record of a body part	To diagnose fractures and dislocations of the bones and joints of the body

Rehabilitation

Part of the healing process following an injury or orthopedic surgery involves **rehabilitation** and **physical therapy**—therapy to develop, maintain, and restore maximum movement to the musculoskeletal tissues. The goal of this type of treatment is to restore as much function and mobility to the patient as possible. For some patients who suffer a permanent loss of function, rehabilitation helps them find a workable solution to assist them with the activities of daily living (ADLs). Many health care professionals play an important role in a patient's recovery.

Physical Therapists and Occupational Therapists

Physical therapists (PTs) and occupational therapists (OTs) are medical specialists who use a variety of treatment methods to help patients recover from injury or surgery and to also cope with chronic illnesses and conditions. **Massage**, which involves the use of pressure, friction, and kneading to promote muscle relaxation, is frequently used. PTs, in general, focus on the lower extremities for strengthening and ambulation. OTs, in general, focus on the upper extremities, for the activities of daily living such as dressing, grooming, and bathing. The therapy goals of the OT and PT are to

- reduce the extent of damage to an injured or diseased limb or other related structure,
- assist in recovering lost functions,
- aid the patient in adapting to the current level of activity,
- help the patient to remain physically fit, and
- assist the patient in performing ADLs with little or no help from others.

The OT assists patients with learning how to perform ADLs with the least amount of strain on the impaired body part. The OT can also make suggestions for modifying the home or workplace and even recommend assistive devices to help with bathing, driving, dressing, and housekeeping.

The PT utilizes physical agents or **modalities** such as heat, cold, water, massage, and exercise to improve or restore lost function. The PT may also suggest the use of an **assistive device** like a cane, walker, or crutches to help the patient with mobility.

The role of the medical assistant in physical therapy may be to administer a variety of modalities including thermotherapy, hydrotherapy, and ultrasound treatments. The provider will prescribe the exact treatment necessary and the medical assistant will follow the provider's instructions. Remember: never administer any type of treatment without a direct order from the provider.

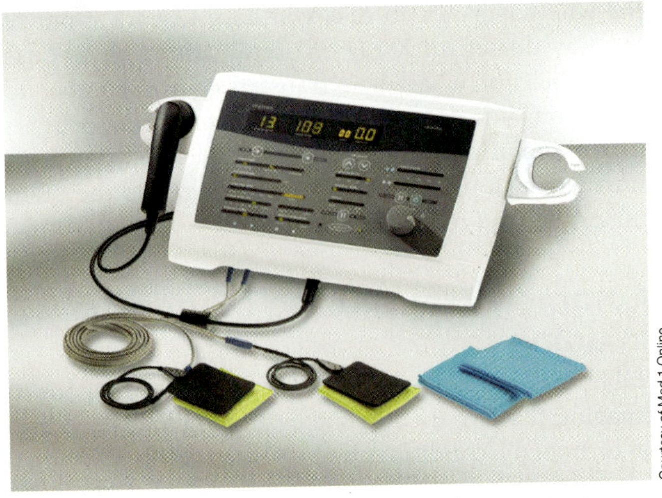

Courtesy of Med 1 Online

Figure 22-16 ■ Metron Vectorsonic VU270 ultrasound unit.

Ultrasound

A deep-tissue modality such as therapeutic ultrasound (Figure 22-16) is used to promote healing of the deeper tissues. **Ultrasound** uses high-frequency sound waves to create heat deep in soft tissues such as muscles and tendons. Ultrasound works best on tissues with a high water concentration and does not penetrate the bone at all.

The medical assistant may be trained to administer an ultrasound treatment in the provider's office under the direction of the provider; however, the laws governing medical assisting duties can vary by state, and it is a good idea to check the Medical Practice Act in the state where you are employed.

Electrical Stimulation of Muscles

Muscles that have been injured or those that have not functioned for a prolonged period of time may need to be stimulated in order for the muscle to be able to move. Low-voltage electric current is delivered directly into a muscle, which causes it to involuntarily contract and relax. This helps to prevent muscle atrophy and stimulates healing. A transcutaneous electrical nerve stimulation (TENS) unit (Figure 22-17) can be worn by patients with spinal cord injuries to help them ambulate and can also be worn to aid in pain control.

Hydrotherapy

This type of therapy, which uses circulating water, is usually performed in hospitals and large clinics, but may also be used in orthopedic and podiatry offices. Hydrotherapy is used to treat injuries, burns, and other

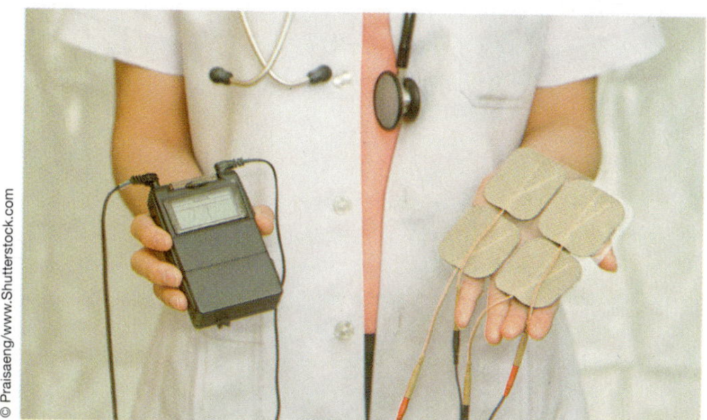
© Praisaeng/www.Shutterstock.com

Figure 22-17 ■ A transcutaneous electrical nerve impulse (TENS) unit.

physical problems. The different forms of hydrotherapy include the following:

- Whirlpools: This therapy consists of a tank filled with constantly moving water. Pressurized air shoots from jets located in the walls of the tank that keep the water circulating. The moving water creates a gentle massage, which increases circulation and relaxes muscles. Whirlpools may range in size from small models that will accept one body part, to those large enough to immerse the entire body. This type of treatment facilitates the removal of necrotic tissue from burn patients, through a process known as **debridement** to remove dead tissue.
- Contrast baths: This method is most often used to treat the hands and feet. The hand or foot is first immersed in hot water for 1 minute and then cold water for 30 seconds. The process is repeated for the prescribed amount of time. The contrast bath should end with cold immersion. This type of hydrotherapy promotes circulation and relaxation.
- Medicated baths: The body is soaked in a bath to which a substance such as oatmeal or Epsom salts has been added.
- Water exercises: Exercises are performed in a warm swimming pool, in water that is shoulder-deep. Exercising in water relieves pain and relaxes muscles, which is ideal for patients with joint problems. The water supports the body and makes movement more tolerable by taking pressure off the joints.

Thermal Modalities

Thermal modalities include the use of heat (**thermotherapy**), cold (cryotherapy), and deep heat therapy achieved through the use of ultrasound. The following factors should be considered before applying any hot or cold modality.

- The age of the patient should be considered. Infants and the elderly are more sensitive to heat and cold and may be unable to report painful sensations.
- Use caution when administering treatment to particularly sensitive areas.
- Avoid areas with broken skin.
- Patients with impaired circulation or sensation, such as those with diabetes or cardiovascular disease, may be unable to distinguish the degree of heat or cold.
- Do *not* apply heat during the first 24 hours of an acute injury or when edema or inflammation is present.
- Always wrap hot or cold articles in a cloth before applying them to the skin.

Thermotherapy

Thermotherapy entails applying dry or moist heat to a body part to promote healing and restore function. Heat increases circulation by creating **vasodilation** (expansion of blood vessels). Increased circulation accelerates tissue metabolism, which promotes healing. Heat is used to

- relax muscles and alleviate muscle spasms,
- relieve pain,
- increase flexibility,
- provide comfort, and
- promote drainage from an infected area.

Heat therapy is categorized as dry or moist. Dry heat modalities include those listed in Table 22-8.

Moist heat modalities penetrate better than dry heat modalities and include those listed in Table 22-9.

Table 22-8 Examples of Dry Heat Modalities

Modality	Description
Heating pads	Always cover the pad with a cloth or towel and adjust the temperature to the level prescribed by the provider. Do *not* adjust the temperature to a higher level if requested by the patient, as this could result in a severe burn.
Hot packs	Chemical hot packs (Figure 22-18) become hot when activated by following the manufacturer's directions. These disposable, flexible packs easily adjust to fit different body parts.
Hot water bottles	The water temperature should not exceed 110°F (43°C). After filling, cover the bottle with a cloth before applying to the body. Refill as needed to maintain the proper temperature level.

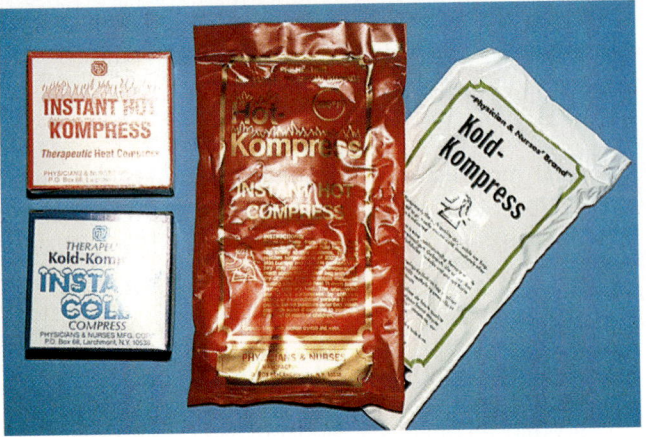

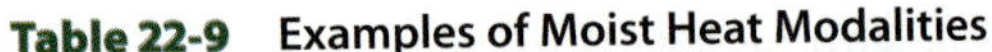

Figure 22-18 ■ Examples of chemical heat and cold packs.

Table 22-9 **Examples of Moist Heat Modalities**

Modality	Description
Hot compresses (Figure 22-19)	A gauze pad or soft cloth is soaked in water no hotter than 110°F (43°C), wrung out, and applied gradually over the affected area. This modality can easily be administered at home.
Hot packs	The pack is soaked in hot water no greater than 110°F (43°C), covered with a pad, and placed on larger areas of the body, such as the back and shoulders.
Hot soaks	The body part is immersed in plain or medicated water that is no hotter than 110°F (43°C) for approximately 15 minutes. This treatment is usually used for the extremities.
Paraffin baths	Used to treat chronic joint diseases, like rheumatoid arthritis. The affected body part is dipped into a mixture of melted paraffin and water until a thick coating of wax is achieved. After 30 minutes, the paraffin is peeled away.

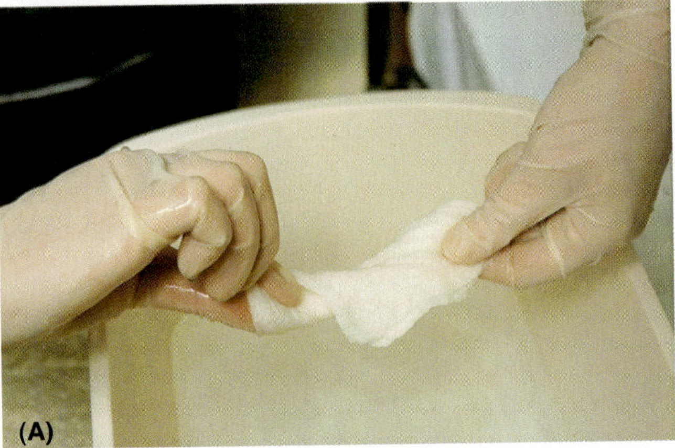

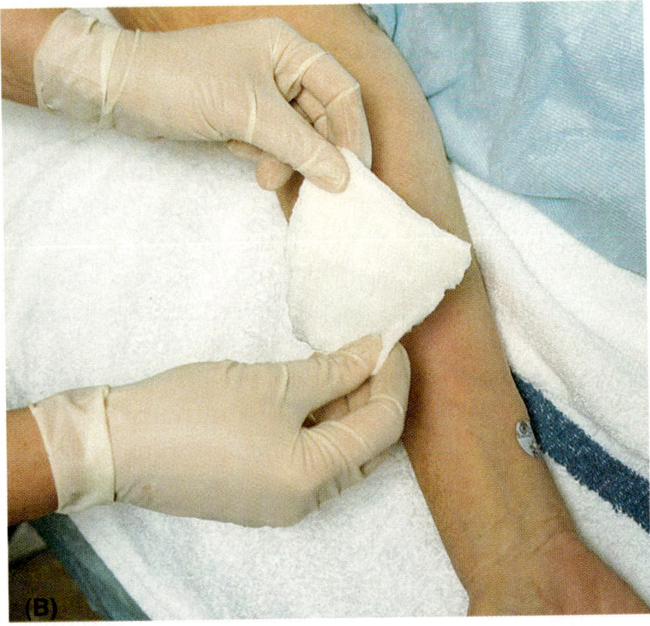

Figure 22-19 ■ (a) Dip the compress in the heated water and wring out excess water before application. (b) Carefully apply moist hot compresses directly to the affected area. *Note:* Once the compress is applied to the skin, wrap a waterproof drape around the area to keep the warmth in.

Refer to Procedure 22-6 for a procedure on applying heat.

Cryotherapy

Cryotherapy involves the application of dry or moist cold to the affected area of the body. Application of cold constricts the blood vessels and induces contraction of the involuntary muscles. Cold application can also produce a numbing affect, which can help to reduce pain.

The applications of cryotherapy are as follows:

- Prevent swelling by decreasing the accumulation of fluid in the tissue
- Provide pain relief
- Decrease inflammation
- Decrease pus formation by suppressing microbial growth
- Decrease body temperature
- Help to control bleeding

Cryotherapy is most effective if used frequently during the first 48 hours after an injury. Dry cold modalities include those listed in Table 22-10.

If the patient does not have a commercial ice pack available, a bag of frozen vegetables will work as a cold pack. As the bag thaws a bit, it contours around the patient's limb. Instruct the patient to lay a towel or cloth between the skin and the frozen vegetables.

Moist cold modalities are usually used for smaller areas of the body and include those listed in Table 22-11.

Refer to Procedure 22-7 for a procedure on applying cold therapy.

Table 22-10 Examples of Dry Cold Modalities

Modality	Description
Ice bags	The bag should be covered with a cloth before applying it to the body and can be left on the area for approximately 20–30 minutes.
Commercial ice packs	This type of pack is filled with materials that can be chilled in the freezer. Commercial ice packs usually contain a type of gel that does not freeze into a solid, which makes the pack more flexible and able to easily conform to any body part. This pack should be left in place according to the manufacturer's directions.
Chemical ice packs	These packs must be activated by squeezing or shaking the contents. The pack will stay cold for approximately 30–60 minutes.

Table 22-11 Examples of Moist Cold Modalities

Modality	Description
Cold compresses	These are created by dipping a cloth or gauze into ice water, which is then applied to the affected area. The cloth must be remoistened frequently throughout the treatment to maintain the proper temperature.
Ice massages	This modality is used following physical therapy, and consists of massaging the body area with a large ice cube, created by freezing water in a paper cup.

Arthritis Treatments

There are a variety of treatments for arthritis. Treatment plans will be based on the type of arthritis and the patient's symptoms. Weight loss plans, exercise, and physical therapy are often initial measures to treat arthritis. Medications such as nonsteroidal anti-inflammatories and corticosteroid injections help to control or relieve patient symptoms; however, there are a variety of other treatments available for the management of arthritis.

Viscosupplementation can help to relieve the severe knee pain associated with osteoarthritis for some individuals. This treatment consists of injecting a preparation of hyaluronic acid—made from rooster combs or bacterial cultures—directly into the knee joint. This lubricates the joint and keeps the dry bone ends from rubbing together, which causes intense pain. The injections are administered in three doses given one week apart. Patients should be informed that they will not feel the full effects of the treatment until approximately one month after the last injection. Some patients do very well with this treatment, which can delay surgery as long as the treatment proves to be beneficial, while others experience little or no relief at all.

New techniques are being developed to restore cartilage in joints where it has been lost. Cartilage grafting involves transplanting cartilage from a healthy area into the joint that has little or no cartilage left. A patient's own tissue (**autograft**) or a donor graft (**allograft**) may be used. To prevent rejection of the grafted tissue, however, a tissue match must be found.

Another technique used to replace lost cartilage is stem cell regeneration. Stem cells harvested through bone marrow aspiration (the withdrawing bone marrow) and under the right circumstances can regenerate articular cartilage. This technique is still being developed, but has shown a lot of promise in treating particular injuries and arthritis.

Exercises

Therapeutic exercise may be prescribed as a treatment for arthritis and fractures, to promote healing and flexibility following an injury, surgery, amputation, and even for patients who have suffered a stroke.

Most exercise programs are designed by the provider to accommodate each patient's individual needs. Therapeutic exercise is used for a variety of reasons including the following:

- Helping a patient to regain mobility after an accident, injury, or surgery
- Preventing muscle atrophy during a prolonged period of immobilization
- Developing or improving neuromuscular coordination
- Developing muscle tone and strength
- Improving circulation
- Strengthening the heart and lungs

Table 22-12 lists some of the different types of exercises commonly prescribed. Figure 22-20 illustrates some of the range of motion (ROM) exercises, and

Table 22-12 Forms of Strengthening Exercises

Type	Description	Uses	Required Equipment
Active	Performed by the patient without assistance	Increases muscle strength and function	Treadmill Stationary bike
Passive	Physical therapist moves the body part without any voluntary movement by the patient	Treats neuromuscular problems, helps to maintain range of motion, and increases circulation	Machines designed specifically to assist with different body movements
Assisted	Self-directed, aided mobility	Improves muscle strength	Walking in a swimming pool
Active resistance	Voluntary movement by the patient against pressure created by the physical therapist or a machine	Increases muscle strength	Refer to equipment for passive exercises
Range of motion (ROM)	Gentle movement of a joint through its normal range of motion	Relieves stiffness, improves joint movement, and increases flexibility Recommended to treat joint injuries and the elderly	None needed

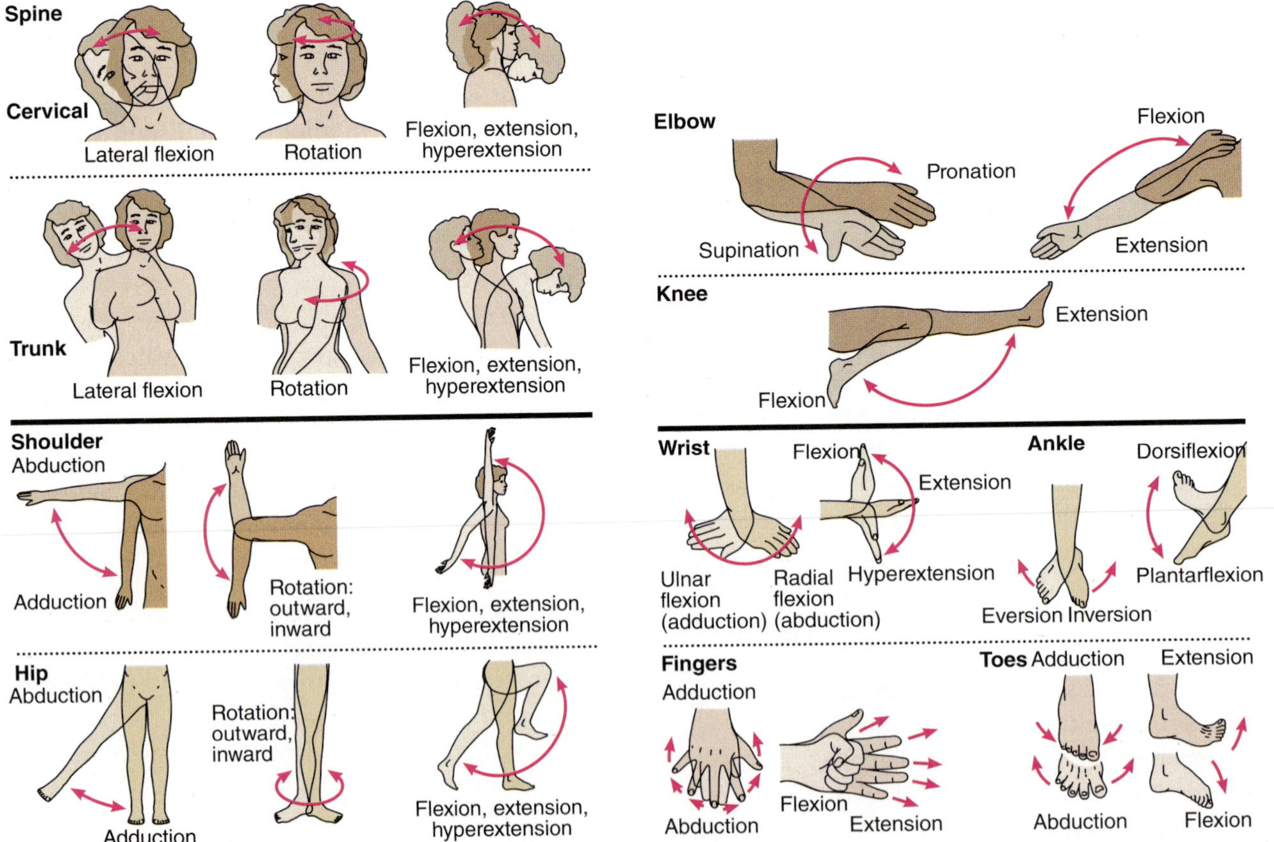

Figure 22-20 ■ Examples of range of motion (ROM) exercises and movements, which are performed to improve circulation, flexibility, and muscle tone.

Table 22-13 lists the terms used to describe the different forms of movement used in ROM.

COMMON ORTHOPEDIC MEDICATIONS

There are also several medications used in the treatment of orthopedic disorders. Table 22-14 features some of the most common orthopedic medications.

Table 22-13 Joint Movement Terms

Technical Term	Description
Abduction	Movement away from the midline of the body
Adduction	Movement toward the midline of the body
Circumduction	To move a body part in a circular motion
Dorsiflexion	Posterior movement of a body part at the joint
Eversion	Turning outward
Extension	To straighten; the opposite of flexion
Flexion	To bend; the opposite of extension
Hyperextension	Abnormal or extreme extension (beyond normal limits)
Inversion	To turn inward
Plantar flexion	Pointing the foot downward at the ankle
Pronation	Turning the palm downward; lying face down
Rotation	Turning a body part on its axis
Supination	Turning the palm upward; lying flat on the back

COMMON DIAGNOSTIC TESTS THAT COINCIDE WITH ORTHOPEDIC DISORDERS

Several lab tests can be performed to evaluate specific orthopedic disorders. Table 22-15 features some of the common diagnostic tests that coincide with these disorders.

Table 22-15 Common Diagnostic Tests That Coincide with Orthopedic Disorders

Test	Clinical Significance
Antibody test	Used to measure the RA factor. An elevation is diagnostic for rheumatoid arthritis.
Arthroscopy	Insertion of a lighted scope into a joint. Used to inspect the inside of the joint for abnormalities (Figure 22-21).
Bone/muscle biopsy	Used to identify bone infection, cancer, or muscle atrophy. Microscopic analysis can detect infections, cancer, and muscle atrophy.
Creatine phosphokinase (CPK)	Measures the levels of CPK in the blood. Elevation indicates damage to muscles.
Electromyography	Needle electrodes are placed on different muscles to detect electrical activity.
Serum calcium, phosphorus, and potassium	Used to determine if mineral levels are within normal limits. Abnormal levels can explain abnormal musculoskeletal conditions.
Urine and blood testing	Measures the amount of minerals in the body (i.e., calcium and phosphorous). These amounts are increased with any disorder that breaks down bones or muscles.
Uric acid	Measures the level of blood uric acid. These levels are elevated when gout is present.

Table 22-14 Common Orthopedic Medications

Medication Classification	Description	Medication Examples
Anti-inflammatory agents	Drugs used to decrease inflammation.	Cortisone, nonsteroidal anti-inflammatory drugs (NSAIDs) such as ibuprofen products.
Bisphosphonates	A class of drugs to prevent loss of bone mass, most commonly prescribed to treat osteoporosis.	Fosamax, Boniva, Actonel, Novartis
Calcitonin	A hormone that reduces blood calcium for the treatment of hypercalcemia or osteoporosis.	Calcitonin/Thyrocalcitonin
Selective estrogen receptor modulators (SERMS)	A class of compounds that act on the body's estrogen receptors, to treat osteoporosis as well as certain cancers.	Femarelle, Raloxifene, Lasofoxifene
Parathyroid hormone (PTH)	Modulates calcium and phosphate homeostasis, improving bone mass as a prescription for osteoporosis. Also used off-label as therapy to speed fracture repair.	Teriparatide
Intra-articular injections	Injections to treat or reduce inflammation (e.g., tendinitis, bursitis, arthritis, fasciitis, and ligament injuries).	Cortisone
Muscle relaxants	Drugs that cause a decrease or relaxation in smooth muscle tone, reducing pain from the spasms.	Flexeril, Robaxin, Soma, Zanaflex, Valium
Narcotics	Drugs used to treat acute pain for a limited time.	Morphine, Codeine
Non-narcotic substitutes	Non-narcotic pain relievers.	Tramadol

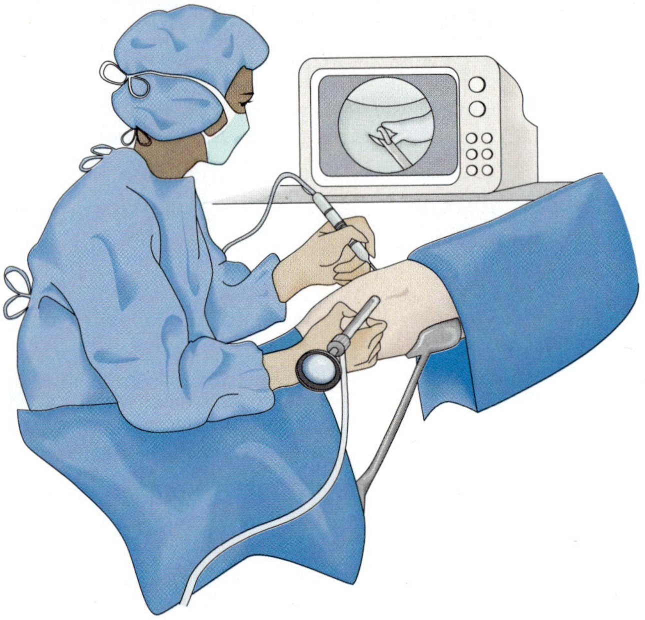

Figure 22-21a ■ The provider is using an arthroscope to view the internal structures of the knee.

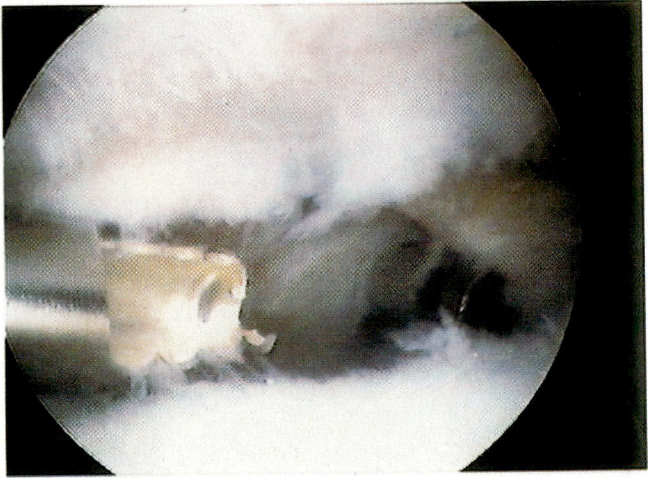

Figure 22-21b ■ An inside view of a joint through an arthroscope.

22-2 Solve the Case

Dr. Bumgardner applied a fiberglass cast to Mr. Conklin's arm and asked the patient to wear a Velcro sling to keep the arm elevated. Mr. Conklin was quite distressed and voiced concern about how he would manage his farm during the next six to eight weeks. He phoned the office three weeks following his visit complaining of burning and tingling under the cast and also reports "a funny smell" coming from the cast. He tells you that he can't get anything done with the cast and is considering removing the cast himself.

1. **What advice can you give Mr. Conklin to eliminate the smell?**
2. **Should Mr. Conklin be concerned about the burning and tingling sensations?**
3. **What should you tell Mr. Conklin about removing his own cast?**
4. **When should Mr. Conklin see Dr. Bumgardner again?**

PROCEDURE 22-1

Splint an Arm

Objective:

To appropriately splint a patient's arm who has a suspected fracture.

Equipment/Supplies:

- Splint
- Sling (if applicable)
- Patient's chart/EHR

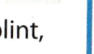

PROCEDURAL STEPS	DETAILS AND/OR RATIONALE
1. Wash hands.	
2. Assemble equipment and supplies.	Gathering equipment prior to the procedure will save time.
3. Identify the patient using two identifiers, identify yourself, and ***explain the rationale for the performance of the procedure, showing awareness of the patient's concerns. Recognize the physical and emotional effects on persons involved in an emergency situation.***	Explaining the rationale for the procedure will assist the patient in knowing why treatment is necessary.
4. Follow the steps on the commercial splint for preparing the splint.	Each commercial splint is different, so you will need to follow the instructions on the packing to apply the splint.
5. Place the arm in the position that will be used for splinting (Figure 22-22). Be sure to stabilize the injured area by stabilizing the joint above and below the injury.	Stabilizing the joints above and below the injury will secure the injured site to prevent further injury.
6. Check the pulse point distal to the injury, checking the strength of the pulse.	You need to determine if the new position is causing any obstruction to the blood flow.
7. Check for sensation and movement while the arm is in the splint position.	A lack of sensation or movement could indicate a nerve injury.
8. Apply the splint following the manufacturer's instructions (Figure 22-23). If arm is to be totally immobilized, place the arm with the splint in a sling as well.	A sling will keep the arm stationary in one position.

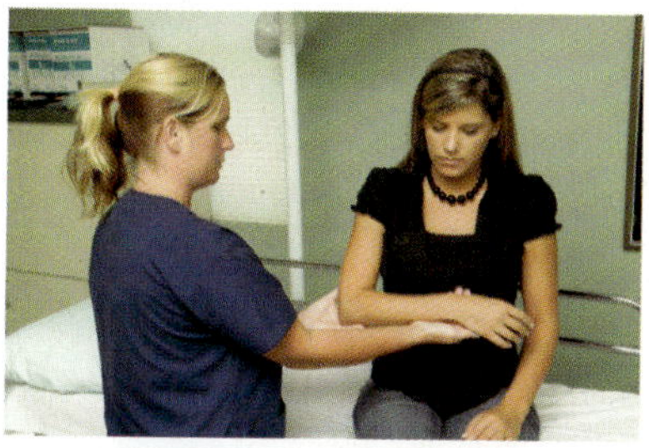

Figure 22-22 ■ Place the arm in the appropriate position for splinting.

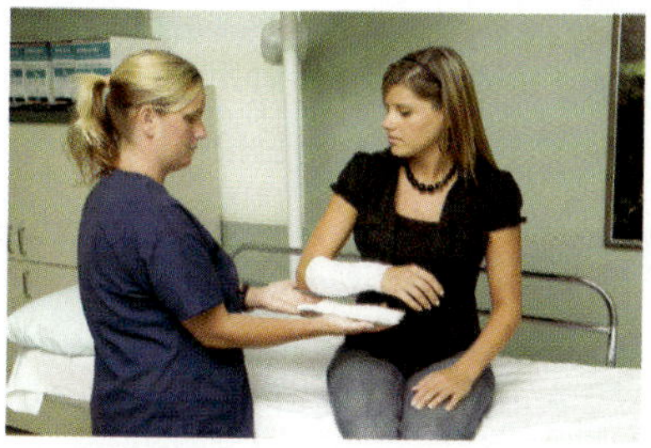

Figure 22-23 ■ Apply the splint, following the manufacturer's instructions.

continues

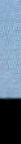

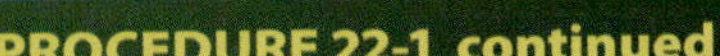

PROCEDURE 22-1 continued

PROCEDURAL STEPS	DETAILS AND/OR RATIONALE
9. Check distal pulse point, check fingers for sensation and movement after applying the splint (Figure 22-24).	Once the splint is on, circulation and nerve reflexes may be altered.
10. Apply ice to help reduce swelling.	Applying ice will help to decrease the swelling.
11. Wash your hands.	
12. Document the procedure.	Documentation is necessary for legal purposes.

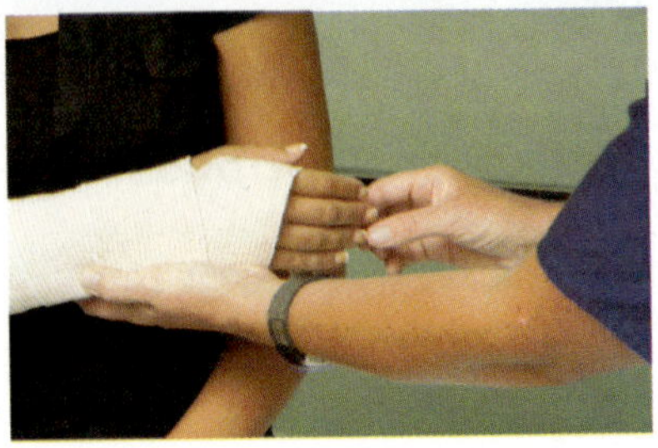

Figure 22-24 ■ Check the distal pulse point, sensation, and movement after applying the splint.

DOCUMENTATION EXAMPLE:

05-14-XX 1230	Pt. entered the office during the lunch session. Dr. Woo stepped out for lunch and was not available when the pt. first arrived. Pt. fell off of his porch hitting his R. forearm on the grill. ⊕tenderness, ⊕swelling, ⊖discoloration. Pt. had good strong pulse, movement, and sensation prior to splinting. Splinted R. forearm with commercial air splint in first aid kit and placed arm in a sling. Checked circulation, sensation, and movement once again after splinting. Good strong pulse, color was slightly pink, and temperature was warm. Pt. still able to move fingers. Applied ice and waited for Dr. Woo to return. Dr. Woo returned at 1300 and took over the management of the pt. Martin Ford, RMA (AMT)----------------

PROCEDURE 22-2
Instruct a Patient to Use a Cane

Objective:

To properly adjust the height of the cane, and to instruct the patient in the proper use of the cane.

Equipment/Supplies:

- Cane (prescribed by provider or physical therapist)
- Patient's chart/EHR

PROCEDURAL STEPS	DETAILS AND/OR RATIONALE
1. Check the provider's orders, assemble the equipment, and wash your hands.	Gathering equipment prior to the procedure will save time.
2. Identify the patient using two identifiers, identify yourself, and ***explain the rationale for the performance of the procedure, showing awareness of the patient's concerns related to the procedure being performed.***	Explaining the procedure will assist the patient in knowing what to expect during the education.

continues

PROCEDURE 22-2 continued

PROCEDURAL STEPS	DETAILS AND/OR RATIONALE
3. Inspect the tip of the cane to be sure there is a rubber tip.	The rubber tip keeps the cane from slipping on the floor.
4. Adjust the cane height so that the handle of the cane is even with the patient's hip joint and the patient's elbow is flexed at a 25°–30° angle.	
5. Demonstrate the correct usage of the cane:	
a. Hold the cane on the strong side.	Holding the cane on the strong side gives better support and balance.
b. Move the cane and the affected leg forward at the same time (Figure 22-25).	The patient should transfer the weight to the cane to avoid too much weight on the weak extremity.
c. Move the strong leg forward, slightly in front of the cane.	
d. Take slow, small steps.	Walking slowly decreases the chance of falling.
e. Repeat b and c.	
6. Apply a gait belt (an added precaution) to the patient and ask the patient to practice the procedure.	The gait belt will make it easier to hold the patient to prevent a fall in case the patient loses balance. The patient must be able to successfully walk with the cane before leaving the office.
7. Document the patient education in the patient's chart.	All educational sessions must be documented in the patient's chart.

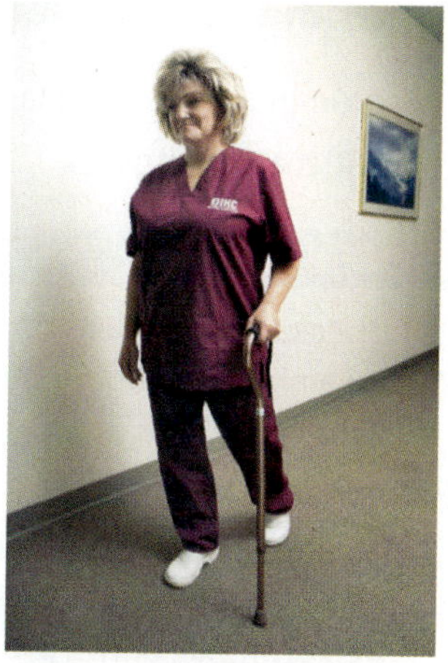

Figure 22-25 ■ The medical assistant demonstrates how to move the cane and the affected leg forward at the same time.

DOCUMENTATION EXAMPLE:

01-11-XX 2:00 p.m.	Demonstrated proper use of cane and adjusted the height to the correct level. Pt. demonstrated proper technique using the cane. Gave patient educational handout on cane use. Ben Jancowski, CMA (AAMA)--

PROCEDURE 22-3
Instruct a Patient to Use Axillary Crutches

Objective:

To properly measure a patient for axillary crutches and to teach the patient how to use the five different crutch gaits.

Equipment/Supplies:

- Aluminum/wood axillary crutches
- Patient's chart/EHR

PROCEDURAL STEPS	DETAILS AND/OR RATIONALE
1. Check the provider's orders, assemble the equipment, and wash your hands.	The provider's orders must be followed as to the type of crutches and gait used.
2. Identify the patient using two identifiers, identify yourself, and ***explain the rationale for the performance of the procedure, showing awareness of the patient's concerns related to the procedure being performed.***	Explaining the procedure will assist the patient in knowing what to expect during the education.
3. Inspect rubber tips at the bottom of each crutch and tighten wing nuts. Check pads on the hand grips and the axillary bars.	Inspecting these items and making any necessary adjustments will help to ensure patient safety and comfort.
4. Instruct the patient (Figure 22-26) to stand erect and place the crutches into the axillary space. The tip of each crutch should be held about 4 to 6 inches to the side of each foot.	This position will ensure correct measurement.
5. Adjust the crutches so there is a two-finger width space between the axillary bar and the armpits (Figure 22-27). The elbows should be flexed at a 25°–30° angle.	Correct height ensures more stability and prevents injury to the nerves of the arms and hands.

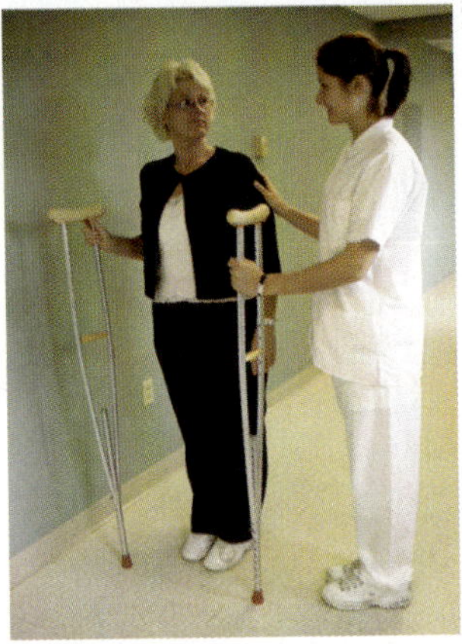

Figure 22-26 ■ The medical assistant gives the patient instructions about how to use the crutches before getting started.

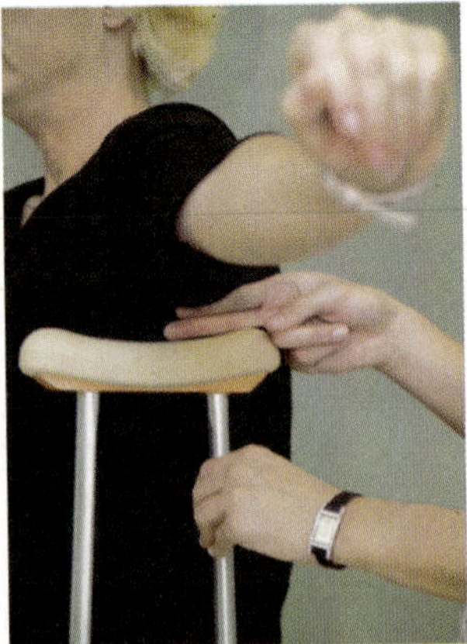

Figure 22-27 ■ The medical assistant measures the patient with the crutches to make certain that the crutches are approximately two finger widths below the patient's armpits.

continues

PROCEDURE 22-3 continued

PROCEDURAL STEPS	DETAILS AND/OR RATIONALE
6. Demonstrate the proper gait (Figure 22-28) and inform the patient not to move the crutches more than 6 inches in front of the body.	Demonstrating the procedure first will help the patient understand the instructions.
7. Allow the patient to practice. Be sure the patient is supporting her weight on the hand grips and not the axillary bar (Figure 22-29).	Supporting the weight on the axilla can cause nerve damage.
8. Instruct the patient to inspect the crutches regularly for damage to the rubber tips and pads and to check the tightness of the wing nuts.	Damaged parts or loose crutches could cause the patient to fall.
9. Document the patient education in the patient's chart.	All patient education sessions must be documented in the patient's chart.

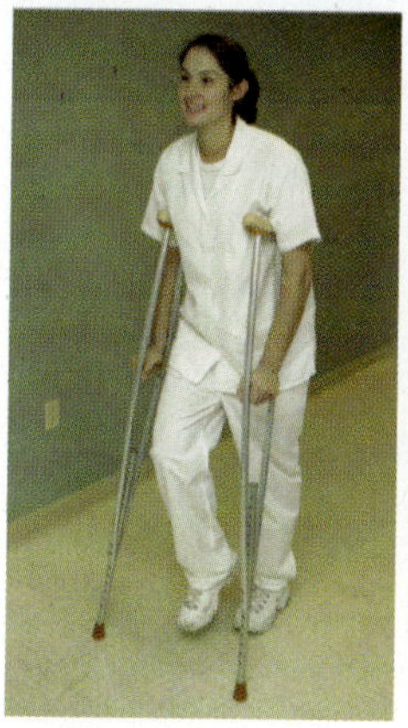

Figure 22-28 ■ The medical assistant demonstrates how to use the crutches.

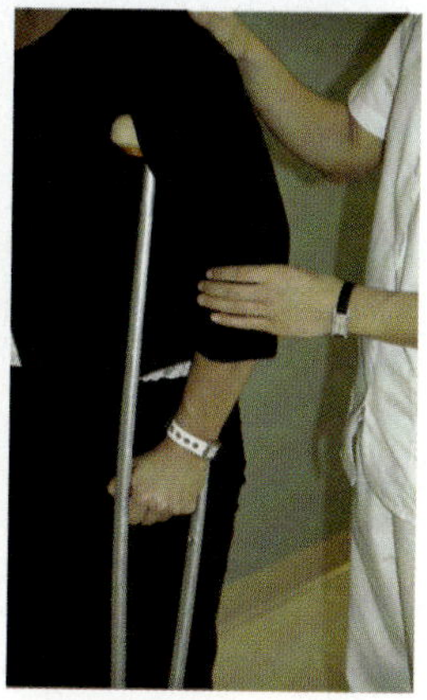

Figure 22-29 The patient supports the weight on the hands, not the axilla, to avoid damaging the nerves of the arm.

DOCUMENTATION EXAMPLE:

05-16-XX 10:00 a.m.	Pt. was fitted for axillary crutches per Dr Ansel. Demonstrated proper use of crutches. Pt. was able to successfully demonstrate back how to use the crutches. I. Crawford, CMA (AAMA)---

PROCEDURE 22-4

Instruct a Patient to Use a Walker

Objective:

To properly adjust a walker to the correct height and instruct the patient in its use.

Equipment/Supplies:

- Walker
- Patient's chart/EHR

continues

PROCEDURE 22-4 continued

PROCEDURAL STEPS	DETAILS AND/OR RATIONALE
1. Assemble the equipment and wash your hands.	Hands must be washed before each patient contact.
2. Identify the patient using two identifiers, identify yourself, and ***explain the rationale for the performance of the procedure, showing awareness of the patient's concerns related to the procedure being performed.***	Explaining the procedure will assist the patient in knowing what to expect during the education.
3. Inspect the walker to be sure the rubber tips and hand grips are in place.	Rubber tips keep the walker from slipping on the floor.
4. Adjust the height of walker (Figure 22-30), so that the hand grips of the walker are at the patient's hip level.	The walker must be at the correct height to ensure maximum stability.
5. After demonstrating the proper procedure, instruct the patient to stand inside the walker and grip the handles. (When gripping the handles, the patient's elbows should be flexed at a 25°–30° angle.) Ask the patient to pick the walker up (not slide it), move it forward about 6 inches, and walk into it (Figure 22-31).	Many patients learn easier by seeing a skill demonstrated first.
6. Inform the patient that all four walker legs should be on the ground before moving forward.	All four walker legs must be on the ground before moving to keep the walker from tipping.
7. Have the patient demonstrate the procedure.	The patient must be able to use the walker correctly before leaving the office.
8. Document the patient education in the patient's chart.	All educational sessions must be documented in the patient's chart.

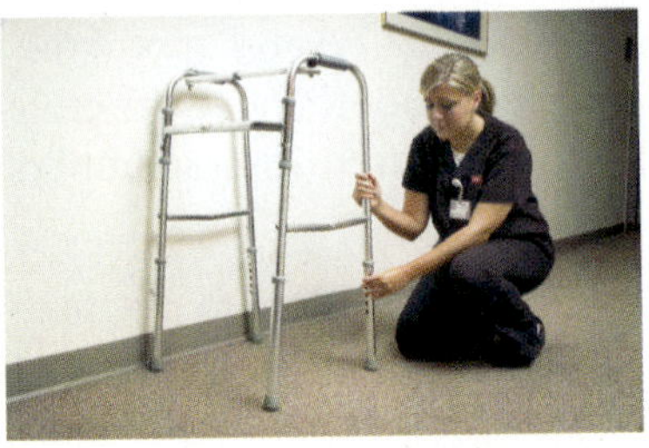

Figure 22-30 ■ The medical assistant adjusts the walker to the proper height for the patient.

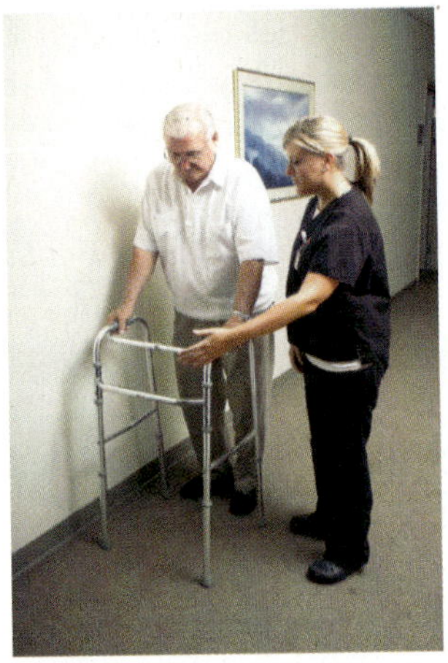

Figure 22-31 ■ The medical assistant instructs the patient to move the walker forward first and then walk into it.

DOCUMENTATION EXAMPLE:

11-08-XX 10:00 a.m.	Adjusted walker to correct height and demonstrated proper procedure for using the walker, per Dr. Raymond's orders. Pt. demonstrated correct usage. Erin Speck, CMA (AAMA)-------

PROCEDURE 22-5

Assist a Patient from the Wheelchair to the Exam Table and Back to the Wheelchair

Objective:

To correctly assist a patient from a wheelchair to the exam table and from the exam table back to the chair.

Equipment/Supplies:

- Wheelchair
- Stool
- Exam table
- Gait belt

PROCEDURAL STEPS	DETAILS AND/OR RATIONALE
1. Wash your hands.	Hands must be washed before each patient contact.
2. Identify the patient using two identifiers, identify yourself, and apply the gait belt around the patient's waist (Figure 22-32). Explain that you will assist them onto the exam table. ***Show awareness of the patient's concerns related to the procedure being performed.***	An explanation can help to alleviate the patient's fear of falling and help the patient know what to expect.
3. Place the wheelchair close to the exam table and lock the wheels (Figure 22-33). Pull out the extension or place a step stool close to the exam table (if necessary).	Locking the wheels keeps the chair from moving.
4. Release the footrests and move them out of the way.	Footrests that are not placed out of the way can catch on the patient's clothing and may cause a fall.
5. Instruct the patient to slide forward to the edge of the wheelchair and place both feet on the floor.	Being close to the edge will allow the patient to have the best momentum when attempting to stand.
6. Stand in front of the patient and place your feet apart with one foot slightly out front.	This position gives you the best balance for lifting the patient.
7. Bend your knees (Figure 22-34) and instruct the patient to place his hands on the armrests of the wheelchair. Place your hands around the patient's waist, grasping the gait belt. Signal the patient to stand, pushing himself upward as you lift upward on the gait belt. Pause for a few seconds after the patient is standing before proceeding.	Bending your knees allows you to lift with your legs and not your back. Pausing allows the patient to gain balance.

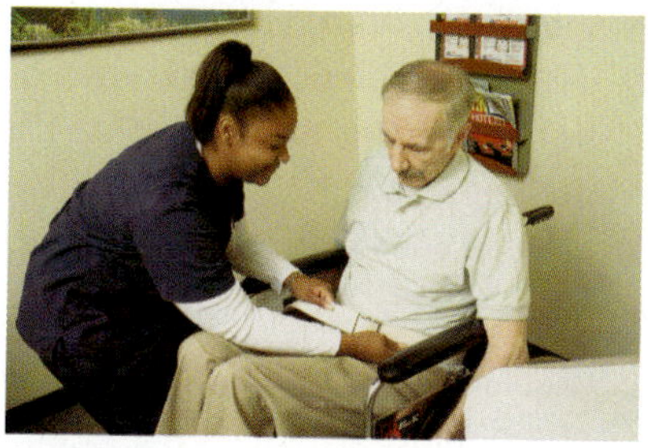

Figure 22-32 ■ The medical assistant places a gait belt around the patient's waist.

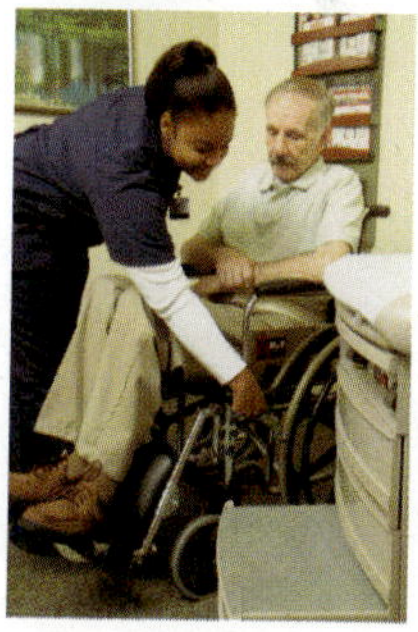

Figure 22-33 ■ The medical assistant locks the wheels of the wheelchair and puts the foot rests up and out of the way.

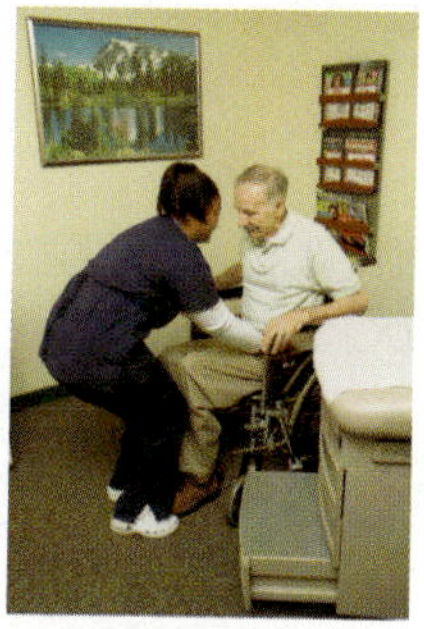

Figure 22-34 ■ The medical assistant bends her knees to avoid injury to her back.

continues

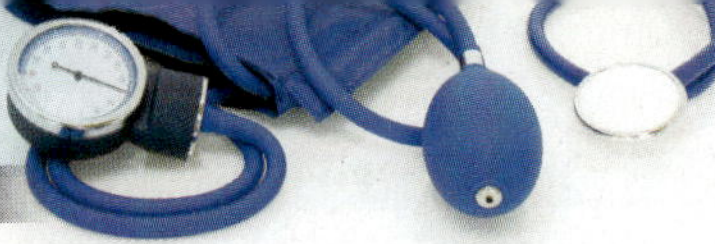

PROCEDURE 22-5 continued

PROCEDURAL STEPS	DETAILS AND/OR RATIONALE
8. Assist the patient up onto the footrest one foot at a time. Pivot the patient so that the backside of the body is against the exam table. Help the patient get into a sitting position (Figure 22-35). Move the wheelchair out of the way.	Helping the patient get into a sitting position assures that the patient is stable before you let go. Moving the chair out of the way eliminates a hazard for falling.
9. After the exam, reapply the gait belt and move the wheelchair close to the exam table. Lock the wheels.	This will keep the wheelchair from moving when the patient is transferred back to the wheelchair.
10. Pull out the extension. Grasp your hands underneath the gait belt and ask the patient to grasp you around your shoulders. Help the patient to step down onto the foot extension and then onto the floor one foot at a time. If the patient is very tall, the patient may step directly onto the floor.	Do not let go of the patient. The patient may be unstable after sitting on the exam table for a period of time.
11. Instruct the patient to reach behind for the arms of the chair and slowly lower the patient into the chair.	Lowering patient slowly helps to eliminate the chance of falling or injury.
12. Reposition the patient's feet on the patient's feet on the footrests and unlock the wheels.	It is easier to move a patient in a wheelchair if the feet are on the footrests.

Figure 22-35 ■ The medical assistant helps the patient onto the table and makes certain that the patient is stable.

PROCEDURE 22-6

Administer Heat Therapy Treatments

Objective:

To correctly apply heat modalities to different areas of the body as prescribed by the provider.

Equipment/Supplies:

- Basin
- Plain warm water or soaking solution, if ordered by the provider
- Thermometer
- Gauze
- Washcloths
- Towels
- Heating pad with protective cover
- Hot water bottle
- Patient's chart/EHR

continues

PROCEDURE 22-6 continued

PROCEDURAL STEPS	DETAILS AND/OR RATIONALE
1. Assemble the supplies and wash your hands.	This is for infection control purposes.
2. Identify the patient using two identifiers, identify yourself, and ***explain the rationale for the performance of the procedure, showing awareness of the patient's concerns related to the procedure being performed.***	Explaining the procedure helps the patient know what to expect so that there are no surprises.
3. Instruct the patient to remove clothing and put on a gown, if necessary, exposing the area to be treated.	The patient's modesty should be protected.
4. Place the patient in the proper position for the treatment.	The body part being treated must be easily accessible and the patient should be in a comfortable position during the treatment.
5. Administer heat therapy as ordered:	
Heating pad:	
a. Place the protective covering over the heating pad.	The pad must be covered to protect the patient's skin and to absorb perspiration.
b. Connect the cord to an electrical outlet and set the control to the setting indicated by the provider.	The setting is usually low or medium.
c. Place the heating pad on the affected area (do not allow the patient to lie on the heating pad) and ask the patient how the temperature level feels.	Instruct the patient not to adjust the temperature to a higher level, as this could result in an injury or burn.
Hot water bottle:	
a. Fill the hot water bottle approximately half full with water [the water temperature should be between 105°F and 110°F (40.5°C and 43°C)].	The provider will indicate the correct temperature of the water to be used, which will depend on the body area being treated.
b. Compress the air out of the bottle and close the lid tightly.	Leakage of the hot water could cause a burn.
c. Cover the water bottle with a cloth or towel.	Placing the surface of the hot water bottle directly on the patient's skin could result in damage or a burn.
d. Leave in place for the prescribed amount of time.	Prolonged treatment may result in tissue damage to the area.
Hot compress:	
a. Fill a basin with hot water [between 105°F and 110°F (40.5°C and 43°C)].	The water must be the correct temperature to be effective and decrease possibility of damage to the skin.
b. Soak cloth or gauze in hot water and wring out excess moisture.	The compress should be wet, but not dripping.

continues

PROCEDURE 22-6 continued

PROCEDURAL STEPS	DETAILS AND/OR RATIONALE
c. Place the compress over the affected area. Cover the compress with a plastic covering.	Covering the pack with plastic helps to maintain the temperature.
d. Re-wet the compress to maintain the correct temperature.	A compress that is not the correct temperature will not be as effective.
e. Replace the compress every few minutes for the amount of time prescribed by the provider.	The provider will determine the amount of time the treatment should be administered.
Hot pack:	
a. Hot packs are soaked in hot water, allowed to drain, and covered with a pad. They are used on larger areas of the body, such as the back or shoulder (Figure 22-36).	
Hot soak:	
a. Fill an appropriate-sized container with hot water [approximately 105–110ºF (40.5–43°C)] and add medication to the water if ordered by the provider.	Check the temperature of the water with a thermometer to ensure accuracy.
b. Place the body part in the water for the prescribed amount of time.	The provider's orders should always be followed.
c. After the prescribed amount of time, remove the body part from the soak and dry with a towel. Inspect the area for any redness or damage.	The part should be inspected for any signs of damage following the treatment.
Paraffin bath:	
a. A paraffin bath, composed of melted paraffin and mineral oil, should be heated to approximately 127ºF (53ºC).	
b. Dip the affected body part in the paraffin until a thick coating of wax builds up.	A thick coat will hold the temperature for a longer period of time.
c. Wrap the body part in foil, plastic wrap, or a cloth for 30 minutes.	The paraffin must be left on for prescribed amount of time to gain the desired effect of the treatment.
d. Take the covering off and peel away the wax.	
6. Check with the patient periodically during any heat treatment. The patient may feel chilled during the treatment, so cover the patient with a sheet or blanket.	Applying heat to the body dilates the blood vessels, which causes heat loss and can produce a chilled feeling.
7. Check the treatment area for signs of damage such as redness, blisters, or irritation.	If any signs of problems are observed, stop the treatment and inform the provider.

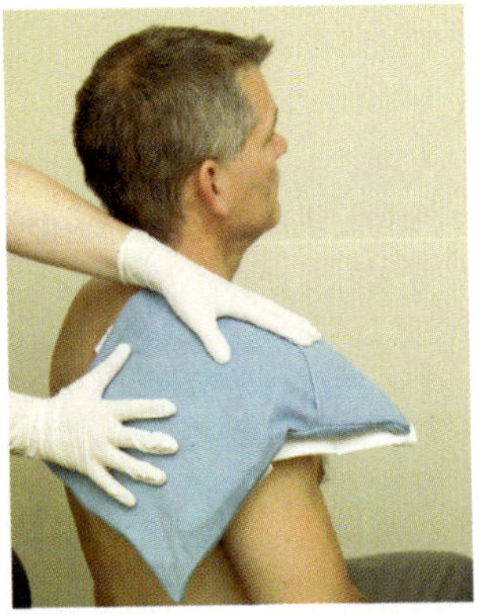

Figure 22-36 ■ The medical assistant applies a commercial heat pack to the patient's shoulder (gloves are optional).

continues

PROCEDURE 22-6 continued

PROCEDURAL STEPS	DETAILS AND/OR RATIONALE
8. Assist the patient with dressing, if needed.	
9. Clean the area and wash hands.	
10. Document treatment in the patient's chart.	This confirms that the procedure was performed.

DOCUMENTATION EXAMPLE:

08-12-XX 1:30 p.m.	Hot compress applied to right forearm x 10 minutes per Dr. Cho's orders. No blistering or redness observed after treatment. Pt. tolerated procedure well. Ryan Leonard, CMA (AAMA)--

PROCEDURE 22-7
Administer Cold Therapy Treatments

Objective:

To correctly administer cold modalities to different areas of the body, as prescribed by the provider.

Equipment/Supplies:

- Basin
- Water
- Ice cubes
- Gauze
- Washcloths
- Ice bag
- Commercial cold pack
- Chemical cold pack
- Large ice cube frozen in a paper cup
- Patient's chart/EHR

PROCEDURAL STEPS	DETAILS AND/OR RATIONALE
1. Assemble the supplies and wash your hands.	This reduces the spread of microorganisms from one patient to another.
2. Identify the patient using two identifiers, identify yourself, and ***explain the rationale for the performance of the procedure, showing awareness of the patient's concerns related to the procedure being performed.***	Explaining the procedure helps the patient know what to expect so that there are no surprises.

continues

PROCEDURE 22-7 continued

PROCEDURAL STEPS	DETAILS AND/OR RATIONALE
3. Instruct the patient to remove clothing and put on a gown, if necessary, exposing the area to be treated.	The patient's modesty should be protected.
4. Place the patient in the proper position for treatment.	The body part being treated must be easily accessible and the patient should be in a comfortable position during the treatment.
5. Administer the cold therapy as ordered:	
Ice bag:	
a. Check the ice bag for damage or leaks.	A leaky bag can cause the patient to become wet and chilled.
b. Fill the bag approximately two-thirds full with small ice chips or cubes; refill as needed (Figure 22-37).	Small ice chips help the bag to conform to the body part better.
c. Squeeze the bag to expel excess air and screw the top into place.	Air in the bag can create spaces, which will not allow for good conduction of the cold and can also cause the bag not to conform easily to the body part.
d. Cover the pack with a towel for patient comfort and to help absorb any moisture.	Covering the pack helps to keep the area from becoming too cold.
e. Keep the ice bag in place for the amount of time ordered by the provider (usually 15 to 30 minutes).	The area should feel numb, but there should not be pain or extreme paleness.
Commercial ice pack:	
a. Place the gel pack in the freezer for the amount of time recommended by the manufacturer.	This ensures that the pack is completely cooled and will retain the correct temperature for the amount of time indicated.
b. If pack has a protective covering over it, place it on the affected area.	Placing a cold pack directly on the patient's skin could cause damage.
c. If there is no covering on the pack, cover the pack with a cloth or towel before applying.	
d. Leave the pack in place for the prescribed amount of time.	Exceeding the prescribed amount of time could result in damage to the area.
e. Place the bag in the freezer after use.	The bag must be cooled before using again.

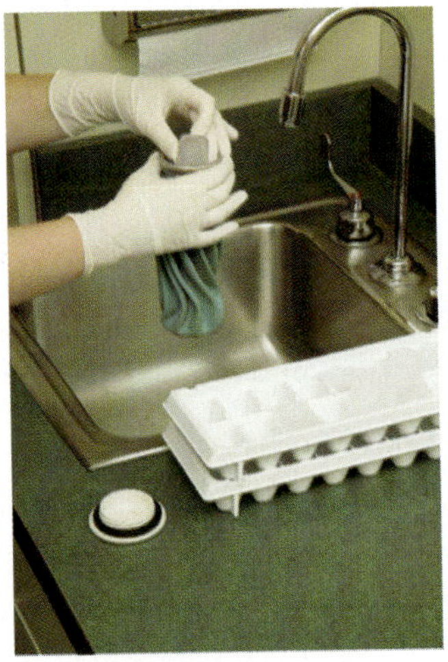

Figure 22-37 ■ The medical assistant fills an ice bag with ice cubes (gloves are optional).

continues

PROCEDURE 22-7 continued

PROCEDURAL STEPS	DETAILS AND/OR RATIONALE
Chemical ice pack:	
a. Inspect the bag for leaks.	Leaking chemicals can cause damage to the skin.
b. Squeeze the bag and shake.	Squeezing and shaking activates the pack so it becomes cold.
c. Cover the pack with a protective covering.	Covering protects the skin in the area being treated.
d. Apply the pack to the affected area for the amount of time prescribed by the provider.	
e. Discard the pack after use.	Chemical cold packs are for single use only.
Cold compress:	
a. Place a small volume of water in a basin, and add large ice cubes to the water.	Large ice cubes melt more slowly and will maintain the cold temperature of the water for a longer period of time.
b. Soak a washcloth or gauze pad in the water and wring out any excess.	Excess cold water can drip on the patient and cause the patient to become chilled.
c. Place an ice pack over the compress.	Covering the compress with an ice pack keeps it colder longer.
d. Re-wet, as needed, to maintain the temperature of the compress.	Re-wetting the compress helps to maintain the proper temperature.
e. Repeat application every 2 to 3 minutes for the amount of time prescribed by the provider.	
Ice massage:	
a. Fill a paper cup three-fourths full of water and place in the freezer.	A large ice cube is needed to perform an ice massage.
b. Expose the area to be treated and squeeze the paper cup so the ice cube is exposed.	Holding the ice cube by the paper cup keeps it from melting quickly and also protects the hands of the person administering the treatment.
c. Move the ice cube in a circular motion over the affected area for the prescribed amount of time, or until the patient reports numbness and burning in the area.	Continuously moving the ice keeps the cold temperature evenly distributed and prevents damage.
6. Check the treatment area following the procedure for paleness, redness, blueness, or any other signs of damage.	The patient should not be permitted to leave the office until the area is inspected. If damage is observed, the provider should be informed immediately.
7. Assist the patient with dressing if needed.	
8. Clean the work area and wash hands.	
9. Document the treatment in the patient's chart.	

DOCUMENTATION EXAMPLE:

08-16-XX 12:30 p.m.	Applied cold compress to left forearm, as per Dr. May's orders. Pt. tolerated procedure well. Notable decrease in swelling. Pt. noted a definite decrease in pain as well. Dawn Carter, RMA (AMT)---

CHAPTER SUMMARY

- Orthopedics deals with injuries and disorders of the musculoskeletal system, including bones, muscles, joints, tendons, and ligaments.
- The function of the skeletal system is to provide support, protect internal organs, serve as an anchor for muscles to enable movement, store minerals, and to serve as the site for blood cell formation.
- Muscles enable movement; give the body shape and maintain posture, as well as generate heat.
- The physician orthopedist treats diseases and disorders of the bones and muscles, working with a team of specialists.
- Common orthopedic disorders include the development of osteoporosis, fractures, osteoarthritis, gait changes, and a loss of balance.
- Bone fractures are classified as simple or closed, or compound or open. Fractures are reduced through closed or open reduction and then immobilized using splints or casts.
- New treatments for arthritis include injections into the joint, and techniques to restore cartilage in joints.
- Minimally invasive surgery, using an arthroscope vs. standard open procedures, has revolutionized orthopedic surgery. There is less postoperative swelling and pain, a decreased risk of complications and a more rapid recovery. Almost all arthroscopic procedures can be performed in an outpatient setting.
- Rehabilitation following an injury or orthopedic surgery may include the application of modalities such as the use of heat and cold treatments, electrical muscle stimulation, hydrotherapy, massage, and the use of assistive devices for mobility. Exercises are prescribed to increase strength and mobility.
- Primary ambulatory assistive devices include canes, crutches, walkers, and wheelchairs. All devices must be modified to fit the individual properly.

CERTIFICATION REVIEW QUESTIONS

1. The human skeleton functions to:
   a. provide heat.
   b. store proteins.
   c. protect internal organs.
   d. form muscle cells.

2. The muscles of the body are responsible for:
   a. generating heat.
   b. forming blood cells.
   c. storing nutrients.
   d. developing glycogen.

3. The term *atrophy* means:
   a. increase in muscle strength.
   b. shrinkage of the muscle due to inadequate nutrition or other factors.
   c. increase in muscle mass.
   d. decrease in muscle strength.

4. Screening questions for musculoskeletal issues include:
   a. age, ROM, and flexion.
   b. strength, bruising, and endurance.
   c. height, sex, and weight.
   d. pain, loss of feeling, and weakness.

5. Osteoporosis is defined as:
   a. loss of joint mobility and general ROM.
   b. malformation of weight-bearing bones.
   c. brittle bones with loss of bone calcium.
   d. softening of the skeleton.

6. Aging changes in the musculoskeletal system can include:
   a. loss of appetite.
   b. increase in joint flexibility.
   c. shrinkage of intervertebral cartilage, resulting in a decrease in height.
   d. increase in calcium deposits in bones.

7. Treatment of arthritis includes:
   a. viscosupplementation.
   b. a decrease in dietary protein.
   c. cartilage removal.
   d. calcium injections.

8. Cortisone is classified as:
   a. a calcium antagonist.
   b. an estrogen.
   c. an intra-articular injection.
   d. an appetite stimulant.

9. Physical therapists, in general, focus on:
   a. upper extremity issues.
   b. aerobic exercises.
   c. restoring function, improving mobility, and decreasing pain.
   d. instrumental activities of daily living.

10. Which of the following statements regarding heat treatments is correct?
    a. Apply heat treatment to an injury when inflammation is present.
    b. Do not apply heat treatment in the first 24 hours of an injury.
    c. Never apply heat at a temperature greater than 98.6°F.
    d. Do not apply heat when edema is present.

STUDY RESOURCES

Resources to Test and Reinforce Your Knowledge:	
Certification Review Questions	Take this end-of-chapter quiz
Workbook	• Complete the activities for Chapter 22 • Perform the procedures for Chapter 22 using the Competency Checklists
Resources to Promote Critical Thinking:	
***Solve the Case* Activities**	• Consider these case studies and discuss your conclusions
Learning Lab	• Module 15: Skeletal and Muscular Systems
MindTap	• Complete Chapter 22 readings and activities

REFERENCES

Goldman, L. and Schafer, A.I. (2012). *Goldman's Cecil Medicine* (24th ed.). St. Louis, MO: Elsevier Saunders.

Mayo Clinic. (2014, December 13). *Diseases and Conditions: Osteoporosis*. Retrieved December 15, 2014, from http://www.mayoclinic.org/diseases-conditions/osteoporosis/basics/definition/con-20019924

Medical Abbreviations: Muscles. (n.d.). Retrieved December 10, 2014, from http://www.medicabbreviations.com/cat/muscles.html

MedlinePlus. (2012, September 3). *Aging Changes in the Bones—Muscles—Joints*. Retrieved December 5, 2014, from http://www.nlm.nih.gov/medlineplus/ency/article/004015.htm

National Institute of Arthritis and Musculoskeletal and Skin Diseases. (2012, January). *Osteoporosis: Peak Bone Mass in Women*. Retrieved December 12, 2014, from http://www.niams.nih.gov/health_info/bone/osteoporosis/bone_mass.asp

Orthopaedic & Neurosurgery Specialists. (n.d.). *Conditions & Treatments Orthopedics*. Retrieved December 13, 2014, from http://onsmd.com/orthopedics/conditions-treatments/

Scott, A.S. and Fong, E. (2014). *Body Structures and Functions* (12th ed.). Clifton Park, NY: Cengage Learning.

Whiting, Steven E. (n.d.). *Osteoporosis: A Factor of Aging*. Retrieved December 10, 2014, from http://www.healingwithnutrition.com/odisease/osteoporosis/calcium_estrogen.html

Fundamentals of the Medical Laboratory

23

CHAPTER OUTLINE

Rationale for Laboratory Tests

Laboratory Regulations
- Clinical Laboratory Improvement Amendment (CLIA '88)
- Testing Categories

Implications of CLIA '88 for the Medical Assistant

Other Accreditation Options for POLs

Classifications of Laboratories

Laboratory Departments

Quality Assurance
- Quality Control
- Test Logs
- Orientation of Personnel
- Maintenance Checks on All Equipment and Instruments
- Required Calibration of Instruments
- Temperature Checks
- Proficiency Testing
- Reference Ranges

Safety in the Laboratory

Hazards

Processing Requests for Laboratory Tests
- The Laboratory Requisition Form

Preparing the Patient for Laboratory Testing

General Guidelines for Specimen Collection, Handling, and Transport
- Specimen Collection
- Preserving Specimens
- Sources of Contamination

The Laboratory Report
- Abnormal or Panic Test Values

Flow Sheets

The Microscope
- Parts of the Microscope
- Care and Maintenance

The Centrifuge
- Operating the Centrifuge

ESSENTIAL TERMS

Assessment Based Recognition in Order Entry (ABR-OE)
asymptomatic
baseline value
centrifuge
Clinical Laboratory Improvement Amendments of 1988 (CLIA '88)
clinical diagnosis
Commission on Office Laboratory Accreditation (COLA)
computerized provider order entry (CPOE)
differential diagnosis
external controls
flow sheets
high-complexity testing
internal controls
lab requisition form
laboratory report form
microscope
moderate-complexity tests
normal value
ocular
physician's office laboratory (POL)
point-of-care testing (POCT)
procurement station
proficiency testing
profile
provider-performed microscopy (PPM) procedures
qualitative
quality assurance (QA)
quality control (QC)
quantitative
reference ranges
waived tests

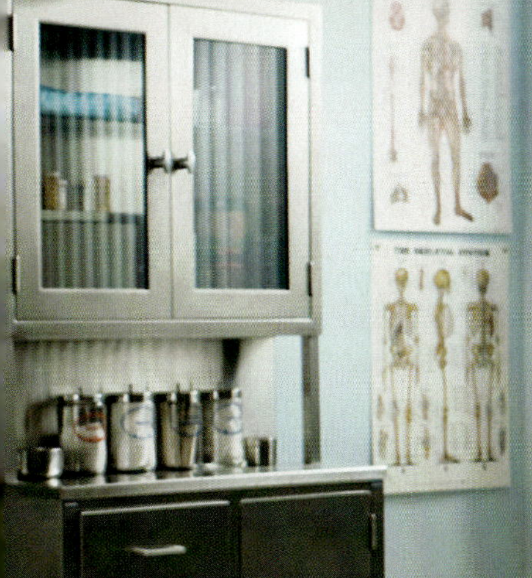

DEVELOPMENTAL OBJECTIVES

After completing this chapter, you should be able to:

1. Correctly spell and define the essential terms.
2. Explain the reasons for performing laboratory tests.
3. Describe the different classifications of laboratories.
4. List the different departments of the laboratory and at least three examples of the tests performed within each department.
5. Discuss the three levels of testing regulated by CLIA '88.
6. List the level of testing that the medical assistant can perform in regards to CLIA '88 and justify why medical assistants can perform testing in this category.
7. Identify common CLIA-waived tests and common disorders associated with testing.
8. Identify quality assurance practices in health care.
9. Compare and contrast quantitative and qualitative results.
10. Explain the need for maintenance checks, calibration of instruments, temperature checks, and proficiency testing.
11. List basic safety rules for the laboratory and explain the PPE necessary when working with all body fluids, blood, nonintact skin, and mucous membranes.
12. Correctly complete a laboratory requisition form and explain who can place orders in the Computerized Provider Order Entry (CPOE) system.
13. Discuss the importance of normal reference ranges.
14. Discuss the importance of proper patient preparation.
15. Identify five general guidelines for proper specimen collection and guidelines for preserving specimens.
16. Assess the use of flow sheets and explain how they can improve tracking.
17. Label the parts and state the functions of each part of the microscope.
18. Describe the use and balancing technique of a centrifuge.
19. Perform a control.
20. Review and report laboratory results.
21. Properly collect a specimen for offsite testing.
22. Properly use a microscope.

INTRODUCTION

The medical laboratory performs a vast array of tests that assist providers in diagnosing, treating, and following the progression of patients with acute and chronic illnesses. There are a variety of personnel who work in laboratories. Medical assistants may work in an onsite **physician's office laboratory (POL)**, or may even work in a hospital or reference laboratory performing specific services.

The medical assistant's responsibilities in regards to lab testing may be any of the following: Preparing patients for lab testing, specimen collection and processing, performance of waived or noncomplex lab tests, and sending specimens to outside laboratories.

Proper specimen collection and processing is vital to ensure that test results are accurate. Careful specimen collection and handling can make the difference in whether the provider receives timely and accurate results or receives an error message stating that the specimen was rejected and must be collected again.

Being familiar with commonly ordered lab tests, rationale for ordering the tests, and normal values for each test can assist the medical assistant with patient education and appropriate test follow-up.

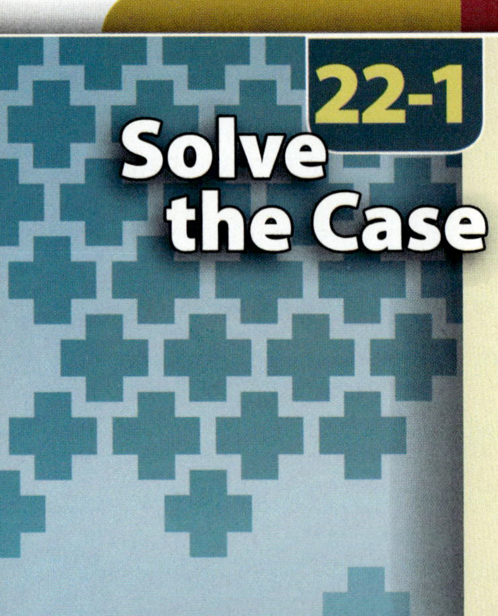

Mrs. Baker, 78 years old, comes in to the office complaining of severe fatigue and mild dyspnea (shortness of breath) upon exertion. After questioning the patient, you discover that the symptoms have been present for three months. After further questioning and examination, Dr. Dorado is concerned that the patient may be bleeding internally. He orders a battery of tests on the patient to obtain better insight as to the cause of Mrs. Baker's symptoms.

1. **Why do you think it took Mrs. Baker three months to schedule an appointment?**
2. **Based on your current understanding of physiological processes, why do you think Dr. Dorado suspects Mrs. Baker may have internal bleeding? What vital signs may be good indicators of internal bleeding?**
3. **What can you do to help Mrs. Baker feel more relaxed while waiting for the doctor?**

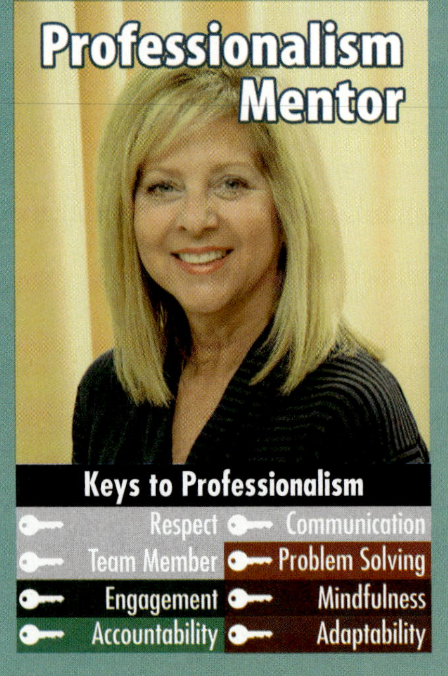

Medical Assistants will perform many CLIA-regulated tests requiring accuracy in both performance and documentation. Attention to detail is vital when handling and labeling specimens. Imagine getting the wrong lab results leading to a wrong or delayed diagnosis. Mistakes like these happen and sometimes the consequences are severe. Medical assistants also need to be especially careful when entering lab orders in the EHR. While mistakes happen, the key to your success is to establish a personal accountability to your patient by being dependable and always double checking your work to reduce the likelihood of making an error. This is a work ethic I encourage all MAs to strive for, and I look for that work ethic when recommending MAs for a position with the company. Medical assistants are also responsible for assuring that patients comprehend instructions for specific laboratory tests to ensure accuracy. What will you do if you do not understand the test instructions yourself? How will you establish that the patient has a clear understanding of the instructions? How will you handle patients with limited English? Take a minute to answer these questions in your journal. ■

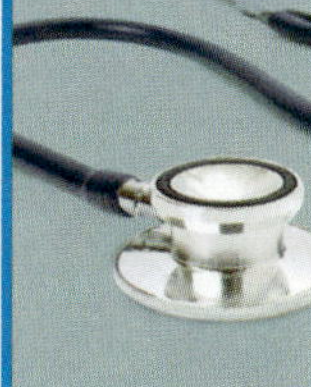

RATIONALE FOR LABORATORY TESTS

Laboratory tests are usually ordered in conjunction with other diagnostic tests to assist in diagnosing a patient's condition. However, there are a number of reasons for requesting laboratory testing. The rationale for lab testing includes the following:

- Determining **baseline values**: All laboratory values have normal ranges for particular patient populations; however, some patients may run at the lower or higher end of a range. Baseline readings establish a starting point for monitoring a patient's lab results. These values may be ordered during a complete physical exam or during a first office visit to establish a point of reference for future testing.
- For legal purposes: Insurance companies and many employers require individuals to submit to testing for alcohol and drug screenings. Individuals who have been involved in a vehicular accident or who are named in a crime may also be required to submit to testing. Another legal reason for laboratory testing includes the determination of paternity.
- To screen for pathologic conditions: Sometimes patients present with very vague or general symptoms, while others are **asymptomatic** (no symptoms at all). Laboratory tests can steer the provider in the right direction when general symptoms alone, such as fatigue, cannot provide a diagnosis. Oftentimes, the provider will order a **profile** (a group of related tests) to assist with a diagnosis based on vague signs and symptoms.
- To confirm a clinical diagnosis: Many times, the provider can arrive at a **clinical diagnosis** based solely on observing the patient's signs and listening to the patient's description of the symptoms. To confirm the diagnosis, the provider will order lab tests. For example, a patient presents with classic symptoms of mononucleosis: swollen lymph nodes, extreme fatigue, sore throat, and low-grade fever. By obtaining laboratory results, the diagnosis can be confirmed.
- To obtain a differential diagnosis: Sometimes patients will present with symptoms that can be attributed to more than one disease or condition. Laboratory tests can provide the provider with results that will help him to arrive at a **differential diagnosis**. An example would be a patient who exhibits signs and symptoms of strep throat. The provider must determine whether or not the patient has a viral or streptococcal infection in order to implement an appropriate treatment plan.

Field Smarts

Performing baseline readings not only assists the provider with knowing what is "normal" for a particular patient, but it can also help to forecast future disease. By performing a patient's baseline readings for tests such as glucose, cholesterol, and blood urea nitrogen (BUN) levels, the provider can determine if the patient is at a higher risk for future diseases such as diabetes, heart attack, or kidney problems.

- To assess treatment methods and patient progress: Conditions such as diabetes must be followed on a continuous basis. The provider will order a battery of tests at predetermined intervals to follow the progression of a disease and to evaluate the effectiveness of a prescribed treatment.

LABORATORY REGULATIONS

Health care facilities, including medical laboratories, must adhere to strict rules and regulations. Federal regulations were developed to protect the public by improving the quality of laboratory testing. These regulations govern all facilities and personnel performing laboratory tests on human specimens that are used for diagnosis, treatment, and prevention of disease.

Clinical Laboratory Improvement Amendment (CLIA '88)

Under the protection of the agency formally known as the Health Care Financing Administration (HCFA) (now referred to as the Center for Medicare and Medicaid Services (CMS) and the Department of Health and Human Services [DHHS]), the **Clinical Laboratory Improvement Amendments of 1988 (CLIA '88)** was enacted by Congress as an amendment to the original Act of 1967. CLIA '88 includes standards and laboratory practice guidelines created to ensure quality laboratory testing in order to protect patients from actions based on inaccurate results.

CLIA '88 established federal standards for all lab tests in order to ensure test accuracy, reliability, and timeliness, regardless of what type of laboratory performs the test. The regulations consist of four sets of

Table 23-1 Three Federal Agencies That Administer CLIA and Their Responsibilities

Federal Agency	Responsibilities
CMS	• Approves private accreditation organizations and state exemptions • Collects fees • Conducts inspections • Enforces compliance • Issues laboratory certificates • Publishes CLIA rules and regulations • Monitors laboratory performance on proficiency testing and approves proficiency testing (PT) programs
FDA	• Categorizes tests based on complexity • Develops rules and guidance for CLIA complexity categorization • Reviews requests for Waiver by Application
CDC	• Conducts laboratory quality improvement studies • Develops and distributes professional information and educational resources • Develops technical standards and laboratory practice guidelines • Provides analysis, research, and technical assistance • Manages the CLIA Advisory Committee (CLIAC) • Monitors proficiency testing practices

Source: Centers for Medicare and Medicaid Services, www.cms.gov.

rules: laboratory standards, user and application fees, procedures for enforcement, and approval of accreditation programs.

Three federal agencies administer CLIA: the Centers for Medicare and Medicaid Services (CMS), the Food and Drug Administration (FDA), and the Centers for Disease Control and Prevention (CDC). Table 23-1 categorizes the responsibilities of each agency.

Testing Categories

The final CLIA regulations were published on February 28, 1992, based on the complexity of the test method—the more complex the test, the more rigid the requirements. CLIA regulations established three test categories: waived testing, moderate-complexity (which includes provider-performed microscopy [PPM]), and high-complexity. Each category of testing has different requirements for personnel performing the testing and for quality control.

The FDA considers the following when categorizing tests:

- Amount of interpretation involved
- Calibration and quality control requirements of the instruments used
- Degree of independent judgment involved
- Difficulty of the calculations involved
- Examinations and procedures performed and the methodologies employed
- Type of training required to operate the instruments used in methodology.

Waived Tests

Waived tests (low-complexity) are simple to perform, require a minimum of quality control and documentation, and a minimum of judgment and interpretation. Many waived tests are available for home use. Medical assistants are permitted to perform waived tests; however, the provider must be able to confirm that test results are accurate and precise and were performed on the appropriate patient sample. Performance of waived tests does not require the laboratory to participate in proficiency testing (described later in the chapter) by outside inspectors or to employ specially trained personnel. The laboratory is required, however, to obtain a "Certificate of Waiver" in order to perform low-complexity tests. Table 23-2 provides a general listing of CLIA-waived tests.

Moderate-Complexity Tests

Of all tests in the United States including PPM procedures, 75% fall into the moderate-complexity category. Performance of **moderate-complexity tests** requires an understanding of test methodology, quality control, and instrument calibration. Unlike waived tests, tests for moderate-complexity are not available for home use. Detailed record keeping, proficiency testing, and biannual inspections are required.

Provider-Performed Microscopy (PPM) Procedures

The **provider-performed microscopy (PPM) procedures** are a subgroup of moderate-complexity testing. Any laboratory that has a waived certificate may also

Table 23-2 General List of CLIA-Waived Tests and Common Disorders Associated with Testing

CLIA-Waived Test	Common Clinical Conditions Associated With Testing
Certain drug levels	Screen for drugs of abuse and alcohol
Cholesterol (total, HDL, and LDL)	Screen for risk of developing coronary heart disease
Erythrocyte sedimentation rate	Screen for inflammation or monitor treatment of inflammatory diseases such as rheumatoid arthritis
Fecal occult blood	Screen for gastrointestinal disorders and colon cancer
Gastric occult blood	Screen for gastrointestinal disorders such as ulcers or malignancy
Glucose monitoring devices (cleared by FDA for home use)	Monitor glucose levels of diabetics
hCG, urine	Test for pregnancy
Hgb A1c (glycosolated hemoglobin)	For baseline or monitoring estimated average glucose levels of diabetics over a three-month period
Helicobacter pylori whole blood test	Screen for gastrointestinal disorders such as ulcers
Hematocrit	Screen for anemia caused by many factors such as nutritional deficiency and blood loss
Hemoglobin (single analyte instrument)	Screen for anemia caused by many factors such as nutritional deficiency and blood loss
Infectious mononucleosis rapid whole blood test	Test for infectious mononucleosis
Ovulation test by color comparison	Test for ovulation to assist with conception
Prothrombin time (PT)	Screen for coagulation disorders or for monitoring oral anticoagulant therapy
Rapid strep test	Detects *Streptococcus pyogenes* pharyngitis (commonly known as "strep throat")
Triglycerides	Screen for risk of developing coronary heart disease
Urine reagent strip testing (qualitative)	Urine chemical evaluation that is helpful in screening for disorders such as cystitis or kidney disease
Vaginal pH	Screen for possible vaginal infection

**Note*: This is not a complete listing of all waived tests. For a more complete list, visit the CMS website (www.cms.gov) and search for "waived tests."

apply for a PPM certificate as long as the following general criteria are met:

1. Personnel performing the test must complete appropriate training, either by formal schooling or on-the-job training, per state requirements.
2. The test must be performed during the patient's visit by a physician, or a mid-level provider (such as nurse practitioner, nurse midwife, or physician assistant) under the supervision of a physician or a dentist.
3. The test must be performed on the actual patient of the provider and the provider must be a member or employee of the practice.
4. The test must be categorized as moderately complex.
5. The microscope is the primary instrument used to perform the procedure.
6. If testing is delayed on the specimen, it could produce inaccurate results.
7. The test requires limited handling and processing of the specimen.

Table 23-3 lists examples of tests that may be performed by a laboratory with a PPM certificate.

High-Complexity Tests

High-complexity testing is similar to moderate-complexity testing with respect to not being available for home use. In addition, regulations require detailed record keeping, proficiency testing, and biannual inspections. High-complexity testing personnel are required to have more specialized education and/or experience and credentialing than those performing waived and some moderate-complexity testing. Examples of high-complexity testing include cytologic evaluation (Pap smears), cytogenetic testing, tests in histopathology, and histocompatibility.

Registration Requirements

All laboratories are required to register with CLIA regardless of the number or category of tests performed. A laboratory must meet performance essentials based on the complexity of the test method used and risk factors associated with incorrect results. A laboratory enrolling in the CLIA program must complete a registration application, pay fees, be surveyed (if applicable), and become certified.

Table 23-3 Examples of PPM Tests

Name of Test	Purpose of the Test
Direct wet mounts	Identify yeasts, trichomoniasis, bacterial vaginosis, and the presence of semen in possible rape cases
Potassium hydroxide preparations	Identify types of fungal infections such as *Candida* yeast infections (oral thrush, vaginitis, and skin candidiasis) and dermatophyte infections such as ringworm, athlete's foot, and jock itch
Pinworm examinations	Detect pinworms
Fern tests	Monitor fertility or to determine if a patient's amniotic membranes are leaking
Post-coital direct, qualitative examinations, or vaginal cervical mucus	Evaluate infertility
Urine sediment examinations	Diagnose urinary tract infections
Nasal smears for eosinophils	Distinguish between allergic and nonallergic rhinitis
Fecal leukocyte examinations	Detect colon inflammation or disruption
Qualitative semen analysis (limited to detection of absence of sperm and sperm motility)	Detection of absence of sperm and sperm motility

IMPLICATIONS OF CLIA '88 FOR THE MEDICAL ASSISTANT

The medical assistant must be familiar with the regulations mandated in the CLIA '88 amendment and must continually monitor any related changes that may occur in the future. Record keeping is an important component of the amendment. The medical assistant may be responsible for collecting and storing this important information. Types of documentation required as a result of CLIA '88 include the following:

1. Personnel credentials: Any licensing, national certifications, or registrations as well as continuing education units (CEUs) acquired by each individual performing lab testing must be kept in each employee's file.
2. Employee hepatitis B vaccine records.
3. Equipment maintenance logs for each instrument that include information on calibration, quality control, and quality assurance.
4. Procedure manual that includes how each test is performed must be available to all employees. Changes should be made as procedures change and should be reviewed annually.

OTHER ACCREDITATION OPTIONS FOR POLS

The **Commission on Office Laboratory Accreditation (COLA)** was established in 1988 as a private alternative to assist clinical laboratories in complying with the CLIA '88 standards. In 1993, the Health Care Financing Administration (HCFA, now known as the Centers of Medicare and Medicaid Services, or just "CMS") granted COLA authority under CLIA '88 to provide accreditation to POLs and in 1998 the Joint Commission also recognized COLA as an accreditation program.

After establishing itself as an accreditation agency for POLs, COLA expanded its program to include hospitals, medical facilities, and independent laboratories. Because of this expansion, the Commission on Office Laboratory Accreditation shortened its name to just COLA. COLA provides onsite reviews of laboratory facilities, as well as choices for accreditation, consultation, and education.

CLASSIFICATIONS OF LABORATORIES

Laboratories are classified according to their size, the categories of tests performed, and with whom they are affiliated. Many labs are independently owned and located within larger clinics or medical facilities, while others are located in hospitals or providers' offices. Larger reference laboratories usually have procurement stations located throughout the community for the purpose of specimen collection only. Table 23-4 lists the different classifications and locations of laboratories and the test categories performed by each.

LABORATORY DEPARTMENTS

Laboratories are usually categorized into different departments, each performing tests that are specific to their area of expertise. It should be noted that there may be subdepartments in each area that involve more specialized testing. For example, special chemistry and

Table 23-4 Laboratory Classifications

Type	Location	Test Capabilities
Reference lab	Regional/large service area	Routine/complex/expensive specialty tests. Does not include a blood bank department.
Hospital	Within area hospitals	Most tests required by the hospital (this will vary with each hospital depending on patient population).
Physician's Office Laboratory (POL)	Within the physician's office	Common waived tests including blood glucose testing, rapid strep testing, hemoglobin/hematocrit testing, PT/INR testing, and urinalysis testing. Some POLs also have PPM certification so the provider can perform some microscopic testing.
Point-of-care testing (POCT)	Bedside or near the patient testing. Performed in hospitals, nursing homes, POLs, or ambulatory care centers	The intention of POCT is to deliver rapid and accurate results so medical treatment can be promptly implemented. Most often common waived tests. Rapid tests such as glucose, cholesterol, strep screening, and hemoglobin.
Procurement station/satellite lab	Suburban areas/near isolated medical facilities throughout the community	Patients are often sent to a procurement station from a clinic or provider's office that does not have the capability to collect specimens. These labs just collect specimens, they do not perform testing.

toxicology may be subspecialties found in the clinical chemistry department. Larger laboratories may have more specialized areas.

Refer to Table 23-5 for common laboratory tests listed by department and the specimen requirements for each.

Table 23-5 Common Laboratory Tests and General Specimen Requirements

Laboratory Department	Tests Performed	Specimen Requirements
Hematology	*Routine Hematology* Complete blood count (CBC): white blood cell count, red blood cell count, hemoglobin, hematocrit, platelet count, and RBC indices and WBC differential Erythrocyte sedimentation rate (ESR)	EDTA whole blood for CBC, WBC differential, and ESR
Subdepartments of hematology may include: *Coagulation*	Prothrombin time PT/INR, and other coagulation studies	Citrated plasma for PT/INR and other Coagulation studies
Body Fluid Analysis	Urinalysis; Physical, chemical, and microscopic testing, and other body fluids	Urine Cerebrospinal fluid, synovial fluid, and bone marrow aspirates
Clinical chemistry	*Routine Chemistry* Glucose, sodium, potassium, chloride, calcium, protein, albumin, globulin, blood urea nitrogen (BUN), creatinine, bilirubin, cholesterol, triglycerides, uric acid, liver enzymes	Serum or plasma, or other body fluids
Subdepartments of clinical chemistry may include: *Special Chemistry*	Looks for specific diseases or conditions such as heart attacks, stroke, kidney failure, and other organ failures.	Serum or plasma, or other body fluids
Toxicology	Therapeutic drug monitoring and drugs of abuse	Serum or plasma, or other body fluids
Immunology or serology	VDRL/RPR: syphilis detection tests, C-reactive protein (CRP), Rheumatoid factor (RA), Mono test, heterophile antibody test, hepatitis tests, HIV testing, antistreptolysin titer (ASO), pregnancy tests	Serum
Subdepartments of immunology or serology may include: *Immunohematology (Blood Bank)*	ABO and Rh blood typing, antibody screening, compatibility testing of blood and blood products, direct Coombs	Clot tube without additive or EDTA

continues

Table 23-5 Common Laboratory Tests and General Specimen Requirements (*continued*)

Laboratory Department	Tests Performed	Specimen Requirements
Microbiology	Growth and identification of many different pathogenic organisms that can cause diseases such as the organisms that cause strep throat, pharyngitis, whooping cough, diphtheria, chlamydia, gonorrhea, or tuberculosis	Specimens from any area of the body including but not limited to: throat, wound, blood, urine, and other body fluids, sputum, and genital areas
Subdepartments of microbiology may include:		
Parasitology	Determining the presence of parasites and their eggs, which can cause diseases such as amoebic dysentery and malaria. Testing also confirms the presence of pinworm, hookworm, scabies, or trichomonas	Blood, skin, feces, or other body fluids
Virology	Identifies specific viruses such as mumps, measles, hepatitis, CMV, and HIV.	Serum, culture swabs, CSF, and other body fluids
Mycology	Determines the presence of fungi in the body. Examples include Aspergillus PCR, pneumocystis, and histoplasmosis.	Serum and urine
Cytotechnology	Testing for the presence of cancer cells	Cervical specimens, urine, and lung tissue
Histology	Biopsy tissue analysis	Tissue samples derived from surgical procedures or biopsy procedures

CRITICAL THINKING CHALLENGE

You have just assisted the provider during removal of a suspicious growth from a patient's face. You prepare the specimen to be sent to the reference lab.

1. Which department will perform the testing on this specimen?

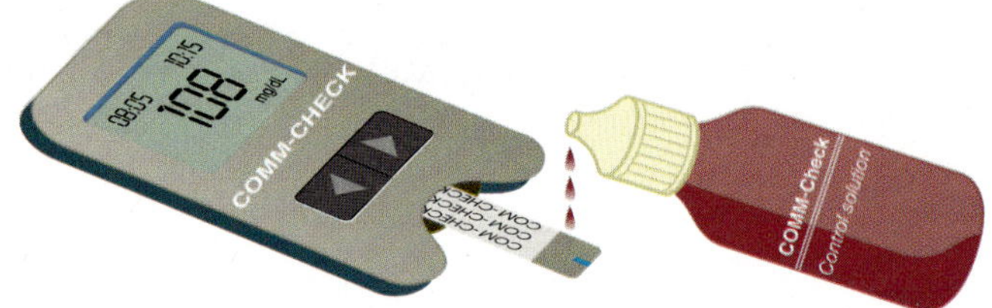

Figure 23-1 ■ A control is performed to make certain the glucometer is working properly.

QUALITY ASSURANCE

Quality assurance (QA) is a set of policies and procedures designed to ensure the accuracy and reliability of laboratory testing and should include the following.

Quality Control

Quality control (QC) procedures are designed to ensure the accuracy and precision of laboratory tests and to discover and eliminate human error. Every laboratory, including physician's office labs, is required by law to have a carefully performed, documented, and ongoing QC program in place.

Quality Control Testing

Quality control testing confirms that test kits and lab instruments are working properly. There are usually two types of controls found in waived offices:

- **Internal controls**: These evaluate whether or not the test is working as it was designed, the correct amount of sample was added, the sample moving through the test correctly, or whether the instrument is in good working order.
- **External controls**: Evaluates the entire testing process and that the control results are in the expected ranges. Figure 23-1 features a glucose control used to check the accuracy of glucose testing performed in the medical office.

Controls should be performed according to manufacturer's instructions; however, kits or equipment typically should be checked with each new shipment of reagents or lot numbers, when there is a change in lot numbers, or when a new operator is using the kit or equipment. If control readings are not within the accepted range or the expected result, the medical assistant should do the following:

- Check to see if he or she followed the manufacturer's instructions correctly.
- Recheck the expiration dates on all reagents and testing items.
- Check to see if reagents were stored properly.

- Make certain that reagents actually go with the testing kit.
- Rerun the control.
- Follow manufacturer's troubleshooting instructions.

If troubleshooting doesn't resolve the problem, the analyzer should not be used until it is properly serviced or if the problem is with a testing kit, it should be disposed of and a new kit should be used in its place.

Refer to Procedure 23-1 to learn how to run a control.

Documentation of Controls in a Quality Control Log

Anytime a control is performed, it needs to be documented in a log. This validates that the lab took the proper steps to ensure test accuracy. Logs may be paper or electronic. Figure 23-2 is an example of a paper quality control log.

Test Logs

The medical assistant should perform and interpret all test results exactly as described by the manufacturer. Timing is imperative when interpreting tests, so always set a timer or use a watch to make certain results are interpreted at the right time intervals. Use reference guides when available for test interpretation.

There are two types of results:

- **Quantitative** results provide an actual measurement of the substance in specific units. Always write out the result and unit when documenting the value.
- **Qualitative** results usually identify the presence or absence of a substance and are interpreted as positive or negative. Do not use symbols when recording these types of results, either write the result or use accepted abbreviations.

Whenever you perform a lab test, the result should be documented in a testing or performance log. The testing log provides a record of every person that had testing on a particular test kit or piece of equipment. In the event there is a recall on any of the associated items, the practice will know which patients had testing so that follow up is easier. Paper testing logs are not necessary when logs are electronic. When you create the lab order and select lot numbers or instrument identification numbers associated with testing, reports can easily be generated by selecting specific

GLUCOSE METER QUALITY CONTROL LOG

Name and Address of Facility	Manufacturer's Name
Riverside Family Practice *1026 Riverside Drive* *Columbus, GA.*	*Optum Diagnostics*
Instrument Name: *Optum GC 165*	Instrument Serial Number: *A36259V*

Test Strip Lot #	Test Strip Open Date	Test Strip Exp. Date
1587952	*07/16/2020*	*08/01/2021*
Control Manuf. & Lot #	**Control Open Date**	**Control Exp. Date**
Optum 96873	*07/12/2020*	*06/15/2021*

Category	Date	Date	Date	Date	Date
	07/16/2020	*07/17/2020*	*07/18/2020*	*07/19/2020*	*07/20/2020*
Type of Control	*HI*	*HI*	*Low*	*Low*	*Normal*
Acceptable Range	*285-335 mg/dL*	*285-335 mg/dL*	*30-60 mg/dL*	*30-60 mg/dL*	*70-110 mg/dL*
Today's Reading	*310 mg/dL*	*305 mg/dL*	*35 mg/dL*	*37 mg/dL*	*85 mg/dL*
Technician's Initials	*MH*	*BV*	*MH*	*BV*	*MH*
Category	**Date**	**Date**	**Date**	**Date**	**Date**
	07/23/2020	*07/24/2020*			
Type of Control	*Normal*	*HI*			
Acceptable Range	*70-110 mg/dL*	*285-335 mg/dL*			
Today's Reading	*92 mg/dL*	*320 mg/dL*			
Technician's Name	*BV*	*MH*			

Figure 23-2 ■ An example of a glucose quality control log.

Test Log for the GC 165					
Test Strip Lot Number		Test Strip Expiration Date			
1587952		08/01/2021			
Today's Date	Ordering Provider	Patient's Chart #	Result	Name of Person Performing Test	
07/16/2020	Dr. Dorado	986523	320 mg/dL	Marcy Harris	
07/16/2020	Dr. Dorado	475239	108 mg/dL	Mary Harris	
07/16/2020	Dr. Dorado	228745	86 mg/dL	Marcy Harris	
07/17/2020	Dr. Anderson	026587	96 mg/dL	Blake Verhoff	
07/17/2020	Dr. Anderson	475254	162 mg/dL	Blake Verhoff	

Figure 23-3 ■ An example of a glucose test log.

testing parameters. Figure 23-3 illustrates a manual testing log.

Reagents and Expiration Dates

When conducting testing or running controls, expiration dates should be checked on all items used for testing, including reagents. Reagents are chemicals that are used to process tests and should be stored according to the manufacturer's instructions. Some reagents need to be refrigerated but may need to be brought to room temperature prior to testing. Reagents not stored or processed correctly may lose their effectiveness resulting in inaccurate test results.

Orientation of Personnel

Medical staff members responsible for lab testing should be oriented to laboratory procedures and policies. Each test performed in the POL should have a written standard operating procedure (SOP) and employees that perform testing should be tested on each procedure prior to conducting patient testing. Employees also need to be trained on the lab's quality assurance and quality control programs. Any time new test kits or instruments are purchased employees should be updated on their training. Documentation of training should be electronically recorded or kept in a training notebook and available for surveyors and auditors.

Maintenance Checks on All Equipment and Instruments

Lab equipment should have routine maintenance inspections to ensure they stay in proper working order. Labs should follow the maintenance schedule that is called for by the manufacturer. Maintenance journals should be kept to illustrate the dates of maintenance and any concerns. Maintenance stickers should be placed on equipment by technicians that service the equipment. Stickers should indicate when the service took place and when the next servicing date is due. Maintenance logs should be available for surveyors when accreditation visits occur.

Required Calibration of Instruments

Some lab equipment will need to be calibrated. CLIA describes calibration as the process of testing and adjusting an instrument or test system readout to establish a correlation between the instrument's measurement of the substance being tested and the actual concentration of the substance. The majority of CLIA-waived analyzers do not need calibration; however, there are some analyzers that do. Always follow the manufacturer's instructions for calibration.

Temperature Checks

Refrigerators and freezers used to store reagents, test kits, and patient samples need to have daily temperature checks to make certain the temperature is appropriate. Acceptable temperature ranges for refrigeration typically runs between 2 and 8°C or 35.6 and 46.4°F and ranges for freezers should be –25 to –15°C or –13 to 5°F. Always make certain thermometers are in good working order and that there are no cracks or bubbles. Refrigeration monitoring systems are available, which may include Web-enabled data logging and annunciation solutions. Logs should appear on the refrigerator and placed in a notebook when completed. If the refrigerator or freezer temperatures fall below the acceptable ranges, reagents may need to be discarded. Follow manufacturer's instructions for specifics.

Proficiency Testing

Proficiency testing is a program designed to evaluate the quality of a laboratory's performance. It is a form of external quality control. Several times a year, moderate- and high-complexity laboratories receive specimens from an approved proficiency testing agency. These samples are evaluated along with patient samples using the same test methodology. Results are then forwarded to the proficiency testing agency for evaluation.

Reference Ranges

Another component of QA is the development of **reference ranges** (also known as **normal values**, expected values, or reference intervals). Every laboratory establishes references ranges for their lab. Read more about reference ranges in the lab report section of the chapter.

SAFETY IN THE LABORATORY

Safety is of critical importance in preventing accidents in the lab. Hazards in the laboratory are not only biological in nature but chemical and physical as well. In 1983, OSHA published the *Hazard Communications Standard,* which it expanded in 1992, with the development of *The Occupational Exposure to Hazardous Chemicals in the Laboratory Standard.* This law was designed to make employees aware of the risks involved with exposure to chemicals in the laboratory. Chapter 8 expands on these standards.

Health care workers not only handle patient samples, but also chemicals, known as reagents. These chemicals can be toxic, corrosive, and even carcinogenic. The use of specialized protective equipment may be required to protect personnel from toxic fumes and vapors from these chemicals. Many of the chemicals used in the laboratory are highly volatile and flammable. Proper storage, handling, and labeling are required.

Electrical hazards in the laboratory can be the cause of burns and electrical shocks as well as fire. Caution must be taken when working around laboratory equipment and other sources of electricity.

In the event of fire or other emergencies, evacuation routes should be clearly posted and marked. All emergency phone numbers should be clearly posted near each telephone. These numbers should include: 911 or emergency medical services (EMS), police and fire department, hospital emergency room, and poison control center. To learn more about these topics refer to the Emergency Preparedness materials in MindTap.

HAZARDS

Hazards in the laboratory are divided into physical, chemical, and biological categories. Each category requires its own specific set of guidelines for safe handling.

Physical hazard cautions include the following:

- Ground all electrical equipment with UL-approved three-pronged plugs.
- Do not use extension cords.
- Avoid overloading electrical circuits.
- Inspect all plugs and cords for possible damage on a regular basis.
- Use surge protectors on equipment and computers to protect against electrical power surges.
- Before servicing, make sure electrical equipment is unplugged from the power source.
- Post signs or labels indicating electrical hazards and high voltage.
- Always follow manufacturer's directions for use of equipment.
- Know the location of the eye wash, chemical shower, fire blanket, and fire extinguisher.

Chemical hazard cautions include the following:

- Label all bottles of hazardous chemicals. Be sure to include a safety data sheet (SDS) for each chemical stored in the lab in the SDS manual. Sheets should include instructions for proper storage, handling, and disposal of each individual chemical.
- Immediately recap bottles containing toxic substances.
- Immediately clean all chemical spills following the required protocol established by OSHA.
- If skin or eyes are splashed with a chemical, the area should be flushed with water for at least five minutes. (For a procedure on using an emergency eye wash refer to the Emergency Preparedness materials in MindTap.)
- Never pipette anything by mouth.
- Use a safety hood (not generally used in POLs) when working with toxic, flammable, or volatile chemicals.
- Store flammable or volatile chemicals following manufacturer's guidelines. Figure 23-4 shows some of the labels that help identify the category of a chemical.

Biological hazard cautions include the following:

- Wash hands before and after each patient.
- Always wear gloves and other PPE where appropriate.

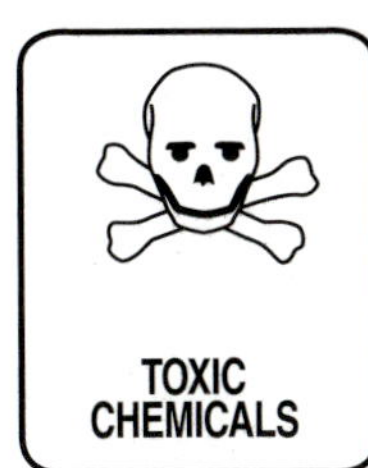

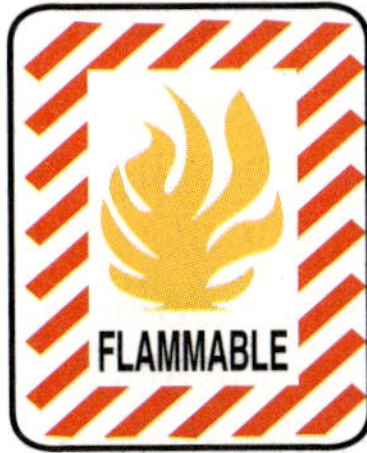

Figure 23-4 ■ Hazard symbols used on chemicals found in the laboratory.

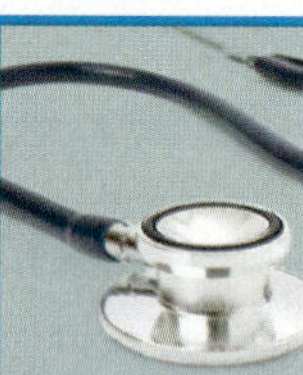

Field Smarts

Questions often arise regarding the application of PPE. Different types of PPE that you apply to your body include gloves, gown, mask, goggles, head covers, and shoe covers.

- Gloves should be worn whenever there is a risk of coming into contact with biological fluids, mucous membranes, non-intact skin, or handling any type of specimens or chemicals.
- Gowns, eye protection, and masks should be worn whenever there is a *significant* risk of splash to body fluids or chemicals. Surgical bonnets may also be worn to protect hair from splash. (Examples of when splash may occur include the following: When removing lids from specimens, when removing stoppers from blood tubes, when collecting specimens such as throat swabs and when performing certain tests such as erythrocyte sedimentation rates [ESRs] due to the potential of splash.)
- Shoe covers should be worn when cleaning up biological or chemicals spills.

- Follow Standard Precautions. (Refer to Chapter 8 for a complete list of Standard Precautions.)
- Do not eat, drink, smoke, or apply cosmetics or contact lenses in the lab.
- Disinfect all work surfaces after each procedure to control the growth of microorganisms.
- Dispose of biohazardous material in proper waste receptacles and all sharps in the sharp's container.

PROCESSING REQUESTS FOR LABORATORY TESTS

It is usually the medical assistant's responsibility to process the provider's requests for laboratory tests. Some tests are performed in office while others are sent to outside facilities. In-office CLIA-waived tests do not usually require a laboratory requisition form. In the few offices still using paper charts, the request is documented in the patient's chart along with the provider's name. Specimens to be sent to an outside lab for testing must be properly collected, processed, and documented in both the patient's chart and in a specimen log. A **lab requisition form**, containing all pertinent information and tests requested, must accompany each specimen.

The Laboratory Requisition Form

The requisition form (Figure 23-5) must be accurately completed. Each laboratory supplies its own forms, which may vary slightly from one lab to another. Several tests can be ordered on a single form, which may mean sending more than one specimen container with a single requisition. Label each specimen with all the information requested by the contracted laboratory. Careful attention to detail is crucial when completing laboratory requisition forms. Mistakes or omissions in documentation may result in delays in receiving critical test results. The following information must be accurately completed on the requisition form:

1. Provider information: Name, address, telephone number, and laboratory account number. This information is needed in order to contact the office to report results or to clarify test requests. Some laboratories provide forms that are preprinted with the provider's information; however, if the form is electronically generated, the doctor's information will automatically generate on the form.
2. Patient information: Name, address, telephone number, age, date of birth, and gender. Some tests results are influenced by age and gender. Once again, this is automatically generated when using electronic health records.
3. Specimen source: The source of the specimen is important to the lab, especially when a visual inspection cannot reveal its source. For example, a swab containing a specimen for a throat culture would be tested differently than a wound specimen.
4. Date and time of collection: Some laboratory tests must be performed within a certain amount of time following collection, while others need to be performed after a period of time has elapsed. Fasting may also be required for some types of testing in order to be accurate.
5. Requested tests: Each test or profile requested must be marked with a check mark or an "X" in the box beside the test name and number. For those tests not listed, additional space is provided to fill in the test ordered.
6. Patient medications: Certain medications can affect results, so it is important for the lab to have accurate information.

7. Clinical diagnosis: Diagnostic and procedural codes are required for billing purposes. This information may also be useful if abnormal test results or discrepancies are encountered.
8. Results requested: The provider may want a result immediately (stat or ASAP). The time requested for results must be clearly indicated.

Generating Orders in the CPOE

Many labs can now integrate with the practice's EHR or PM software by way of an interface that automates the transfer of patient demographics and lab orders/results. This allows lab orders and result information to be shared electronically between the lab and the practice.

Prior to 2012, the CMS stated that only licensed health care professionals had the authority to enter orders into EHR. However, on August 23, 2012, the CMS issued a final rule on Stage 2 Meaningful Use of the Medicare and Medicaid EHR incentive program stating that credentialed medical assistants also qualify to enter medication orders into the **computerized provider order entry (CPOE)** system. This was later changed to include lab and radiology orders as well.

According to the CMS, credentialed medical assistants are any medical assistants who take a credentialing test from a third party organization not connected to the employer. Examples of credentialed medical assistants include graduates of CAAHEP or

N7708

BILL
☐ ACCOUNT
☐ PATIENT SEE ①
☐ 3RD PARTY SEE ②

PLEASE LEAVE BLANK
AREA ________
DEPT. ________
BILL CD ________

C-3 REQUEST FORM
INSTRUCTIONS ① FOR PATIENT BILLING, COMPLETE BOX A.
② FOR 3RD PARTY BILLING, COMPLETE BOX A AND FILL IN DIAGNOSIS, THEN EITHER B, C, or D.

USA Biomedical Labs
957 Central Avenue
Heartland, NY 11112

PATIENT NAME (LAST) | (FIRST) | SPECIES | SEX | AGE YRS. MOS. | DATE COLLECTED MO. DAY YR. | TIME COLLECTED
PATIENT ADDRESS | STREET | MISC. INFORMATION | DR. I.D. | MEDICARE: #
CITY | STATE | ZIP | DIAGNOSIS
PHYSICIAN | WELFARE: # | CASE NAME:
PROGRAM: | PATIENT 1ST NAME: | DATE OF BIRTH ALL CLAIMS MO. DAY YR.
INSURANCE GR. # | I.D. | SERVICE CODE:
SUBSCRIBER NAME: | RELATION: | PHONE

STANDARD PROFILES

2987 ( ) Diagnostic (Multi-Chem) Profile
2804 ( ) Health Survey (SMA-12)
2824 ( ) Executive Profile A
2825 ( ) Executive Profile B
2826 ( ) Executive Profile C
2858 ( ) Amenorrhea Profile
7330 ( ) Anticonvulsant Group
2927 ( ) Autoimmune Profile
2801 ( ) Calcium Metabolism Profile
2859 ( ) Diabetes Management Profile
7701 ( ) Drug Abuse Screen
( ) Drug Analysis Comprehensive (S & U or G)
( ) Drug Analysis, Qual (U/G)
7340 ( ) Drug Analysis, Quant. (S)
2022 ( ) Electrolyte Profile
( ) Exanthem Group
( ) Glucose/Insulin Response
2871 ( ) Hepatitis Profile I
2872 ( ) Hepatitis Profile II
2873 ( ) Hepatitis Profile III
2874 ( ) Hepatitis Profile IV
2875 ( ) Hepatitis Profile V
2876 ( ) Hepatitis Profile VI
2879 ( ) Hepatitis Profile VII
2864 ( ) Hirsutism Profile
2865 ( ) Hypertension Screen

8350 ( ) Immunologic Evaluation*
2814 ( ) Lipid Profile A
2817 ( ) Lipid Profile B
2003 ( ) Lipid Profile C
2805 ( ) Liver Profile A
2867 ( ) Liver Profile B
2868 ( ) MMR Immunity Panel
2869 ( ) Myocardial Infarction Profile
2585 ( ) Parathyroid Panel A (Mid-Molecule)
2586 ( ) Parathyroid Panel B (Dialysis)
2587 ( ) Parathyroid Panel C (Adenoma)
2818 ( ) Prenatal Profile A
2819 ( ) Prenatal Profile B
2820 ( ) Prenatal Profile C
2877 ( ) Prenatal Profile D
( ) Respiratory Infection Profile A
( ) Respiratory Infection Profile B
( ) Respiratory Infection Profile C
( ) Respiratory Infection Profile D
2821 ( ) Rheumatoid Profile A
2878 ( ) Rheumatoid Profile B
2882 ( ) T & B Lymphocyte Differential Panel
2883 ( ) Testicular Function Profile
2832 ( ) Thyroid Panel A
2032 ( ) Thyroid Panel B
2833 ( ) Thyroid Panel C

SINGLE TESTS

5165 ( ) ABO and Rho (B) (S)
6555 ( ) Alpha-Fetoprotein RIA (S)
3015 ( ) Alk. Phosphatase (S)
3041 ( ) Amylase (S)
5163 ( ) Antibody Screen ( ) If pos. ID & Titer (S) (B)
5166 ( ) Antibody ID (B&S)
5164 ( ) Antibody Titer (B&S) (Previous Pat. #________)
5208 ( ) ANA. Fluorescent (S)
5169 ( ) ASO Titer (B) (S)
3147 ( ) Bilirubin, Direct (S)
3010 ( ) BUN (S)
3018 ( ) Calcium (S)
6472 ( ) CEA (RIA) (Plasma Only)
2995 ( ) CBC with Automated Diff. (Abnormal Follow-Up Studies) (B) (SL)
2996 ( ) CBC less Diff. (B)
3022 ( ) Cholesterol (S)
3042 ( ) CPK (S)
6500 ( ) Digoxin (S)
6501 ( ) Digitoxin (S)
3606 ( ) GGT (S)
3006 ( ) Glucose (S) Fasting
3009 ( ) Glucose (P) Fasting
3023 ( ) Glucose P.P. (P) Hrs. ________
3650 ( ) HDL Cholesterol (S)
5180 ( ) Heterophile Screen (Mono) (S)
5179 ( ) Heterophile Absorption (S)
3342 ( ) Hemoglobin A_{1C} (B)
6416 ( ) IgE (S)
3078 ( ) Iron and T.I.B.C. (S)

6526 ( ) Neonatal T_4 (S)
6525 ( ) Neonatal TSH (S)
7941 ( ) Neonatal T_4 Blood Spot
3019 ( ) Phosphorus (S)
4132 ( ) Platelet Count (B) (S)
3026 ( ) Potassium (S)
( ) Pregnancy Test, (S or U)
5187 ( ) Premarital RPR (S)
6505 ( ) Prostatic Acid Phosphatase (RIA) (S)*
2992 ( ) Protein Electrophoresis (S) IEP if Abnormal ( ) 9085
4149 ( ) Prothrombin Time (P)*
4144 ( ) Reticulocyte Count (B)
5207 ( ) RA Latex Fixation (S)
5194 ( ) RPR
5195 ( ) Rubella H.I. (S)
3016 ( ) SGOT (S)
3045 ( ) SGPT (S)
3031 ( ) T-3 Uptake (S)
3032 ( ) T-4 (S)
2832 ( ) Thyroxine Index, Free (T_7) (S)
3036 ( ) Triglycerides (S)
4111 ( ) Urinalysis (U)
5277 ( ) Urogenital GC Assay

UNLISTED TESTS OR PROFILES

* FROZEN • (B) BLOOD • (P) PLASMA • (U) URINE • (S) SERUM • (SL) SLIDES

(Rev. 1-84)

FOLD THIS FORM IN HALF SO TEST(S) ORDERED IS CLEARLY VISIBLE

Figure 23-5 ■ An example of a lab requisition form.

EHR Application

In order to generate a lab order in most EHRs, the medical assistant goes into the patient's record and clicks on the lab icon. The lab screen comes up and the medical assistant completes the requested information. For an example of a screen shot of a CPOE from Harris CareTracker, refer to Figure 23-6. Labels to place on specimen containers and tubes (Figure 23-7) may also be generated at the time of order implementation, making labeling of specimens much easier.

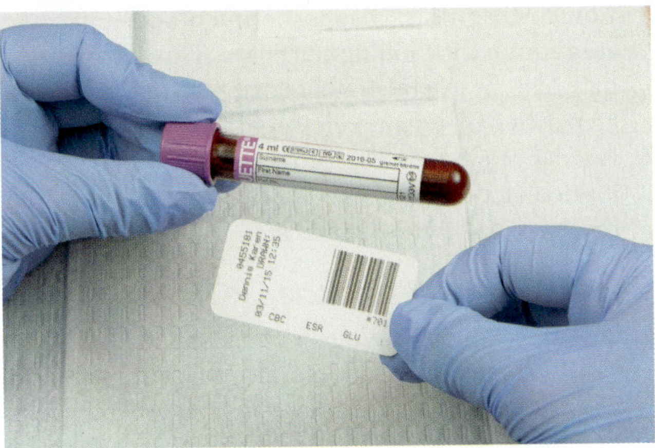

Figure 23-7 ■ An electronically generated label that can be placed on patient specimens.

ABHES accredited programs who have passed the CMA exam through the AAMA or the RMA exam through the AMT; however, other medical assisting credentials in which testing is required also meets the standard. The AAMA now offers a pathway for noncredentialed medical assistants to qualify to enter orders into the CPOE. Noncredentialed medical assistants may apply to take the **Assessment Based Recognition in Order Entry (ABR-OE)** program. By taking the program and passing the test, noncredentialed medical assistants will meet the qualifications of "Credentialed Medical Assistant" so that they may place orders in the EHR. To learn more about this program, refer to the AAMA website at www.aama-ntl.org.

All specimens sent to outside laboratories should be documented in a special log when using paper charts. This may be referred to as an "outside lab log."

This log should be checked daily for tracking purposes. Once the results are sent back to the medical office, the medical assistant or other appropriate personnel will document that the results were received. Pending laboratory results should be followed up with a phone call to the lab to determine the cause for the delay in reporting.

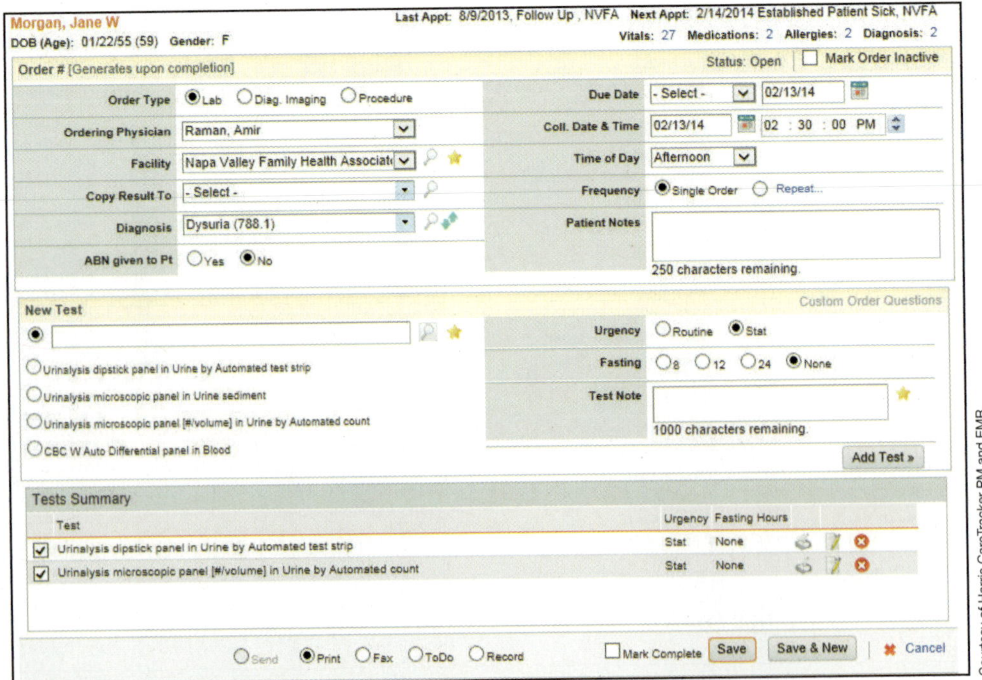

Courtesy of Harris CareTracker PM and EMR.

Figure 23-6 ■ An example of an Order Entry Screen in Harris CareTracker.

Open Orders

Show Inacti

Order #	Due Date	Patient	Type	Test Description	Provider	Enc Date	Status
973761	05/09/14	Morgan, Jane W	Lab	Urinalysis dipstick panel in Urine by Automated test strip (S)	Raman, Amir	05/09/14	Open
973793	05/09/14	Morgan, Jane W	Diag Imag	Patient information entered into a reminder system with a target due date for the next mammogram (RAD) (S)	Raman, Amir	05/09/14	Open
973794	05/09/14	Thompson, Adam	Lab	CBC W Auto Differential panel in Blood (S); Electrolytes 1998 panel in Serum or Plasma	Brockton, Anthony	05/09/14	Open
973981	05/09/14	Morgan, Jane W	Lab	Urinalysis microscopic panel [#/volume] in Urine by Automated count	Raman, Amir	05/09/14	Open
974223	05/21/14	Hernandez, Julia	Lab	Basic metabolic panel in Blood	Ayerick, Rebecca	05/21/14	Open
989589	08/29/14	Patient, Claire	Lab	Urinalysis dipstick panel in Urine by Automated test strip (S); CBC W Auto Differential panel in Blood (S)	Raman, Amir	08/29/14	Open
999875	11/02/14	Sweeney, Caroline	Proc	12-Lead Electrocardiogram Performed	Raman, Amir	11/03/14	Open

Courtesy of Harris CareTracker PM and EMR.

Figure 23-8 ■ An Open Orders screen in Harris CareTracker. Notice the second column features the due date of the test. The red font signals to the MA that these tests have been ordered but there are no results associated with the order.

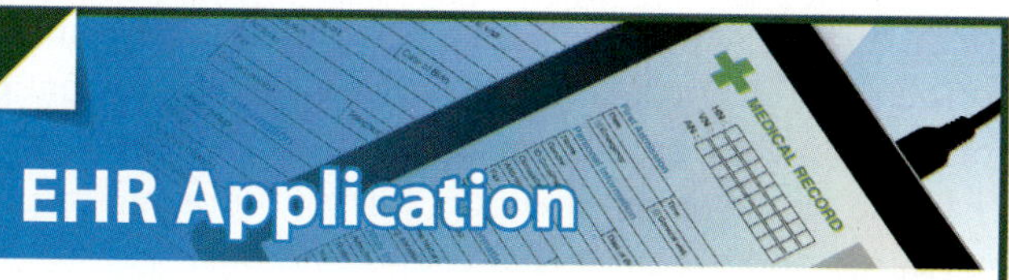

EHR Application

Many EHR programs are able to track open orders for lab, radiology, and other diagnostic procedures. In Harris CareTracker, this tool is located in the task section of the EHR (Figure 23-8); therefore, a written outstanding lab log is not necessary. Once results are electronically uploaded or scanned into the chart, they will appear in the provider's and MA's task or electronic mail box. Anything of high priority is flagged for the provider's immediate attention. The results are generally linked to the original order, reviewed, and signed by the provider. Once the provider electronically signs off on the results, the open order is removed from the ordering provider's task list and the results can be made available for viewing in the results section of the patient's EHR.

PREPARING THE PATIENT FOR LABORATORY TESTING

Proper specimen collection is crucial in order to obtain accurate laboratory results. Patients must clearly understand the collection process, especially if they will be collecting the specimen themselves. For example, a 24-hour urine specimen is collected by the patient at home. Clear, printed instructions should be given to the patient and reviewed before the patient leaves the office. An improperly collected specimen can create a delay in obtaining results due to rejection of the specimen by the laboratory. In addition to the delay in test results, the patient will be inconvenienced if they need to recollect the specimen at home or return to the office for another collection.

Keep in mind that many patients are apprehensive about what tests may reveal, or may be in pain, or feeling very ill, and may not be able to process the instructions given to them. Medical assistants should give patients a copy of their contact information in the event they have questions during the collection process.

GENERAL GUIDELINES FOR SPECIMEN COLLECTION, HANDLING, AND TRANSPORT

Outside laboratories will provide the medical office with a catalog or instruction manual of the tests performed at their facility. The catalog includes information on the correct type of specimen needed for each test as well as proper collection, handling, and transport instructions. It is important to double check specimen information in each catalog because specimen requirements differ from one lab to another. If there are any questions concerning the type of specimen to be collected, it is best to contact the laboratory directly.

Insurance companies contract with different laboratories to perform patient testing. It is not unusual for several labs to pick up specimens at one office; therefore, it is important to be sure that the specimen is sent to the correct facility. If the patient must go to an outside laboratory to have a specimen collected, there are usually satellite labs or procurement stations conveniently located throughout the community.

Specimen Collection

Specific specimen collection techniques will be discussed in related chapters.

Procedure 23-3 lists step-by-step instructions for specimen collection for offsite testing.

Preserving Specimens

Each clinical laboratory will maintain a laboratory manual that lists the specimen requirements along with procedures to follow to maintain specimen integrity. For example, specimens for urinalysis that cannot be tested within two hours should be refrigerated. Serum samples for routine clinical chemistry tests must be allowed to clot, and then centrifuged to quickly separate the cells from the serum. If the tube does not contain a gel separator, the serum must be removed and placed in another tube. If testing will be delayed, the new tube with the serum added should be capped and placed in the refrigerator. Some tests, such as bilirubin, must be protected from light if testing is delayed. In addition, reference laboratories may require that serum or plasma be frozen if testing is delayed.

Sources of Contamination

Proper specimen collection will reduce potential for sample contamination. For example, the medical assistant should explain to the patient how to properly collect a clean-catch midstream urine for a culture in order to avoid contamination with normal skin flora. Patients should be discouraged from submitting culture samples such as urine in containers found at home (empty jars, or any other). Even if washed, these containers will contain interfering substances (including the soap used) that will contaminate the original specimen.

THE LABORATORY REPORT

A **laboratory report form** is received by the provider's office after testing is completed. Laboratory report forms may reach the office electronically, be phoned to the practice, or faxed to the practice. The format of forms may vary by laboratory. Figure 23-9 shows one example of a laboratory report form. Abnormal results are in red and green so that they stand out.

Service Laboratories
734 Dunlap Street
Chicago, IL 60171
Telephone: 312-824-6925
Fax: 312-824-5829

Patient: Samuels, Annette (ID #ICH 041309)
Female, Age 22

Referred by: Inner City Health Care
Susan Rice
#10004086

SAMP COLL: 04/24/XX 10:40 AM SAMP RECD: 04/24/XX 12:10 PM

TEST	RESULTS		REFERENCE RANGE	UNITS	*
CBC					
Col: 04/26/XX 11:30					(1)
WBC	5.3		5.0-11.0	X10-3	
RBC	4.5		3.9-5.3	X10-6	
HGB	12.8		11.5-13.5	G/DL	
HCT	37.2		34.0-40.0	%	
MCV	83		79-99	FL	
MCH	28		27-32	PG	
MCHC	34		32-37	G/DL	
RDW	13		11-15	%	
PLT	290		130-400	X10-3	
MPV	7		7-11	FL	
AUTO DIFF					
Col: 04/26/XX 11:30					(1)
DIFFERENTIAL (MAN)					
Col: 04/26/XX 11:30					(1)
SEGS	34	L	41-85	%	
LYMPHS	56	H	15-48	%	
MONOS	9		2-15	%	
EOS	1		0-55	%	
RBC MORPH	RBC NORM				
URINALYSIS (ROUTINE)					
Col: 04/26/XX 11:31					(1)
SP GRVTY	1.025		1.003-1.030		
PH	6.5		5.0-8.0		
PROTEIN	NEGATIVE		<= TRACE		
GLUCOSE	NEGATIVE		NEGATIVE		
KETONES	NEGATIVE		NEGATIVE		
BILIRUBIN	NEGATIVE		NEGATIVE		
UROBILINOGEN	0.2 E.U./dL		0.2-1.0		
BLOOD/HGB	NEGATIVE		NEGATIVE		
NITRITE	NEGATIVE		NEGATIVE		
LEUKOCYTES	NEGATIVE		NEGATIVE		

Figure 23-9 ■ An example of a lab report. Notice how the abnormal results are in red.

Whatever the format, specific information appearing on the report form will include the following:

1. Laboratory's name, address, and phone number
2. Provider's name, address, and identification number
3. Patient's name, age, gender, and identification/accession number assigned by the lab
4. Date the specimen was collected
5. Date the specimen was received by the testing laboratory
6. Date and time the results were reported
7. Name of tests performed
8. Test results and time reported
9. Normal reference ranges for each test

Each office will have its own policy for handling patient lab reports and for providing patients with the results. If the office is completely electronic, the medical assistant will just track labs through the EHR. Once the provider reviews the results, he or she will send a message to the medical assistant with special instructions for the patient. Depending on the EHR and the preferences of the provider, the medical assistant may need to make the results assessable in the patient's portal by clicking on a specific link. In offices still using paper charts, the medical assistant is usually responsible for receiving reports, reviewing the results, checking for abnormal values, attaching the report form to the patient's chart, and delivering the chart to the provider for review. (*Note*: Never give out any lab results without the provider's permission unless office protocol dictates that normal results can be given to patients without the provider's permission.)

When calling to give patients lab results, use the phone number listed on the privacy form indicating where messages and test results can be left. Oftentimes this is a personal cell phone number. Never leave results on an answering machine or with another individual unless the patient specified it was okay to do so this has been documented in the patient's chart communication preference and authorization section. Once you connect with the patient, provide the results and give an explanation of what the results mean if applicable. Give the patient any instructions from the provider such as medication or dietary changes or the need to set up an appointment. Have patient repeat back instructions to verify comprehension and document the information in the chart. Patients may question the validity of the results; if so reassure the patient of the accuracy of the results. Refer to Figure 23-10 for a screen shot of a follow-up to a lab report in Harris CareTracker and refer to Procedure 23-2 for a complete procedure on handling and following up on lab reports.

Abnormal or Panic Test Values

The laboratory usually flags abnormal results on the report form. For example, an increased value will have an "H" beside the results indicating a high value, while a decreased value will have an "L" beside the results indicating a low value. Some labs also make abnormal lab results a different color or mark with an "A". Each office will have its own protocol for handling abnormal results. Some laboratory results are so abnormal

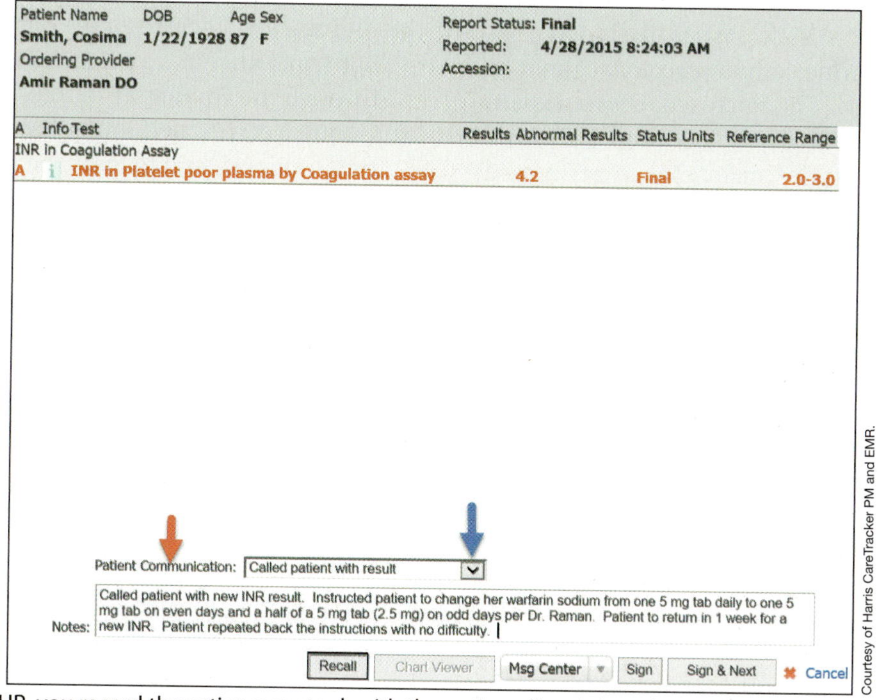

Figure 23-10 ■ With EHR, you record the actions you took with the patient directly into the results screen.

they can pose an immediate health threat to the patient. These results are known as critical lab values or panic values. A panic value or critical value may be sent electronically to the provider's task portal or may be telephoned to the office by the laboratory. Providers usually like to handle their own panic values, but may give the medical assistant instructions on what to relay to the patient.

FLOW SHEETS

Flow sheets contain data collected on patients that can be reviewed and updated each time the patient visits their health care provider. These can be found in paper form in the chart, or can be tracked electronically. Lab results are a great example of tracking a patient over time. An example of how flow sheets are helpful for tracking is their use with the diabetic patient. A diabetic patient may come to the office complaining of flu-like symptoms, but in addition, the flow sheet will show what the $HbA1_c$ results had been trending in past visits. This way the health care provider can determine if the care given previously had been effective, while also treating the cause for the recent visit. Electronic charts can be displayed in a variety of formats including horizontal and vertical tables and in a graphing chart.

Figure 23-11 illustrates an electronic flow sheet featuring a group of $HbA1_c$ results in Harris CareTracker illustrating a graphing chart.

THE MICROSCOPE

The **microscope** is a valuable piece of equipment in the laboratory. It is utilized to view objects like blood cells, microorganisms, and urine components that cannot be seen with the naked eye. The microscope is an expensive piece of equipment that requires proper use and maintenance. Any service or maintenance performed on the microscope must be recorded in a maintenance log. This log should be available for viewing during a laboratory inspection.

Even though medical assistants do not perform microscopic work, they should be able to identify the parts of the microscope, explain their function, and demonstrate their proper usage and care (see Procedure 23-4).

There are different types of microscopes, but the most common type used in the POL is the compound microscope, which is named for its two different lenses. One lens increases the magnification produced by the other lens.

Parts of the Microscope

Each part of the microscope has a unique function. A health care professional using the microscope should be familiar with each part and its function. A listing of each part and its function follows. Refer to Figure 23-12 for the location of the different parts.

- Base: Supports the upper components of the microscope
- Arm: Used to carry the microscope
- Stage: Large, flat plate or platform that holds the specimen slide to be viewed. The slide is held in place with a spring-loaded device called the stage clip. The stage can be stationary, which means the slide must be moved by hand, or mechanical, which means the slide can be moved forward, backward, and side-to-side by using the mechanical stage knobs. The stage has a hole in the center that allows the light to pass from the light source through the specimen.
- Illuminator: Located in the base, consisting of a light bulb and an on-off switch. The light passes through the condenser to the slide.
- Condenser: Located under the stage, it concentrates, directs, and focuses the light from the

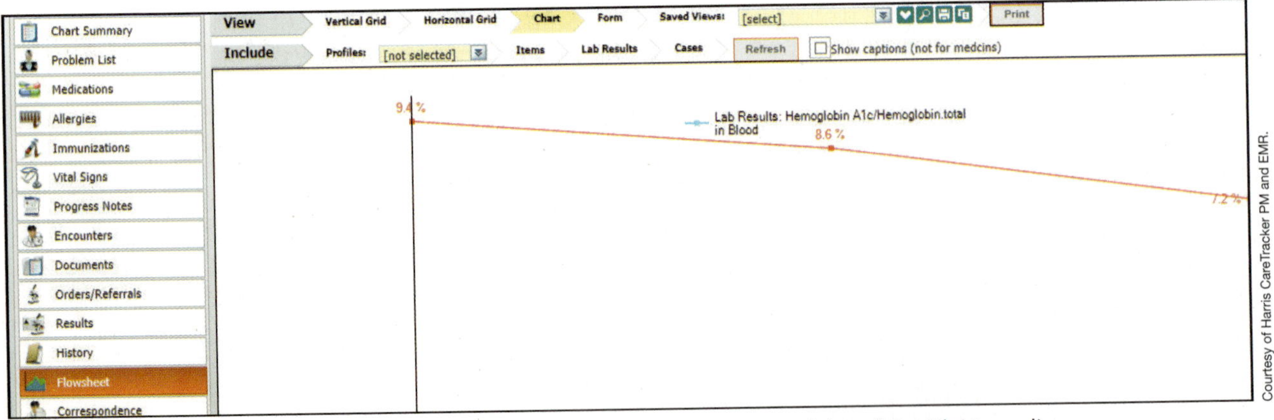

Figure 23-11 ■ An example of a flow sheet in Harris CareTracker featuring the patient's last three $HbA1_c$ readings.

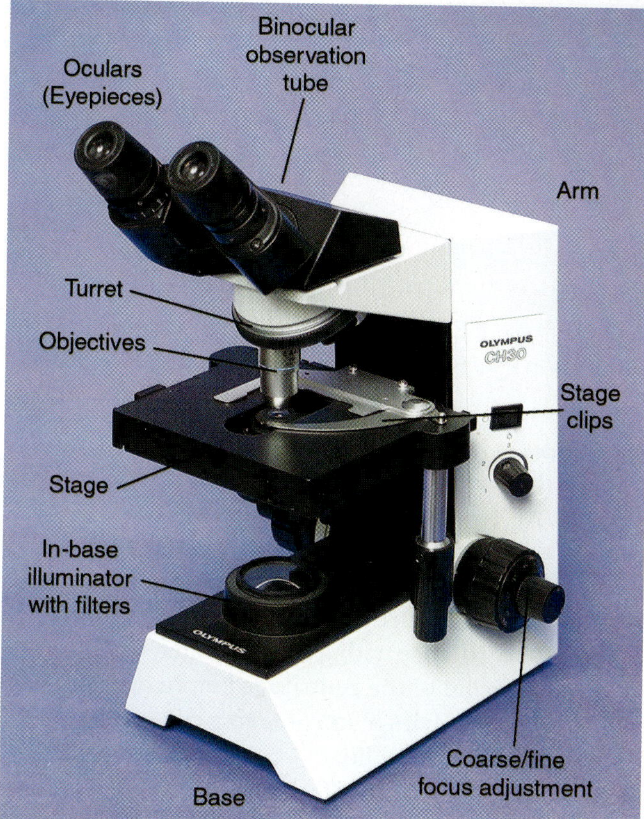

Figure 23-12 ■ The parts of a microscope.

illuminator on the object being viewed. The condenser can be moved up or down by using the control knob, which will increase or decrease the intensity of the light.

- Diaphragm: Located within or beneath the condenser, the iris diaphragm, which resembles the iris of the eye, can be opened or closed to increase or decrease the intensity of the light.
- Coarse and fine adjustment knobs: Located on either side of the arm, the coarse adjustment knob is used to initially bring the specimen into focus and the fine adjustment knob is used to fine tune the focus to produce a clear, sharp image.
- Objectives: Often, there are three objectives, or lenses, attached to the revolving nosepiece. The low-power objective magnifies by a power of 10 (indicated as "10×") and is the shortest lens. The high-power objective has a magnification of 40×, and the oil immersion objective has a magnification of 100×. The oil immersion objective is the longest of the lenses. A drop of clear immersion oil is placed on the slide for viewing when using this objective.
- Ocular/eyepiece: Microscopes are equipped with either one eyepiece (monocular) or two eyepieces (binocular). The width of the eyepieces of a binocular microscope can be adjusted to fit each individual user. Each **ocular** contains a lens with a magnification power of 10×. Thus, the total magnification of an object is obtained by multiplying the ocular magnification by the objective magnification. For example, on low power, the magnification is 100 times (10 × 10).

Care and Maintenance

The microscope is an expensive and delicate instrument that can be easily damaged if not handled and used properly. Proper care and maintenance will lengthen the life of the microscope. Following these guidelines will help to maintain the microscope and guarantee its longevity:

1. Always carry the microscope by lifting it by the arm and placing the other hand under the base for support. The microscope is top heavy and carrying it by this method will ensure that it is moved safely from one location to the next.
2. Keep the microscope covered with a plastic dust cover when not in use.
3. Clean all lenses with lens paper. Using tissues, paper towels, or gauze could scratch the lenses.
4. Enamel surfaces should be cleaned with mild soap and water and dried with a soft cloth. The oil immersion objective and the stage should be wiped off after use to remove any oil residue.
5. A malfunctioning microscope should be repaired by a qualified service technician.

THE CENTRIFUGE

The **centrifuge** is an instrument that spins tubes at high speeds to separate the liquid portion of the sample from the cells and other formed elements. By spinning a tube containing a sample in a centrifuge, the different components separate into layers. For example, when centrifuging a urine sample, the heavier solid matter found in the urine is concentrated in the bottom of the tube. The lighter liquid portion is then poured off and the sediment that remains is examined under the microscope. Spinning a tube of blood in the centrifuge will separate the blood into several layers with the red blood cells in the bottom, the serum or plasma on top, and the white blood cells and platelets in the middle (Figure 23-13).

The medical assistant will use the centrifuge to process samples to be sent to outside laboratories for testing. There are different sizes of centrifuges for different uses. Figure 23-14 shows a centrifuge used to spin blood or urine tubes. An example of a microhematocrit centrifuge can be found in Chapter 25.

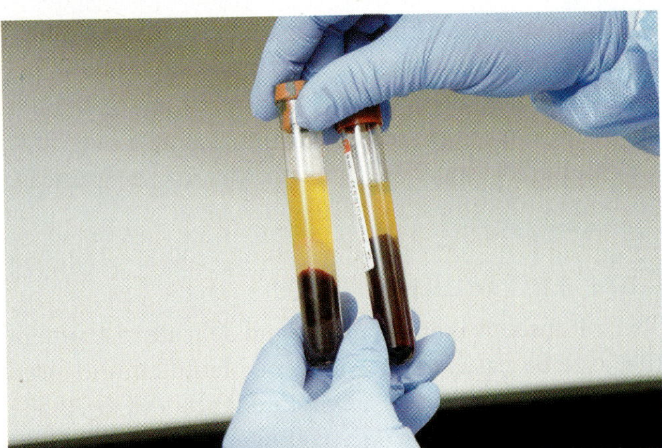

Figure 23-13 ■ Notice how the red cells are now all at the bottom of the tube and the serum is at the top of the tube.

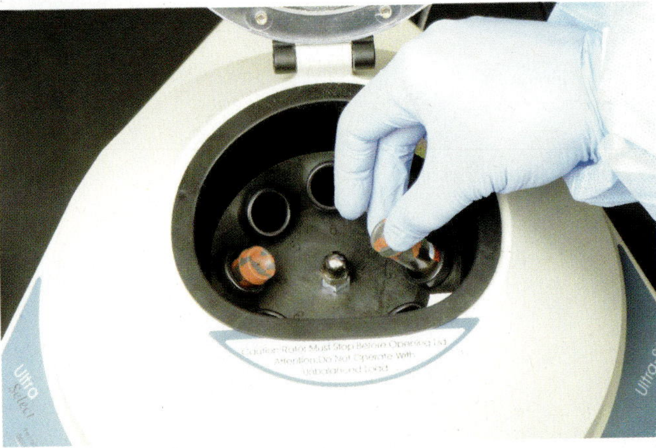

Figure 23-14 ■ Like tubes must be at the same volume and placed across from each other to properly balance the centrifuge.

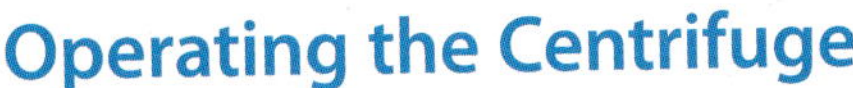

Operating the Centrifuge

Several different models of centrifuges are available from various manufacturers. Medical assistants should always follow the manufacturer's directions for operation of the model in their office. The following are general guidelines that apply to the operation of any centrifuge:

- Use only the type of tube designed for that specific centrifuge.
- To prevent creation of an aerosol contamination, spin tubes with caps securely in place.
- Always balance the centrifuge by placing tubes with an equal amount of sample across from one another (see Figure 23-14). If centrifuging only one tube, balance with a tube of water.
- Secure the lid of the centrifuge before operating.
- Allow the centrifuge to come to a complete stop before opening the lid.
- Always clean and disinfect all surfaces after any tube breakage or spill.

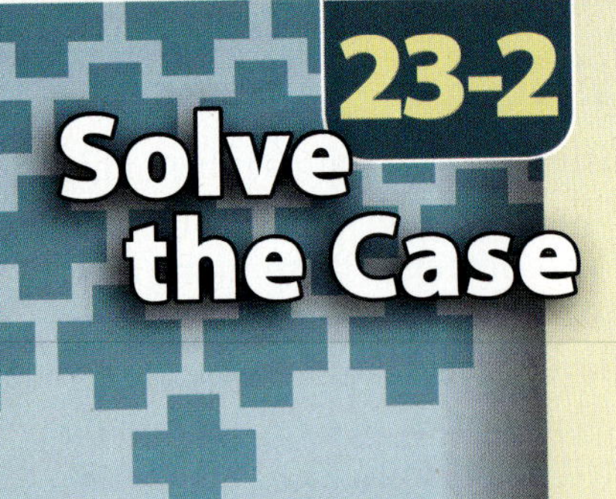

Dr. Dorado orders a comprehensive metabolic panel which is a battery of chemistry tests that looks at the health of several organs and possible disease processes. He also orders a CBC and differential.

1. **When collecting the blood sample, what type of PPE should be worn to protect you during the blood draw?**
2. **Which departments in the lab processed and performed Mrs. Baker's lab tests?**
3. **Mrs. Baker's chemistry panel values were normal; however, her CBC results were abnormal. Her hematocrit, hemoglobin, and red count were critically low. Mrs. Baker is on the phone wanting to know her results but the provider has not reviewed them yet. The values were just loaded into the provider's electronic task box before the patient called. The doctor is making rounds at the hospital right now. What should you do?**

PROCEDURE 23-1

Run a Control

Objective:

To use quality control data to determine if it is safe to report patient results.

Special Note: Gown and goggles icons are shown here; however, these items only need to be worn when the control uses biological reagents or chemicals that may splash upon opening.

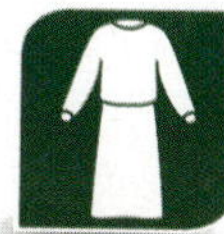

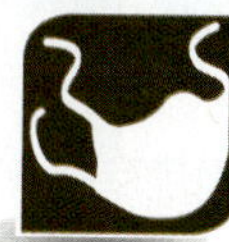

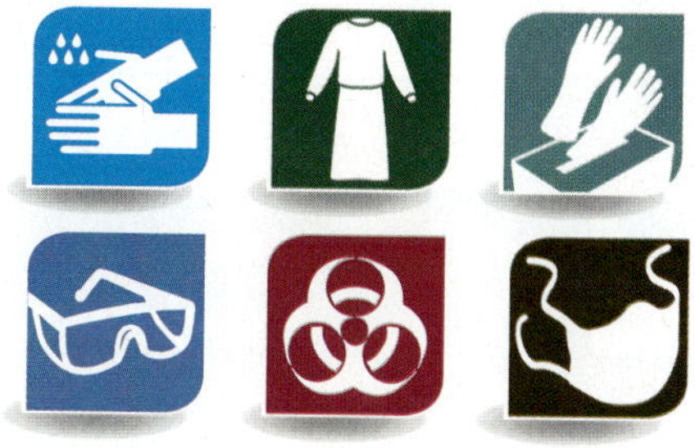

Equipment and Supplies

- Control
- Any necessary equipment, test strips or test kits to run the control on
- Directions for running control
- Necessary reagents if applicable
- Quality Control Log

PROCEDURAL STEPS	DETAILS AND/OR RATIONALE
1. Wash hands and put on appropriate PPE (Figure 23-15).	Applying appropriate PPE will protect you from chemicals in the control and working with equipment that has been contaminated with biological reagents.
2. Gather all equipment and supplies needed to run control.	Gathering equipment and supplies before performing the control will help the procedure to run much more efficiently.
3. Check expiration date on control and any reagents to be used.	Using controls, reagents, and testing strips after the expiration date may result in erroneous results.
4. Read manufacturer's instructions for running the control.	Reading the instructions insures you are performing the control correctly.
5. Run control according to manufacturer's instructions.	Same as above
6. Record results in control log, as well as the expected results.	If results did not turn out as expected, perform the test again using the same control, if results still are not within the reference range, get a new control and start the test all over again. If results are not within range after using a new control, you know that there is something wrong with the equipment or test kit. Report findings to manager and do not use equipment with patient samples until it has been properly serviced. Test kits that are not working properly should be disposed of in proper waste receptacle.
7. Dispose of testing items in the proper trash receptacle.	Controls may contain biologics. (Follow manufacturer's instructions so that you dispose of the control properly.)

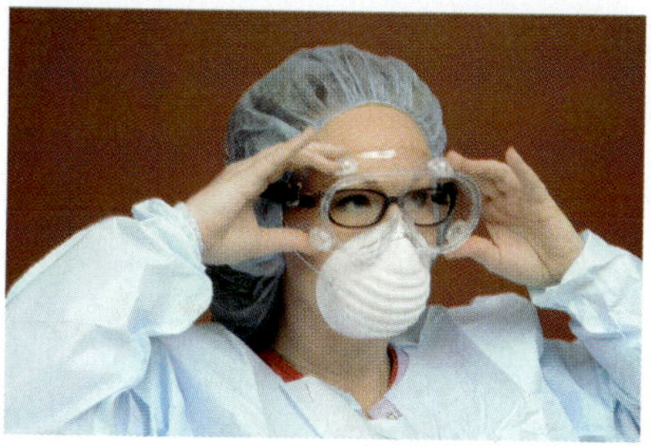

Figure 23-15 ■ Medical assistant dons her PPE before running control.

QUALITY CONTROL LOG FOR THE ABBOT GLUCOMETER 720:

Date and Time	Lot # and Expiration date on control	Lot # and Expiration date on strips	Type of Control	Reference Range	Results and Initials of person running the control
07/07/XX	Lot: 598732V EXP: 02/01/XX	Lot: 9314VD- Exp: 06/15/XX	High	285 mg/dL to 345 mg/dL	315 mg/dL, CL

PROCEDURE 23-2
Review and Report Laboratory Results

Objective:
To check laboratory test results for abnormal values and relay results to the provider for review.

Equipment/Supplies:

- Laboratory report form
- Patient's chart/EHR

PROCEDURAL STEPS	DETAILS AND/OR RATIONALE
1. Check open orders in tasks pane of the EHR. If you notice any open orders that are past due, contact the lab to see when the results will be available. (If using paper charts, check outstanding lab log and contact lab as above.)	Orders that are delayed may be a signal that there was something wrong with the specimen or that the specimen was not received.
2. Check electronic tasks pane to review results that were electronically delivered from the night before. If results need to be scanned into the EHR, do so. (If using paper charts, pull labs off of printer and attach reports to the corresponding patient charts.)	Lab results need to be reviewed as soon as possible. A delay in reviewing results will mean a delay in treatment.
3. If using paper charts, review the laboratory report form, verifying all patient and provider information. Verify that all tests ordered were performed. Follow up with lab if missing any results. (Results delivered electronically are usually initially reviewed by provider.)	Just because you received a lab report on a patient doesn't mean that all tests were performed. Always check to make certain all tests were performed that were ordered.
4. If using paper charts, check the test results with laboratory reference ranges and immediately report any panic values to the provider. Stack charts with lab reports on provider's desk, making certain that abnormal results are on top of the pile.	Panic values could indicate a life-threatening medical condition requiring immediate medical intervention.
5. After the provider has reviewed the results, check to see if there are any special instructions for the patient.	Often times, the provider will want the patient to make dietary or medication changes when results are abnormal.

continues

PROCEDURE 23-2 continued

PROCEDURAL STEPS	DETAILS AND/OR RATIONALE
6. Report the results to the patient according to office protocol. (Verify you are speaking with patient or that you can leave results with someone listed on the patient's privacy statement.) If using EHR, make tests available in patient portal. Call patients who are not electronically connected or patients who have abnormal lab results. If patient questions the validity of the results, ***reassure patient of the accuracy of the results.***	Reporting results to anyone not listed on the privacy statement is a violation of HIPAA. Many patients are electronically connected via their patient portal, but don't assume everyone is. Call patients who are not electronically connected with lab results. This may be a good time to discuss how to create a patient portal account.
7. Have patient repeat back any special instructions that need to be followed.	It's important to verify that patients have a good understanding of any changes or follow up visits.
8. Document the call in the chart and any special instructions given to patient.	Documentation verifies that the patient was given the results and any special instructions.
9. Make certain that flow sheets were completed if applicable.	Flow sheets are electronically generated in the EHR but need to be manually created in paper charts. Flow sheets allow the provider to see at a glance any unique patterns.

DOCUMENTATION EXAMPLE:

Patient Communication: Called patient with result

Notes: Called patient with new INR result. Instructed patient to change her warfarin sodium from one 5 mg tab daily to one 5 mg tab on even days and a half of a 5 mg tab (2.5 mg) on odd days per Dr. Raman. Patient to return in 1 week for a new INR. Patient repeated back the instructions with no difficulty.

Recall | Chart Viewer | Msg Center | Sign | Sign & Next | Cancel

Courtesy of Harris CareTracker PM and EMR

PROCEDURE 23-3
Specimen Collection for Offsite Testing

Objective:

To provide the laboratory with the best quality specimen and a lab requisition form that contains all pertinent information.

Special note: Gown, goggles, and masks are only necessary when collecting specimens in which there may be splashing such as when collecting a throat swab or following collection during the processing stage of the collection (i.e., removing the stopper from a tube to separate serum).

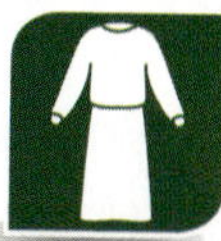

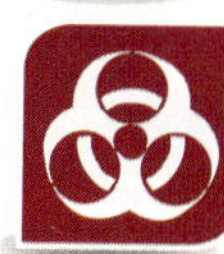
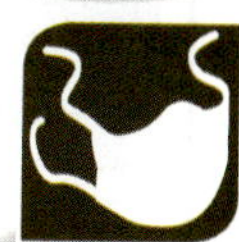

continues

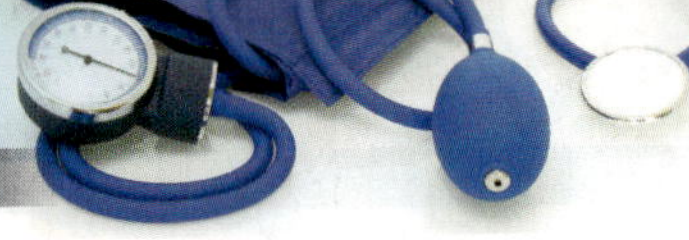

PROCEDURE 23-3 continued

PROCEDURAL STEPS	DETAILS AND/OR RATIONALE
11. Properly dispose of wastes in the correct trash receptacle, clean and disinfect the area. Remove PPE and dispose of according to facility policy.	Disposing of wastes in the correct trash receptacle protects trash handlers from exposure to biological wastes.
12. Wash hands and document the collection in the patient's chart and lab log if applicable.	Documenting the specimen collection proves that the collection was performed and provides specific details about the collection.

DOCUMENTATION EXAMPLE:

04-01-XX 1:10 p.m.	Venipuncture—R. arm antecubital area for blood glucose and potassium levels per Dr. Kelly. Verified pt. fasting. 1 red top and 1 gray top picked up by courier for Lab, Inc. 04-01-XX. Trey Miller, CMA (AAMA)--

LABORATORY SPECIMEN LOG:

DATE	TIME COLLECTED	PATIENT NAME	TEST ORDERED	ORDERED BY	SPECIMEN SENT TO:	INTIALS
04-01-XX	1:10 p.m.	Brown, John	FBS and POT.	Dr. Kelly	Lab, Inc.	TM

PROCEDURE 23-4

Use the Microscope

Objective:

To correctly use and maintain the microscope and to become proficient in the use of the coarse and fine adjustments as well as all objectives.

Equipment/Supplies:

- Microscope
- Lens paper
- Specimen slide
- Immersion oil
- Tissue
- Gloves

continues

PROCEDURE 23-3 continued

PROCEDURAL STEPS	DETAILS AND/OR RATIONALE
5. Assemble the proper equipment.	Appropriate containers must be used as specified by the lab to ensure specimen integrity.
6. Label all specimen tubes and containers with the patient's name, the date and time of collection, your initials, and any other information required by the lab. (Figure 23-17 illustrates a bar code label.)	Properly labeled containers prevent specimen mix-ups.
7. Wash your hands and put on the required PPE.	Both the specimen and the medical assistant should always be protected from contamination.
8. Identify the patient using two identifiers, identify yourself, and ***explain the rationale for the performance of the procedure, showing awareness of the patient's concerns related to the procedure being performed.*** Verify fasting compliance, and properly collect the specimen according to lab directions.	Providing the lab with the best quality specimen prevents delays in the testing and reporting process.
9. Properly engage safety device on needle if a needle was used and dispose of in sharp's container. Care for your patient and dismiss according to institutional policies.	Engaging the safety device will protect you from an accidental needle stick.
10. Process, prepare, and store specimen according to the protocol of the lab. Be sure to include the requisition in the outside pocket of the transfer bag and place the specimen in the middle pocket of the bag (Figure 23-18a and b).	Improper storage of the specimen prior to pickup could damage the specimen and cause erroneous results.

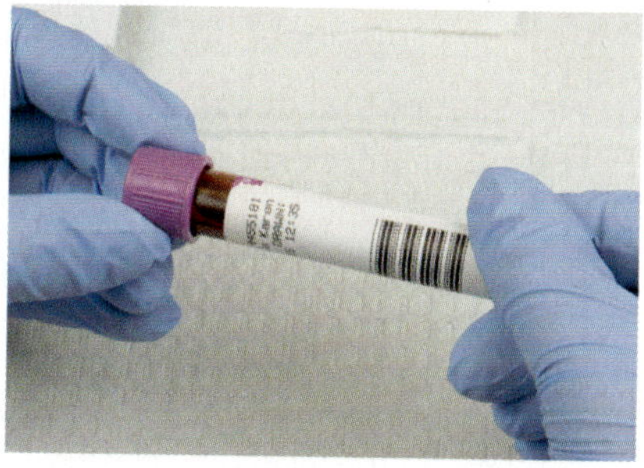

Figure 23-17 ■ The MA labels the tube using a barcode label which includes all requested information.

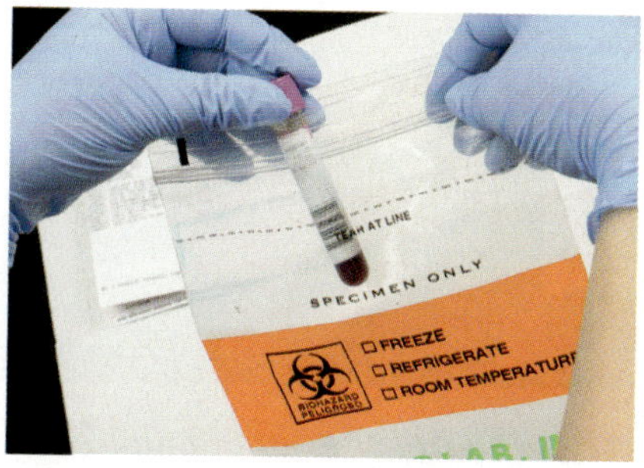

Figure 23-18a ■ The blood tubes go in the center sleeve of the transfer bag.

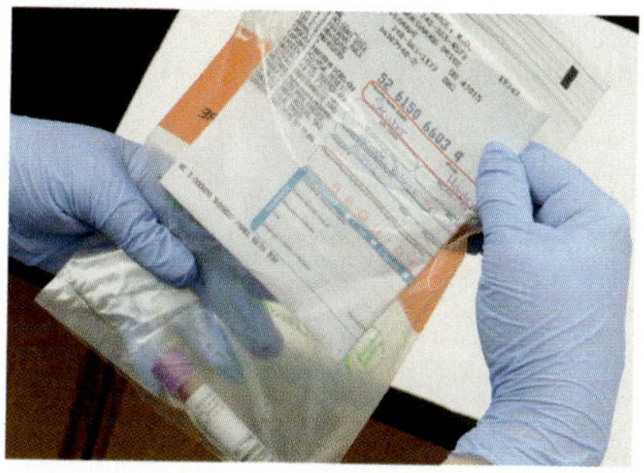

Figure 23-18b ■ The MA puts the lab requisition form in the outside sleeve of the transfer bag to prevent it from becoming contaminated by the tubes of blood.

continues

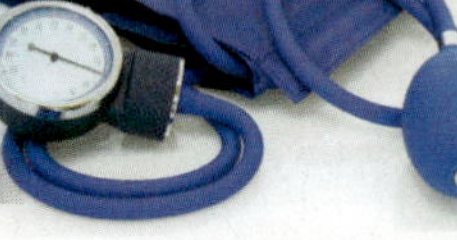

PROCEDURE 23-3 continued

PROCEDURAL STEPS	DETAILS AND/OR RATIONALE
11. Properly dispose of wastes in the correct trash receptacle, clean and disinfect the area. Remove PPE and dispose of according to facility policy.	Disposing of wastes in the correct trash receptacle protects trash handlers from exposure to biological wastes.
12. Wash hands and document the collection in the patient's chart and lab log if applicable.	Documenting the specimen collection proves that the collection was performed and provides specific details about the collection.

DOCUMENTATION EXAMPLE:

04-01-XX 1:10 p.m.	Venipuncture—R. arm antecubital area for blood glucose and potassium levels per Dr. Kelly. Verified pt. fasting. 1 red top and 1 gray top picked up by courier for Lab, Inc. 04-01-XX. Trey Miller, CMA (AAMA)--

LABORATORY SPECIMEN LOG:

DATE	TIME COLLECTED	PATIENT NAME	TEST ORDERED	ORDERED BY	SPECIMEN SENT TO:	INTIALS
04-01-XX	1:10 p.m.	Brown, John	FBS and POT.	Dr. Kelly	Lab, Inc.	TM

PROCEDURE 23-4

Use the Microscope

Objective:

To correctly use and maintain the microscope and to become proficient in the use of the coarse and fine adjustments as well as all objectives.

Equipment/Supplies:

- Microscope
- Lens paper
- Specimen slide
- Immersion oil
- Tissue
- Gloves

continues

PROCEDURE 23-2 continued

PROCEDURAL STEPS	DETAILS AND/OR RATIONALE
6. Report the results to the patient according to office protocol. (Verify you are speaking with patient or that you can leave results with someone listed on the patient's privacy statement.) If using EHR, make tests available in patient portal. Call patients who are not electronically connected or patients who have abnormal lab results. If patient questions the validity of the results, ***reassure patient of the accuracy of the results***.	Reporting results to anyone not listed on the privacy statement is a violation of HIPAA. Many patients are electronically connected via their patient portal, but don't assume everyone is. Call patients who are not electronically connected with lab results. This may be a good time to discuss how to create a patient portal account.
7. Have patient repeat back any special instructions that need to be followed.	It's important to verify that patients have a good understanding of any changes or follow up visits.
8. Document the call in the chart and any special instructions given to patient.	Documentation verifies that the patient was given the results and any special instructions.
9. Make certain that flow sheets were completed if applicable.	Flow sheets are electronically generated in the EHR but need to be manually created in paper charts. Flow sheets allow the provider to see at a glance any unique patterns.

DOCUMENTATION EXAMPLE:

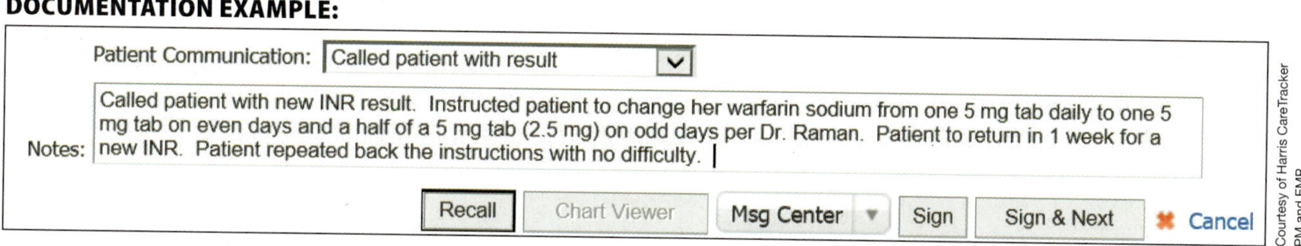
Patient Communication: Called patient with result

Notes: Called patient with new INR result. Instructed patient to change her warfarin sodium from one 5 mg tab daily to one 5 mg tab on even days and a half of a 5 mg tab (2.5 mg) on odd days per Dr. Raman. Patient to return in 1 week for a new INR. Patient repeated back the instructions with no difficulty.

Courtesy of Harris CareTracker PM and EMR

PROCEDURE 23-3
Specimen Collection for Offsite Testing

Objective:

To provide the laboratory with the best quality specimen and a lab requisition form that contains all pertinent information.

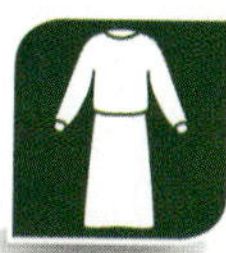

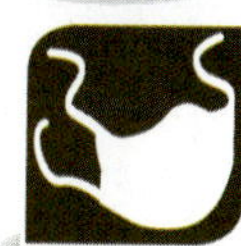

Special note: Gown, goggles, and masks are only necessary when collecting specimens in which there may be splashing such as when collecting a throat swab or following collection during the processing stage of the collection (i.e., removing the stopper from a tube to separate serum).

continues

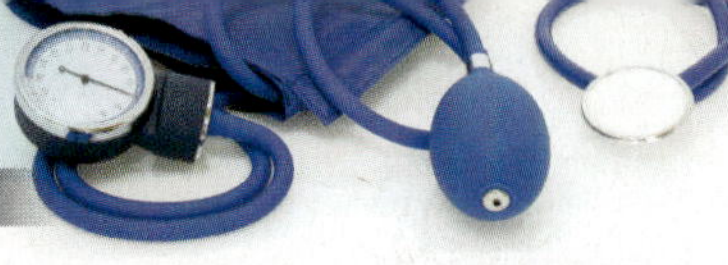

PROCEDURE 23-3 continued

Equipment/Supplies:

- Laboratory requisition form, if applicable
- Necessary collection equipment
- Proper specimen containers
- Personal protective equipment (PPE)
- Sharps container
- Patient's chart/EHR

PROCEDURAL STEPS	DETAILS AND/OR RATIONALE
1. Verify the provider's order in the patient's chart.	Always check to be sure the specimen collection matches the provider's orders.
2. Review the requirements of the laboratory manual for specimen collection and transport.	Requirements may vary by lab. Always check the catalog to prevent errors in collection and handling of the specimen.
3. If the patient is collecting the specimen at home, gather materials with any special preparation instructions, such as fasting, diet or medication restrictions, and home collection instructions.	Improper preparation by the patient can result in inaccurate results and the need to collect the specimen again.
4. Create lab order in CPOE if electronic (Figure 23-16) or, if using paper charts, complete lab requisition with all important information before collecting the specimen.	A completed requisition provides the lab with the essential information necessary to complete the testing process.

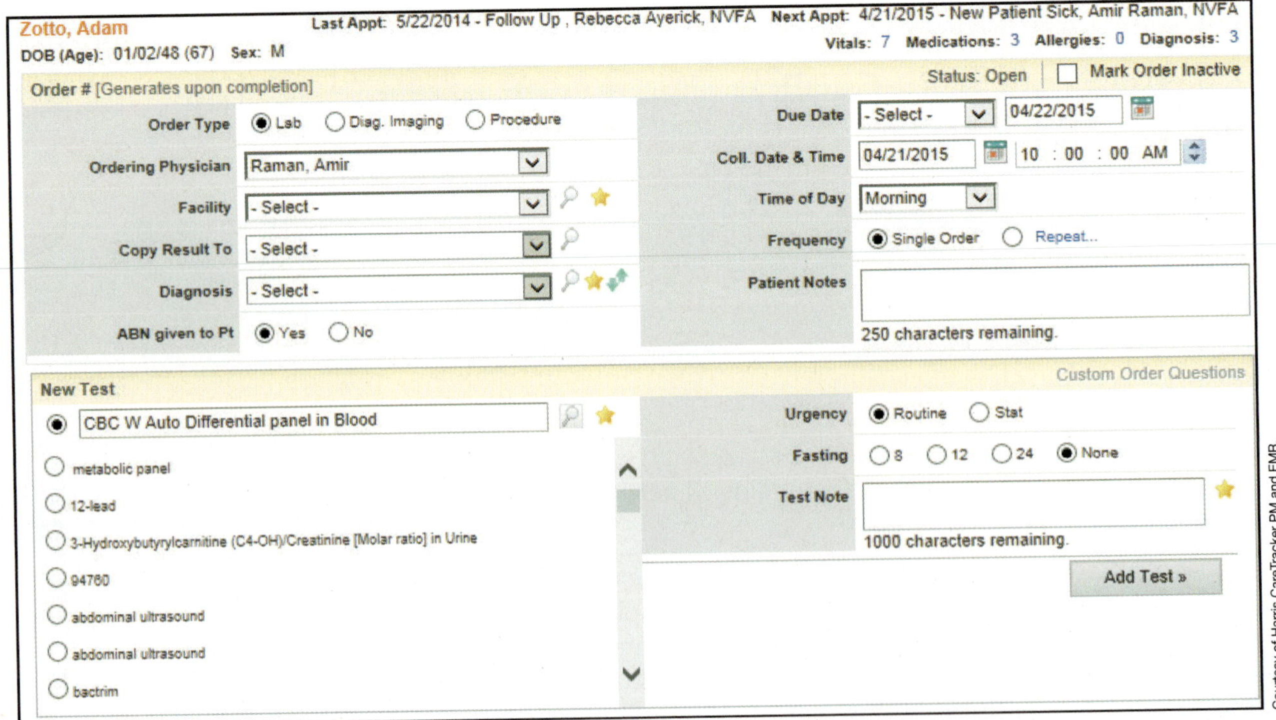

Courtesy of Harris CareTracker PM and EMR.

Figure 23-16 ■ Create your order in the electronic lab entry screen when using EHR.

continues

PROCEDURE 23-4 continued

PROCEDURAL STEPS	DETAILS AND/OR RATIONALE
1. Wash your hands, apply gloves, and assemble all the equipment.	Gloves must be worn to protect the user from possible exposure to materials that may be present on the microscope or specimen slide.
2. Clean the oculars and the objectives with lens paper (Figure 23-19).	Lenses may be soiled from the previous user. Clean lenses produce a clearer, sharper image.
3. Turn on the light source and adjust the light to a low-level.	Low light intensity helps to prolong the life of the bulb.
4. Rotate the nosepiece to the low-power (10×) objective or high power (40×) objective according to type of specimen and provider's order and click it into place.	Whether you use the low or high power objective will be according to the type of specimen and provider's preference. In today's POL, the majority of microscopic analysis will be of urine.
5. Place the specimen slide on the stage (Figure 23-20) and move the stage upward using the stage adjustment knobs, so the objective is in its lowest position. Observe the stage movement so that the objective does not come in contact with the slide.	The slide could be damaged if the objective strikes the slide.
6. Adjust the eyepieces to a comfortable width. View the slide through the oculars, and using the coarse adjustment knob (larger knobs) to bring the specimen into focus.	Initial focusing is accomplished using the coarse adjustment knob only.
7. Adjust light intensity as needed.	The light intensity must be correct in order to properly view the specimen. Light that is too bright may shine through certain objects, making them invisible. Light that is too dim may make some items impossible to see.
8. Using the fine adjustment knob (Figure 23-21), bring the specimen into sharp, clear focus.	As the specimen slide is moved on the stage, the image seen will become blurry and must be refocused.
9. After observation of the specimen is complete, notify provider that the specimen is ready to be viewed under the scope.	

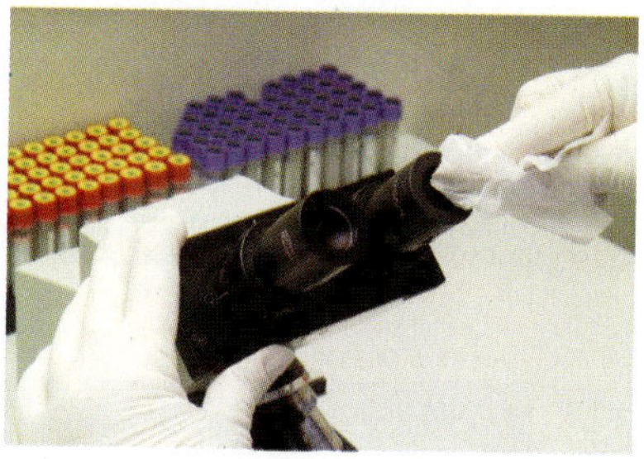

Figure 23-19 ■ Lens paper is used to clean the oculars of the microscope.

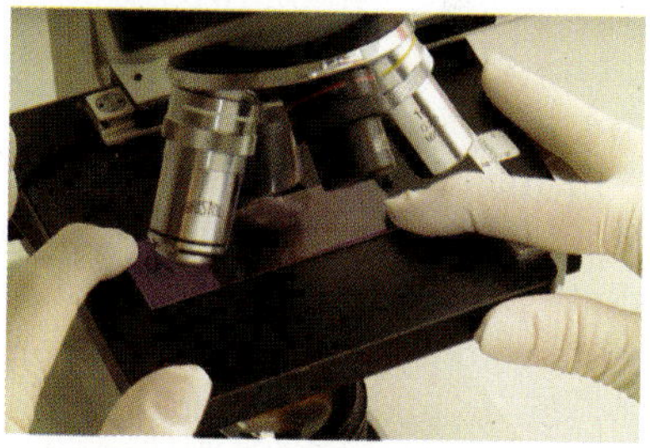

Figure 23-20 ■ The specimen slide is placed on the stage of the microscope.

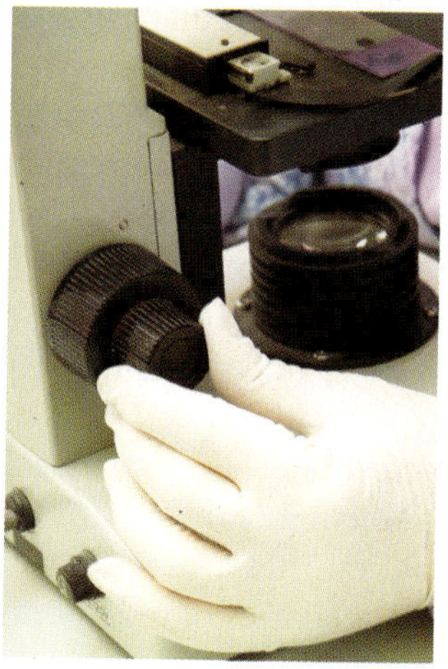

Figure 23-21 ■ The microscope must be focused to make the image crisp and clear.

continues

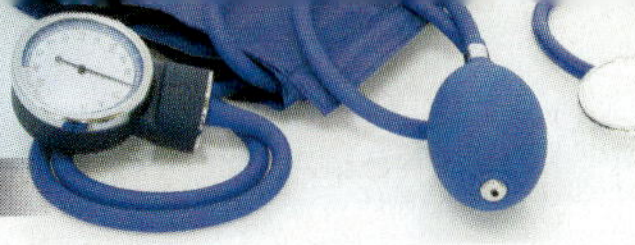

PROCEDURE 23-4 continued

PROCEDURAL STEPS	DETAILS AND/OR RATIONALE
10. When provider is done, remove slide from the stage and clean the objective with lens paper and wipe the stage clean with tissue or gauze.	Objectives should be cleaned immediately to prevent oil from collecting and drying on the lens.
11. Turn off the light source and cover the scope with a protective dust cover.	Turning off the light source between uses helps to prolong the life of the bulb. Keeping a cover on the scope between uses prevents a buildup of dust and debris.

CHAPTER SUMMARY

- The medical laboratory performs a vast array of tests that assist providers in diagnosing and treating disorders.
- The majority of doctor's office labs are referenced as physician's office laboratories (POLs).
- Rationale for ordering lab testing includes determining baseline values, for legal purposes, to screen for pathological conditions, to confirm a clinical diagnosis, or to obtain a differential diagnosis.
- Federal regulations that regulate medical laboratories include the Clinical Laboratory Improvement Act of 1967 and its 1988 amendments.
- Final CLIA regulations were published on February 28, 1992, based on the complexity of the test method—the more complex the test, the more rigid the requirements. CLIA regulations established three test categories: waived testing, moderate-complexity (which includes PPM), and high-complexity.
- The Commission on Office Laboratory Accreditation (COLA) was established in 1988 as a private alternative to assist clinical laboratories in complying with the CLIA '88 standards.
- Laboratories are classified according to their size, the categories of tests performed, and with whom they are affiliated and include reference labs, hospital labs, physician's office labs, point-of-care testing lab, and procurement stations.
- Laboratory departments consist of the following departments: Urinalysis, hematology, clinical chemistry, microbiology, immunology, cytology, histology, parasitology, and immunohematology, or blood bank.
- Quality assurance is a set of policies and procedures designed to ensure the accuracy and reliability of laboratory testing and should include: quality control testing, testing and control logs, orientation of personnel, maintenance checks on all equipment and instruments, required calibration of instruments, refrigerator and freezer temperature checks, proficiency testing, and reference ranges.
- Safety is of critical importance in preventing accidents in the lab. The Occupational Exposure to Hazardous Chemicals in the Laboratory Standard was designed to make employees aware of the risks involved in exposure to chemicals in the laboratory.
- Hazards in the laboratory are divided into physical, chemical, and biological categories. Each category requires its own specific set of guidelines for safe handling.
- The medical assistant usually processes lab requests in the POL. A lab requisition form is an order for the lab on tests that need to be performed. Only licensed health care personnel and credentialed medical assistants can enter orders into the computerized provider order entry (CPOE) system.
- Noncredentialed medical assistants may apply to take the Assessment Based Recognition in Order Entry (ABR-OE) program through the American Association of Medical Assistants (AAMA).
- Proper specimen collection is crucial in order to obtain accurate laboratory results. Patients must clearly understand the collection process, especially if they will be collecting the specimen themselves.

- The medical assistant should check the lab catalog for instructions on patient preparation, specimen collection, handling, and proper transport. Always check the patient's insurance to see which lab contracts with the insurance company.
- Laboratory report forms provide the results for lab testing and normal ranges.
- Medical assistants should be familiar with the policies of the office regarding sharing results with patients.
- Flow sheets can be reviewed and updated each time the patient visits their provider. Flow sheets track a patient's progress in regards to lab values.
- The microscope views objects that cannot be seen with the naked eye.
- The centrifuge is an instrument that spins tubes at high speeds to separate the liquid portion of the sample from the cells and other formed elements.

CERTIFICATION REVIEW QUESTIONS

1. Lab tests are performed to:
   a. obtain a baseline value.
   b. obtain a differential diagnosis.
   c. confirm a clinical diagnosis.
   d. All of the above

2. Tests that the medical assistant can perform in the POL are known as:
   a. waived tests.
   b. CLIA '88.
   c. proficiency testing.
   d. nonwaived tests.

3. The medical assistant's responsibilities in laboratory testing include all of the following except:
   a. having a working knowledge of normal reference ranges.
   b. proper patient preparation.
   c. specimen collection.
   d. performing waived and moderately-complex lab testing.

4. The form that accompanies all specimens to the lab is the:
   a. report form.
   b. lab specifications form.
   c. lab requisition form.
   d. data form sheet.

5. When performing a glucose control, you notice that the results are not within the ranges specified by the manufacturer. What should you do?
   a. Relay the information to your supervisor
   b. Record results and go on about your daily activities
   c. Throw the kit out
   d. Make certain that reagents, test strips and glucometer all match and rerun the control

6. The analysis of abnormal cells is performed in which department of the laboratory?
   a. Hematology
   b. Serology
   c. Microbiology
   d. Cytology

7. All microscope lenses should be cleaned with:
   a. acetone.
   b. tissue.
   c. gauze.
   d. lens paper.

8. The Pap smear test is performed in this department:
   a. Hematology
   b. Chemistry
   c. Microbiology
   d. Cytology

9. Which of the following tests is performed by the medical assistant?
   a. Nasal smear for eosinophils
   b. Urine sediment examination
   c. Urine reagent strip test
   d. Fecal leukocyte examination

10. The waived test used to detect inflammation is the:
    a. hematocrit test.
    b. hemoglobin test.
    c. occult blood test.
    d. erythrocyte sedimentation rate.

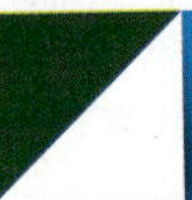

STUDY RESOURCES

Resources to Test and Reinforce Your Knowledge:	
Certification Review Questions	Take this end-of-chapter quiz
Workbook	• Complete the activities for Chapter 23 • Perform the procedures for Chapter 23 using the Competency Checklists
Resources to Promote Critical Thinking:	
***Solve the Case* Activities**	• Consider these case studies and discuss your conclusions
Learning Lab	• Module 22: Laboratory Procedures
MindTap	• Complete Chapter 23 readings and activities

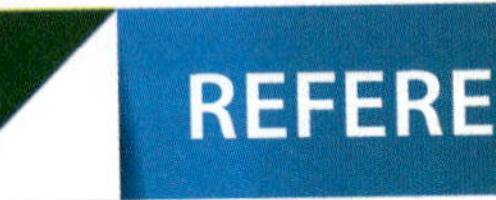

REFERENCES

Clinical Laboratory Improvement Amendments (CLIA). (n.d.). Retrieved March 10, 2015, from https://www.cms.gov/Regulations-and-Guidance/Legislation/CLIA/index.html?redirect=%2Fclia

Hazard Communication Safety Data Sheets. (n.d.). Retrieved March 10, 2015, from https://www.osha.gov/Publications/HazComm_QuickCard_SafetyData.html

Testing Tips. (n.d.). Retrieved March 8, 2015, from http://www.aafp.org/practice-management/regulatory/clia/tips.html

Waived Tests. (n.d.). Retrieved March 10, 2015, from http://wwwn.cdc.gov/clia/resources/waivedtests

Washington State Dept. of Health. (n.d.). Retrieved March 10, 2015, from http://www.doh.wa.gov/

24

Blood Collection Techniques

CHAPTER OUTLINE

Why Do We Collect Blood?

Venipuncture
- Equipment and Supplies

Vacuum Tube System
- Multisample Needles
- Holders and Adapters
- Vacuum Tubes

Winged Infusion (Butterfly) System

Blood Collection Tray

Performing the Venipuncture
- Assembling Equipment and Supplies
- Identifying the Patient
- Positioning the Patient
- Selecting the Site

Specimen Collection by the Syringe Method

Specimen Collection by the Vacuum Tube Method

Specimen Collection by the Butterfly Method

Patient Response and Complications

The Failed Venipuncture

Criteria for Specimen Rejection
- Improper Labeling of Specimen Tubes
- Use of Incorrect Specimen Tubes
- Incorrect Collection Time
- Incorrect Specimen Handling
- Hemolyzed and Lipemic Specimens

The Capillary Puncture
- Equipment
- Common Sites for Collection
- Preparing the Site
- Collecting the Specimen
- Order of Draw

General Guidelines for Specimen Handling

Drawing Blood Cultures

ESSENTIAL TERMS

additive
aliquot
antecubital space
anticoagulant
butterfly
capillary puncture
constrict
evacuated tube
gauge
hematoma
hemoconcentration
hemolysis
integrity
lancet
lipemia
palpate
phlebotomist
phlebotomy
plasma
primary container
quantity not sufficient (QNS)
serum
thixotropic separator gel
tourniquet
vacuum tube
venipuncture
winged infusion

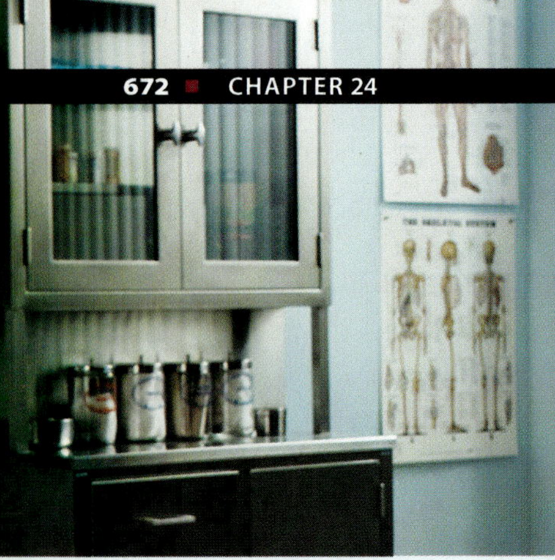

DEVELOPMENTAL OBJECTIVES

After completing this chapter, you should be able to:

1. Correctly spell and define essential terms.
2. Assess the different types of equipment used to perform venipuncture when using a syringe, evacuated tube holder and butterfly.
3. Name the additives or anticoagulants contained in each of the tube top colors and state their functions.
4. List the equipment found in a well-stocked blood collection tray.
5. List the general steps for performing a venipuncture.
6. Explain the importance of proper patient education when performing the venipuncture.
7. Decide which tubes to draw first when multiple tubes are necessary based on the order of draw for both capillary and venous specimens.
8. Analyze reasons for blood specimen rejection and recommend steps that can be taken to avoid rejection.
9. List the general guidelines for specimen handling.
10. Perform a capillary puncture, and collect a venous blood specimen using a syringe blood vacuum tube blood and butterfly.

INTRODUCTION

Phlebotomy is the name given to the procedure of collecting blood samples. Each health care facility will have specific professionals (**phlebotomists**) designated to perform phlebotomy. In many health care settings, the medical assistant will be the health care worker that collects blood samples.

Proper collection techniques must be followed to ensure that the laboratory receives the highest-quality specimen for testing. An improperly collected blood specimen can lead to inaccurate results that can, in turn, lead to a misdiagnosis.

Correct procedures for performing venipuncture and capillary puncture will be discussed in this chapter. Each method requires training and rigorous practice. Proper specimen collection is critical for obtaining accurate test results.

WHY DO WE COLLECT BLOOD?

As blood is circulated throughout the body, it transports oxygen, carbon dioxide, nutrients, waste products, and hormones. Because of its role in transporting these

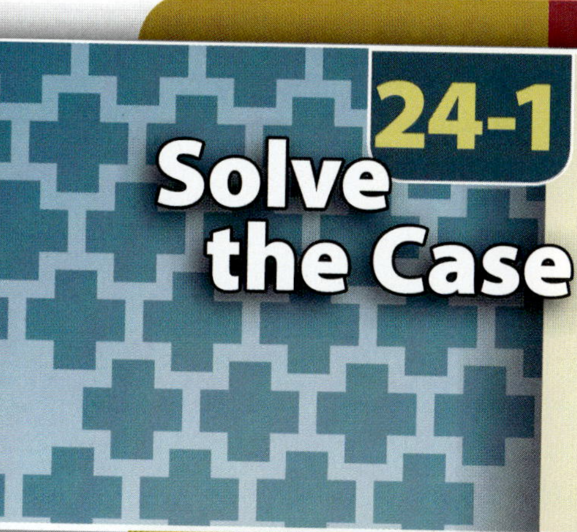

Abby Hunter is a 16-year-old patient with an appointment for a physical that requires a blood draw. Abby shares with you that she is very nervous about having her blood drawn. Her mother is with her and finds the whole thing quite humorous and teases her about her fear. The doctor still needs to examine the patient prior to the blood draw.

1. **What factors are making this process difficult for Abby?**
2. **Is there anything you can do to help reduce the fear Abby is experiencing?**
3. **Should you mention your observations to the physician?**

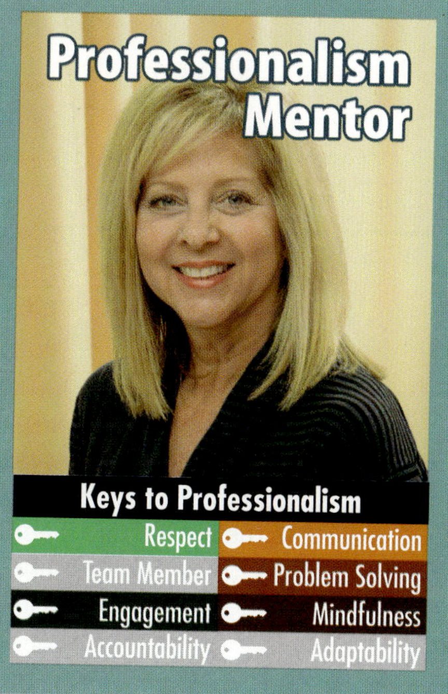

Having blood drawn is probably one of the least favorite procedures a patient has done during a medical office visit. Some patients are not afraid of having their blood drawn while others may have considerable anxiety over the thought of being stuck by a needle. Patients expect the medical assistant drawing their blood to be proficient in this task. Demonstrating professionalism and self-confidence is key to putting your patient at ease. Having a positive attitude and showing compassion will help patients who are nervous get through the procedure. As with any procedure, especially an invasive one such as a blood draw, it's important to gain the patient's trust. They may not like having blood drawn but they will know you are doing your job to maintain their health and well-being. Looking ahead to when you will do this skill on a patient, think about what you might say to a patient who is fearful of needles. What would you say to your patient to help put them at ease? Jot your ideas down in your journal. These will be very useful to you in your practice as a medical assistant. ■

components, a multitude of information can be obtained by analyzing the blood to determine the number and type of cells present and the amounts of different types of elements such as electrolytes, cholesterol, and glucose.

Every system in the body can be evaluated by performing an analysis of the blood and quantifying specific chemical components. The provider uses information obtained from this analysis to establish baseline values for patients and to diagnose disease states.

Information provided by the laboratory is only as good as the specimen received for testing. It is critical that the specimen be obtained by following the proper procedure.

VENIPUNCTURE

Venipuncture is an invasive procedure in which a vein is punctured to obtain a blood sample. It can be performed using any of the following types of equipment: **vacuum tube** or **evacuated tube** and holder, syringe, or **butterfly** and related equipment.

Venipuncture requires special equipment, training, and supervision. Practice makes the medical assistant proficient at venipuncture and helps to make the procedure less painful for the patient.

Equipment and Supplies

Specialized equipment is necessary to perform each method of venipuncture. Using the right equipment is essential to obtain the best possible specimen.

Tourniquets

A **tourniquet** is applied to the patient's arm 3 to 4 inches above the puncture site to **constrict** blood flow and enlarge the veins. This makes the veins easier to **palpate**, or feel. The tourniquet must be tight enough to decrease venous blood flow to the area, but not so tight that it affects arterial blood flow to the area.

Several different types of tourniquets are available for use and can be purchased in both pediatric and adult sizes. One-use tourniquets are safer than multiple use tourniquets due to exposure from other patients' skin or blood. Once a tourniquet is used, it is considered contaminated and must be disinfected between patients. If tourniquets become soiled with blood or any other contaminants, they should definitely be disposed of. The most common type used is a flat vinyl or latex strap approximately 15 to 18 inches in length (Figure 24-1). Vinyl tourniquets are preferred over latex because of patients with latex sensitivity. Many of the new latex-free tourniquets are designed for one time use, come in rolls of different colors, and are pre-notched for easy removal. Figure 24-2 shows the proper way to tie a flat tourniquet to the patient's arm.

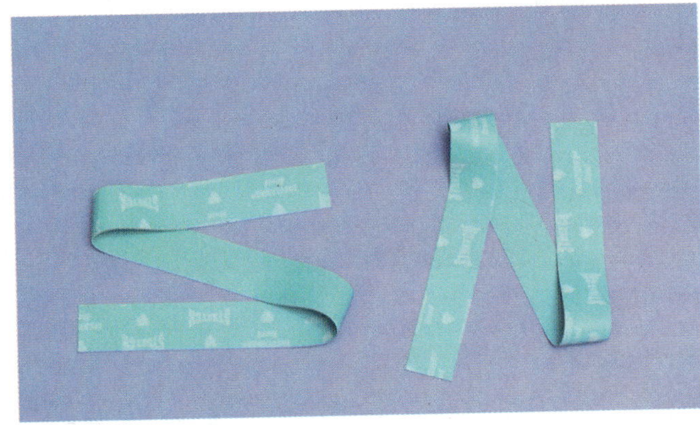

Figure 24-1 ■ A Vinyl Tourniquet.

Health Coach

Venipuncture

It is important to fully explain the venipuncture procedure to the patient, especially if it is the patient's first time having blood drawn. Whenever possible, instruct the patient before the day of the appointment to drink lots of water prior to the appointment. This will assist in making the patient's veins more prominent. Answer all patient questions honestly. Try to put the patient at ease. Many patients are concerned about the amount of blood being drawn. Explain to the patient that there are several pints of blood in the body and that the blood you are taking will automatically be replaced in just a few hours.

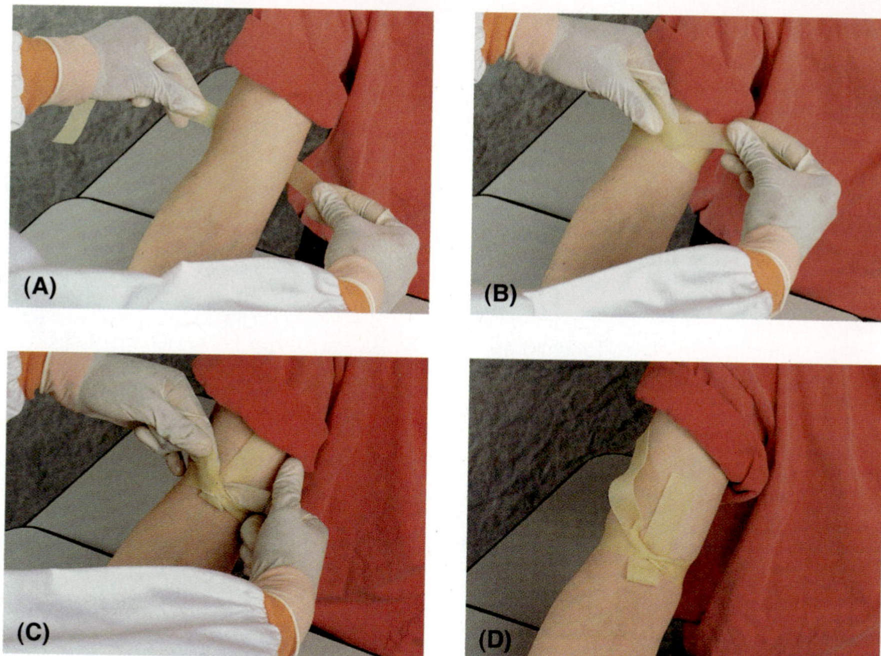

Figure 24-2 ■ Applying a tourniquet: (a) Keep the tourniquet flat and wrap it around the arm 3 to 4 inches above the puncture site. (b) While stretching the tourniquet tight, cross one end over the other. (c) While keeping tension on the ends and keeping the tourniquet tight, tuck one end under the other. (d) Check to be sure the tourniquet is tight enough so it won't loosen. The ends should point up and not hang down over the puncture site.

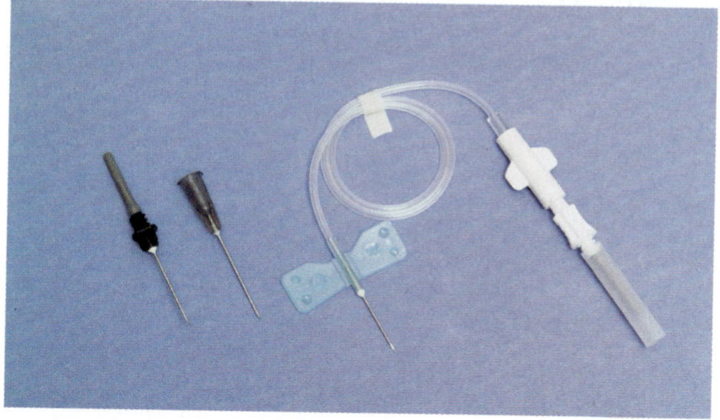

Figure 24-3 ■ Different types of needles used to perform venipuncture (Pictured left to right): multisample needle, hypodermic needle for use with a syringe, butterfly needle for use with a syringe or vacuum tube system. (Safety devices have been intentionally left off so that you can see the entire needles.)

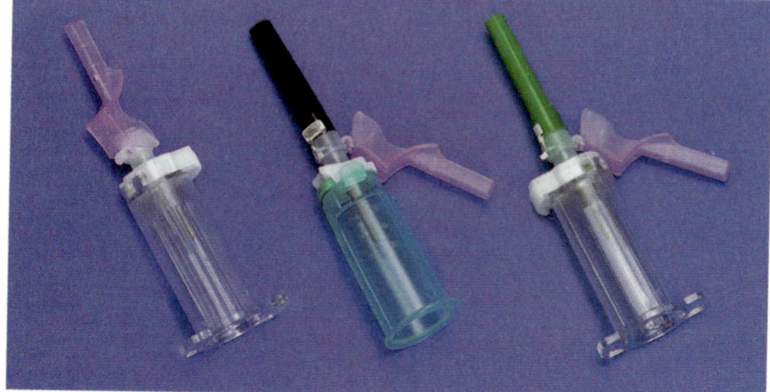

Figure 24-4 ■ Examples of phlebotomy safety needles.

Needles

The different types of needles used to perform venipuncture include multisample needles for use with the evacuated tube system, hypodermic needles for use with a syringe, and winged infusion (butterfly) needles used for both systems (Figure 24-3). Occupational Safety and Health Administration (OSHA) regulations require needles to have safety features to decrease the chances of accidental needle sticks. Refer to Figure 24-4 for examples of safety needles that can be used when using performing phlebotomy using the evacuated tube method.

Needles are individually wrapped in sterile packaging, disposable, and designed for a single use only. Hypodermic needles (needles that attach to a syringe) and butterfly needles (smaller needles used typically for hand sticks) are packaged in sterile pull-apart packages. Multisample needles (needles that allow several tubes to be drawn during one blood draw) are sealed in a tube with a twist-off cap that covers both ends of the needle. Refer to the vacuum tube system later in the chapter to learn more about multisample needles.

Needles are available in a variety of sizes and are classified by their **gauge** (G) and length. The gauge is a number that indicates the diameter of the lumen: the larger the number, the smaller the diameter. The gauge of the needle will be determined by the amount of blood to be withdrawn, the size and condition of the patient's vein,

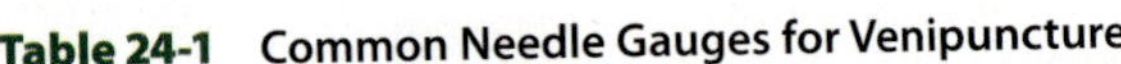

Table 24-1 Common Needle Gauges for Venipuncture

Gauge	Type	Application
20	Multisample or hypodermic	For collection using large-volume vacuum tubes or large-volume syringes. Used for patients with normal-sized veins.
21	Multisample or hypodermic	Standard gauge used for routine venipuncture for patients with normal-sized veins.
22	Multisample or hypodermic	Gauge used for syringe draws on difficult veins. Used for children and adults with small veins.
23	Butterfly	Gauge used for infants and children. Used for difficult hand veins of adults. This gauge may cause hemolysis, use small tubes with little vacuum.

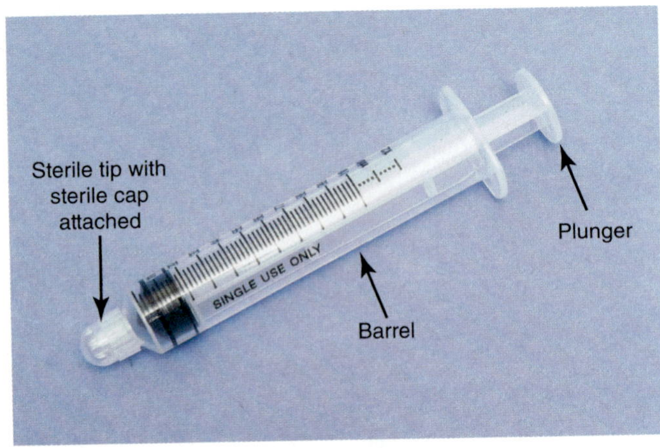

Figure 24-5 ■ Parts of a syringe (this is a 10 mL syringe).

and the procedure used to perform the phlebotomy. The usual range of gauges for phlebotomy is 21G to 23G; however, when working in a blood donation center, a 16G needle may be used because of the amount of blood being taken from the patient. See Table 24-1 for a listing of needle gauges used for venipuncture.

The length of the needle used for venipuncture usually depends on the depth of the vein selected and user preference. Multisample needles are available in lengths of 1 to 1½ inches. Syringe needles come in a wide variety of lengths; however, needles 1 to 1½ inches long are commonly used for venipuncture. A 1-inch needle can be much less intimidating to the patient. Butterfly needles are usually ½ to ¾ inch long.

Most manufacturers color-code needles for easier identification, but beware: Color codes are not universal and may vary by manufacturer.

Syringes

The syringe method is used to obtain blood from patients with fragile or small veins that tend to collapse when using the vacuum tube method. Pediatric or geriatric patients are likely to have these types of veins.

Syringes used to perform venipuncture are disposable, made of plastic, and vary in size. The syringe has three main parts: the barrel, with graduated markings in mL, the sterile tip where the needle attaches, and the plunger, which fits tightly inside the barrel (Figure 24-5).

The range of syringe volumes most commonly used for blood collection is 2 to 10 mL. The size of the syringe selected for use is determined by the amount of blood required for collection and the size and condition of the patient's veins. One disadvantage of the syringe method is that the capacity of the syringe limits the amount of blood that can be collected with one venipuncture.

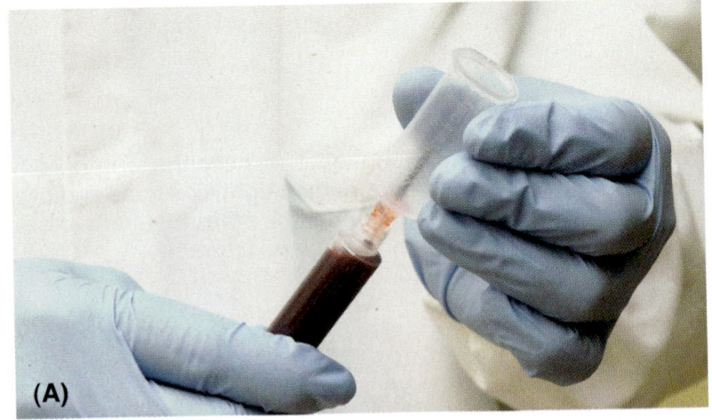

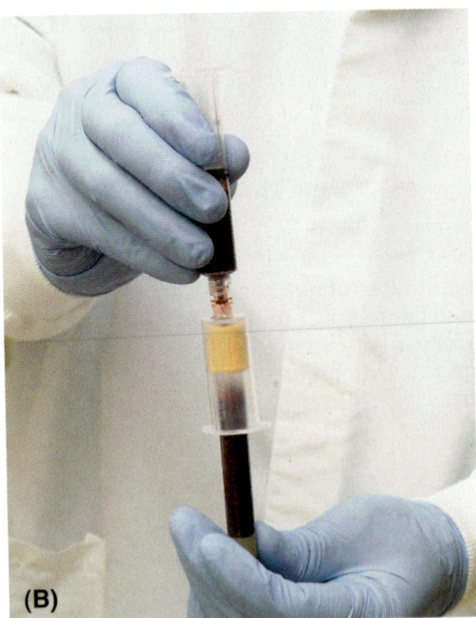

Figure 24-6 ■ (a) The medical assistant attaches the safety device to the syringe once the needle is removed. (b) The medical assitant pushes the tube into the safety device.

Another disadvantage of the syringe method is that the blood must be transferred from the syringe to evacuated tubes, which requires extra time. Safety transfer devices, such as the one in Figure 24-6, are now available for safer transfer.

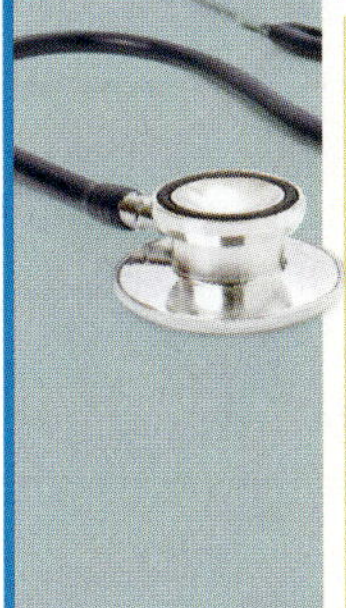

Field Smarts

When using a transfer device, immediately remove the external needle from the syringe used to draw the blood. To transfer blood from the syringe to the tubes, push each tube up into the sheathed needle of the transfer device. Invert each tube as you remove it from the transfer device prior to filling a new tube. Once the tubes are done filling, carefully place the transfer device and syringe into the sharps container as one unit.

VACUUM TUBE SYSTEM

The most common method of collecting a blood sample is by using the evacuated or vacuum tube method. This method facilitates the collection of numerous tubes of blood with one stick. The vacuum tube system also has the advantage of being a closed system. The blood flows from the patient through the needle and into a closed collection tube. This closed system greatly diminishes the risk of exposure to blood for the health care worker.

Three main components comprise the vacuum tube system. A specially designed needle attaches to a disposable plastic holder or adapter that holds the vacuum tubes and various types of evacuated tubes. Figure 24-7 shows an example of the components used in the vacuum tube method of venipuncture.

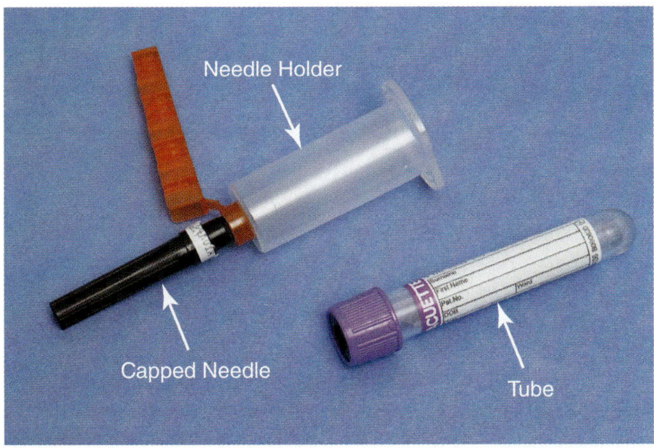

Figure 24-7 ■ The components of a vacuum tube collection system.

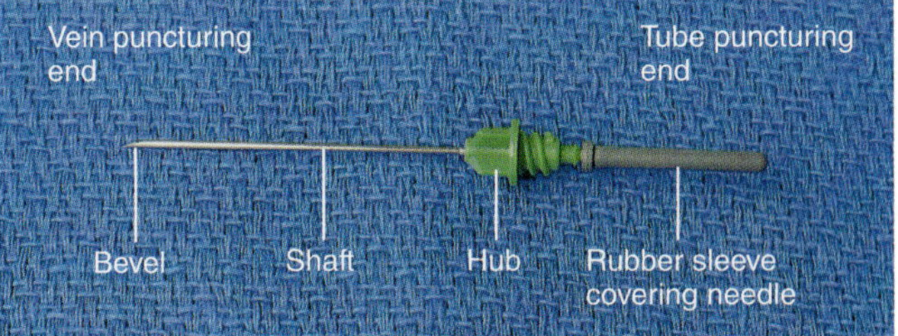

Figure 24-8 ■ The parts of a multisample needle.

Multisample Needles

Special needles are used with the vacuum tube system to allow multiple tubes of blood to be collected with a single venipuncture. The multisample needle consists of a double needle with a bevel on each end and a threaded hub near the center (Figure 24-8). The threaded hub of the needle screws into the plastic needle or tube holder. When properly assembled, the longest portion of the needle is exposed and used to puncture the patient's vein, while the shortest portion fits inside the tube holder and punctures the rubber stopper on the vacuum tube.

Multidraw needles are designed with a beveled point and have a silicon-coated shaft to facilitate easy penetration of the skin. Parts of the needle include the bevel (slanted tip), shaft, lumen (internal core), hub (attaches to collection system), and the rubber sleeve covering at the distal end of the needle where the tube is inserted.

The portion of the needle that punctures the rubber stopper of the tube is covered with a rubber sleeve. When the tube is pushed onto the needle, the sleeve retracts and exposes the point of the needle, allowing the blood to flow into the tube. When the tube is removed, the sleeve moves back over the needle, stopping the flow of blood. The sleeve prevents leakage of blood both when changing tubes and when the tube is removed prior to withdrawing the needle from the vein.

Multisample needles are manufactured with safety features to be used with a traditional tube holder.

Holders and Adapters

A plastic holder or adapter is a cylinder with a small opening at one end where the needle screws into place and a large opening at the opposite end that holds the vacuum tube. Holders are available in an adult size (for regular tubes) and a pediatric size (for small tubes). The large end of the holder is equipped with extensions known as flanges, which aid insertion and removal of the blood collection tubes.

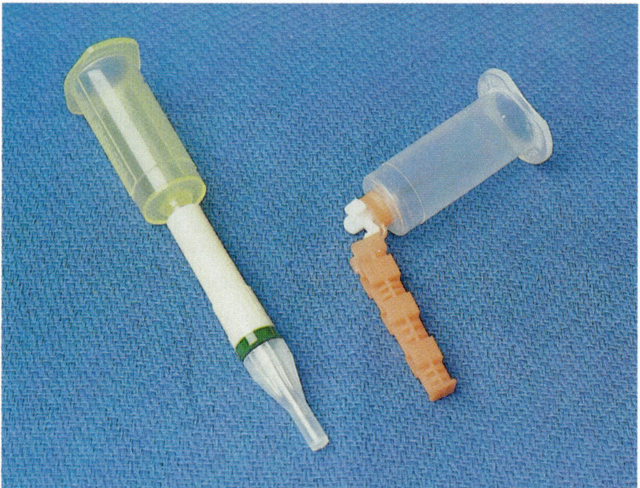

Figure 24-9 ■ Examples of tube holders with safety devices that cover the needle after use.

Safety holders, such as the ones in Figure 24-9, are either equipped with sleeves that slide over the needle after use, or with covers that snap closed over the contaminated needle. These safety features protect the medical assistant from accidental needlesticks until the equipment can be properly discarded.

Vacuum Tubes

Blood collection tubes used with the vacuum tube method are designed to automatically withdraw a precise, premeasured volume of blood. During the manufacturing process, a vacuum is created inside the tube and is released when the stopper is punctured. The release of the vacuum causes the blood to flow into the tube. When the appropriate volume has been collected, the flow stops and the tube is removed. Collection tubes are available in different sizes and volumes (2 to 15 mL). The size of the tube selected depends on several factors, including the volume of blood required for the test, the size of the needle, the condition of the patient's veins, and the age of the patient.

Vacuum tubes are available in both glass and plastic. Glass tubes are sometimes coated with silicon on the inside to create a smooth surface, which prevents red blood cell destruction.

Vacuum tubes may contain special **additives** that perform different functions. These are discussed in more depth later in the chapter. Vacuum tubes that contain additives must be filled to capacity. An underfilled tube can create an incorrect ratio of blood to additive, resulting in inaccurate test results due to dilution of the specimen.

Vacuum tubes come with special tube stoppers made of either rubber or plastic. During the blood draw procedure, the needle pierces the stopper, delivering the blood into the tube from the vein. The stopper may be removed once full, in order to retrieve the specimen for testing. Benton Dickinson manufactures both conventional rubber stoppers and plastic closures referred to as Hemogard™ Closures. These special safety closures are designed to protect personnel by preventing the specimen from splattering when the closure is removed. Both types of stoppers are color-coded, indicating which type of anticoagulant or additive is contained in each tube. Tube stopper colors may vary by manufacturer and depend on whether the stopper is made of rubber or plastic. Table 24-2 lists the different tube top colors, the additive contained in each, and the types of testing requiring each of the additives. Additionally, the table illustrates the order in which tubes should be drawn, which is explained later in the chapter.

An **anticoagulant** added to a collection tube prevents the blood from clotting. Many types of anticoagulants are available. The most common types used include EDTA, heparin, oxalates, and citrates. The choice depends on which type of laboratory testing is being performed.

Additives inside the vacuum tube can be used to preserve certain blood components until testing can be performed. Some additives are used to accelerate specimen processing for faster testing. Some tubes, used to collect **serum** (the liquid portion of clotted blood) samples, are available with a clot activator that helps the clotting process to begin more quickly. Thrombin is a type of clot activator added to speed the clotting process for *STAT* test results. Another additive found in serum tubes is a gel-like substance, **thixotropic separator gel**, which forms a barrier between the cells and serum upon centrifugation (Figure 24-10a and b).

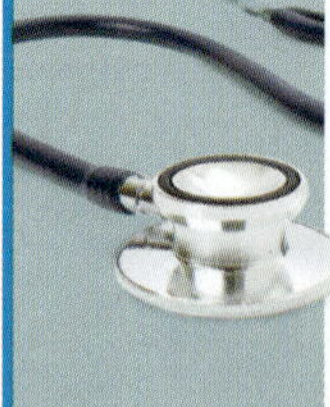

Field Smarts

Manufacturers guarantee the tube vacuum and the stability of the additive until the expiration date shown on the tube. *Never* use a tube that has an expired date for patient samples. Laboratories will not accept specimens drawn in expired tubes. When the expiration date is listed as month and year, it is good until the last day of the month.

Table 24-2 Common Vacuum Tube Color Guide

Order of draw	Hemogard Closure	Rubber Stopper	Additive	Additive Function	Laboratory Use	Number of Inversions
#1 Blood Cultures or SPS tubes		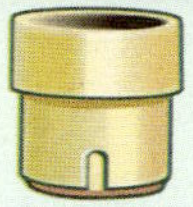	Sodium polyanetholesulfonate (SPS)	Binds calcium to prevent clotting and inhibits bacterial growth	Blood or body fluid cultures	8-10 inversions
# 2 Citrate Tubes	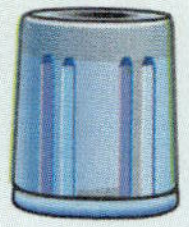	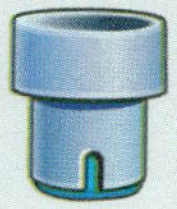	Sodium citrate	Binds calcium to prevent clotting	Coagulation studies: Prothrombin time (PT), Activated partial thromboplastin time (aPTT), and International normalized ratio (INR)	3-4 inversions
# 3 Serum Separator Tubes (SST)	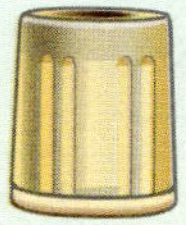	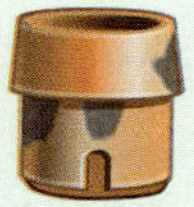	Clot activator and gel for serum separation (SST)	Serum separation; allows technician to pour off serum	Serum testing: hormone studies, organ panels, cholesterol testing, medication levels, and so on.	5 inversions
# 4 Serum Tubes	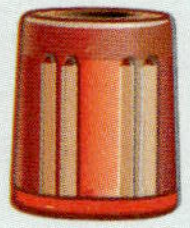	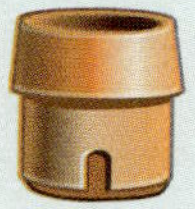	No additive	Promotes blood clot formation	Serum testing: hormone studies, organ panels, cholesterol testing, medication levels, and so on.	None
# 5 Plasma Separator Tube (PST)	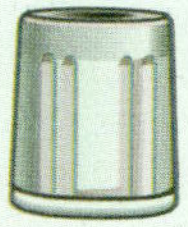	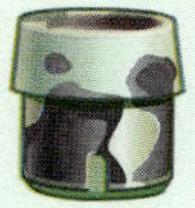	Lithium heparin and gel for plasma separation (PST)	Heparin prevents the release of potassium by platelets during clotting and the gel separates the plasma from the red cells.	*STAT* chemistry plasma studies: electrolytes, arterial blood gases, and many of the same tests you can do on serum.	8-10 inversions
# 6 Heparin Tube	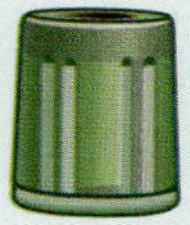	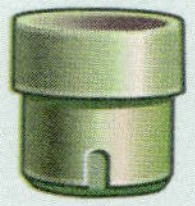	Lithium or sodium heparin	Inhibits formation of thrombin and prevents clotting	Chemistry plasma studies electrolytes, arterial blood gases, and so on. Same testing as PST tube.	8-10 inversions
# 7 EDTA Tubes	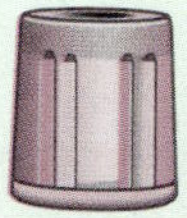	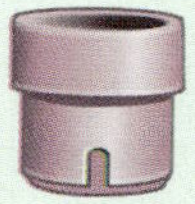	EDTA (ethylenediaminetetraacetic acid)	Binds calcium to prevent clotting	Hematology testing: complete blood count (CBC), differential, and erythrocyte sedimentation rate (ESR)	8-10 inversions
# 8 Fluoride tubes	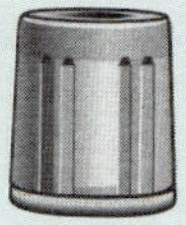	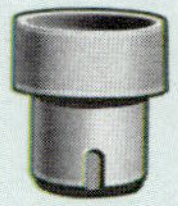	Potassium oxalate and sodium fluoride	Binds calcium and stabilizes glucose	Glucose testing and alcohol levels	8-10 inversions

**Note*: Each tube containing an additive of any kind must be inverted a specified number of times immediately following blood collection. Refer to the manufacturer's directions for the correct number of inversions.

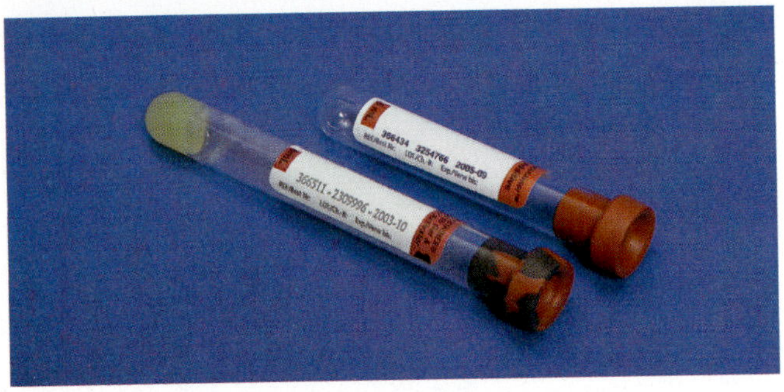

Figure 24-10a ■ An SST tube containing thixotropic gel and a plain red top tube without any blood.

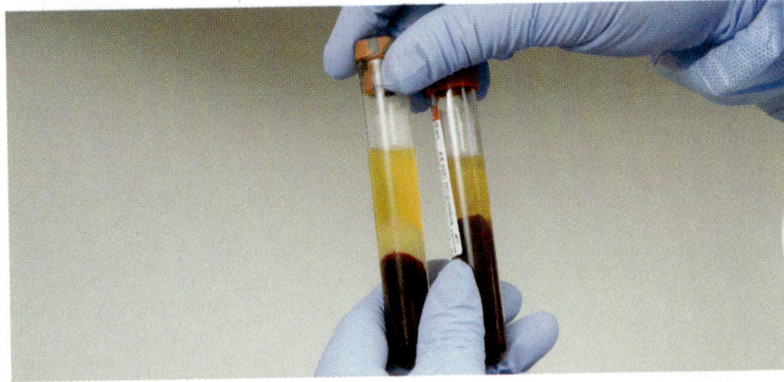

Figure 24-10b ■ An SST and plain tube once they have been filled with blood and centrifuged.

When centrifuged, the gel becomes liquid and moves up the sides of the tube to form a solid plug between the cells and serum (Figure 24-11). Once the plug is in place, the serum can easily be poured off into another tube. This type of tube is referred to as a serum separator tube (SST).

Some vacuum tubes do not contain an additive; blood collected in a nonadditive tube takes approximately 20 to 30 minutes to clot. Once the blood has clotted, the specimen must be centrifuged to separate the serum from the clotted blood. The serum is then removed by pipette and transferred to another tube to be sent to the lab for testing. Figure 24-12 shows a specimen in a nonadditive tube after centrifugation. The serum must be carefully removed before transport to prevent remixing of cells and serum.

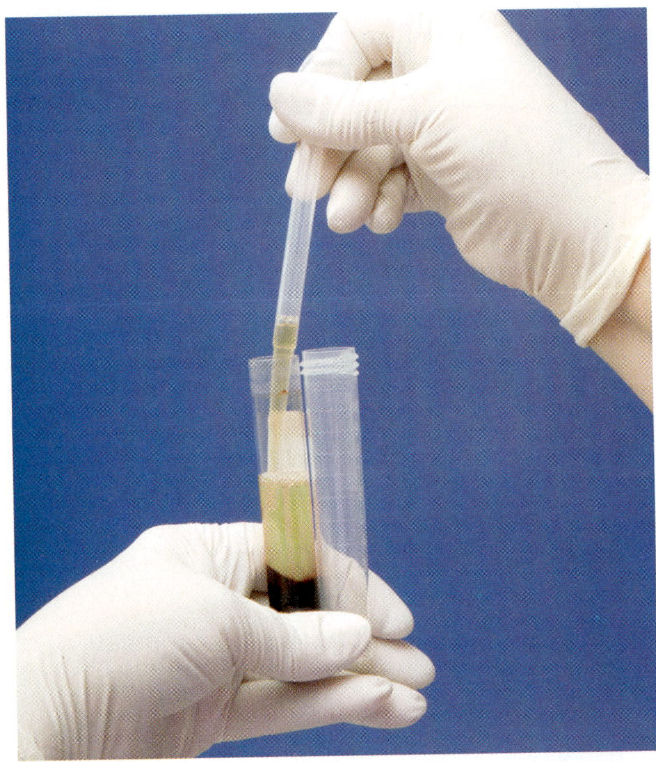

Figure 24-12 ■ The medical assistant removes the serum from a plain red-topped tube using a pipette.

WINGED INFUSION (BUTTERFLY) SYSTEM

The **winged infusion** or butterfly set is used to collect blood from small or difficult veins, usually in the hand. These sets are commonly used on pediatric and

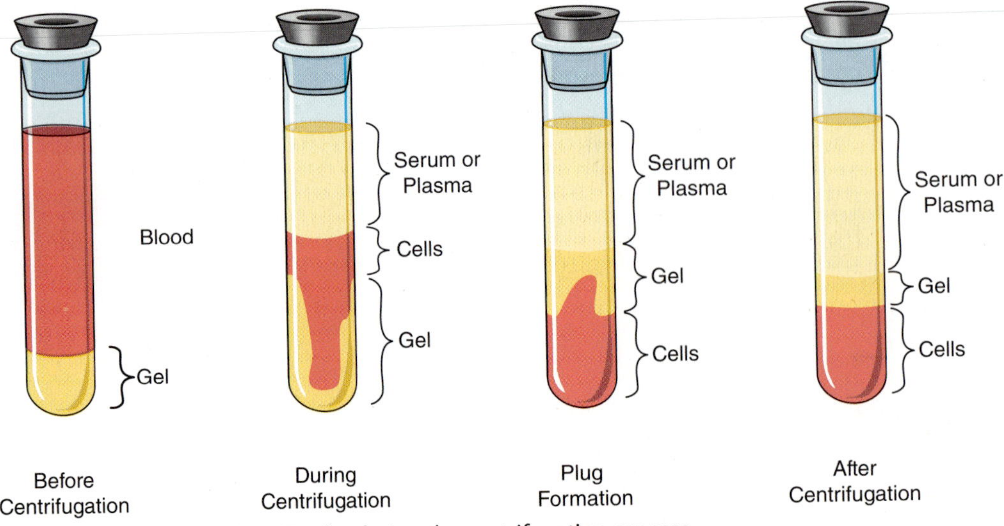

Figure 24-11 ■ Changes that occur in the SST tube during the centrifugation process.

geriatric patients. The set includes a 23 gauge, ½- to ¾-inch needle connected to a 5- to 12-inch length of plastic tubing. At the end of the tubing is either a hub that attaches to a syringe or a needle that is covered by a rubber sleeve that attaches to a vacuum tube holder (Figure 24-13).

The needle has plastic projections attached to it that resemble butterfly wings. By grasping the wings together between the thumb and index finger, the medical assistant can enter the smaller vein at a lower angle.

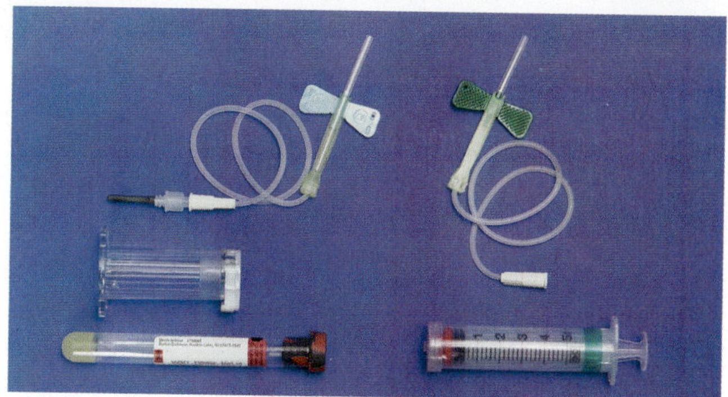

Figure 24-13 ■ Two butterfly needles: one that attaches to a vacuum tube adapter and one that attaches to a syringe.

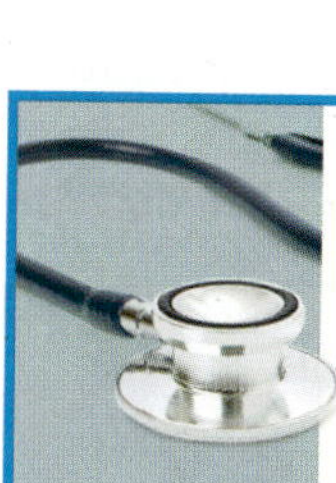

Field Smarts

Tube selection is not just about obtaining the correct color; it is also about matching up the right tube with the right needle. Choosing the correct tube size is very important to preserve the integrity of the specimen. When using a larger tube, a larger gauge needle should be used. This is because a larger tube has a greater vacuum; if combined with a smaller needle, cells are forced through the lumen of the needle at a much greater force than what the lumen can handle. This practice causes the cells to be destroyed as they pass through the lumen, resulting in hemolysis (destruction/rupture of blood cells).

BLOOD COLLECTION TRAY

Venipuncture equipment may be located in a special blood-drawing area or stored in a blood collection tray, which can be moved from room to room. Trays can vary in design, but because they are used to transport blood specimens, OSHA requires the tray to be red in color or to have the biohazard symbol prominently displayed on the outside of the tray (Figure 24-14). The type of equipment stocked in each tray will depend on the type of specimen that is to be collected. General items contained in most trays include the following:

- Antiseptic wipes
- Gauze
- Bandages/tape
- Multisample and single-use needles, hypodermic needles for use with a syringe, and winged infusion needles
- Syringes and vacuum tube adapters of various sizes
- Transfer devices

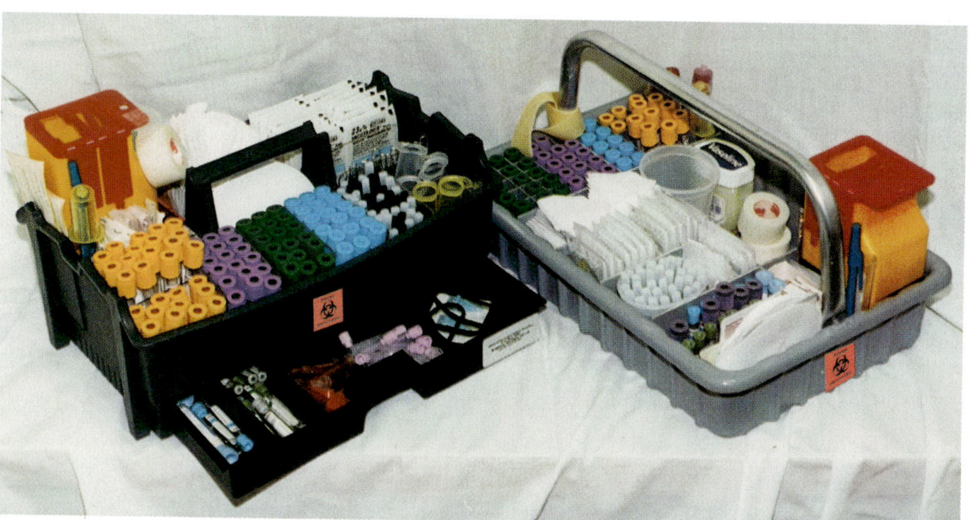

Figure 24-14 ■ Examples of fully stocked blood collection trays.

- Evacuated tubes of different sizes and types
- Tourniquets
- Sharps container

Always replace used equipment and dispose of contaminated wastes from the blood collection tray after each use.

PERFORMING THE VENIPUNCTURE

Venipuncture is the process of puncturing a vein with a needle to obtain a blood specimen and is the most common method used to collect blood. It is a specialized procedure that requires numerous steps that must be precisely performed. Table 24-3 lists the general steps to be followed when performing a venipuncture by any of the three methods previously mentioned. Specific procedural steps for each method can be found in Procedures 24-1, 24-2, and 24-3.

Assembling Equipment and Supplies

It is important to assemble all necessary equipment before beginning the venipuncture. All supplies should be within easy reach to avoid crossing over the patient's arm during the procedure. Several spare tubes should be available in case a tube has a defective vacuum and will not fill completely. Table 24-4 lists the necessary equipment for performing the venipuncture.

Identifying the Patient

Proper identification of the patient is vital to confirm that the testing is performed on the correct patient. Occasionally, when the medical assistant calls a patient's name, an anxious or distracted patient may answer in error. Some names sound alike and it is even possible to have two patients with the same name. Ask the patient to give a full name and to provide a second identifier, such as date of birth or the last four digits of the social security number. This will help to avoid a mix-up. The second identifier should not be checked until you are in the exam room.

Positioning the Patient

Positioning of the patient will depend on the vein selected. Patients are usually seated for blood draws unless there is a risk of the patient fainting. The arm should be supported on the arm of a phlebotomy chair, the exam table, or a table/countertop and should extend downward in a straight line. By placing the arm in a

Table 24-3 General Steps for Performing a Venipuncture

Check the provider's orders for testing.
Assemble and inspect the equipment.
Label the tubes.
Identify the patient using two identifiers, identify yourself, and explain the procedure and rationale for the procedure.
Verify restrictions such as fasting and check to see if there is any reason you can't draw blood on a particular side of the body such as on patients that have had mastectomies, patients with shunts or ports, or on areas of the skin that has been damaged.
Wash hands and apply the appropriate personal protective equipment (PPE). (For the best protection, the medical assistant should wear a mask, goggles, waterproof lab coat, apron or gown, and gloves.)
Properly position the patient. (Arm should be straightened.)
Visually inspect the patient's skin and veins in both arms and ask patient if he or she has a preference.
Apply tourniquet and clean the area with alcohol using a circular motion.
Palpate the veins using the pad of your index finger. (The vein should feel spongy. Do not use if the area feels hard, as it may be a tendon. Notice the direction and depth of the vein as you palpate.)
Perform venipuncture.
Withdraw needle and engage safety device.
Follow specimen handling instructions.
Check the site and apply pressure dressing.
Properly dispose of sharps and contaminated equipment according to OSHA guidelines.
Use a 10% bleach solution for cleaning spills and the work area.
Remove gloves and wash hands.
Log the specimen and process the paperwork.
Document the procedure in the patient's chart.

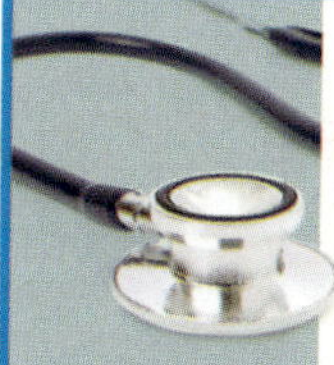

Field Smarts

What you should know prior to the procedure: If a patient's medical history is unfamiliar to you, there are specific questions that you should ask prior to performing phlebotomy. They include the following:

- Do you have any latex allergies? (If yes, wear nonlatex gloves during the procedure.)
- Have you ever had a reaction to an adhesive bandage? (If yes, apply a gauze square to the site following the venipuncture, and secure it with a piece of paper tape, or wrap with Coban wrapping material.)
- Is there any reason I shouldn't draw blood on one side or the other (patient has had a mastectomy, has a shunt or port, and so on)? If the answer is yes, draw the blood on the opposite side.
- Are you taking any blood thinners such as Coumadin or warfarin, or are you on aspirin therapy? (If yes, be especially careful about moving the needle around. Injury to the vessels may cause prolonged bleeding under the skin. Apply pressure for a minimum of two to five minutes following the blood draw and apply a pressure bandage.)
- Do you have a history of fainting associated with having your blood drawn? (If yes, position the patient in a supine or semi-Fowler's position.)

If at all possible, review the patient's history prior to escorting the patient back to the room. The patient will have more confidence in you if you already know the information because you reviewed the chart first. Any new information gained during questioning should be placed in the patient's health record.

Table 24-4 **Venipuncture Equipment**

Gloves/Personal protective equipment (PPE)
Tourniquet
Sterile/clean gauze squares
Alcohol wipes
Needle
Needle/tube holder or syringe
Tubes, including extras
Bandage

downward position, the veins will enlarge and become more prominent. The downward position also helps the blood tubes to fill from the bottom up and helps prevent reflux. While reflux is uncommon, it can occur if blood flows back into the patient's vein from the vacuum tube. If the tube contains an additive, especially EDTA, the patient could have an adverse reaction.

The arm should be straight, not bent, which makes the vein easier to locate. Placing the fist of the other hand under the elbow will help with straightening the arm.

Some patients become quite nervous prior to having their blood drawn and will find it difficult to remain still if seated. Extremely anxious patients and those who have a history of syncope (fainting) should be placed on the exam table in a supine or semi-Fowler's position. A pillow with a disposable waterproof covering may be placed under the patient's arm for support and proper positioning.

Selecting the Site

An examination of the skin should be performed before selecting the actual vein. Avoid areas with extensive scarring or burns when selecting a site. Blood should not be collected from an edematous region (area that is swollen), an area where a hematoma (blood clot) is located, or an area on the skin that appears infected.

The most common site for venipuncture is the **antecubital space** of the arm. This area is located where the upper arm and the forearm meet at the bend of the elbow. Three prominent veins are located in this area: the median cubital, cephalic, and basilic veins (Figure 24-15a). Arteries can also be found in this area and should be avoided if at all possible (Figure 24-15b).

The median cubital is usually the vein of choice. It is a large vein located in the middle of the antecubital area; it is close to the surface and easily accessible. If the median cubital vein is not suitable, the cephalic vein (located on the thumb side) should be the second vein of choice, and if neither of those are available, the basilic vein (located toward the inner portion of the arm) may be used, but with caution. The median nerve runs in this area which can become damaged if accidentally pierced.

The first step in selecting a vein is to apply a tourniquet 3 to 4 inches above the venipuncture site. It should be tight enough to slow the flow of blood in the veins but not so tight that it stops the blood flow

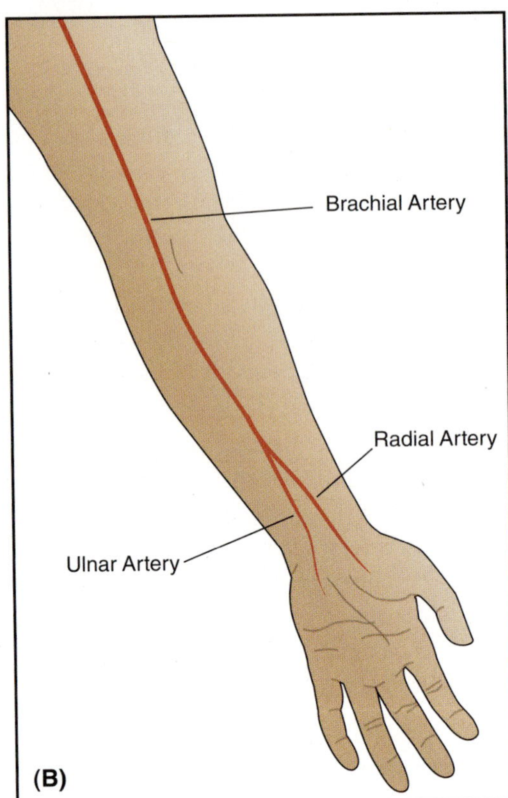

Figure 24-15 ■ (a) Surface veins used for venipuncture; (b) Major arteries of the arm that should be avoided during a venipuncture.

in the arteries. By slowing the flow, the blood will pool in the veins, causing them to dilate (enlarge) and making them easier to palpate. The tourniquet should feel tight but not painful. *Never leave the tourniquet on the arm longer than one minute.* This can cause a condition known as **hemoconcentration**, which is caused by pooling of blood; this can increase the concentration of certain blood components and result in inaccurate test results.

Once the tourniquet is properly applied, the medical assistant should use the index finger to palpate the vein by firmly pressing and releasing the vein several times. The thumb should not be used for palpating veins. A vein will feel similar to a spongy rubber tube. If the vein is difficult to palpate, it can be made more prominent by tapping the area with the index and middle finger, which will cause the vein to dilate. Rubbing the arm from wrist to elbow to force the blood into the vein or covering the area with a warm compress can also increase the blood flow and make the vein easier to feel. Veins that feel hardened or scarred should not be selected due to inadequate blood flow.

If a pulse is felt in the vessel, it could be the brachial artery, which is also located in the antecubital space. Puncturing an artery should be avoided. It is painful and can produce inaccurate test results.

When trying to locate a proper vein for venipuncture, remember that tendons and nerves also run the length of the arm and can be quite painful if punctured. Tendons located near the surface will feel hard and cord-like and should not be mistaken for a vein. Nerves cannot be seen or felt, but can usually be avoided by not performing deep or probing venipunctures. If the patient experiences unusual pain during the venipuncture, the process should be stopped immediately and another site selected.

Both arms should be inspected for a suitable site before proceeding. If neither arm appears appropriate, alternative sites are located on the back of the hand, the back of the wrist, the ankle, or the foot. Veins on the back of hand and the back of the wrist are small and tend to roll easily, so a collection system with a small gauge needle should be used. *Veins of the ankle or foot should only be used when directed to do so by the provider.*

SPECIMEN COLLECTION BY THE SYRINGE METHOD

Venipuncture by the syringe method is commonly performed for difficult draws, such as those performed on patients with fragile or weak veins. By using a syringe, the blood may be drawn more slowly than with the vacuum tube method and can prevent the vein from collapsing.

Blood collection tubes must be filled in a specific order, according to the order of draw established by the National Committee of Clinical Laboratory Standards (NCCLS), now referred to as the Clinical and Lab Standards Institute (CLSI). The purpose of the order is to prevent possible cross-contamination from the collection tube additives, which could result in erroneous test results. The order of draw has been revised several times; the CLSI currently recommends the same order of draw for both the syringe method and the vacuum tube method. Refer back to Table 24-2, which lists the order of draw.

When blood is drawn into a syringe, microclot formation can begin quickly while the blood is still in the syringe. For this reason, some facilities still prefer to use a separate order of draw for syringe collection to prevent microclots from forming in tubes with additives. These small clots can become lodged in automated laboratory equipment and can also affect test results. Refer to Procedure 24-1 for complete step-by-step instructions on collecting a blood sample by the syringe method.

SPECIMEN COLLECTION BY THE VACUUM TUBE METHOD

The vacuum tube method is usually the method of choice for routine blood specimen collection. This method has several advantages over the syringe method. Multiple tubes of blood for a variety of tests can easily be collected with one needlestick. Blood is drawn directly into collection tubes containing an additive, and can be mixed immediately to prevent microclot formation. The risk of accidental needlestick is also reduced because the blood does not need to be transferred from the syringe to a collection tube. Procedure 24-2 supplies the necessary information and steps for collecting a blood sample by the vacuum tube method.

SPECIMEN COLLECTION BY THE BUTTERFLY METHOD

The butterfly or winged infusion collection system has the advantages of both the vacuum tube system and the syringe method. Two types of winged infusion systems are available: one for use with a syringe and one for use with the vacuum tube system.

This system was designed to be used for veins that are difficult to puncture with a standard size needle. The winged needle is easy to slide into the surface veins of the hand, wrist, or foot. The butterfly can also be used for very small veins in the antecubital area, but should not be used routinely for this purpose. Procedure 24-3 lists the steps required to perform a venipuncture using a butterfly or winged infusion set.

CRITICAL THINKING CHALLENGE

Three patients are waiting to have their blood drawn. After reviewing their histories you see that Patient A has a history of veins that collapse easily, Patient B can only be stuck in the hand, and Patient C doesn't have any history of problems from blood draws.

1. **Which collection setup would you most likely use for each patient?**

PATIENT RESPONSE AND COMPLICATIONS

Many patients are fearful of having their blood drawn. Complications may arise as a result of venipuncture such as a hematoma, prolonged bleeding from the puncture site, infection, nerve damage, reflux, vein damage, and collapsed veins. The medical assistant must be prepared to deal with different situations and know how to correctly respond in the event the patient suffers an adverse reaction or complication. Table 24-5 lists some possible reactions the patient may experience and how the medical assistant can best prevent or handle the situation.

Hematoma is one of the most common complications resulting from a venipuncture. It is a swelling or bruising resulting from an accumulation of blood at the puncture site. This accumulation of blood is usually caused by leakage from the vessel that was punctured. Table 24-6 lists some hematoma prevention tips.

THE FAILED VENIPUNCTURE

There are numerous reasons for a failed venipuncture. By instituting preventive measures to avoid complications, the medical assistant is usually successful during the first blood draw attempt. Table 24-7 lists potential problems and the steps necessary to correct them.

Table 24-5 Venipuncture Adverse Reaction Responses

Patient Reaction	Medical Assistant's Response
Pain during venipuncture	*Gently* reposition the needle. If pain persists, remove the needle and stop venipuncture immediately.
Nausea	Instruct the patient to breathe slowly and deeply through the mouth. Apply a cold damp compress to the patient's forehead. Give the patient an emesis basin.
Fainting (syncope)	Patients with a history of syncope should lie down while having their blood drawn. If the patient feels faint or does faint while lying down, remove the tourniquet and needle and elevate the patient's feet. If the patient feels faint while seated, immediately remove the tourniquet and needle and have the patient lower the head between the knees if conscious. If unconscious, call for help and gently lower the patient to the floor. Elevate the patient's feet. Whether the patient is seated or lying down: Once the patient is properly positioned, apply cool compresses to the forehead and the back of the neck, manage the puncture site, and obtain instruction from the provider.
Seizures and convulsions	Remove the tourniquet and needle immediately. Apply pressure to the venipuncture site without restricting the patient's arm movement. Lower the patient to the floor and move objects out of the way to prevent injury to the patient. Notify the provider immediately.
Hematoma	Stop the venipuncture immediately. Apply firm pressure to the site for five minutes. Apply an ice pack to the site. See Table 24-6 for hematoma prevention tips.
Prolonged bleeding	Apply pressure for a minimum of five minutes. If bleeding continues, apply pressure until bleeding stops. Notify the provider.
Nerve damage	Avoid excessive probing with the needle, especially if there is no blood flow or if the patient complains of pain. *Gently* reposition the needle and if no blood flow appears, stop the venipuncture and choose an alternative site.
Infection	Infection is rare, but can occur. Following aseptic technique will help prevent infections from occurring.
Reflux	Reflux is a condition in which the blood is able to re-enter the vein due to poor positioning of the arm. The patient's arm should be positioned so that the blood flows downward. Do *not* allow the tube contents to move back and forth while the needle is in the patient's vein.
Vein damage	Avoid repeated venipunctures in the same vein. Avoid excessive probing or using improper technique when repositioning the needle.
Collapsed vein	If the vein is no longer visible and blood stops flowing into the tube, discontinue the venipuncture.

Table 24-6 Hematoma Prevention Tips

Use smaller needles for small or fragile veins. Consider using a syringe for these types of veins.
Avoid going through the vein, partially penetrating a vein, or excessive movement while the needle is in the vein.
The bevel of the needle should be completely covered.
Use smaller size tubes when using smaller needle gauges.
Avoid excessive probing.
Remove the tourniquet prior to withdrawing the needle.
Have the patient apply direct pressure for a minimum of two minutes following the draw and instruct the patient not to lift anything heavy with the affected arm for several hours following the draw.

CRITERIA FOR SPECIMEN REJECTION

When collecting a blood specimen, one of the medical assistant's first responsibilities is to provide the laboratory with an adequate specimen that has been properly collected and processed. Poor specimen quality can affect test results and in turn delay treatment. Specimens can be rejected for a variety of reasons, such as improper labeling, using incorrect tubes, improperly filled tubes, incorrect collection time, incorrect specimen handling, or sending a hemolyzed or lipemic specimen. If a specimen is rejected or inaccurate test results are suspected, the specimen will need to be redrawn.

Table 24-7 Causes of Failed Venipuncture

Possible Causes	Steps to Correct
Needle Position:	
• Bevel against wall of vein	Slightly rotate the bevel. Slowly advance the needle until blood begins to flow.
• Bevel partially exposed	Advance the needle inward until bevel is completely covered.
• Needle too deep	Gently pull back on the needle until blood starts flowing into the tube.
• Needle to the side of the vein	Gently pull back on the needle until the bevel is just under the skin, anchor the vein and redirect the needle into the vein. Use a new tube after redirecting the needle.
Collapsed vein	The tourniquet may be too tight—remove it. Pressure from the vacuum in the tube can cause the vein to collapse. Using a syringe or a smaller tube with a reduced vacuum may help to prevent the vein from collapsing.
Tube vacuum insufficient	Try another tube first. Do *not* use tubes that have expired or that have been dropped.

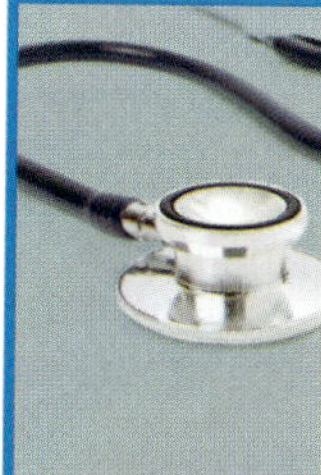

Field Smarts

Most practices have what is referred to as a two-stick rule: Never attempt more than two sticks per patient. It is hard on the patient, hard on you, and makes the practice look bad when multiple attempts occur. Ask someone with more experience to take over. If possible, watch to see if that individual has a different technique. Don't feel bad if you miss a vein occasionally; even the most experienced phlebotomists miss from time to time.

Improper Labeling of Specimen Tubes

A specimen can be rejected for reasons as simple as an error in labeling. Each specimen must have a label that contains the following information:

- Patient's full name and identification number, if applicable
- Date and time of collection
- Initials of person collecting the specimen
- Type of specimen if not obvious

Use of Incorrect Specimen Tubes

Specimens must be collected in the correct tube containing the proper additive. An incorrect additive can adversely affect test results. For example, if **plasma** is required for testing, the specimen must come from a tube with an anticoagulant. If serum is required, the specimen must come from a clot tube. Because serum and plasma look the same to the naked eye, proper tube choice is critical. Always check the lab manual for collection requirements.

Vacuum tubes must be filled to the proper volume in order to provide a good quality specimen for testing. If the tube is only partially filled, known as a short draw, the ratio of additive to blood will be insufficient and can be the source of inaccurate test results. Improperly filled tubes used for coagulation studies (light blue top) are rejected by most laboratories due to the increased amount of additive, which dilutes the specimen and can lead to a falsely elevated partial thromboplastin time (PTT). A partially filled tube with EDTA (lavender top) will affect the hematocrit and mean cell volume (MCV). A partially filled plain red top tube with no additive can still be used for testing, as serum is not affected by a short draw. A sufficient amount of specimen must be available for testing. If there is an insufficient amount, the specimen will be referred to as **quantity not sufficient (QNS)** and must be redrawn.

Incorrect Collection Time

Specimens for some laboratory tests, such as some glucose tolerence tests and therapeutic drug monitoring, must be collected at specific times or the lab will reject the specimen. If a specimen is collected at the wrong time, it must be noted on the requisition form and the laboratory will make the determination if it is adequate for testing.

Incorrect Specimen Handling

Specimens must be collected and stored in the proper environment until the test can be performed. It is important for the medical assistant to check the lab manual prior to collecting a blood specimen for special collection and handling instructions. Certain components such as bilirubin are photosensitive and must be protected by wrapping the tube in a foil following the collection or pouring the substance into a special amber-colored tube. Another component is temperature sensitivity. Some specimens must be frozen or refrigerated while others must be kept at room temperature until testing can be performed.

Hemolyzed and Lipemic Specimens

Hemolysis occurs when the red blood cells rupture and release hemoglobin into the liquid portion of the specimen. The serum or plasma may appear light orange (slight hemolysis) to red (gross hemolysis) in color. Hemolyzed specimens will affect the accuracy of certain laboratory tests, such as the complete blood count (CBC), potassium levels, and certain enzyme levels. Hemolysis is most commonly caused by errors in the collection process, but may also be the result of liver disease and hemolytic anemia. The most common collection errors resulting in hemolysis include the following:

- Collecting a specimen from a vein with a hematoma
- Using a needle gauge that is too small for venipuncture
- Using a large vacuum tube with the butterfly system or a smaller needle
- Vigorous mixing of additive tubes
- Blood frothing caused by incorrect fitting of the needle on the syringe
- Pulling back too quickly on the plunger during a syringe draw

A lipemic specimen is one that has a cloudy or milky appearance. **Lipemia** can be caused by ingesting fatty foods prior to specimen collection or by certain physiological conditions. Since lipemia can appear anywhere from 1 to 10 hours after ingestion of fats, a 12-hour fast is required for accurate cholesterol and triglyceride levels. Because a lipemic specimen is cloudy, it may interfere with certain chemistry tests. Figure 24-16 illustrates the appearance of a hemolyzed and lipemic specimen.

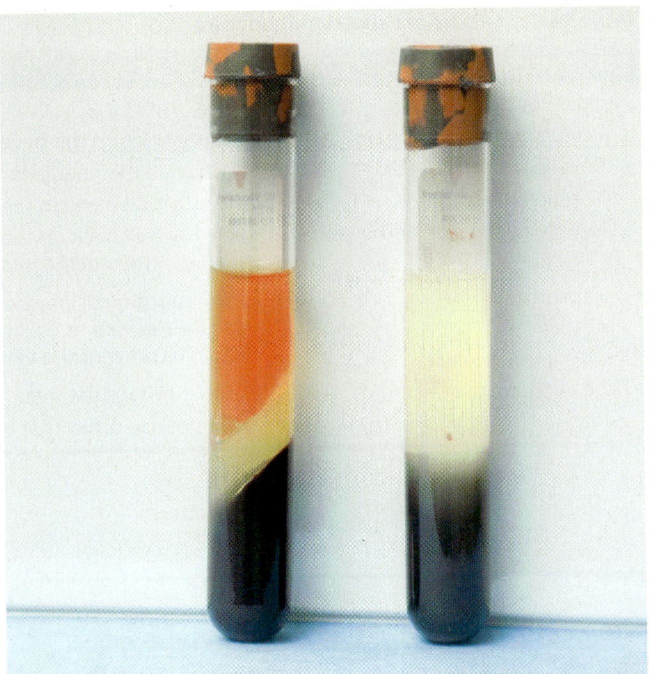

Figure 24-16 ■ An example of the appearance of both a hemolyzed specimen (left) and a lipemic specimen (right).

THE CAPILLARY PUNCTURE

The **capillary puncture**, also known as a skin or dermal puncture, is used when a venipuncture is not the preferred method of specimen collection. It is the method of choice for infants and children under the age of two due to their extremely small veins and low blood volume. The capillary puncture is also used for adults whose veins are fragile and weak due to age or illness. Many test methodologies have been developed that require only micro amounts of blood, which can be easily obtained by capillary puncture. Capillary samples can be tested at the location of collection for point-of-care testing (POCT). POCT produces immediate results and eliminates the need for specimen processing and transport. Examples of POCT tests include hemoglobin and hematocrit, blood glucose, cholesterol, and coagulation studies.

If a specimen is collected by capillary puncture and sent to an outside laboratory for testing, the collection method must be noted on the specimen container and on the requisition form because certain tests such as glucose, calcium, and potassium will have different results than those of a venous blood sample. Blood collected by the capillary method is primarily made up of undetermined proportions of blood from arterioles, venules, plus interstitial and intracellular blood.

Equipment

The equipment used to perform the capillary puncture is very similar to that used to perform a venipuncture

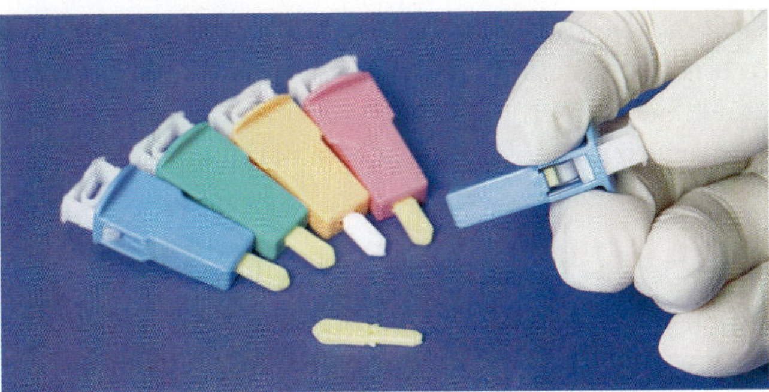

Figure 24-17 ■ Examples of Microtainer Genie brand lancets that come in different sizes for different uses. They are color-coded according to their use.

with a few exceptions. The following is a list of the necessary supplies and equipment needed to perform this procedure:

- Alcohol wipes
- Gauze squares
- Gloves
- Adhesive bandage
- **Lancets**
- Micro collection containers

Some of the lancets are self-contained, such as those in Figure 24-17, and have the plunger device already attached, while others must be used with a spring-loaded device.

Common Sites for Collection

The most common sites for capillary collection in adults and children are the tips of the middle (great) or ring finger. For specimen collection from an infant, the medial or lateral plantar surface of the heel is used, as this is the area that has the most soft tissue and is the safest area to reduce the possibility of striking the heel bone during the puncture. When selecting a site, it is important to choose an area that is warm and pink, and not edematous, cyanotic, or cold. Figure 24-18a illustrates the most common sites used for capillary blood collection.

Preparing the Site

A warm puncture site is one that has adequate blood flow for capillary collection. If the skin is cool, circulation can be increased by warming the site with a heat pack, warm, moist towel or through gentle massage.

The site must be disinfected with 70% isopropyl alcohol and then allowed to air dry or immediately wiped with a sterile piece of gauze. If alcohol is carried into the puncture site because of inadequate drying time after cleansing, it can cause hemolysis of the specimen as well as discomfort for the patient.

Collecting the Specimen

The skin puncture is performed on the tip of the finger, off to the side across the grain of the fingertip, not along the grain (Figure 24-18b). The first drop of blood is wiped away before collection of the specimen because it is diluted with tissue fluid, which can dilute the levels of the components being tested. The site may be gently squeezed and released to promote an adequate drop of blood.

One end of the collection container (often a capillary tube) is positioned so that the open end of the tube is advanced to the drop of blood, not to the skin itself. Refer to Procedure 24-4 for the complete, detailed steps for collecting a capillary sample.

Order of Draw

The order of draw for capillary collection differs from that of specimens collected by venipuncture. Platelets can accumulate at the puncture site resulting in erroneous test results. The CLSI recommends the following order of draw for capillary punctures:

1. Lavender-topped (EDTA) tubes for hematology studies
2. Other additive tubes such as green-topped (heparin) tubes, gray, and serum-separator tubes (gel)
3. Nonadditive tubes (red-topped), which contain no anticoagulants, gels, or clot activators

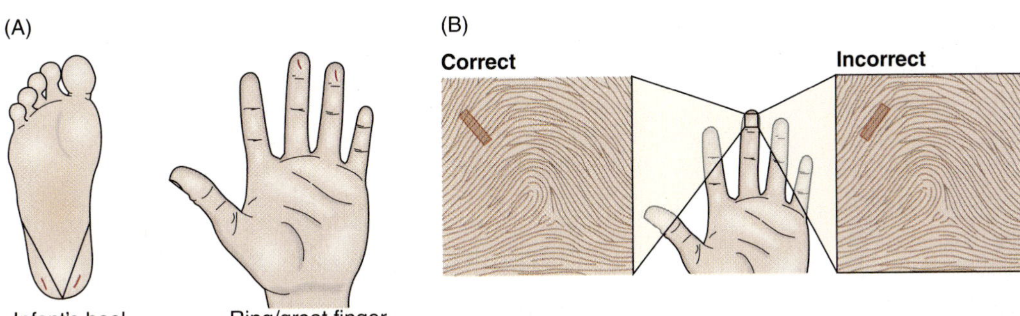

Figure 24-18 ■ (a) Common sites used for capillary puncture; (b) Correct puncture pattern—across the grain of the fingertip, not along the grain.

GENERAL GUIDELINES FOR SPECIMEN HANDLING

Because different laboratories employ different testing procedures, it is critical that the medical assistant follow specimen handling guidelines outlined in the laboratory user manual in the medical facility. Errors that affect patient results often occur during collection, processing, storage, and transport of specimens. Specific specimen-handling guidelines will be discussed in related lab chapters. General guidelines are as follows:

- Vacuum tubes containing an additive should be gently inverted *immediately* following collection to completely mix the additive with the specimen. Each additive requires a specific number of inversions. Vigorous mixing can cause hemolysis. Insufficient mixing can cause microclot formation, which will produce erroneous test results.
- Transport all tubes containing blood with the stopper in the upright position to prevent hemolysis.
- According to CLSI and OSHA, specimens other than blood must be transported in leak-proof containers with tight lids and placed in a sealed plastic bag displaying the biohazard symbol. All paperwork should be attached to the outside of the bag.
- Specimen-handling guidelines for temperature and protection from light must be followed exactly.
- The CLSI recommends that serum or plasma be separated from the cells within two hours after collection. Some specimens must be separated in a quicker time frame. The laboratory used by each facility will supply specific information on this process.

Some specimens are collected in a **primary container**, or original container. Following collection and processing, an **aliquot**, or portion, of the specimen is taken from the primary container for transport to the laboratory.

DRAWING BLOOD CULTURES

When the provider suspects that the patient may have bacteremia (bacteria in the blood), a culture may be ordered. When drawing blood for a culture (Figure 24-19), sterile measures must be taken to ensure that the special container used for blood cultures is not contaminated in any way. The skin must be cleansed with a surgical cleanser such as Betadine and the stoppers on the containers used for collections should also be cleansed with Betadine. Sterile gloves should be worn throughout the procedure. Two bottles may be used for culturing. The aerobic bottle is filled before the anaerobic bottle.

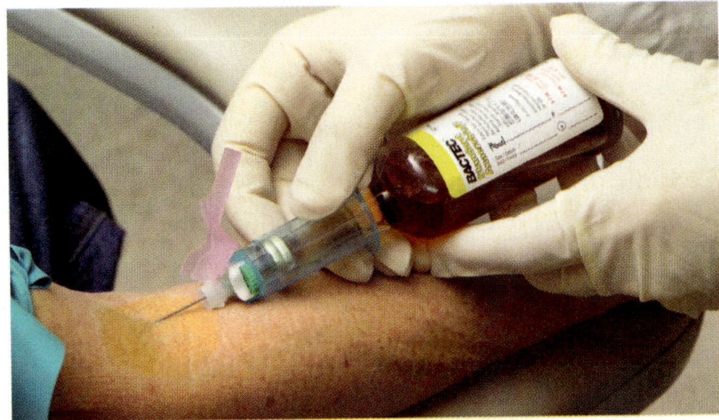

Figure 24-19 ■ Medical assistant is drawing blood for culturing on the patient.

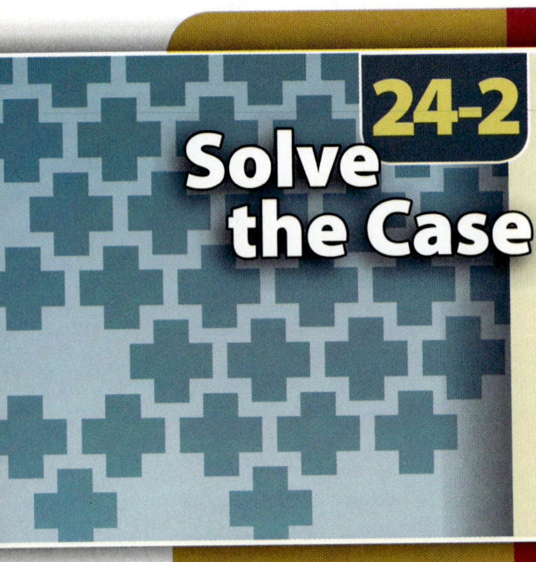

The doctor has ordered Abby to have a complete blood count (CBC) and a basic metabolic panel (BMP), which is a chemistry panel that looks at fluid levels, electrolytes, and the health of different organs. Abby is still very fearful about the blood draw and Abby's mom is really frustrated with her daughter.

1. **What color top tubes will you need to use for the blood draw?**
2. **What order of draw will you use?**
3. **What method of blood draw should you use with Abby knowing she is fearful of needles?**
4. **Is there anything you can do to decrease the stress that Abby's mom is creating?**

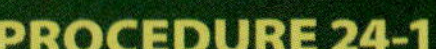

PROCEDURE 24-1

Perform Venipuncture (Syringe Method)

Objective:

To withdraw a venous blood sample for laboratory testing as requested by the provider. (This method is most often used for fragile or weak veins and those that could collapse when using the vacuum tube method.)

Equipment/Supplies:

- Gloves
- Personal protective equipment (PPE)
- Alcohol wipes
- Gauze squares (sterile or clean depending on facility guidelines)
- Syringe (10 to 20 mL)
- Syringe needle (21 to 22 G)
- Transfer device
- Tourniquet
- Vacuum tubes
- Adhesive bandage
- Sharps container
- Patient's chart/EHR

PROCEDURAL STEPS	DETAILS AND/OR RATIONALE
1. ***Incorporating critical thinking skills when performing patient care,*** check the provider's order and complete the laboratory requisition form.	Verification of tests ordered ensures the correct tests are performed.
2. Wash your hands and apply PPE.	The types of PPE worn will vary from office to office; however, wearing a full set of PPE will provide you with the most protection possible.
3. Assemble all the necessary equipment, and loosen the plunger by pulling it all the way back and pushing it all the way in at least one time. Label all tubes.	Loosening the plunger before beginning the blood draw will prevent the plunger from sticking during the procedure. Labeling tubes before the draw eliminates the possibility of error later.
4. Identify the patient using at least two identifiers and identify yourself.	Always clearly identify the patient using two identifiers (for example, name and date of birth) before collecting the blood sample to be sure you are collecting the specimen from the correct person.
5. ***Explain the rationale for the procedure, showing awareness of the patient's concerns related to the procedure being performed.***	If the patient is informed about the procedure, the patient will be more relaxed and less fearful.
6. Verify compliance of fasting instructions and other restrictions (for instance, the need to draw blood from one side or another due to a mastectomy or the presence of a shunt).	If the patient is not compliant with fasting instructions, the sample will have to be drawn at another time or test results could be adversely affected. Drawing blood from the side on which a patient has had a mastectomy may result in lymphedema.

continues

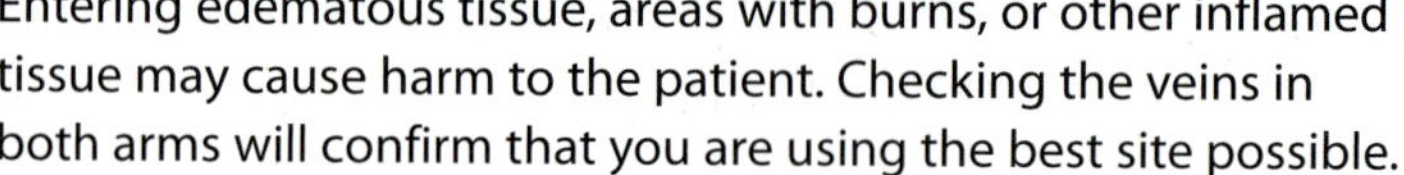

PROCEDURE 24-1 continued

PROCEDURAL STEPS	DETAILS AND/OR RATIONALE
7. Visually inspect the patient's skin and veins in both arms, ***incorporating critical thinking skills when performing patient assessment.*** Always ask if the patient has a preference. Patients usually know which veins produce the best results.	Entering edematous tissue, areas with burns, or other inflamed tissue may cause harm to the patient. Checking the veins in both arms will confirm that you are using the best site possible.
8. Select the potential site and apply the tourniquet 3 to 4 inches above the elbow. The tourniquet should not remain in place longer than one minute.	Applying the tourniquet too close to the puncture site can cause a decrease in the flow of blood, making the blood sample more difficult to obtain. A tourniquet left in place too long can cause hemoconcentration.
9. Palpate the vein using your index finger, moving in an upward and downward direction and side to side (Figure 24-20).	Palpating the vein moving in an upward and downward direction and side to side helps to inflate the vein and helps to determine its direction and depth.
10. Straighten and place the arm and hand in a downward position.	This helps to keep the blood flowing in a downward direction and prevents reflux.
11. Ask the patient to make a slight fist and hold. (Do not pump the fist, as this can cause erroneous results.)	Making a fist helps to enlarge the vein.
12. Cleanse the site with alcohol using a circular motion (Figure 24-21).	This cleanses the skin of surface bacteria in the puncture area and decreases the risk of infection from the puncture.
13. Allow the area to air dry, or dry wipe the area with a clean/sterile gauze square.	Dry wiping the area decreases the waiting time before puncturing and also decreases the chances of carrying alcohol into the puncture site, which could sting.
14. Pull the skin taut to anchor the vein.	Anchoring the vein keeps it from rolling.
15. Insert the needle using a 15° to 30° angle and make certain that the bevel is upward (Figure 24-22).	The needle must be bevel up for easy blood flow.

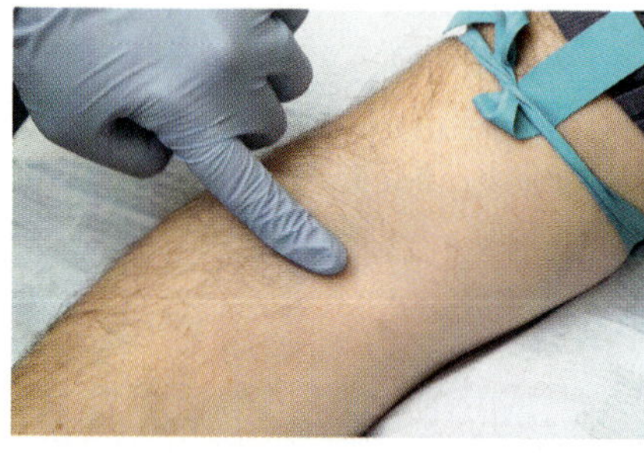

Figure 24-20 ■ Palpate the vein and check its direction.

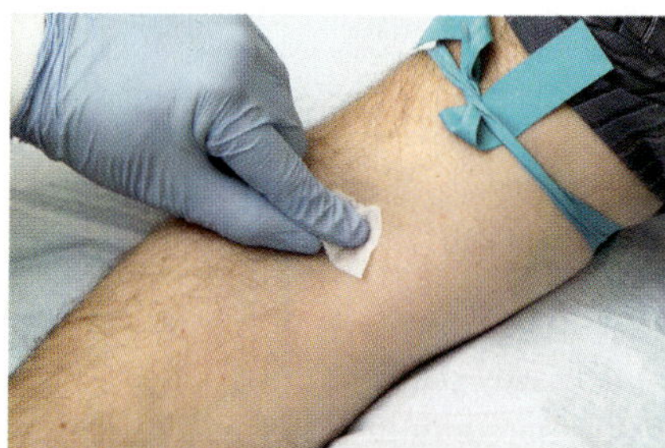

Figure 24-21 ■ Cleanse the area with alcohol and either wipe dry or allow to air dry.

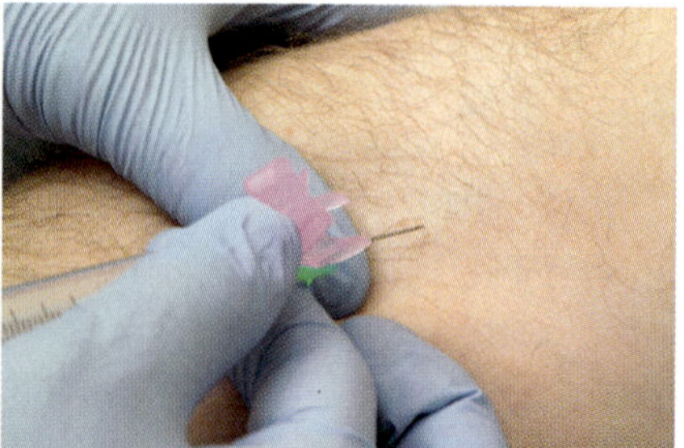

Figure 24-22 ■ Pull the skin taut and insert the needle.

continues

PROCEDURE 24-1 continued

PROCEDURAL STEPS	DETAILS AND/OR RATIONALE
16. When blood appears in the hub of needle, pull back on the plunger at a slow steady rate using the opposite hand (Figure 24-23).	Using the other hand to pull back on the plunger eliminates movement of the needle. Slow, steady pressure on the plunger prevents hemolysis.
17. Allow the syringe to fill completely.	
18. When the syringe is full, instruct the patient to open the hand.	
19. Release the tourniquet (Figure 24-24).	The tourniquet should be released before removing the needle from the vein to eliminate blood squirting due to the pressure of the tourniquet.
20. Place a dry piece of (clean or sterile) gauze above the site, withdraw the needle, and ask the patient to apply firm pressure to the site for two to three minutes (Figure 24-25).	Placing gauze above the site keeps the patient from seeing the needle as it is withdrawn. Continuous pressure must be applied to stop the bleeding and prevent hematoma.
21. Push the sheath over the needle and carefully remove it from the syringe. Discard the needle into the sharps container.	Activating the safety device will help to protect you from harm when removing the needle.
22. Carefully transfer the blood from the syringe to vacuum tubes using a safety transfer device (Figure 24-26).	OSHA regulations require the use of a safety transfer device to reduce the possibility of needlestick injury.
23. Immediately mix each filled tube according to the manufacturer's instructions.	Mixing the tubes immediately reduces the possibility of microclot formation.
24. Discard used equipment according to OSHA standards.	Proper disposal of contaminated equipment reduces the possibility of accidental exposure to the health care worker.

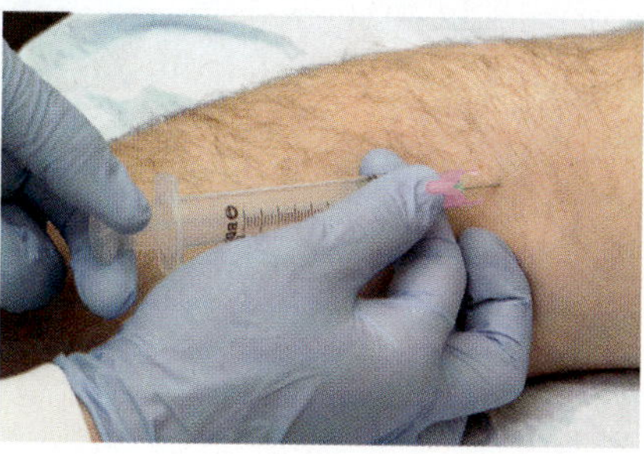

Figure 24-23 ■ Pull back on the plunger at a steady rate to withdraw the blood.

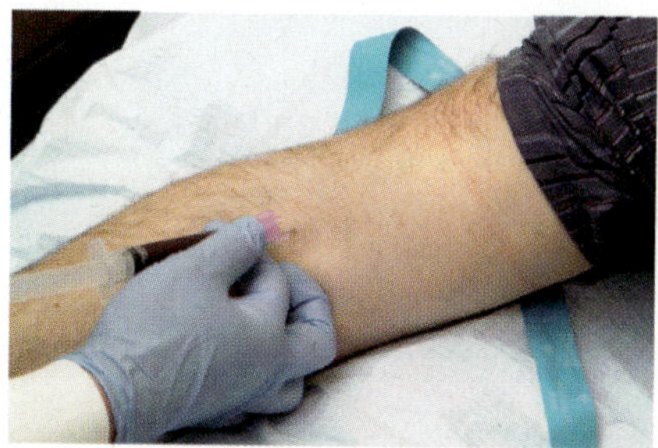

Figure 24-24 ■ Release the tourniquet.

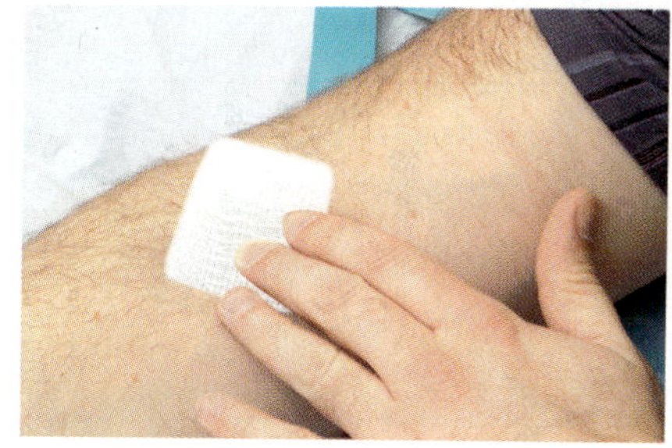

Figure 24-25 ■ Instruct the patient to apply firm pressure to the site until bleeding has stopped.

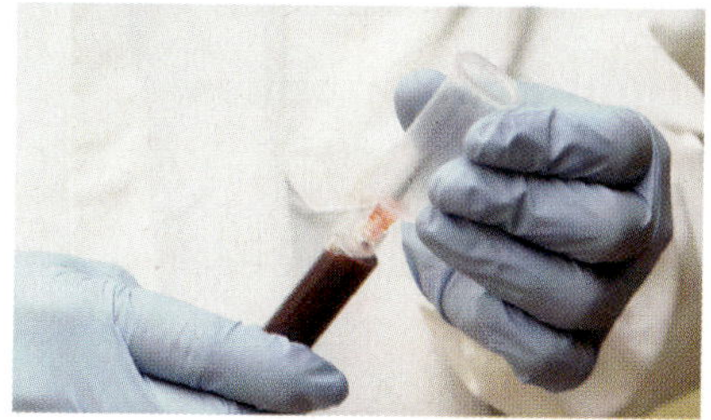

Figure 24-26 ■ The medical assistant attaches the needleless syringe to the safety device.

continues

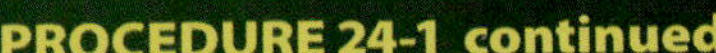

PROCEDURE 24-1 continued

PROCEDURAL STEPS	DETAILS AND/OR RATIONALE
25. Check the puncture site and apply a pressure bandage (Figure 24-27).	Always check the site before applying the bandage to be sure that bleeding has subsided.
26. Dismiss the patient.	
27. Clean the work area and process the specimen.	Process the specimen following the lab's specifications in regard to centrifugation, and proper storage and handling.
28. Remove gloves and wash your hands.	
29. Document the procedure in the patient's chart and in the lab log.	Include the phlebotomy method, location, tests ordered, types of tubes drawn, and the name of the laboratory where tests were sent.

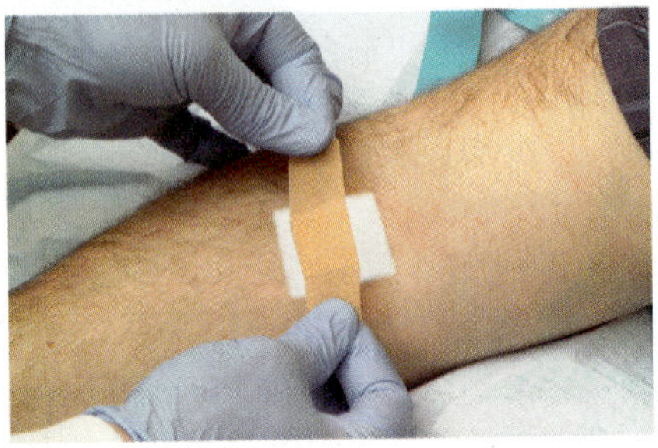

Figure 24-27 ■ The medical assistant places an adhesive bandage on the patient's arm.

DOCUMENTATION EXAMPLE:

02-24-XX 10:30	Phlebotomy (syringe method), L. antecubital for CBC and ESR per Dr. Leonard. 2 lavender tops sent to ABC Labs. No complications. Abisha Hood, CMA (AAMA)----------------------------------

PROCEDURE 24-2
Perform Venipuncture (Vacuum Tube Method)

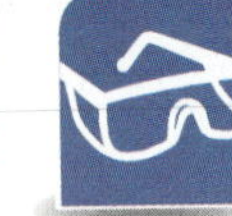

Objective:

To collect multiple tubes of venous blood for testing with one needlestick to the patient.

Equipment/Supplies:

- Gloves
- Personal protective equipment (PPE)
- Tourniquet
- Alcohol wipes
- Gauze squares (clean or sterile according to office policy)
- Adhesive bandage
- Multisample needle (20 to 22 gauge)
- Vacuum tube holder with needle safety shield
- Vacuum tubes
- Sharps container
- Patient's chart/EHR

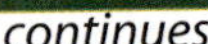

continues

PROCEDURE 24-2 continued

PROCEDURAL STEPS	DETAILS AND/OR RATIONALE
1. ***Incorporating critical thinking skills when performing patient care,*** check the order and complete the laboratory requisition form.	Always verify that tests being drawn are correct according to provider's orders.
2. Wash your hands and apply PPE. Remember the amount of PPE worn may vary from one facility to the next.	PPE must be worn to protect the individual collecting the sample.
3. Assemble all the necessary equipment and label all tubes.	Assembling all equipment before beginning the procedure helps the procedure to go a lot more smoothly. Labeling tubes before the draw eliminates the possibility of error later.
4. Identify the patient using at least two identifiers. Identify yourself.	Always use two identifiers to be certain that you have the correct patient.
5. ***Explain the rationale for performance of the procedure, showing awareness of the patient's concerns related to the procedure being performed.***	If the patient is informed about the procedure, the patient will be more relaxed and less fearful.
6. Verify compliance of fasting instructions and other restrictions (for instance, the need to draw blood from one side or another due to a mastectomy or the presence of a shunt).	If the patient is not compliant with fasting instructions, the sample will have to be drawn at another time, or test results could be adversely affected. Drawing blood from the side on which a patient has had a mastectomy may result in lymphedema.
7. Visually inspect the patient's skin and veins in both arms, ***incorporating critical thinking skills when performing patient assessment.*** Always ask if the patient has a preference. Patients usually know which veins produce the best results.	Going into edematous tissue, areas with burns, or other inflamed tissue may cause harm to the patient. Checking the veins in both arms will confirm that you are using the best site possible.
8. Apply a tourniquet 3 to 4 inches above the elbow. The tourniquet should not remain in place longer than one minute.	Applying the tourniquet too close to the puncture site can cause a decrease in the flow of blood, making the blood sample more difficult to obtain. Leaving the tourniquet in place too long can cause hemoconcentration.
9. Straighten and place the arm and hand in a downward position.	This helps to keep the blood flowing in a downward direction and prevents reflux.
10. Ask the patient to make a fist and hold. (Do not pump the fist, as this can cause erroneous results.)	Making a fist helps to enlarge the vein.
11. Palpate the vein and select final site. Check the direction the vein is running and the vein's depth (Figure 24-28).	Checking the direction of the vein and the vein's depth helps you to line the needle up correctly as you enter the vein.

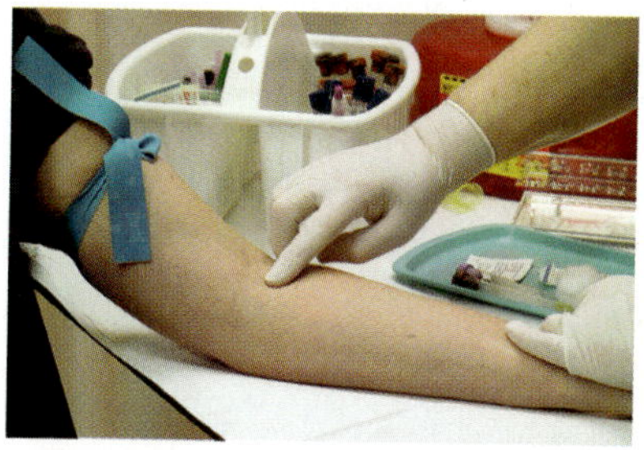

Figure 24-28 ■ Palpate the vein in an up–and-down direction.

continues

PROCEDURE 24-2 continued

PROCEDURAL STEPS	DETAILS AND/OR RATIONALE
12. Cleanse the site with alcohol using a circular motion (Figure 24-29).	This cleanses the skin of surface bacteria in the puncture area and decreases the risk of infection from the puncture.
13. Allow the area to air dry, or dry wipe the area with a clean/sterile piece of gauze.	Dry wiping the area decreases the waiting time before puncturing and also decreases the chances of carrying alcohol into the puncture site, which will sting.
14. Pull the skin taut to anchor the vein.	Anchoring the vein keeps it from rolling.
15. Using a 15° to 30° angle, insert the needle with the bevel up (Figure 24-30) and tube label down.	The needle must be bevel up for easy blood flow. The tube label down makes it easier to see the blood flow into the tube.
16. Using the hand that anchored the vein, grasp the flanges of the holder and push the tube until the needle punctures the stopper and blood flows into the tube (Figure 24-31).	Using the other hand to change tubes eliminates movement of the needle in the patient's arm.
17. Allow the tube to fill completely before changing the tube. Withdraw the tube and mix the additive tubes immediately.	Tubes are designed to fill to a predetermined volume. This ensures the correct ratio of blood to additive. Immediate mixing of the additive tubes prevents the formation of microclots.
18. Change tubes until all tubes have been collected (Figure 24-32). Instruct the patient to open the hand.	Opening the hand releases some of the pressure on the vein before removing the tourniquet.
19. Release the tourniquet and remove the tube before removing the needle.	Removing the tube before removing the needle from the arm prevents blood from dripping from the end of the needle. The tourniquet should be released before removing the needle from the vein to eliminate blood squirting due to the pressure of the tourniquet.

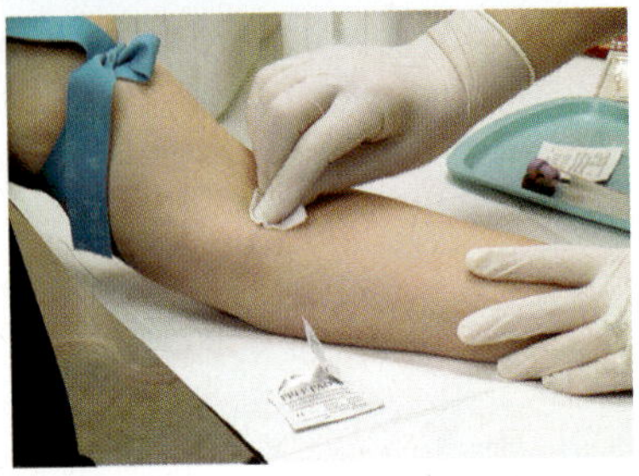

Figure 24-29 ■ Cleanse the site with alcohol, moving in a circular motion.

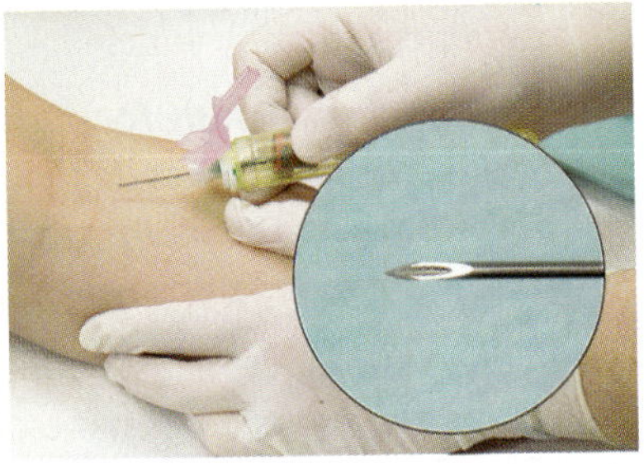

Figure 24-30 ■ Insert the needle using a 15° to 30° angle with the bevel up.

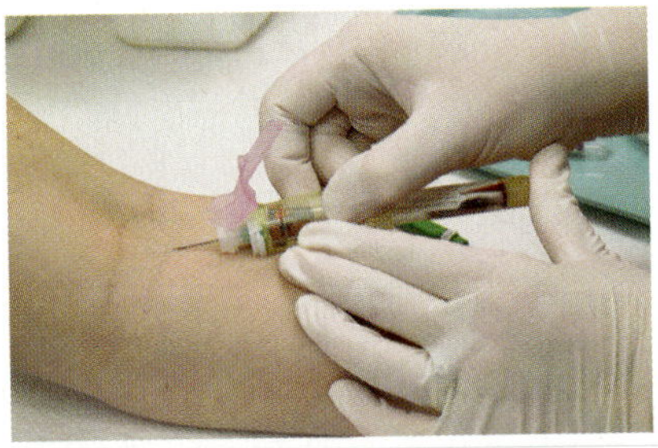

Figure 24-31 ■ With your nondominant hand, push the vacuum tube onto the needle, allowing it to completely fill.

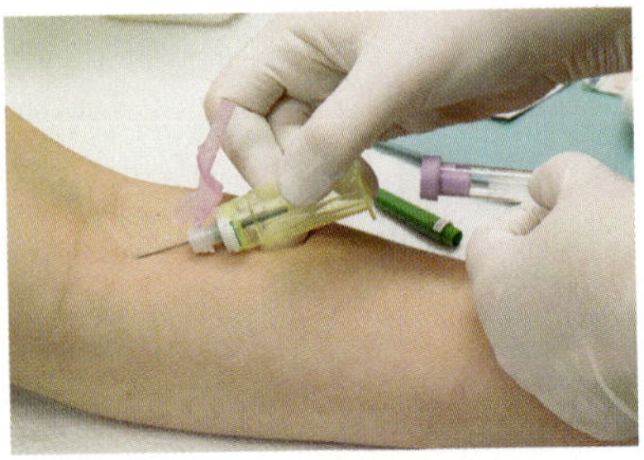

Figure 24-32 ■ Change tubes as needed until all tubes have been collected.

continues

PROCEDURE 24-2 continued

PROCEDURAL STEPS	DETAILS AND/OR RATIONALE
20. Place a dry sterile or clean piece of gauze above the site, withdraw the needle, and ask the patient to apply firm pressure to the site for two to three minutes.	Continuous pressure must be applied to stop the bleeding and prevent hematoma.
21. Engage the safety device and discard the used equipment according to OSHA standards (Figure 24-33).	Proper disposal of contaminated equipment reduces the possibility of accidental exposure to the health care worker.
22. Check the puncture site and apply a pressure bandage.	Always check the site before applying the bandage to be sure that bleeding has subsided.
23. Dismiss the patient.	
24. Clean the work area and process specimen.	Processing the specimen means to follow the lab's specifications in regard to centrifugation, and storage and handling.
25. Remove gloves and wash your hands.	
26. Document the procedure in the patient's chart.	Include the phlebotomy method, location, tests ordered, types of tubes drawn, and the name of the laboratory where tests were sent.

Figure 24-33 ■ Close the safety sheath over the needle and deposit the entire unit into the sharps container.

DOCUMENTATION EXAMPLE:

02-12-XX 10:30 a. m	Phlebotomy, (vacuum tube method) R. antecubital for CBC and Executive profile per Dr. Smith. 2 red tops and 1 lavender top sent to ABC Labs. No complications. Carson O'Brien, CMA (AAMA)--

PROCEDURE 24-3

Perform Venipuncture (Butterfly Method)

Objective:

To obtain a venous blood sample for laboratory testing from small, fragile veins that could easily collapse using other methods.

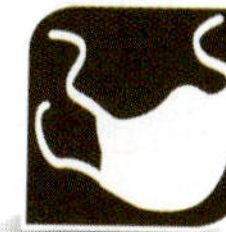

Equipment/Supplies:

- Gloves
- Personal protective equipment (PPE)
- Tourniquet
- Alcohol wipes
- Gauze squares (clean or sterile according to office policy)

continues

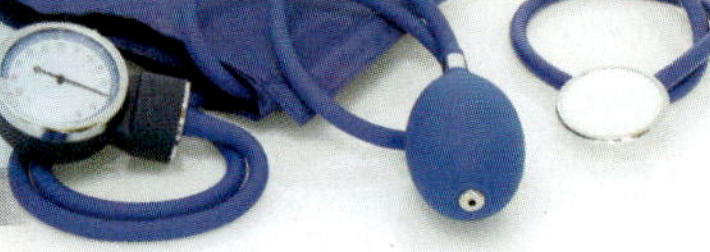

PROCEDURE 24-3 continued

- Adhesive bandage
- Vacuum tube holder/syringe
- Vacuum tubes, usually short draw or pediatric size
- Safety device (if performing the syringe method)
- Butterfly needle (21 to 25 gauge, ½ to 1 inch)
- Sharps container
- Patient's chart/EHR

PROCEDURAL STEPS	DETAILS AND/OR RATIONALE
1. ***Incorporating critical thinking skills when performing patient care,*** check the provider's order and complete the laboratory requisition form.	Always verify that tests being drawn are correct according to provider's orders.
2. Wash your hands and apply PPE. Remember that the types of PPE worn during a blood draw may vary from one facility to another.	PPE must be worn to protect the individual collecting the specimen. The more types of PPE worn, the more you will be protected.
3. Assemble all the necessary equipment and label all tubes.	Labeling tubes before the draw eliminates the possibility of error later.
4. Identify the patient using two identifiers, and identify yourself.	Always clearly identify the patient before collecting the blood sample to be sure you are collecting the specimen from the correct person.
5. ***Explain the rationale for performance of the procedure, showing awareness of the patient's concerns related to the procedure being performed.***	If the patient is informed about the procedure, the patient will be more relaxed and less fearful.
6. Verify compliance of fasting instructions and other restrictions (for instance, the need to draw blood from one side or another due to a mastectomy or the presence of a shunt).	If the patient is not compliant with fasting instructions, the sample will have to be drawn at another time, or test results could be adversely affected. Drawing blood from the side on which patient has had a mastectomy may result in lymphedema.
7. Visually inspect the patient's skin and veins in both arms or hands, ***incorporating critical thinking skills when performing patient assessment.*** Always ask if the patient has a preference. Patients usually know which veins produce the best results.	Entering the needle in edematous tissue, areas with burns, or other inflamed tissue may cause damage to the patient. Checking the veins in both arms will assure that you are using the best site possible.
8. Select the appropriate arm or hand and apply a tourniquet 3 to 4 inches above the elbow or wrist when drawing from the hand (Figure 24-34). The tourniquet should not remain in place longer than one minute.	Applying the tourniquet too close to the puncture site can cause a decrease in the flow of blood, making the blood sample more difficult to obtain. Leaving the tourniquet in place too long can cause hemoconcentration.
9. Ask the patient to make a fist.	Making a fist helps to enlarge the vein.

Figure 24-34 ■ Tie a tourniquet around the patient's wrist and ask him to make a fist.

continues

PROCEDURE 24-3 continued

PROCEDURAL STEPS	DETAILS AND/OR RATIONALE
10. Place the fist of the patient's other hand under the elbow when drawing from the arm, or under the wrist when drawing from the hand.	This helps to keep the arm or hand positioned correctly.
11. Palpate the vein and selected final site.	Always palpate the vein upward and downward and side to side to determine its direction and depth.
12. Cleanse the site with alcohol using a circular motion.	This cleanses the skin of surface bacteria in the puncture area and decreases the risk of infection from the puncture.
13. Allow the area to air dry, or dry wipe the area with a clean/sterile gauze square.	Dry wiping the area decreases the waiting time before puncturing and also decreases the chances of carrying alcohol into the puncture site, which may sting.
14. Pull the skin taut.	This keeps the vein from rolling.
15. Grasp the wings of the butterfly and insert the needle bevel up, at a 5° to 10° angle (Figure 24-35).	The needle must be bevel up for easy blood flow. When performing hand sticks, the degree is much shallower than in other methods of venipuncture to facilitate entry into the surface veins of the hand.
16. *Vacuum tube method* Once blood enters the tubing, push the tube onto the needle inside the tube adapter and allow it to fill completely. Remove the tube and invert additive tubes to mix before pushing in additional tubes. When the last tube is filling, release the tourniquet. When the tube is completely full, withdraw the tube and then withdraw the needle. Engage the safety device (Figure 24-36).	Mixing additive tubes immediately before beginning to fill another tube will prevent the possibility of microclot formation. Relaxing the hand and releasing the tourniquet before removing the needle helps to eliminate the possibility of blood squirting.
Syringe method Once blood enters the hub of the needle, start pulling back on the plunger. Fill the syringe completely and ask the patient to relax the hand. Release the tourniquet, withdraw the needle, engage the safety device, and remove the needle, placing it in a sharps container. Fill the tubes using a safety transfer device, and immediately invert them to mix.	
17. Place a dry sterile or clean gauze square over the site and instruct the patient to apply firm pressure to the site for two to three minutes.	Continuous pressure must be applied to stop bleeding and prevent hematoma.

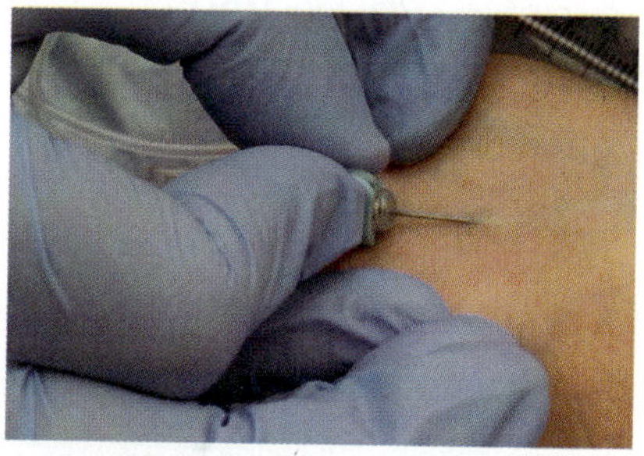

Figure 24-35 ■ Hold the skin taut, grasp the wings of the butterfly together and insert the needle at a five to ten degree angle.

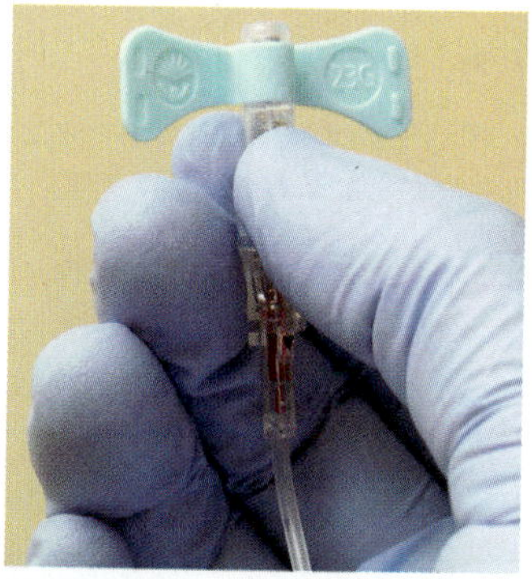

Figure 24-36 ■ Engage the safety device on the butterfly needle.

continues

PROCEDURE 24-3 continued

PROCEDURAL STEPS	DETAILS AND/OR RATIONALE
18. Discard used equipment according to OSHA standards.	Proper disposal of contaminated equipment reduces the possibility of accidental exposure to the health care worker.
19. Check the puncture site and apply a pressure bandage.	Always check the site before applying the bandage to be sure that bleeding has subsided.
20. Dismiss the patient.	
21. Clean the work area and process the specimen.	Processing the specimen means to follow the lab's specifications in regard to centrifugation, and storage and handling.
22. Remove gloves and wash your hands.	
23. Document the procedure in the patient's chart.	Include the phlebotomy method, location, tests ordered, types of tubes drawn, and the name of the laboratory where tests were sent.

DOCUMENTATION EXAMPLE:

02-12-XX 11:25 a.m.	Phlebotomy (butterfly method) R. hand for a PT, APTT, and INR per Dr. Price. 1 blue top sent to ABC Labs. Addison Miller, CMA (AAMA)--

PROCEDURE 24-4
Perform a Capillary Puncture

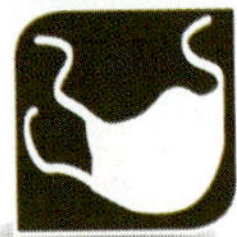

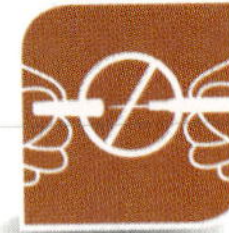

Objective:

To collect a capillary blood sample by the correct method to be used for laboratory testing.

Equipment/Supplies:

- Gloves
- Personal protective equipment (PPE)
- Alcohol wipes
- Gauze squares (sterile or clean according to office policies)
- Adhesive bandage
- Sterile disposable lancet
- Collection tubes or containers
- Sharps container
- Equipment and supplies to perform testing
- Patient's chart/EHR

PROCEDURAL STEPS	DETAILS AND/OR RATIONALE
1. ***Incorporating critical thinking skills when performing patient care,*** check the provider's order and complete the laboratory requisition form.	Always verify that tests being drawn are correct according to provider's orders.

continues

PROCEDURE 24-4 continued

PROCEDURAL STEPS	DETAILS AND/OR RATIONALE
2. Wash your hands and apply PPE. The types of PPE worn during a capillary stick may vary from one facility to another.	PPE must be worn to protect the individual collecting the specimen. Wearing all PPE will decrease your risk of contamination.
3. Assemble all the necessary equipment and label all tubes.	Always assemble extra equipment in case of a problem to eliminate the need for a second capillary stick. Labeling tubes before the puncture helps to eliminate error later.
4. Identify the patient using two identifiers and identify yourself.	Always clearly identify the patient before collecting the sample to be sure you are collecting the specimen from the correct person.
5. ***Explain the rationale for performance of the procedure, showing awareness of the patient's concerns related to the procedure being performed.***	If the patient is informed about the procedure, the patient will be more relaxed and less fearful.
6. Select the fleshy portion of the patient's distal middle or ring finger on the nondominant hand.	Using the nondominant hand will result in less pain for the patient throughout the day.
7. Apply a warm compress to the area or have the patient run the hands under warm water.	This will open up the blood vessels in the area, promoting better blood flow.
8. Clean the site with alcohol and allow it to air dry, or dry wipe with a gauze square (Figure 24-37).	Sticking the finger while it is wet with alcohol will sting the patient.
9. Grasp the finger securely and puncture the fingertip perpendicular to the whorls of the fingerprint (Figure 24-38).	Puncturing the fingertip across the fingerprints, not parallel to them, will provide a better blood sample.
10. Dispose of the lancet in the sharps container according to OSHA guidelines (Figure 24-39).	Proper disposal of sharps reduces the possibility of accidental needlesticks.
11. Wipe away the first drop of blood before beginning the sample collection.	The first drop of blood can be diluted with tissue fluid, resulting in an erroneous result.
12. Hold the finger, applying pressure by gently squeezing and releasing the fingertip.	Gentle pressure to the finger will increase blood flow.

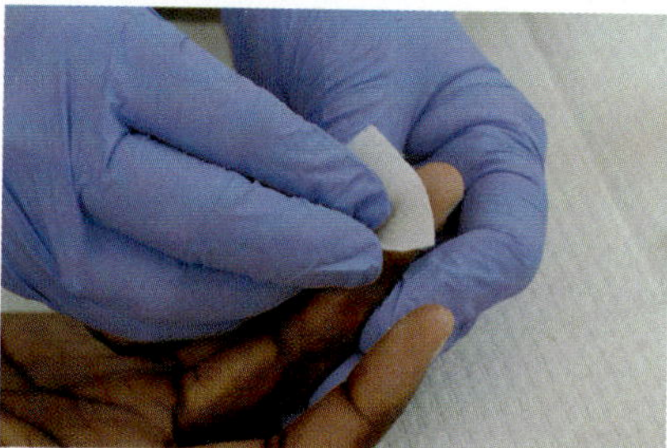

Figure 24-37 ■ Cleanse the tip of the finger with alcohol.

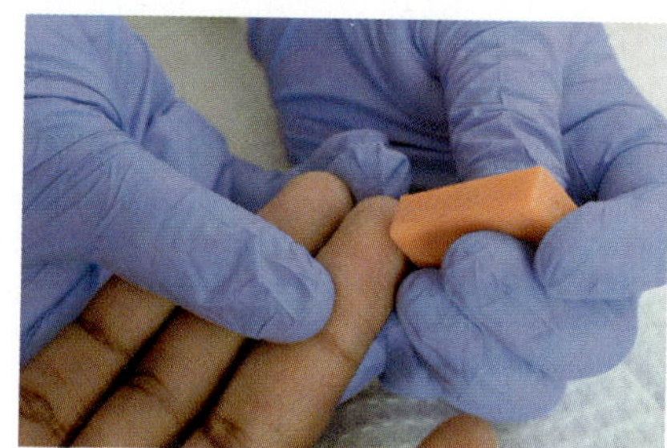

Figure 24-38 ■ Firmly grasp the distal portion of the finger and lance the tip of the finger perpendicular to the whorls of the fingerprint.

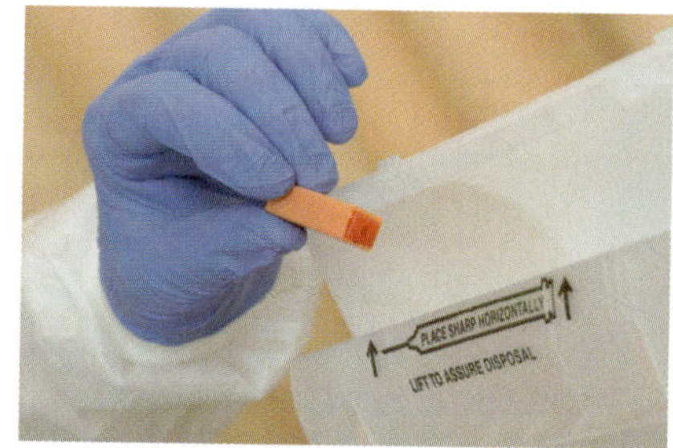

Figure 24-39 ■ Immediately dispose of the used lancet.

continues

PROCEDURE 24-4 continued

PROCEDURAL STEPS	DETAILS AND/OR RATIONALE
13. Collect needed samples either in a capillary tube or microcollection tube (Figures 24-40 and 24-41).	
14. Ask the patient to apply gentle pressure with a clean or sterile gauze square to the puncture site.	Pressure will help to stop bleeding and decrease bruising at the puncture site.
15. Check the puncture site and apply a bandage, if necessary.	Never allow the patient to leave before checking the site to make sure the bleeding has stopped.
16. Dismiss the patient.	
17. Properly dispose of all used equipment according to OSHA standards.	Disposing of contaminated equipment reduces the possibility of accidental exposure to the health care worker.
18. Clean the work area.	
19. Remove gloves and wash your hands.	
20. Document the procedure in the patient's chart.	Include the collection method, location, and tests performed.

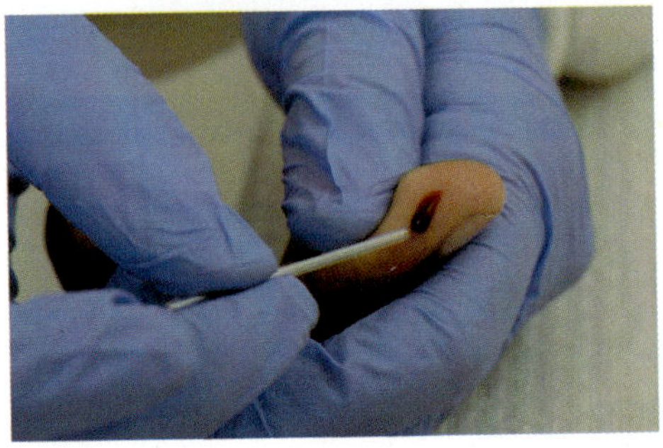

Figure 24-40 ■ Collect the specimen into a capillary tube.

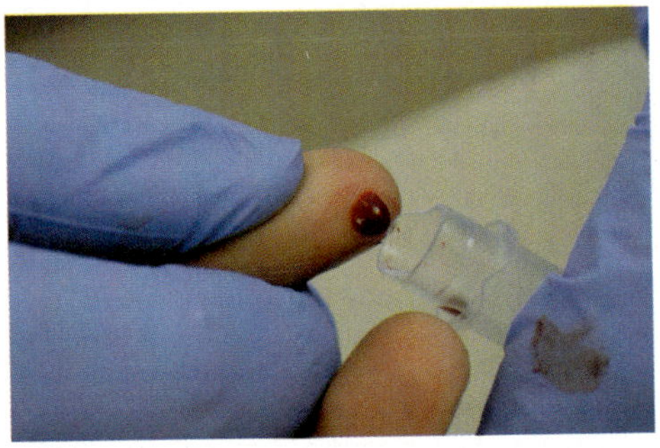

Figure 24-41 ■ Collect the specimen into a Microtainer tube.

DOCUMENTATION EXAMPLE:

11-08-XX 12:30 p.m	Capillary puncture, R.middle finger. 2 heparinized capillary tubes collected for microhematocrit per Dr. Christoper. Hct. 28%. Jessica Hunnicutt, CMA (AAMA)----------

CHAPTER SUMMARY

- Phlebotomy is the name given to the procedure of collecting blood samples. Each health care facility will have specific professionals.
- As blood is circulated throughout the body, it transports oxygen, carbon dioxide, nutrients, waste products, and hormones.
- Venipuncture is an invasive procedure in which a vein is punctured to obtain a blood sample.
- A tourniquet is applied to the patient's arm 3 to 4 inches above the puncture site to constrict blood flow and enlarge the veins.

- The different types of needles used to perform venipuncture include multisample needles for use with the evacuated tube system, hypodermic needles for use with a syringe, and winged infusion (butterfly) needles used for both systems.
- The syringe method is used to obtain blood from patients with fragile or small veins that tend to collapse when using the vacuum tube method.
- The syringe has three main parts: the barrel, with graduated markings in mL or cc; the sterile tip where the needle attaches; and the plunger, which fits tightly inside the barrel.
- The most common method of collecting a blood sample is by using the evacuated or vacuum tube method. This method facilitates the collection of numerous tubes of blood with one stick.
- Blood collection tubes used with the vacuum tube method are designed to automatically withdraw a precise, premeasured volume of blood. Vacuum tubes may contain special additives that perform different functions.
- An anticoagulant added to a collection tube prevents the blood from clotting.
- The winged infusion or butterfly set is used to collect blood from small or difficult veins, usually in the hand.
- The median cubital vein is usually the vein of choice for blood draws. If that vein is not available, your second choice should be the cephalic vein (located on the thumb side of the arm). The basilic vein (located on the inner side of the arm) should not be used unless the other two veins are not available due to nerves that run on the inside of the arm.
- Blood collection tubes must be filled in a specific order, according to the order of draw established by the National Committee of Clinical Laboratory Standards (NCCLS), now referred to as the Clinical and Lab Standards Institute (CLSI).
- When drawing multiple tubes the following order of draw should be followed: Blood cultures, clear/discard tube, light blue top tube, plain red top, gold (SST), green, lavender, and gray. The same order of draw should be used for the syringe method.
- Adverse reactions that may occur during a blood draw include the following: pain, nausea, syncope, seizures, hematoma, prolonged bleeding, nerve damage, infection, reflux, and vein damage or collapse.
- A hematoma is swelling or bruising resulting from an accumulation of blood at the puncture site.
- Medical assistants should be aware of reasons for venipuncture failure and take the proper steps to prevent failure from occurring.
- Criteria for specimen rejection includes: improper labeling, improperly filled tubes, using the wrong tubes, incorrect collection time, incorrect specimen handling, or sending hemolyzed or lipemic specimens.
- The capillary puncture, also known as a skin or dermal puncture, is used when a venipuncture is not the preferred method of specimen collection. Examples of testing that can be performed from a capillary sample of blood includes: hemoglobins and hematocrits, blood glucose, cholesterol studies, and coagulation studies.
- When the provider suspects that the patient may have bacteremia (bacteria in the blood), a culture may be ordered.

CERTIFICATION REVIEW QUESTIONS

1. When transporting vacuum tubes to the laboratory, they should be:
   a. protected from light.
   b. placed on ice.
   c. placed in a heating block.
   d. kept in an upright position.
2. A failed venipuncture can occur for all the following reasons except:
   a. insufficient tube vacuum.
   b. collapsed vein.
   c. needle inserted bevel up.
   d. needle bevel is against the wall of the vein.
3. Failure to invert additive tubes can result in:
   a. hematoma.
   b. hemolysis.
   c. lipemia.
   d. microclot formation.
4. The anticoagulant of choice for most hematology studies is:
   a. sodium citrate.
   b. EDTA.
   c. sodium fluoride.
   d. lithium heparin.

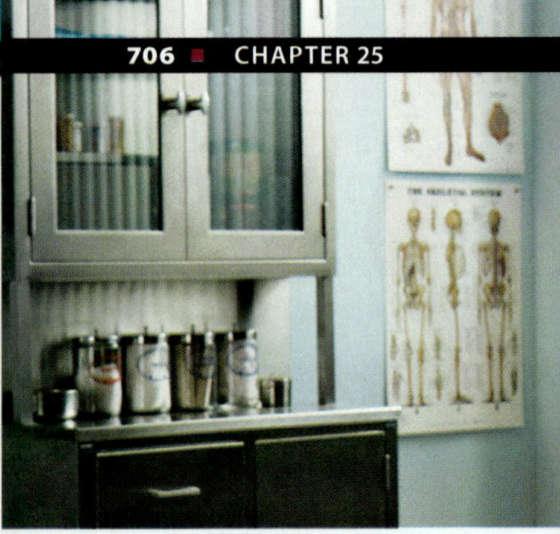

DEVELOPMENTAL OBJECTIVES

After completing this chapter, you should be able to:

1. Correctly spell and define the essential terms.
2. Instruct a patient in the collection of clean-catch midstream urine specimen and 24-hour specimen, and ensure that she understands.
3. Discuss the importance of quality control and proper record keeping.
4. List the three parts of a complete urinalysis and describe the test methods employed in each.
5. Perform a physical and chemical examination of urine.
6. Demonstrate preparing a slide for microscopic examination.
7. Record the normal values for a physical and chemical urinalysis and state the clinical significance of abnormal readings of all three parts of the urinalysis.
8. State the medical assistant's role in urinalysis and the scope of practice according to state laws.
9. Perform urinary catheterization if allowed to by state law.
10. Demonstrate steps for preparing a urine specimen for transport.

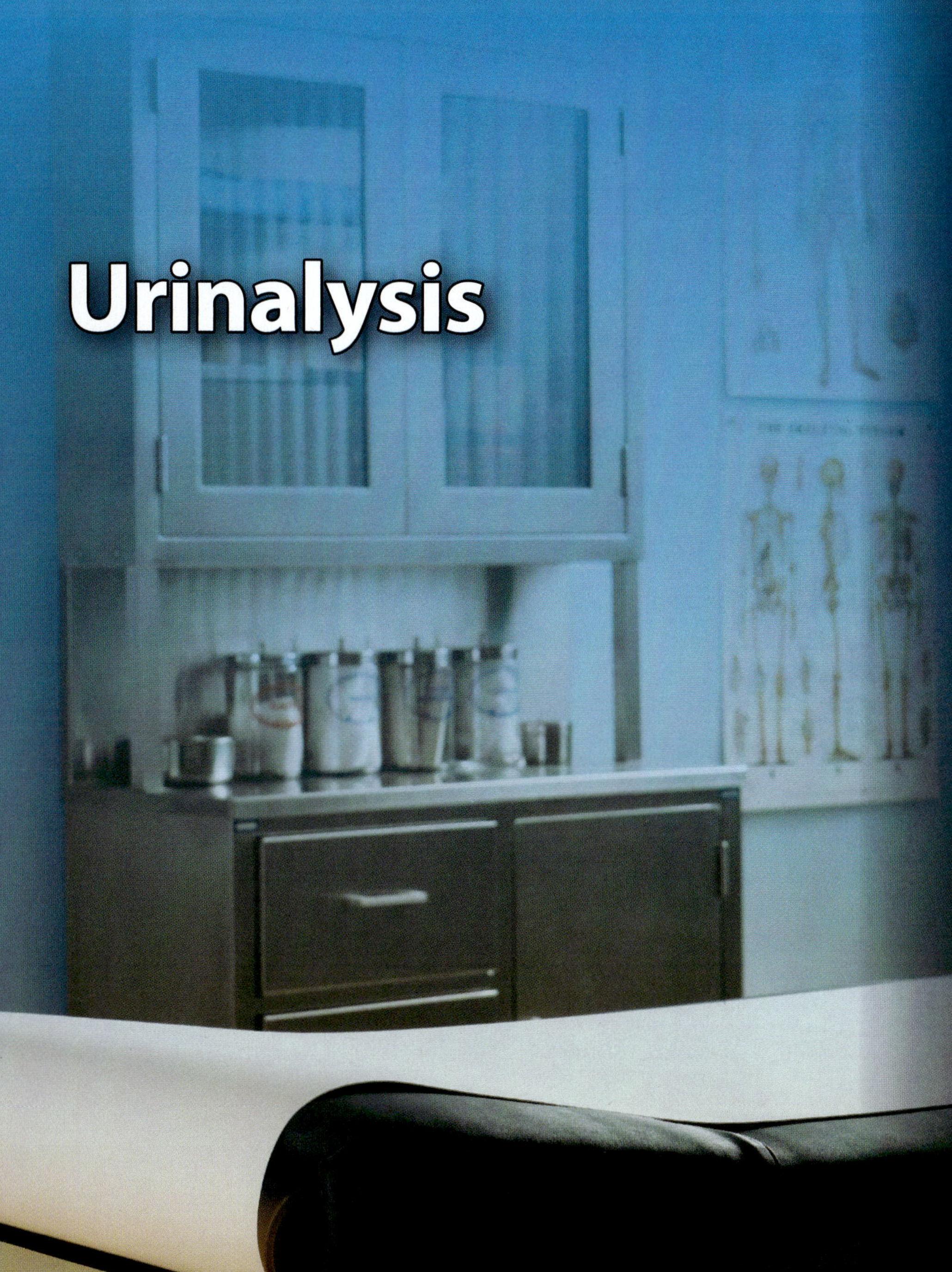

25 Urinalysis

ESSENTIAL TERMS

bilirubin
casts
catheterize
clean-catch midstream (CCMS) specimen
hematuria
hemoglobinuria
ketones
pH
random collection
reagent test strip
refractometer
renal threshold
sediment
specific gravity
supernatant
turbid
urea
urochrome
voiding

CHAPTER OUTLINE

Urinalysis Medical Terms and Abbreviation Review

Composition of Urine

Specimen Collection
- General Collection Guidelines
- Urine Specimen Containers
- Methods of Collection
- Types of Urine Specimens

Quality Control

Routine Urinalysis
- Physical Examination
- Chemical Urinalysis

Microscopic Examination

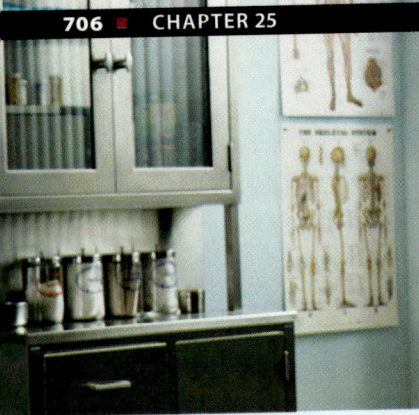

DEVELOPMENTAL OBJECTIVES

After completing this chapter, you should be able to:

1. Correctly spell and define the essential terms.
2. Instruct a patient in the collection of clean-catch midstream urine specimen and 24-hour specimen, and ensure that she understands.
3. Discuss the importance of quality control and proper record keeping.
4. List the three parts of a complete urinalysis and describe the test methods employed in each.
5. Perform a physical and chemical examination of urine.
6. Demonstrate preparing a slide for microscopic examination.
7. Record the normal values for a physical and chemical urinalysis and state the clinical significance of abnormal readings of all three parts of the urinalysis.
8. State the medical assistant's role in urinalysis and the scope of practice according to state laws.
9. Perform urinary catheterization if allowed to by state law.
10. Demonstrate steps for preparing a urine specimen for transport.

- The different types of needles used to perform venipuncture include multisample needles for use with the evacuated tube system, hypodermic needles for use with a syringe, and winged infusion (butterfly) needles used for both systems.
- The syringe method is used to obtain blood from patients with fragile or small veins that tend to collapse when using the vacuum tube method.
- The syringe has three main parts: the barrel, with graduated markings in mL or cc; the sterile tip where the needle attaches; and the plunger, which fits tightly inside the barrel.
- The most common method of collecting a blood sample is by using the evacuated or vacuum tube method. This method facilitates the collection of numerous tubes of blood with one stick.
- Blood collection tubes used with the vacuum tube method are designed to automatically withdraw a precise, premeasured volume of blood. Vacuum tubes may contain special additives that perform different functions.
- An anticoagulant added to a collection tube prevents the blood from clotting.
- The winged infusion or butterfly set is used to collect blood from small or difficult veins, usually in the hand.
- The median cubital vein is usually the vein of choice for blood draws. If that vein is not available, your second choice should be the cephalic vein (located on the thumb side of the arm). The basilic vein (located on the inner side of the arm) should not be used unless the other two veins are not available due to nerves that run on the inside of the arm.
- Blood collection tubes must be filled in a specific order, according to the order of draw established by the National Committee of Clinical Laboratory Standards (NCCLS), now referred to as the Clinical and Lab Standards Institute (CLSI).
- When drawing multiple tubes the following order of draw should be followed: Blood cultures, clear/discard tube, light blue top tube, plain red top, gold (SST), green, lavender, and gray. The same order of draw should be used for the syringe method.
- Adverse reactions that may occur during a blood draw include the following: pain, nausea, syncope, seizures, hematoma, prolonged bleeding, nerve damage, infection, reflux, and vein damage or collapse.
- A hematoma is swelling or bruising resulting from an accumulation of blood at the puncture site.
- Medical assistants should be aware of reasons for venipuncture failure and take the proper steps to prevent failure from occurring.
- Criteria for specimen rejection includes: improper labeling, improperly filled tubes, using the wrong tubes, incorrect collection time, incorrect specimen handling, or sending hemolyzed or lipemic specimens.
- The capillary puncture, also known as a skin or dermal puncture, is used when a venipuncture is not the preferred method of specimen collection. Examples of testing that can be performed from a capillary sample of blood includes: hemoglobins and hematocrits, blood glucose, cholesterol studies, and coagulation studies.
- When the provider suspects that the patient may have bacteremia (bacteria in the blood), a culture may be ordered.

CERTIFICATION REVIEW QUESTIONS

1. When transporting vacuum tubes to the laboratory, they should be:
   a. protected from light.
   b. placed on ice.
   c. placed in a heating block.
   d. kept in an upright position.
2. A failed venipuncture can occur for all the following reasons except:
   a. insufficient tube vacuum.
   b. collapsed vein.
   c. needle inserted bevel up.
   d. needle bevel is against the wall of the vein.
3. Failure to invert additive tubes can result in:
   a. hematoma.
   b. hemolysis.
   c. lipemia.
   d. microclot formation.
4. The anticoagulant of choice for most hematology studies is:
   a. sodium citrate.
   b. EDTA.
   c. sodium fluoride.
   d. lithium heparin.

5. The butterfly method should be used:
   a. routinely.
   b. for hand sticks.
   c. rarely.
   d. for large veins.

6. The medical assistant should only attempt a venipuncture on a patient:
   a. three times.
   b. two times.
   c. once.
   d. as many times as necessary.

7. When filling the following tubes from a syringe draw, which tube should be filled first?
   a. Lavender
   b. Red
   c. Green
   d. Blue

8. The most common vein selected to perform a venipuncture is:
   a. cephalic.
   b. median cubital.
   c. antecubital.
   d. brachial.

9. Leaving the tourniquet in place longer than one minute can cause:
   a. hematoma.
   b. hemostasis.
   c. hemoconcentration.
   d. viscosity.

10. The vein or veins that should only be used if absolutely necessary for blood draws includes which of the following?
   a. Cephalic
   b. Medial
   c. Basilic
   d. Both a and b

STUDY RESOURCES

Resources to Test and Reinforce Your Knowledge:	
Certification Review Questions	Take this end-of-chapter quiz
Workbook	• Complete the activities for Chapter 24 • Perform the procedures for Chapter 24 using the Competency Checklists
Resources to Promote Critical Thinking:	
***Solve the Case* Activities**	• Consider these case studies and discuss your conclusions
Learning Lab	• Module 21: Clinical Procedures
MindTap	• Complete Chapter 24 readings and activities

REFERENCES

Estridge, B. & Reynolds, A. (2012). *Basic clinical laboratory techniques* (6th ed.). Clifton Park, NY: Cengage Learning.

Lindh, W., Pooler, M., Tamparo, C., Dahl, B., & Morris, J. (2014). *Delmar's comprehensive medical assisting: Administrative & Clinical Competencies* (5th ed.). Clifton Park, NY: Cengage Learning.

INTRODUCTION

The term *urinalysis* literally means an analysis of the urine. It can offer the provider a multitude of information about different body systems, disease states, and metabolic processes occurring within the body. Urine is plentiful, easily collected, and results can often be obtained quickly right in the medical office. However, the test results are only as good as the specimen collected. Correct specimen collection and handling are critical to ensuring accurate results. Along with technical skills, you must use your best interpersonal communication skills when assisting patients through the urinalysis procurement procedures.

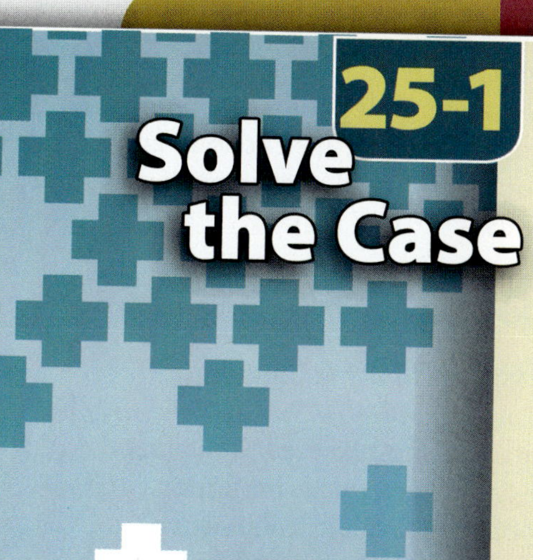

Mrs. Pankey, an 84-year-old established patient in otherwise good health, has complained of bladder irritation and blood in her urine for several months. Dr. Shapiro, her family doctor, has treated her with antibiotics that seem to relieve the irritation but she continues to see blood in her urine. Dr. Shapiro now recommends that she see a specialist and his medical assistant sets up an appointment for a referral.

1. **What type of specialist do you think Mrs. Pankey is being referred to?**
2. **What interpersonal skills would you use when assisting Mrs. Pankey in her care?**
3. **Since Mrs. Pankey's bladder irritation has subsided, do you think the infection is gone?**

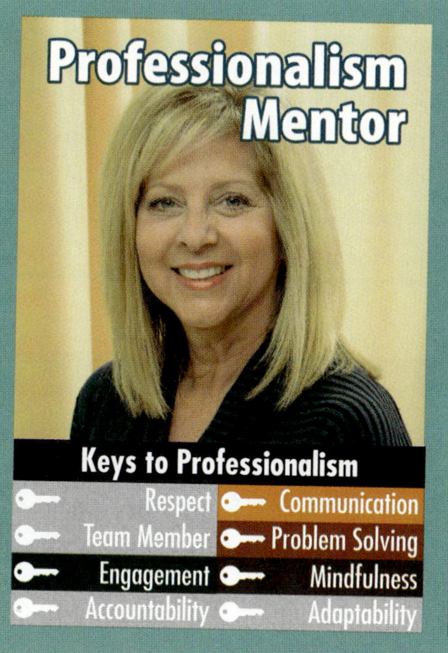

During a recent orientation, I asked my group of medical assistants why they perform urine testing? Most answered to help detect certain disorders, some said to look for abnormal results, and one medical assistant stated that urine can be used as a screening tool for pregnancy or drug testing. When I asked the group what they could do to ensure the most accurate results, the room became silent. It seems they were so used to performing this "routine" test that they had forgotten that even the most routine test has specific criteria that should be followed each time testing is performed in order to ensure accuracy, a key component of being a successful medical assistant. Throughout this text, we have discussed the importance of being mindful as you perform tasks that assist the provider in formulating a diagnosis. Will you become complacent when performing routine tasks or will you demonstrate excellence by being vigilant to the fine details of each test you perform? My advice: choose excellence! ■

URINALYSIS MEDICAL TERMS AND ABBREVIATION REVIEW

Medical assistants who perform urinalysis testing should be familiar with the medical terms associated with urinary flow and other urinary conditions in Table 25-1. Common abbreviations associated with urinary testing can be found in Table 25-2.

COMPOSITION OF URINE

Urine is produced in the kidneys as they filter the blood. Once it is formed, it consists of approximately 95% water and 5% dissolved substances. The following are the primary dissolved substances found in the urine:

- Urea: end product of protein metabolism
- Uric Acid: end product of dietary purines
- Creatinine: end product of muscle breakdown
- Ammonia: a smell in concentrated urine from bacterial breakdown of urea
- Calcium: excess dietary calcium is excreted through urine
- Magnesium: excess dietary magnesium is excreted through urine
- Phosphorus: excess dietary phosphorus is excreted through urine

Other substances can also be found in urine, depending on a person's diet and general state of health. If there are pathological conditions present, substances such as glucose, albumin, ketones, blood, bilirubin, pus, casts, and bacteria may also be found in the urine. See Table 25-3 featured later in the chapter to learn more about these components.

Certain substances such as glucose are usually entirely reabsorbed by the body if they are present in the blood at normal levels. However, if the concentration of a substance in the blood is so high that the kidneys cannot reabsorb all of it, a **renal threshold** s reached and the excess spills into the urine and is detected by chemical urinalysis. Surpassing the renal threshold usually indicates the presence of an abnormal condition or disease.

SPECIMEN COLLECTION

Many professional attributes are used when performing urinalysis. The interaction with patients is important so they clearly understand the instructions and are comfortable with your tactfulness, professionalism, and communication skills.

General Collection Guidelines

- Collect a sufficient volume of urine (minimum of 10 mL).
- Appropriate lab containers must be used. Containers brought from home are not acceptable for testing.
- Properly label the specimen container (not the cap). Labeling should include patient name, date, and time.
- If a specimen must be collected during menses, it must be noted on the laboratory requisition form (e.g., patient menstruating).
- List all current medications, supplements, and herbals being taken by the patient.

Table 25-1 Medical Terms That Describe Urinary Symptoms

Term	Description	Term	Description
Anuria	Inability to make urine	Incontinence	Inability to control urine flow
Dysuria	Painful urination	Nocturia	The need to urinate during the night
Frequency	The need to urinate frequently	Oliguria	Scanty urination
Hematuria	Blood in the urine	Polyuria	Excessive urination
Hesitancy	Difficulty in beginning urine flow	Urgency	The urgent need to urinate

Table 25-2 Common Abbreviations Used for Urinalysis Testing and Diagnosis

Abbreviation	Meaning	Abbreviation	Meaning
C&S	Culture and sensitivity	RBC	Red blood cells
CCMS	Clean-catch midstream	RTE	Renal tubular epithelial cells
CLIA	Clinical Laboratory Improvement Amendments	SG or SpGr	Specific gravity
HPF	High-power field	UA	Urinalysis
LPF	Low-power field	U/C	Urine culture
PPM	Provider performed microscopy	UTI	Urinary tract infection
QNS	Quantity not sufficient	WBC	White blood cells

- Make sure the patient fully understands the collection procedure. The instructions should be given verbally and written instructions should be posted in the restroom.
- Be patient and sensitive to patient embarrassment when explaining the collection procedure.
- Specimens must be refrigerated if testing cannot be completed while the urine is still warm. Refrigerated urine should be tested within two hours of collection.

Urine Specimen Containers

A variety of different containers are available for urine collection (an example is shown in Figure 25-1). A urine specimen cup is used for random specimen testing and consists of a clean, dry container with a tight-fitting lid. Urine specimen cups must be sterile when there is a probability that a urine culture will be ordered, such as when a patient displays urinary symptoms. A sterile container is always used for **catheterized** specimens. A 24-hour urine collection requires a container into which a preservative has been added.

All urine containers ***(not the lids)*** must be properly labeled before the specimen is collected. (Lids are removed for testing, so if the lid were labeled, the label could be lost.) Labeling requirements may vary by facility, but generally include the following:

- Patient's name
- Date and time of collection

Additional information on the label might be required in large facilities and/or to outside laboratories:

- Age
- Gender
- Provider's name

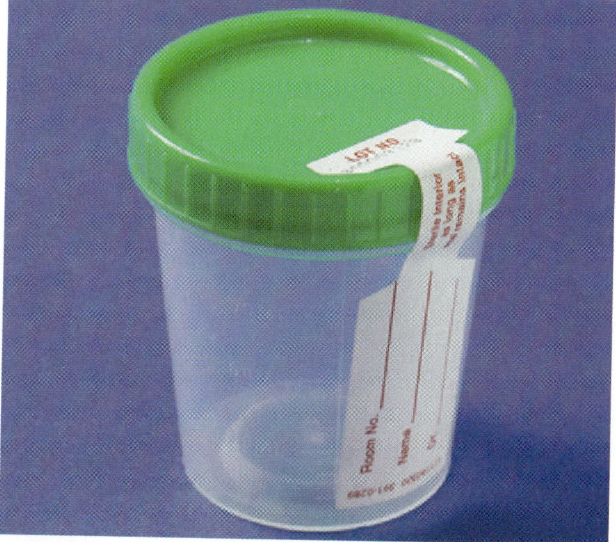

Figure 25-1 ■ An example of a clean-catch collection container.

Methods of Collection

Urine may be collected in a sterile manner as with catheterized specimens or, more frequently, collected by the patient as a clean-catch midstream specimen.

Clean-Catch Midstream Specimen

The distal urethra and the urinary meatus usually contain normal flora (nonpathogenic bacteria normally present), which can interfere with test results. For this reason, providers will usually request a **clean-catch midstream (CCMS) specimen**. This method flushes the normal flora from the urethra and urinary meatus before the specimen is collected. This method should be used for all urine specimen collections in the outpatient settings except for sterile collection by catheterization. The clean-catch midstream method can often be used for bacterial culture and sensitivity testing, avoiding the need to collect a sterile specimen by catheterization.

The initial step in collecting a clean-catch midstream specimen is to cleanse the genital area. After thoroughly cleansing the genital area, the patient should be instructed to collect the midstream portion of the urine flow (males by maintaining the foreskin retraction and females while still spreading the labia folds). The patient should begin voiding into the toilet, then catch a portion of the stream in a sterile specimen container, and finish **voiding** (urinating) into the toilet. A specimen collected by this method should be as free of contamination as possible. Specific oral instructions for men and women should be explained so the patient clearly understands the rationales and printed instructions should be posted in patient restrooms where collection takes place. Instructions for males should be posted on the wall behind the toilet, and instructions for females should be posted as viewed from a sitting position on the door of the stall. Laminating or otherwise protecting the paper instructions is useful for keeping the documents clean. Refer to Procedure 25-1 for a full procedure and photographs of proper collection technique.

Pediatric Urine Collection

Occasionally a parent is asked to collect a pediatric urine sample at home from an infant or a toddler who is still wearing diapers. Detailed oral and written instructions should be provided to avoid problems with the collection process. A special collection bag that attaches to the infant's skin over the genital area (Figure 25-2) is used to collect the urine. This process is sometimes difficult for the parent so the medical assistant may apply the pediatric urine collection bag to the patient in the

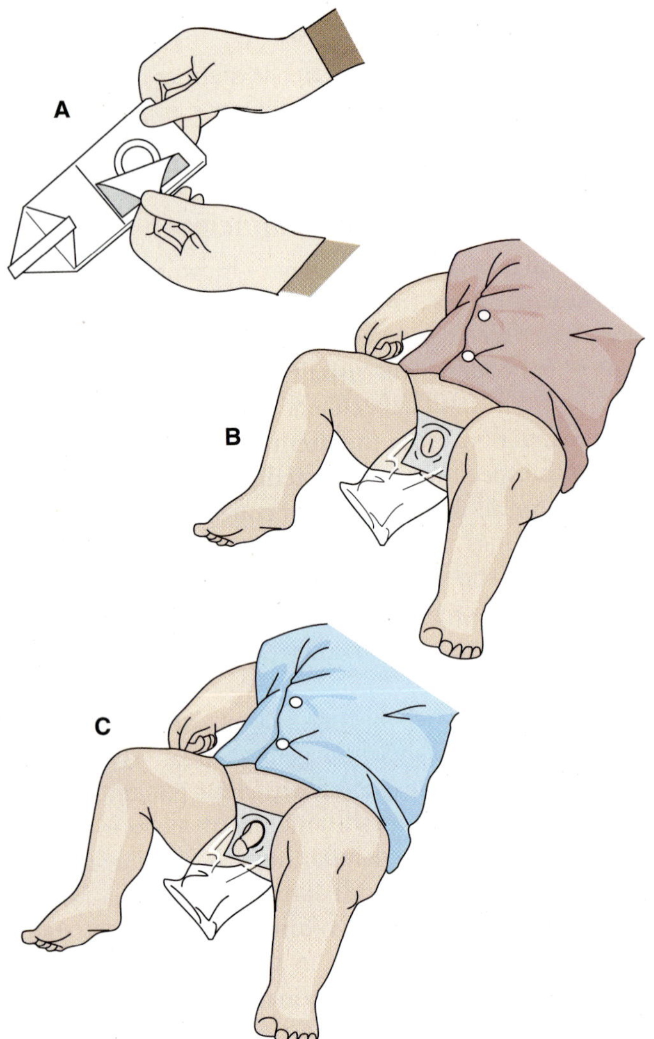

Figure 25-2 ■ An example of a pediatric urine collection system.

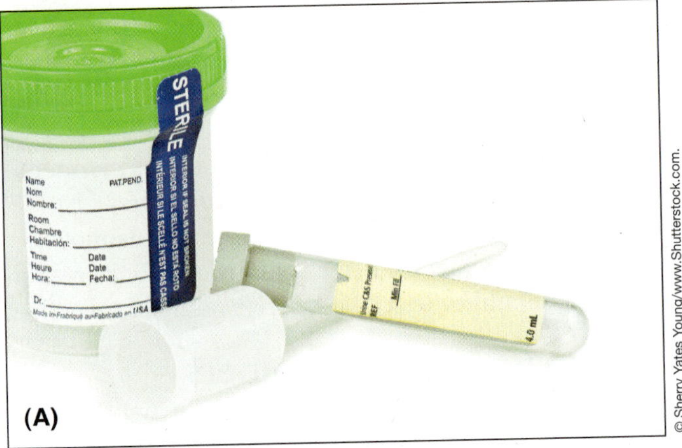

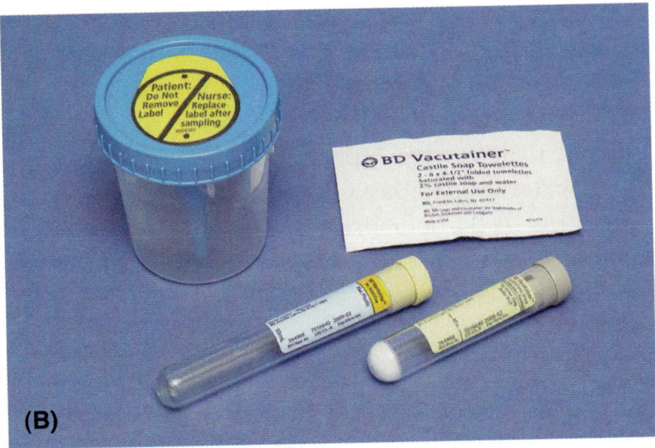

Figure 25-3 ■ Examples of two different C&S urine collection kits. The tube is placed in the tube adapter and the straw is placed in the urine.

office and is often able to collect the specimen right away. Once the specimen has been collected, it is transferred to a specimen container for transport.

Catheterization

Collecting a urine specimen by catheterization requires passing a soft, flexible sterile tube (catheter) through the urethra into the bladder to obtain a sterile specimen for culture and sensitivity.

Urinary catheterizations may be within the scope of practice for the medical assistant, depending on individual state law. Many medical assistant programs provide urinary catheterization training and education or the skill may be acquired on the job.

Because this type of specimen collection is invasive into a sterile area, strict sterile procedures must be adhered to and, as with all sterile procedures, extra care should be taken when handling the patient, supplies, and specimen to avoid contaminating the sterile specimen. The provider will usually order a culture and sensitivity test on this type of specimen. The medical assistant is responsible for preserving the urine and preparing the specimen for transport to the lab. A special transport kit (Figure 25-3) for a urine culture and sensitivity test is used when sending the specimen to the laboratory. Refer to Procedure 25-4 for the full procedure.

Types of Urine Specimens

Different types of specimens and methods of collection will depend on the substance being measured or studied. Common methods of collection used in provider's offices include random collection and 24-hour specimens.

Random Collection Specimen

A **random collection** method is used to collect urine that requires no special preparation and in lab-provided sterile containers with tight-fitting lids. Random collection is the easiest of all urine collections and is used when only a dipstick reading is necessary.

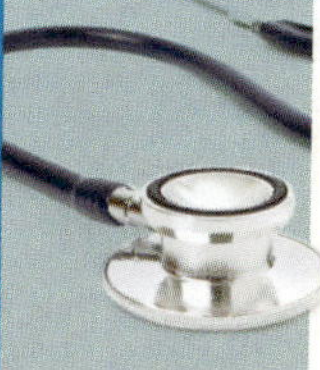

Field Smarts

Urine specimen containers should be handled following the precautions below:

- All body fluid specimens, including urine, should be considered potentially infectious.
- PPE such as a face mask, goggles, and especially gloves should be worn to protect the medical assistant against possible contamination.
- Urine should be tested as soon as possible, preferably while still warm.
- Food and drinks should never be stored in the same refrigerator as urine and other lab specimens.
- Properly dispose of urine specimens by pouring the specimen down the drain of the "dirty" sink while running water. A "dirty" sink is used to dispose of specimens such as urine, while a "clean" sink should only be used for hand washing and cleaning. Some facilities request all urine specimens be flushed down the toilet.

24-Hour Urine Collection

Certain substances, such as protein, sodium, creatinine, potassium, and urea nitrogen, can vary in concentration in the urine over a 24-hour period. Factors such as exercise, metabolism, and food and water intake can affect the amount of a substance present in a randomly collected urine sample, but the 24-hour urine collections are quantitative tests measuring the specific amount of a substance the body is excreting over the 24-hour period. Detailed verbal and written instructions must be provided to the patient to ensure an accurate collection of the 24-hour urine sample.

A large, opaque container is provided by the laboratory for the patient to collect all urine voided over a 24-hour period (Figure 25-4). A preservative may be included in the container to ensure the integrity of the specimen. Once the patient returns the 24-hour specimen to the laboratory, the total volume of urine is measured and recorded on the laboratory requisition form. An aliquot (portion) of the well-mixed specimen is sent to the laboratory for quantitative analysis, and the remaining urine is discarded.

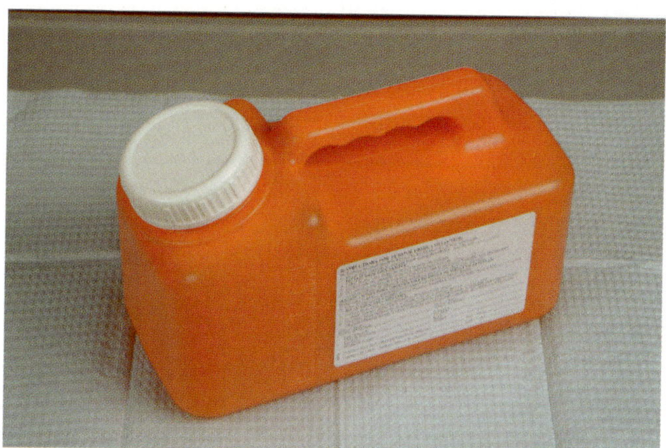

Figure 25-4 ■ A 24-hour urine specimen collection container.

QUALITY CONTROL

Quality control is important to ensure safe and accurate test results in every area of laboratory testing, including urine testing. CLIA requires all physician office laboratories (POLs), including waived category labs, to perform quality control tests and to maintain documentation.

According to CLIA regulations, the manufacturer's directions should be followed regarding how often controls should be performed on test strips, reagents, or automated urine analyzers. Multistix, as with most reagent test strip manufacturers, requires quality controls be run every 24 hours once a container is opened. Results from control testing should be recorded on a quality control log.

Figure 25-5 shows a quality control kit and several control urines. Controls must be prepared and stored according to specific manufacturer's directions. Each manufacturer will provide an acceptable value range for the specific control sample. If the control does not fall within the acceptable range of results, patient results cannot be reported until the problem is corrected. All chemicals, including control reagents, can become compromised and can result in inaccurate quality control tests. Because controls generally expire one month after opening, sometimes, starting with a fresh package of controls can solve the problem.

Digital, electronic, and automated medical instruments need to be calibrated to make sure that they are within normal parameters. Calibrations should be performed at the beginning of each procedure using the instrument.

Health Coach

24-Hour Collection

Advise the patient that early morning is the most common time to begin a 24-hour collection. She is to drink and eat as she normally does during the 24 hours of collection. Instruct the patient to label the large container with her name and any other required information on the form. Instruct the patient to empty her bladder without saving the urine from the first voiding of the day. All urine for the next 24 hours is to be collected. She is to note the time the collection begins on the form provided. A smaller container is used to collect each specimen and is then poured into the large container following collection. The patient is cautioned to use care during this process to avoid splashing and possible exposure to the chemical preservative in the large container. At the end of the 24-hour period, the first specimen of the second morning is collected and added to the collection bottle and the time is noted (the time the collection ended). Labs may have different procedures for storing the urine. Some analytes need to be stored at room temperature, while others need refrigeration. Make certain the patient knows the proper way to store the urine to avoid any problems. The large specimen container should be returned to the laboratory as soon as possible.

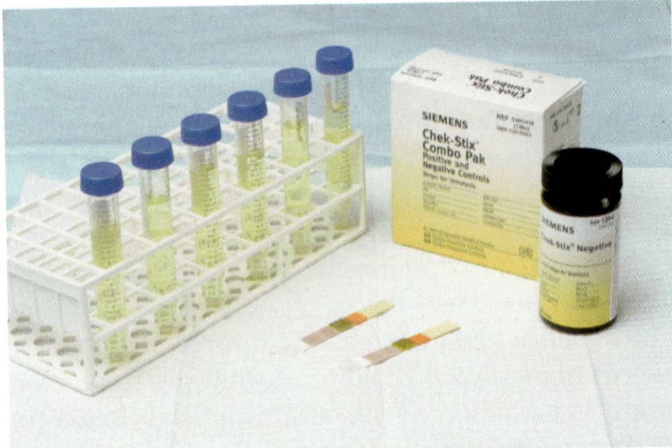

Figure 25-5 ■ An example of a urine control collection kit and control urines.

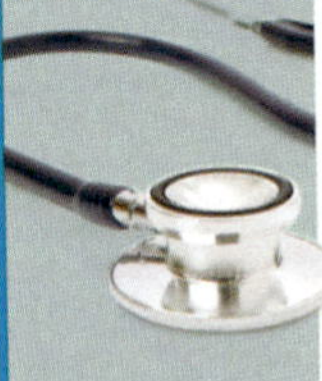

Field Smarts

Troubleshooting in the POL is a necessary skill attainable by all medical assistants if logical step-by-step protocol is followed. When a problem arises, such as a control result that is not within range, an unexpected test result on a patient sample, or an instrumentation problem, you must be able to recognize and solve the problem. The best protocols are written and involve a step-by-step detailed investigation of all phases of the testing process. Patience and perseverance are required. Review every aspect of the test method, procedure, instrumentation, and reagents, until the problem is resolved.

ROUTINE URINALYSIS

The routine urinalysis is one of the most commonly performed tests in the medical office. This simple test can supply the provider with information about the urinary tract as well as other body systems. It is often performed as part of a complete physical exam or used as a diagnostic tool when a specific condition is suspected.

A fresh, well-mixed urine specimen must be used for testing. If the specimen has been refrigerated it must be brought to room temperature before testing. Table 25-3 lists possible changes that can occur if urine is allowed to be unpreserved or unrefrigerated at room temperature. A routine urinalysis consists of three parts: physical, chemical, and microscopic examination.

Physical Examination

The physical portion of the urinalysis consists of observing the color and clarity and measuring the specific gravity of the urine. Volume should also be assessed to determine if the quantity is sufficient for testing. For

Table 25-3 Changes in Unpreserved/Unrefrigerated Urine Specimens

Component	Possible Changes
Clarity	Becomes cloudy due to bacterial growth
Odor	Can become stronger due to bacterial growth and the breakdown of **urea** to ammonia
pH (acidity or alkalinity)	Increases due to bacterial growth
Glucose	Decreases due to utilization of glucose as a food source by bacteria
Ketones (normal products of fat metabolism)	Decrease due to the conversion of ketones to acetone, which is not detectable by the reagent strip
Bilirubin (product of the breakdown of red blood cells)	Decreases due to breakdown when exposed to light
Urobilinogen	Decreases due to breakdown as a result of oxidation
Nitrite	Increases due to multiplication of bacteria
Red blood cells (RBCs) and white blood cells (WBCs)	Decrease due to the breakdown of the cells
Casts (structures formed due to accumulation of protein, cells, and fats in the renal tubules)	Decrease due to decomposition
Bacteria	Increase due to perfect conditions for multiplication

accurate testing, a minimum of 10 mL of urine is necessary. If the volume is found to be less than 10 mL, a notation of QNS (quality not sufficient) should be made on the report form. The physical and chemical examination of urine can still be performed (clearly noting the QNS), but the microscopic examination is often difficult for the provider to assess accurately. Nevertheless, follow clinic policy about testing the QNS sample because special considerations may be given to pediatric samples.

Urine odor is not usually recorded as part of the physical urinalysis; however, any abnormal odor should be noted on the report. A foul odor could indicate an increase in bacteria, which could indicate infection, whereas a sweet, fruity odor could indicate a potentially serious condition known as ketoacidosis (a condition that occurs in patients with uncontrolled diabetes).

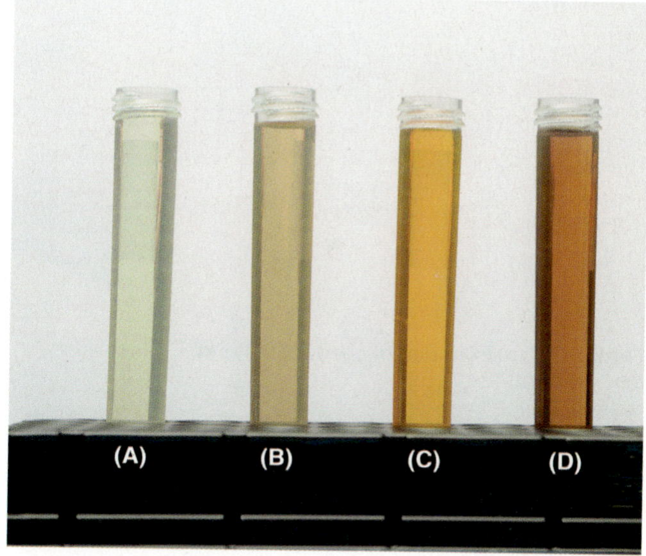

Figure 25-6 ■ Different urine colors: (a) Straw, (b) Light yellow, (c) Yellow, (d) Amber.

Color

The color of urine is produced by an orange-yellow pigment known as **urochrome**. Normal colors of urine range from straw (almost colorless, diluted) to amber (deep yellow/orange, concentrated) (see Figure 25-6).

Abnormal colors may indicate an infection or disease or may simply be caused by certain drugs or foods. Table 25-4 lists urine colors and their possible significance.

Clarity/Turbidity

Freshly voided urine should be clear, but may become cloudy upon standing. Cloudy urine can have a nonpathological cause, such as squamous epithelial cells or mucous (especially in female patients). The most common pathologic causes of urine cloudiness are bacteria, white blood cells, red blood cells, protein, or lipids. Semen, fecal contamination, vaginal creams, and powder can also affect the clarity of the urine.

To evaluate the clarity of the urine, the specimen should be mixed well, placed in a clear container, and held in front of a light source. Common terms used to describe urine clarity are clear, hazy, cloudy, or **turbid** (opaque or unable to see through the specimen).

Table 25-4 Urine Colors and Potential Causes

Color	Potential Cause
Colorless	Very dilute urine due to increased fluid intake; chronic renal disease
Straw to yellow	Normal color
Dark yellow/amber	Very concentrated urine; first-morning void; dehydration (as seen with vomiting, diarrhea, excess fluid loss)
Bright yellow	Vitamin B_{12}
Orange	Some medications such as Pyridium used to treat bladder irritation, Coumadin (blood thinner), vitamin C, excessive dietary beta-carotene
Cloudy pink, red, or reddish/brown	Red cells present in the urine (**hematuria**) due to kidney stones, UTI, or menstrual contamination **Hemoglobinuria**: red cells have ruptured and hemoglobin has been released into the urine
Yellow/brown or yellow/green	Bilirubin present; bilirubin converted to biliverdin, such as in liver disease
Green or blue/green	Urinary tract infection caused by *Pseudomonas* bacteria; various medications
Brown	RBCs aged and oxidized to methemoglobin; various medications and some foods
Black	Various medications, liver conditions

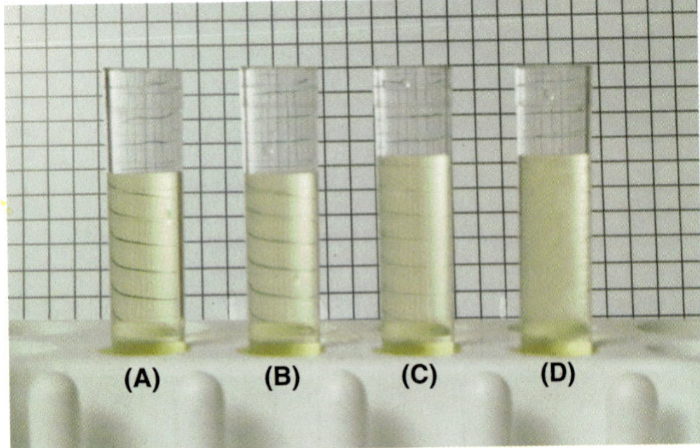

Figure 25-7 ■ Examples of clarity of urine: (a) Clear, (b) Hazy, (c) Cloudy, (d) Turbid.

The medical assistant should become proficient at determining urine clarity. Figure 25-7 shows examples of urine clarity.

Specific Gravity

The **specific gravity** of urine provides information on the kidneys' ability to concentrate and dilute urine. It measures the concentration of dissolved substances present in the urine by comparing the weight of the urine to the weight of an equal volume of distilled water. The more concentrated the urine, the higher the specific gravity. For instance, in diabetes mellitus, the presence of dense (heavy) glucose molecules in the urine causes the specific gravity to be high. Specific gravity of distilled water is 1.000. Specific gravity of urine can range from 1.005 (dilute urine) to 1.030 (concentrated urine).

The three most common methods to measure urine specific gravity are the refractometer, which gives either a scale or digital readout; reagent test strips, which are color assessed; and the automated urine analyzer. All three methods are classified in the Waived Tests Category by CLIA.

Refractometer

The **refractometer** is a device used to measure the refractive index of urine, which is directly related to its specific gravity. The digital instrument (Figure 25-8) and the more commonly used handheld refractometer (Figure 25-9) require only a drop of urine and are the most cost-effective for smaller primary care clinics. The digital refractometer results are shown in a window and the handheld refractometer results are read directly from a calibrated scale. Figure 25-10 shows the scale within the handheld refractometer.

Refractometers are calibrated before each use by measuring a drop of distilled water and adjusting the instrument to read 1.000. A small screwdriver is provided with the handheld refractometers for making the adjustments.

Chemical Urinalysis

The second part of a complete urinalysis is the chemical exam. Results from this part of the analysis can provide the practitioner with valuable information about the patient's kidney and liver function, carbohydrate metabolism, and acid–base balance.

The chemical exam is performed using either a reagent test strip or an automated urine analyzer. The **reagent test strip** consists of a narrow plastic strip with

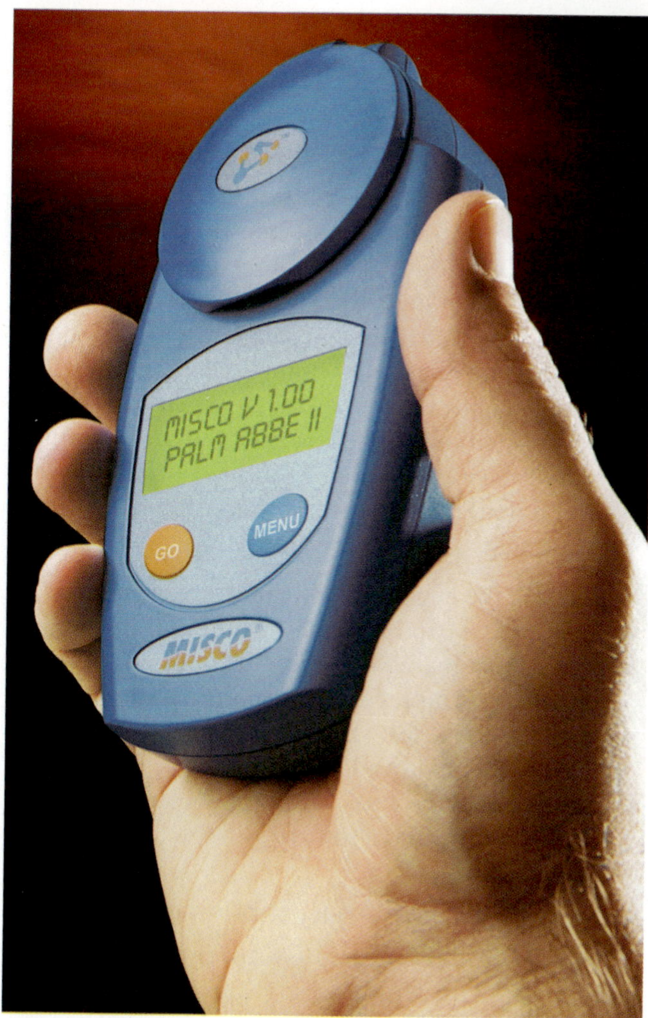

Courtesy of MISCO Refractometer

Figure 25-8 ■ A digital refractometer.

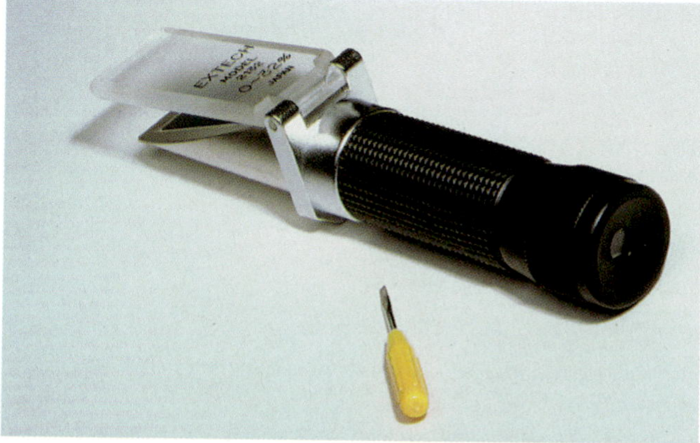

Figure 25-9 ■ A handheld refractometer with a screwdriver to make adjustments.

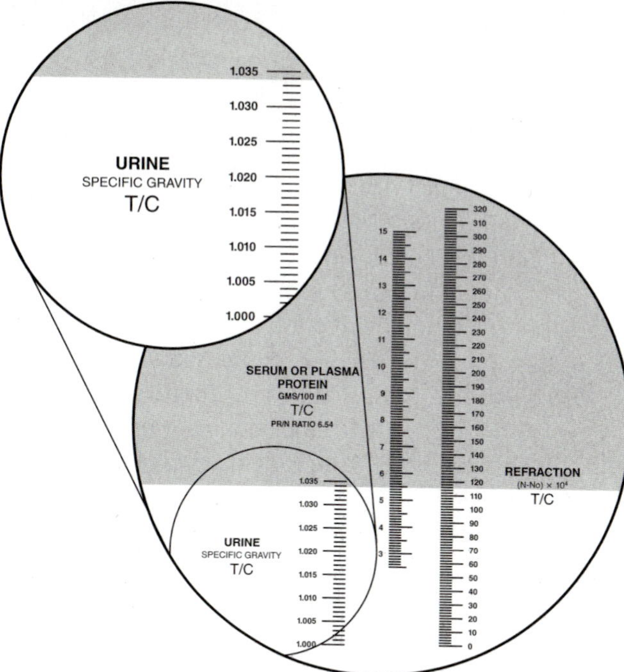

Figure 25-10 ■ A handheld refractometer scale.

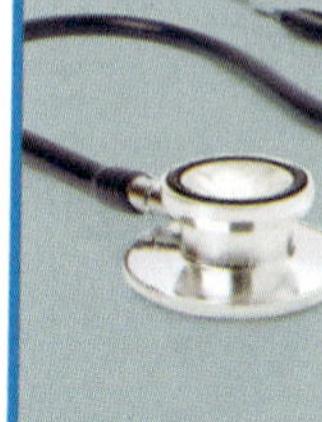

Field Smarts

Several factors can impact the integrity of chemical reagent strips, including expiration, light, moisture, and temperature. Always check the expiration date on the bottle before using. Rotate stock when new stock comes in to avoid expiration. Store test strip containers in a clean dry environment at the temperature listed on the bottle. One sure indicator that the strips have been compromised is any color change on the test pads. Always check the test pads on the test strips upon removing them from the bottle. If the color of the pads of the strips does not match the first row on the color chart on the bottle, the test strips should not be used.

pads. When dipped in urine, the pads will change color due to a chemical reaction, indicating the presence of certain substances in the urine. Reagent strips come in an opaque bottle (to protect the test pads from light), must be stored at a specific temperature range, and must be protected from moisture. When performing the reagent strip test, only the number of strips to be used should be removed. The bottle should be

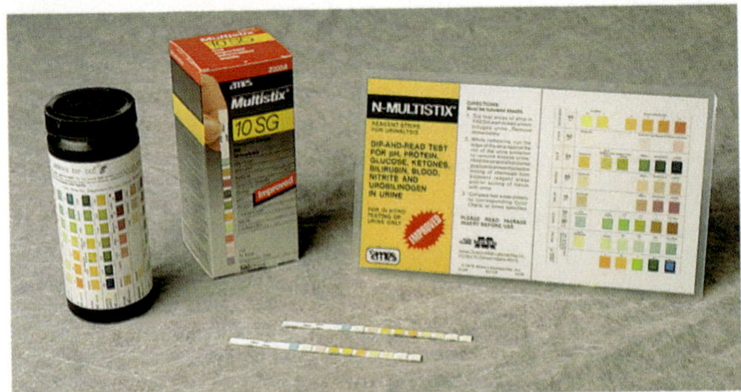

Figure 25-11 ■ Chemical reagent test strips with color-coded chart.

recapped immediately to protect the strips from moisture and light.

Reagent test strips are available from several different manufacturers and each type may vary slightly. Always follow individual manufacturers' recommendations for handling the strips and the timing of test results. We will reference the Multistix 10 SG® brand in this text. The "10" indicates that there are 10 tests included on the strips and the SG indicates that specific gravity is included in this option. There are many brands of reagent test strips available and many test choices within each brand. Figure 25-11 shows the Multistix 10 SG® reagent strip and the reference chart found on the bottle.

Chemical analysis of urine using a reagent test strip requires precise timing of the readings to ensure accurate results. Table 25-5 lists the chemical tests available on the Multistix 10 SG® reagent test strips, the normal values, and the clinical significance of positive results. When using paper charts, the results should be recorded on a testing form provided by the manufacturer, and in the lab section of the EHR when using electronic charts.

See Procedure 25-2 for the steps necessary to perform a physical and chemical urinalysis, which includes plating a specimen for microscopic analysis.

Quality Control for Reagent Test Strips

Reagent test strips must be tested using a commercially prepared control sample with known value ranges to ensure that the test strips and automated urine analyzer are in good working order. Control samples should provide both positive and negative results. Results of all controls and reagent lot numbers must be recorded in a quality control log. Remember, patient results cannot be reported unless the results of the control sample fall within the expected range. If the control sample is tested and does not fall within the acceptable range, the following steps should be performed:

- Recheck the expiration date of the reagent strips.
- Recheck the expiration date of the control sample.
- Be sure that manufacturer's directions were followed when preparing the control sample.
- Ensure that the test strips and controls have been properly handled and stored.
- Repeat the control test, using a new set of controls and/or new bottle of test strips.

Automated Urine Analyzers

Automated urine analyzers are accurate, easy to use, and becoming more affordable (Figure 25-12a–h). The health care worker dips the reagent strip into the urine, blots it, and places it into the instrument. The instrument automatically reads the reagent strip and prints out the results. Figure 25-13 illustrates examples of reports from an automated analyzer.

Table 25-5 Multistix 10 SG® Results

Component	Normal Value	Clinical Significance of Positive or Elevated Results
pH	4.5–7.0	Specimen not fresh; UTI
Protein	Negative/trace	Renal disease; extreme exercise; high fever; dehydration
Glucose	Negative	Diabetes; pancreatic disease; advanced kidney disease
Ketones	Negative	Starvation; low-carbohydrate/high-fat diet; uncontrolled diabetes
Blood (hemolyzed and nonhemolyzed)	Negative	Hemolytic anemia; kidney or urinary tract damage; kidney stones; UTI; menstrual contaminant
Bilirubin	Negative	Hepatitis or liver disease; possible bile duct obstruction
Urobilinogen	0.1–1.0	Liver dysfunction; hemolytic diseases
Nitrite	Negative	UTI; presence of bacteria
Leukocytes	Negative	Urinary tract infection and inflammation
Specific gravity	1.005–1.030	Kidney dysfunction; diabetes

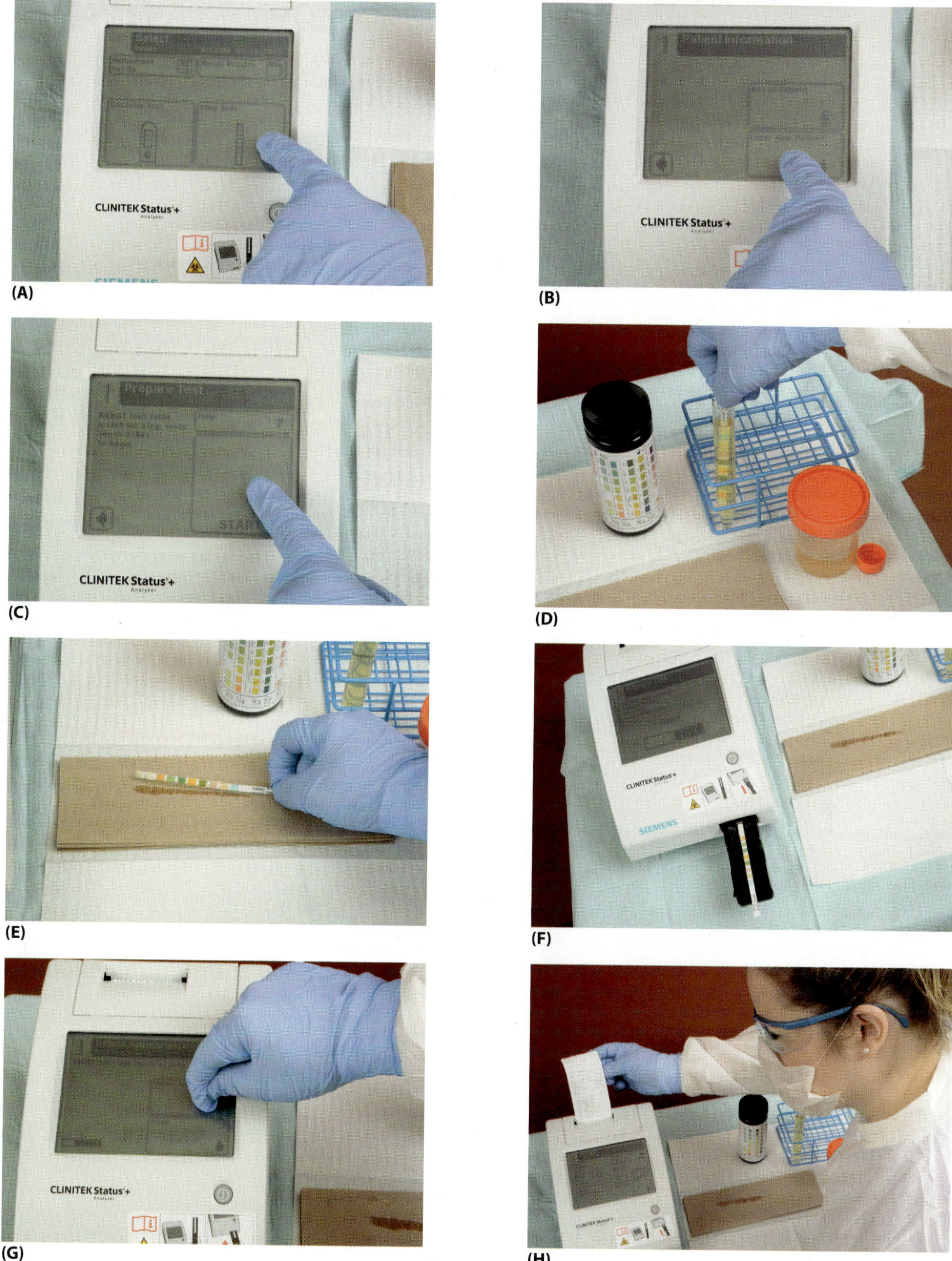

Figure 25-12 ■ (a) After mixing urine in tube, turn machine on and select "Strip Test." (b) Enter the operator and patient information. (c) Select the "Start Button." (d) Immediately dip the test strip into the urine. (e) Place strip on its side against paper towel so that the pads don't run onto each other, or blot the pads with a gauze square. (f) Immediately place the strip on the test strip holder. (g) Enter the color and clarity of the urine. (h) At the end of testing, results will appear in the LCD or will print directly from the analyzer.

(A) Brenda Stoaks 03-18-20XX

Test	Result	Flag
GLU	Negative	
BIL	Negative	
KET	Negative	
SG	<=1.005	
*BLO	Trace-intact*	
PH	5.5	
PRO	Negative	
URO	0.2 E.U./dL	
NIT	Negative	
LEU	Negative	

(B) Katie Oberleitner 06-18-20XX

Test	Result	Flag
GLU	Negative	
BIL	Negative	
KET	Negative	
SG	>=1.030	
*BLO	Trace-intact*	
PH	5.5	
*PRO	100 mg/dL	*
URO	0.2 E.U./dL	
NIT	Negative	
LEU	Negative	

(C) Janie Carter 12-02-20XX

Test	Result	Flag
GLU	Negative	
BIL	Negative	
KET	Negative	
SG	1.015	
*BLO	Large	*
PH	5.5	
*PRO	100 mg/dL	*
URO	0.2 E.U./dL	
*NIT	Positive	*
*LEU	Moderate	*

Figure 25-13 ■ Example of automated reports from a chemical analyzer.

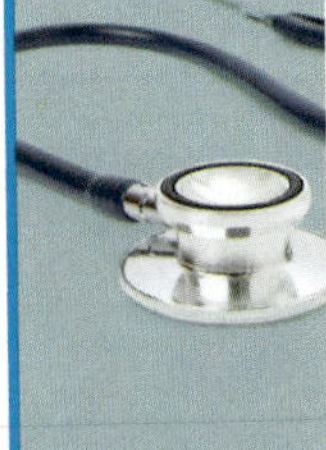

Field Smarts

Care must be taken to understand each brand of test strips, as they will all differ slightly. The strip must be read in the correct order and at the proper timing intervals to ensure accurate results. Also, when testing urine for possible infection, collect specimen in a C&S transport kit and prepare culture tubes before testing urine (see Procedure 25-3). If not using a C&S transport kit, pour urine from the original container into a test tube. Dip the urine dipstick into the test tube rather than the cup. This keeps the urine as sterile as possible in the event the urine is sent out for a culture and sensitivity test.

MICROSCOPIC EXAMINATION

The microscopic exam of the urine sediment is the third part of a complete urinalysis. CLIA categorizes the microscopic examination as a PPM (provider-performed microscopy) procedure, which means that the medical assistant may not perform this portion of the urinalysis. However, the medical assistant may prepare the slide and place it on the microscope for the physician to read. In order to prepare the slide, the medical assistant will pour 10–12 mL of urine into a clear plastic tube and spin it in the centrifuge at 1500–2000 rpm for five minutes. Refer to Figure 25-14 to see a urine centrifuge properly balanced. Tubes should be placed directly across from each other and have equal volumes of urine (or water if a balance tube is used). Label the tube prior to filling it with the patient's last name and label the slide with the patient's initials, especially if more than one sample is being tested. After centrifugation, the medical assistant will remove the tube from the unit and pour the **supernatant** (the clear liquid that remains after spinning the urine; Figure 25-15) out into the designated sink, leaving about 0.5–1 mL in the tube to re-suspend the sediment. The **sediment** (the solid material in the bottom of the tube) is mixed to re-suspend it, and a drop is placed on the labeled microscope slide. A cover slip is applied and the slide is ready for the microscopic examination. Leave the microscope's light turned off (the lamp's heat will dry the specimen) and notify the provider that the slide is ready to be read. If the provider cannot read the slide within a few minutes, prepare a fresh slide for analysis. Procedure 25-2 lists the steps for preparing a urine sediment slide.

Urine sediment can be viewed under the microscope either with or without the use of a sediment stain such as Sedi-Stain® (see Figure 25-16). Many of the elements found in urine are very light and almost colorless when viewed under the microscope. A stain added to the sediment can make things easier to see by adding color to the elements. Whether or not to use a sediment stain is

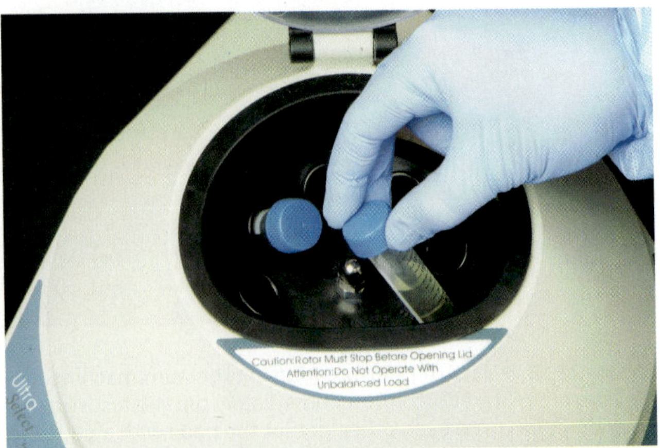

Figure 25-14 ■ Example of a properly balanced centrifuge.

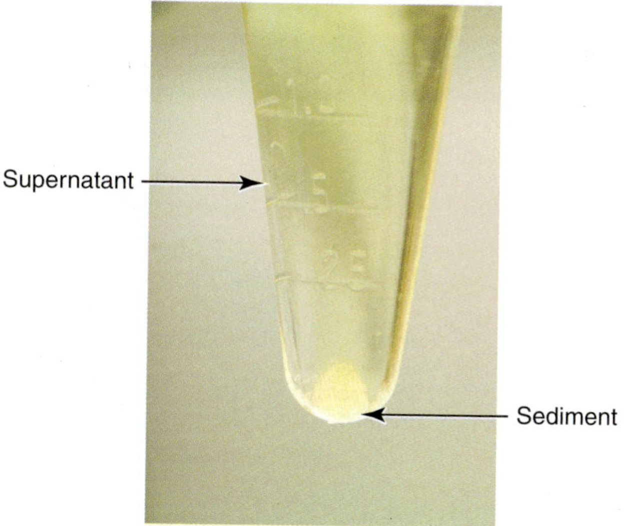

Figure 25-15 ■ Example of a tube of urine after centrifugation.

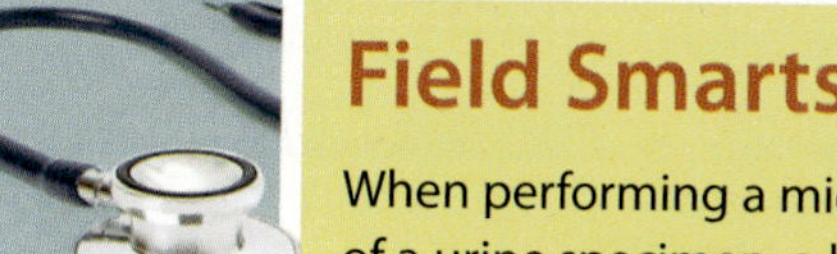

Field Smarts

When performing a microscopic exam of a urine specimen, a handy tool to have available is a color atlas of urinary sediment. Medical assistants do not perform the microscopic portion of the urinalysis but should be familiar with the location of the atlas in the office if the provider requests it. Table 25-6 features pictures with the most common elements found in urine, along with significant information about each one.

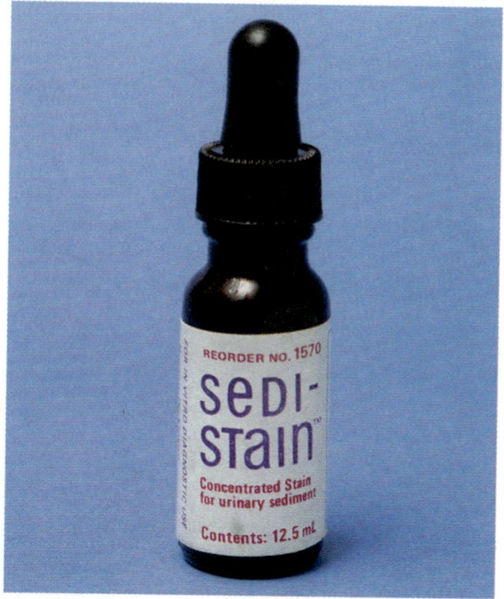

Figure 25-16 ■ A bottle of Sedi-Stain®.

up to individual provider preferences. If your provider requests the use of a sediment stain, it should be added to the sediment prior to mixing.

Another important factor to consider is the correlation of the reagent strip findings with the microscopic findings. For instance, if the reagent strip is positive for leukocytes, then white blood cells should be seen and reported during the microscopic exam. Another factor is the correlation of one chemistry result to another. A positive glucose almost always correlates with positive ketones, and a positive nitrite frequently correlates with white blood cells. Blood might be positive on the test strip, but red blood cells might not be seen under microscopic examination. If the red blood cells have hemolyzed, which can happen in very alkaline urine, the provider performing the microscopy might only see the ruptured membranes, or "ghost red blood cells."

Table 25-7 is a reagent strip/microscopic correlation chart that illustrates the connection between reagent strip findings and the anticipated microscopic results.

Table 25-6 Mini Atlas of Urinary Sediment

Element	Reported As	Normal Value	Pathological Conditions	Distinctive Features	Causes of Identification Error
Hyaline cast	Range of numbers/LPF*	0–2/LPF	Congestive heart failure Acute glomerulonephritis Chronic renal pyelonephritis	Colorless with rounded ends	Hair Mucus Fiber

*Abbreviations used in this table:
LPF: Low-power field
HPF: High-power field
RTE: Renal tubular epithelial cell

continues

Table 25-6 Mini Atlas of Urinary Sediment *(continued)*

Element	Reported As	Normal Value	Pathological Conditions	Distinctive Features	Causes of Identification Error
Red blood cell (RBC) cast	Range of numbers/LPF	0/LPF	Damage to glomerulus Nephron bleeding Proteinuria In a healthy individual, following strenuous exercise	Orange/red color	Clumps of RBCs
White blood cell (WBC) cast	Range of numbers/LPF	0/LPF	Upper UTI Pyelonephritis Differentiates upper UTI from lower UTI	Granular appearance/ white cells have multilobed nuclei	Clumps of WBCs
Granular cast	Range of numbers/LPF No longer differentiated as coarse or fine	0/LPF	Pyelonephritis Glomerulonephritis Stress and exercise	Coarse/fine granules contained within the cast	Clumps of crystals
Red blood cells (RBC)	Range of numbers/HPF	0–3/HPF	Damaged glomerular membrane Malignancy Renal calculi Trauma	No nucleus Biconcave disk	Yeast Oil droplets Air bubbles
White blood cells (WBC)	Range of numbers/ HPF	0–5/HPF	Infection/inflammation Cystitis Bacterial infection Urethritis Prostatitis	Cells possess granules Multilobed nucleus	Renal tubular epithelial cell
Squamous epithelial cell	Rare, few, moderate, many/HPF	Few/HPF	Many might indicate a contaminated specimen and might include mixed bacteria	Largest cell found in urine Large irregular cytoplasm Distinct nucleus approximately the size of a red cell	If folded, may be mistaken for a cast
Transitional epithelial cell	Rare, few, moderate, many/HPF	Rare/HPF	Increased after recent catheterization and tubule injury Malignancy	Sphere-shaped Polyhedral Caudate (tail) Distinct nucleus	Sphere-shaped can resemble RTE
Renal epithelial cell	Rare, few, moderate, many/HPF	More than 2/HPF indicates tubular injury and the specimen should be sent for cytology exam	Tubular injury Tissue destruction	Not totally round Columnar-shaped Cuboidal Large nucleus	Sphere-shaped Granular casts

Table 25-6 Mini Atlas of Urinary Sediment *(continued)*

Element	Reported As	Normal Value	Pathological Conditions	Distinctive Features	Causes of Identification Error
Bacteria	Rare, few, moderate, many/HPF	Rare to few due to contamination during collection method	Lower or upper UTI	Cocci- or bacilli-shaped	Amorphous urates or phosphates
Yeast	Rare, few, moderate, many/HPF	Small amount may be present due to contamination	Diabetes Immunosuppressed patients Vaginal yeast infections	Small, oval Refractive May have a bud	RBCs
Trichomonas vaginalis (parasite)	Rare, few, moderate, many/HPF	None	Sexually transmitted vaginal infection	Pear-shaped with whipping tail Darting movement	WBCs
Mucus thread	Rare, few, moderate, many/HPF	Frequently present in the urine of females	None	Thread-like	Hyaline cast
Spermatozoa	According to lab protocol	May be found following intercourse or nocturnal emission	None	Oval head with long tail	None

Normal Crystals Found in Acid pH	Characteristic Color and Shape	Seen in
Amorphous urates (Not pictured)	Yellow-brown Granular Clumped	Specimens that have been refrigerated, causing a pink sediment that resembles "brick dust" No pathology
Calcium oxalate (may also be found in slightly alkaline urine)	Colorless squares with "X" shape in center Resembles an "envelope"	Renal calculi Foods high in oxalic acid After ingesting tomatoes and asparagus
Uric acid	Yellow-brown Rhombic flat plate with four sides Rosettes	Gout Renal calculi Metabolic disorder
Amorphous phosphate (Not pictured)	Colorless Looks exactly like amorphous urates Has a yellowish-brown color under the microscope	Specimens that have been refrigerated, causing a white precipitate Not associated with pathology

continues

Table 25-6 Mini Atlas of Urinary Sediment *(continued)*

Normal Crystals Found in Acid PH	Characteristic Color and Shape	Seen in
Triple phosphate	Colorless Resemble "coffin lids"	Found in neutral alkaline urine
Calcium carbonate	Colorless "Dog bone" or "dumbbell" shaped	No pathology
Ammonium biurate	Yellow-brown Spicules	Old specimen Ammonia produced by bacteria
Abnormal Crystals	**Color and Shape**	**Pathology**
Cystine	Colorless Hexagon-shaped plates	Cystine reabsorption metabolic disorder Renal calculi
Tyrosine	Colorless to yellow Needles Clumps of rosettes	Severe liver disorders
Leucine	Yellow spheres with central circle and stripes	Severe liver disorders

Courtesy of Bayer Diagnostics

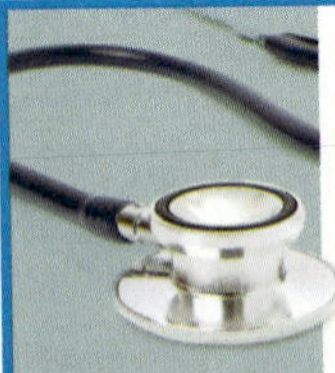

Field Smarts

Important facts to remember when performing a urinalysis:

- Glove before assembling equipment. The outside of the reagent strip bottle and the outside of the specimen container could be contaminated with urine.
- An appropriate urine cup with a tight-fitting lid should be used to obtain the specimen.
- Label the cup, not the lid, with patient name and date/time. Label the tube and slide as well with the patient's initials.
- If a specimen is tested during a female's menses, a notation should be made.
- The specimen must be refrigerated if not tested within two hours of collection and should be brought to room temperature prior to testing.
- *Never* store urine, or any lab specimens, in the same refrigerator with food items.
- Mix the specimen well before beginning the urinalysis.

- Do *not* allow excess urine to run from one reagent pad to the next. This can cause inaccurate readings.
- Proper sequencing and timing when reading results is critical for accurate results.
- Do *not* touch a reagent strip that has been dipped in urine to the outside of the reagent strip bottle.
- Inform the physician when the sample is ready for microscopic examination. Allowing the slide to sit for any length of time, especially with the microscope light on, can dry out the specimen.

Table 25-7 Urinalysis Reagent Strip/Microscopic Correlation Chart

Substance/Related if Found in Urine	Normal Value	Clinical Significance	Correlation	Causes of Error/Interference
Glucose/glucosuria	Negative	Diabetes mellitus Pancreatitis Gestational diabetes Hyperthyroidism	+Ketones (in patients with diabetes)	*False-positive:* Specimens contaminated with bleach or peroxide *False-negative:* Increased specific gravity Increased levels of ascorbic acid/ vitamin C Increased ketones
Bilirubin/bilirubinuria	Negative	Hepatitis Cirrhosis Bile duct obstruction	+Urobilinogen (in patients with liver disease)	*False-positive:* Lodine and Thorazine *False-negative:* Exposure to light Ascorbic acid Increased nitrites
Ketones/ketonuria	Negative	Starvation Diabetic acidosis Vomiting Strenuous exercise	+Glucose (in patients with diabetes)	*False-positive:* Certain medications (Levodopa) Red dyes *False-negative:* Breakdown of bacteria Incorrect timing of reading
Specific gravity (SG or SpGr)	1.005–1.030	Measure of the kidneys' concentrating ability ↑ in diabetes mellitus ↓ in diabetes insipidus		*Increased SG:* Increased protein *Decreased SG:* pH above 6.5
Blood: Hematuria Hemoglobinuria Myoglobinuria	Negative	Glomerulonephritis Calculi Trauma Severe burns Strenuous exercise Muscle wasting	RBCs present on microscopic exam unless the condition is hemoglobinuria, in which case the red cells have lysed and released hemoglobin + Protein	*False-positive:* Menses Bleach peroxidases from bacteria *False-negative:* Increased specific gravity Increased nitrites Captopril use Vitamin C use Unmixed specimens
pH (7.0—Neutral) (Below 7.0—Acidic) (Above 7.0—Alkaline)	4.5–7.0	Metabolic/respiratory acid/base disorders Renal calculi UTI treatment Crystals	pH identification of crystals +Nitrites	*Inaccurate readings:* Allowing urine to run from one test pad to another
Protein/Proteinuria	Negative	Early renal disease Muscle injury Severe infection and inflammation Glomerular problems	+Blood +WBCs +Nitrites	*False-positive:* Disinfectants Detergents *False-negative:* Proteins other than albumin Dilute urines
Urobilinogen/ Urobilinogenuria	0.1–1.0	Hemolytic diseases Hepatitis Cirrhosis Cancer of the liver	+Bilirubin (liver disease)	*False-positive:* Highly pigmented urine *False-negative:* Old specimen Formalin used as a preservative Patients with nitrates Improper storage

Medical assistants are often responsible for placing orders in the EHR for diagnostic testing. Figure 25-17 illustrates a screen shot of an order entry screen with an order for a dipstick panel urinalysis and a microscopic urinalysis. Figure 25-18 illustrates what the order looks like when printed out. This replaces the manual paper lab requisition form that was used in the past.

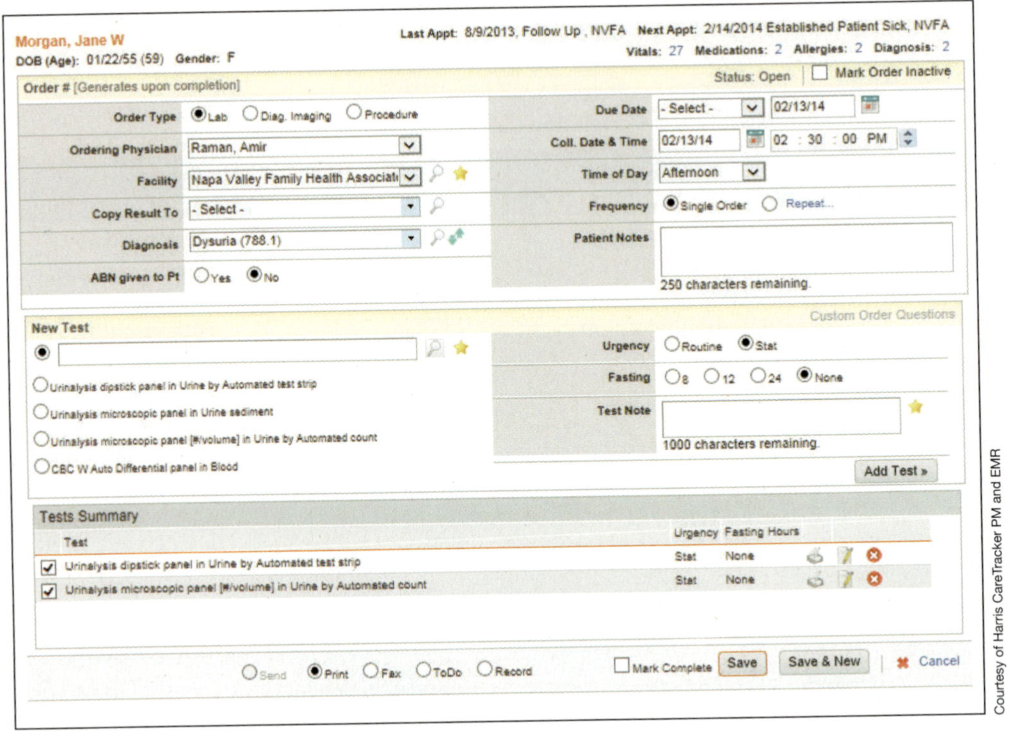

Courtesy of Harris CareTracker PM and EMR

Figure 25-17 ■ An example of an order's screen in an EHR featuring a urine dipstick and microscopic order.

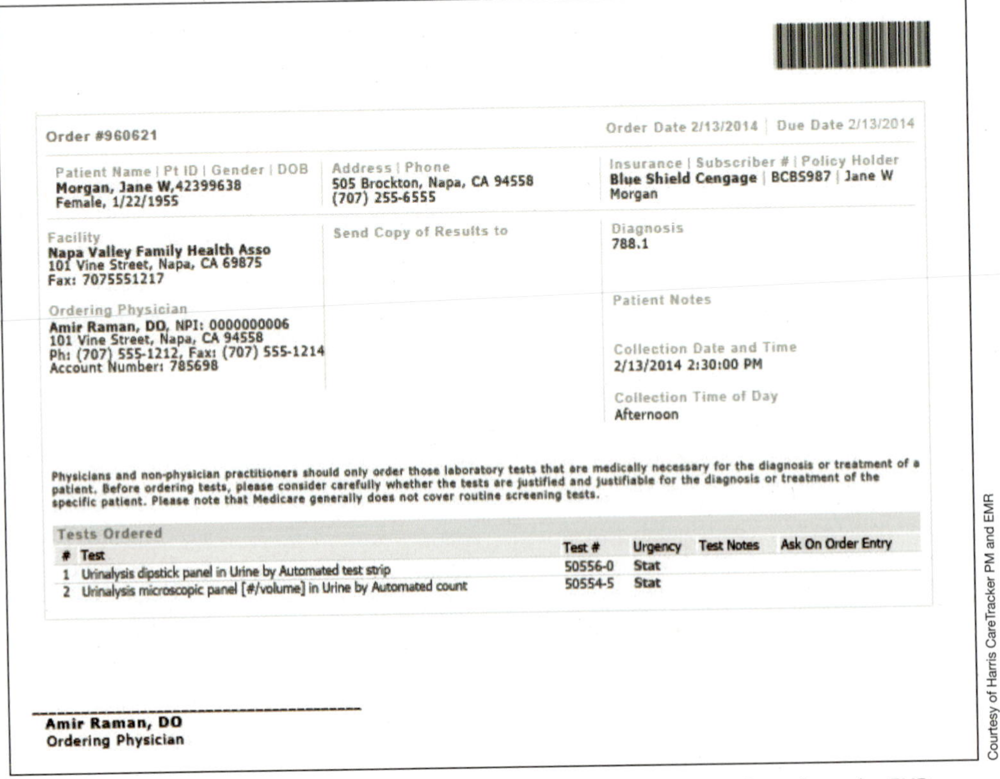

Order #960621

Order Date 2/13/2014 | Due Date 2/13/2014

Patient Name | Pt ID | Gender | DOB
Morgan, Jane W,42399638
Female, 1/22/1955

Address | Phone
505 Brockton, Napa, CA 94558
(707) 255-6555

Insurance | Subscriber # | Policy Holder
Blue Shield Cengage | **BCBS987** | **Jane W Morgan**

Facility
Napa Valley Family Health Asso
101 Vine Street, Napa, CA 69875
Fax: 7075551217

Send Copy of Results to

Diagnosis
788.1

Ordering Physician
Amir Raman, DO, NPI: 0000000006
101 Vine Street, Napa, CA 94558
Ph: (707) 555-1212, Fax: (707) 555-1214
Account Number: 785698

Patient Notes

Collection Date and Time
2/13/2014 2:30:00 PM

Collection Time of Day
Afternoon

Physicians and non-physician practitioners should only order those laboratory tests that are medically necessary for the diagnosis or treatment of a patient. Before ordering tests, please consider carefully whether the tests are justified and justifiable for the diagnosis or treatment of the specific patient. Please note that Medicare generally does not cover routine screening tests.

Tests Ordered

#	Test	Test #	Urgency	Test Notes	Ask On Order Entry
1	Urinalysis dipstick panel in Urine by Automated test strip	50556-0	Stat		
2	Urinalysis microscopic panel [#/volume] in Urine by Automated count	50554-5	Stat		

Amir Raman, DO
Ordering Physician

Courtesy of Harris CareTracker PM and EMR

Figure 25-18 ■ An example of the lab requisition form that can be printed out from the EHR after entering the order for a urinalysis.

25-2 Solve the Case

Review the following notes from Mrs. Pankey's visit with Dr. Shapiro:

Chief Complaint: Mrs. Pankey complains of bladder irritation and visible blood in her urine over the past several months. Dr. Shapiro has treated her with antibiotics but symptoms remain.

Current Medications: Mrs. Pankey's current medications include Synthroid (25 mcg/daily), Crestor (5 mg/day), and Diovan (160/12.5 mg/day).

Vital Signs: BP of 138/78, a pulse rate of 88, and respiration of 16. Patient's height is 5′3″ and weight is 142 pounds.

Assessment Information: The doctor diagnoses the patient today with chronic hematuria.

Lab Report: Today's urinalysis was normal with the exception of moderate blood on the UA dipstick.

Provider's Plan: Refer patient to Dr. John Pettit (urologist), give patient a 30-day refill on her BP medicine, and a handout on chronic hematuria.

Based on the patient's symptoms, the diagnosis, and treatment plans, answer the following questions.

1. **How does Dr. Shapiro's diagnosis and dipstick result correlate with one another?**
2. **Why didn't Dr. Shapiro give the patient a prescription for an antibiotic today?**
3. **A positive result for which pads on the dipstick may have indicated the need for more antibiotic therapy?**
4. **What are your communication concerns when assisting Mrs. Pankey in her care?**
5. **Go to the Internet and look up educational materials for chronic hematuria, and the prescription the doctor asked to be renewed today. Print off the materials and role-play with a classmate discharging the patient and going over educational materials.**

PROCEDURE 25-1

Instruct a Patient on a Clean-Catch Midstream Urine Collection

Objective:

To instruct a patient how to collect a clean-catch midstream urine specimen in order to obtain a specimen appropriate for urinalysis

Equipment/Supplies:

- Urine specimen cup with tight-fitting lid
- Waterproof marking pen
- Cleansing towelettes (3)
- Patient's chart/EHR
- Gloves

continues

PROCEDURE 25-1 continued

PROCEDURAL STEPS	DETAILS AND/OR RATIONALE
1. Wash your hands.	
2. Assemble the necessary equipment.	Assembling all supplies keeps things organized and saves time.
3. Identify the patient using at least two identifiers, and introduce yourself by name and credentials.	Identifying the patient ensures that you are instructing the proper person on specimen collection. Identifying yourself and stating your credentials demonstrates professionalism and reassures the patient.
4. ***Show awareness of a patient's concerns related to the procedure being performed. Incorporate critical thinking skills when performing patient care.***	The patient may be anxious about the testing or embarrassed in regards to the collection procedure. Do your best to make the patient feel comfortable. Consider language, physical, or cognitive limitations that may impair the patient's ability to collect the specimen correctly. Do what you can to assist patients who have limitations or do not understand English well.
5. Label the specimen cup with the patient's name and date/time.	Labeling the cup ensures the sample will be identified as belonging to the right patient.
6. Give the patient gloves (optional), towelettes, and a labeled urine specimen cup and lid.	Gloves may be offered to the patient to keep the hands clean during the collection. Towelettes are used for cleansing the genital area prior to collection, and the lid is placed on the specimen cup after collection.
7. Assuring privacy, and using language that enables the patient's understanding, explain the clean-catch process. ***Explain the rationale for performing the procedure, displaying sensitivity to the patient's rights*** and feelings when explaining the process.	The purpose of cleansing the area before collecting the specimen is to remove any epithelial cells and surface bacteria that could contaminate the specimen. Using language that the patient can understand and explaining the rationale for the procedure will assure that she is able and willing to follow the instruction.
Instruct the female patient to:	
■ Open the towelettes so they are readily available.	
■ Spread the labia apart with nondominant hand to expose the urinary meatus, use one towelette to wipe down one side of the meatus from front to back (Figure 25-19a), and discard the towelette into the toilet.	Keeping the labia spread apart will prevent contamination of the area that was just cleansed.
■ With the second towelette wipe down the other side of the meatus (Figure 25-19b) from front to back and discard the towelette into the toilet.	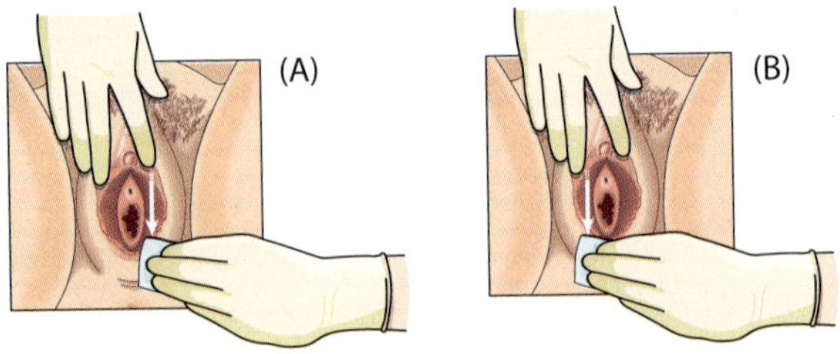

Figure 25-19a and b ■ Proper cleansing method for females: (a) Clean down one side of the labia from top to bottom. (b) Clean down opposite side of labia.

continues

PROCEDURE 25-1 continued

PROCEDURAL STEPS	DETAILS AND/OR RATIONALE
■ Using the third towelette, wipe down the center of the meatus (Figure 25-19c) from front to back and discard the towelette. ■ Caution the patient to hold the labia apart during urination.	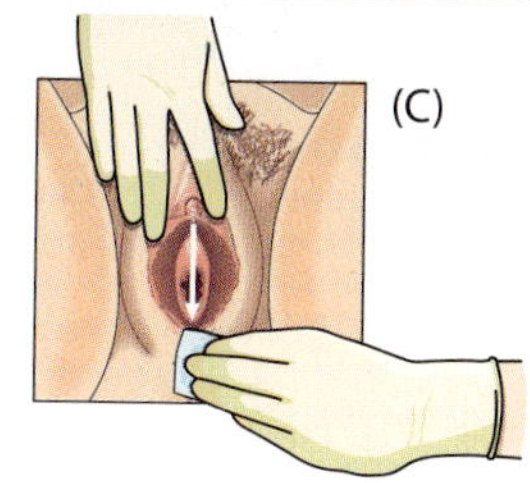 **Figure 25-19c** ■ Clean down the center of the meatus.
Instruct the male patient to: ■ Retract the foreskin (if applicable) and cleanse the tip and the urethral opening from the tip of the penis toward the ring of the glans twice, with two separate towelettes (Figure 25-20). Discard into the toilet and keep foreskin retracted while urinating into the cup.	Keeping the foreskin retracted will prevent contamination of the area that was just cleansed. 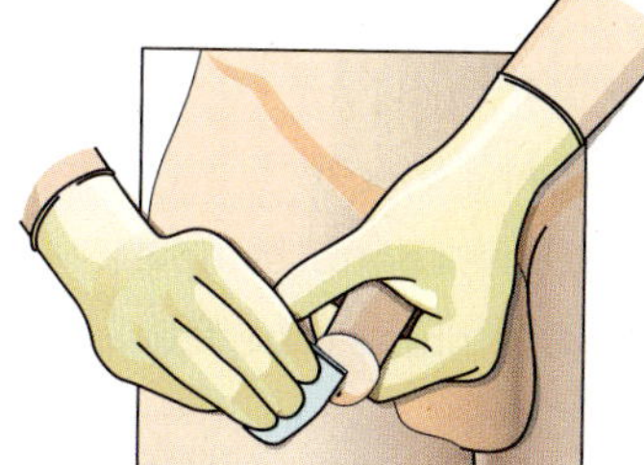 **Figure 25-20** ■ Proper cleansing method for males. Cleanse from the tip to the ring of the penis.
For all patients: **8.** After beginning to urinate into the toilet, catch the middle portion of the urine in the specimen cup, then withdraw the cup, and finish urinating into the toilet.	If the patient were to collect the first portion of the urine flow, it could be contaminated with epithelial cells and bacteria that are in the urethra. Contamination may make the specimen difficult to read upon microscopic examination.
9. Instruct the patient to place the lid tightly on the specimen container and wipe the outside of the container with a paper towel.	A tight lid will prevent spills. Cleansing the outside of the cup decreases the contaminants.
10. Show the patient where to leave the sample, where they may wash their hands, and where to wait for further instructions.	The patient will need to know what to do with the specimen and what to do after giving the specimen. Mentioning the hand washing supplies to the patient will remind them to wash their hands.
11. Document the clean-catch order.	The collection method and patient instructions should be documented on the laboratory report form.

DOCUMENTATION EXAMPLE:

CC/HPI

HX

PROCEDURE NOTE

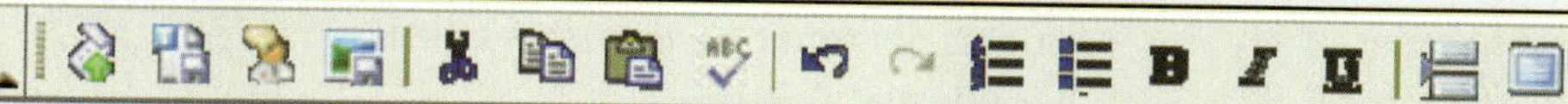

Instructed patient on collecting a clean-catch midstream urine sample per Dr. Samuals. Specimen sent to Qwest Laboratory for a complete urinalysis and sensitivity. Lilly Karnes, CMA (AAMA)

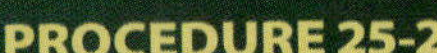

PROCEDURE 25-2

Perform a Physical and Chemical Urinalysis and Prepare a Microscope Slide for the Provider

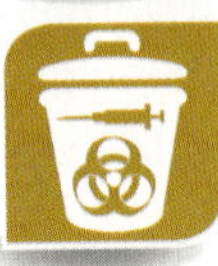

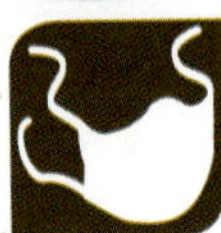

Objective:

To perform a physical and chemical urinalysis (using dip strip method) and prepare a slide of urinary sediment for microscopic examination.

Equipment/Supplies:

- Personal protective equipment (PPE)
- Urine specimen with secure lid, labeled
- Urine control sample
- Centrifuge tube, labeled
- Centrifuge
- Disposable pipettes
- Microscopic slide, labeled
- Cover slip
- Reagent strips
- Refractometer
- Laboratory report form
- Laboratory log sheet
- Biohazard container
- Patient's chart/EHR

PROCEDURAL STEPS	DETAILS AND/OR RATIONALE
1. Wash your hands and apply appropriate PPE.	Urine is a body fluid, and PPE, especially gloves, must be worn when handling a body fluid specimen.
2. Assemble the necessary equipment.	Having all equipment readily available saves time.
3. Gently mix the specimen.	The specimen must be well mixed to evenly distribute all components present.
4. Pour 10 mL of the specimen into a clear, labeled centrifuge tube (Figure 25-21).	If less than 10 mL is available, make a notation on the report form. QNS indicates you have less than needed to perform the chemical analysis. Follow your office policy on how to proceed. A labeled tube assures that patient samples will not be mixed up.
5. While holding the specimen in front of a light source, assess and record the color of the urine.	Viewing the specimen in front of a light source makes it easier to assess the true color.
6. Observe the clarity of the urine by holding a printed sheet of paper behind the specimen (Figure 25-22).	Observing printed material through the specimen makes it easier to determine the presence or degree of cloudiness.
7. Note any unusual odor, if present.	Odor is not routinely assessed, unless it is unusual.
8. Measure the specific gravity using method of choice, following manufacturer's instructions.	Following manufacturer's instructions ensures accuracy of results.

Figure 25-21 ■ Pour urine specimen into clear tube over the sink.

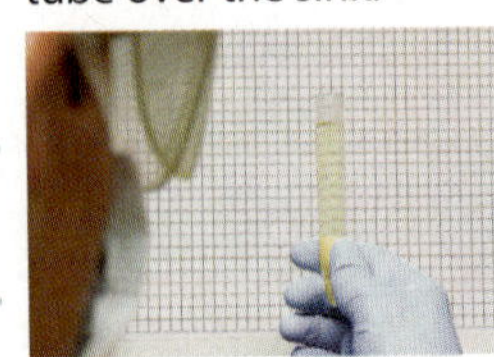

Figure 25-22 ■ Assess the clarity of the urine.

continues

PROCEDURE 25-2 continued

PROCEDURAL STEPS	DETAILS AND/OR RATIONALE
9. Cap the tube and remix the urine. Remove cap and dip the reagent strip into the tube, being certain to cover the entire strip with urine (Figure 25-23).	The entire strip must be covered with urine for a reaction to occur on all test pads. Dipping the urine into the original container contaminates the specimen in the event in needs to be sent to the lab for a culture and sensitivity.
10. After removing the strip from the cup, place the strip on its side on a paper towel to allow excess urine to be removed (Figure 25-24).	Excess urine can run down the strip, carrying the chemicals from one test pad to another and producing inaccurate results.
11. Hold the strip next to but not against the color chart on the bottle (Figure 25-25).	Holding the strip against the bottle will contaminate the outside of the container.
12. Accurately time all readings and read the results.	Timing is critical to obtain accurate results.
13. Record all results. Follow office protocol for all abnormal results.	Results must be recorded immediately to ensure accuracy.
14. Centrifuge the tube of urine for five minutes at 1500 rpm. Remove tube from the centrifuge.	Centrifugation concentrates all elements in the sediment at the bottom of the tube (Figure 25-26a).
15. Invert the tube upside down without shaking to pour the supernatant off (Figure 25-26b). Exactly 1 mL should remain in the tube. Add sediment stain if directed by provider. Mix the sediment well.	Urine centrifuge tubes are specially built to reserve 1 mL of the sample as long as the tube isn't shaken while upside down. Sediment stain highlights sediment during microscopic examination. Mixing the sediment well ensures good distribution of the elements present.

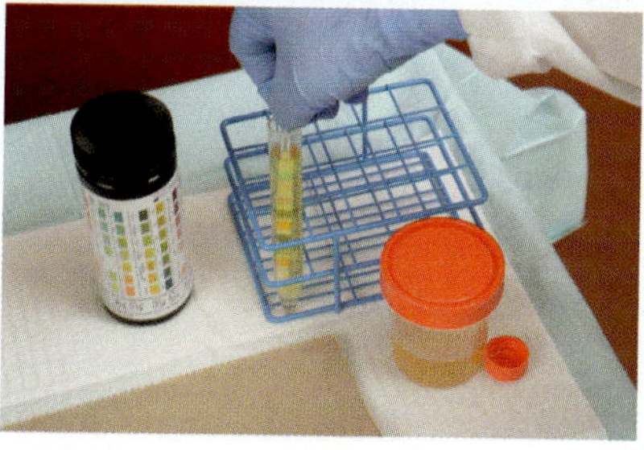

Figure 25-23 ■ Carefully dip the reagent strip into the tube of the well-mixed specimen. Make certain all test pads are covered by urine.

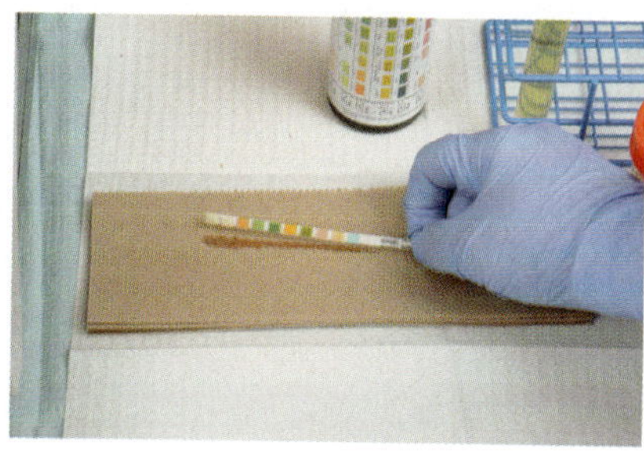

Figure 25-24 ■ Hold strip on its side on the paper towel and allow excess urine to drain onto the paper towel.

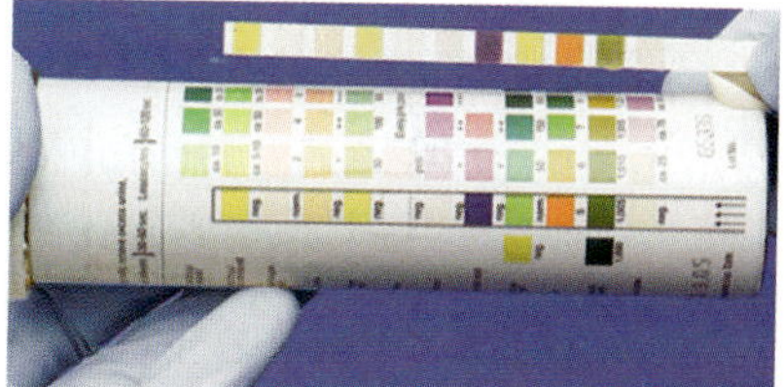

Figure 25-25 ■ Hold the strip next to the bottle, keeping the strip vertical so that the test pads strip matches the test pads on the bottle.

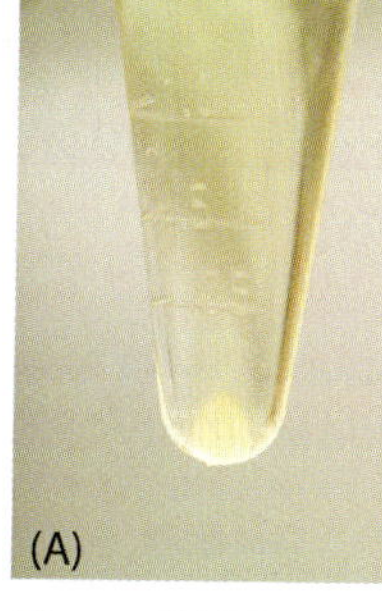

(A)

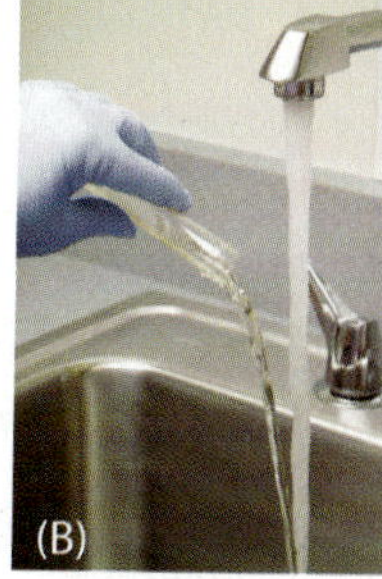

(B)

Figure 25-26 ■ (a) A small amount of sediment forms after centrifugation. (b) Gently pour off the supernatant, being careful not to shake or tap the tube in the inverted position.

continues

PROCEDURE 25-2 continued

PROCEDURAL STEPS	DETAILS AND/OR RATIONALE
16. Place one drop of well-mixed sediment onto a labeled glass slide and carefully place a cover slip over the drop of urine (Figure 25-27).	The labeled slide ensures patient identification. The cover slip spreads the drop of urine evenly, making examination more accurate.
17. Place the slide under the microscope, leaving the light off, and inform the provider that the specimen is ready to examine.	Microscopic examination of urine is not a CLIA-waived test and must be performed by a qualified provider.
18. Properly dispose of all equipment and specimens into the biohazard container, and the slide and cover slip into the sharps container.	Biohazard materials and glass/sharp items must be disposed of properly to assure safety and contamination control.
19. Remove gloves and wash your hands.	Hands must be washed both before and after wearing gloves.
20. Document the procedure.	Proper and timely documentation ensures accuracy.

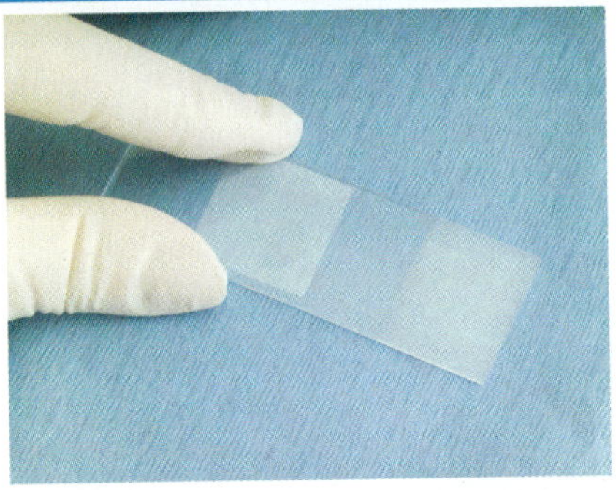

Figure 25-27 ■ Place the coverslip over the drop of urine.

DOCUMENTATION EXAMPLE:

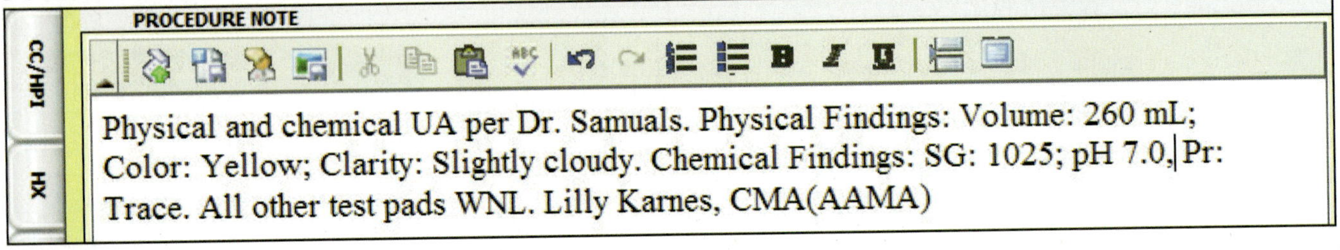

CC/HPI | HX

PROCEDURE NOTE

Physical and chemical UA per Dr. Samuals. Physical Findings: Volume: 260 mL; Color: Yellow; Clarity: Slightly cloudy. Chemical Findings: SG: 1025; pH 7.0, Pr: Trace. All other test pads WNL. Lilly Karnes, CMA(AAMA)

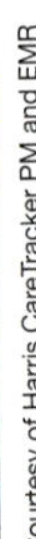

PROCEDURE 25-3

Utilizing a Urine Transport System for Culture and Sensitivity

Objective:

Using a urine transport system to prepare a urine specimen for an outside lab for a culture and sensitivity test.

Equipment/Supplies:

- Personal protective equipment (PPE)
- Urine transport system
- Urine specimen in a sterile container
- Gloves
- Lab requisition
- Patient's chart/EHR

continues

PROCEDURE 25-3 continued

PROCEDURAL STEPS	DETAILS AND/OR RATIONALE
1. Wash your hands, and apply gloves and the appropriate PPE. Check the provider's order and complete the lab requisition form.	PPE protects you from exposure to pathogenic organisms contained in the specimen. Checking the provider's order while completing the lab requisition form helps to assure that you order the correct tests.
2. Assemble the equipment.	Being organized prevents confusion and possible errors.
3. Check the expiration date on the transport system. Check that the urine specimen is properly labeled.	The integrity of the transport system cannot be guaranteed if the unit has expired. Proper labeling can prevent errors.
4. Open the urine transport kit (Figure 25-28a) and assemble it according to the manufacturer's directions.	Following the manufacturer's directions will ensure proper use of the kit. Piercing the stopper before the unit is in the urine can destroy the vacuum.
5. Label the tubes. Insert the urine tube into the holder without piercing the stopper (Figure 25-28b).	
6. Put the straw of the transport system into the urine specimen and push the vacuum tube onto the needle inside the tube holder (Figure 25-29).	Pushing the vacuum tube onto the needle will allow the vacuum in the tube to draw the urine in automatically.
7. Allow the tube to fill completely.	Allowing the tube to fill completely will provide the lab with an adequate amount of specimen.
8. Remove the tube from the holder and properly dispose of the unit.	The transport unit contains a body fluid and must be disposed of according to Occupational Safety and Health Administration (OSHA) guidelines.
9. Place the specimen tube into the laboratory transport bag and seal that compartment. Clean and disinfect the work area and properly dispose of contaminated supplies.	Sealing the specimen into the bag helps prevent contamination. Disinfecting all surfaces and properly disposing of contaminated supplies into biohazard container prevents contamination to others.

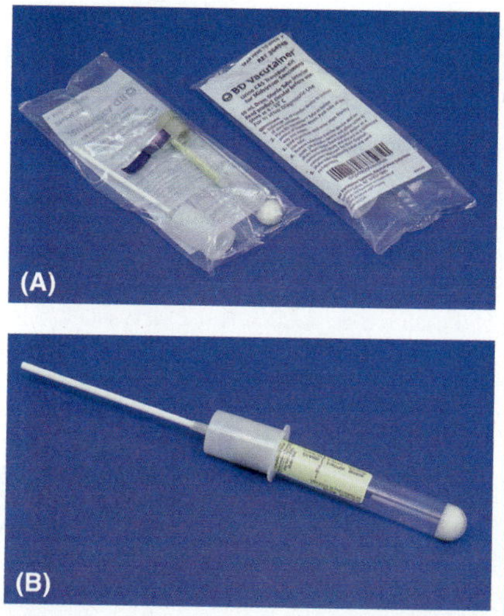

(A)

(B)

Figure 25-28 ■ (a) Packaged transport system. (b) Insert the vacuum tube into the holder, taking care not to puncture the tube with the needle.

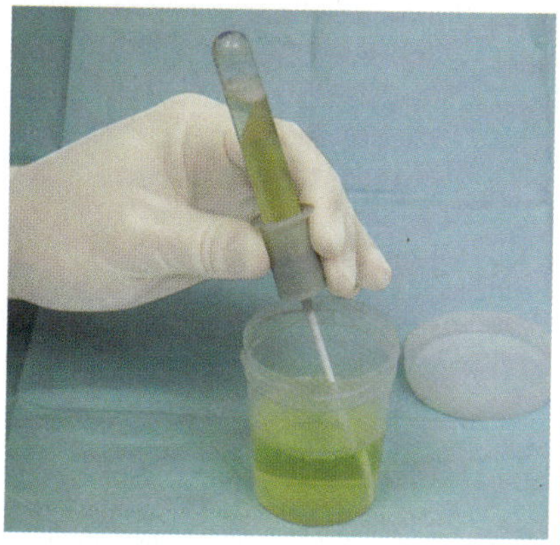

Figure 25-29 ■ Push the tube onto the needle, piercing the stopper.

continues

PROCEDURE 25-3 continued

PROCEDURAL STEPS	DETAILS AND/OR RATIONALE
10. Remove gloves and wash your hands.	Washing hands prevents possible contamination.
11. Complete the requisition and place it into its own compartment of the transport bag.	Placing the requisition into its own compartments protects separates the paperwork from the contaminated specimen tube.
12. Document the procedure in the patient's chart.	Documentation is proof of completion of the procedure and confirms to which laboratory the specimen was sent.

DOCUMENTATION EXAMPLE:

PROCEDURE NOTE

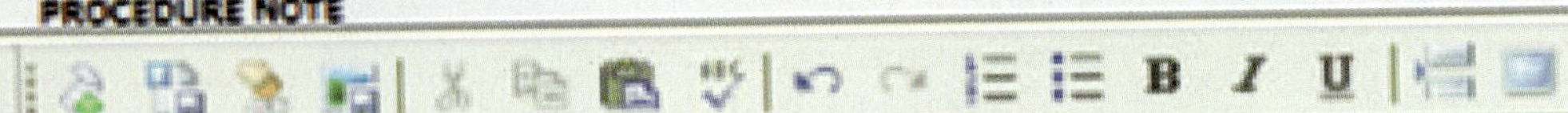

Sent sterile urine specimen for C & S per Dr. Anderson, to Lab of America. L. Karnes, CMA (AAMA)

PROCEDURE 25-4

Urinary Catheterization

Objective:

To obtain a sterile urine specimen by inserting a sterile catheter into the bladder while observing strict sterile technique. (Note: If catheter is to be indwelling, a Foley kit is used and a urine bag is attached to the leg [Figure 25-30].)

Equipment/Supplies:

- Sterile gloves
- Sterile urethral catheter (size ordered by the provider)
- Sterile disposable catheter kit (includes receptacle, fenestrated and nonfenestrated drapes, sterile wipes or sterile gauze pads, gauze, antiseptic cleanser, sterile lubricant)
- Sterile specimen container with lid (may be included in kit)
- Mayo stand/tray
- Adjustable lamp
- Patient's chart/EHR

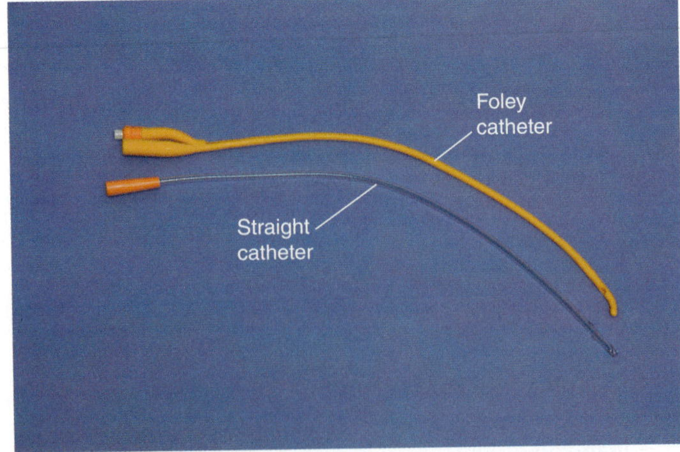

Figure 25-30 ■ Straight urethral catheter and indwelling Foley catheter.

continues

PROCEDURE 25-4 continued

PROCEDURAL STEPS	DETAILS AND/OR RATIONALE
1. Identify the patient using two identifiers, introduce yourself using your credentials, and ***explain the rationale for performance of the procedure***.	Using two identifiers will prevent performing the procedure on the wrong patient, introducing yourself increases patient confidence and establishes a professional relationship, and explaining the procedure will help the patient understand what to expect.
2. Wash your hands and assemble the supplies. Place the catheter kit on the Mayo stand or a nearby counter surface.	Washing hands is an effective way to prevent from spreading microorganisms to other patients.
3. ***Showing awareness of a patient's concerns related to the procedure being performed***, instruct the patient to remove clothing from the waist down, providing privacy. Give the patient a drape, ***demonstrating the principles of self-boundaries***. Assist as needed.	The patient may be anxious about the testing or embarrassed in regards to the collection procedure. Do your best to make the patient feel comfortable. The patient will appreciate the privacy and assistance.
4. Position the patient in a comfortable dorsal recumbent position, draping with only the external genitalia exposed.	This position provides the visualization necessary for the procedure, and helps the patient to relax.
5. Adjust the light as needed.	Good lighting is helpful for viewing during the procedure, especially with female patients.
6. Place the catheter kit on the Mayo stand at a right angle to the patient. Open the external covering of the catheter kit. (The inside of the outer covering of the kit will now become a sterile field.)	The catheter kit needs to be near the working area so the supplies are accessible. Having the Mayo stand at a right angle assures that you do not turn your back on the sterile field.
7. Carefully reach inside the kit without contaminating the field or contents of the kit and place the waterproof sterile drape from the kit underneath the penis for a male patient (Figure 25-31a), or underneath the buttocks for a female patient. Touch only the corners of the drape.	The waterproof drape will help protect the patient and the surrounding area from becoming wet.
8. Wash hands and put on sterile gloves, using caution not to contaminate gloved hands. (From this point on, you will touch only the sterile materials inside the kit and the surface to be catheterized. If anything outside the kit is needed, ask for assistance.)	Touching anything outside the kit will contaminate the sterile field and could prove harmful to the patient.

continues

PROCEDURE 25-4 continued

PROCEDURAL STEPS	DETAILS AND/OR RATIONALE
9. Open the fenestrated drape and place the drape over the external genitalia (Figure 25-31b).	The drape provides extra modesty for the patient and helps to focus on the working area, and lessens the chances of contaminating sterile supplies. 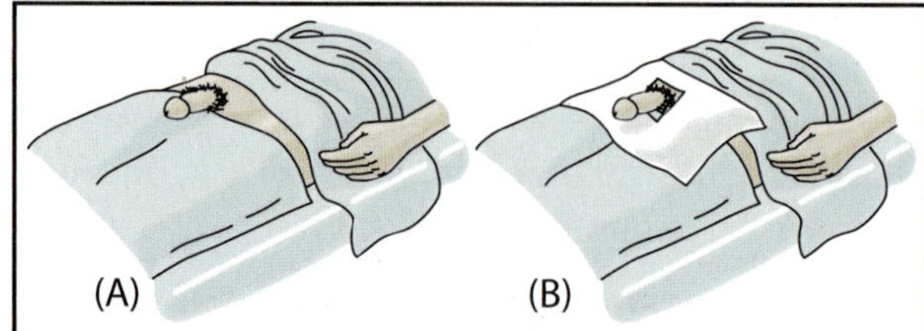 **Figure 25-31** ■ (a) Place a sterile waterproof drape underneath the male patient's penis. (b) Place fenestrated drape over the penis.
10. Prepare a cleaning solution (either sterile wipes or sterile gauze pads with an antiseptic cleanser) and apply some lubricant onto the sterile gauze pad.	The cleansing wipes or gauze pads and lubrication must be prepared prior to starting the procedure; once you start the procedure, you will have no free hands.
11. Insert the tip of the catheter into the sterile lubricant and leave the catheter on the sterile field until ready for use. Open the specimen container and place within reach.	Lubrication will provide easier insertion. The catheter tubing is not very long, so the specimen container must be nearby to receive the urine.
12. For a female, spread the labia with nondominant hand and cleanse the genital areas (right side, left side, and middle) from front to back with the other hand. For males, cleanse the urinary meatus in a circular motion working from the center outward (Figure 25-32). Repeat two more times.	Wipe only from front to back once per wipe. This will prevent contamination to the area. Keep the labia spread in order to prevent contaminating the cleaned area. Note: The hand holding the labia open is no longer sterile.
13. Resting the distal end of the catheter in the urine receptacle, insert the well-lubricated tip of the catheter *slowly* into the urinary meatus as seen in Figure 25-33. Proceed slowly and do not force the catheter in. If an obstruction is noted or pain or bleeding is present, stop the insertion.	Placing the distal end of the catheter into the urine receptacle, provide a place for the urine to flow into. Generously lubricating the catheter will ease insertion. Forcing the insertion past an obstruction or pain could cause damage to the area and result in later complications.
14. ***Display sensitivity to the patient's rights*** and feelings when collecting the specimen.	The patient may be anxious about the testing or embarrassed in regards to catheterization procedure. Do your best to make the patient feel comfortable by asking him to relax and breathe deeply.

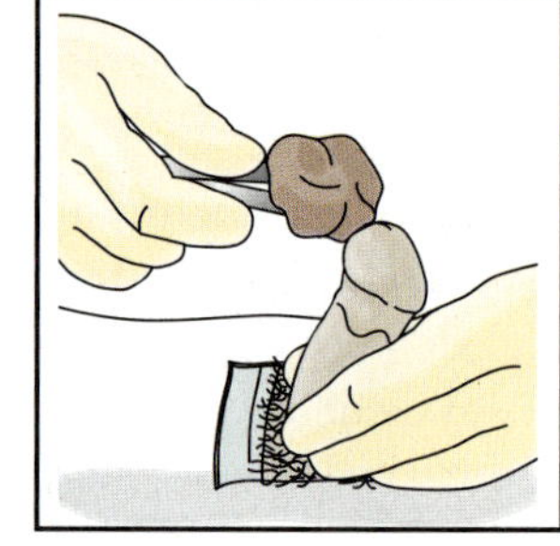

Figure 25-32 ■ Scrub the tip of the penis with an antiseptic cleanser before inserting the catheter.

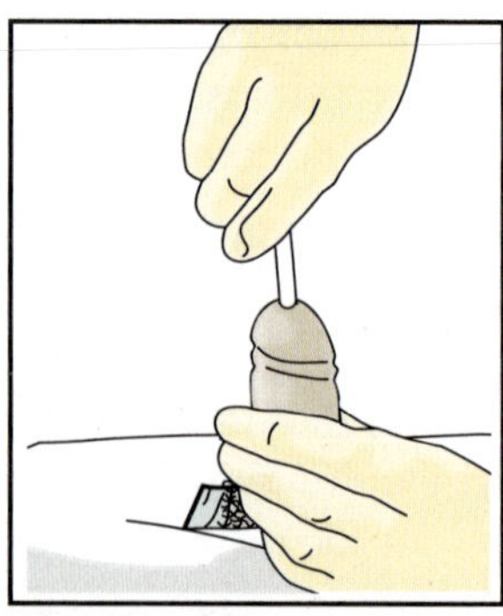

Figure 25-33 ■ Insert the catheter into the urinary meatus.

continues

PROCEDURE 25-4 continued

PROCEDURAL STEPS	DETAILS AND/OR RATIONALE
15. Progress the catheter into the bladder until urine flows. Collect the initial stream in the receptacle basin (Figure 25-34), and then obtain the sample in the specimen container.	The initial urine may contain bacteria. Midstream is a better specimen for accurate analysis.
16. After adequate collection, empty the remainder of the urine inside the bladder into the receptacle basin. Never leave the bladder partially full after catheterization.	Emptying the bladder completely allows for a measurement of total urine if requested by the provider and relieves the patient of residual pressure.
17. Slowly remove the catheter from the meatus and place on the table.	Slowly removing the catheter is more comfortable and gentle for the patient.
18. Gently clean the genital region as needed and provide tissues for the patient.	Cleaning the meatus and area provides comfort for the patient.
19. Remove gloves and wash hands. Assist the patient into a sitting position as needed.	The patient may need assistance to sit up following this procedure.
20. Discard the materials in the appropriate waste containers.	Following biohazard guidelines can prevent cross-contamination.
21. Label the urine specimen container and attach a lab requisition form that has been filled out with all pertinent information.	An improperly documented requisition form could delay testing and treatment.
22. Document the procedure on the patient's record. Include any adverse reactions from the patient.	Thorough and accurate documentation is essential for continuity of care.

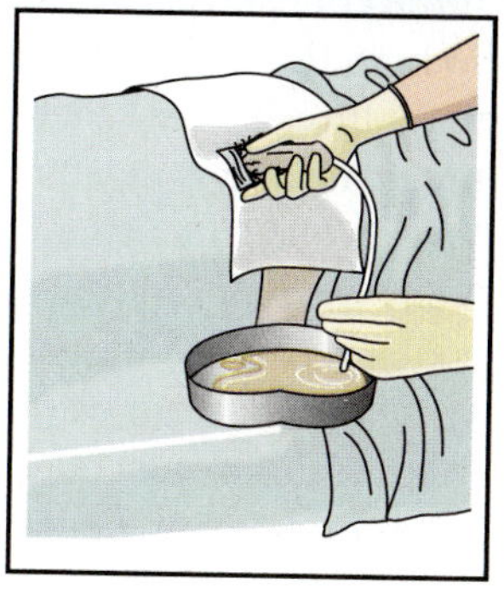

Figure 25-34 ■ Collect the first part of the urine stream into the basin.

DOCUMENTATION EXAMPLE:

CC/HPI | HX

PROCEDURE NOTE

Patient catheterized without difficulty and tolerated the procedure well. Urine clear and light yellow, 200 mL return. Specimen sent to lab for C&S per Dr. J. Pettit. Helen Chung, CMA (AAMA)

CHAPTER SUMMARY

- Urinalysis is a complete analysis of the urine and can provide important information about different body systems, diseases, and metabolic processes.
- Urine is produced in the kidneys as they filter the blood. Once it is formed, it consists of approximately 95% water and 5% dissolved substances.

- Primary substances found in the urine include urea, uric acid, creatinine, ammonia, calcium, magnesium, and phosphorus. Other substance can also be found in urine, depending on a person's diet and general state of health.
- If the concentration of a substance in the blood is so high that the kidneys cannot reabsorb all of it, a renal threshold is reached and the excess spills into the urine and is detected by chemical urinalysis.
- When collecting urine, a nonsterile container is generally used for random specimen testing and a sterile container is used for patients who exhibit urinary symptoms or from patients that are catheterized.
- Methods of urine collection include clean-catch midstream, pediatric urine collection, and catheterization.
- Types of urine specimens include random collection specimens and 24-hour specimens. Quality control is important to ensure safe and accurate test results in every area of laboratory testing, including urine testing.
- CLIA requires all physician office laboratories (POLs), including waived category labs, to perform quality control tests and to maintain documentation.
- The routine urinalysis is one of the most commonly performed tests in the medical office. Parts of a complete urinalysis include the physical, chemical, and microscopic findings.
- The physical portion of the urinalysis consists of observing the color and clarity and measuring the specific gravity of the urine.
- The specific gravity of urine provides information on the kidneys' ability to concentrate and dilute urine. The three most common methods to measure urine specific gravity are the refractometer, which gives either a scale or digital readout; reagent test strips, which are color assessed; and the automated urine analyzer.
- Results from the chemical analysis of urine can provide the practitioner with valuable information about the patient's kidney and liver function, carbohydrate metabolism, and acid–base balance. The chemical exam is performed using either a reagent test strip or an automated urine analyzer. Refer to Table 25-7 for normal values for Multistix results and the significance of results that are abnormal.
- The microscopic exam of the urine sediment is the third part of a complete urinalysis. CLIA categorizes the microscopic examination as a PPM (provider-performed microscopy) procedure, which means that the medical assistant may not perform this portion of the urinalysis.

CERTIFICATION REVIEW QUESTIONS

1. Which part of a urinalysis gives information on the protein content of the urine?
   a. Physical
   b. Microscopic
   c. Volume
   d. Chemical

2. The pigment that gives urine its color is:
   a. urobilinogen.
   b. urochrome.
   c. amorphous.
   d. bilirubin.

3. Liver disorders may yield a positive reagent strip test for:
   a. blood.
   b. protein.
   c. bilirubin.
   d. nitrites.

4. Which of the following would be considered abnormal if found in the urine?
   a. RBC casts
   b. 0–2 WBCs/hpf
   c. 15–20 epis/hpf
   d. Few calcium oxalate crystals

5. The presence of tyrosine crystals in the urine would be considered:
   a. abnormal.
   b. normal.
   c. suspicious.
   d. expected if the patient is pregnant.

6. A positive test for albumin (protein component) could be an early indicator of:
   a. diabetes.
   b. kidney dysfunction.
   c. liver disease.
   d. hypertension.

7. What is the difference between a urine specimen collected through a CCMS and one collected through catheterization?
   a. They are the same.
   b. The CCMS is more useful than a catheterized specimen.
   c. The catheterized specimen is sterile whereas the CCMS is considered clean.
   d. The CCMS is more difficult to perform for the patient.
8. What is the purpose of asking the patient to try to relax and to breathe deeply while performing a urinary catheterization?
   a. The urine will flow more quickly.
   b. The procedure will be more comfortable if the patient's muscles are relaxed.
   c. The urine specimen will be more useful for testing.
   d. The procedure will go more quickly.
9. Why is the microscopic examination of urine a PPM procedure?
   a. Because the medical assistant might not set up the slide properly.
   b. Because the provider has more time and experience with using a microscope.
   c. Because reading the microscopic contents is a higher level of expertise than a nonprovider has within her scope of practice.
   d. Because CLIA wants to keep records of who is doing each part of the procedure.
10. What is the minimum amount of urine ideal for a complete urinalysis?
   a. 10 mL
   b. 12 mL
   c. 15 mL
   d. There is no minimum amount needed.

STUDY RESOURCES

Resources to Test and Reinforce Your Knowledge:	
Certification Review Questions	Take this end-of-chapter quiz
Workbook	• Complete the activities for Chapter 25 • Perform the procedures for Chapter 25 using the Competency Checklists
Resources to Promote Critical Thinking:	
***Solve the Case* Activities**	• Consider these case studies and discuss your conclusions
Learning Lab	• Module 18: Urinary, Endocrine, and Reproductive Systems
MindTap	• Complete Chapter 25 readings and activities

REFERENCES

Centers for Disease Control and Prevention. (2014, August 28). *Clinical Laboratory Improvement Amendments (CLIA)*. Retrieved from http://www.cms.gov/Regulations-and-Guidance/Legislation/CLIA/index.html?redirect=/clia/

26

Hematology and Coagulation Studies

CHAPTER OUTLINE

Medical Abbreviation Review

Hematopoiesis

Blood Components
- Serum and Plasma
- Erythrocytes
- Leukocytes
- Thrombocytes

Coagulation

Basic Hematology Studies

The Complete Blood Count (CBC)
- Red Blood Cell Count
- White Blood Cell Count
- Platelet Count
- Hemoglobin
- Hematocrit
- Differential Count
- Red Blood Cell Morphology
- Complete Blood Count Normal Values

Erythrocyte Sedimentation Rate (ESR)

Automated Hematology Analyzers

Coagulation Tests

ESSENTIAL TERMS

activated partial thromboplastin time (aPTT)
anisocytosis
basophil
coagulation cascade
complete blood count (CBC)
differential count
eosinophil
erythrocyte
erythrocyte sedimentation rate (ESR)
fibrin
hematocrit
hematopoiesis
hemoglobin
hemostasis
international normalized ratio (INR)
leukocyte
lymphocyte
macrocyte
microcyte
monocyte
morphology
neutrophil
normocyte
plasma
poikilocytosis
prothrombin time (PT)
red blood cell indices
reticulocyte
serum
thrombocyte

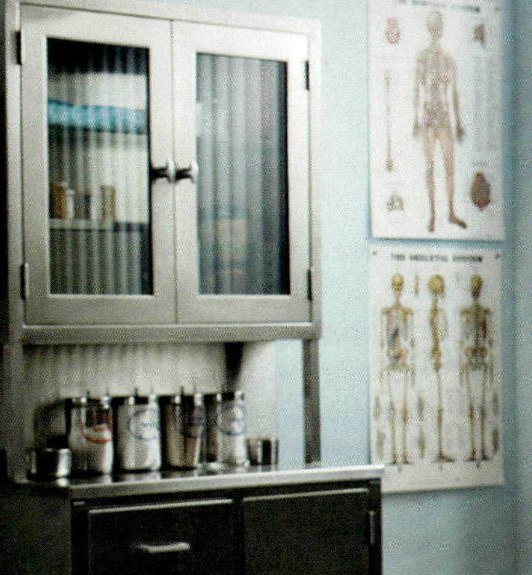

DEVELOPMENTAL OBJECTIVES

After completing this chapter, you should be able to:

1. Correctly spell and define the essential terms.
2. Explain the process of hematopoiesis.
3. Compare plasma to serum.
4. Name the three cellular components found in blood and explain the function of each.
5. Select appropriate personal protective equipment (PPE) for use while performing blood tests.
6. List the tests included in the CBC and the normal values for each individual test.
7. Discuss the function of hemoglobin and its relationship to hematocrit.
8. List the different types of white blood cells found on a differential, their normal values, and probable causes for an increase in each type.
9. Explain the importance of the red blood cell indices.
10. Describe the concept of the erythrocyte sedimentation rate test and what is indicates.
11. Given PT, aPTT, and INR test results, determine which are within normal ranges.
12. Demonstrate how to determine which hematologic tests are CLIA-waived.
13. Perform CLIA-waived hematology tests including hematocrit, hemoglobin, and erythrocyte sedimentation rate.
14. Perform CLIA-waived PT/INR testing.

INTRODUCTION

Hematology is the study of blood and the blood-forming tissues with a primary focus on the formed elements found in the blood, which include red blood cells, white blood cells, and platelets suspended in a liquid called plasma.

The functions of blood include the transportation of both nutrients and waste products, carrying oxygen to the cells of the body, protecting the body against infection, and playing a vital role in the coagulation/clotting process.

Hematologic tests can supply the provider with valuable information about a patient's state of health. An abnormality in these studies may be the first sign that a more serious condition exists, prompting the provider to conduct additional tests.

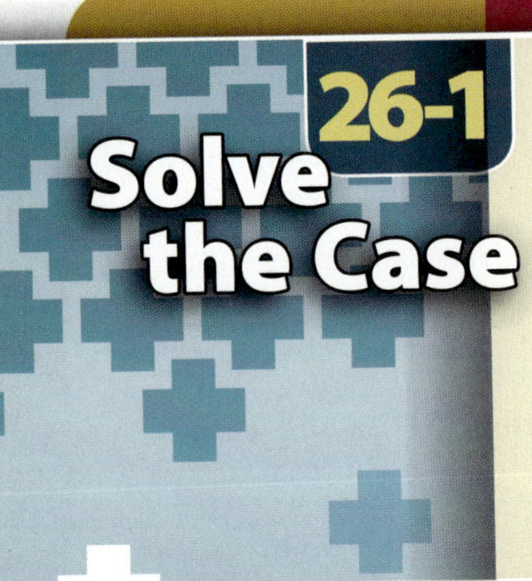

Sarah Walker, a 45 year old, comes into the office because of severe fatigue, shortness of breath, and generalized bruising. She states her periods are horrible and she wonders if she is starting to go through the "change." She is not overly concerned with the symptoms but does want answers today and something to make her feel better. Based on your current level of knowledge, answer the following questions.

1. **What other questions may help the provider determine what is wrong with Sarah?**
2. **What vital signs may correlate with Sarah's current symptoms?**
3. **What may Sarah's menstrual symptoms have to do with her other symptoms?**
4. **How would you respond to Sarah's question about advancing menopause?**

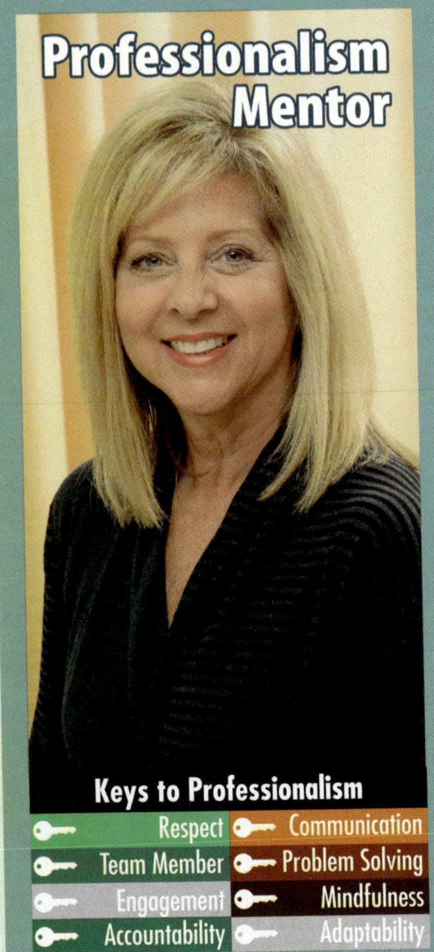

As a medical assistant you have the responsibility of contacting patients with lab results and providing education based on those lab results. In this chapter, you will learn about coagulation tests referred to as prothrombin time (PT) and international normalized ratio (INR). These two tests measure how quickly the blood clots. Patients who have atrial fibrillation (Afib), suffered a heart attack or a stroke, or have a history of blood clots are often put on anticoagulants (blood thinners) to prevent new clots from forming. If the patient's PT and INR are too high, it makes the patient more at risk for internal bleeding, if the patient's PT and INR are too low, the patient has a higher risk for forming new blood clots.

One of the medical assistant's in our network received a message from the doctor to call a patient regarding a critically low PT and INR level and instructions for changing the patient's medication regimen. The order was given on a Thursday afternoon. The medical assistant couldn't get a hold of the patient so she just stuck the chart in a drawer in her desk and left, knowing that she wouldn't return until the following Tuesday. This put the patient at serious risk of forming a new blood clot. Thankfully, the patient called back herself on Friday to obtain her results. When we searched the medical assistant's desk, looking for the chart, we saw several other messages related to lab tests that had not been taken care of. As you can guess, the medical assistant was terminated from her position. As a health care professional, you need to take full responsibility for following through with patient assignments. In your workbook journal, write what you would have done if you couldn't get a hold of the patient. Do you think the medical assistant should have been fired? Why or why not? How do the professionalism keys listed in this feature apply to this scenario? ■

MEDICAL ABBREVIATION REVIEW

Medical assistants working in the clinical areas should be familiar with the medical abbreviations associated with hematology and coagulation listed in Table 26-1.

HEMATOPOIESIS

Hematopoiesis, or *hemopoiesis*, is the formation and development of blood cells, which primarily takes place in the bone marrow of the ribs, sternum, and pelvic bone. Initially, blood cells begin their development in the liver of the young fetus. As the fetus matures and develops cartilage and bones, the blood cells form in the bone marrow. **Lymphocytes**, a particular type of white blood cell, are not only produced in the bone marrow, but also in the lymph nodes and spleen.

Blood cell formation and development is a continuous process throughout life. Formation begins with a single cell known as a stem cell. The stem cell begins as a *nondifferentiated* (generic) cell that develops and matures while gradually taking on the characteristics of a specific cell type. When the cell is mature, it is released into circulation. Figure 26-1 shows the development and maturation of different blood cell types and their characteristic traits.

BLOOD COMPONENTS

The average adult has about five liters (L) of blood; approximately half is composed of cells and the other half is the fluid portion.

Serum and Plasma

Serum consists of approximately 90% water with the remaining 10% consisting of noncellular chemical components such as electrolytes, hormones, carbohydrates, lipids, amino acids, protein, and antibodies. Blood tests to measure the levels of these substances in the serum portion of blood are often conducted in the chemistry department of the laboratory. On the other hand, **plasma** is the liquid portion of blood obtained when anticoagulated blood is centrifuged. Since this sample was not "clotted," it will contain components of the clotting process such as fibrinogen. You've no doubt heard of "plasma centers" where people can donate blood for transfusions to individuals who lack certain components in their blood. It is called plasma because the blood in these centers is collected from donors using an anticoagulant. Knowing the difference between serum and plasma samples is important when collecting specimens for laboratory testing.

Erythrocytes

Erythrocytes, or red blood cells (RBC), are the most plentiful cellular components found in the blood. They transport oxygen to the cells of the body and carry carbon dioxide to the lungs to be exhaled. The biconcave shape of the red cells provides a surface area large enough for the oxygen and carbon dioxide exchange to take place and also allows for flexible movement through the small blood vessels. Most of the nucleus of the RBC stays in the bone marrow to be used to make more RBCs. For the first day or two, the RBC will retain a bit of the nuclear material and is referred to as a **reticulocyte**. Normally reticulocytes make up about 1% of all the RBCs. If more reticulocytes are present, it can mean that the body is losing blood somewhere and more RBCs are needed to maintain homeostasis. The biconcave shape of the RBC shows us where the nucleus was originally. Without a nucleus, the RBC cannot duplicate once in circulation so it only lives about 120 days. As it travels through the liver with each circuit through the body, the shape and condition of the RBC is assessed. The liver removes any damaged or aged RBCs, keeping and reusing or storing any useful materials, such as iron.

The RBC contains **hemoglobin**, a protein molecule that contains iron. Hemoglobin can bind to gases such as oxygen, carbon dioxide, and even carbon monoxide. Hemoglobin is the part of the red cell responsible for

Table 26-1 Common Abbreviations Associated with Hematology and Coagulation

Abbreviation	Meaning	Abbreviation	Meaning
CBC	Complete blood count	MCHC	Mean corpuscular hemoglobin concentration
CDC	Centers for Disease Control and Prevention	MCV	Mean corpuscular volume
CLIA	Clinical Laboratory Improvement Act	PPE	Personal protective equipment
ESR	Erythrocyte sedimentation rate	PT	Prothrombin time
Hct	Hematocrit	aPTT	Activated partial thromboplastin time
Hgb	Hemoglobin	RBC	Red blood cell
MCH	Mean corpuscular hemoglobin	WBC	White blood cell

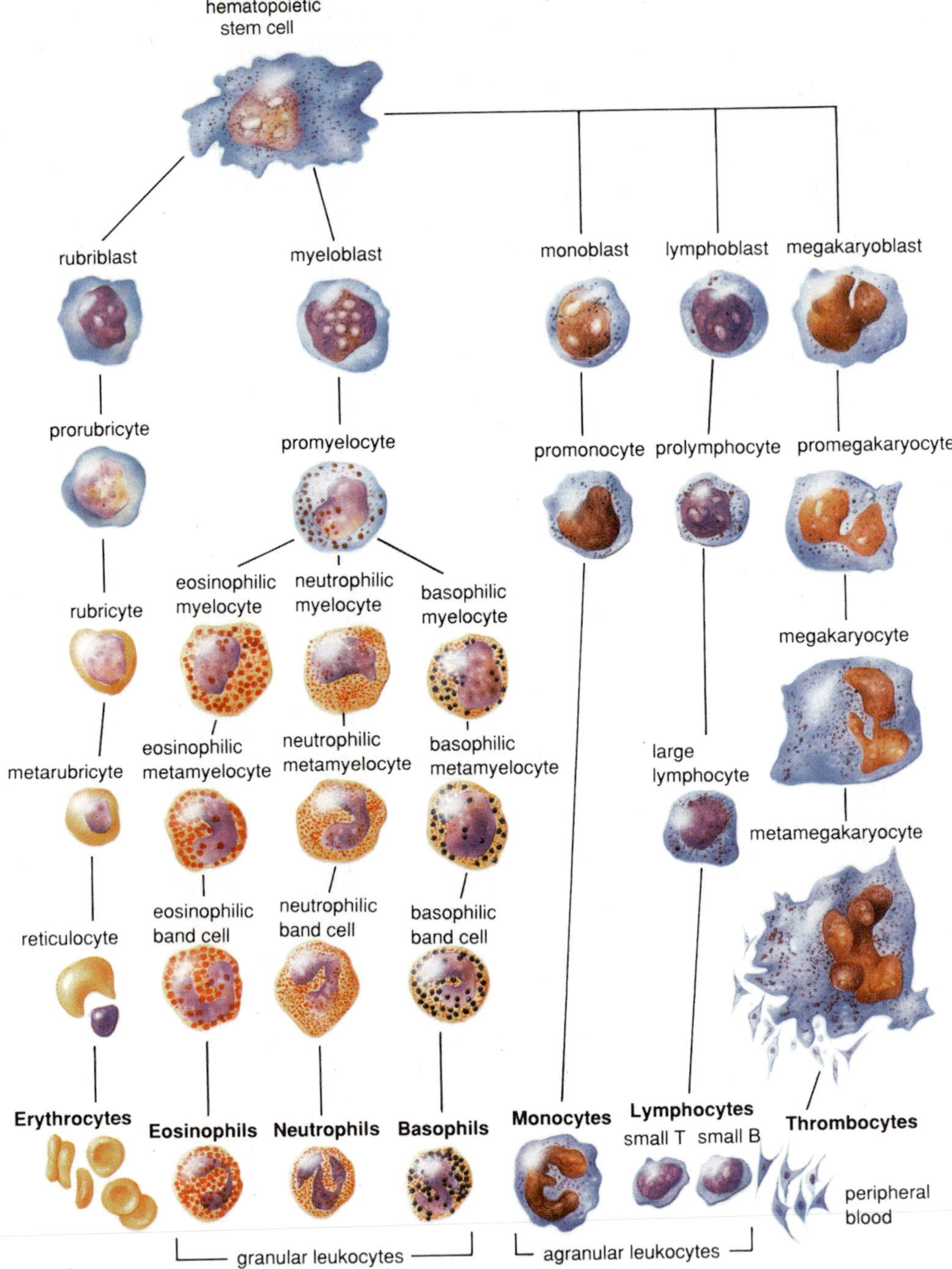

Figure 26-1 ■ The maturation of blood cells and platelets beginning from a single stem cell.

> **CRITICAL THINKING CHALLENGE**
>
> Referring to the information regarding plasma and serum, which liquid contains the clotting factors: plasma or serum? Referring to Chapter 24, which blood collection tubes (when centrifuged) provide the medical assistant with serum and which tubes provide the medical assistant with plasma?

transporting fresh oxygen from our lungs to our cells and transporting cellular waste, mostly carbon dioxide from our cells back to the lungs for disposal. When hemoglobin binds with oxygen, it gives arterial blood its bright red color. After the hemoglobin releases oxygen into the cellular tissues and picks up carbon dioxide, the color of the venous blood is dark red.

Leukocytes

Five different types of **leukocytes**, or white blood cells (WBC), include **neutrophils**, **eosinophils**, **basophils**, lymphocytes, and **monocytes**. Leukocytes guard the body against infection by producing antibodies and functioning in the immune response. White blood cells move through the bloodstream and into the tissues to the site of an infection, where they perform various functions.

Each type of white blood cell has a very specific function; these functions are further explained later in the chapter.

Thrombocytes

Thrombocytes, or platelets, are actually cell fragments. They function mainly in the process of **hemostasis** (stopping the flow of blood). Platelets stop bleeding by forming a sticky plug in the damaged blood vessel wall. Once they adhere to the site of bleeding they release a chemical that attracts other platelets to the site, forming a loose platelet plug and providing a surface for clotting proteins (also known as factors) to form a stable clot.

COAGULATION

Whenever a blood vessel is injured, it contracts, thus slowing the flow of blood so the clotting process can begin. The formation of platelet plug happens next, as mentioned above, followed by the onset of the complex chemical processes of coagulation, involving proteins, called clotting factors. Since these events happen one right after the other, they are often referred to as the **coagulation cascade**. Each factor has an active and inactive form. Once a factor is activated, it will activate the next factor, thus cascading through the process. The factors are numbered using Roman numerals I through XIII, although only a couple are needed for our study here. The first factor, Factor I, is called fibrinogen and is the origin of fibrin. **Fibrin**, just like it sounds, is fiber-like and forms a network of fibers to help form the needed blood clot. Factor II, called prothrombin (meaning before thrombin) makes thrombin with the help of vitamin K. Calcium is needed in the clotting process and is considered Factor IV. Once the bleeding stops, the clot will start to dry, contracting the edges of the wound together and eventually forming a scab on the skin, which turns into a scar. Figure 26-2 shows a diagram of the clot formation.

BASIC HEMATOLOGY STUDIES

Hematologic (blood) tests are among the most common ordered by the provider. Some of the tests can be performed in the physician's office laboratory (POL) and some are performed in outside laboratories. Blood tests can measure each blood cell type individually to determine the relative number present and also for abnormalities to the cells themselves. Through blood tests, the provider can gain valuable information about the general health of the patient as well as particular disease processes occurring within the body. For instance, a patient with a decreased red blood cell count might be diagnosed with anemia. Since there are a number of different types of anemia, an evaluation of the red cell **morphology** (a study of the cell's size, shape, and color) can help to determine the type and cause of the anemia. Then, once the patient is treated for the anemia, further blood tests can help the provider monitor the effectiveness of medications and treatments. The provider can also use blood tests to determine whether an infection is viral or bacterial by evaluating the results of the white blood cell **differential count**. This test, sometimes performed as part of a complete blood count (CBC), determines the percentage of the five different types of white blood cells present and examines their characteristics. Table 26-2 lists some of the blood cell disorders that may be detected by a simple hematology test.

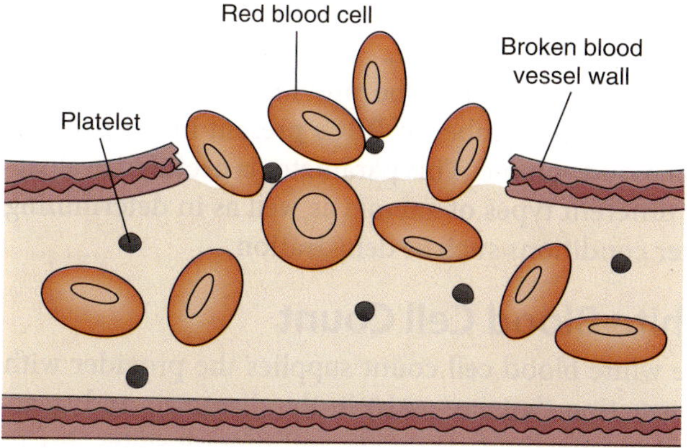

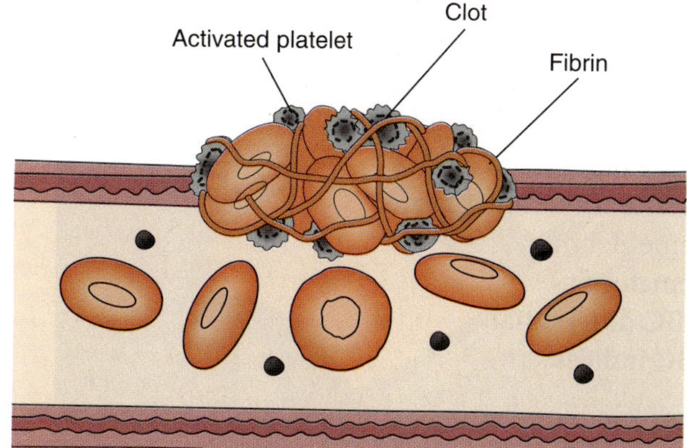

Figure 26-2 ■ With the help of fibrin and platelets, a clot is formed.

received from an outside laboratory. The hemoglobin determination results are reported as grams of hemoglobin per deciliter (g/dL).

Refer to Procedure 26-2 for a full procedure on how to perform a hemoglobin determination.

Hematocrit

The **hematocrit (Hct)**, also a CLIA-waived test, is a quick and easy method for determining the volume of packed red blood cells in a given volume of blood. Hematocrit is reported as a percentage (e.g., a hematocrit reported as 48% means that 48% of the total blood volume is made up of red blood cells).

The hemoglobin and hematocrit tests have a unique relationship and are rarely performed separately. They both provide information about the hemoglobin- and oxygen-carrying ability of the RBCs. Hemoglobin tests indicate the density of hemoglobin within the RBCs and the hematocrit test indicates the percentage of RBCs within the sample of blood. The hemoglobin result is generally one-third of the hematocrit and any deviation from that ratio may be indicative of a disease or condition.

The hematocrit may be performed with an automated analyzer or manually. The manual hematocrit test is performed by centrifuging a small sample of whole blood in a petite narrow tube called a capillary tube. The test is often referred to as a micro-hematocrit test because of the size of the tubes. Either capillary or venous blood may be used for this test.

Heparinized tubes are used when collecting blood from a capillary puncture to prevent the sample from clotting prior to testing. Figure 26-6 shows some examples of plain and heparinized safety capillary tubes with clay sealant.

The tube fills by capillary action, a force that draws a thick liquid, such as blood, into a narrow tube. The tube is held horizontally with the end of the tube placed into a well-rounded drop of blood and then sealed. When using self-sealing tubes, the dry plug in the other end of the tube will expand when the blood reaches it, sealing off the tube. There are other brands and types of safety self-sealing microhematocrit tubes available.

Filled capillary tubes are placed in the microhematocrit centrifuge with the sealed end placed at the bottom of the holders in the unit featured in Figure 26-7. When using tubes that are placed horizontally in the centrifuge, the sealed end should face the gasket or outside of the unit, and spun for two to five minutes. When centrifuged, the cellular components of the blood are separated into three layers with the red blood cells at the bottom, the white blood cells and platelets in the middle (buffy coat), and the plasma on top. Figure 26-8 illustrates the separation of the cellular components after centrifugation. The spun hematocrit tubes are placed on a reading device and the percentage of red blood cells is determined. Two tubes are filled, centrifuged, and read, and the readings are averaged to determine the hematocrit. The two readings must agree within 2% or the test must be repeated. Procedure 26-1 lists the necessary steps for performing a manual microhematocrit.

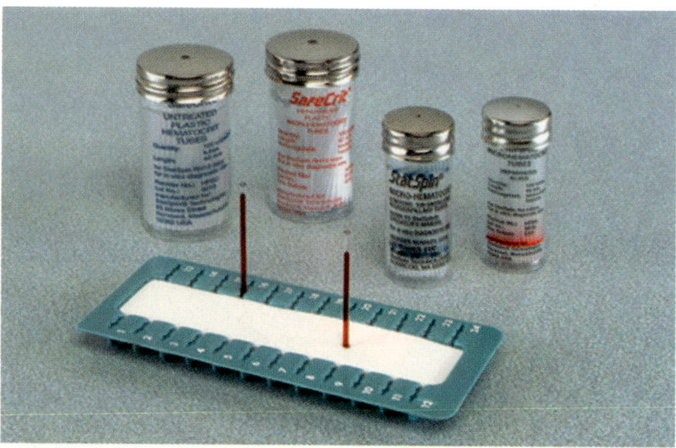

Figure 26-6 ■ Examples of safety capillary tubes and clay sealant.

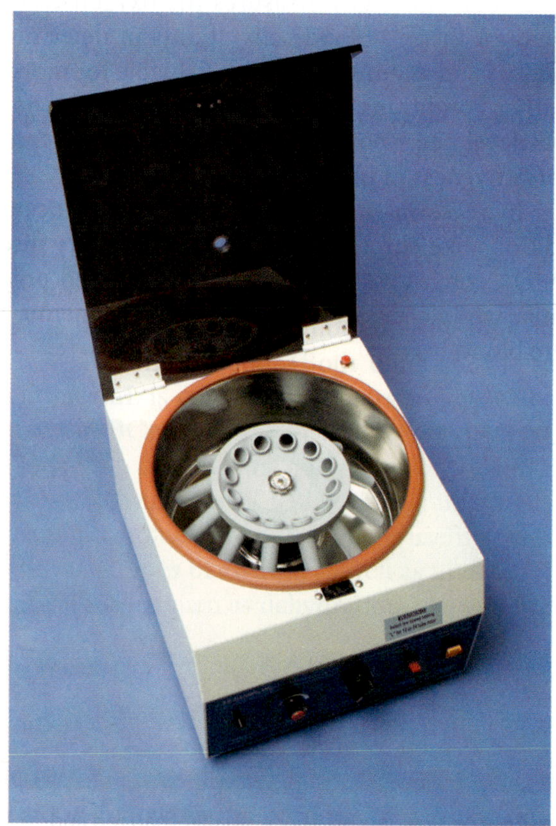

Figure 26-7 ■ A microhematocrit centrifuge.

The white blood cell count measures the number of WBCs present in 1 cu mm of blood; results are reported as the number of WBCs/cu mm of blood or WBCs $\times 10^3$/uL or WBCs $\times 10^9$/L.

An increase in the number of white cells (leukocytosis) may be seen in acute infections such as mononucleosis, chicken pox, and appendicitis, as well as some leukemias. A decrease in the white cell count (leukopenia) can be indicative of a viral infection or can be the result of chemotherapy and radiation.

Platelet Count

Platelets (Figure 26-4) are cells active in blood clotting. Platelet counts are calculated by an automated instrument and the result is reported as the number of platelets/cu mm or platelets $\times 10^9$/L of blood. Since normal platelet counts range in the hundreds of thousands, the count is an estimated calculation. The platelet count is important when evaluating patients for the presence of clotting disorders. A decrease in the number of platelets (thrombocytopenia) can place a patient at risk for bruising and uncontrolled bleeding whereas an increase in platelets (thrombocytosis) will often occur when a patient has cancer. Platelet disorders can be either inherited or acquired.

Hemoglobin

The **hemoglobin** (Hgb) measures the oxygen-carrying capacity of the red blood cells. It aids in determining blood loss and anemia and is also valuable for monitoring other conditions such as dehydration. The hemoglobin level can also provide information concerning the effectiveness of blood transfusions.

An increase in the hemoglobin level can occur in conditions like chronic obstructive pulmonary disease (COPD), congestive heart failure (CHF), and polycythemia, while a decrease can occur with anemia and severe blood loss.

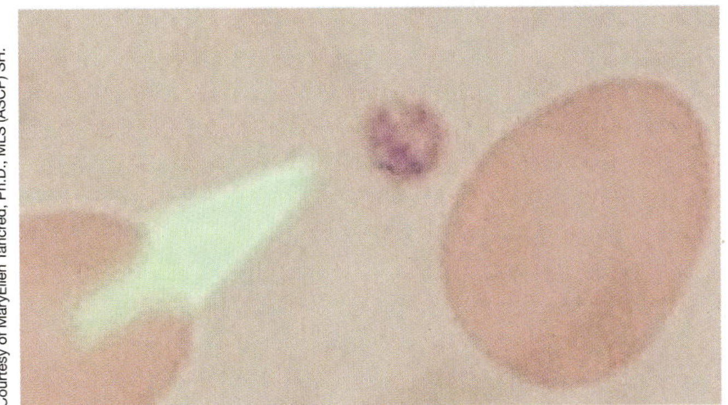

Courtesy of MaryEllen Tancred, Ph.D., MLS (ASCP) SH.

Figure 26-4 ■ Platelets are much smaller than red and white blood cells.

CRITICAL THINKING CHALLENGE

Think about the function of hemoglobin on the red cells. Why might a patient's hemoglobin level be increased in a condition like chronic obstructive pulmonary disease (COPD)?

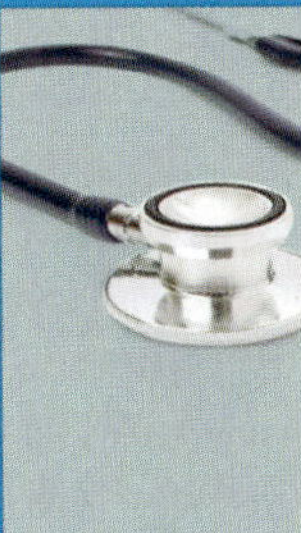

Field Smarts

Because hemoglobin carries oxygen to the cells of the body, it is common for patients to experience both fatigue and shortness of breath when their hemoglobin levels plummet. Be certain to alert the provider prior to examination if the patient is experiencing these symptoms. The provider may want testing performed immediately to determine if a low hemoglobin level is the reason for the patient's symptoms.

A hemoglobin determination can be easily performed using an automated device such as the Hemocue hemoglobin analyzer (Figure 26-5). The Hemocue is waived by CLIA and, therefore, ideal for use in the POL. Several other manufacturers offer analyzers that are also CLIA-waived. By performing this analysis in-house, the provider has the advantage of testing the patient and receiving results while the patient waits. Treatment can be implemented much sooner than if it was necessary to wait for results to be

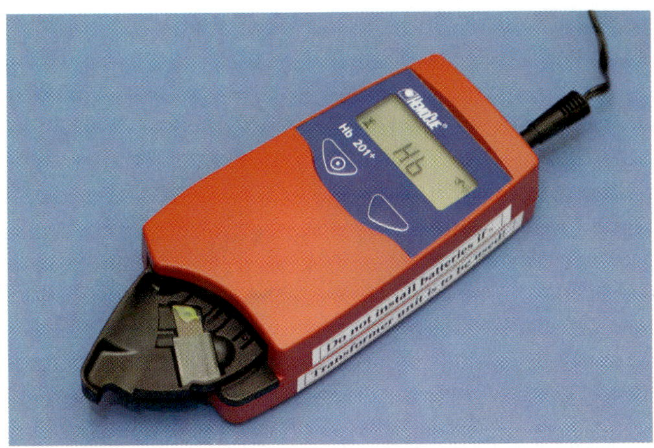

Figure 26-5 ■ A Hemocue automated hemoglobin analyzer.

received from an outside laboratory. The hemoglobin determination results are reported as grams of hemoglobin per deciliter (g/dL).

Refer to Procedure 26-2 for a full procedure on how to perform a hemoglobin determination.

Hematocrit

The **hematocrit (Hct)**, also a CLIA-waived test, is a quick and easy method for determining the volume of packed red blood cells in a given volume of blood. Hematocrit is reported as a percentage (e.g., a hematocrit reported as 48% means that 48% of the total blood volume is made up of red blood cells).

The hemoglobin and hematocrit tests have a unique relationship and are rarely performed separately. They both provide information about the hemoglobin- and oxygen-carrying ability of the RBCs. Hemoglobin tests indicate the density of hemoglobin within the RBCs and the hematocrit test indicates the percentage of RBCs within the sample of blood. The hemoglobin result is generally one-third of the hematocrit and any deviation from that ratio may be indicative of a disease or condition.

The hematocrit may be performed with an automated analyzer or manually. The manual hematocrit test is performed by centrifuging a small sample of whole blood in a petite narrow tube called a capillary tube. The test is often referred to as a micro-hematocrit test because of the size of the tubes. Either capillary or venous blood may be used for this test.

Heparinized tubes are used when collecting blood from a capillary puncture to prevent the sample from clotting prior to testing. Figure 26-6 shows some examples of plain and heparinized safety capillary tubes with clay sealant.

The tube fills by capillary action, a force that draws a thick liquid, such as blood, into a narrow tube. The tube is held horizontally with the end of the tube placed into a well-rounded drop of blood and then sealed. When using self-sealing tubes, the dry plug in the other end of the tube will expand when the blood reaches it, sealing off the tube. There are other brands and types of safety self-sealing microhematocrit tubes available.

Filled capillary tubes are placed in the microhematocrit centrifuge with the sealed end placed at the bottom of the holders in the unit featured in Figure 26-7. When using tubes that are placed horizontally in the centrifuge, the sealed end should face the gasket or outside of the unit, and spun for two to five minutes. When centrifuged, the cellular components of the blood are separated into three layers with the red blood cells at the bottom, the white blood cells and platelets in the middle (buffy coat), and the plasma on top. Figure 26-8 illustrates the separation of the cellular components after centrifugation. The spun hematocrit tubes are placed on a reading device and the percentage of red blood cells is determined. Two tubes are filled, centrifuged, and read, and the readings are averaged to determine the hematocrit. The two readings must agree within 2% or the test must be repeated. Procedure 26-1 lists the necessary steps for performing a manual microhematocrit.

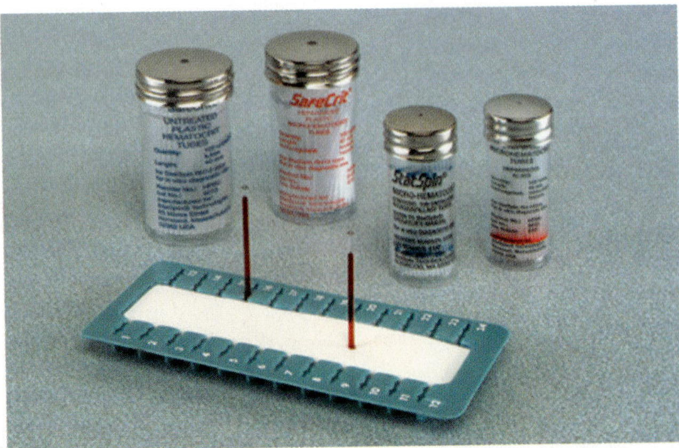

Figure 26-6 ■ Examples of safety capillary tubes and clay sealant.

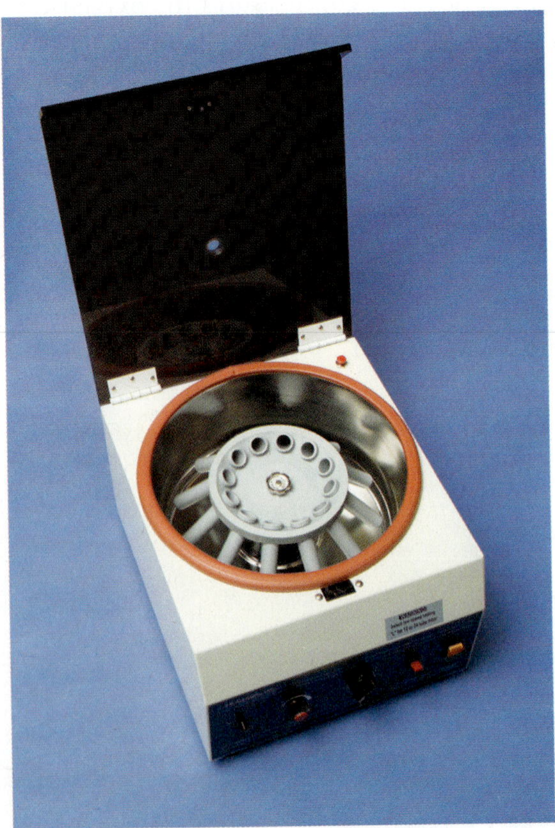

Figure 26-7 ■ A microhematocrit centrifuge.

lymphocytes, and **monocytes**. Leukocytes guard the body against infection by producing antibodies and functioning in the immune response. White blood cells move through the bloodstream and into the tissues to the site of an infection, where they perform various functions.

Each type of white blood cell has a very specific function; these functions are further explained later in the chapter.

Thrombocytes

Thrombocytes, or platelets, are actually cell fragments. They function mainly in the process of **hemostasis** (stopping the flow of blood). Platelets stop bleeding by forming a sticky plug in the damaged blood vessel wall. Once they adhere to the site of bleeding they release a chemical that attracts other platelets to the site, forming a loose platelet plug and providing a surface for clotting proteins (also known as factors) to form a stable clot.

COAGULATION

Whenever a blood vessel is injured, it contracts, thus slowing the flow of blood so the clotting process can begin. The formation of platelet plug happens next, as mentioned above, followed by the onset of the complex chemical processes of coagulation, involving proteins, called clotting factors. Since these events happen one right after the other, they are often referred to as the **coagulation cascade**. Each factor has an active and inactive form. Once a factor is activated, it will activate the next factor, thus cascading through the process. The factors are numbered using Roman numerals I through XIII, although only a couple are needed for our study here. The first factor, Factor I, is called fibrinogen and is the origin of fibrin. **Fibrin**, just like it sounds, is fiber-like and forms a network of fibers to help form the needed blood clot. Factor II, called prothrombin (meaning before thrombin) makes thrombin with the help of vitamin K. Calcium is needed in the clotting process and is considered Factor IV. Once the bleeding stops, the clot will start to dry, contracting the edges of the wound together and eventually forming a scab on the skin, which turns into a scar. Figure 26-2 shows a diagram of the clot formation.

BASIC HEMATOLOGY STUDIES

Hematologic (blood) tests are among the most common ordered by the provider. Some of the tests can be performed in the physician's office laboratory (POL) and some are performed in outside laboratories. Blood tests can measure each blood cell type individually to determine the relative number present and also for abnormalities to the cells themselves. Through blood tests, the provider can gain valuable information about the general health of the patient as well as particular disease processes occurring within the body. For instance, a patient with a decreased red blood cell count might be diagnosed with anemia. Since there are a number of different types of anemia, an evaluation of the red cell **morphology** (a study of the cell's size, shape, and color) can help to determine the type and cause of the anemia. Then, once the patient is treated for the anemia, further blood tests can help the provider monitor the effectiveness of medications and treatments. The provider can also use blood tests to determine whether an infection is viral or bacterial by evaluating the results of the white blood cell **differential count**. This test, sometimes performed as part of a complete blood count (CBC), determines the percentage of the five different types of white blood cells present and examines their characteristics. Table 26-2 lists some of the blood cell disorders that may be detected by a simple hematology test.

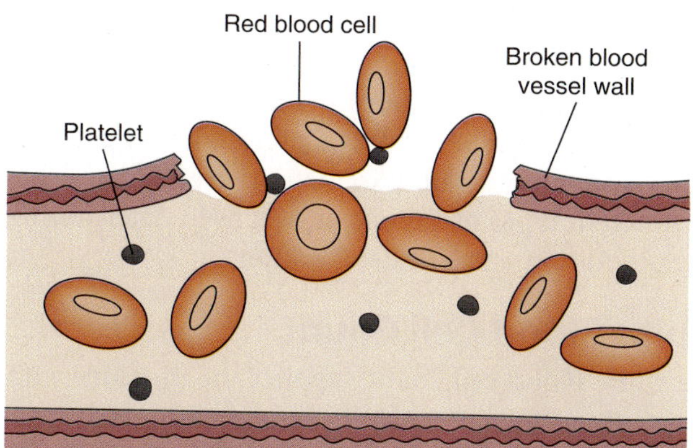

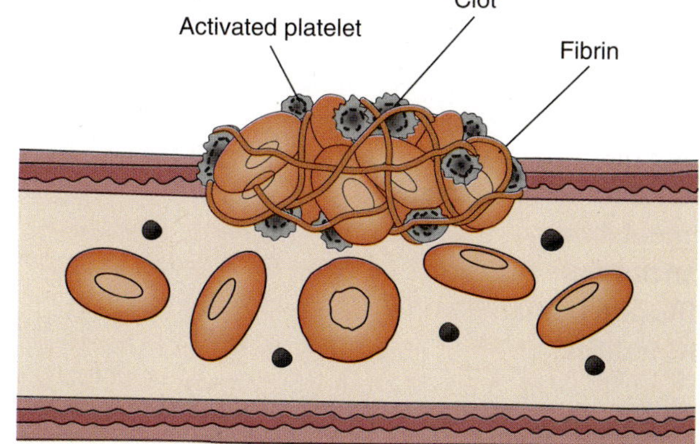

Figure 26-2 ■ With the help of fibrin and platelets, a clot is formed.

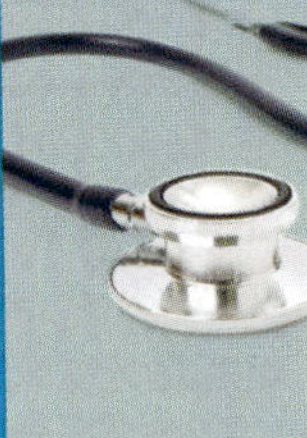

Table 26-2 Disorders of Blood Cells

Disorder	Description
General causes of anemia	Blood loss, insufficient production of RBCs, excessive destruction of RBCs, or deformed/dysfunctional RBCs
Aplastic anemia	Caused by bone marrow disorders that cause red cell production to be decreased or inhibited
Hemolytic anemia	Inherited or acquired disorder that results in the destruction of the red blood cells
Iron deficiency anemia	Most common type of anemia, caused by a decrease in stored dietary iron
Pernicious anemia	Decreased number of RBCs caused by a lack of vitamin B_{12}
Sickle cell anemia	Inherited disorder, which causes a sickle-shaped RBC, interfering with the ability of the cell to carry oxygen
Erythrocytosis	An abnormal increase in the number of RBCs
Leukemia	A malignant cancer of WBCs in which the bone marrow creates abnormal and dysfunctional WBCs
Leukopenia/ Leukocytopenia	A low number of total WBCs
Leukocytosis	An increase in the total number of WBCs
Pancytopenia	A decrease in all blood cell types
Thrombocytopenia	A low platelet count
Thrombocytosis	An overproduction of platelets

Field Smarts

Sickle cell anemia is an inherited disorder caused by the presence of an abnormal hemoglobin (hemoglobin S) in the blood. This abnormal hemoglobin becomes thickened when exposed to a decrease in oxygen, which in turn causes the red cells to be crescent or sickle-shaped. The abnormal shape of the cells (Figure 26-3) interferes with their movement through the capillaries, creating an obstruction that can cause pain in the area.

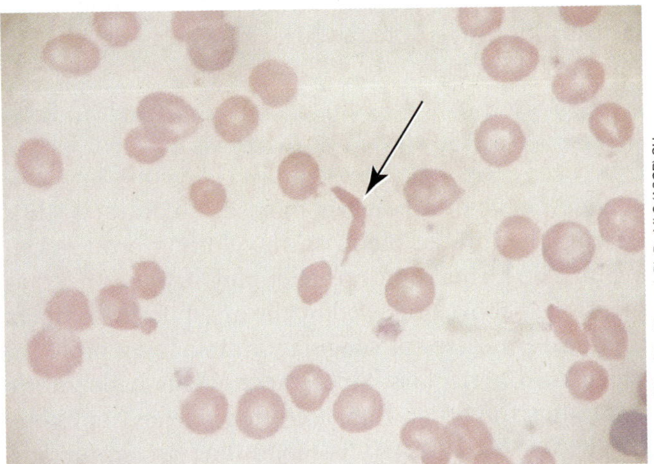

Courtesy of MaryEllen Tancred, Ph.D., MLS (ASCP) SH.

Figure 26-3 ■ Notice how the red cells are sickle shaped in this patient's blood.

THE COMPLETE BLOOD COUNT (CBC)

The **complete blood count (CBC)** is a group of tests that count the number of each type of blood cell (RBCs, WBCs, and platelets), the percentage of the five different types of white blood cells (WBC differential), the specifics of the red blood cells (RBC indices), the hemoglobin content and quality within the red blood cells (hemoglobin and hematocrit), and a listing of any abnormal cells.

CBC parameters can vary by facility, but usually include the following:

- Red blood cell count
- White blood cell count
- Platelet count or estimate
- Hemoglobin
- Hematocrit
- WBC differential
- RBC indices

Complete blood counts and individual parts of the CBC are performed by automated methods using CBC analyzers. Some analyzers and tests are included in the CLIA-waived category.

Red Blood Cell Count

The red blood cell count measures the number of RBCs present in 1 cubic millimeter of blood. The RBC count is reported as the number of RBCs/cu mm or RBCs $\times$ 10^6/uL of blood. (Both units are the same.) Oftentimes uL is converted to liters so you will see it written as RBCs $\times$ 10^{12}/L.

The count supplies the provider with an estimate of the relative number of RBCs present in the patient's total blood volume. This parameter is useful in evaluating different types of anemia as well as in determining other conditions such as dehydration.

White Blood Cell Count

The white blood cell count supplies the provider with information that can assist in the diagnosis and treatment of infectious processes and disease states. It can also aid in following the progress of a disease and the effectiveness of treatments.

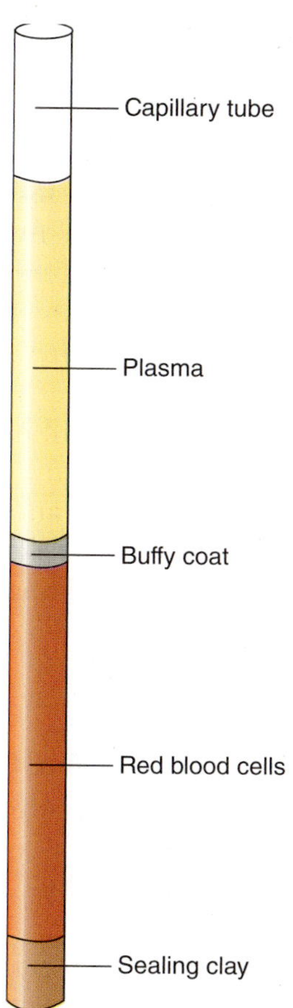

Figure 26-8 ■ An illustration of a hematocrit tube after centrifugation. Note the separation into distinct layers.

CRITICAL THINKING CHALLENGE

What do you suspect would happen to a patient's hematocrit and hemoglobin during periods of dehydration? Why?

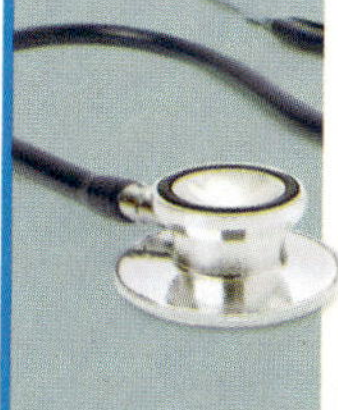

Field Smarts

Correlation of laboratory results is essential to ensure that tests have been performed accurately. A general rule of thumb is that the hematocrit should be approximately three times the result of the hemoglobin (e.g., a sample with 12.5 g/dL of hemoglobin should have a hematocrit result of approximately 36–37%). If this rule does not hold true (e.g., 12.5 g/dL of hemoglobin and a hematocrit of 50%), the test should be repeated.

Differential Count

The white blood cell differential count is a valuable tool used to assess many different patient conditions. Because each WBC performs a different action during an infectious disease, determining which of the five WBCs is activated or elevated can help diagnose the condition or disease.

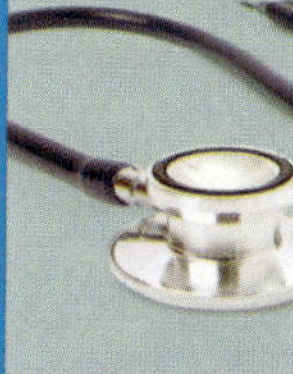

Field Smarts

Neutrophils may be released into the blood stream during times of acute infectious disease before they are fully matured. These immature neutrophils are called bands or stabs due to the shape of the stained cytoplasm. Look at the photo of the band/stab in Figure 26-9. You can see that the nucleus has not yet separated into segments like the mature neutrophil nucleus. When the test reveals an increase in immature neutrophils, the patient is probably dealing with an acute infection and the body is producing large amounts of neutrophils to try to fight the infection. Sometimes the bones will actually ache in response to the marrow activity and certainly the patient will experience a fever.

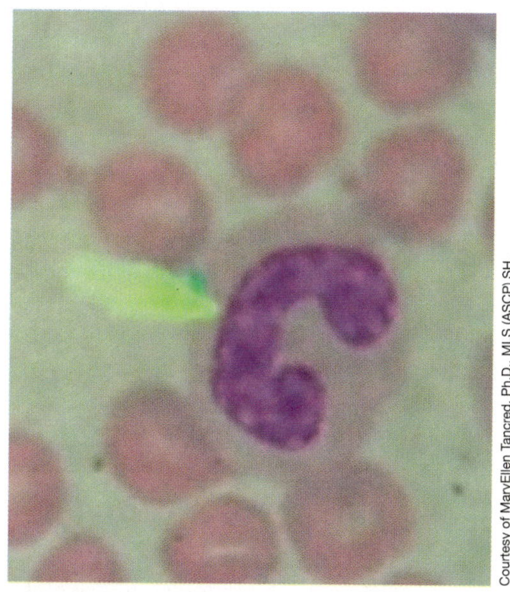

Figure 26-9 ■ A neutrophilic band cell.

Neither the manual nor the automated differential count are CLIA-waived. Manual methods require a slide of a blood smear be prepared, stained, and set before being examined under a microscope.

Neutrophils, eosinophils, and basophils all received their names based on what happens during the staining process. The medical suffix *phil* means an attraction to something. Eosinophils received their name because of their attraction to the eosin dye during the staining process; thus, their granules are orange-red. Basophils received their name because of their attraction to the base dye, or methylene blue stain, causing their granules to be a purplish-black. Neutrophils received their name because they pick up a combination of both dyes, which provides a neutral color or pink to purple granules. Table 26-3 illustrates the different types of white blood cells.

Table 26-3 White Blood Cell Identification

White Blood Cell Type	Illustration
Neutrophil or seg	
Band or stab (immature neutrophil)	
Eosinophil	
Basophil	
Lymphocyte	
Monocyte	

After counting 100 white blood cells, the red blood cells are observed by the lab technician for their morphology.

Differentials are performed in medical laboratories by automated analyzers that sort the WBCs cells by size and separate them into five classifications. Abnormal cells found on a differential are usually flagged by the automated instrument and a manual differential count is performed for specific observation of the cells.

While the medical assistant will not perform a differential, being familiar with terms used to describe the results, and normal values and conditions that can affect the results will assist the medical assistant with priority tasking and in providing education to the patient.

Red Blood Cell Morphology

Red blood cell morphology refers to the study of the form and structure of the red blood cells. This is usually done after identification of the white blood cells during the differential portion of the CBC.

The automated analyzer observes the red blood cells for their size and shape. Variations in the sizes of the red blood cells is known as **anisocytosis** (Figure 26-10a), while variations in the shapes of the red blood cells is known as **poikilocytosis** (Figure 26-10b). Abnormal red cell morphology can be indicative of many different hematologic conditions.

A normal red blood cell (Figure 26-11a) with its biconcave shape will stain a pinkish color and will have no nucleus. Red cells can either be normocytic (from **normocyte**, meaning of normal size), microcytic (from **microcyte** (Figure 26-11b), meaning smaller than normal), or macrocytic (from **macrocyte**, meaning larger than normal), as shown in Figure 26-11c.

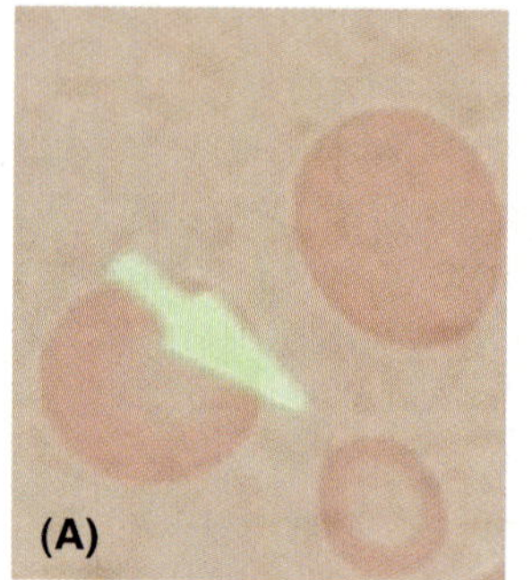

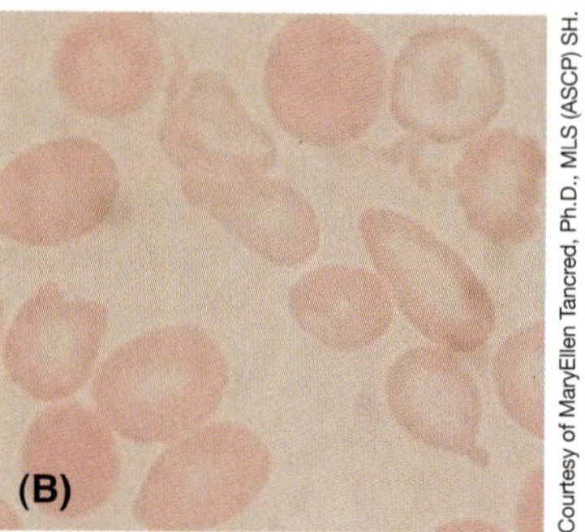

Courtesy of MaryEllen Tancred, Ph.D., MLS (ASCP) SH.

Figure 26-10 ■ (a) A slide illustrating anisocytosis (variation of the size of the RBCs). (b) A slide illustrating poikilocytosis (variation of the shapes of the RBCs).

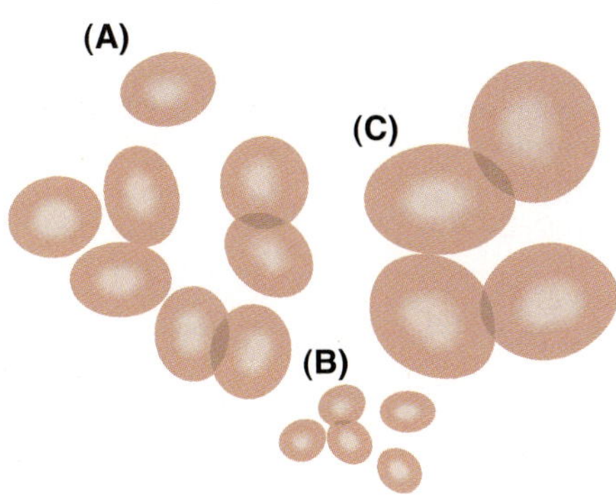

Figure 26-11 ■ (a) A normal-sized red blood cell; (b) a microcyte; (c) a macrocyte.

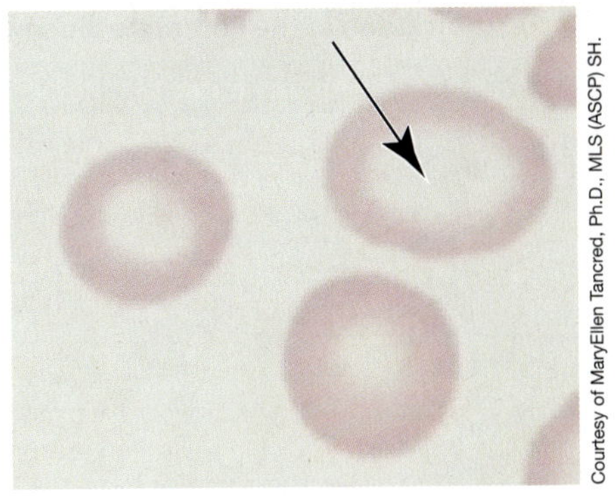

Figure 26-12 ■ A red cell that illustrates a hypochromic center.

The center of a normal red cell is thin and will not pick up as much color as the rest of the cell, creating a pale area described as a "central pallor." The hemoglobin is contained in the pink area of the cell. If the central pallor is large, this means that the hemoglobin content of the red cell is decreased, alerting the provider that an abnormal condition exists (Figure 26-12). The typical biconcave shape of the red cell allows it to easily perform the function of carrying oxygen to the cells and tissues of the body and carbon dioxide away from the cells and tissues of the body. Red cells that are shaped differently cannot perform this vital function and are indicative of a blood disease or disorder.

Red Blood Cell Indices

The final component of the CBC is a group of tests that provides complete information about the red blood cells. This group of tests is known as the **red blood cell indices** (plural for index). The indices are calculated using the values of the red blood cell count with the hemoglobin and the hematocrit. The RBC indices are valuable in diagnosing, evaluating, and treating different types of anemias and bleeding disorders.

The RBC indices include the following:

- Mean (average) corpuscular volume (MCV), per femtoliters
- Mean (average) corpuscular hemoglobin (MCH), per picogram/cell
- Mean (average) corpuscular hemoglobin concentration (MCHC), per grams/deciliter

Table 26-4 provides information about each of the indices, including reference ranges, what the index is actually measuring, and possible reasons for increased or decreased values.

Refer to Table 26-5 for information about all tests included in the CBC.

Table 26-4 RBC Indices

Test	Measurement	Reference Range	Causes for Abnormal Values
MCV	Volume (size) of the average red blood cell in a given sample of blood	80–100 fL	High MCV: cells are macrocytes (larger than normal) Low MCV: cells are microcytes (smaller than normal)
MCH	Estimation of the average weight of hemoglobin in a single red blood cell	27–33 pg	Corresponds with the MCV, smaller cells have lower MCH, larger cells have higher MCH
MCHC	Concentration of hemoglobin in the red blood cells in relation to their size and volume	32–37 g/dL	Low MCHC: hypochromia (pale)

Table 26-5 Tests Included in the Complete Blood Count

Test	Abbreviation	Reference Range*	Abnormal Values Seen In:	
Hematocrit	Hct	Males: 42–52% Females: 36–45% Neonates: 44–64%	High Hct results seen in: • Polycythemia • Vomiting • Diarrhea • Dehydration • Hyperglycemia	Low Hct results seen in: • Anemia • Hemorrhage • Pregnancy
Hemoglobin	Hgb	Males: 13–18 g/dL Females: 12–16 g/dL Neonates: 15–20 g/dL	High Hgb results seen in: • COPD • CHF • Polycythemia • Dehydration	Low Hgb results seen in: • Anemia • Blood loss • Leukemia
Red blood cell count (For red blood cell indices refer to Table 26-6)	RBC count	Males: 4.5–6.0 million $\times 10^{12}$/L Females: 4.0–5.5 million $\times 10^{12}$/L Neonates: 4.0-6.6 million $\times 10^{12}$/L	High RBC count seen in: • Polycythemia • Dehydration • Pulmonary fibrosis	Low RBC count seen in: • Anemias • Leukemia
White blood cell count	WBC count	Adults: 4,500–11,000 $\times 10^9$/L Neonates: 9,000–25,000 $\times 10^9$/L	High WBC count seen in: • Acute infections • Appendicitis • Mononucleosis • Meningitis	Low WBC count seen in: • Viral infections • Chemotherapy • Radiation therapy
Differential cell count				
Neutrophils	Segs	50–65%	High, seen in: • Bacterial infections • Parasitic infections • Leukemia • Inflammation • Liver disease	Low, seen in: • Viral infections • Certain diseases of body fluids • Chemotherapy
Bands	Stabs Juvs	0–7%	High, seen in: • Most infectious diseases • Some leukemias	
Eosinophils	Eos	1–3%	High, seen in: • Allergic reactions • Parasitic infections • Lung and bone cancer	Low, seen in: • Infectious mononucleosis • CHF • Aplastic anemia
Basophils	Basos	0–1%	High, seen in: • Leukemia • Hemolytic anemia • Chronic inflammations	
Lymphocytes	Lymphs	25–40%	High, seen in: • Viral infections • Carcinoma • Hematopoietic disorders	Low, seen in: • HIV infection • Myelocytic leukemia • Hodgkin's disease
Monocytes	Monos	3–9%	High, seen in: • Certain bacterial infections	Low, seen in: • Chemotherapy
Thrombocytes	Platelets	140,000–400,000 $\times 10^9$/L	High, seen in: • Cancers • Major traumas • Surgeries • Anemia	Low, seen in: • Cancer treatments • Drugs • Autoimmune disorders

*Unless otherwise noted, all reference ranges are for adults.

Notes: Reference ranges listed were compiled from several different sources. Laboratory reference values may differ from one lab to another according to test methodology and each laboratory's own "normal patient population."

Complete Blood Count Normal Values

Table 26-5 summarizes the tests included in a complete blood count and their reference ranges.

Medical assistants are often responsible for placing orders in the EHR for diagnostic testing. Figure 26-13 illustrates a screen shot of an order entry screen with an order for a CBC and differential. Figure 26-14

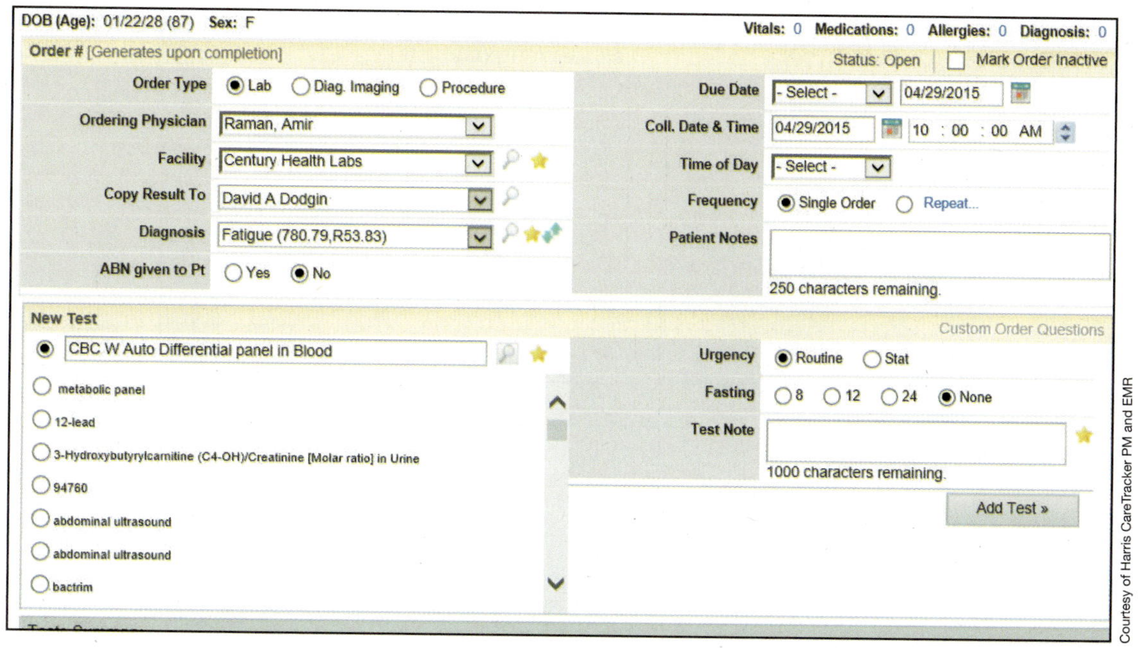

Courtesy of Harris CareTracker PM and EMR

Figure 26-13 ■ A screen shot of an order entry screen for a CBC and differential.

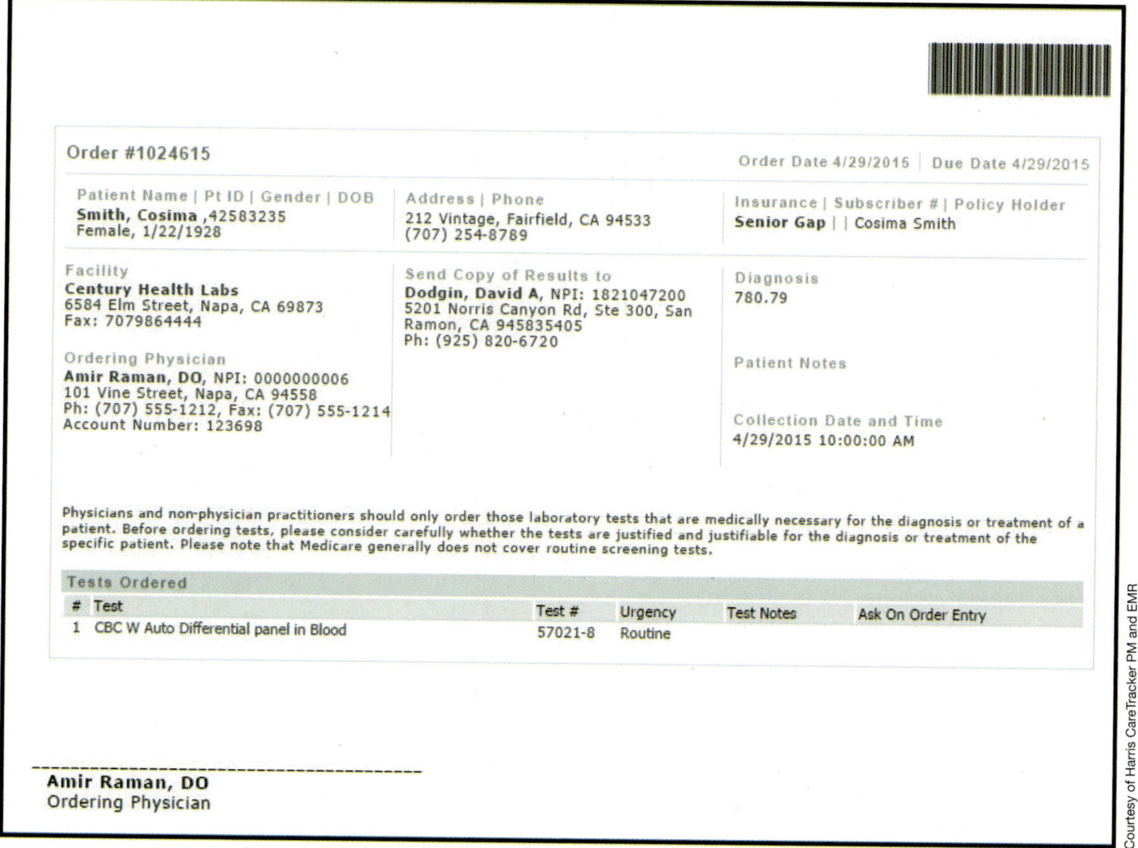

Order #1024615

Order Date 4/29/2015 | Due Date 4/29/2015

Patient Name | Pt ID | Gender | DOB
Smith, Cosima ,42583235
Female, 1/22/1928

Address | Phone
212 Vintage, Fairfield, CA 94533
(707) 254-8789

Insurance | Subscriber # | Policy Holder
Senior Gap | | Cosima Smith

Facility
Century Health Labs
6584 Elm Street, Napa, CA 69873
Fax: 7079864444

Send Copy of Results to
Dodgin, David A, NPI: 1821047200
5201 Norris Canyon Rd, Ste 300, San Ramon, CA 945835405
Ph: (925) 820-6720

Diagnosis
780.79

Ordering Physician
Amir Raman, DO, NPI: 0000000006
101 Vine Street, Napa, CA 94558
Ph: (707) 555-1212, Fax: (707) 555-1214
Account Number: 123698

Patient Notes

Collection Date and Time
4/29/2015 10:00:00 AM

Physicians and non-physician practitioners should only order those laboratory tests that are medically necessary for the diagnosis or treatment of a patient. Before ordering tests, please consider carefully whether the tests are justified and justifiable for the diagnosis or treatment of the specific patient. Please note that Medicare generally does not cover routine screening tests.

Tests Ordered

#	Test	Test #	Urgency	Test Notes	Ask On Order Entry
1	CBC W Auto Differential panel in Blood	57021-8	Routine		

Amir Raman, DO
Ordering Physician

Courtesy of Harris CareTracker PM and EMR

Figure 26-14 ■ A printed order for a CBC and differential.

Allied Health Professions
1122 Sycamore St.
Santa Anna. XY
Mary Smith, M.D.
1(800)555-1122

Patient: Black Doris L
ID: 161111
Birth Date: MAY 22 1924 Age: 90Y Sex: F
Room: ED
Sample ID: 70150072 Collected On: 03/11/XX @ 14:00

Physician: Larkin, Alicia, FNP
Report To: ED

Received: 03/11/XX @ 14:17

Test	Flag	Result	Units	Reference
WHITE BLOOD CELL CT		7.7	X10^9	4.5 - 11.5
RED BLOOD CELLS	H	5.5	x10^12	4.2 - 5.4
HEMOGLOBIN	H	15.2	g/dl	12.0 - 15.0
HEMATOCRIT		48	%	35 - 49
MCV		88	f	80 - 100
MCH		32	X10^9	26.0 - 33.0
MCHC		35	%	32 - 36
PLATELET		327	X10^9	150 - 450
NEUT % - AUTO COUNT		68	%	50 - 70
MIXED CELL % - AUTOL		1	U/L	2 - 12
LYMPH% - AUTO COUNT		19	X10^9	18 - 42
NEUTROPHIL ABSOLUTE		6.5	x10^12	1.5 - 7.1
MIXED CELL ABSOLUTE		0.2	x10^12	0.2 - 1.0
LYMPHOCYTE ABSOLUTE		1.7	x10^12	0.8 - 2.8
RDW-CV		11.4	%	-
MEAN PLT VOLUME	H	13.0		8.6 - 11.7

Original Print Date: 03/11/XX @ 14:47 **Reviewed By:**____________

Figure 26-15 ■ An example of a lab report for a CBC.

illustrates what the order looks like when printed out. This replaces the traditional lab requisition form that was used in the past. Figure 26-15 illustrates a lab report for a CBC.

ERYTHROCYTE SEDIMENTATION RATE (ESR)

The **erythrocyte sedimentation rate (ESR)**, or sed rate, is a test that, with knowledge and practice, can be performed by the medical assistant (see Procedure 26-3). The principle of the ESR is to determine how far the red blood cells descend or settle in a one-hour time frame in a given volume of whole blood.

The ESR is not specific for one particular disease, but can indicate general inflammation and tissue destruction. It is also used to follow treatment of certain conditions. All nonautomated ESR tests are CLIA-waived, specifically the Wintrobe method, the Westergren Sediplast method, as well as the automated BD Sedi-15. In both the Wintrobe and the Westergren methods, well-mixed anticoagulated blood is placed in a calibrated tube and allowed to stand for one hour. The BD Sedi-15 uses an automated analyzer.

The Wintrobe method uses a Wintrobe tube, which holds 1 mL of blood and has graduated markings from 0 to 100 mm. The tube is filled with well-mixed anticoagulated blood to the "zero" line and placed in a rack for one hour. After one hour, the distance the red blood cells have fallen is read and recorded as the ESR. The results are recorded in mm/h. Figure 26-16 shows a magnification of the tube and its markings.

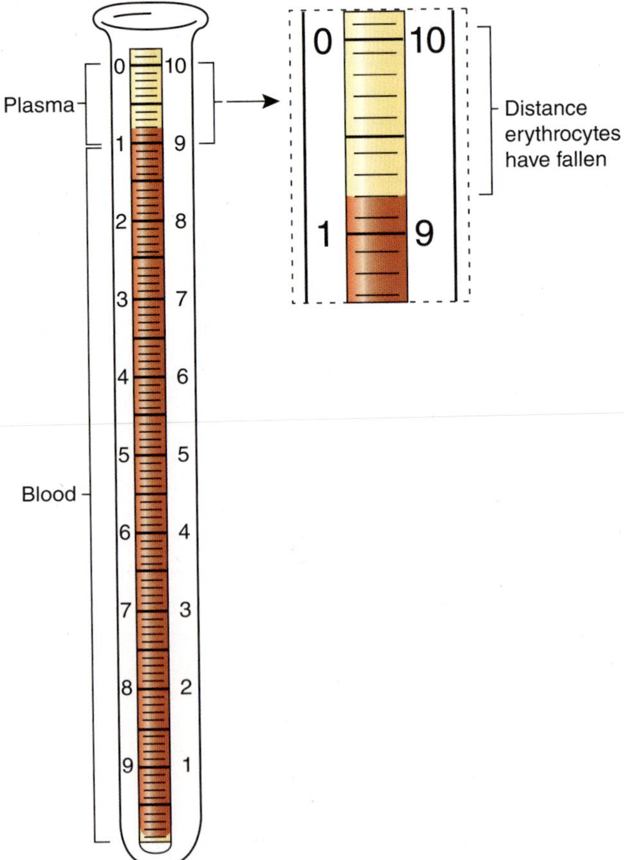

Figure 26-16 ■ A Wintrobe sedimentation tube. Magnification shows an 8 mm/h ESR reading. (Read on the left side going down.)

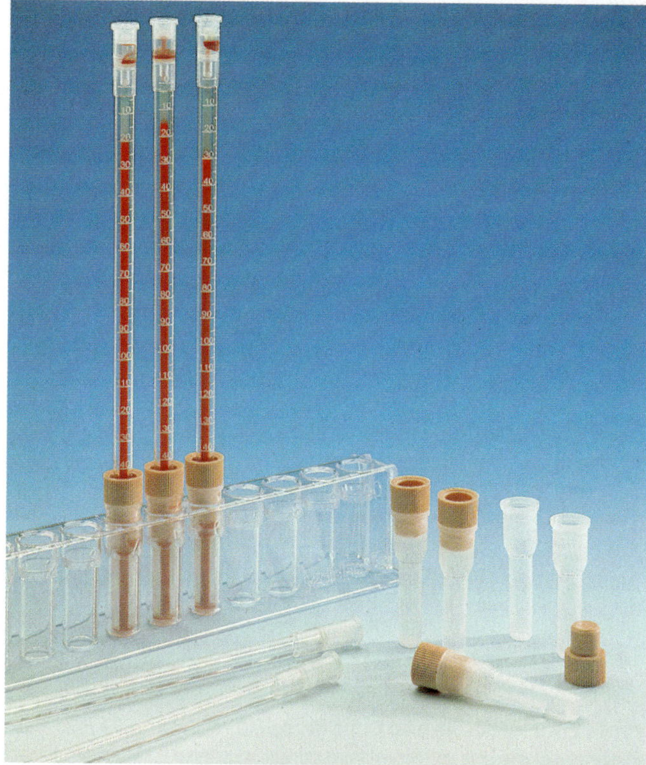

Figure 26-17 ■ The Sediplast ESR system.

An example of an ESR test using the Westergren method is The Sediplast system (Figure 26-17). This is a closed, self-filling system that protects medical personnel from possible exposure. Procedure 26-2 lists the steps necessary to perform the Sediplast method.

General guidelines to follow when performing an ESR by either manual method include the following:

1. Timing is critical. The test must be timed for precisely one hour.
2. The tubes must remain undisturbed in a vertical position for the entire hour.
3. The tube rack should be placed on a counter or table that is free of vibrations.
4. The tubes must not be placed in direct sunlight or draft.
5. The test should be performed at room temperature on well-mixed blood.
6. The test should be performed within two hours of specimen collection.

Table 26-6 lists ESR normal values. Notice how ESR will increase with age. Table 26-7 lists possible causes for both increased and decreased sed rate results.

Table 26-6 ESR Normal Values

Gender and Age	Normal Values
Males:	
<50 years of age	0–15 mm/h
>50 years of age	0–20 mm/h
Females:	
<50 years of age	0–20 mm/h
>50 years of age	0–30 mm/h
Children	0–10 mm/h

Table 26-7 Factors and Conditions Affecting the ESR

Factors That Can Increase the ESR
Plasma proteins that cause RBCs to stick together and fall faster
Macrocytosis
Pregnancy
Anemia
Cancer
Inflammatory diseases like rheumatoid arthritis
Acute and chronic infections
Multiple myeloma
Factors That Can Decrease the ESR
Sickle cell anemia
Spherocytosis
Polycythemia
Microcytosis
Irregularly shaped cells that do not stick together easily and fall more slowly

AUTOMATED HEMATOLOGY ANALYZERS

Hematology tests performed in the POL and outside medical laboratories will usually be performed using automated analyzers. Some are CLIA-waived and some, due to their complexity, are not CLIA-waived.

Automated analyzers are fast, accurate, and often simple to use, but they do require stringent maintenance and controls. Many are equipped with printers that produce a hard copy of the results immediately. Some analyzers are also equipped to store quality control data. Hematology analyzers are available that can perform one or two tests or a complete blood count including RBC indices.

COAGULATION TESTS

Common coagulation tests are the **prothrombin time (PT)** and the **activated partial thromboplastin time (aPTT)**. Both PT and aPTT tests measure clotting times in seconds. They are used as screening tests for deficiencies in the coagulation cascade mentioned earlier, and for monitoring of patients on anticoagulation therapy. Oral anticoagulant therapy such as Coumadin is monitored with the PT and INR tests. The patient's PT result is reported with the **International normalized ratio (INR)** which provides standardization of the PT value. The INR is calibrated by dividing the patient's PT test result by the laboratory's normal value. By using this standardized system, it is easier to ensure both consistent results from one lab to another and the continuity of anticoagulant therapy. In some cases, only the INR is reported. Normal INR ratio for a patient on anticoagulants is between 2.0 and 3.0. A higher INR indicates the patient is at risk for internal bleeding while a lower INR indicates the patient is at risk of developing blood clots. Normal ranges for PT, aPTT, and INR can be found in Table 26-8. Table 26-9 lists factors and conditions affecting the PT.

Patients taking anticoagulants/blood thinners such as Coumadin will have their blood tested at varying intervals to see how they are responding to anticoagulation therapy and to have the medication dosages adjusted as needed by their health care professional. Some of the more recently developed anticoagulants do not require the frequent blood testing and dietary restrictions that Coumadin requires, which are distinct advantages; however, these newer types of anticoagulants are not without their own risks. Examples of uses of anticoagulant therapy include patients with a history of deep vein thrombosis (DVT), stroke (CVA), or myocardial infarction (MI) also known as a heart attack or, most commonly, anticoagulants are used with patients who have atrial fibrillation.

As discussed earlier in this chapter, vitamin K is needed for the synthesis of prothrombin (Factor II) into thrombin. Therefore, the PT test can be useful in screening for vitamin K deficiencies as well as liver function.

Coagulation tests can be performed in the POL within minutes by the medical assistant using a very small amount of blood taken from a fingerstick capillary puncture. There are dozens of CLIA-waived automated handheld or countertop instruments available that perform the coagulation tests. See Figure 26-18 for examples. By having this test performed in the clinic, the provider can counsel the patient and make medication adjustments immediately.

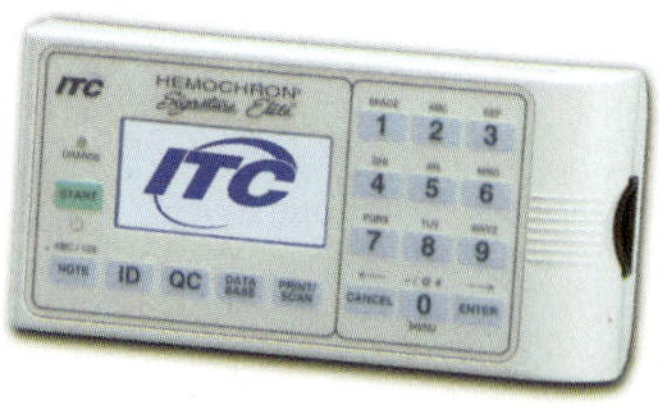

(A)

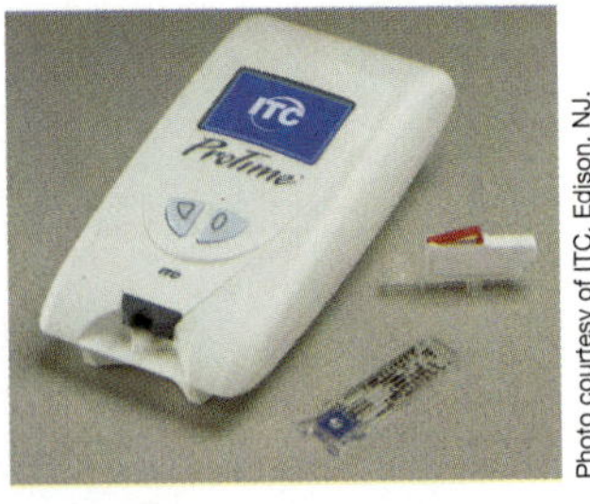

(B)

Photo courtesy of ITC, Edison, NJ.

Figure 26-18 ■ Small point-of-care coagulation analyzers: (a) HEMOCHRON Signtature Elite; (b) ProTime.

Table 26-8 Normal Values for PT, aPTT, and INR

Test	Normal Value	Anticoagulant Therapy
PT	10–13 seconds	2.5 times longer
aPTT	25–40 seconds	2.5 times longer
INR	0.8–1.1	2.0–3.0

Table 26-9 Factors and Conditions Affecting the PT

Factors That Can Increase the PT
Liver disease
Clotting factor deficiency
Vitamin K deficiency
Depression of the bone marrow
Cancer
Collagen disease
Factors That Can Decrease the PT
Medications
High intake of vitamin K in supplements or food source
Pulmonary embolism
Multiple myeloma
Myocardial infarction
Thrombophlebitis

Refer to Procedure 26-4 for performing a PT/INR procedure.

CRITICAL THINKING CHALLENGE

Why is it so important to ask patients on anticoagulants about their diets and which vitamins, minerals, and herbals they are taking?

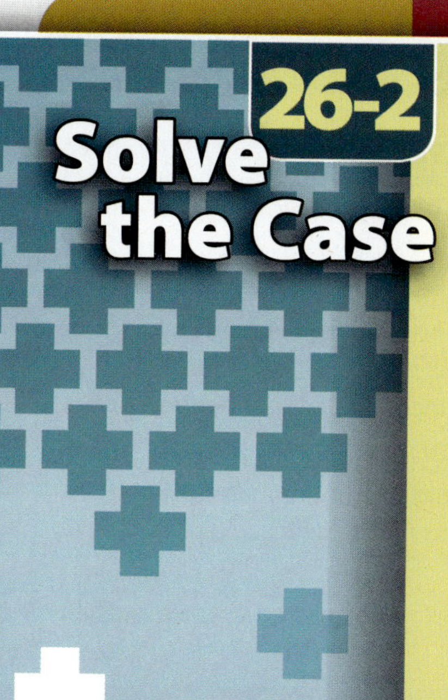

Dr. Dorado orders a stat hematocrit and hemoglobin on Mrs. Walker. Her hematocrit is 21.2% and her hemoglobin is 7.0 g/dL. The doctor is very concerned and orders a complete CBC with a differential. He also orders an FSH level (a hormone associated with estrogen) and asks you to set up an appointment for a uterine ultrasound ASAP on Mrs. Walker.

1. **Are the hematocrit and hemoglobin results high or low? What are the normal values for a hematocrit and hemoglobin?**
2. **Why do you think the doctor ordered an FSH level on the patient?**

You find out that the patient did not keep her appointment for the uterine ultrasound. The doctor asks you to call the patient and find out what happened. He tells you that he suspects the patient has uterine fibroids, which is causing her to have excessive bleeding each month and that he is very concerned about her blood count. When you call the patient she states that her schedule is just too full right now and that she is feeling better.

3. **What type of response can you give to the patient to help her understand the importance of having this test performed?**

PROCEDURE 26-1

Perform a Capillary Puncture and Microhematocrit Test

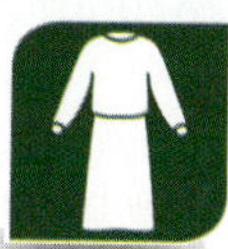

Objective:

Properly perform and determine the microhematocrit value by centrifuging a sample of blood in a capillary tube to separate the cellular components from the plasma.

Equipment/Supplies:

- Personal protective equipment (PPE) (this will vary by facility)
- Safety capillary tubes (heparinized)
- Microhematocrit centrifuge
- Microhematocrit reader
- Fingerstick blood sample
- Tissue wipes, 2 × 2 gauze squares
- Sharps container
- Biohazard container
- Patient's chart/EHR

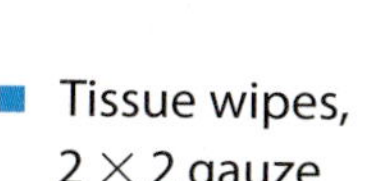

PROCEDURAL STEPS	DETAILS AND/OR RATIONALE
1. Wash your hands and apply PPE.	Hands must be washed before and after each procedure and PPE, especially gloves, must be worn when handling any body fluid specimens to avoid transmission of infectious organisms.

continues

PROCEDURE 26-1 continued

PROCEDURAL STEPS	DETAILS AND/OR RATIONALE
2. Assemble the equipment and supplies.	Having the supplies ready to go will help the procedure efficiency.
3. Identify the patient using two identifiers, identify yourself with your credentials. ***Explain the rationale for the performance of the procedure, showing awareness of the patient's concerns related to the procedure being performed.***	Performing the testing on the wrong patient can result in serious consequences. Introducing yourself and stating your credentials will promote professionalism. Explaining the procedure increases patient cooperation.
4. Perform a capillary puncture and wipe away the first drop of blood with the 2 × 2 gauze.	The first drop of blood could be contaminated with alcohol or diluted with tissue fluid, which will produce inaccurate results.
5. Hold a heparinized capillary tube horizontal to the second drop of blood without touching the skin.	Heparinized capillary tubes must be used to prevent the blood from clotting.
• Allow the capillary tube to fill three-fourths full.	• The tube should be filled three-fourths full for easier reading.
• Seal the end of tube with clay or a sealing cap (Figure 26-19).	• Sealing the tube with clay prevents the blood from exiting the tube. **Figure 26-19** ■ Gently press the end of the capillary tube into the sealing clay.
• After filling the tube to the appropriate level, wipe the outside of the tube with a tissue to remove excess blood.	Cleaning the outside of the tube prevents contaminating the centrifuge.
• Repeat the procedure with a second tube.	• The test results will be obtained by averaging the readings of the two tubes.
• Apply a gauze square to the puncture site.	• Applying pressure will help the area to clot faster.
6. Place tubes in the centrifuge directly opposite each other with the sealed ends pointed outward and pushed against the gasket (Figure 26-20).	The centrifuge must be balanced with equal weight to avoid tube breakage, and the clay must point outward to avoid losing the specimen during centrifugation. **Figure 26-20** ■ Place tubes across from each other to balance the centrifuge.
7. Securely fasten both centrifuge lids.	The fastened lid prevents breakage of the capillary tubes.
8. Set the timer for five minutes and adjust the speed if needed. (Follow manufacturer's instructions.)	Proper timing and speed ensures accurate results.
9. Apply a bandage on the puncture site once the bleeding has stopped.	The puncture site could start bleeding again. The bandage will keep blood from contaminating the patient's clothes and other surfaces.

continues

PROCEDURE 26-1 continued

PROCEDURAL STEPS	DETAILS AND/OR RATIONALE
10. Allow the centrifuge to stop completely before opening both lids.	Stopping the centrifuge manually can dislodge packed cells and cause injury to the medical assistant.
11. Remove both tubes, place them on the reader (Figure 26-21), and follow directions on reader to determine the value.	Both tubes must be read to ensure test accuracy. Each reader is a little different so read the directions to make certain you are reading it correctly.
12. Average the results of both tubes.	Results must agree within 2%; if not, the test should be performed again.
13. Record the results as a percentage.	The hematocrit value is reported as percent of red blood cells in that volume of blood.
14. Capillary tubes should be placed in a sharps container and any contaminated gauze should be placed in the biohazard trash.	Many capillary tubes have glass embedded in them. The sharps container helps to protect individuals from getting stuck.
15. Remove PPE and wash your hands.	Washing hands reduces risk of cross-contamination.
16. Document the procedure both in the chart and in the lab log if applicable.	Documentation proves that the procedure was performed.

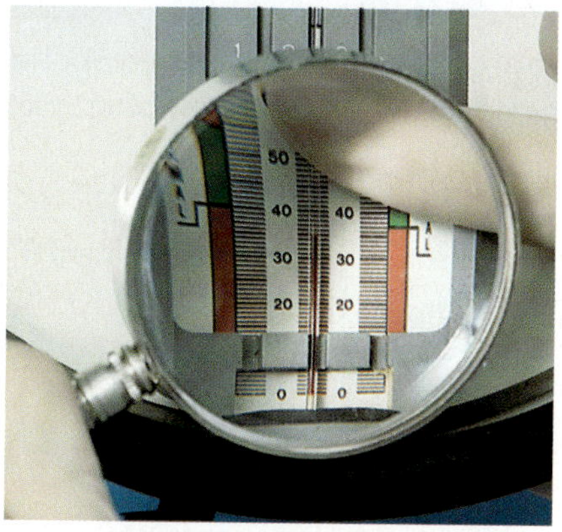

Figure 26-21 ■ Hematocrit Reader: After centrifuging the specimen, line up the tube so that the intersecting portion where the plasma meets the sealant is even with the zero line. To obtain the result, read where the red cells intersect the plasma. This result is 35%.

DOCUMENTATION EXAMPLE:

11-08-XX 11:00 a.m.	Microhematocrit per Dr. Leonard. Result: 48% K. Harding, CMA (AAMA) ----------------------

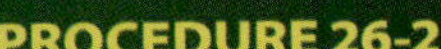

PROCEDURE 26-2

Perform a Hemoglobin Using the Hemocue System

Objective:

To accurately collect a capillary specimen and perform a hemoglobin using the Hemocue System.

Equipment/Supplies

- Personal protective equipment (PPE)
- Hemocue Unit
- EDTA blood sample
- Timer
- Sharps container
- Biohazard waste container
- Patient's chart/EHR

PROCEDURAL STEPS	DETAILS AND/OR RATIONALE
1. Verify test order, wash your hands, and apply appropriate PPE.	PPE reduces the risks of contamination during the procedure.
2. Assemble the equipment, read the manufacturer's instructions, and run a control.	Being organized helps the procedure proceed safely and accurately. Running a control helps to ensure the equipment is in good working order.
3. Identify the patient using two identifiers, identify yourself with your credentials. ***Explain the rationale for the performance of the procedure, showing awareness of the patient's concerns related to the procedure being performed.***	Performing the testing on the wrong patient can result in serious consequences. Introducing yourself and stating your credentials will promote professionalism. Explaining the procedure increases patient cooperation.
4. Make certain the analyzer is in the "ready" loading position. (The display will show a three flashing dashes and the Hemocue symbol.)	Having the analyzer in the loading position allows the procedure to flow without interruption.
5. Remove a cuvette from the vial or individually wrapped package. Recap vial.	Recapping the vial preserves the remaining cuvettes.
6. Perform capillary puncture and wipe away first drop of blood.	The first drop of blood could be contaminated with alcohol or diluted with tissue fluid, which will produce inaccurate results.
7. Position the cuvette so that the open end is facing the drop of blood. Fill the cuvette in one continuous motion. (Do not refill a partially filled cuvette.)	Not filling the blood with one continuous motion could cause bubbles to form resulting in an inaccurate result.
8. Wipe off any excess blood from the outside of the cuvette using a clean, lint-free tissue. (Do not touch the open end with the tissue.)	Excess blood can contaminate the unit and cause problems with future readings.
9. Visually inspect the cuvette for any bubbles.	Air bubbles can result in inaccurate results.
10. Place the cuvette into the cuvette holder and gently slide the holder into the measuring position.	The unit has to be in the measuring position to measure the result.

continues

PROCEDURE 26-2 continued

PROCEDURAL STEPS	DETAILS AND/OR RATIONALE
11. Once a result displays, pull cuvette holder out of the measuring position and remove cuvette.	
12. Dispose of cuvette in biohazard trash or sharp's container.	Cuvette must be placed in biohazardous trash because it contains blood.
13. Remove PPE, wash hands, dispose of supplies, and disinfect area.	Washing hands reduces risk of cross-contamination.
14. Document result in the chart and in the lab log if applicable.	All procedures must be correctly documented in the patient's chart/medical record and the laboratory log to confirm the tests were performed.

DOCUMENTATION EXAMPLE:

02/12/XX, 10:00 a.m.	Capillary puncture, 4th finger, right hand for a hemoglobin determination per Dr. Dorado. Result: 10.2 g/dL (Hemocue System) L. Whalen, CMA (AAMA)------------------------------

PROCEDURE 26-3
Perform an Erythrocyte Sedimentation Rate

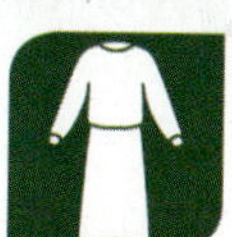

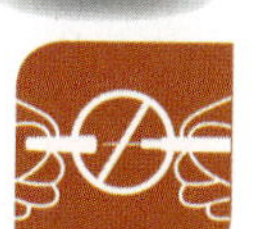

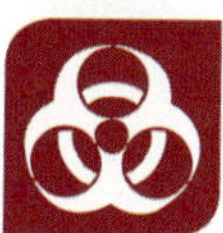
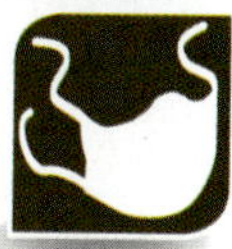

Objective:

To accurately determine the erythrocyte sedimentation rate by the Sediplast (Westergren) method.

Equipment/Supplies:

- Personal protective equipment (PPE)
- EDTA blood sample
- Sediplast kit and rack
- Timer
- Patient's chart/EHR

PROCEDURAL STEPS	DETAILS AND/OR RATIONALE
1. Check the provider's order, wash your hands, and apply PPE.	PPE reduces the risks of contamination during the procedure.
2. Assemble the equipment.	Being organized helps the procedure proceed safely and accurately.
3. Mix the blood gently, but well, for two minutes.	The blood must be well mixed to ensure that all components have been evenly distributed.

continues

PROCEDURE 26-3 continued

PROCEDURAL STEPS	DETAILS AND/OR RATIONALE
4. Remove the stopper from the sedivial and fill with 0.8 mL of blood to the indicated mark (Figure 26-22). Replace the stopper and mix the sodium citrate and blood well.	The correct amount of blood must be used and blood must be well mixed with sodium citrate solution to ensure correct dilution and distribution of cells.
5. Place the sedivial in the Sediplast rack and place the rack on a level surface free of vibrations.	The rack must remain level for accurate results. Vibrations can interfere with the reading.
6. Insert the Sediplast tube through the stopper while pushing down (Figure 26-23) until tube rests on the bottom of the vial and the blood reaches the zero line.	The blood must reach the zero line in order for measurements to be correct.
7. Set the timer for one hour.	Precise timing is critical to accurate results.
8. Read the results of the ESR at exactly one hour.	Reading results too early or too late will produce erroneous results.
9. Clean the work area and properly dispose of used supplies in biohazard waste container and the tube of blood into the sharps container.	Proper disinfection of the work area will prevent contamination to others that use the area.
10. Remove PPE and wash your hands.	Washing hands helps to prevent the transfer of microorganisms to others.
11. Record the results in the patient's chart and the laboratory log.	Recording the results verifies the procedure was completed.

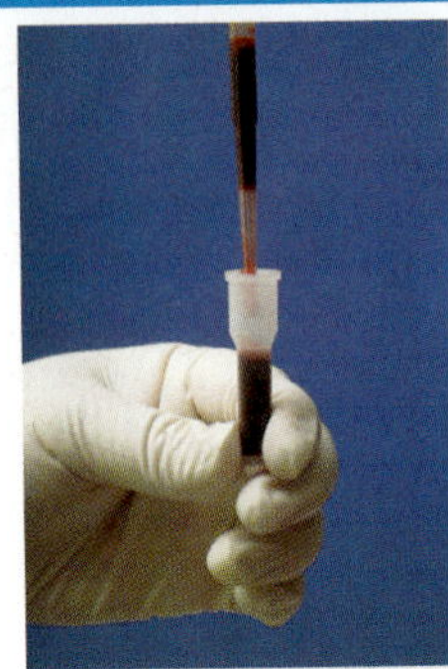

Figure 26-22 ■ Fill the sedivial to the proper level, seal with the lid, and mix well.

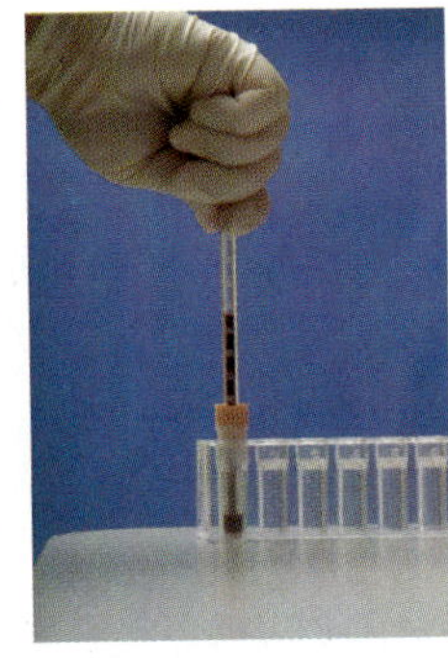

Figure 26-23 ■ Push the Sediplast tube into the sedivial with a firm, twisting motion until the tube fills to the zero line.

DOCUMENTATION EXAMPLE:

DOB: 1/22/1928 Age: (87) Sex: F
Last Appt: 4/28/2015 Established Patient Sick -NVFA
Next Appt: (None)
Smith, Cosima Vitals: 0 Medications: 0 Allergies: 0 Diagnosis: 0

Patient Name DOB Age Sex
Smith, Cosima 1/22/1928 87 U
Ordering Provider
Amir Raman DO

Report Status: **Final**
Reported: **4/28/2015 7:11:34 AM**
Accession:

A	Info	Test	Results	Abnormal Results	Status	Units	Reference Range
		Erythrocyte sedimentation rate					
N	i	Erythrocyte sedimentation rate	12		Final	mm/hr	0-16 mm/hr

PROCEDURE 26-4

Performing a Prothrombin Time (PT) and INR

Objective:

To perform a PT and INR using a CLIA-approved analyzer.

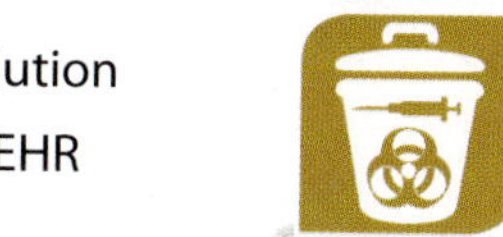

Equipment and Supplies

- Personal protective equipment (PPE)
- Capillary puncture supplies: Lancet, 2 × 2 gauze squares, gauze pads, and adhesive strips
- PT/INR unit/code chip/code strip
- Disinfecting solution
- Patient's chart/EHR

PROCEDURAL STEPS	DETAILS AND/OR RATIONALE
1. Verify provider's order, gather supplies, wash hands, and apply appropriate PPE.	You must verify the order to make certain you are performing the correct test. Applying appropriate PPE protects you from accidental exposure to the patient's blood.
2. Check the expiration date on the test strip label to confirm it hasn't passed its expiration date.	Using test strips that are expired may result in erroneous results.
3. Read the manufacturer's instructions to familiarize yourself with the testing procedure.	Every testing unit has different instructions, so it is imperative that you are familiar with the unit to ensure accurate results.
4. If applicable, run a control according to manufacturer's instructions.	Running a control makes certain that the unit is working properly.
5. Greet your patient, identify yourself and state your credentials. Identify the patient using two identifiers, and ***explain the rationale for the performance of the procedure, showing awareness of the patient's concerns related to the procedure being performed***.	Performing the testing on the wrong patient can result in serious consequences. Introducing yourself and stating your credentials will promote professionalism. Explaining the procedure increases patient cooperation.
6. If the unit has a code chip, insert it into the unit and turn on the coagulation unit by depressing the "On" button. (Make certain the number on the code chip corresponds with the number on the code strip label.)	If the numbers on the code chip and code strips do not match, it may result in erroneous results.
7. Insert the test strip into the test strip guide following manufacturer's instructions. (Make certain that the unit has detected the test strip by listening for a beep or looking for a symbol to appear on the display.)	The test strip must be inserted correctly for the unit to work properly.
8. Perform a capillary puncture and wipe away the first drop of blood.	The first drop of blood could be contaminated with alcohol or diluted with tissue fluid, which will produce inaccurate results.

continues

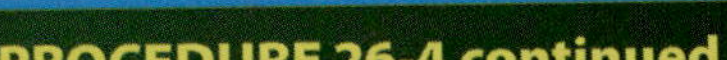

PROCEDURE 26-4 continued

PROCEDURAL STEPS	DETAILS AND/OR RATIONALE
9. Follow the manufacturer's instructions regarding when it is appropriate to apply the drop of blood to the test strip or testing apparatus.	Many units have count down clocks which only allows you to apply blood within a certain time frame.
10. Apply drop of blood to the test strip following the manufacturer's instructions.	Each unit is different so you must check the manufacturer's instructions to make certain you are performing the testing correctly.
11. Wait for the test result to appear and make a mental note of result or write down on a piece of scrap paper. Discard the test strip after removing from unit and place into the biohazardous waste container.	It is important to note the reading or write it down so you don't forget it during the documentation procedure.
12. Disinfect work area, and remove PPE.	Disinfecting the area helps to remove blood contaminants that could infect others.
13. Document the results in the patient's chart and lab log.	Lab logs are only used for paper records so that lab results can be tracked.

DOCUMENTATION EXAMPLE:

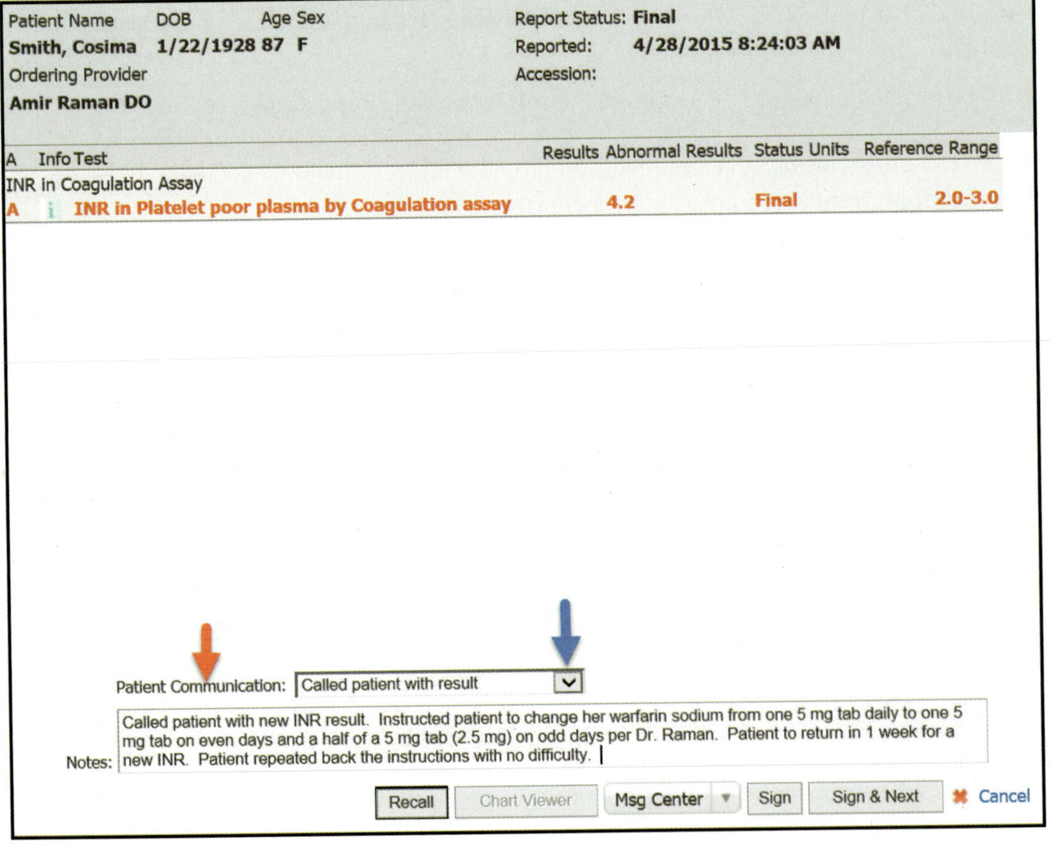
Patient Name DOB Age Sex
Smith, Cosima 1/22/1928 87 F
Ordering Provider
Amir Raman DO
Report Status: **Final**
Reported: **4/28/2015 8:24:03 AM**
Accession:

A	Info	Test	Results	Abnormal Results	Status	Units	Reference Range
		INR in Coagulation Assay					
A	i	INR in Platelet poor plasma by Coagulation assay		4.2	Final		2.0-3.0

Patient Communication: Called patient with result

Notes: Called patient with new INR result. Instructed patient to change her warfarin sodium from one 5 mg tab daily to one 5 mg tab on even days and a half of a 5 mg tab (2.5 mg) on odd days per Dr. Raman. Patient to return in 1 week for a new INR. Patient repeated back the instructions with no difficulty.

Recall | Chart Viewer | Msg Center | Sign | Sign & Next | Cancel

Courtesy of Harris CareTracker PM and EMR

CHAPTER SUMMARY

- Hematology is the study of blood and the blood-forming tissues.
- Functions of blood include the transportation of both nutrients and waste products.
- Hematopoiesis is the formation and development of blood cells, which primarily takes place in the bone marrow of the ribs, sternum, and pelvic bone.
- The average adult has about five liters of blood, approximately half is composed of cells and the other half is the fluid portion.
- Serum is the liquid portion of blood when no anticoagulant is added to the blood; plasma is the liquid portion of blood when anticoagulated blood is centrifuged.
- Erythrocytes are red blood cells and are the most numerous of all formed elements. They live approximately 120 days and contain an iron pigment called hemoglobin which carries oxygen to the body's tissues.
- Leukocytes are the white blood cells and include, neutrophils, eosinophils, basophils, lymphocytes, and monocytes. They guard the body against infection by producing antibodies and functioning in the immune response.
- Thrombocytes are platelets that are active in hemostasis.
- A coagulation cascade is a number of events that happen to stop the flow of blood.
- Hematological tests are among the most common ordered by the provider. They can assist the provider in determining conditions such as anemia, helping to identify the type of infection the patient has, measuring inflammation in the body, and flagging the provider when the patient has certain types of blood cancer.
- The hematocrit determines the volume of packed red blood cells in a given volume of blood and hemoglobin measures the oxygen-carrying capacity of the red blood cells.
- Hemoglobin is a protein molecule that contains iron. It carries oxygen to the body's tissue and CO_2 back to the lungs.
- A differential count is a procedure that identifies the different types of white blood cells in the body. It also includes RBC morphology, which looks at the color, size, and shape of the red cells, and is useful for determining the type and cause of anemia. RBC indices are calculations which use the values from the red blood cell count, hemoglobin, and hematocrit to further evaluate the health of the red blood cells.
- The erythrocyte sedimentation rate (ESR) measures how far the red blood cells descend or settle in a one-hour time frame in a given volume of blood. It is used to measure inflammation and tissue destruction in the body. There are two methods for ESR testing; The Wintrobe method and Westergren method.
- Common coagulation tests are the prothrombin time (PT) and activated partial thromboplastin time (aPTT). The PT result is usually reported with the international normalized ratio (INR), which is calibrated by dividing the patient's PT test by the laboratory's normal value.

CERTIFICATION REVIEW QUESTIONS

1. Which hematology test would be increased with an inflammatory condition?
   a. Hemoglobin
   b. Hematocrit
   c. ESR
   d. Differential

2. The differential count categorizes which type of blood cell?
   a. Red blood cells
   b. White blood cells
   c. Platelets
   d. Thrombocytes

3. The volume of packed red cells in a sample of blood is known as the:
   a. hematocrit.
   b. hemoglobin.
   c. ESR.
   d. WBC.
4. By measuring hemoglobin, we are indirectly measuring the ___ of the red blood cells.
   a. color
   b. shape
   c. size
   d. oxygen-carrying capacity
5. The cellular component responsible for aiding in blood clotting is the:
   a. plasma.
   b. thrombocyte.
   c. leukocyte.
   d. erythrocyte.
6. Which white blood cell is elevated during an allergic reaction?
   a. Monocyte
   b. Lymphocyte
   c. Basophil
   d. Eosinophil
7. What will happen if the sealed end of the hematocrit tube is pointing the opposite direction of the gasket during centrifugation?
   a. Nothing, as this is the direction the tube should be facing.
   b. The blood will spin out of the tube and spray throughout the centrifuge.
   c. The tubes will break.
   d. The results will not be accurate.
8. When testing blood for chemical components, which type of sample is used?
   a. Blood serum
   b. Blood plasma
   c. Any type is appropriate
   d. It depends on the chemical being tested
9. What information is the INR test revealing?
   a. The density of the components that cause blood to clot
   b. The proportion of PT to aPTT
   c. The standardization of the PT result
   d. The national requirements for lab tests
10. RBC morphology studies which of the following?
    a. The size of the RBC
    b. The shape of the RBC
    c. The color of the RBC
    d. All of the above

STUDY RESOURCES

Resources to Test and Reinforce Your Knowledge:	
Certification Review Questions	Take this end-of-chapter quiz
Workbook	• Complete the activities for Chapter 26 • Perform the procedures for Chapter 26 using the Competency Checklists
Resources to Promote Critical Thinking:	
***Solve the Case* Activities**	• Consider these case studies and discuss your conclusions
Learning Lab	• Module 22: Laboratory Procedures
MindTap	• Complete Chapter 26 readings and activities

REFERENCES

Centers for Disease Control and Prevention. (n.d.). *Tests Granted Waived Status Under CLIA*. Retrieved from http://www.cms.gov/Regulations-and-Guidance/Legislation/CLIA/downloads/waivetbl.pdf

WebMD. (2012, June 4). *Sedimentation Rate (Sed Rate)*. Retrieved from http://www.webmd.com/a-to-z-guides/sedimentation-rate?page=2

"Hematocrit": *The Test*. N.p., n.d. Web. August 2, 2015. https://labtestsonline.org/understanding/analytes/hematocrit/tab/test.

"Prothrombin Time Test." *Mayo Clinic*. n.p., n.d. Web. August 2, 2015. http://www.mayoclinic.org/tests-procedures/prothrombin-time/basics/definition/prc-20013300.

"Sed Rate (erythrocyte Sedimentation Rate)."—*Mayo Clinic*. n.p., n.d. Web. August 2, 2015. http://www.mayoclinic.org/tests-procedures/sed-rate/basics/definition/PRC-20013502

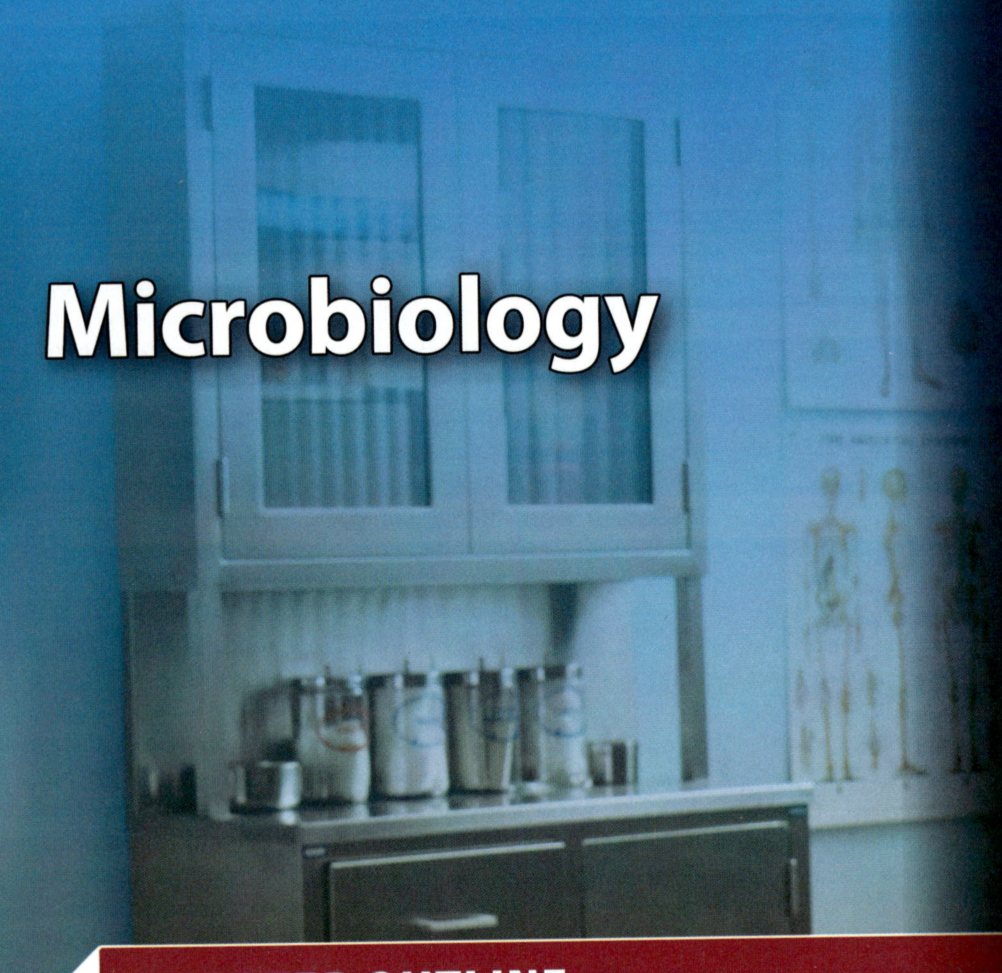

27

Microbiology

CHAPTER OUTLINE

Microbiology Abbreviation Review

Classification of Microorganisms

Divisions of Microbiology

Binomial Nomenclature System for Bacteria

Characteristics of Bacteria
- Basic Bacterial Cell Structure
- Morphology of Bacteria
- Classification by Staining Reaction

Specimen Collection and Safe Handling Requirements
- General Specimen Collection Guidelines
- Specific Specimen Collection Requirements
- Sources of Contamination

Identification of Bacteria
- The Culture
- Growth Media
- *Streptococcus* Identification
- Rapid Strep Tests

Sensitivity Testing

Special Microscopic Techniques
- The Wet Mount

Virology
- Identification of Viruses

Parasitology
- Identification of Parasites

Mycology
- Identification of Fungi

Quality Control

Lab Requisition and Test Report Forms

ESSENTIAL TERMS

aerobic
agar
anaerobic
bacilli
bacteria
cocci
colonies
culture
culture and sensitivity (C&S) test
culture medium
fungi
Gram negative
Gram positive
Gram stain
incubation
inoculation
microbiology
normal flora
opportunistic infection
parasite
pathogen
pathogenic
pure culture
sensitivity testing
taxonomy
virus

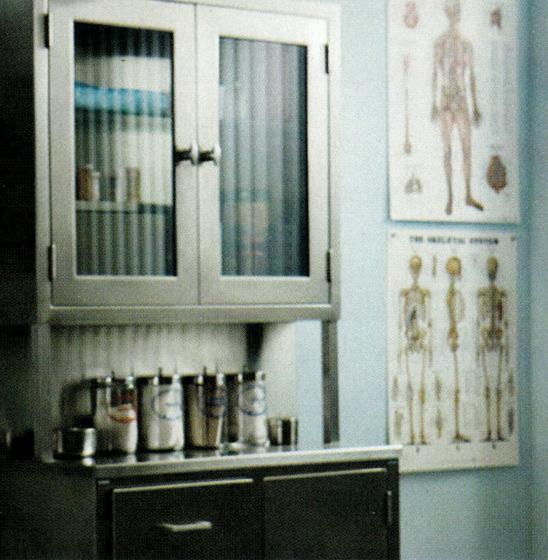

DEVELOPMENTAL OBJECTIVES

After completing this chapter, you should be able to:

1. Correctly spell and define the essential terms.
2. Identify and use common abbreviations associated with microbiological testing.
3. Explain taxonomy.
4. Compare and contrast bacteriology, virology, parasitology, and mycology.
5. List and describe bacterial morphology.
6. Explain the significance of normal flora.
7. Analyze the differences between bacteria that are Gram positive and bacteria that are Gram negative.
8. Collect specimens and perform CLIA-waived microbiology testing.
9. Identify CLIA-waived tests associated with common diseases.
10. Explain the purpose of culture and sensitivity testing.
11. Collect a throat specimen and perform a rapid strep test.
12. Collect a wound specimen.
13. Prepare a wet mount and instruct a patient on fecal specimen collection for ova and parasite testing.

INTRODUCTION

The field of medical **microbiology** includes the study of microscopic organisms such as bacteria, viruses, parasites, and fungi. While many microorganisms are present in nature, only a small percentage are **pathogenic** or disease producing. Some microbes, known as **normal flora**, are actually helpful and necessary to maintain a balance in certain areas of the body.

This chapter will discuss the more common microorganisms and the diseases they cause, along with test methods used to isolate and identify them. Since new microbes are always being discovered, the medical assistant should strive to continuously update his or her knowledge in this ever-expanding area.

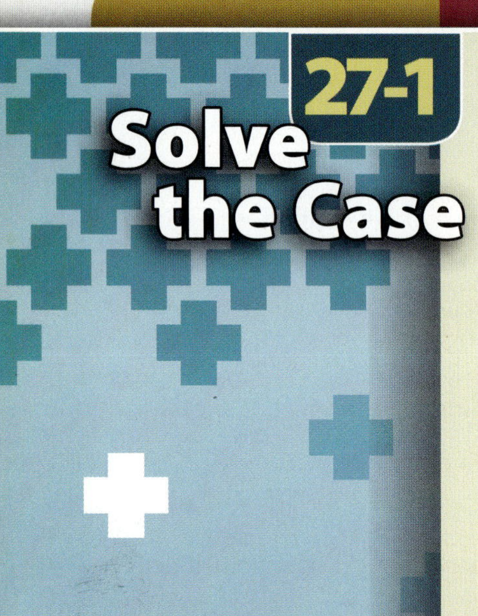

Gabby French came into the office today complaining of a sore throat, fever, and chills. The pain started about two days ago and she has noticed some white spots at the back of her throat. Gabby's twin daughters were just diagnosed with strep throat last week. She is very concerned that she too may have strep throat. Her daughters just finished their antibiotic treatment yesterday, and she is fearful that if she is positive for strep, she may pass it back to her daughters. She goes on to say that she doesn't want her throat swabbed because she has a terrible gag reflex. She wants to know if Dr. Anderson can give her an antibiotic without testing her. Using your current knowledge, answer the following questions:

1. **What type of organism causes strep throat?**
2. **What would you say to Gabby about her question regarding whether or not she can pass the strep throat back to her daughters?**
3. **Do you feel that testing is necessary for Gabby since she probably got the strep throat from her daughters?**

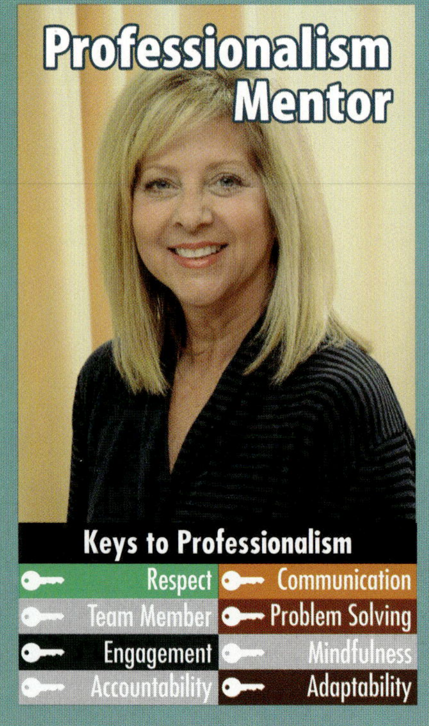

No matter what type of office you will work in, you will most likely be involved with performing some type of microbiological testing. The test that always comes to mind is the dreaded "throat culture." At a very busy family practice care site, I witnessed a medical assistant struggle to swab the throat of a very reluctant six-year-old boy. At one point he refused to open his mouth, even as he was crying! Instead of forcing the boy to comply, the medical assistant explained in a calm and kind voice that by allowing him to swab his throat, the doctor would know the right medicine to give to make him feel better. The medical assistant didn't say it wouldn't hurt, but he did promise it would be very quick. I think the honesty of the medical assistant finally won the little boy over. I was impressed with this medical assistant because he didn't make a false promise to the little boy. To do the swab correctly, the medical assistant knew that it would be uncomfortable. A throat swab is not the type of test that you want to repeat due to improper collection, processing, contamination, or mislabeling. Attention to detail is key to your success with microbiology specimen collection and handling. In your workbook journal, record how the keys listed in this feature apply to this scenario. ■

MICROBIOLOGY ABBREVIATION REVIEW

Medical assistants who perform or prepare specimens for microbiological testing should be familiar with common abbreviations associated with such testing. Refer to Table 27-1 for a listing of these abbreviations.

CLASSIFICATION OF MICROORGANISMS

Microorganisms are usually classified using a set of laws and principles known as **taxonomy**. Since no universal agreement exists on which system is best, several different methods are often used for classification.

Originally, living organisms were divided into two kingdoms: plant and animal. After the invention of the microscope, a new kingdom of microscopic organisms known as *Protista* were discovered. Since most microorganisms are neither plant nor animal, these one-celled organisms were classified as *protists*. Two groups of *protists* are present in medicine: lower protists or *prokaryotes*, which include bacteria and blue-green algae, and higher protists or *eukaryotes* including protozoa, algae, and fungi.

DIVISIONS OF MICROBIOLOGY

Within the microbiology department of a laboratory, a multitude of specimens are processed and tested. The results obtained from these studies aid in the diagnosis, treatment, and prevention of diseases. In larger reference laboratories, the microbiology department is usually divided into the following subdepartments or specialized areas of study:

- *Bacteriology*: This area is usually the largest and is responsible for the growth, isolation, identification, and study of bacteria.
- *Virology*: This is the area responsible for the study of viral diseases.
- *Parasitology*: This is the area responsible for the identification and study of parasites.
- *Mycology*: This subdivision studies fungi, including yeasts and molds.

Table 27-1 Common Abbreviations Used for Microbiological Testing and Diagnosis

Abbreviation	Meaning
BC	Blood culture
C&S	Culture and sensitivity
C-Diff	*Clostridium difficile*
CMV	Cytomegalovirus
CSF	Cerebrospinal fluid
Cx	Culture
O&P	Ova and parasites
RSV	Respiratory syncytial virus

Along with isolating and identifying microorganisms, the microbiology department plays an important role in conjunction with the infection control department of the hospital in determining the causes of nosocomial (hospital acquired) infections. These infections must be quickly identified and closely monitored to prevent their spread. Patients with suppressed immune systems are quite susceptible to these **opportunistic infections**.

The microbiology department also has a responsibility to notify the Public Health Department when certain types of organisms are grown and identified from patient samples. Each state and metropolitan area has its own guidelines for reporting these communicable diseases; health care workers must be aware of the regulations in their area. Common reportable organisms include the following:

- *Salmonella*: The normal causative agent of severe food poisoning
- *Shigella*: The normal causative agent of mild to severe dysentery
- Sexually transmitted infections (STIs): Organisms that cause gonorrhea, syphilis, chlamydia, and genital herpes
- Mumps, measles, and many other infectious diseases.

BINOMIAL NOMENCLATURE SYSTEM FOR BACTERIA

Bacteria (single-celled microbes lacking a nucleus) are named using a binomial (two-name) system. The first name is the genus and is capitalized; the second name is the species and is not capitalized (e.g., in *Escherichia coli*, *Escherichia* is the genus and *coli* is the species).

Bacteria that possess similar characteristics belong to the same genus, or family. For example, *Staphylococcus aureus* and *Staphylococcus epidermidis* are members of the genus *Staphylococcus*, but have different species names due to specific characteristics. Many bacteria are named for people or places related to their discovery; for example, *Legionella pneumophila*, which causes Legionnaire's disease, was first noted following an American Legionnaire's convention in 1976, where 34 attendees died from the disease.

CHARACTERISTICS OF BACTERIA

All bacteria possess individual characteristics that aid in their identification. The features used as criteria for recognition include structure, morphology, and staining characteristics.

Basic Bacterial Cell Structure

Every cell of every living structure contains deoxyribonucleic acid (DNA), which carries the genetic information specific to that entity. A bacterial cell (Figure 27-1) is a single-celled organism that possesses a cell membrane, a cell wall, and a nucleus. This particular type of cell takes in nutrients from the environment for growth, function, and reproduction through cell division. Some bacteria are nonmotile; they do not possess a flagellum, which is necessary for movement. Other forms of bacteria produce a protective covering around the cell wall (known as a capsule) that can make them resistant to certain antibiotics and protect them from attack by white blood cells. Certain bacteria produce spores that can remain inactive for as long as 150,000 years. Spores are extremely hard to kill and are resistant to heat, freezing, radiation, and certain chemicals.

Morphology of Bacteria

The microbes that most commonly cause diseases in humans are bacteria and viruses. Bacteria are categorized according to their morphology, or shape, and their reactions to Gram staining. Bacterial morphology is divided into three basic shapes:

- Cocci: round-shaped
- Bacilli: rod-shaped
- Spirilla: spiral-shaped

The shapes of bacteria may be further identified according to the way they are grouped:

- The prefix *mono-* is used when describing single fragments.
- The prefix *diplo-* is used for bacteria occurring in pairs.
- The prefix *strepto-* is used for bacteria occurring in chains.
- The prefix *staphylo-* is used for bacteria occurring in clusters.

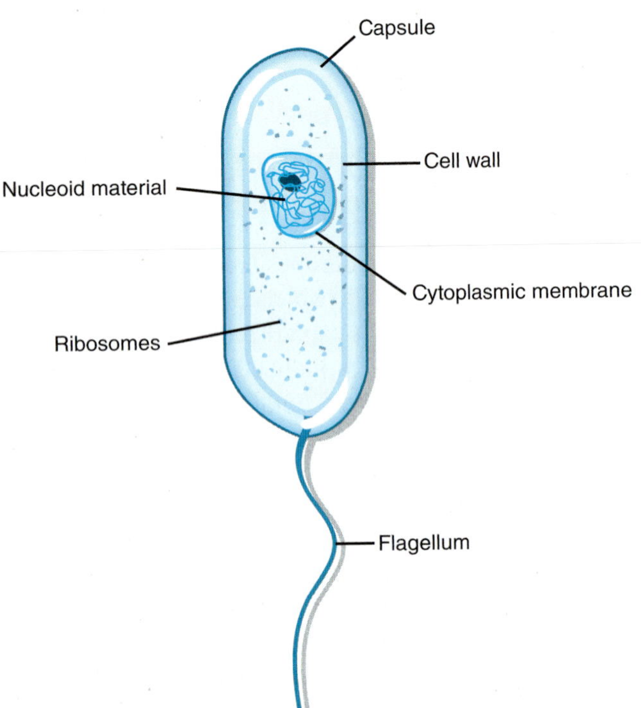

Figure 27-1 ■ Bacterial cell structure.

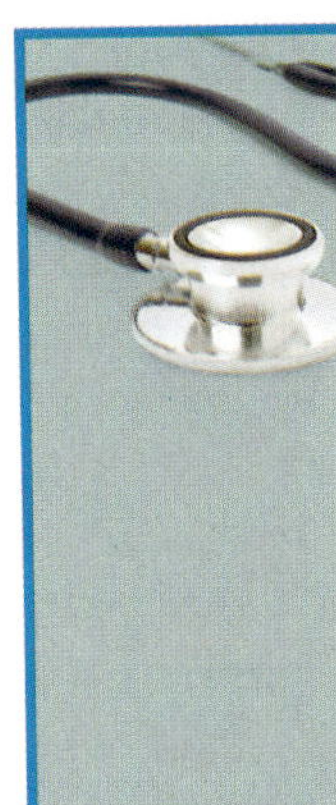

Field Smarts

Because of their tough capsule, spores are resistant to most chemical disinfectants and even boiling temperatures. The best means of destroying spores is by autoclaving. All critical devices that enter nonintact skin must be sterilized in an autoclave to ensure that all microbes—including those that produce spores—have been destroyed. Some chemical sterilants also kill spores.

Cocci

Round-shaped bacteria, or **cocci**, can occur in pairs (diplococci), chains (streptococci), or clusters (staphylococci). Figure 27-2 illustrates the three different types of cocci.

Diplococci (Figure 27-2a) are responsible for diseases such as meningitis, gonorrhea, and pneumonia. Streptococci (Figure 27-2b) are the cause of strep throat, certain types of pneumonia, rheumatic fever, scarlet fever, and some skin conditions like impetigo. A species of staphylococci (Figure 27-2c) known as *Staphylococcus epidermidis* is present as normal flora on the skin, in the mucous membranes of the nose, throat, mouth, and intestines, and normally does not pose a problem. However, a small abrasion or break in the skin can allow the normal flora to enter the tissues

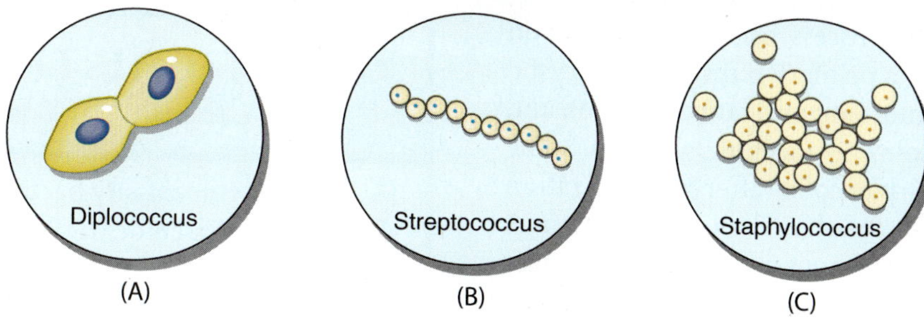

Figure 27-2 ■ Bacteria classified as cocci: (a) occurring in pairs, (b) occurring in chains, (c) occurring in clusters.

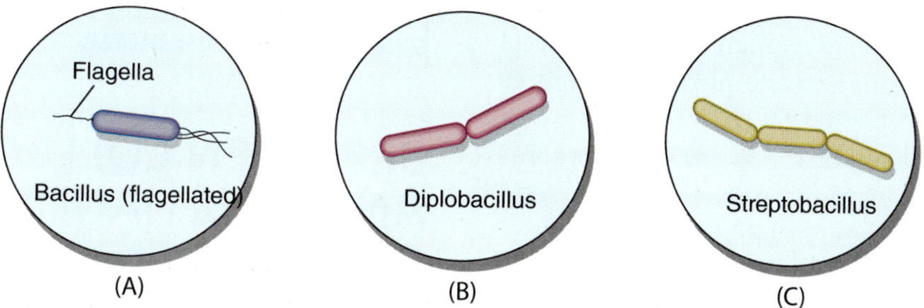

Figure 27-3 ■ Bacteria classified as bacilli: (a) with flagella for motility, (b) occurring in pairs, (c) occurring in chains.

and cause an infection. Another species known as *Staphylococcus aureus* is responsible for infections that produce large amounts of pus, such as abscesses, boils, impetigo, and carbuncles. Staphylococcus bacteria can also cause certain forms of food poisoning.

Bacilli

Rod-shaped bacteria, or **bacilli**, can possess a rounded, straight, or pointed end. They may also possess flagella that make them motile (able to move from one place to another).

One species of bacilli, *Escherichia coli*, is present in the intestinal tract as normal flora; however, it can be the cause of a urinary tract infection (UTI) if it enters the urinary tract due to poor hygiene. Different species of bacilli are also found in the soil and air and are often responsible for serious diseases, such as typhoid fever, pertussis (whooping cough), diphtheria, tuberculosis, botulism, and tetanus. Bacilli may also be spore forming, allowing them to withstand extreme temperatures and particular chemicals in disinfectants, making them viable for decades. Figure 27-3 illustrates the different types of bacilli.

Spirilla

Most spiral-shaped bacteria are motile. They are responsible for a number of diseases, such as syphilis and cholera. The spirochete, *Treponema pallidum*, the causative agent of syphilis, cannot be grown on common culture medium; therefore, syphilis must be diagnosed by testing blood serum for the presence of treponemal antibodies or by expressing fluid from a lesion and staining with a fluorescent antibody stain. Figure 27-4 illustrates the morphology of spirilla.

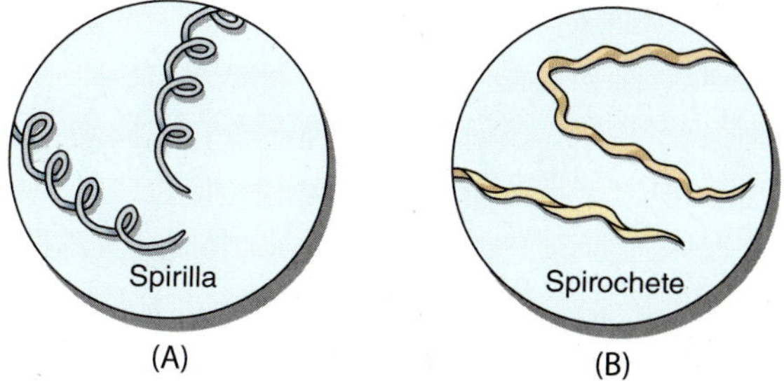

Figure 27-4 ■ Spiral-shaped bacteria: (a) spirilla, (b) spirochete.

Classification by Staining Reaction

Bacteria are often classified by their reaction to different dyes or stains. These stains are used to give color to the bacteria, making them more visible under the microscope. Stains are either basic or acidic and are classified as a simple or differential stain.

A simple stain illustrates the structure and arrangement of the bacterial cells, but does not provide much other information.

A differential stain is one that produces variable results based on the composition of the bacterial cell wall. A common differential staining method, the **Gram stain**, was developed over 100 years ago by Dr. Hans Christian Gram and is still used today. This method differentiates bacteria based on their color reactions to various stains.

During the Gram stain process, bacteria are placed on a slide and stained with a primary purple stain (crystal violet), flushed with a mordant or fixative (iodine), and then treated with a decolorizer (acetone/alcohol). Some bacteria retain the purple color after decolorization and are classed as **Gram positive** (Figure 27-5). Others cannot retain the dye after being decolorized and must be counterstained with a red dye (safranin) to make them visible under the microscope. These bacteria are classed as **Gram negative** and appear pink in color (Figure 27-6). The Gram-staining characteristics along with the morphological arrangement of the bacteria are often the only information the physician requires to begin treatment.

Gram staining in the medical office was rather common years ago; however, most medical offices send their specimens out to reference labs for testing now.

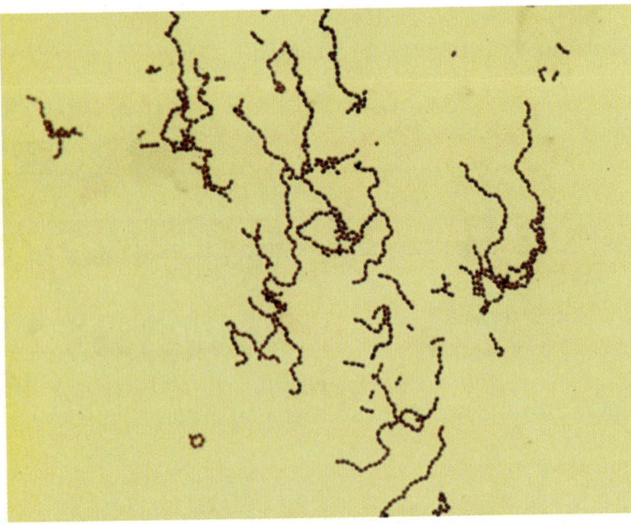

Figure 27-5 ■ Gram-positive *Streptococci* exhibiting the characteristic purple color.

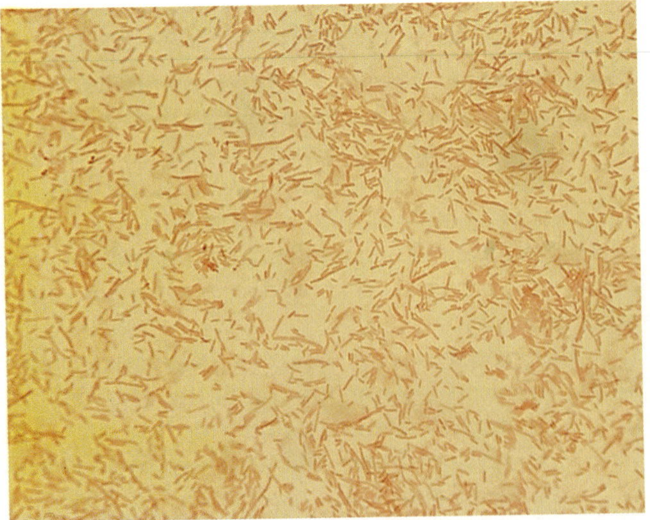

Figure 27-6 ■ Gram-negative rods exhibiting the characteristic pink color.

CRITICAL THINKING CHALLENGE

How would you classify bacteria that are round in shape, purple in color, and appear in chains? How would you classify single rod-shaped bacteria that appear pink in color? If the rod-shaped bacteria also contained a flagellum, it would be further classified as motile, meaning that it has the ability to move from one area to another.

SPECIMEN COLLECTION AND SAFE HANDLING REQUIREMENTS

The physician must identify the **pathogen** causing a specific condition before implementing proper treatment. For example, a sore throat such as one caused by the bacteria *Streptococcus* would be treated with an appropriate antibiotic. If a virus is causing the sore throat, an antibiotic would be ineffective. Proper specimen collection and handling is essential to ensure accurate identification of the pathogen.

When collecting microbiological specimens, growth requirements such as moisture, temperature, oxygen, carbon dioxide, and special nutrients must be considered. Some bacteria require oxygen for growth and are referred to as **aerobic**; others grow only in the absence of oxygen and are referred to as **anaerobic**.

General Specimen Collection Guidelines

The medical assistant is often the person responsible for obtaining specimens for microbiological studies and must follow certain guidelines to ensure accurate results. The following general guidelines will help to ensure proper specimen collection and preservation:

- The specimen should be collected before antibiotics are administered.
- Sterile supplies should be used to collect and preserve the specimen.
- The specimen should be collected from the site of infection, not the surrounding areas. Contamination of the specimen with unrelated bacteria, such as normal flora, may make it difficult to identify.
- Be sure to collect a sufficient amount of the specimen.

- Immediately place the specimen in the appropriate container and transport media, following the directions packaged with the media. Transport media keeps the specimen moist and viable until testing can be performed. Figure 27-7 illustrates a variety of collection and transport systems.
- Appropriately label the specimen with the patient's name, date of collection, source of the specimen, and your initials.
- Send the specimen to the laboratory within the appropriate time limit.

Safe handling of microbiology specimens is crucial to prevent the spread of disease. The following precautions should be observed:

- Handle all specimens as if they contain pathogens.
- Wear appropriate PPE when collecting and handling specimens. PPE should consist of gloves, lab coat or apron, and safety goggles or a face shield.
- PPE should be removed before leaving the work area.
- Check specimen containers for leaks before placing into protective bags.
- Place specimen containers in an outside protective bag to protect those handling the specimen.
- Clean spills and work surfaces with 5% phenol or a 10% bleach solution.

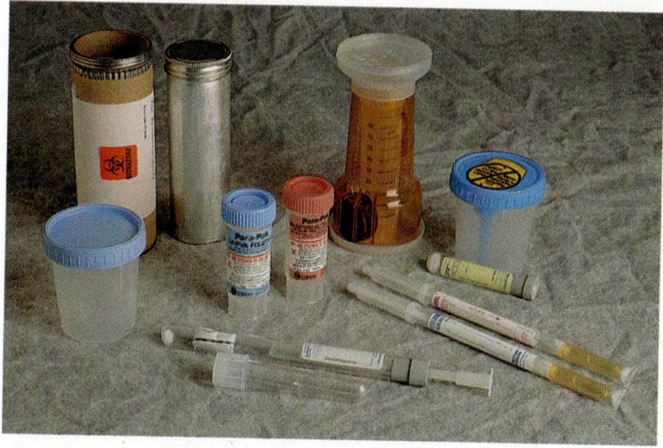

Figure 27-7 ■ Examples of different transport media and specimen collection containers.

Specific Specimen Collection Requirements

When obtaining specimens for microbiology testing, it is necessary to strictly adhere to the collection protocol. The majority of specimens must be placed in a sterile container and properly preserved until testing can be conducted. Table 27-2 lists information on the most common types of specimens collected in the physician's office.

Table 27-2 Specimen Collection Requirements

Specimen Type	Collection Requirements	Presence of Normal Flora	Possible Pathogens
Urine	A clean-catch midstream specimen is preferred. A sterile specimen container should be used to collect the specimen. Catheterization is performed when a sterile specimen is absolutely necessary. The specimen is placed in a sterile container. For a complete procedure on using a C&S transport system for urine samples, refer to Chapter 25.	Yes	*Pseudomonas* species *Klebsiella-Enterobacter* species *Proteus species* *E. coli*
Blood	Collected by venipuncture with a variety of phlebotomy equipment using strict sterile technique.	No	Blood is normally sterile. Anything growing from blood would result in investigating its potential of causing life-threatening illness.
Cerebrospinal fluid (CSF)	Fluid is obtained by lumbar puncture using strict sterile procedure. Usually performed by a physician and placed in a sterile vial.	No	CSF is normally sterile. Anything growing from CSF would result in investigating its potential of causing life-threatening illness.
Sputum	A morning specimen is required, collected from deep cough. Expectorated material is placed in a special container. You can find a complete procedure for collecting a sputum specimen in Chapter 15.	Yes	*Streptococcus pneumoniae* *Staphylococcus aureus* *Klebsiella pneumoniae* *Campylobacter* *Yersinia* *Haemophilus influenzae*

continues

Table 27-2 Specimen Collection Requirements *(continued)*

Specimen Type	Collection Requirements	Presence of Normal Flora	Possible Pathogens
Stool	A sterile container is generally required. The patient may need to submit a series of specimens from different days. Stool specimens must not be contaminated with urine. Chapter 16 includes a full procedure for collecting a stool specimen for C&S testing and a procedure for occult blood testing. Procedure 27-4 lists steps for collecting stool specimens for ova and parasite (O&P) testing.	Yes	*Salmonella* species *Shigella* species *Giardia lamblia* *Entamoeba* species C-difficile
Wound	A provider may aspirate a specimen from a pus filled wound with a sterile needle or collect the specimen with a sterile swab. The medical assistant may assist with the collection of a wound specimen or more rarely, collect the specimen. Refer to Procedure 27-2 for a full procedure for collecting a wound specimen.	No	*Staphylococcus aureus* *Streptococcus pyogenes* *Pseudomonas aeruginosa* *Clostridium* species
Genital	The provider usually collects the specimen with a sterile swab or thin wire. The medical assistant usually assists with the procedure. Refer to Procedure 27-3 for a direction on how to set up a wet mount.	Yes	*Trichomonas vaginalis* *Neisseria gonorrhoeae* *Chlamydia trachomatis* *Candida albicans*
Nasal	A sterile swab or thin wire is gently inserted into each nostril and then placed into a sterile tube for transport. A separate swab is used for each nostril. This is usually performed by the provider.	Yes	*Bordetella pertussis* *Staphylococcus aureus*
Throat	Use a sterile tongue depressor to hold down the tongue and swab the back portion of the throat and tonsils, if present. Do not swab the sides of the mouth or the tongue. The swab is immediately placed in transport media or container supplied by the lab. Procedure 27-1 has a full procedure for collecting a throat swab and performing a rapid strep test.	Yes	*Streptococcus pyogenes* or group A strep
Eye	Specimens from the eye are usually obtained by the provider using a pre-moistened swab with sterile saline. Two different swabs should be used when culturing organisms from each eye.	Yes	*Staphylococcus aureus* *Pseudomonas aeruginosa* *Haemophilus influenzae*
Ear	Outer ear: A moistened swab is used to remove debris or crust from the outer ear canal. (Vigorous swabbing may be required.) The provider may perform a tympanocentesis to obtain a sample from the inner ear.	Yes	*Staphylococcus aureus* *Streptococcus pneumoniae* *Pseudomonas aeruginosa* *Haemophilus influenzae*

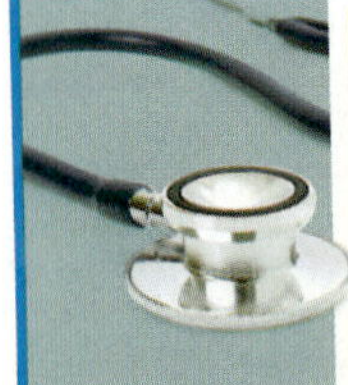

Field Smarts

Proper Area for Swabbing When Collecting a Throat Specimen

Ask the patient to open his mouth, stick out the tongue, and say "ahh." Saying "ahh" helps to lift the back of the throat away from the tongue. In order to obtain a good specimen, direct the swab to the back of the throat. Vigorously rotate the swab in a circular motion over the oropharynx and tonsillar regions on one side of the throat. Move the swab across the throat to the center, behind the uvula, and then over to the other side of oropharynx and tonsillar region. Be sure to swab any areas that are reddened or that contain pustules. Avoid touching or swabbing the hard and soft palate, uvula, buccal area, teeth, tongue, or lips, particularly when directing the swab in or out of the oral cavity. Figure 27-8 illustrates the parts of the throat. If your practice regularly collects two swabs, collect both specimens at the same time, rather than performing two separate collections. Make certain that the swab being sent out is immediately placed in the swab transport medium to prevent it from drying out.

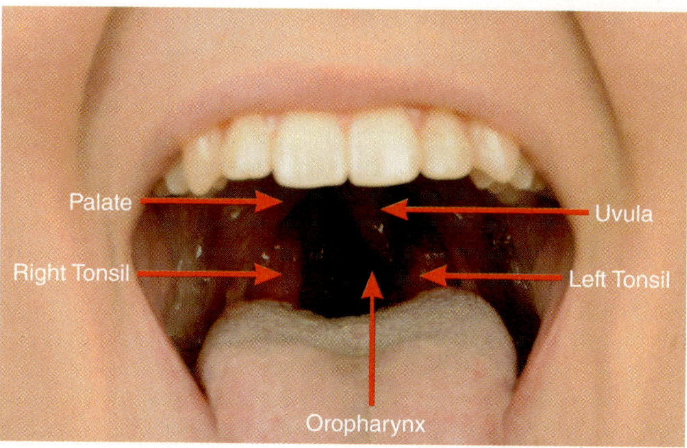

Figure 27-8 ■ When swabbing the throat, swab the posterior wall of the oropharynx and tonsillar areas on each side of the throat. Avoid the tongue, buccal areas, and palate.

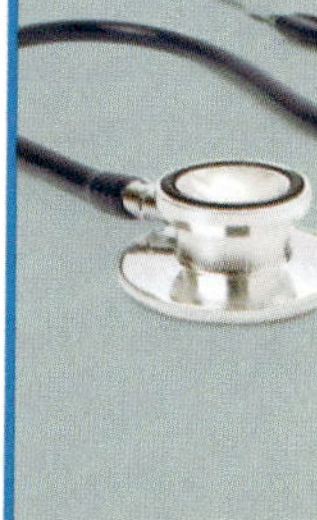

Field Smarts

Avoiding or Minimizing the Gag Reflex during a Throat Swabbing

Many people feel the need to gag during throat specimen collection. One of the biggest culprits of gagging is the depression of the tongue with the tongue depressor. Using a flavored tongue depressor may help the patient concentrate more on the flavoring rather than the tongue being depressed. Another little trick is to slightly moisten the tongue depressor before insertion. A moistened tongue depressor helps to alleviate the "dry wood" sensation over the tongue.

Sources of Contamination

There are many ways that specimens can become contaminated, which may delay or interfere with identifying the cause of disease or discomfort. For example, when collecting blood cultures, sterile technique must followed to avoid normal skin flora found on the skin around the puncture site. To avoid contamination of urine cultures, the patient must be instructed how to collect a clean-catch midstream sample to avoid contaminating the urine with normal urogenital skin flora. In addition, the patient who is instructed to collect a stool for ova and parasites should be cautioned to avoid contaminating the sample with urine and to avoid ingesting interfering substances such as barium, and anti-diarrheal medications that will make finding the parasites practically impossible. Following the protocols and procedures found in the laboratory manual for specimen collection and storage will help to avoid contamination and delays in appropriate treatment.

IDENTIFICATION OF BACTERIA

Many microorganisms dwell in nature within soil and water. Some reside in areas of the human body as normal flora. These microorganisms do not pose any threat to the host and, in fact, provide protection by competing for nutrients that might otherwise be used by pathogenic organisms. They are therefore helpful to the body. Normal flora is found on the skin, in the mouth, in the respiratory tract, and in the intestines.

Only a small quantity of the bacteria in existence are actually pathogenic. Proper identification and isolation of a pathogen is essential in determining the diagnosis of a condition and the desired treatment method.

In order to identify which pathogen is causing the patient's condition and which antibiotic will most likely destroy the organism, the provider will order a **culture and sensitivity (C&S) test**. The culture grows and identifies the organism and the sensitivity portion of the test determines which antibiotic is most effective against the organism. Most specimens such as wound, blood, and sputum may be collected in the medical office, but are generally sent to an outside reference laboratory for identification. Throat and urine cultures are also usually sent out for testing; however, some physician office labs (POLs) that are moderately-complex may still perform them in-house.

Identification of some common bacteria can often be made from a simple smear and Gram stain, while other species may be more difficult to identify. Some organisms require special growth media, stains, and biochemical tests.

The Culture

The **culture** is defined as a group of microbes growing on nutrient-rich media. Following specimen collection, microorganisms must be placed on an appropriate **culture medium** to facilitate proper growth and isolation for identification purposes. Cultures are usually grown in a Petri dish, which is a small, shallow circular plate made of clear plastic (Figure 27-9). The Petri dish is covered with a lid to help protect its contents. The Petri dish or culture plate holds a growth medium that contains special nutrients to support and encourage microbial growth. Because the plate is clear, a culture can be observed without removing the lid. This prevents possible contamination of the culture and helps to prevent any pathogens from being released into the air as an aerosol.

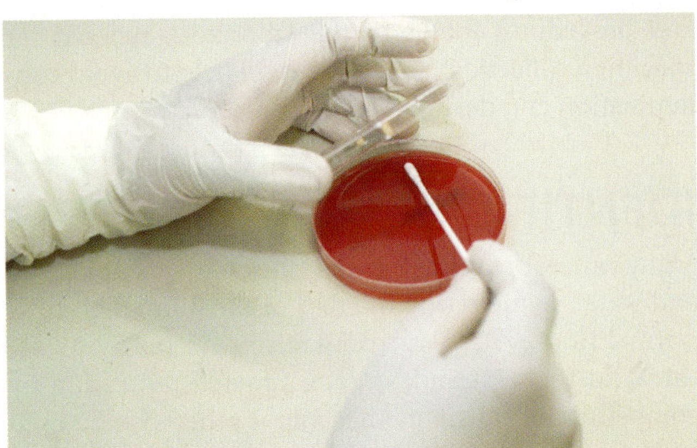

Figure 27-9 ■ A Petri dish containing blood agar.

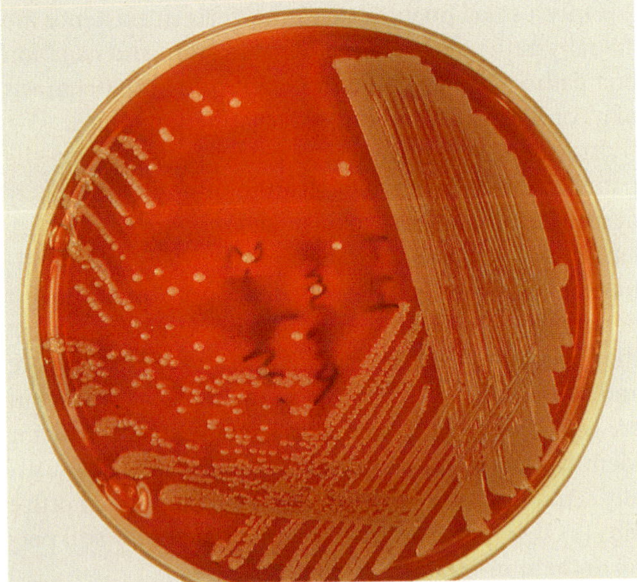

Figure 27-10 ■ Bacterial growth on sheep's blood agar (note the individual colonies).

Figure 27-10 illustrates a bacterial culture after growth has been established. The visible areas of growth are known as **colonies**. Colonies of different microorganisms often have a characteristic appearance, which can be observed on the culture. This can be the first or preliminary step in identifying the microbe.

The first or original culture is known as the *primary culture*. After 24 to 48 hours of **incubation** and growth, the colonies are observed for differing characteristics. If the culture contains more than one organism, known as a "mixed culture," each organism is separated and plated on the appropriate media. This new culture is known as a *subculture*. The object of subculturing is to yield a **pure culture** that contains only one organism.

Growth Media

The media used to grow microorganisms can be a liquid broth, a semisolid, or a solid known as **agar** (Figure 27-11). Agar is a gelatin-like substance containing additives and nutrients that will support the growth and multiplication of microorganisms. Some organisms require additives such as vitamins, minerals, sugars, salts, amino acids, eggs, potatoes, meat, blood, and certain dyes to grow well in a laboratory environment.

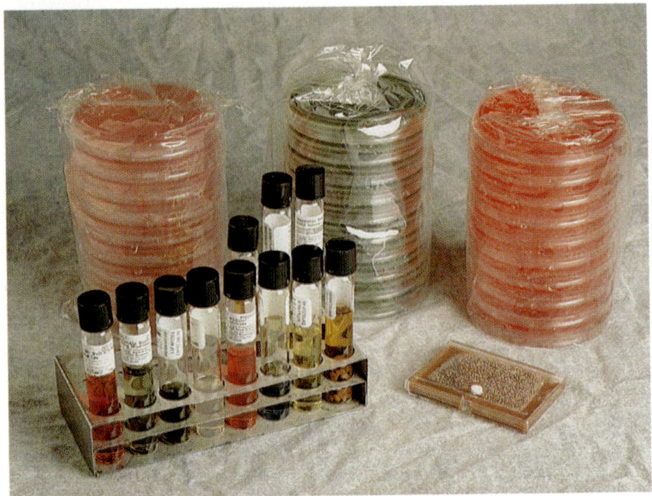

Figure 27-11 ■ Different types of growth media including broth, semisolid tube media, and agar plates.

Commercially prepared culture plates usually come in protective plastic sleeves to prevent the media from drying out and should always be stored in a refrigerator. Condensation tends to form on the lid of the Petri dishes, so the plates should be placed in the refrigerator with the lids facing down to prevent moisture from dripping onto the agar.

Growth media contained in culture plates is classified into the following general categories:

- *Enriched*. Enriched media contains additives that encourage the growth of some bacteria, while inhibiting the growth of others. It is used for cultures from sites that contain normal flora, like the throat or mouth. Enriched media will inhibit the growth of the normal flora, while promoting the growth of the pathogenic organism.
- *Selective*. Selective media promotes the growth of one type of bacteria while inhibiting the growth of others. Chemicals, dyes, salts, and even antibiotics are added to selective media.
- *Differential*. Differential media is also known as indicator media. It contains certain substances that will alter the appearance of the colonies, usually in the form of a color change. For example, MacConkey agar contains the sugar lactose, and will distinguish between lactose-fermenting organisms, which appear pink, and non-lactose-fermenting organisms, which will appear clear.

Inoculating the Media

Microbiology specimens must be placed on culture media through a process known as **inoculation**. Quite simply, inoculation is transferring some of the microorganism onto growth media from the original collection swab. Once the specimen has been inoculated onto the media, it must be dispersed or streaked on the plate. A common streaking method involves dividing the plate into four quadrants.

The specimen is inoculated onto the plate by rolling the original swab over the center of the first quadrant. A sterile loop is then used to spread the specimen over the media to the remaining three quadrants (greatly thinning out the cells from one quadrant to the next). The loop is sterilized by inserting the loop (Figure 27-12a) into the incinerator (Figure 27-12b). The process of incineration should be performed both before and after inoculation.

The four-quadrant method of streaking the culture plate is illustrated in the subculture found in Figure 27-13.

The following guidelines should be followed when performing the four-quadrant streaking method:

- Remove the culture plate from the refrigerator and allow it to warm to room temperature. (Plating a specimen on a cold plate will destroy microorganisms that may be present on the specimen swab.)
- Culture plates have an expiration date. Always check the expiration date before plating a specimen and do not use expired plates.
- When streaking the plate using the four-quadrant method, hold the plate in the nondominant hand and perform the streaking with the dominant hand. (Remember that the initial inoculation will be with the original swab, while the remainder of inoculating will be performed with a sterile loop.)

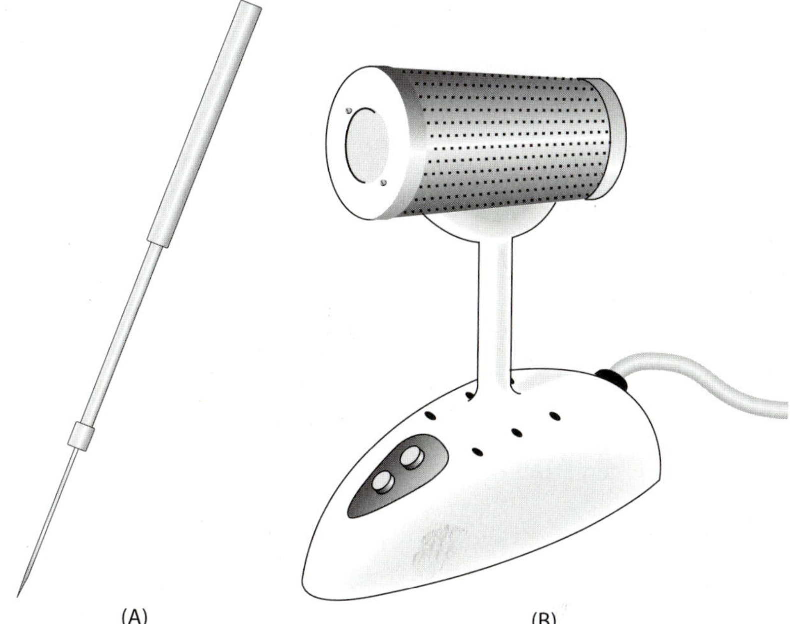

Figure 27-12 ■ The inoculating loop (a) is passed through the electric incinerator (b) before and after inoculation.

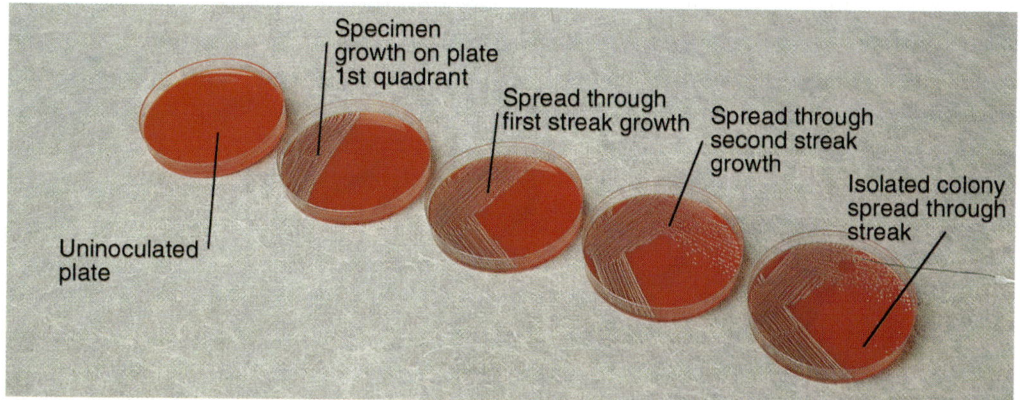

Figure 27-13 ■ Blood agar plates showing examples of the four-quadrant streaking method when plating a subculture. Notice how the bacteria is being pulled from one quadrant to another to isolate the colonies.

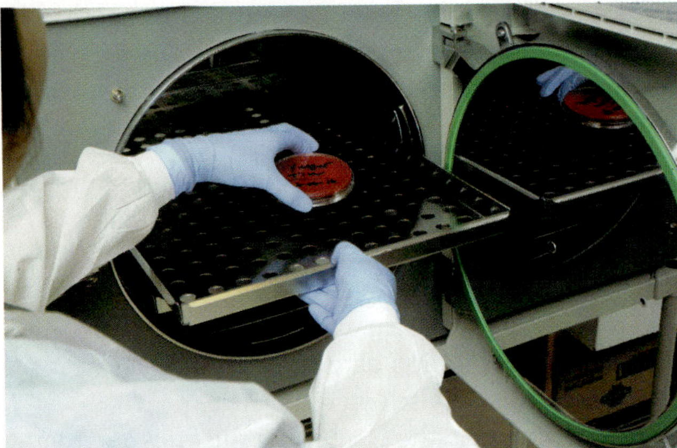

Figure 27-14 ■ The medical assistant labeled the agar plate on the bottom of the dish and placed it in the incubator (agar side up) to prevent condensation from dripping on the agar material.

- Replace the lid immediately after streaking. Agar should not be unnecessarily exposed to the air. Drying and contamination may result.
- Label the bottom of the plate and place in the incubator bottom or agar side-up for the prescribed amount of time (24 to 48 hours). Placing the plate agar side-up prevents the condensation that forms on the lid from dripping onto the culture (Figure 27-14).

The most common culture media used in offices that still perform cultures is blood agar. This agar promotes the growth of most Gram positive and Gram negative organisms, and exhibits hemolysis, or destruction, of the red cells. It is the agar of choice when strep throat is suspected.

Special streaking techniques are used for antibiotic sensitivity testing and urine colony counts. These techniques involve spreading the specimen across the entire plate. Antibiotic sensitivity testing will be discussed later in the chapter.

Streptococcus Identification

Because several species of *Streptococcus* exist, it is necessary to identify which of the species is causing a particular condition.

The most common condition caused by a *Streptococcus* species is strep throat, which is caused by *Streptococcus pyogenes*, a group A beta-hemolytic *Streptococcus*. Positive identification of this species will ensure that the proper treatment is implemented quickly. Some patients can develop serious secondary post-strep infections (such as rheumatic fever), making rapid identification paramount.

Streptococcus species are categorized into several groups and may be classified by the type of hemolysis exhibited on blood agar. The different species of *Streptococcus* can produce three types of hemolysis:

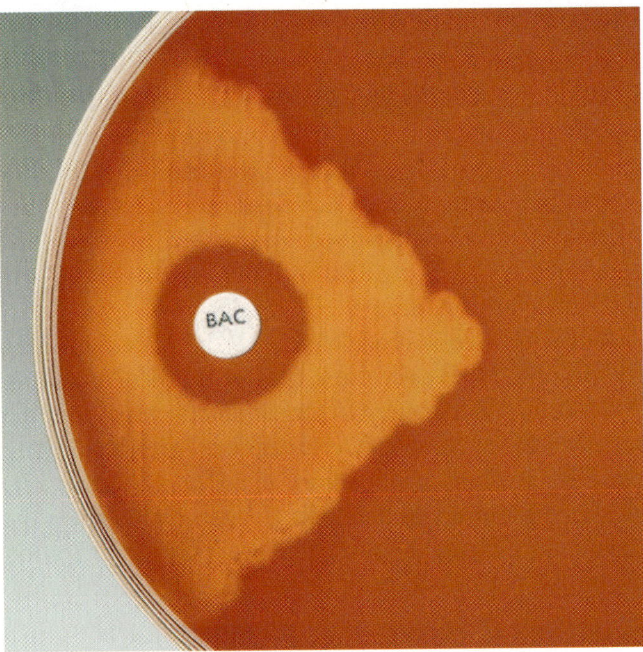

Figure 27-15 ■ A clear zone of inhibition around the bacitracin disk indicates a positive for strep. If the bacteria grows up to the disk, it is negative for strep.

- Alpha hemolysis: Indicated by a greenish halo around the bacterial colonies on blood agar
- Beta hemolysis: Indicated by a wide clear zone around the colonies
- Gamma hemolysis: Indicated by no reaction on the blood agar

Bacitracin Testing

A paper disc impregnated with bacitracin and designated with “A” or “BAC” is then placed on top of the agar and the plate is incubated for the prescribed amount of time. Following incubation, the plate is observed for hemolysis and a clear zone of inhibition around the disc. Figure 27-15 shows a zone of inhibition around the bacitracin disk, indicating susceptibility and the presence of group A strep. Bacterial growth up to the disk would indicate resistance to bacitracin and the presence of a different species of strep.

Bacitracin testing can easily be performed in the POL; however, with the development of rapid strep testing, it is used less frequently in the POL due to the time required to obtain results. The provider may request a culture to be sent out to confirm the results of a rapid strep test, particularly if the rapid strep test was negative.

Another type of test that can be performed utilizes a “P” disc impregnated with optochin. This test will detect the presence of *Streptococcus pneumoniae* in patients with pneumonia.

QUICKVUE DIPSTICK STREP A PROCEDURE

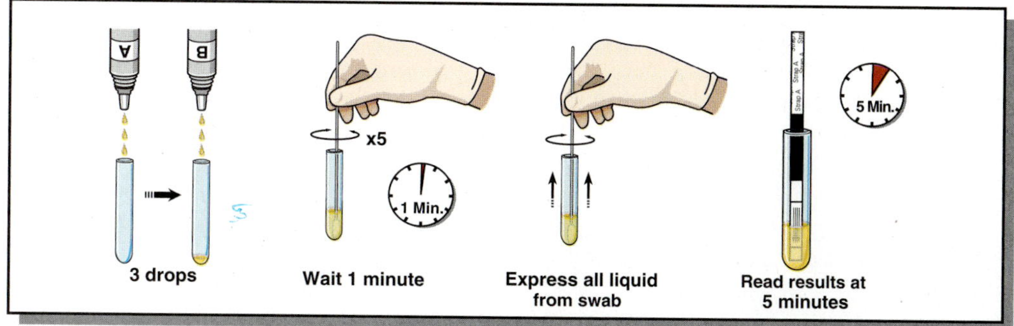

QUICKVUE+ STREP A PROCEDURE

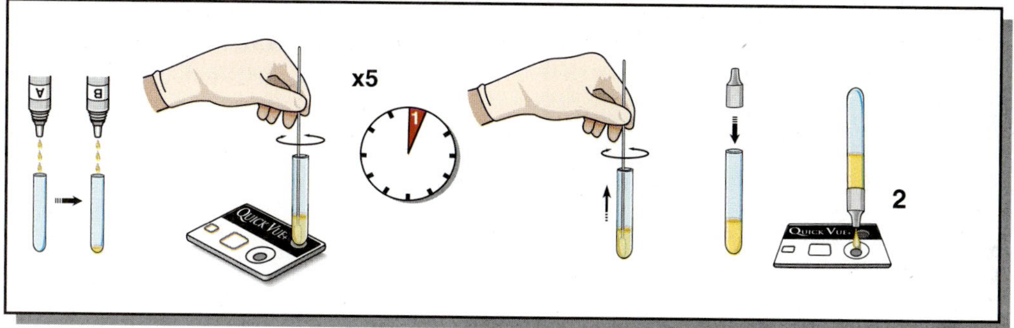

QUICKVUE IN-LINE STREP A PROCEDURE

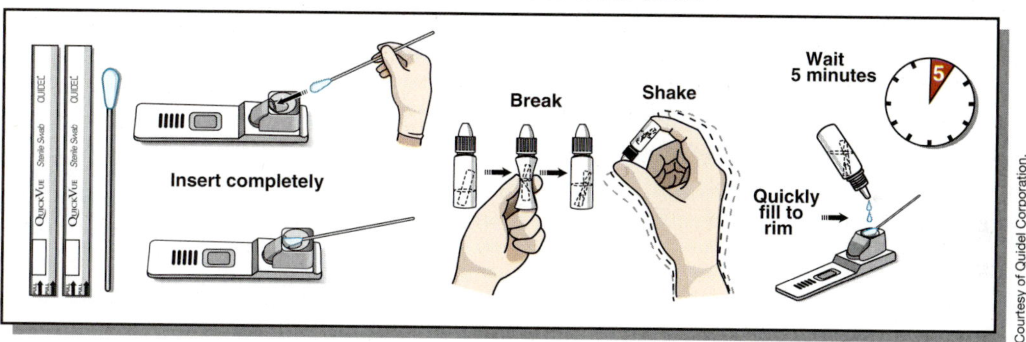

Courtesy of Quidel Corporation.

Figure 27-16 ■ Three methods of the QuickVue rapid strep test by Quidel.

Rapid Strep Tests

As mentioned, strep throat can now be diagnosed quickly while the patient is still in the office by performing a rapid strep test. The rapid test can produce results in five minutes or less, may be Clinical Laboratory Improvement Amendments (CLIA) waived, and can easily be performed by the medical assistant. Several companies manufacture rapid strep tests, but this text features the QuickVue® test method by Quidel. Figure 27-16 illustrates the three QuickVue CE, add (R) symbol as in previous reference. methods for the detection of group A strep. Refer to Procedure 27-1 for instructions on how to properly perform the tests.

A throat swab is collected (see Procedure 27-1) and tested by one of the methods shown. Each kit includes controls to ensure test accuracy. Interpretation is quick and easy, and treatment can begin immediately.

SENSITIVITY TESTING

Once the pathogen has been identified, the provider must determine which antibiotic will work best to destroy the pathogen. The answer often comes from the results of susceptibility or **sensitivity testing**.

Several automated test methods are used to determine the sensitivity of a microorganism to an antimicrobial agent or antibiotic. One manual method is a disc-diffusion method known as the Kirby–Bauer method. This test is performed by placing paper discs containing a known concentration of an antibiotic on top of a plate that has been inoculated with the pathogen. The plate is then incubated for 24 hours while the antibiotics diffuse into the agar. If an antibiotic inhibits the growth of the organism, a clear zone of no growth will appear around the disk (Figure 27-17a) and it is said that the organism is susceptible or sensitive to that

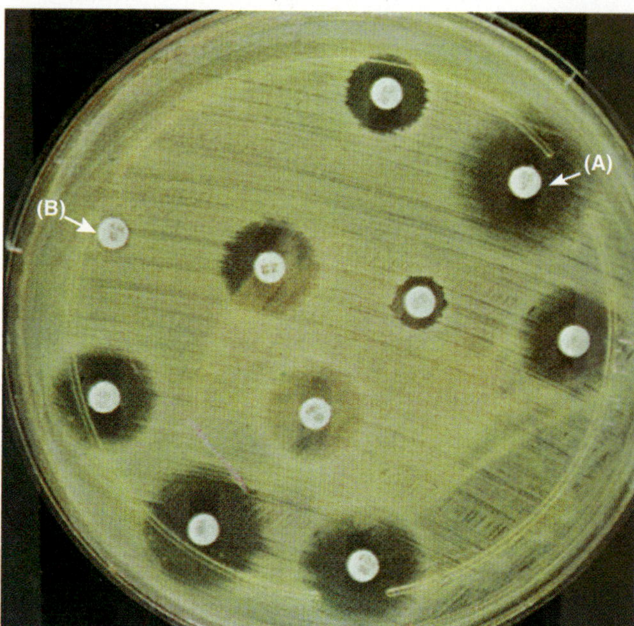

Figure 27-17 ■ Sensitivity testing indicating varying sizes of zones of inhibition for different antibiotics: (a) sensitive and (b) resistant.

particular antibiotic. If the organism is resistant to or unaffected by the antibiotic, it will grow up against the disc with no clear zone present (Figure 27-17b).

The zones of inhibition are measured in millimeters and the organisms are classified according to the width of the zones and are reported as follows:

- (R) resistant
- (I) intermediate
- (S) sensitive/susceptible

In general, treatment is based on the results of the antibiotic susceptibility result, the organism, and the site where the organism was isolated from.

Manufacturers' guidelines should be followed for determining the zone sizes for resistant, intermediate, and sensitive/susceptible.

SPECIAL MICROSCOPIC TECHNIQUES

Microorganisms are usually examined microscopically in either a living state or a fixed state. A fixed state exam involves the preparation of a smear made directly from the specimen or from the culture itself. The smear is then heat-fixed so the cells will adhere to the slide. Then the smear is stained with special dyes to make the organism more visible. A living state exam requires the organism to first be suspended in a liquid, such as normal saline. The suspension itself is then examined microscopically by using preparation methods known as the wet mount procedure or the hanging drop procedure.

The Wet Mount

The wet mount procedure involves placing a drop of bacterial suspension on a slide and gently covering the drop with a cover slip.

The wet mount procedure is commonly used to diagnose the cause of vaginosis. The specimen is examined for the presence of "clue cells," or epithelial cells covered with coccobacilli. The motility (movement) of *Trichomonas vaginalis* may also be observed by this method. Examination is performed under high-power,

Health Coach

Antibiotic-Resistant Bacteria

In recent years, several strains of antibiotic-resistant bacteria have emerged. Scientists believe that microbes learn to adapt to their environment, making changes over time to their genetic structure so that drugs that were once effective are no longer effective. As more and more individuals take antibiotics for specific organisms, those organisms continue to make changes in their DNA and eventually become known as super microbes (microbes resistant to antibiotics). The Centers for Disease Control and Prevention (CDC) and other world health organizations caution physicians to only prescribe antibiotics if it is absolutely necessary. Patients should avoid taking leftover medication from a previous illness, or accepting medication from a friend or family member. In addition, patients should be instructed to take all of their medication, even if symptoms start to subside. The antibiotic may have wiped out enough organisms to relieve symptoms, but the bacteria may not be fully destroyed. They still live in the body, changing their chemical structures so that eventually the patient becomes ill again—but may not respond to the same medication during the next bout.

Table 27-3 Common Bacteria and Related Diseases

Microorganism	Disease
Staphylococcus aureus	Skin and wound infections, UTI, pneumonia, food poisoning, toxic shock syndrome, nosocomial infections
Staphylococcus epidermidis (may enter blood stream from skin via an inserted A-line)	Nosocomial infections
Streptococcus pyogenes (group A strep)	Acute pharyngitis; sequelae (an abnormal condition that results from a previous disease or injury): scarlet fever, rheumatic heart disease, glomerulonephritis; necrotizing fasciitis
Streptococcus pneumonia	Pneumonia
Streptococcus agalactiae (group B strep)	Bacterial sepsis, meningitis in newborns
Enterococci	Nosocomial infections
Escherichia coli	UTI, sepsis, neonatal meningitis
Neisseria species	Meningitis, gonorrhea, urethritis, pelvic inflammatory disease (PID)
Proteus species	UTI
Haemophilus influenzae	Sinusitis, pneumonia, meningitis, otitis media
Klebsiella pneumonia	Lobar pneumonia
Salmonella species	Typhoid fever, bacteremia, food poisoning, diarrhea
Shigella species	Dysentery
Bordetella pertussis	Whooping cough
Citrobacter	Opportunistic infections, UTI, neonatal meningitis
Gardnerella vaginalis	Bacterial vaginosis
Yersinia enterocolitica	Diarrhea
Legionella	Pneumonia or Legionnaire's disease
Bacillus species	Anthrax, endocarditis, food poisoning, septicemia, meningitis
Pseudomonas species	Opportunistic infections, drug-resistant nosocomial infections, wound and burn infections
Listeria species	Listeriosis, food poisoning, encephalitis, meningitis
Helicobacter pylori	Gastritis, peptic ulcer
Corynebacterium diphtheriae	Diphtheria
Vibrio cholerae	Cholera

low-intensity light. Procedure 27-3 lists the steps necessary to prepare a wet mount.

Since a multitude of bacteria exist in nature and are capable of causing many different conditions, Table 27-3 was developed as a quick reference for some of the most common bacteria found in patients, and the diseases they cause.

VIROLOGY

The term virology means the study of viruses. A **virus** is a common cause of infectious diseases in humans. They are responsible for such maladies as influenza (flu), measles, mumps, and the common cold. Viruses are known as obligate intracellular parasites because they can only duplicate or multiply after entering another living cell. Viruses are also the smallest of all microorganisms and therefore must be viewed with an electron microscope.

Diagnostic virology is performed in larger clinical laboratories. Lab tests have been developed to facilitate prompt diagnosis of human immunodeficiency virus (HIV), human papillomavirus (HPV), hepatitis B (HBV) and hepatitis C (HCV) viruses.

Identification of Viruses

Several methods are employed to isolate and identify viruses. The following are utilized for identification:

- Cell culture: The cell culture is the standard identification method. Viruses are grown in a layer or suspension of living tissue cells.
- Direct detection: The viral antigen is detected in a patient specimen.
- Serodiagnosis: Virus antibodies are detected in the patient's serum by enzyme-linked immunosorbent assay (ELISA) or enzyme immunoassay (EIA) techniques.

- Newer molecular tests allow for quick and early detection of some viruses and other pathogens.

Diagnostic kits are available that detect common viruses such as influenza, rubella, and herpes simplex. While most small laboratories do not perform viral testing, specimens are often collected in the medical office. Most viruses will generally survive for 24 to 48 hours after collection if refrigerated, but some may require freezing for preservation. Instructions for specimen collection and transport are provided by the reference laboratory and should be strictly followed to ensure accurate identification.

Table 27-4 lists some of the common specimens collected and tested for viral conditions.

Refer to Table 27-5 for a listing of some common viruses, the pathogenic conditions they cause, and whether or not there is currently a vaccine available to prevent those diseases.

PARASITOLOGY

The clinical aspect of parasitology focuses on the study and identification of pathogenic parasites, the diseases they cause, and appropriate treatment methods.

A **parasite** is an organism that lives in, on, or at the expense of another organism or host without assisting in its survival. A pathogenic parasite can cause illnesses spanning from infections that produce no symptoms,

Table 27-4 Common Viral Specimen Types

Specimen Type	Disease or Complaint	Commonly Associated Virus
Stool sample	Gastroenteritis	Rotavirus is the most common cause of diarrhea in children; calicivirus (Norwalk-like virus) is more common in adults
Serum	Acute or chronic hepatitis	Most commonly caused by hepatitis A, hepatitis B, and hepatitis C viruses
	Shingles	Varicella-zoster virus (VZV)
	Immune deficiency	Human Immunodeficiency virus (HIV)
	Infectious mononucleosis	Epstein-Barr virus (EBV)
Scrapings	Genital warts and tumors	Human papillomavirus (HPV)
Cerebrospinal fluid (CSF)	Central nervous system conditions: Meningitis/encephalitis	Meningitis: Echovirus Encephalitis: Herpes simplex 1
Tracheal aspirate, lung aspirate, or biopsy	Pneumonia	Influenza A
Nasopharyngeal aspirate	Croup	Parainfluenza 1, 2, and 3 viruses
Aspirate of vesicle fluid or swab	Skin conditions: vesicular rash	Herpes simplex 1 and 2 virus
Nasopharyngeal aspirate plus feces	Maculopapular rash	Echovirus

Table 27-5 Viral Diseases

Virus	Disease	Immunizations
Rhinovirus and coronavirus	Common cold	None
Influenza A, B, C	Influenza	Yes
Epstein-Barr virus (EBV)	Infectious mononucleosis	In progress
Human immunodeficiency virus (HIV)	Acquired immune deficiency syndrome (AIDS)	None
Human papillomavirus (HPV)	Genital warts and tumors	Yes
Respiratory syncytial virus (RSV)	Bronchiolitis	None
Calicivirus	Adult gastroenteritis	None
Rotavirus	Gastroenteritis in infants and children	Yes
Herpes simplex type 1	Fever blisters	None
Herpes simplex type 2	Genital herpes	In progress
Varicella-zoster virus	Chicken pox	Yes
Varicella-zoster virus	Shingles	Yes
Hepatitis B virus (HBV)	Hepatitis B	Yes
Hepatitis C virus (HCV)	Hepatitis C	In progress

Health Coach

Human Papillomavirus (HPV)

It should be noted that over 40 genetic types of HPV exist. Some of these types are associated with cervical cancer and genital warts. The genetic types that are most often associated with cervical cancer are HPV-16 and HPV-18. HPV-6 and HPV-11 are most often associated with genital warts. There are two manufacturers that produce a vaccine against HPV-16 and HPV-18. One of these vaccines also targets HPV-6 and HPV-11.

Patients need to understand that just because they have received the HPV vaccine doesn't mean that they are immune from all forms of HPV. The vaccine only covers the strains listed above.

to gastrointestinal disorders with mild symptoms, to systemic infections that are life-threatening. Parasites can be unicellular or multicellular and may exist in any organ or system such as the blood, bone marrow, liver, spleen, skin, hair, or intestinal tract. The most common parasites found in the United States inhabit the blood, urogenital system, intestinal tract, skin, and hair.

Identification of Parasites

Parasites are identified by name first and further identified by stage of development. The stages include the following:

- Trophozoite: Motile, multiplying form of protozoan (feeding and growing stage)
- Cyst: Dormant, nonmotile protozoan
- Ova: Eggs of the parasite
- Larvae: Immature form
- Adult: Mature worm

Visit the CDC's website at http://www.cdc.gov or search for "CDC PDP" for a great collection of parasite images. Click on "professional" pages and PDx lab assistance.

Proper specimen collection and preservation is essential for accurate identification of a parasite. The medical assistant must explain proper collection procedures to the patient for those specimens collected at home. The following are some common specimen requirements for parasite testing.

- Stool specimen (ova and parasites): Stool is usually collected in a wide-mouth container, then a small aliquot, or portion, is placed in a vial with a preservative. Specimens are collected each day for three days. See Procedure 27-4, which lists the steps for proper collection of a fecal specimen for ova and parasite studies.
- Urine: A clean-catch midstream specimen is required.
- Vaginal/urethral discharge: A swab from the affected area is obtained. The specimen is set up for a wet mount.
- Blood: Draw a lavender top tube. The test is performed on stained smears.
- Pinworm: Cellophane tape test (Figure 27-18).

Refer to Table 27-6 for a listing of some common parasites, specimen requirements, how they are transmitted, and the diseases or conditions they cause.

CRITICAL THINKING CHALLENGE

A patient brings in a stool sample in a plastic bowl. Upon examination, you see that there is also a small amount of yellow fluid resembling urine in the container.

1. Is the specimen appropriate for testing?

MYCOLOGY

Mycology is the study of **fungi**, which includes yeasts and molds. Most fungi are nonpathogenic. Only a small group are capable of causing disease. Most fungi are characterized as opportunistic and only cause disease

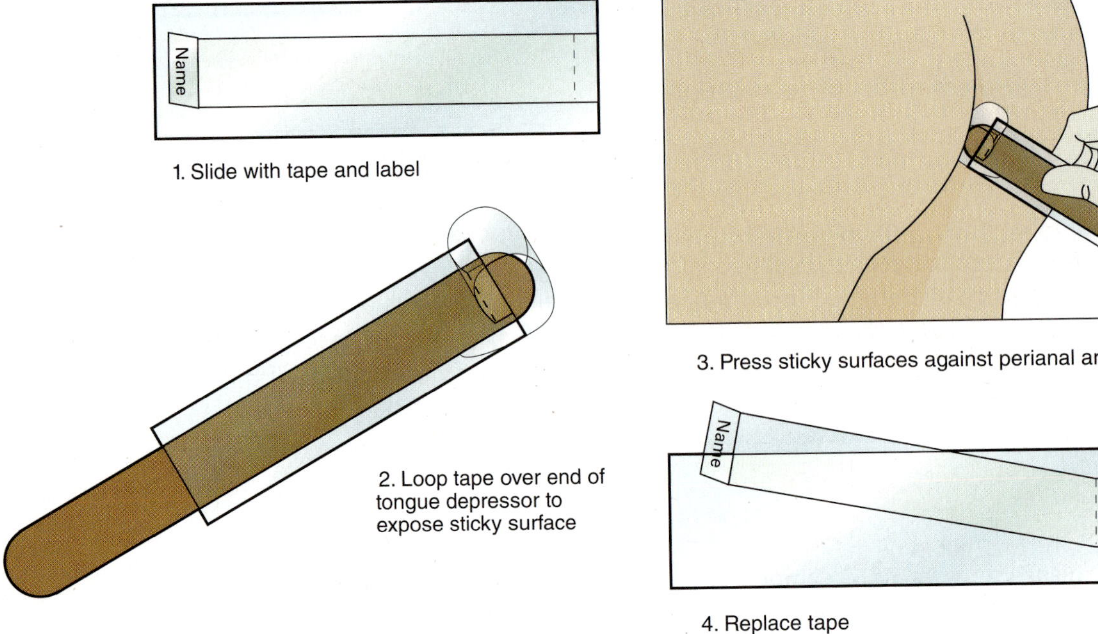
Name
1. Slide with tape and label
2. Loop tape over end of tongue depressor to expose sticky surface
3. Press sticky surfaces against perianal areas
Name
4. Replace tape

Figure 27-18 ■ The steps required to prepare a cellophane tape slide for detection of pinworms.

Table 27-6 Common Parasites

Parasite	Specimen Required	Means of Transmission	Disease/Condition
Trichomonas vaginalis	Urine Vaginal/prostatic Secretions Urethral discharge	Sexually transmitted Common during pregnancy and following vaginal surgery	Vaginitis and discharge Prostatitis
Entamoeba histolytica	Feces	Ingested in contaminated food or water	Amoebic dysentery
Giardia lamblia	Feces	Ingestion of water or food contaminated with feces	Severe diarrhea
Necator americanus or hookworm	Feces	Larvae in soil can penetrate the bare skin of the foot	Iron deficiency anemia–impaired growth in children
Cryptosporidium parvum	Feces	Ingestion of food or water contaminated with feces; oral-anal sexual contact; direct contact with an infected person or animal	Opportunistic infections in AIDS patients
Enterobius vermicularis or pinworm	Cellophane tape prep	Ingestion of infected food; contaminated hands; soiled clothing or bedding; most common in children	Anal itching and irritation
Plasmodium (malarial parasite)	Blood	Bite of infected anopheles mosquito	Malaria

in the following compromised patients and those taking certain medications:

- Patients on antibiotic therapy
- Patients on corticosteroids
- Trauma patients
- Patients with diabetes mellitus
- Patients with lymphoid malignancies
- Patients with immune deficiencies like HIV
- Patients taking immunosuppressive drugs
- Patients who have had organ transplants

Identification of Fungi

Fungal infections caused by yeasts often develop in patients on antibiotic therapy. Some yeasts are normal flora and are kept at a low-level by the bacteria in that area of the body, which are also considered to be normal flora. As an antibiotic decreases the level of the pathogenic organisms, the level of normal flora is also decreased and the yeast can proliferate, causing an infection. The pathogenic *Candida* species is the common fungus responsible for vaginal yeast infections.

Many yeast infections are often superficial and the causative agent can be identified by culturing and examining skin scrapings and hair and nail clippings. The fungi that cause skin, hair, and nail infections are classified as dermatophytes.

Both yeasts and molds have specific identifying characteristics that can be viewed in Figure 27-19. Molds produce a characteristic branching filament known as hyphae and reproduce by forming spores. Yeasts appear in an egg-shaped unicellular form and reproduce by a process known as budding.

Yeasts can be identified by microscopic observation and biochemical reactions. Molds are identified by both macroscopic observation of their growth and microscopic examination for morphology and spores. Molds are known to produce aerosols and should be examined under a safety hood.

KOH Prep

A test known as the KOH (potassium hydroxide) prep is used to identify certain fungi. The reagent potassium hydroxide is added to the specimen on a slide to clear away cellular debris. This makes the fungal characteristics, such as hyphae and spores, more visible microscopically. Table 27-7 lists some common fungi and the conditions they cause.

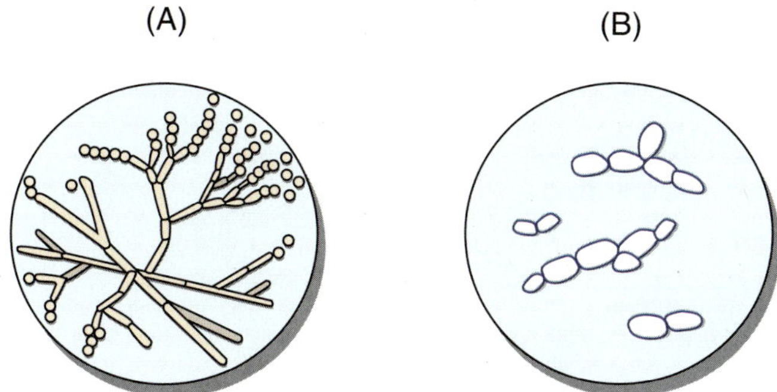

Figure 27-19 ■ Identifying characteristics of yeasts and molds: (a) mold-producing hyphae, (b) budding yeast.

Table 27-7 Common Fungi

Fungi	Disease/Condition
Histoplasma capsulatum	Histoplasmosis
Coccidioides immitis	Coccidioidomycosis (valley fever)
Tinea species	Dermatomycosis (ringworm)
Candida	Candidiasis Vaginal infections Thrush
Aspergillus and *Cryptococcus*	Systemic infections in immunocompromised patients

QUALITY CONTROL

Quality control must be performed in every department of the laboratory, including microbiology. Specimens and equipment must be properly checked and maintained. Reagents and media need to have quality control checks as well. The following guidelines are suggested as part of microbiology quality control:

- Microscopes must be cleaned and maintained in proper working order.
- Refrigerators and incubators must be checked daily for proper temperature levels, and a log must be maintained listing the daily readings.
- Culture media must be stored properly and must not be used past the expiration date.
- A positive or negative control must be performed with each test kit and the results entered and maintained in a quality control log.
- Proficiency testing should be performed according to the level of the laboratory.

LAB REQUISITION AND TEST REPORT FORMS

As with any laboratory, each specimen should include a lab requisition form. When using paper charts, these are forms supplied by the laboratory. When using electronic health records, the medical assistant will create an electronic order (Figure 27-20). Once the order is created, a lab requisition order can be printed to include with the specimen (Figure 27-21).

An example of a test report form can be seen in Figure 27-22. It usually will include the test name, results, and reference ranges.

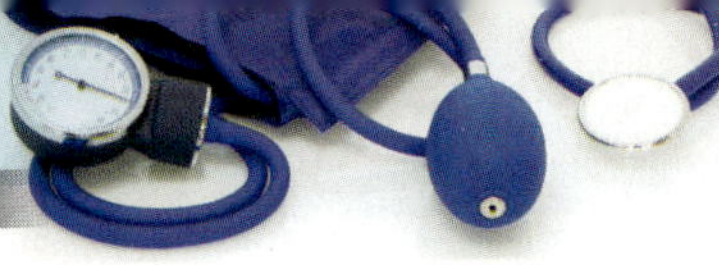

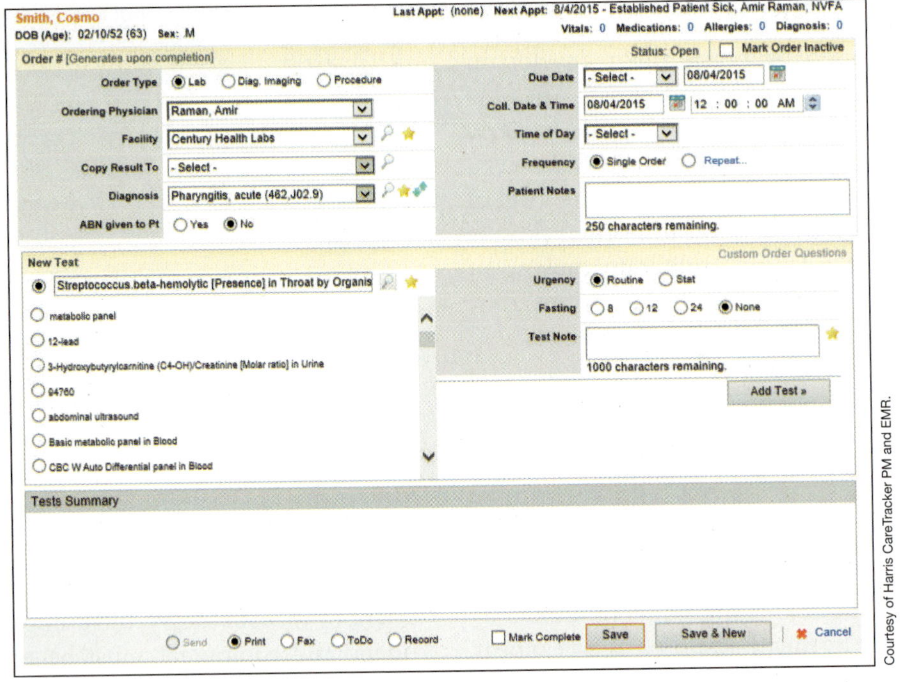

Courtesy of Harris CareTracker PM and EMR.

Figure 27-20 ■ An Order's entry screen from Harris CareTracker. The medical assistant enters a request for a strep culture via the provider's order.

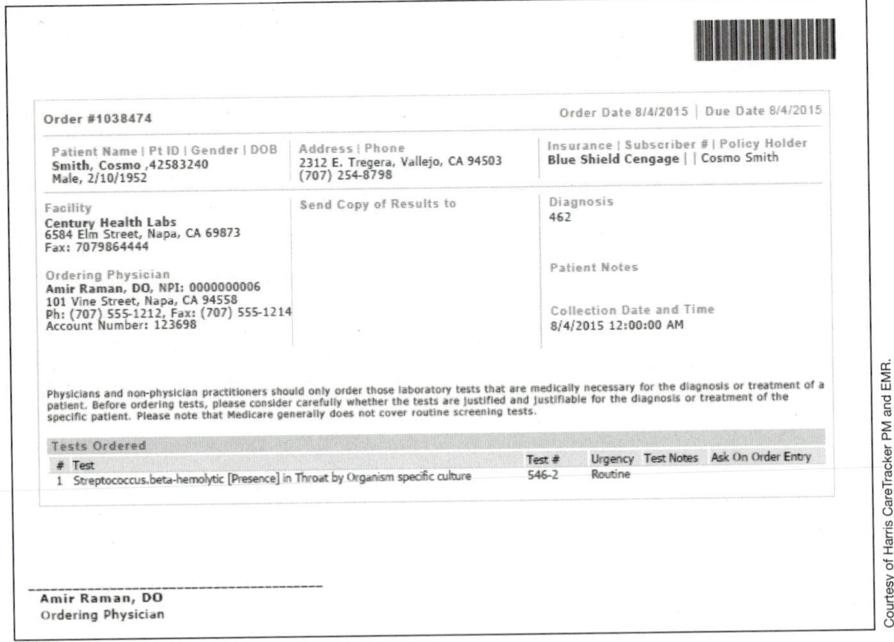

Order #1038474

Order Date 8/4/2015 | Due Date 8/4/2015

Patient Name | Pt ID | Gender | DOB	Address | Phone	Insurance | Subscriber # | Policy Holder
Smith, Cosmo ,42583240 Male, 2/10/1952	2312 E. Tregera, Vallejo, CA 94503 (707) 254-8798	**Blue Shield Cengage** | | Cosmo Smith

Facility
Century Health Labs
6584 Elm Street, Napa, CA 69873
Fax: 7079864444

Send Copy of Results to

Diagnosis
462

Ordering Physician
Amir Raman, DO, NPI: 0000000006
101 Vine Street, Napa, CA 94558
Ph: (707) 555-1212, Fax: (707) 555-1214
Account Number: 123698

Patient Notes

Collection Date and Time
8/4/2015 12:00:00 AM

Physicians and non-physician practitioners should only order those laboratory tests that are medically necessary for the diagnosis or treatment of a patient. Before ordering tests, please consider carefully whether the tests are justified and justifiable for the diagnosis or treatment of the specific patient. Please note that Medicare generally does not cover routine screening tests.

Tests Ordered

#	Test	Test #	Urgency	Test Notes	Ask On Order Entry
1	Streptococcus.beta-hemolytic [Presence] in Throat by Organism specific culture	546-2	Routine		

Amir Raman, DO
Ordering Physician

Courtesy of Harris CareTracker PM and EMR.

Figure 27-21 ■ This is the requisition order that is printed out and sent with the specimen.

```
                Allied Health Professions
                     Santa Anna, XY
                     1(800)555-1122

PATIENT NAME:   Black Doris L          SAMPLE ID #    :   70150072
DOB:            SEX:  F                DRAW DATE/TIME:         @
PATIENT ID #:   161111                 PHYSICIAN      :   Larkin, Alicia, FNP
================================================================================
STREPAPOS
STREP A CULTURE        POS      -      1
Beta Strep, presumptive Group A isolated
```

Figure 27-22 ■ An example of a lab report showing a positive result for strep.

27-2 Solve the Case

The doctor is pretty certain by the looks of Gabby's throat and the recent history of her twin daughters that she has strep throat. He still wants you to try to swab Gabby's throat for a rapid strep test and culture. Gabby starts to panic before you start the throat swab process. She refuses to open her mouth.

1. **What can you do to help Gabby relax both before and during the procedure?**
2. **What should you do if Gabby just won't cooperate at all with the procedure?**

The doctor asks you to give Gabby a prescription for Amoxicillin, 500 mg tablets, three times a day for 10 days. Gabby informs you that she is not good with taking prescriptions and doesn't trust herself to complete the treatment.

3. **What is the best way to handle Gabby's request?**

PROCEDURE 27-1

Collect a Throat Specimen and Perform a Rapid Strep Test

Objective:

To collect a specimen from the pharynx and tonsillar area to be used when performing a rapid strep test or sending out a culture.

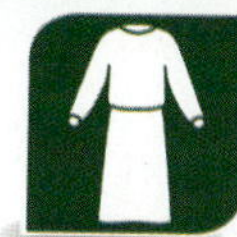

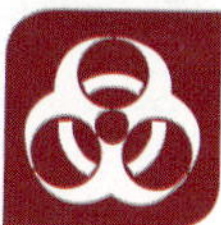
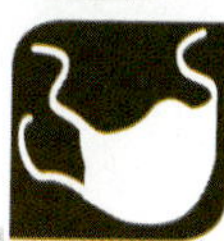

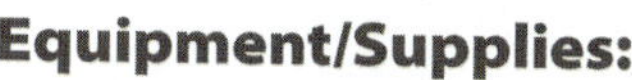

Equipment/Supplies:

- Personal protective equipment (PPE)
- Tongue depressor
- Culture collection system (Culturette)
- Sterile swabs
- Patient's chart/EHR

PROCEDURAL STEPS	DETAILS AND/OR RATIONALE
1. Assemble the equipment (Figure 27-23a) and check the order, ***incorporating critical thinking skills when performing patient care***. Check expiration date on all supplies (Figure 27-23b).	Always have the needed equipment ready before beginning the collection to avoid delays in the procedure.

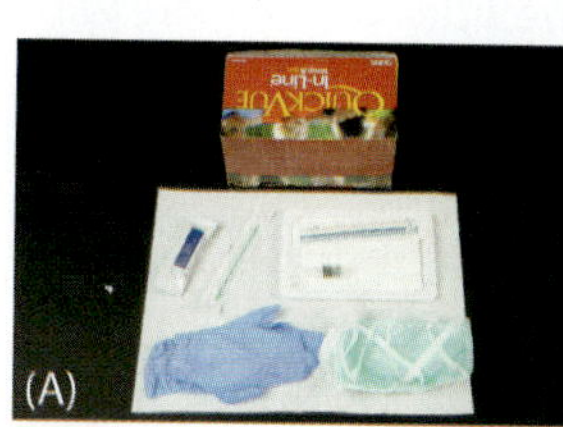

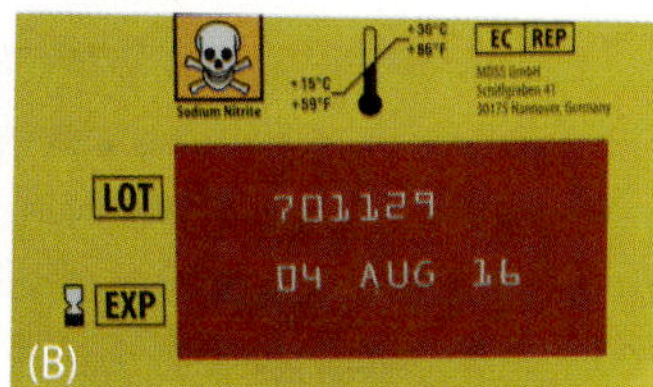

Figure 27-23 ■ (a) The equipment supplies you will need for testing. (b) Always check the expiration date to make certain it hasn't passed.

continues

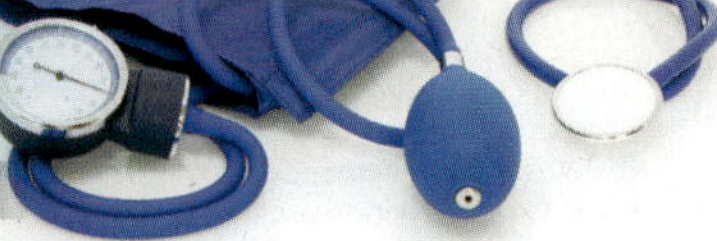

PROCEDURE 27-1 continued

PROCEDURAL STEPS	DETAILS AND/OR RATIONALE
2. Run an external control for the rapid strep kit if necessary.	Running a control helps to confirm that the kit's reagents and supplies are working properly.
3. Wash your hands and apply all PPE except mask and goggles.	Having the mask and goggles on while explaining the procedure may make it difficult for the patient to understand you.
4. Identify the patient using at least two identifiers, identify yourself, and ***explain the rationale for performance of the procedure, showing awareness of the patient's concerns related to the procedure being performed***.	Explaining the procedure helps the patient know what to expect.
5. Adjust the light source so the throat is clearly visible.	The entire throat must be clearly visible in order to see the proper area for collection.
6. Instruct the patient to stick out the tongue and say "ahh" while depressing the tongue with the tongue depressor.	Holding the tongue down with the tongue depressor keeps it out of the way and makes the area of the throat to be swabbed more visible.
7. Carefully insert the swab into the oral cavity being careful not to touch the lips, teeth, tongue, or inside cheeks. Vigorously rotate the swab in a circular motion over the back of the throat swabbing the oropharynx on both sides of the throat (Figure 27-24), and the tonsillar area, being sure to swab any reddened areas or pustules.	Rolling the swab over inflamed areas ensures maximum coverage of the swab with material from areas where pathogens may be present. Rotating the swab in a circular motion helps to cover the entire swab and not just a section of the swab.
8. While still holding the tongue down, carefully withdraw the swab from the mouth being sure not to touch the sides of the mouth, tongue, teeth, or lips.	Touching the swab to the sides of the mouth or the tongue will contaminate the swab with normal flora that may interfere with test results.
9. Place swabs in appropriate wrapper or transport media and provide patient with instructions for what they should do while waiting for the results.	

Figure 27-24 ■ (a) The medical assistant rolls the swab along the posterior wall of the oropharynx on both sides of throat and, (b) if applicable the swab is rolled over both sets of tonsils.

continues

PROCEDURE 27-1 continued

PROCEDURAL STEPS	DETAILS AND/OR RATIONALE
10. If sending the specimen to the lab for a culture, make certain it is accompanied by a lab requisition form. If performing a rapid strep test, follow the manufacturer's directions.	The requisition form contains all of the identifying information and the tests requested. If it is not with the specimen, the specimen will be rejected.
11. Properly dispose of used equipment.	Proper disposal of contaminated articles will help to prevent cross-contamination.
12. Remove PPE and wash your hands.	Washing your hands after a procedure helps to prevent self and cross-contamination.
13. Document the procedure in the patient's chart.	Always document specimen collection in the patient's chart, even if the specimen is not tested in the POL.

DOCUMENTATION EXAMPLE:

04-22-XX 12:30 p.m.	*Collected throat swab for C & S testing per Dr. Samuel's orders. Sent specimen to Qwest labs for testing. C. Leonard, RMA (AMT)--*

PROCEDURE 27-2

Collect a Wound Specimen

Objective:

To collect a specimen free from normal flora and from deep within the wound to ensure accurate culture results.

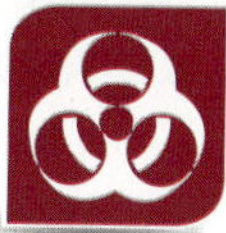
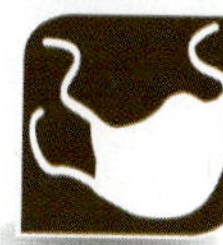

Equipment/Supplies:

- Disposable gloves/sterile gloves
- Gown
- Face shield
- Sterile saline
- Sterile drapes/bandaging supplies
- Sterile swab/Transport media
- Patient's chart/EHR

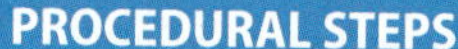

PROCEDURAL STEPS	DETAILS AND/OR RATIONALE
1. Assemble the equipment, wash your hands, and apply PPE.	Apply PPE before beginning specimen collection to prevent self-contamination.
2. ***Incorporating critical thinking skills when performing patient care***, check the provider's order, and complete lab requisition form.	Checking the order ensures that you are ordering the correct test.

continues

PROCEDURE 27-2 continued

PROCEDURAL STEPS	DETAILS AND/OR RATIONALE
3. Identify the patient using at least two identifiers, identify yourself, and ***explain the rationale for performance of the procedure, showing awareness of the patient's concerns related to the procedure being performed***.	Patients are often more cooperative if they know what to expect.
4. Wash your hands, set up a sterile tray (Figure 27-25), and drape the patient. Wash your hands again and apply sterile gloves.	Because this is an open wound, sterile technique must be followed to prevent contamination of wound bed.
5. Cleanse the wound by irrigating with sterile saline prior to collection.	Irrigating the wound will help to remove normal flora from the surface, which could interfere with test results.
6. If wound is dry, moisten swab with sterile saline before collection. Without touching skin or wound edges, rotate tip of swab over a 1 cm area for five seconds (Figure 27-26).	Moistening the swab will help the bacteria to adhere to the swab. Touching the skin or edges of the wound could contaminate the swab with normal flora which can interfere with the results.
7. Immediately place the swab in the appropriate transport media (Figure 27-27). Remove gloves, wash hands, and put on new gloves. Clean and dress the wound (Figure 27-28) according to the provider's instructions.	The swab must be protected from drying. The swab should also be transported under anaerobic conditions, as many wound infections are caused by anaerobic microorganisms. The wound is dressed to keep out microorganisms.
8. Properly dispose of contaminated equipment.	Proper disposal of contaminated articles will help to prevent cross-contamination.
9. Remove PPE and wash your hands.	Washing your hands after a procedure helps to prevent self and cross-contamination to other patients.
10. Document the collection procedure in the patient's chart.	Always document specimen collection in the patient's chart, indicating the laboratory that will be testing the specimen.

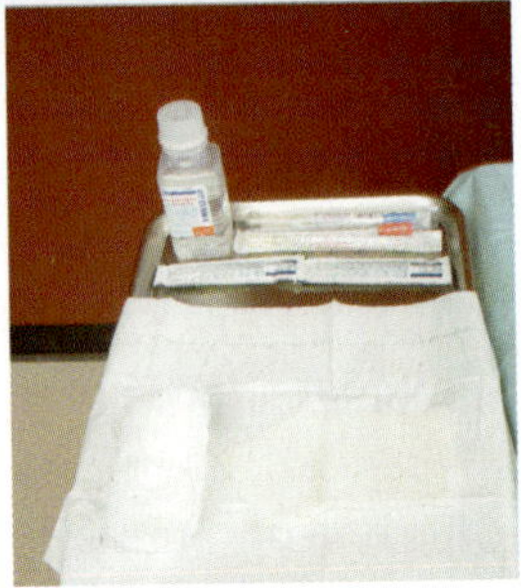

Figure 27-25 ■ A sterile tray is set up for placement of sterile items and a side tray is set up for items that are not sterile.

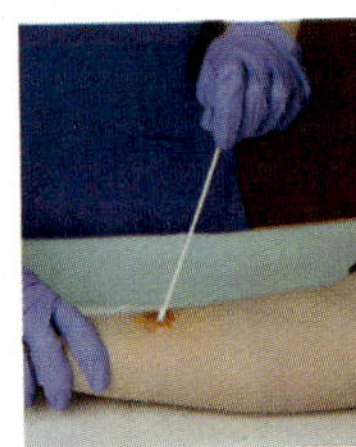

Figure 27-26 ■ The medical assistant inserts the swab deep into the center of the wound over a 1 cm area for five seconds.

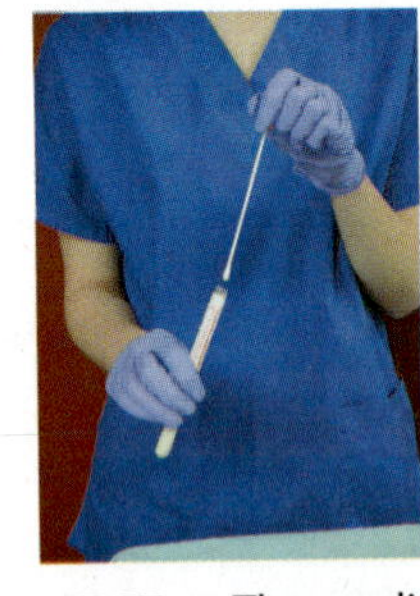

Figure 27-27 ■ The medical assistant immediately inserts the swab into the transport media, following the manufacturer's instructions for preservation.

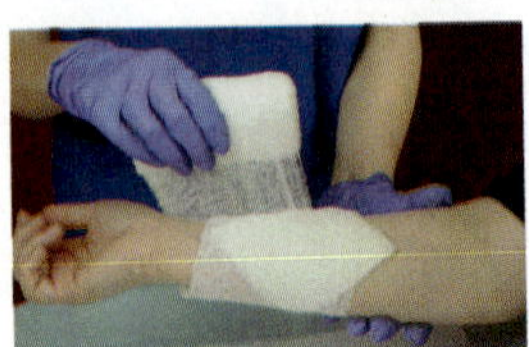

Figure 27-28 ■ Dress the wound according to provider's instructions.

DOCUMENTATION EXAMPLE:

02-24-XX 10:10 a.m.	Collected wound culture specimen from lesion on right forearm, per Dr. Leonard's orders. Specimen sent to Qwest labs for C & S. Lilian Karnes, CMA (AAMA) -----------------------------

PROCEDURE 27-3

Prepare a Wet Mount

Objective:

To prepare a slide for observation of organisms in a living state to view motility and other identifying characteristics.

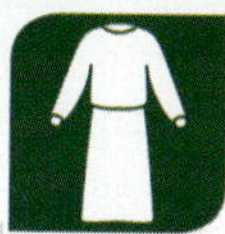

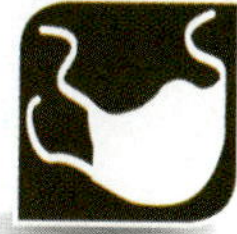

Equipment/Supplies:

- Personal protective equipment (PPE)
- Glass slide
- Cover slips
- Dropper
- Bacterial suspension

PROCEDURAL STEPS	DETAILS AND/OR RATIONALE
1. Assemble the equipment and supplies.	Assembling all equipment and supplies before beginning a procedure helps to eliminate delays.
2. Wash your hands and apply PPE.	Washing your hands helps to eliminate contamination and PPE offers personal protection.
3. *Wet mount slide preparation:* **a.** Place the swab in a test tube with 0.5 mL of saline and mix well. Deposit a drop of bacterial suspension in the middle of a clean glass slide **b.** Place the slide on the microscope stage and focus on high power. Alert provider the slide is ready for viewing.	Suspending the bacterial specimen in a liquid, like normal saline, makes viewing easier.

PROCEDURE 27-4

Instruct a Patient on Fecal Specimen Collection for Ova and Parasite Testing

Objective:

To instruct the patient on proper collection and preservation of a fecal specimen to ensure accurate test results.

Equipment/Supplies:

- Printed instructions
- Appropriate collection container
- Appropriate sets of O&P kits
- Gloves for all collections
- Patient's chart/EHR

continues

PROCEDURE 27-4 continued

PROCEDURAL STEPS	DETAILS AND/OR RATIONALE
1. Wash your hands and assemble the equipment.	Hands should be washed before and after each patient to prevent contamination.
2. Identify the patient using at least two identifiers, and identify yourself.	
3. Provide patient with proper instructions on medications that should be avoided prior to testing.	Patient shouldn't use any antacids, anti-diarrheals, or oily laxatives 7–10 days prior to collection, and should wait 2–3 weeks following antibiotic therapy before collection. These could interfere with the results.
4. Give the patient the appropriate specimen collection kits and gloves (Figure 27-29). ***Explain the rationale for performance of the procedure.*** Explain that the specimens will be collected at home. Patients are given 1–3 sets of O&P collection kits. Each kit contains two to three small vials containing a preservative to hold an aliquot of the original specimen.	The preservative will preserve the specimen until it can be tested. Explaining the procedure will help the patient understand how to properly collect the specimen.
5. Instruct the patient to: (*Note*: Instructions may vary depending on manufacturer. Always check before providing patient with instructions.) **a.** Wash hands and put on gloves. Collect the specimen in a collection hat (without contaminating the fecal specimen with urine or toilet paper). **b.** Start with the pink capped vial, using the collection spoon built into the vial cap (Figure 27-30), collect samples from both ends and middle of the sample. Continue adding sample into vial until you have reached the red line (Figure 27-31). Mix the contents with spoon. Recap and put the lid on the vial, making certain the lid is tight. Shake the vial until contents are fully mixed. **c.** Now repeat step b for the gray capped vial (Figure 27-32). **d.** If applicable, for empty white capped vial, fill with sample as directed. No mixing or shaking is necessary. **e.** Complete the requested information on each vial, remove gloves, and wash hands thoroughly.	Using a wide-mouthed container makes collection much easier. Urine can destroy protozoan trophozoites. Each collection system has its own specific instructions. Following the manufacturer's directions will help to ascertain that the collection was performed properly.

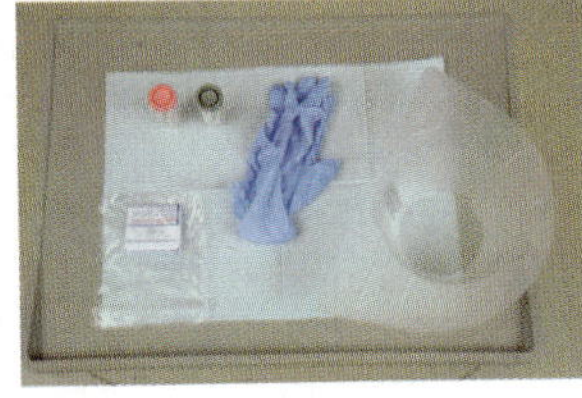

Figure 27-29 ■ Equipment and supplies to be given to the patient.

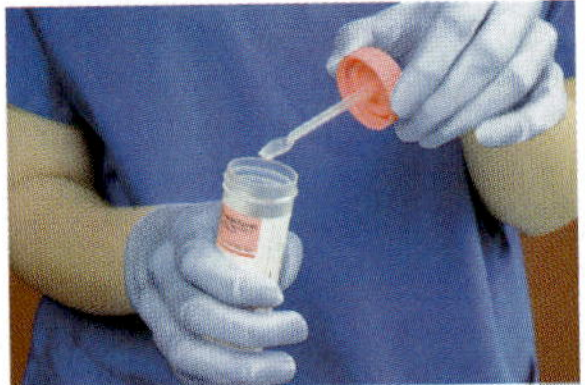

Figure 27-30 ■ The medical assistant illustrates that the bottle with the pink cap is filled first.

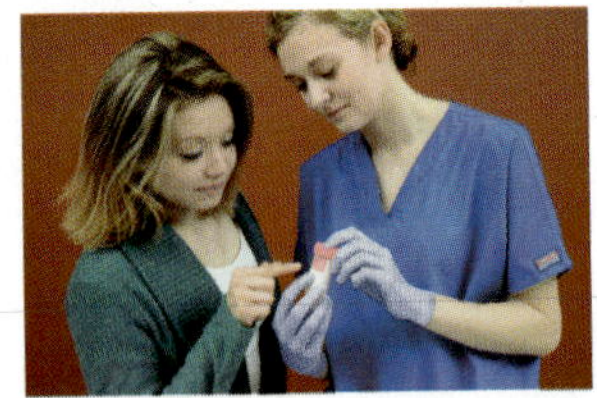

Figure 27-31 ■ The medical assistant points to the fill line so that the patient knows when to stop adding stool contents.

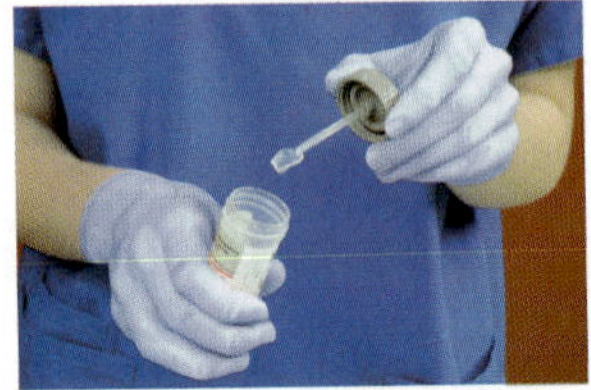

Figure 27-32 ■ The medical assistant shows the patient to fill the gray top vial next.

continues

PROCEDURE 27-4 continued

PROCEDURAL STEPS	DETAILS AND/OR RATIONALE
f. If doctor ordered more than one set of vials, you should wait at least 48 hours but within ten days to collect next set of specimens. **g.** Transfer each vial into the plastic sealable storage bag following collection. Store at room temperature.	Refrigeration could kill the parasites.
6. Encourage the patient to ask questions and give ample time for answers, ***showing awareness of the patient's concerns related to the procedure being performed***.	It is vitally important that the patient clearly understands all aspects of the collection process to ensure accurate test results.
7. Supply the patient with written instructions.	Written instructions eliminate the need to rely on memory.
8. Make sure the patient understands the collection process before leaving the office and when and where to return the specimens.	Some patients are reluctant to call the office with questions.

DOCUMENTATION EXAMPLE:

08-12-XX 2:30 p.m.	Provided instructions and appropriate containers for O&P fecal specimen collection per Dr. Gent. Pt. instructed to RTO with specimens within 24 hours of collection for each set. M. Leonard, CMA (AAMA) --

CHAPTER SUMMARY

- Microorganisms are usually classified using a set of laws and principles known as taxonomy.
- Since most microorganisms are neither plant nor animal, these one-celled organisms were classified as *protists*. Two groups of *protists* are present in medicine: lower protists or *prokaryotes*, which include bacteria and blue-green algae, and higher protists or *eukaryotes* including protozoa, algae, and fungi.
- The microbiology department is usually divided into the following subdepartments: bacteriology, virology, parasitology, microbiology, and mycology.
- Bacteria (single-celled microbes lacking a nucleus) are named using a binomial (two-name) system. The first name is the genus and is capitalized; the second name is the species and is not capitalized (e.g., in *Escherichia coli*, *Escherichia* is the genus and *coli* is the species).
- All bacteria possess individual characteristics that aid in their identification. The features used as criteria for recognition include structure, morphology, and staining characteristics.
- Bacterial morphology is divided into three basic shapes: Cocci (round), bacilli (rod), and spirilla (spiral).
- Stains are used to give color to the bacteria making them more visible under the microscope; A common differential staining method is the Gram stain. Gram-positive bacteria retain the purple color from crystal violet and Gram-negative

bacteria retain the safranin stain so appear pink in color.

- Some bacteria require oxygen for growth and are referred to as aerobic; others grow only in the absence of oxygen and are referred to as anaerobic.
- The medical assistant must follow general and specific collection guidelines to ensure proper specimen collection and preservation.
- Many microorganisms dwell in nature within soil and water. Some reside in areas of the human body as normal flora. Normal flora is found on the skin, in the mouth, in the respiratory tract, and in the intestines.
- In order to identify which pathogen is causing the patient's condition and which antibiotic will most likely destroy the organism, the provider will order a culture and sensitivity (C&S) test.
- The culture is defined as a group of microbes growing on nutrient-rich media. Following specimen collection, microorganisms must be placed on an appropriate culture medium to facilitate proper growth and isolation for identification purposes. The media used to grow microorganisms can be a liquid broth, a semisolid, or a solid known as agar. Microbiology specimens must be placed on culture media through a process known as inoculation.
- Because several species of *Streptococcus* exist, it is necessary to identify which of the species is causing a particular condition. One method of identifying group A beta strep is by performing a bacitracin test. A throat swab is obtained and the specimen is inoculated onto a blood agar plate. A faster method is the rapid strep test.
- Sensitivity testing is performed to determine the sensitivity of microorganisms to an antimicrobial agent or antibiotic.
- Microscopic techniques performed in the office to identify microorganisms include the wet mount and hanging drop tests.
- Virology means the study of viruses; parasitology is the study of parasites; mycology is the study of fungi.

CERTIFICATION REVIEW QUESTIONS

1. Bacteria that are normally present in the body and usually pose no health threat to the host are called:
   a. obligate parasites.
   b. microbes.
   c. normal flora.
   d. pathogens.
2. The method used to grow and isolate microorganisms is:
   a. sensitivity testing.
   b. culture.
   c. Gram stain.
   d. wet mount.
3. A KOH prep is used to identify:
   a. viruses.
   b. parasites.
   c. rickettsiae.
   d. fungi.
4. Bacteria that appear round and occur in bunches are known as:
   a. diplococci.
   b. streptococci.
   c. staphylococci.
   d. cocci.
5. Culture media that supports the growth of one type of organism while inhibiting the growth of another is known as:
   a. basic.
   b. selective.
   c. differential.
   d. enriched.
6. Rod-shaped bacteria occurring in pairs are known as:
   a. bacilli.
   b. diplococci.
   c. streptobacilli.
   d. diplobacilli.
7. Bacteria that stain purple with Gram stain are classified as:
   a. Gram negative.
   b. Gram variable.
   c. Gram positive.
   d. Gram absolute.
8. To preserve a swabbed specimen after collection, it should be placed in the:
   a. refrigerator.
   b. transport media.
   c. sterile container.
   d. incubator.

9. Another name for "pinworm" is:
   a. Giardia lamblia.
   b. Enterobius vermicularis.
   c. Necator americanus.
   d. Entamoeba histolytica.

10. The fungi that cause skin, hair, and nail infections are classified as:
   a. yeasts.
   b. molds.
   c. dermatophytes.
   d. Candida.

STUDY RESOURCES

Resources to Test and Reinforce Your Knowledge:	
Certification Review Questions	Take this end-of-chapter quiz
Workbook	• Complete the activities for Chapter 27 • Perform the procedures for Chapter 27 using the Competency Checklists
Resources to Promote Critical Thinking:	
***Solve the Case* Activities**	• Consider these case studies and discuss your conclusions
Learning Lab	• Module 19: Infection Control and Medical Asepsis
MindTap	• Complete Chapter 27 readings and activities

REFERENCES

How to Collect a Throat Swab Specimen [VIDEO]. (n.d.). Retrieved from http://blog.puritanmedproducts.com/bid/345721/How-to-Collect-a-Throat-Swab-Specimen-VIDEO

Microbiology. (n.d.). Retrieved August 5, 2015, from http://www.questdiagnostics.com/home/physicians/testing-services/specialists/hospitals-lab-staff/specimen-handling/infectious-diseases-microbiology.html

Submitting Specimens to CDC Test Directory. (2015, April 13). Retrieved from http://www.cdc.gov/laboratory/specimen-submission/list.html

28

Clinical Chemistry and CLIA-Waived Testing

CHAPTER OUTLINE

Chemistry Abbreviation Review

Clinical Chemistry Tests

- Quality Control

Specimen Requirements

- Serum
- Plasma
- Whole Blood
- Arterial Blood

Appearance of Serum and Plasma

Profiles and Panels

- Hepatic (Liver) Profile
- Renal Profile
- Lipid Profile
- Cardiac Biomarkers
- Thyroid Panel

Glucose Testing

- Fasting Blood Glucose Level
- Two-Hour Postprandial Blood Glucose Level
- Oral Glucose Tolerance Test (OGTT)
- Glycosylated Hemoglobin ($HbA1_c$)

Additional Chemistry Tests

Serology and Immunology Tests

- Rapid Tests
- Common Serology Tests

Blood Typing

- ABO Blood Typing
- Rh Blood Typing

Drug Testing

- Chain of Custody

Chemistry Tests Normal Values

Lab Requisition and Test Report Forms

ESSENTIAL TERMS

agglutination
analyte
antibody
antigen
antiserum
bilirubin
blood urea nitrogen (BUN)
cholesterol
Clinical Laboratory Improvement Act (CLIA)
high-density lipoprotein (HDL)
homeostasis
human chorionic gonadotropin (hCG)
hyperglycemia
hypoglycemia
lipoprotein
low-density lipoprotein (LDL)
triglyceride

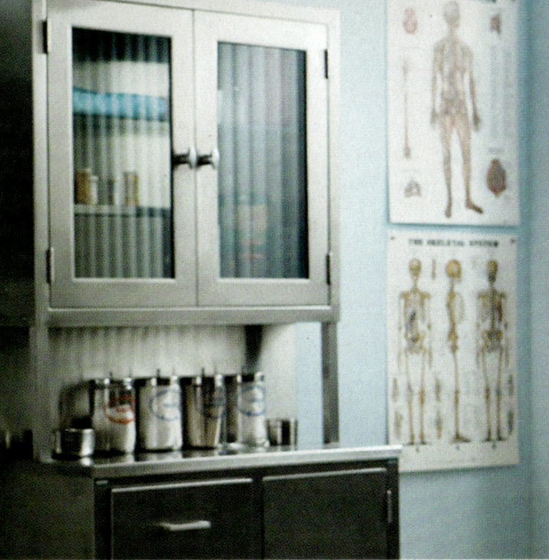

DEVELOPMENTAL OBJECTIVES

After completing this chapter, you should be able to:

1. Correctly spell and define the essential terms.
2. Identify CLIA-waived tests associated with common diseases.
3. Be able to recognize and use common abbreviations used in chemistry testing.
4. List the normal values and clinical significance of common chemistry tests.
5. Explain the importance of proper specimen collection and preservation.
6. Describe the appearance of lipemic, icteric, and hemolyzed serum and the clinical significance of each.
7. Describe the purpose of a laboratory profile.
8. Name the electrolytes and explain their function.
9. List three tests commonly included in a thyroid panel.
10. Explain the difference between type 1 and type 2 diabetes.
11. Discuss the role of the $HbA1_c$ test in the management of diabetes.
12. List the antigens and antibodies present in the four ABO blood types.
13. Explain chain of custody and list the steps that are taken to ensure the validity of a specimen.
14. Obtain specimens and perform CLIA-waived chemistry tests including a fasting blood glucose, pregnancy test, and rapid mononucleosis test.

INTRODUCTION

The numerous analyses performed in the chemistry and serology departments comprise the bulk of all laboratory tests performed. Elevated or diminished levels of certain chemical substances in the blood can be an early indicator of disease or serve as an assessor of the function of a particular organ in a body system. Test results are a fast and useful tool for the physician to determine a diagnosis and implement a proper treatment plan.

Several laboratory tests are often grouped together and ordered as a profile or panel, eliminating the need to order each test separately. For example, a thyroid panel, which commonly includes three separate tests—the T_3, T_4, and TSH—can be ordered as one profile instead of three separate tests. The tests included in a profile may vary from one lab to the next—this chapter lists the general tests included in each type of profile.

The most common CLIA-waived rapid tests are also addressed in this chapter along with their descriptions and normal values.

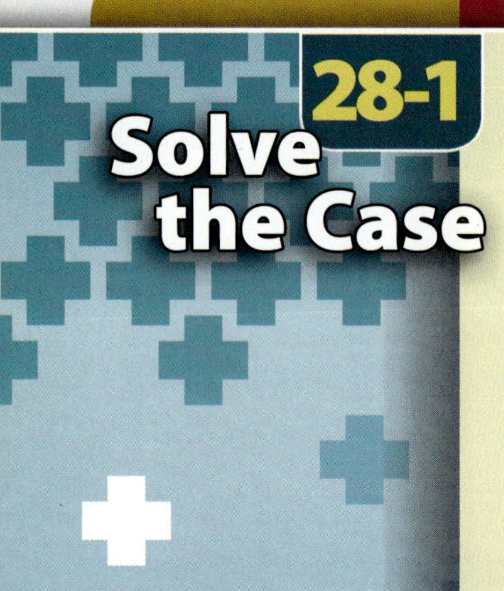

Mr. Wheeler is the president of a large company and is here for a complete physical. He just turned 50 and states that he has been feeling sluggish lately and has a hard time concentrating. When you take Mr. Wheeler to the scale he refuses to be weighed. He states that he knows his weight is up and he doesn't want the doctor to see how much weight he has gained. He asks you to just write in a weight that is five pounds heavier than last year's weight. He goes on to say he is disgusted with himself and the condition his body is in. He has always had great blood pressure but today it is 156/96.

1. **How should you handle Mr. Wheeler's refusal to get on the scale?**
2. **How will you respond to Mr. Wheeler's request to just write in a weight, rather than actually weighing him?**
3. **Is there anything you can say or do to help Mr. Wheeler's frame of mind?**

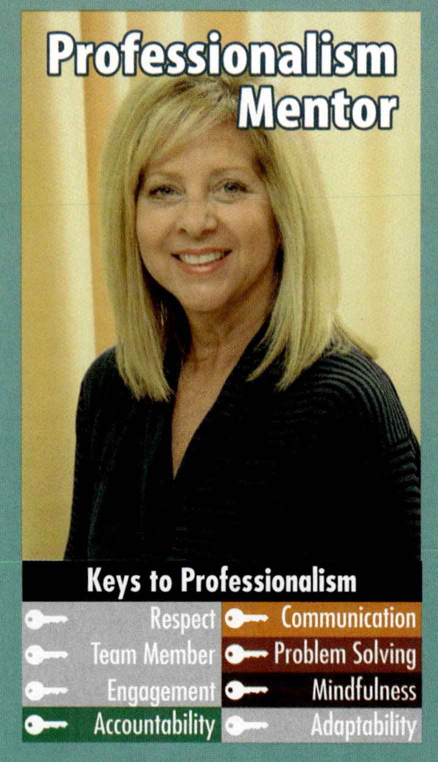

In today's society, we want what we want when we want it! It's no different in health care. Patients want to know their diagnosis, obtain the appropriate treatment, and get on with their lives as quickly as possible. CLIA-waived testing equipment and kits provide us with the ability to give patients instantaneous results; however, there is something you should know before performing waived testing. These tests require the same amount of detail and precision that more complicated tests require. The provider and patient are counting on you to follow the exact steps listed by the manufacturer. Instituting higher level thinking is also necessary when performing testing on patients. If a result doesn't come out as expected, use critical thinking measures to determine possible flaws in testing preparation or performance. For example, if a blood glucose is elevated on a patient with no history of diabetes, go back through the fasting instructions to make certain the patient was truly fasting. If the patient states he followed the fasting instructions, double check the glucose strips you are using and make certain they are the strips manufactured for the unit you are using. Continue troubleshooting until you are certain the result is accurate. After all, a fast result is of no value if it is not accurate. Paying attention to detail and being able to think on your feet is what separates good medical assistants from great medical assistants. ■

CHEMISTRY ABBREVIATION REVIEW

Medical assistants who perform or prepare specimens for chemistry testing should be familiar with common abbreviations associated with such testing. Refer to Table 28-4 for a list of the most common chemistry tests, normal values, and their abbreviations.

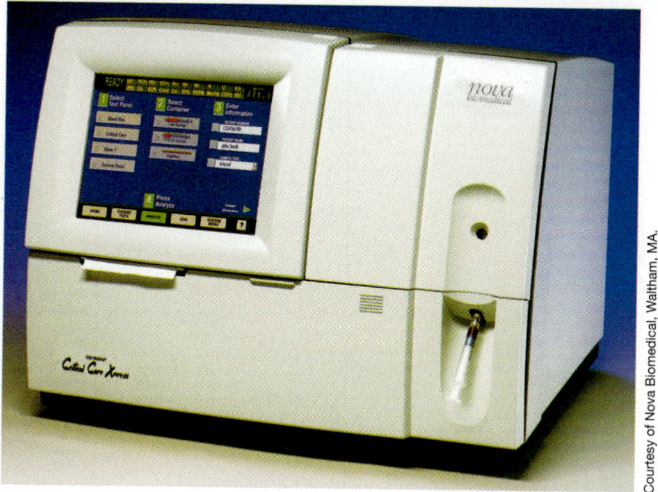

Courtesy of Nova Biomedical, Waltham, MA.

Figure 28-1 ■ The Nova CCX analyzer provides chemistry profiles that include commonly ordered STAT chemistry tests.

CLINICAL CHEMISTRY TESTS

In a healthy body, specific mechanisms monitor and make adjustments to the internal environment to help maintain a constant state of balance known as **homeostasis**. When homeostasis is disrupted, the body responds by making adjustments to either lower or increase chemicals that are out of normal range. These chemical elements can be found in the blood in both health and disease. A change in the level of one of these substances can be indicative of a disease process or how well a particular treatment method is working.

Any body fluid may be chemically analyzed, but this text will address specimens such as serum, plasma, urine, and whole blood. In clinical chemistry, chemical elements, or **analytes**, are measured by many different quantitative methods, using both countertop and handheld instruments.

There are a variety of chemistry analyzers on the market that measure chemical elements in the blood. The majority of these analyzers are considered moderately complex; however, more and more medical manufacturers are developing analyzers that meet the necessary specifications to be CLIA-waived. An example of an automated blood chemistry analyzer is shown in Figure 28-1. These instruments can perform tests that are specific to a particular specialty in a short period of time.

Quality Control

Quality control is performed on all types of laboratory tests, regardless of whether the test is performed manually or through automated methods. Many test kits have internal and external controls to ensure the test is reading accurately and precisely. In addition an instrument must be calibrated using a standard to check the accuracy of its results. Both normal and abnormal controls should be analyzed prior to reporting patient results. If control results do not fall within the acceptable range established by the manufacturer, patient test results should be considered inaccurate and should not be reported.

Any health care worker operating an analyzer must troubleshoot problems and determine if the error exists within the instrument, the reagents, or the way the procedure is being performed. All control results should be documented in a quality control log (Figure 28-2) and should be kept for the appropriate amount of time required by law.

SPECIMEN REQUIREMENTS

Test results are greatly affected by the quality of the specimen that is sent to the lab. It is important to follow all laboratory guidelines for specimen collection and handling. Collection and handling techniques are addressed throughout the remainder of this chapter.

Many chemistry and serology tests are performed on serum; however, other samples such as plasma, whole blood, and arterial blood may be required.

Serum

Serum is the liquid portion of the blood that remains after the blood has clotted. To obtain serum, blood is usually collected in a serum separator tube (SST), which contains a clot activator for faster processing.

After collection, the blood is allowed to sit for 20 to 30 minutes and then centrifuged. During centrifugation, the separator gel moves up the tube to form a

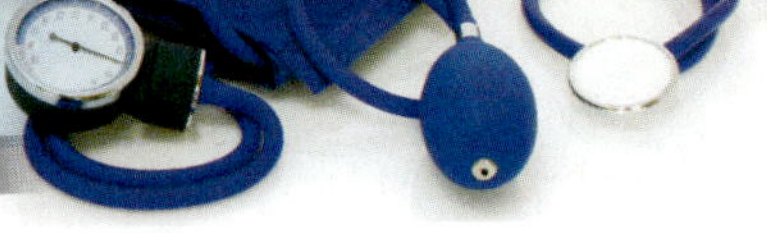

GLUCOSE QUALITY CONTROL LOG
Cholesterol Analyzer (KLM Diagnostics)

Date	Time	Lot#	Type of Control	Reference Range	Results	Initials
10-10-XX	1:30 p.m.	852514789	High Control	300–360 mg/dL	320 mg/dL	LMV

Figure 28-2 ■ An example of a quality control log sheet. Each type of control should have a separate log sheet.

barrier between the cells and the serum (Figure 28-3). Serum is then transferred to a properly labeled transfer tube and sent to the laboratory for testing.

Plasma

There are some chemistry tests that may also be performed on plasma. In a lab setting, plasma is the liquid portion of the blood to which an anticoagulant has been added. Blood is collected into a tube containing an appropriate anticoagulant for a particular chemistry test. Lithium heparin is usually the anticoagulant of choice, as ethylenediaminetetraacetic acid (EDTA) and sodium heparin can destroy some components being analyzed.

Once the tube has been centrifuged, the plasma should be transferred to a separate transfer tube and properly labeled as plasma. When placed in a transfer tube, plasma and serum have the same appearance; therefore, the only way to determine the specimen type is through proper labeling.

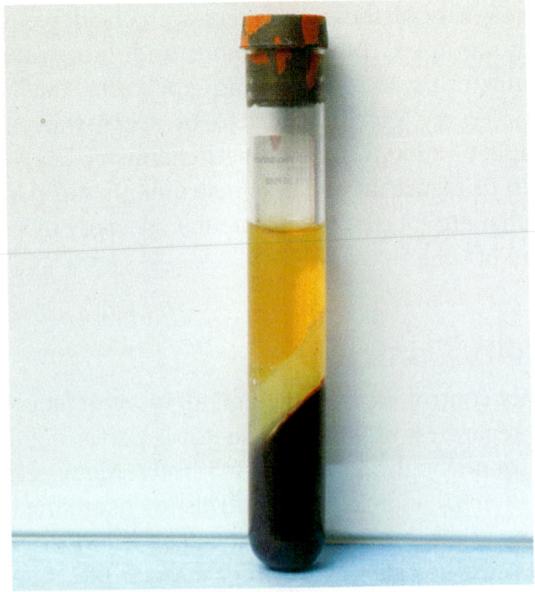

Figure 28-3 ■ An SST that has been centrifuged. The gel forms a barrier between the serum and cells.

Whole Blood

A whole blood sample contains the appropriate anticoagulant and is not separated into its components.

Arterial Blood

Some tests require whole arterial blood. A test known as an arterial blood gas (ABG) is one example of such a test. This test is usually performed in the hospital laboratory, not the POL, and requires specialized training to obtain the sample.

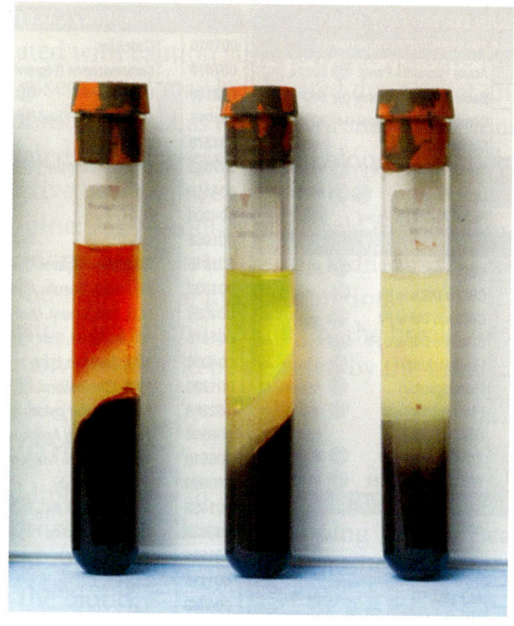

Figure 28-4 ■ Examples of both normal and abnormal appearances of serum (from left to right): (a) hemolyzed, (b) icteric, (c) lipemic.

APPEARANCE OF SERUM AND PLASMA

The appearance of serum and plasma should be observed after collection and processing for any signs of discoloration. Both serum and plasma are normally pale yellow in color and clear in transparency. Improper collection and some diseases may alter the appearance of the specimen. Figure 28-4 illustrates serum samples with different appearances. Table 28-1 lists possible reasons for abnormal specimen appearance. Specimens that are hemolyzed may be rejected. Refer to Chapter 24 for measures that should be instituted to avoid hemolysis.

PROFILES AND PANELS

Instead of ordering each chemistry test individually, the provider can order a group of tests known as a profile or panel. Multiple tests are included in a profile and can be performed on a small sample of blood. General chemistry profiles, such as those shown in Figure 28-5, includes tests that furnish the provider with a general overview of the patient's state of health.

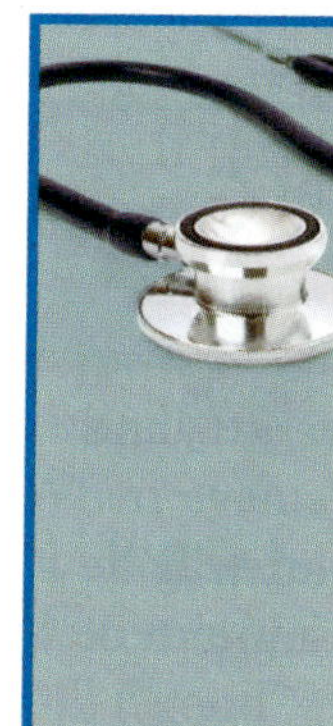

Field Smarts

In order to obtain the required amount of plasma or serum necessary for a particular test, you will need to draw at least 2.5 times that volume in blood. For example, a 10 mL tube of blood will yield approximately 4 mL of serum or plasma following centrifugation. So to figure out how many milliliters of blood you will need, just multiply the required volume of serum or plasma by 2.5 mL.

Table 28-1 Color/Appearance of Serum Specimens

Descriptive Term	Color/Appearance	Possible Cause
Hemolyzed	Pink/red	Collection error Processing error Hemolytic diseases
Lipemic	Milky or cloudy	Lipid metabolism disorders Non-fasting specimen
Icteric	Deep yellow to orange Green tint Pale/watery	Jaundice due to liver disease Obstructive jaundice Jaundice due to hemolytic anemia

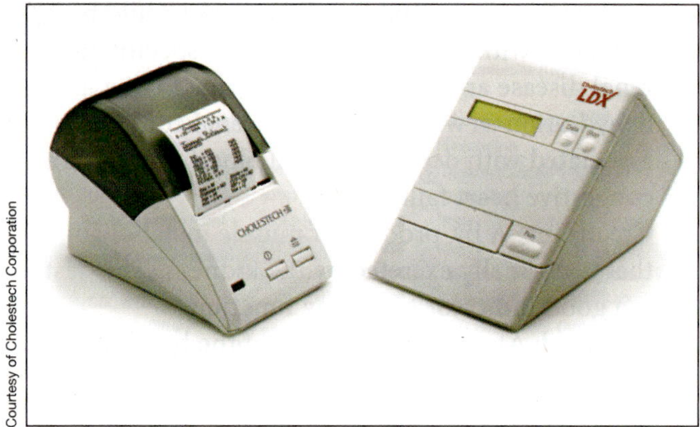

Courtesy of Cholestech Corporation

Figure 28-6 ■ Cholestech LDX system, which provides a full lipid profile, glucose, or ALT-AST.

Triglycerides are another type of lipid or fat found in the blood. While these fats are a source of energy, if present in increased amounts they are stored in the body as adipose tissue. Elevated triglyceride levels can increase a patient's risk of developing cardiovascular disease.

CLIA-waived portable lipid testing systems, such as the one pictured in Figure 28-6, are now available for use in the medical office. The LDX system by Cholestech can complete a lipid panel plus a glucose determination in just five minutes. Testing by this method requires only a small drop of blood, which can be obtained by capillary puncture. This system meets guidelines of the National Cholesterol Education Program (NCEP) for precision and accuracy, and is certified accurate by the CDC's Cholesterol Reference Method Laboratory Network (CRMLN) for total and HDL cholesterol. It also provides an alanine aminotransferase (ALT) and aspartate aminotransferase (AST) test to monitor liver function and determine possible side effects of cholesterol-lowering or diabetes medications. HS-CRP testing is also available with the Cholestech LDX system for moderate-complexity labs.

Cardiac Biomarkers

Cardiac biomarkers include tests that help to determine if the patient has experienced a myocardial infarction (heart attack). These tests are usually performed in free-standing emergency departments (similar to urgent care centers but a little more upscale) and in hospitals. Cardiac biomarkers include the following:

- Cardiac troponin: Considered the most reliable biomarker for a heart attack. It is detectable soon after a heart attack and remains elevated several days following a heart attack.
- Creatinine kinase isoenzymes: These include CK-MM (muscle subunits), CK-BB (brain subunits), and CK-MB (found mainly in the heart). The enzymes can be measured several times during the first day or two from the onset of chest pain but return to normal levels after one or two days. These enzymes are not specific for heart attack.
- Myoglobin: This protein is released more rapidly than troponin (usually within an hour of the onset of symptoms) but may be elevated for conditions other than myocardial infarction.

Thyroid Panel

A thyroid panel may be ordered to evaluate the function of the thyroid gland. The thyroid gland (an endocrine gland) is important because of the role it plays in metabolism. T3 (triiodothyronine) and T4 (thyroxine) are the two hormones produced by the thyroid gland that affect metabolism. Iodine is necessary for the thyroid gland to produce these hormones and can be obtained from seafood, iodized salt, or by consuming vegetables grown in soil containing iodine. A third hormone, thyrocalcitonin, stimulates calcium to be stored in the bones. A thyroid panel usually includes TSH, T3, and T4 levels.

GLUCOSE TESTING

Glucose is the cells' primary source of energy; it must stay within a particular range, or complications will arise. Excess glucose is transformed into glycogen, which is then stored in muscle and the liver tissue for future use. If glucose levels in the blood diminish, the liver converts glycogen back into glucose so that it can be used by cells for energy. If the tissues can no longer hold the excess glucose, the glucose is converted to fat and stored in the form of adipose tissue.

Glucose cannot enter cells without the hormone insulin. Insulin is secreted by the beta cells of the pancreas and is the key that unlocks the door for the glucose to enter the cell. If insulin is not being produced, or the patient has a condition known as insulin resistance, glucose is unable to enter the cell and the body will use other sources of energy such as fats and proteins to feed the cell. The increased levels of glucose will build up in the blood stream, causing an array of problems for organs such as the heart and kidneys.

By measuring the level of glucose in the blood, problems with carbohydrate metabolism, such as diabetes, may be detected, along with **hypoglycemia**, or low blood sugar. High blood glucose levels (or **hyperglycemia**) are

Some laboratories also offer profiles that include tests that are specific for the different types of hepatitis. These tests detect not only the presence of the disease, but the type of hepatitis as well.

Renal Profile

A renal profile can provide a rapid assessment of a patient's general health and is, therefore, one of the most frequently requested groups of tests. This profile can also provide information about the progression of kidney disease and complications that may arise due to other conditions, such as diabetes mellitus. Tests included in a renal profile can furnish the provider with important diagnostic information. The following analytes are usually included in a renal profile because the kidney helps to keep these chemicals in balance through processes known as filtration, reabsorption, and secretion. Abnormal levels of these analytes may indicate kidney disease:

- Sodium: This substance is vital to life and helps to control the acid–base balance in the body, along with transmitting nerve impulses. It also indirectly regulates water levels in the body.
- Potassium: This analyte affects the acid–base balance and aids in the reactions that take place during carbohydrate and protein metabolism. Potassium also has a significant influence in conducting electrical impulses in heart and skeletal muscles.
- Chloride: Chloride maintains water and acid–base balance in the body. ***(Note: Sodium, potassium, and chloride [Na, K^+, and Cl] can be grouped together and requested as an electrolyte panel.)***
- **Blood urea nitrogen (BUN)**: This test measures the nitrogen portion of urea, which is the end product of protein metabolism. This compound should be excreted by the kidneys, so an elevation of this waste product in the bloodstream may be due to impaired renal function. BUN results should be evaluated with caution since it is not specific for renal disease and may be elevated due to diet and dehydration as well as other nonrenal conditions associated with decreased renal blood flow such as congestive heart failure.
- Creatinine: A by-product of muscle metabolism that is normally excreted by the kidneys. This test is a good indicator of kidney function.
- Uric acid: Also an end product of the breakdown of protein that should be excreted by the kidneys.

Lipid Profile

Increased lipids or fats in the blood can be an indicator of an increased risk of developing heart disease. **Cholesterol** and **triglycerides** are the lipids generally found in the blood.

When fats are combined with protein in the blood it is termed as a **lipoprotein**. Cholesterol is important in order for many life functions to take place, such as the synthesis of steroid hormones. Although the body easily produces cholesterol, it is not easily broken down and may build up in different tissues, especially the blood vessels. If this buildup occurs, a condition known as atherosclerosis may develop, which places the patient at a higher risk of heart attack. Because the body produces enough cholesterol to meet its needs, dietary intake is not usually necessary.

When evaluating the level of lipids in the blood, a total cholesterol level is determined. Additionally, the cholesterol level is divided into **high-density lipoprotein (HDL)** ("good" cholesterol) and **low-density lipoprotein (LDL)** ("bad" cholesterol). HDL is the lipoprotein that removes cholesterol from the body by taking it to the liver, where it is excreted in bile. LDL is deposited as fat in the tissues of the body and in the walls of the blood vessels, which increases the risk of coronary artery disease.

Health Coach

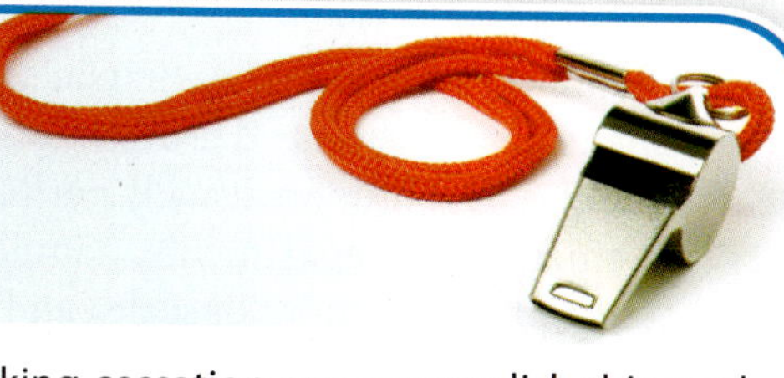

Cholesterol

It is possible to decrease the level of LDL or "bad" cholesterol in the blood and at the same time raise the level of HDL or "good" cholesterol in the blood. A combination of weight loss, exercise, a diet low in saturated fats, and smoking cessation can accomplish this goal. Consumption of foods with polyunsaturated fats, like corn, safflower, and many fish oils, in place of foods high in saturated fat can also lower blood cholesterol levels.

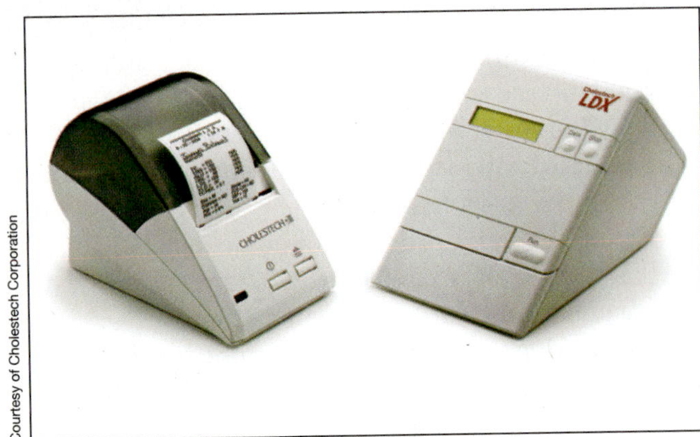

Courtesy of Cholestech Corporation

Figure 28-6 ■ Cholestech LDX system, which provides a full lipid profile, glucose, or ALT-AST.

Triglycerides are another type of lipid or fat found in the blood. While these fats are a source of energy, if present in increased amounts they are stored in the body as adipose tissue. Elevated triglyceride levels can increase a patient's risk of developing cardiovascular disease.

CLIA-waived portable lipid testing systems, such as the one pictured in Figure 28-6, are now available for use in the medical office. The LDX system by Cholestech can complete a lipid panel plus a glucose determination in just five minutes. Testing by this method requires only a small drop of blood, which can be obtained by capillary puncture. This system meets guidelines of the National Cholesterol Education Program (NCEP) for precision and accuracy, and is certified accurate by the CDC's Cholesterol Reference Method Laboratory Network (CRMLN) for total and HDL cholesterol. It also provides an alanine aminotransferase (ALT) and aspartate aminotransferase (AST) test to monitor liver function and determine possible side effects of cholesterol-lowering or diabetes medications. HS-CRP testing is also available with the Cholestech LDX system for moderate-complexity labs.

Cardiac Biomarkers

Cardiac biomarkers include tests that help to determine if the patient has experienced a myocardial infarction (heart attack). These tests are usually performed in free-standing emergency departments (similar to urgent care centers but a little more upscale) and in hospitals. Cardiac biomarkers include the following:

- Cardiac troponin: Considered the most reliable biomarker for a heart attack. It is detectable soon after a heart attack and remains elevated several days following a heart attack.
- Creatinine kinase isoenzymes: These include CK-MM (muscle subunits), CK-BB (brain subunits), and CK-MB (found mainly in the heart). The enzymes can be measured several times during the first day or two from the onset of chest pain but return to normal levels after one or two days. These enzymes are not specific for heart attack.
- Myoglobin: This protein is released more rapidly than troponin (usually within an hour of the onset of symptoms) but may be elevated for conditions other than myocardial infarction.

Thyroid Panel

A thyroid panel may be ordered to evaluate the function of the thyroid gland. The thyroid gland (an endocrine gland) is important because of the role it plays in metabolism. T3 (triiodothyronine) and T4 (thyroxine) are the two hormones produced by the thyroid gland that affect metabolism. Iodine is necessary for the thyroid gland to produce these hormones and can be obtained from seafood, iodized salt, or by consuming vegetables grown in soil containing iodine. A third hormone, thyrocalcitonin, stimulates calcium to be stored in the bones. A thyroid panel usually includes TSH, T3, and T4 levels.

GLUCOSE TESTING

Glucose is the cells' primary source of energy; it must stay within a particular range, or complications will arise. Excess glucose is transformed into glycogen, which is then stored in muscle and the liver tissue for future use. If glucose levels in the blood diminish, the liver converts glycogen back into glucose so that it can be used by cells for energy. If the tissues can no longer hold the excess glucose, the glucose is converted to fat and stored in the form of adipose tissue.

Glucose cannot enter cells without the hormone insulin. Insulin is secreted by the beta cells of the pancreas and is the key that unlocks the door for the glucose to enter the cell. If insulin is not being produced, or the patient has a condition known as insulin resistance, glucose is unable to enter the cell and the body will use other sources of energy such as fats and proteins to feed the cell. The increased levels of glucose will build up in the blood stream, causing an array of problems for organs such as the heart and kidneys.

By measuring the level of glucose in the blood, problems with carbohydrate metabolism, such as diabetes, may be detected, along with **hypoglycemia**, or low blood sugar. High blood glucose levels (or **hyperglycemia**) are

Whole Blood

A whole blood sample contains the appropriate anticoagulant and is not separated into its components.

Arterial Blood

Some tests require whole arterial blood. A test known as an arterial blood gas (ABG) is one example of such a test. This test is usually performed in the hospital laboratory, not the POL, and requires specialized training to obtain the sample.

APPEARANCE OF SERUM AND PLASMA

The appearance of serum and plasma should be observed after collection and processing for any signs of discoloration. Both serum and plasma are normally pale yellow in color and clear in transparency. Improper collection and some diseases may alter the appearance of the specimen. Figure 28-4 illustrates serum samples with different appearances. Table 28-1 lists possible reasons for abnormal specimen appearance. Specimens that are hemolyzed may be rejected. Refer to Chapter 24 for measures that should be instituted to avoid hemolysis.

PROFILES AND PANELS

Instead of ordering each chemistry test individually, the provider can order a group of tests known as a profile or panel. Multiple tests are included in a profile and can be performed on a small sample of blood. General chemistry profiles, such as those shown in Figure 28-5, includes tests that furnish the provider with a general overview of the patient's state of health.

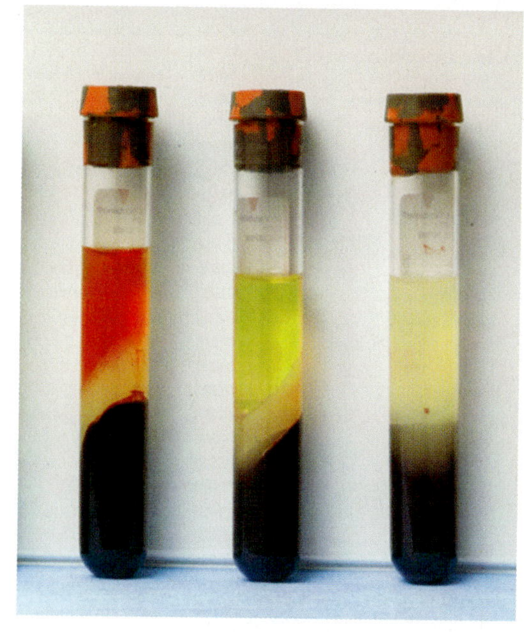

Figure 28-4 ■ Examples of both normal and abnormal appearances of serum (from left to right): (a) hemolyzed, (b) icteric, (c) lipemic.

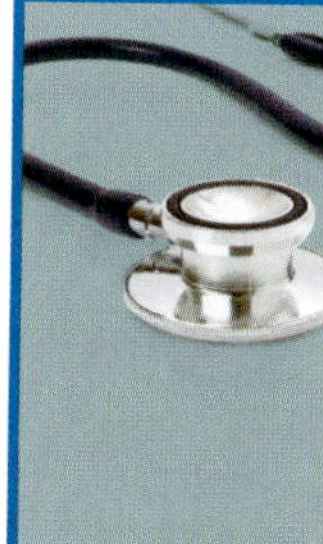

Field Smarts

In order to obtain the required amount of plasma or serum necessary for a particular test, you will need to draw at least 2.5 times that volume in blood. For example, a 10 mL tube of blood will yield approximately 4 mL of serum or plasma following centrifugation. So to figure out how many milliliters of blood you will need, just multiply the required volume of serum or plasma by 2.5 mL.

Table 28-1 Color/Appearance of Serum Specimens

Descriptive Term	Color/Appearance	Possible Cause
Hemolyzed	Pink/red	Collection error Processing error Hemolytic diseases
Lipemic	Milky or cloudy	Lipid metabolism disorders Non-fasting specimen
Icteric	Deep yellow to orange Green tint Pale/watery	Jaundice due to liver disease Obstructive jaundice Jaundice due to hemolytic anemia

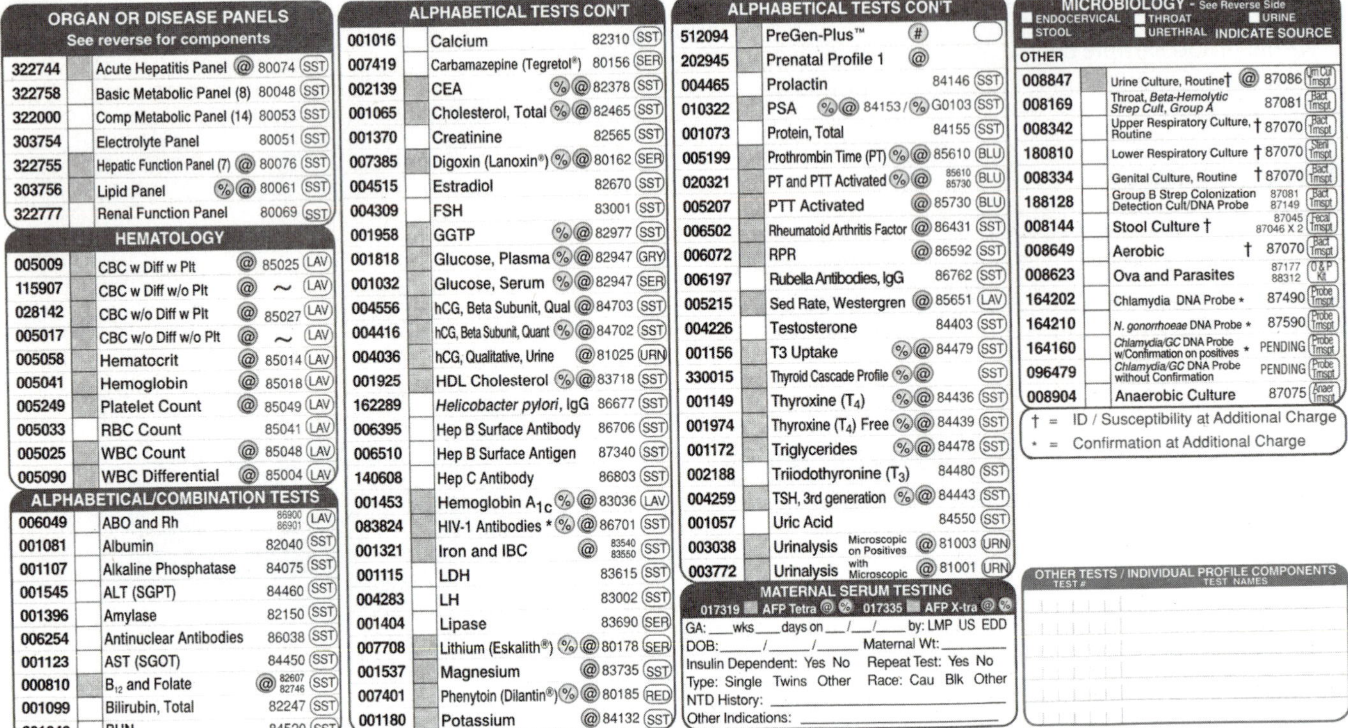

ORGAN OR DISEASE PANELS
See reverse for components

Code	Test		CPT	Tube
322744	Acute Hepatitis Panel	@	80074	SST
322758	Basic Metabolic Panel (8)		80048	SST
322000	Comp Metabolic Panel (14)		80053	SST
303754	Electrolyte Panel		80051	SST
322755	Hepatic Function Panel (7)	@	80076	SST
303756	Lipid Panel	% @	80061	SST
322777	Renal Function Panel		80069	SST

HEMATOLOGY

Code	Test		CPT	Tube
005009	CBC w Diff w Plt	@	85025	LAV
115907	CBC w Diff w/o Plt	@	~	LAV
028142	CBC w/o Diff w Plt	@	85027	LAV
005017	CBC w/o Diff w/o Plt	@	~	LAV
005058	Hematocrit	@	85014	LAV
005041	Hemoglobin	@	85018	LAV
005249	Platelet Count	@	85049	LAV
005033	RBC Count		85041	LAV
005025	WBC Count	@	85048	LAV
005090	WBC Differential	@	85004	LAV

ALPHABETICAL/COMBINATION TESTS

Code	Test		CPT	Tube
006049	ABO and Rh		86900 86901	LAV
001081	Albumin		82040	SST
001107	Alkaline Phosphatase		84075	SST
001545	ALT (SGPT)		84460	SST
001396	Amylase		82150	SST
006254	Antinuclear Antibodies		86038	SST
001123	AST (SGOT)		84450	SST
000810	B_{12} and Folate	@	82607 82746	SST
001099	Bilirubin, Total		82247	SST
001040	BUN		84520	SST

ALPHABETICAL TESTS CON'T

Code	Test		CPT	Tube
001016	Calcium		82310	SST
007419	Carbamazepine (Tegretol®)		80156	SER
002139	CEA	% @	82378	SST
001065	Cholesterol, Total	% @	82465	SST
001370	Creatinine		82565	SST
007385	Digoxin (Lanoxin®)	% @	80162	SER
004515	Estradiol		82670	SST
004309	FSH		83001	SST
001958	GGTP	% @	82977	SST
001818	Glucose, Plasma	% @	82947	GRY
001032	Glucose, Serum	% @	82947	SER
004556	hCG, Beta Subunit, Qual	@	84703	SST
004416	hCG, Beta Subunit, Quant	% @	84702	SST
004036	hCG, Qualitative, Urine	@	81025	URN
001925	HDL Cholesterol	% @	83718	SST
162289	*Helicobacter pylori*, IgG		86677	SST
006395	Hep B Surface Antibody		86706	SST
006510	Hep B Surface Antigen		87340	SST
140608	Hep C Antibody		86803	SST
001453	Hemoglobin A_{1c}	% @	83036	LAV
083824	HIV-1 Antibodies *	% @	86701	SST
001321	Iron and IBC	@	83540 83550	SST
001115	LDH		83615	SST
004283	LH		83002	SST
001404	Lipase		83690	SER
007708	Lithium (Eskalith®)	% @	80178	SER
001537	Magnesium	@	83735	SST
007401	Phenytoin (Dilantin®)	% @	80185	RED
001180	Potassium	@	84132	SST

ALPHABETICAL TESTS CON'T

Code	Test		CPT	Tube
512094	PreGen-Plus™	#		
202945	Prenatal Profile 1	@		
004465	Prolactin		84146	SST
010322	PSA	% @	84153 / G0103	SST
001073	Protein, Total		84155	SST
005199	Prothrombin Time (PT)	% @	85610	BLU
020321	PT and PTT Activated	% @	85610 85730	BLU
005207	PTT Activated	@	85730	BLU
006502	Rheumatoid Arthritis Factor	@	86431	SST
006072	RPR	@	86592	SST
006197	Rubella Antibodies, IgG		86762	SST
005215	Sed Rate, Westergren	@	85651	LAV
004226	Testosterone		84403	SST
001156	T3 Uptake	% @	84479	SST
330015	Thyroid Cascade Profile	% @		SST
001149	Thyroxine (T_4)	% @	84436	SST
001974	Thyroxine (T_4) Free	% @	84439	SST
001172	Triglycerides	% @	84478	SST
002188	Triiodothyronine (T_3)		84480	SST
004259	TSH, 3rd generation	% @	84443	SST
001057	Uric Acid		84550	SST
003038	Urinalysis Microscopic on Positives	@	81003	URN
003772	Urinalysis with Microscopic	@	81001	URN

MATERNAL SERUM TESTING
017319 ■ AFP Tetra @ % 017335 ■ AFP X-tra @ %
GA: ___wks___days on ___/___/___ by: LMP US EDD
DOB:______/______/______ Maternal Wt: ________
Insulin Dependent: Yes No Repeat Test: Yes No
Type: Single Twins Other Race: Cau Blk Other
NTD History: ______________
Other Indications: ______________

MICROBIOLOGY - See Reverse Side
■ ENDOCERVICAL ■ THROAT ■ URINE
■ STOOL ■ URETHRAL INDICATE SOURCE

OTHER

Code	Test		CPT	Tube
008847	Urine Culture, Routine†	@	87086	Urn Cul Trnspt
008169	Throat, *Beta-Hemolytic Strep Cult, Group A*		87081	Bact Trnspt
008342	Upper Respiratory Culture, Routine	†	87070	Bact Trnspt
180810	Lower Respiratory Culture	†	87070	Steri Trnspt
008334	Genital Culture, Routine	†	87070	Bact Trnspt
188128	Group B Strep Colonization Detection Cult/DNA Probe		87081 87149	Bact Trnspt
008144	Stool Culture †		87045 87046 X 2	Fecal Trnspt
008649	Aerobic	†	87070	Bact Trnspt
008623	Ova and Parasites		87177 88312	O & P Kit
164202	Chlamydia DNA Probe *		87490	Probe Trnspt
164210	*N. gonorrhoeae* DNA Probe *		87590	Probe Trnspt
164160	*Chlamydia/GC* DNA Probe w/Confirmation on positives *		PENDING	Probe Trnspt
096479	*Chlamydia/GC* DNA Probe without Confirmation		PENDING	Probe Trnspt
008904	Anaerobic Culture		87075	Anaer Trnspt

† = ID / Susceptibility at Additional Charge
* = Confirmation at Additional Charge

OTHER TESTS / INDIVIDUAL PROFILE COMPONENTS
TEST # TEST NAMES

Figure 28-5 ■ An example of a laboratory form listing different types of profiles.

CRITICAL THINKING CHALLENGE

A test calls for 7 mL of serum. You have 3, 6, and 10 mL tubes available.

1. How many total milliliters of blood will be necessary to obtain the proper amount of serum requested?
2. What color tube tops will you use to obtain the serum?
3. What combination of tube sizes will you draw to obtain the required amount of serum?

General chemistry profiles include the basic metabolic panel (BMP) or the comprehensive metabolic panel (CMP). The BMP comprises seven different tests that check items such as acid–base balance and calcium levels. The CMP is more comprehensive, as its name indicates, and is comprised of 14 tests—the seven included in the BMP, plus other tests that screen particular organ functions. Chemistry profiles may also be organ-specific, such as a renal or liver profiles. Providers often order these profiles during a physical to obtain a baseline; however, they are also ordered on patients with hypertension and other unknown causes of illness.

Hepatic (Liver) Profile

A hepatic profile can evaluate the general condition of the liver as well as assess a particular disease or disorder. Tests included in a hepatic profile will vary depending on which lab is used, but generally the following tests are included:

- Total and direct bilirubin: **Bilirubin** is a waste product of hemoglobin breakdown formed in the liver and excreted in bile. Total and direct bilirubin look at the different types of bilirubin found throughout the body. Knowing the percentages of each type assists the provider with diagnosing particular types of liver or gallbladder disease.
- Total protein: This test evaluates the level of albumin and globulin in the blood and the albumin/globulin ratio; decreased in liver disease.
- Alanine aminotransferase (ALT): Found in high concentrations in liver cells; increased in liver disease.
- Aspartate aminotransferase (AST): Found in cardiac muscle and liver cells; increased levels indicate cell damage.
- Lactate dehydrogenase (LDH): Found in almost all body tissues and released after tissue damage.
- Gamma-glutamyl transpeptidase (GGT): An enzyme found in the liver; increased in liver disease.
- Alkaline phosphatase (ALP): A liver enzyme; this test is performed to assist with the diagnosis of hepatic disease; also elevated in diseases of the bone in adults.

Table 28-2 Types of Diabetes

Classification	General Facts
Type 1 (previously known as insulin-dependent diabetes mellitus (IDDM) or juvenile-onset)	Usually diagnosed before age 25. Patients require insulin therapy.
Type 2 (previously known as non-insulin dependent diabetes mellitus (NIDDM) or adult onset diabetes)	Usually occurs after the age of 40 due to insulin resistance or a deficiency of insulin. Can be controlled with diet, exercise, and oral hypoglycemics. Patients occasionally need insulin therapy.
Gestational	A form of diabetes which begins during pregnancy, usually in the second or third trimester. It often subsides after delivery, but a third of women with this type of diabetes will eventually develop type 2 diabetes.

commonly seen in diabetes mellitus but may be seen in other diseases such as pancreatitis and hyperthyroidism. Refer to Table 28-2 for a description of the different types of diabetes.

Blood glucose levels can be measured by several different test methods, including the fasting blood sugar (FBS), the two-hour postprandial blood glucose (2HPP), and the oral glucose tolerance test (OGTT). Blood glucose determination is one of the most common chemistry tests performed in the laboratory. Patients can also monitor their blood glucose levels at home. Numerous models of handheld glucose monitors are available for use. Figure 28-7 is a photograph of a glucometer and glucose strips. Many of the newer monitors only require a tiny drop of blood for testing and may be obtained from the palm of the hand, upper arm, forearm, thigh, and calf instead of the fingertips. Procedure 28-1 outlines the steps involved in measuring a blood glucose level using a handheld monitor.

Fasting Blood Glucose Level

Since diet can affect the amount of glucose in the blood, screening levels are usually measured when a patient is fasting. To be in a fasting state, the patient must not eat or drink anything (except water) for 8 to 12 hours prior to testing. Some medications can affect the accuracy of test results. The physician should be consulted regarding medications prior to the delivery of fasting instructions. A fasting specimen is usually obtained in the morning so the patient will not need to go without food for a prolonged period of time. A fasting plasma glucose level of >126 mg/dL (usually confirmed on separate occasions) is indicative of diabetes mellitus.

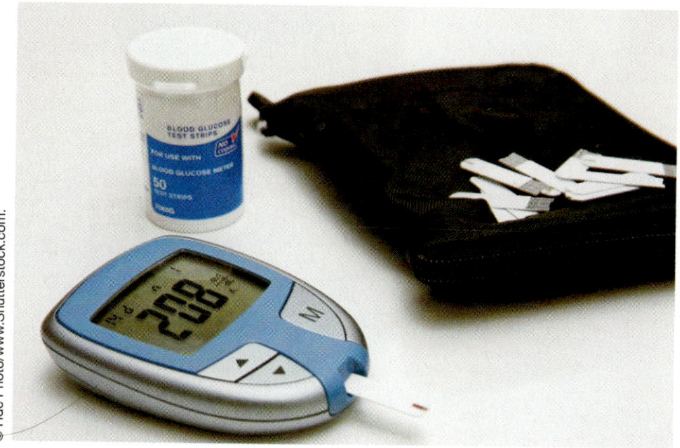

Figure 28-7 ■ An example of a blood glucose monitor and glucose strips.

Two-Hour Postprandial Blood Glucose Level

The two-hour postprandial (2HPP) blood glucose level may also be used to screen for diabetes mellitus and is also used to determine insulin dosage. A 2HPP glucose measures the blood glucose level two hours after the patient ingests a high-carbohydrate meal, or in place of the meal the patient may be asked to drink a glucose solution. The patient should be in a fasting state before the meal is ingested or the glucose liquid is consumed. Two hours following consumption of the meal or liquid glucose, the patient is asked to return to the office for the testing.

Many providers believe that the 2HPP glucose level is the most critical of all glucose tests. In a nondiabetic patient, the glucose level should return to normal within two hours. A level of 140mg/dL is indicative of impaired glucose tolerance.

Oral Glucose Tolerance Test (OGTT)

A glucose tolerance test may be requested following an elevated blood glucose result or 2HPP blood glucose result. During OGTT testing, a 75-gram load of glucose is given to the patient. Afterward, blood samples are collected from the patient at specified intervals. The glucose level of the blood is determined and recorded. A 2HPP glucose equal to 200 mg/dL or above is indicative of diabetes.

Whenever possible, the use of the oral glucose tolerance test is discouraged in favor of the fasting plasma glucose for practical reasons such as inconvenience to the patient and cost.

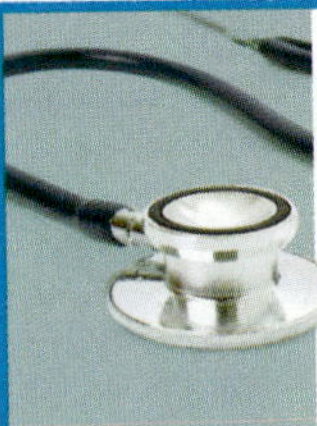

Field Smarts

The following are tips regarding the administration of a glucose supplement.

- You should never administer the glucose supplement until a fasting specimen is obtained and tested. If the fasting specimen is high, the provider should be alerted to determine if the glucose supplement should be administered.
- Chilling the glucose supplement before administering will make it easier to drink.
- The sugary glucose supplement may be hard to get down. Finding a flavor that the patient likes will aid in helping the patient to keep the glucose down once it has been ingested.
- If the patient vomits, the test will need to be stopped and the patient will need to be rescheduled for a new test.

For three days prior to testing, the patient is instructed to follow a normal to high carbohydrate diet. The patient is then instructed to fast for 10 hours prior to testing. Some providers will also ask the patient to refrain from smoking and strenuous activity during the fasting period and testing period, as these activities can also affect blood glucose level.

After collection of a fasting blood sample, the patient is given a maximum of 75 grams of liquid glucose. A blood sample may be collected 30 minutes, one hour, two hours, or three hours following the ingestion of the glucose drink. The patient may consume water during the test, but nothing else.

The patient may experience the normal side effects of weakness, perspiration, and feeling faint during the second or third hour of the test; this is typically the time period that the glucose bottoms out. Reassure the patient that this is normal and should pass. If the patient exhibits symptoms of severe hypoglycemia, the provider should be alerted immediately. The symptoms of hypoglycemia may include the following:

- Headache
- Senseless speech
- Irrational behavior
- Cold, clammy skin
- Paleness
- Profuse sweating
- Fainting

Translating OGTT Results

During an OGTT, a nondiabetic patient's glucose level will peak at around 160 to 180 mg/dL about 30 to 60 minutes after ingesting the glucose load, and will return to the fasting level two to three hours following consumption. A patient with diabetes will have glucose levels that peak at a higher level and remain elevated throughout the test. An OGTT is not necessary for diagnosing diabetes in patients with a fasting blood glucose greater than or equal to 126 mg/dL or a 2HPP glucose level greater than or equal to 200 mg/dL, usually confirmed on two different occasions.

Glycosylated Hemoglobin ($HbA1_c$)

Approximately 98% of normal adult hemoglobin is HbA. A subgroup known as $HbA1_c$ is formed when glucose and hemoglobin bind together. $HbA1_c$, or glycosylated hemoglobin, aids in determining how well blood glucose levels have been controlled over the past 8 to 12 weeks, because the life span of red blood cells (RBC) can be up to 120 days. The information gleaned from this test will tell the provider how diligent the diabetic patient has been about adhering to the prescribed diet and medication regimen, or the overall effectiveness of the treatment plan.

$HbA1_c$ testing can now be performed in the medical office using an analyzer like the DCA 2000+® by Bayer (Figure 28-8). This CLIA-waived analyzer utilizes a

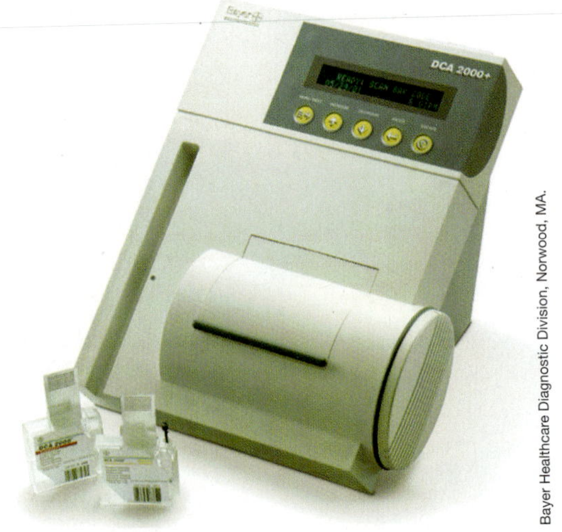

Bayer Healthcare Diagnostic Division, Norwood, MA.

Figure 28-8 ■ DCA 2000+ by Bayer, which performs a $HbA1_c$ within six minutes.

CRITICAL THINKING CHALLENGE

Mr. Brown's fasting blood glucose was in the normal range today; however, when his $HbA1_c$ results came back, they were highly elevated.

1. **List two different theories as to why the results may not match.**

simple three-step procedure and requires only a small sample of blood, with results available in six minutes. The DCA 2000+ can also provide a microalbumin/creatinine result in seven minutes, which helps to detect diabetic nephropathy in its early stages. This simple in-office testing furnishes the provider with fast results while the patient is still in the office. This allows the physician to make the appropriate adjustments in the patient's medication from the point of care.

ADDITIONAL CHEMISTRY TESTS

There are dozens of chemistry tests performed in the laboratory. Many tests were discussed in the profile section of this chapter. The medical assistant needs to have a basic knowledge of other tests as well, including the following:

- Magnesium (Mg): Magnesium is a mineral that is widely distributed in foods such as whole grains, fruits, and vegetables. It is found in soft tissue, bones, muscles, and body fluids. Increased levels are not common, but can occur in patients with chronic diarrhea or malabsorption disorders. Severe muscle spasms, weakness, and mental depression can result from decreased magnesium levels. Decreased blood pressure and bradycardia may occur with increased levels. Certain medications can interfere with magnesium results.
- Phosphorous: A nonmetallic element contained in bone and skeletal muscles. Levels are controlled by parathyroid hormone and calcium metabolism. Phosphorous contributes to acid–base balance, glucose and lipid metabolism, and osteogenesis. Increased levels are most often caused by renal failure, while decreased levels may be found in different disease states and with the administration of diuretics.
- Calcium (Ca): This is the most abundant mineral in the body. Ninety percent of calcium is found in the bones and teeth. It is essential to cellular fluid exchange, blood clotting, regulation of heartbeat, and bone formation. Increased levels are present in diseases such as metastatic cancer, multiple myeloma, and dehydration. Decreased levels can be found in patients with alcoholism, acute pancreatitis, and malnutrition.
- Alkaline phosphatases (ALPs): This is a group of enzymes found in the liver, gall bladder, intestines, and bones. This test is ordered to help with the diagnosis of hepatic and bone diseases. Increased levels are present in liver cancer, cirrhosis, biliary obstruction, and bone infections. Decreased levels may be present in malnutrition, congestive heart failure, and pernicious anemia.
- Amylase: An enzyme responsible for the breakdown of starches and sugars, produced primarily in the pancreas. Increased levels are seen in patients with pancreatitis, bile stones, or obstruction, and decreased levels may be found in patients with hepatitis, cirrhosis, and liver cancer.
- Lipase: This enzyme is responsible for fat digestion and the breakdown of triglycerides. It is secreted into the blood when there is damage to the pancreas. Levels can be increased in patients with acute pancreatitis and pancreatic cancer, acute cholecystitis, and early renal failure. Decreased levels can be found in patients with chronic pancreatitis, viral hepatitis, and cystic fibrosis.
- Carcinoembryonic antigen (CEA): A tumor marker present in certain types of cancer, such as colorectal cancer.
- Prostate-specific antigen (PSA): This marker determines the amount of an enzyme produced by the prostate gland and indicates possible prostate cancer. It can also be increased in patients with benign prostatic hypertrophy, prostatitis, and osteoporosis.

SEROLOGY AND IMMUNOLOGY TESTS

Tests performed under the heading of serology and immunology evaluate antigen–antibody reactions and the body's immune response. Analyses performed in this area include detecting the presence of antibodies to bacteria and viruses, discovering **antibody** production against one's own body (autoimmune), diagnosis of diseases like AIDS and infectious mononucleosis, and determining the presence of an antigenic substances (substances that stimulate an antibody response) such as the ABO antigens. Many rapid tests fall into this category.

Rapid Tests

Commercially prepared rapid test kits are available for use at home and in the medical office. Examples of rapid tests include a test to detect infectious mononucleosis and pregnancy.

Pregnancy Tests

Pregnancy testing may be performed in the medical office on urine. The presence of the hormone **human chorionic gonadotropin (hCG)**, released by the placenta, may be detectable in the patient's sample as early as one to five days after the first missed menstrual cycle. Many urine test kits are now available for home use. The rapid kit featured in this text is the QuickVue® by Quidel (Figure 28-9). This test is easy to perform and read, and results are ready within three minutes. Each test features a built-in control, as do most kits, to ensure test accuracy; however, external controls may also be used. Refer to Procedure 28-2 for an explanation of how to perform a urine pregnancy test. Many pregnancy test kits are available from different manufacturers.

Mono Test

Mononucleosis is a contagious disease caused by the Epstein-Barr virus. It is often passed through saliva during kissing or when drinking after another individual. Infectious mononucleosis develops most often in children and young adults 15 to 25 years of age. Symptoms often begin with a fever, swollen lymph nodes, and fatigue, and can last as long as two to four weeks.

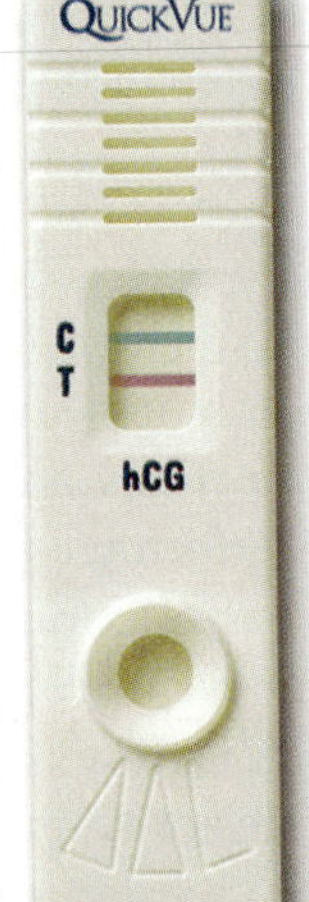

Courtesy of Quidel Corporation.

Figure 28-9 ■ QuickVue One-Step hCG test by Quidel.

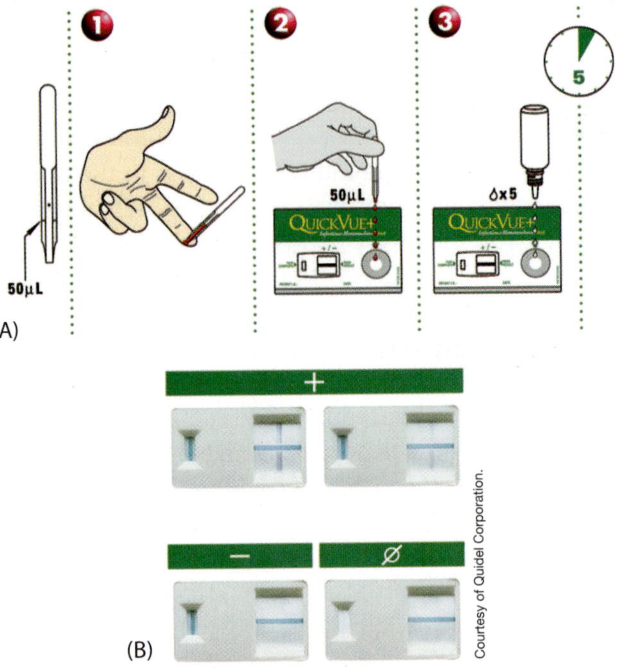

Courtesy of Quidel Corporation.

Figure 28-10 ■ (a) QuickVue+® Infectious Mononucleosis test; (b) The top reaction windows show two positive reactions; the bottom left shows a negative reaction; the bottom right shows an invalid test result.

The QuickVue+® Mononucleosis test by Quidel is one of several rapid tests available for use in the medical office (Figure 28-10). It is simple to perform and highly accurate. This test produces results in as little as three minutes. Some kits are not CLIA-waived because they require testing to be performed on serum or plasma. (Remember that in order for a test kit to be waived by CLIA, it has to be performed on whole blood.) Refer to Procedure 28-3 for instructions on performing a mono test.

Other Rapid Test Kits

New test kits are constantly being developed for use in the medical office and laboratory. Many of these rapid kits are CLIA-waived and testing can be performed by the medical assistant. Rapid results can give the physician an immediate diagnosis, and treatment can begin before the patient leaves the office.

Quidel has developed a rapid test for the detection of influenza (Figure 28-11). Flu symptoms are very vague and can mimic other types of viruses or infections, making it difficult to diagnose. Approximately one third of all respiratory infections are caused by influenza. By performing a rapid test, the physician can have results within 10 minutes and can begin treatment immediately.

Another rapid test kit is the QuickVue One-Step H. pylori Test®. This test detects the presence of the *Helicobacter pylori* bacteria, which is the most common cause of peptic ulcers. The provider can now test

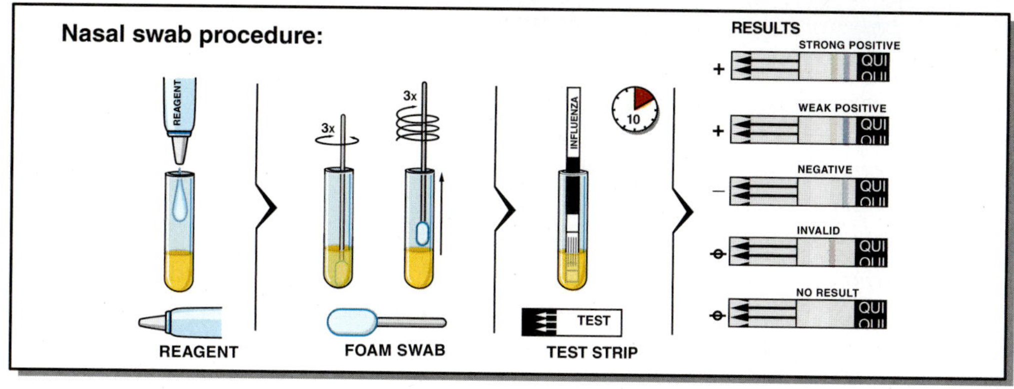

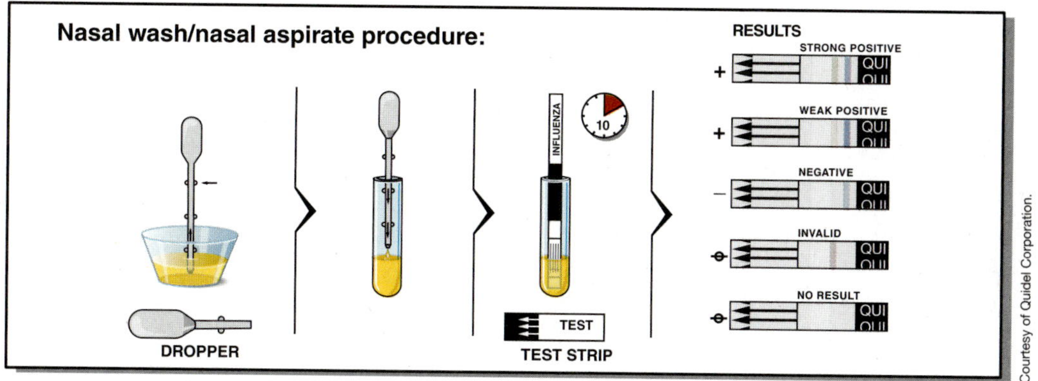

Figure 28-11 ■ CLIA-waived QuickVue® influenza test by Quidel.

patients in the office without the need for a more invasive procedure and a positive result can be obtained within 10 minutes from a simple finger stick. With quick in-house results, treatment can begin immediately.

Common Serology Tests

Common serology tests include the following:

- Venereal Disease Research Laboratory (VDRL) test or rapid plasma reagin (RPR): Screening tests for syphilis. A positive test requires further testing to confirm a diagnosis.
- HIV test: Determines the possible presence of the antibody to HIV virus, the virus that causes AIDS. A positive HIV test requires further testing to confirm that the patient has been exposed to HIV.
- C-Reactive Protein (CRP): Determines the presence of an abnormal protein that is released into the bloodstream as a result of tissue destruction and inflammation. The CRP is nonspecific, but may be increased in rheumatoid arthritis, bacterial infections, metastatic malignancies, and acute rheumatic fever. The CRP test may also be used to track the progression of a condition and its response to medications.
- Rheumatoid factor (RF or RA): The rheumatoid factor is an antibody present in the blood of individuals with rheumatoid arthritis, a chronic inflammatory arthritis that affects the joints. The RA test is an early diagnostic tool for rheumatoid arthritis and other autoimmune disorders that enables the physician to begin early treatment that can inhibit the progression of the disease.

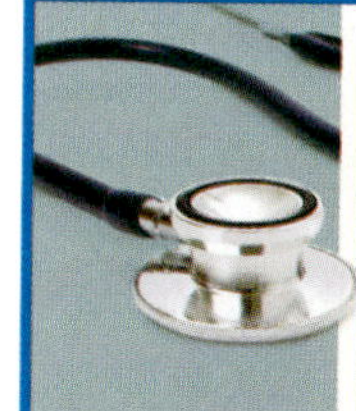

Field Smarts

Once your body produces an antibody to a particular antigen, you will always have antibodies stored in your bloodstream to fight that antigen. Therefore, patients who test positive for mononucleosis will continue to test positive during future testing. In order to determine if the patient has active mononucleosis, the patient will need to have a titer performed that will not only determine the presence of the antibody but the amount of antibodies present in the bloodstream.

Health Coach

H. Pylori

Research has determined that a large percentage of all peptic or stomach ulcers are caused by the bacteria *Helicobacter (H.) pylori*. A rapid *H. pylori* test can confirm this within minutes, enabling the physician to prescribe immediate treatment for the patient. Treatment is generally in the form of antibiotics instead of proton pump inhibitors or antacids that are typically used to treat ulcer symptoms. Once the bacteria is eliminated, the ulcer heals and there is no need for further treatment.

BLOOD TYPING

Every individual has what is known as an ABO and Rh blood type. The red blood cells have a specific protein or **antigen** attached to their surface that determines which ABO blood type an individual has. When typing blood, the antigen on the red blood cells reacts with an antibody in a test serum, causing a reaction known as **agglutination**. Agglutination occurs when the antibody in a typing serum attaches to the antigen on the red blood cells and causes a clumping reaction.

When typing a patient's blood, commercially prepared **antiserum** is mixed with whole blood and observed for agglutination. Anti-A antiserum contains the "A" antibody and Anti-B antiserum contains the "B" antibody. Figure 28-12 illustrates the different reactions that may occur during testing. For example, a patient's blood that is type A will demonstrate clumping when mixed with Anti-A typing serum because the antibodies in the test serum attach to the "A" antigens on the red blood cells and cause clumping. A patient with type B blood will react with Anti-B test serum. If the patient has type AB blood, then the patient's cells will clump when mixed with both Anti-A and Anti-B test serum. Since red cells in type O blood have no antigens, there will be no clumping reaction when type O blood is mixed with Anti-A or Anti-B test serum.

Blood typing plays a critical role when transfusing blood and blood products and when performing organ transplants. For example, a person with one type of blood will have antibodies against another blood type. If the incompatible blood type is transfused, the antibodies of the recipient will react with the antigens on the donor cells and destroy them, causing a life-threatening reaction to occur. ABO and Rh typing does not guarantee that a reaction will not take place. There are many subgroups that can cause mild reactions to occur.

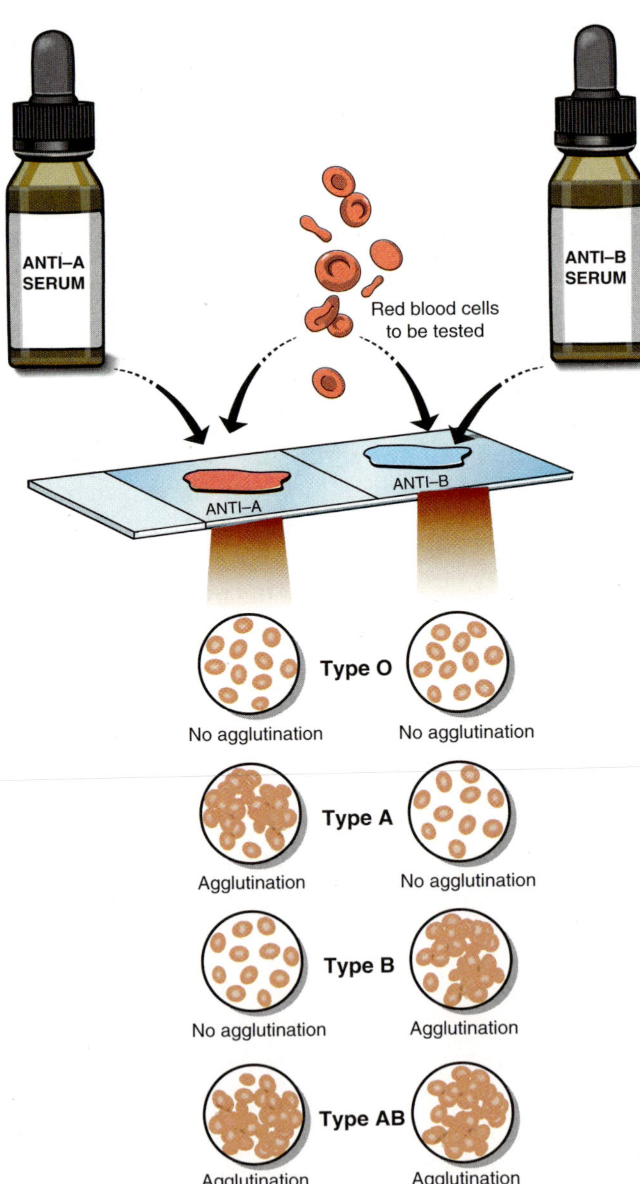

Figure 28-12 ■ Agglutination reactions that occur during ABO blood typing.

Table 28-3 Antigens and Antibodies of the ABO Blood Group

ABO Blood Type	Antigen Present on the RBCs	Antibody Present in the Plasma
Type A	"A"	Anti-B
Type B	"B"	Anti-A
Type AB	Both "A" and "B"	No ABO antibodies
Type O	Neither antigen is present	Both Anti-A and Anti-B

ABO Blood Typing

Two major antigens, A and B, can be present on the red blood cells. The presence or absence of these antigens determines an individual's ABO blood type. The four ABO blood types are A, B, AB, and O. If an individual has the "A" antigen on the red cells, the patient has type A blood; the "B" antigen, type B blood; both the "A" and "B" antigen, type AB blood; neither antigen, type O blood. Naturally occurring antibodies to the opposite type of blood are present in an individual at birth. For example, people who have the "A" antigen on their red blood cells have the "B" antibody in their plasma, and those with the "B" antigen have the "A" antibody. Table 28-3 further explains this process.

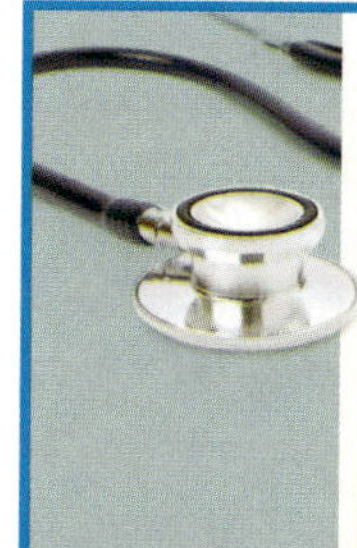

Field Smarts

Type O blood is known as the "universal donor" because the surface of the red cells does not have either of the A or B antigens that can react with the naturally occurring antibodies. Therefore, type O can be given to individuals with any type of blood. Type AB blood is known as the "universal recipient" because individuals with this type blood have no naturally occurring AB antibodies in their serum to react with the antigens on the transfused red cells. Therefore, individuals with type AB blood may receive any ABO blood type.

Rh Blood Typing

Another major blood type that must be considered in transfusions, organ transplants, and in pregnancy is the Rh blood group, named for the Rhesus monkey. A person either has the Rh antigen (Rh positive, Rh+) or does not (Rh negative, Rh–). Approximately 85% of North Americans are Rh positive. This typing is usually performed along with ABO typing using the test serum Anti-D.

While the ABO antibodies are naturally occurring, the Rh antibodies are not. Antibody production against the Rh factor must be stimulated. When an Rh negative person receives a transfusion of Rh positive blood, there will usually be no reaction with the first transfusion; however, antibodies to the Rh factor will begin to develop in about two weeks post-transfusion. A second transfusion of Rh positive blood can result in a life-threatening reaction.

During pregnancy, the Rh factor must be considered if the mother is Rh negative and the father is Rh positive. If the baby inherits the Rh factor from the father and has Rh positive blood, future pregnancies for the mother can be affected. The baby's red cells enter the mother's blood stream during delivery and the mother's body will recognize the cells as "foreign" and will begin to make antibodies against the Rh positive invader soon after delivery.

A medication known as RhoGAM is administered by injection to the mother at around 28 weeks gestation and again within 72 hours following delivery of the baby. This prevents her from forming antibodies that could develop if the baby she is carrying is Rh positive and will prevent any incompatibility problems with subsequent pregnancies. If the antibodies are allowed to form, they will attack future babies' blood cells and can cause a serious disease known as hemolytic disease of the newborn (HDN). Therefore, when collecting specimens for blood typing tests for prenatal screenings, it is essential that the identification of the patient and the sample be 100% correct. Mislabeling the sample will cause the reporting of incorrect blood type results and has the potential for serious harm.

DRUG TESTING

On-the-job drug use is becoming a growing problem in the workplace, accounting for increased absenteeism and on-the-job accidents. Many places of employment are developing a no-tolerance policy, and now require drug testing as a prerequisite for employment and also require random drug testing throughout employment. Employers may conduct drug testing at the following intervals:

- During preemployment testing
- When an incident or irrational behavior occurs on the job
- During random screenings

A blood sample is more precise when testing for the presence of drugs, but also quite costly and time consuming. Therefore, urine drug testing is usually performed. It is less costly, easier to perform, and non-invasive. Urine drug screenings test for the most commonly abused drugs such as:

- Marijuana
- Amphetamines
- PCP
- Cocaine
- Opiates
- Barbiturates
- Benzodiazepines

Initial testing is only a screening and a positive result must be confirmed with more precise tests.

Because some individuals fear the discovery of illegal substances in their drug screen, they may attempt to tamper with their specimen. Some people have even attempted to have a drug-free person provide the sample to avoid detection. Therefore, strict security measures must be followed to ensure the integrity of the specimen.

Alcohol and drug testing may also be performed immediately following a vehicular accident or during criminal investigations. This testing is normally performed in a hospital environment or special reference laboratory.

Chain of Custody

Steps must be taken to ensure the validity of a specimen for alcohol and drug testing. This procedure is known as the "chain of custody." A specific protocol must be followed during collection and handling of the specimen; if not, the chain is broken. Steps usually included in the chain of custody are the following:

1. Complete the chain of custody form provided by the lab or employer (Figure 28-13).
2. Identify the patient and check a photo ID.
3. Thoroughly explain the collection process to the patient and have the patient sign a consent form. The consent is sometimes part of the chain of custody form. The consent form explains the purpose of the test and gives the health care professional permission to collect and handle the specimen. Consent also gives permission to send the specimen for testing and to give the results to the requesting agency.
4. Explain to the patient that prescription and OTC drugs will be detected in the sample and instruct the patient to list all medications or substances taken within the last 30 days.
5. Instruct the patient to remove all outer clothing and empty pockets. Females must leave purses outside the collection area.
6. Ask the patient to wash and dry the hands prior to collecting the specimen. No water may be running during specimen collection.
7. Explain the collection process to the patient and supply the patient with a specimen container. Sometimes, the health care professional may need to witness the collection procedure (occurs most often in cases where a crime has been committed).
8. After collection, check the specimen for any signs of alteration such as unusual color or odor.
9. Measure the temperature of the urine within four minutes of collection. Variations in temperature could indicate tampering with the specimen.
10. Transfer the specimen to a transport container while the patient witnesses the transfer. Place an identification label on the container, and instruct the patient to initial the label.
11. Check the chain of custody form to ensure all information is complete.
12. Note the date and time of collection and sign and print your full name.
13. Give the patient a copy of the chain of custody form.
14. Seal the specimen in a leak-proof bag.
15. Give the specimen to the lab courier.

CHEMISTRY TESTS NORMAL VALUES

Table 28-4 lists common tests performed in the clinical chemistry lab and their normal values.

LAB REQUISITION AND TEST REPORT FORMS

As with any laboratory, each specimen should include a lab requisition form. When using paper charts, these are forms supplied by the laboratory. When using

USA LABS
ID#

Referred by

Health Care Provider
Address
Phone

DO NOT WRITE IN THIS AREA

CHAIN OF CUSTODY

STEP 1 — TO BE COMPLETED BY EMPLOYER/COLLECTOR.
DONOR IDENTIFICATION—PLEASE PRINT

LAST NAME

FIRST NAME M.I.

SOC. SEC. NO. ____ — ____ — ____

EMPLOYEE NO. ____

DONOR I.D. VERIFIED ☐ PHOTO I.D. ☐ EMPLOYER REPRESENTATIVE

SIGNATURE OF EMPLOYER REP.

REASON FOR TEST (CHECK ONE)
☐ (1) PRE-EMPLOYMENT ☐ (2) POST ACCIDENT ☐ (3) RANDOM
☐ (4) PERIODIC ☐ (5) REASONABLE SUSPICION/CAUSE
☐ (6) RETURN TO DUTY
☐ (99) OTHER (SPECIFY)

TESTS REQUESTED:

TOTAL TESTS ORDERED ☐

SPECIMEN ☐ Urine ☐ Blood (SUBMIT ONLY ONE SPECIMEN WITH EACH REQUISITION)

STEP 2—COLLECTOR, FOR URINE SPECIMENS, READ TEMPERATURE WITHIN FOUR MINUTES OF COLLECTION.
CHECK THE BOX IF TEMPERATURE IS WITHIN THE SPECIFIED RANGE ☐ 90°–100°F / 32°–38°C

OR RECORD ACTUAL TEMPERATURE HERE: ____

STEP 3—TO BE COMPLETED BY COLLECTOR.

COLLECTION SITE

COLLECTION DATE ____ TIME ____ ☐ AM PM

ADDRESS

REMARKS ____

CITY STATE ZIP

( )
PHONE

I certify that the specimen identified on this form is the specimen presented to me by the employee identified in Step 1 above, and was collected, labeled and sealed in the donor's presence.

COLLECTOR'S NAME PRINT (FIRST, M.I., LAST) SIGNATURE OF COLLECTOR

STEP 4—TO BE INITIATED BY THE DONOR AND COMPLETED AS NECESSARY THEREAFTER.

PURPOSE OF CHANGE	RELEASED BY SIGNATURE	RECEIVED BY SIGNATURE	DATE
A. PROVIDE SPECIMEN FOR TESTING			
B. SHIPMENT TO LABORATORY			
C.			

COMMENTS:

Self-stick identification
Labels for sealing specimen:

(123) (123) (123) (123)

SPECIMEN PACKAGE INTEGRITY WAS ☐ACCEPTABLE ☐UNACCEPTABLE WHEN RECEIVED IN LAB.

RECEIVER'S INITIALS

FOR OFFICE USE

Figure 28-13 ■ An example of a chain of custody form.

Table 28-4 Quick Reference for Common Chemistry and Waived Tests

Test Name	Test Abbreviation	Reference Range*	Clinical Significance
Albumin	ALB	3.0–5.0 g/dL	Liver, kidney, and nutritional status
Alkaline phosphatase	ALP	< 130 mU/L	Hepatobiliary and bone disease
Amylase	AMS	25–125 IU/L	Pancreatic disease
Bilirubin			
Total	TBil, Tbili, Bili	0.2–1.0 mg/dL	Liver disease and hemolytic anemia
Direct	DBil, Dbili	0.0–0.2 mg/dL	
Indirect	IBil, Ibili	<0.8 mg/dL	
Blood urea nitrogen	BUN	8–25 mg/dL	Kidney function
Calcium	Ca	8.5–10.5 mg/dL	Parathyroid disorders
Cancer detection			
Carcinoembryonic antigen	CEA	<2.5 ng/mL	Mainly used to monitor response to chemotherapy of colon cancer patients.
Prostate-specific antigen	PSA	< 4 ng/mL	Prostate cancer and prostate disorders
Creatine kinase	CK, CPK	< 130 U/L	Cardiac muscle, skeletal muscle, or brain damage
Creatinine	Creat	0.4–1.5 mg/dL	Renal function
C-Reactive protein	CRP	< 10 mg/L	Bacterial infections, acute rheumatic fever, SLE (systemic lupus erythematosus), active rheumatoid arthritis
Electrolytes	Analytes		
Sodium	Na	136–145 mEq/L	Diabetes insipidus, diarrhea, and dehydration
Potassium	K	3.5–5.0 mEq/L	Diuretic therapy, starvation, and liver disease
Chloride	Cl	96–110 mEq/L	Renal disease, CHF, anemia, dehydration
Gamma-glutamyl transpeptidase	GGT, GGTP	< 70 U/L	Pancreatitis and liver disorders
Glucose			
Fasting blood sugar	FBS	70–105 mg/dL	FBS and $HbA1_c$ help to diagnose and follow the management of diabetes.
Hemoglobin A1c or glycosylated hemoglobin	$HbA1_c$	4.5–6.5	Indicates blood glucose control over the previous three-month period
Lipids			
Total cholesterol	Chol	< 200 mg/dL	Coronary artery disease and also assesses the risk of developing coronary heart disease (CHD)
High-density lipoprotein	HDL (good)	> 40 mg/dL	
Low-density lipoprotein	LDL (bad)	< 100 mg/dL	
Triglycerides	Trig	< 150 mg/dL	
Magnesium	Mg, Mag	1.2–2.4 mEq/L	Malnutrition, diarrhea, pancreatitis
Phosphorous	P	2.5–4.5 mg/dL	Parathyroid, renal, and diabetic disorders
Total protein	TP, TPRO	6.0–8.0 g/dL	Dehydration, multiple myeloma, nephrotic syndrome, severe burns
Aspartate aminotransferase	AST	5–40 U/L	MI, muscular dystrophy, infectious mononucleosis, and liver disease
Alanine aminotransferase	ALT	7–56 U/L	Liver disorders, MI, and muscular dystrophy
Thyroid stimulating hormone	TSH	0.3–4.5 mU/L	Thyroid disorders
Uric acid	UA	Males: 3.5–7.2 mg/dL Females: 2.6–6.0 mg/dL	Renal failure, gout, leukemia, and lymphomas

*Unless otherwise noted, all reference ranges are for adults.
Note: Reference values were compiled from several different sources and can vary according to test methodology.

electronic health records, the medical assistant will create an electronic order (Figure 28-14). Once the order is created, a lab requisition order can be printed to include with the specimen (Figure 28-15).

An example of a test report form can be seen in Figure 28-16. It usually will include the test name, results, and reference ranges.

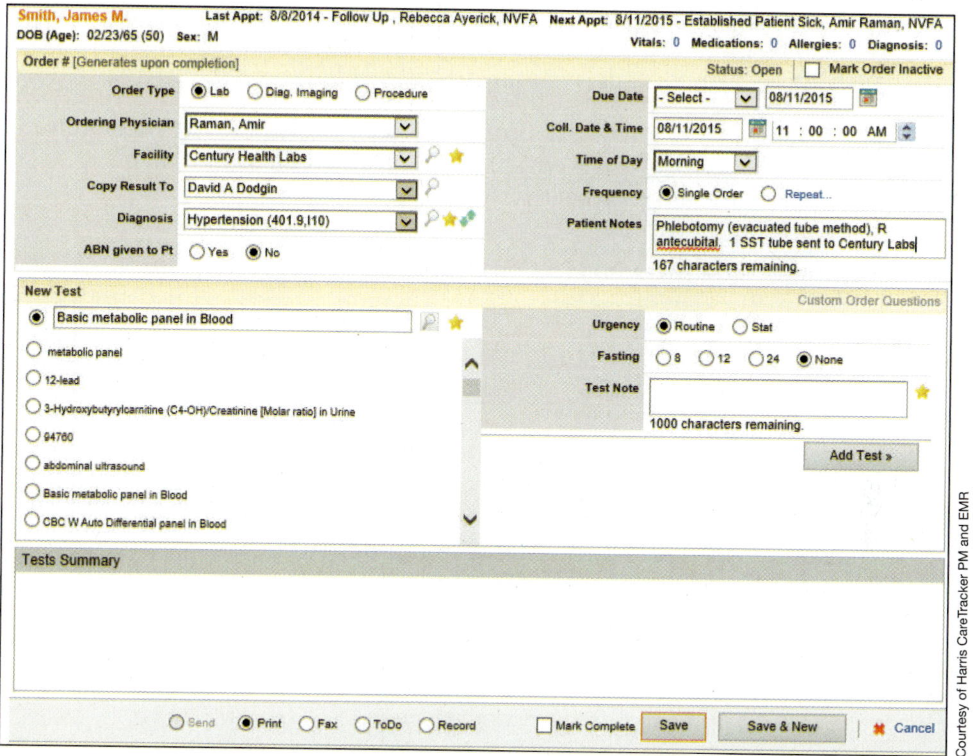

Courtesy of Harris CareTracker PM and EMR

Figure 28-14 ■ An example of a Lab Order Screen in Harris CareTracker.

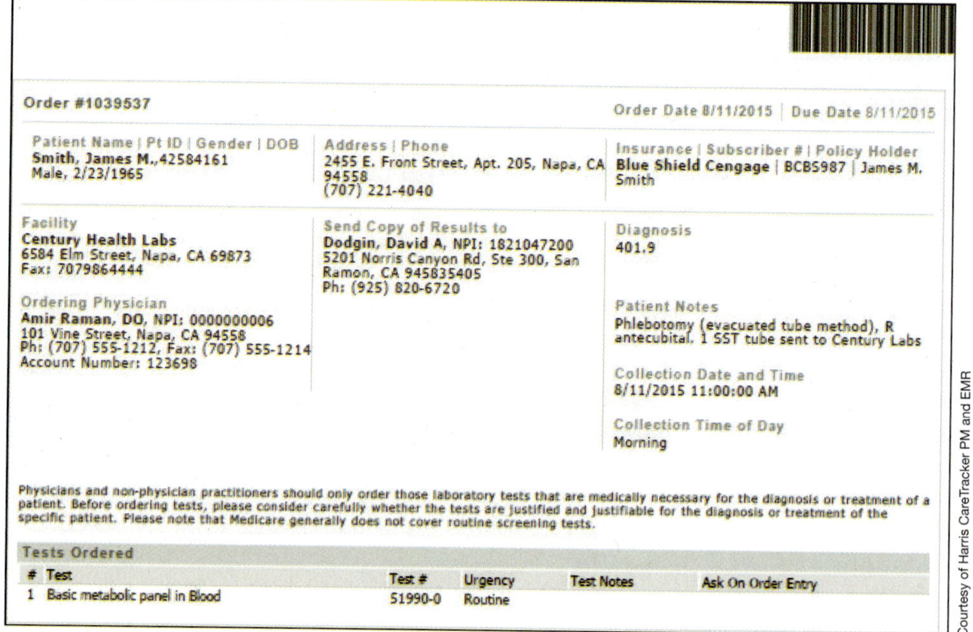

Order #1039537

Order Date 8/11/2015 | Due Date 8/11/2015

Patient Name | Pt ID | Gender | DOB
Smith, James M.,42584161
Male, 2/23/1965

Address | Phone
2455 E. Front Street, Apt. 205, Napa, CA 94558
(707) 221-4040

Insurance | Subscriber # | Policy Holder
Blue Shield Cengage | BCBS987 | James M. Smith

Facility
Century Health Labs
6584 Elm Street, Napa, CA 69873
Fax: 7079864444

Send Copy of Results to
Dodgin, David A, NPI: 1821047200
5201 Norris Canyon Rd, Ste 300, San Ramon, CA 945835405
Ph: (925) 820-6720

Diagnosis
401.9

Ordering Physician
Amir Raman, DO, NPI: 0000000006
101 Vine Street, Napa, CA 94558
Ph: (707) 555-1212, Fax: (707) 555-1214
Account Number: 123698

Patient Notes
Phlebotomy (evacuated tube method), R antecubital, 1 SST tube sent to Century Labs

Collection Date and Time
8/11/2015 11:00:00 AM

Collection Time of Day
Morning

Physicians and non-physician practitioners should only order those laboratory tests that are medically necessary for the diagnosis or treatment of a patient. Before ordering tests, please consider carefully whether the tests are justified and justifiable for the diagnosis or treatment of the specific patient. Please note that Medicare generally does not cover routine screening tests.

Tests Ordered

#	Test	Test #	Urgency	Test Notes	Ask On Order Entry
1	Basic metabolic panel in Blood	51990-0	Routine		

Courtesy of Harris CareTracker PM and EMR

Figure 28-15 ■ An electronic generated lab requisition form from the EHR.

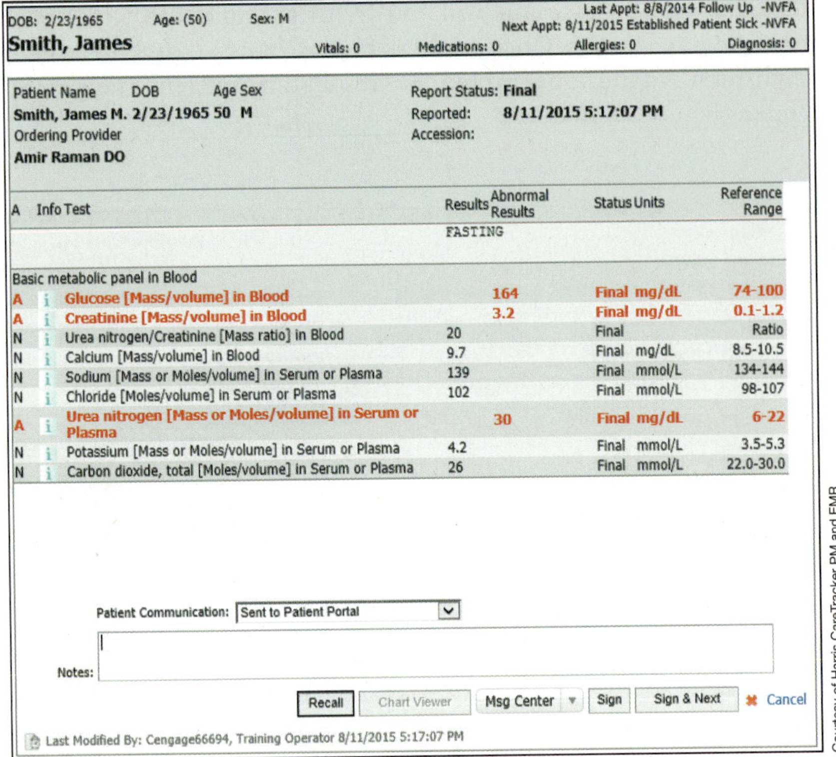

DOB: 2/23/1965 Age: (50) Sex: M
Last Appt: 8/8/2014 Follow Up -NVFA
Next Appt: 8/11/2015 Established Patient Sick -NVFA
Smith, James
Vitals: 0 Medications: 0 Allergies: 0 Diagnosis: 0

Patient Name DOB Age Sex
Smith, James M. 2/23/1965 50 M
Ordering Provider
Amir Raman DO

Report Status: **Final**
Reported: **8/11/2015 5:17:07 PM**
Accession:

A	Info	Test	Results	Abnormal Results	Status	Units	Reference Range
			FASTING				
		Basic metabolic panel in Blood					
A	i	Glucose [Mass/volume] in Blood		164	Final	mg/dL	74-100
A	i	Creatinine [Mass/volume] in Blood		3.2	Final	mg/dL	0.1-1.2
N	i	Urea nitrogen/Creatinine [Mass ratio] in Blood	20		Final		Ratio
N	i	Calcium [Mass/volume] in Blood	9.7		Final	mg/dL	8.5-10.5
N	i	Sodium [Mass or Moles/volume] in Serum or Plasma	139		Final	mmol/L	134-144
N	i	Chloride [Moles/volume] in Serum or Plasma	102		Final	mmol/L	98-107
A	i	Urea nitrogen [Mass or Moles/volume] in Serum or Plasma		30	Final	mg/dL	6-22
N	i	Potassium [Mass or Moles/volume] in Serum or Plasma	4.2		Final	mmol/L	3.5-5.3
N	i	Carbon dioxide, total [Moles/volume] in Serum or Plasma	26		Final	mmol/L	22.0-30.0

Patient Communication: Sent to Patient Portal

Notes:

Recall | Chart Viewer | Msg Center | Sign | Sign & Next | Cancel

Last Modified By: Cengage66694, Training Operator 8/11/2015 5:17:07 PM

Courtesy of Harris CareTracker PM and EMR

Figure 28-16 ■ An electronic chemistry report.

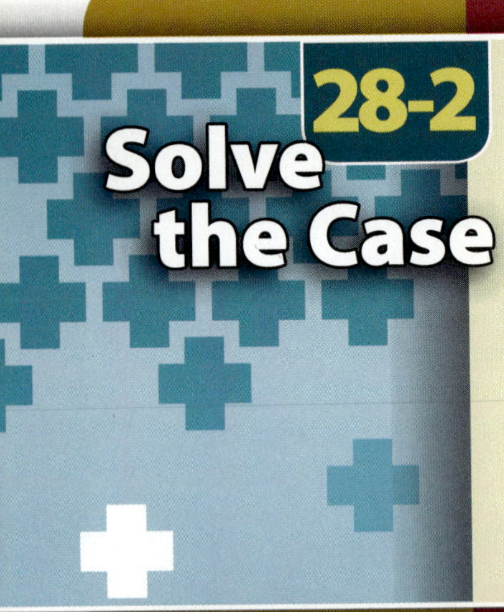

Dr. Dorado has completed his examination and has talked the patient into allowing you to weigh him. The doctor also requests the patient have a comprehensive metabolic panel and a thyroid panel. He sent an electronic prescription to the patient's pharmacy for lisinopril (antihypertensive) and he wants you to give educational materials to Mr. Wheeler for both hypertension and obesity.

1. **What color top tubes do you need to draw for the requested tests?**
2. **Go on the Internet and print off the educational materials the provider requested.**
3. **Practice going over the materials with a classmate. Keep in mind the patient's frame of mind. What professionalism keys will be necessary when educating Mr. Wheeler?**

PROCEDURE 28-1

Measure Blood Glucose Using a Handheld Monitor

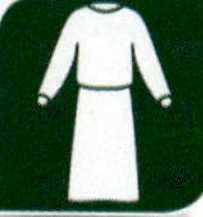

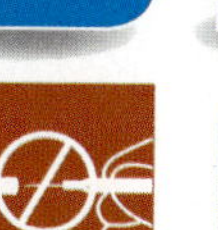

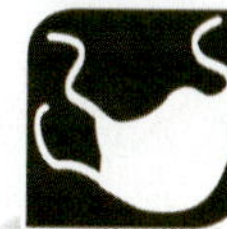

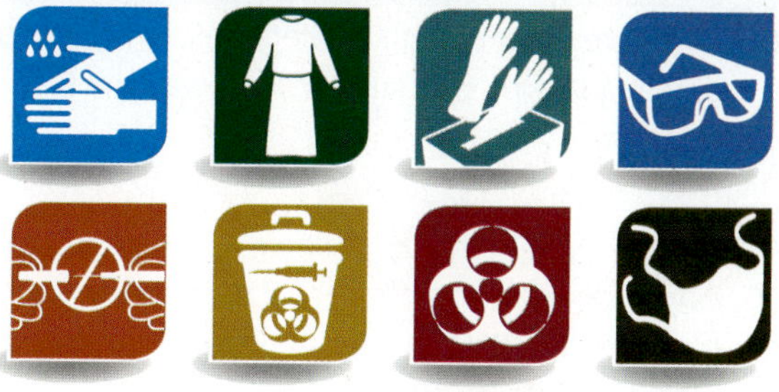

Objective:

To determine blood glucose levels at intervals requested by the provider to aid in the management of diabetes.

Equipment/Supplies:

- Gloves
- Personal protective equipment (PPE)
- Glucose monitor
- Glucose test strips/Code key
- Sterile lancet and lancing device
- Control solution
- Antiseptic wipe and gauze square
- Biohazard waste container/Trash receptacle
- Sharps container
- Patient's chart/EHR

PROCEDURAL STEPS	DETAILS AND/OR RATIONALE
1. ***Incorporating critical thinking skills when performing patient care***, check the provider's order, and assemble the equipment and supplies. Check the expiration date on the reagent strip and control containers.	Incorporation of critical thinking skills illustrates to the provider and patient that you are competent in your skill level and have the ability to think through problems when they arise. Expired strips can cause inaccurate test results.
2. Wash your hands and apply PPE.	PPE should always be worn whenever exposure to blood is possible for protection against splatters.
3. Calibrate the instrument and run a control sample according to the manufacturer's instructions.	Calibrating the instrument and running controls help to ensure that both the unit and strips are working properly.
4. Identify the patient using two identifiers and identify yourself. ***Explain the rationale for performance of the procedure, showing awareness of the patient's concerns related to the procedure being performed.*** Verify if the patient is fasting or not.	Using two identifiers assures you have the correct patient. Explaining the rationale for the procedure helps the patient understand why the procedure needs to be performed. Showing awareness of the patient's concerns demonstrates a caring attitude on the part of the medical assistant. Determining if the patient is fasting assists with interpretation of the results.
5. Ask the patient to wash and dry his hands.	Washing the hands with warm water reduces microorganisms and stimulates blood flow to the area.
6. Cleanse the puncture site with an antiseptic wipe, allowing the site to dry before puncturing.	Puncturing before allowing the antiseptic to dry may cause stinging and the wet alcohol could interfere with the results.
7. Turn the unit on and check to make certain that the code number on the monitor matches the code number on the reagent strip container (Figure 28-17).	If the codes do not match, accurate results cannot be guaranteed.
8. Wait until the blood drop icon appears on the monitor screen (this may vary in some units) and then puncture the site.	Placing the blood on the strip before the unit is ready may cause a malfunction to occur.

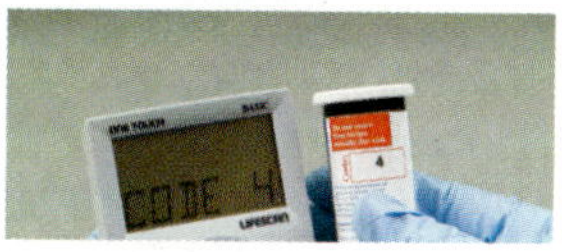

Figure 28-17 ■ The medical assistant inserts a test strip into the monitor and verifies that the code number on the bottle matches the code number on the meter.

continues

PROCEDURE 28-1 continued

PROCEDURAL STEPS	DETAILS AND/OR RATIONALE
9. Puncture the site with a safety device and dispose of it in a sharps container. Wipe away the first drop of blood.	Using the first drop of blood may produce an inaccurate reading because of the increase in tissue fluid.
10. Advance one edge of the test strip to the drop of blood and allow the strip to absorb the drop of blood (Figure 28-18).	Advancing the strip into the drop of blood rather than the patient's skin will produce a more accurate result.
11. Instruct the patient to apply pressure to the puncture site with a gauze pad.	Applying pressure helps to stop the bleeding and reduces bruising.
12. Wait for the reading to appear on the screen (Figure 28-19).	If the test did not read properly, an error code will appear instead of the results.
13. Remove the reagent strip from the monitor and dispose of properly. Throw bloody gauze square and other waste into trash receptacle following the office policy.	Every office has its own guidelines for the disposal of items that contain blood. According to OSHA, anything that isn't saturated with blood may go into the regular trash and anything saturated with blood should go into the biohazardous trash.
14. Remove gloves and wash your hands.	Cleansing the hands after removing gloves helps to reduce cross-contamination.
15. Document the test results in the patient's chart and the lab log if applicable.	Documenting in the patient's chart verifies that the procedure was performed. When using EHR, it is not necessary to document in a separate log because reports can be generated with log information.

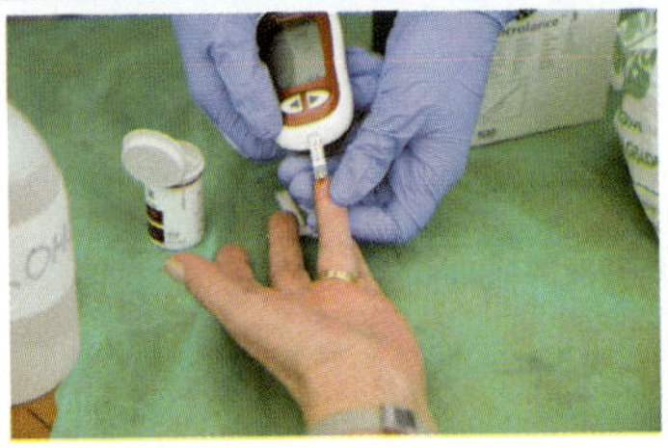

Figure 28-18 ■ The test strip is gently advanced to the drop of blood.

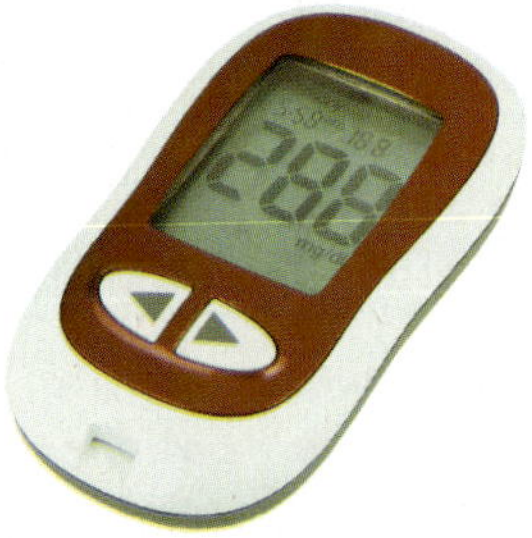

Figure 28-19 ■ The result is automatically displayed.

DOCUMENTATION EXAMPLE:

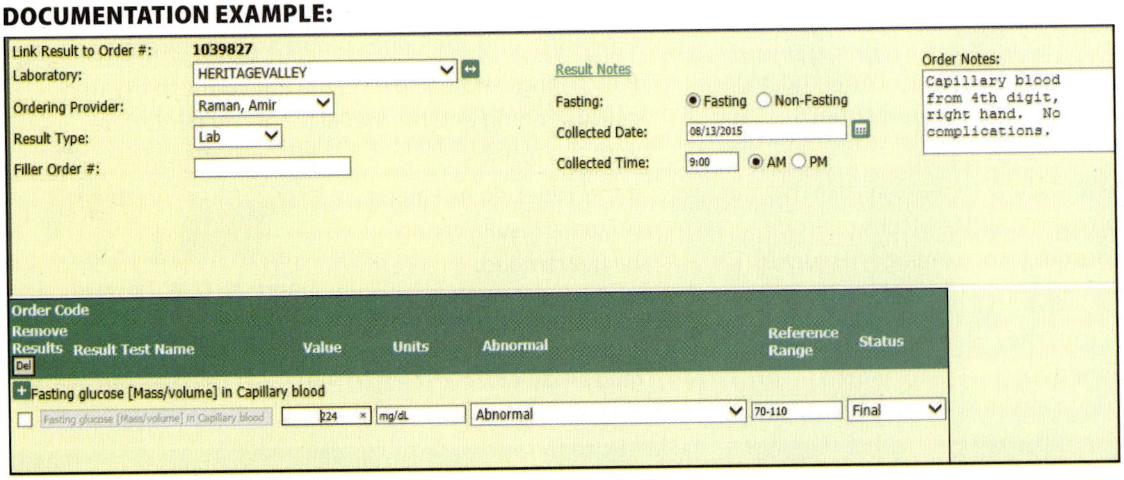

Link Result to Order #: 1039827
Laboratory: HERITAGEVALLEY
Ordering Provider: Raman, Amir
Result Type: Lab
Filler Order #:

Result Notes
Fasting: (•) Fasting ( ) Non-Fasting
Collected Date: 06/13/2015
Collected Time: 9:00 (•) AM ( ) PM

Order Notes:
Capillary blood from 4th digit, right hand. No complications.

Order Code Remove Results	Result Test Name	Value	Units	Abnormal	Reference Range	Status
Del						
+ Fasting glucose [Mass/volume] in Capillary blood						
☐	Fasting glucose [Mass/volume] in Capillary blood	224	mg/dL	Abnormal	70-110	Final

PROCEDURE 28-2

Perform a Urine Pregnancy Test

Objective:

To determine the presence of hCG in the urine, indicating pregnancy.

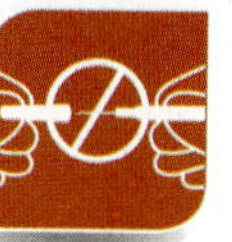

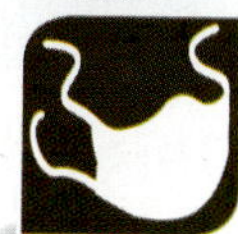

Equipment/Supplies:

- Gloves
- Personal protective equipment (PPE)
- Urine specimen
- QuickVue One-Step hCG urine test kit
- Timer
- Biohazard waste container
- Patient's chart/EHR

PROCEDURAL STEPS	DETAILS AND/OR RATIONALE
1. ***Incorporating critical thinking skills when performing patient care***, check the order and assemble the test kit, the patient urine sample, and all necessary supplies. Read the test kit directions.	Incorporation of critical thinking skills illustrates to the provider and patient that you are competent in your skill level and have the ability to think through problems when they arise. All test kits are different so reading the directions will ensure proper performance of the test.
2. Wash your hands and apply gloves and other required PPE.	PPE helps to prevent you from becoming contaminated from the patient's urine.
3. Perform a control.	A control confirms the kit is working properly.
4. Open the test unit, and using the dropper provided in the test kit, add the number of drops of urine recommended by the manufacturer to the test well (Figure 28-20).	The dropper from the kit must be used, because it is designed to deliver the precise amount of urine required for the test.
5. Allow the test to develop for precisely the recommended time. Set a timer for accurate timing of the test.	Accurate timing is crucial for accurate results.
6. Read the test window and determine if the results are positive or negative (Figure 28-21). Check for a line beside the control display.	If there is no line by the control, the unit may not be functioning properly.
7. Properly dispose of used equipment, test unit, and specimen.	
8. Remove gloves, wash your hands, and record results in the patient's chart and the appropriate logs if applicable.	Removing gloves and cleansing the hands before documenting in the patient's chart helps to prevent contamination. Documentation verifies the procedure was performed. Manual logs are not necessary when using EHR because logs can be automatically generated in the EHR.

Figure 28-20 ■ Add three drops of urine to the test well.

Courtesy of Quidel Corporation

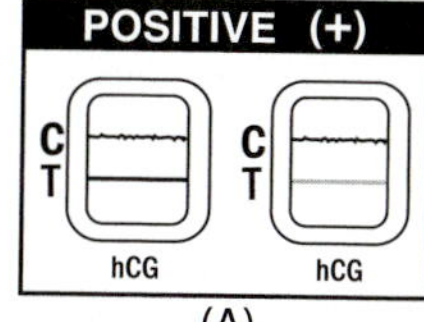

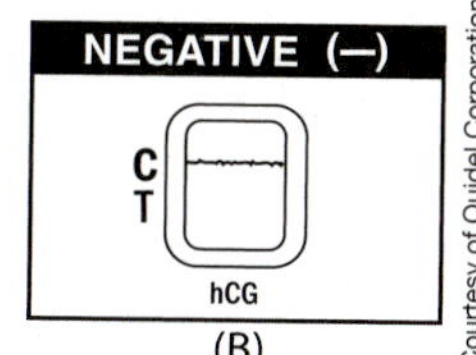

Figure 28-21 ■ (a) A positive result; (b) a negative result (note the control line).

Courtesy of Quidel Corporation

DOCUMENTATION EXAMPLE:

06-01-XX 11:30 a.m.	Performed QuickVue hCG test per Dr. Stevens, Result⊕Lot # 123456. Exp. 01/01/XX Melanie Maren, CMA (AAMA)----------

PROCEDURE 28-3

Perform a CLIA-Waived Mono Test

Objective:

To perform a CLIA-waived test to confirm or rule out a diagnosis of infectious mononucleosis.

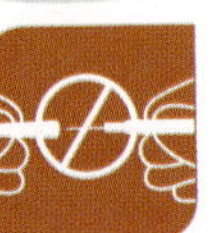

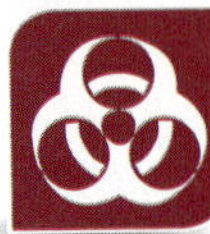

Equipment/Supplies:

- Patient specimen
- Control (if necessary)
- Gloves
- Personal protective equipment (PPE)
- Mono test kit
- Biohazard waste container
- Patient's chart/EHR

PROCEDURAL STEPS	DETAILS AND/OR RATIONALE
1. ***Incorporating critical thinking skills when performing patient care***, check the order and assemble the test kit, the patient sample, and all necessary supplies.	Incorporation of critical thinking skills illustrates to the provider and patient that you are competent in your skill level and have the ability to think through problems when they arise. Having the patient sample and all supplies readily accessible saves time.
2. Wash your hands and apply gloves and other required PPE.	PPE must be worn when working with any body fluids to prevent possible contamination.
3. Perform a finger puncture and then perform the test following the manufacturer's directions. Be sure to run a control along with the test.	Each test kit may differ slightly, so the manufacturer's directions must be read and followed exactly each time the test is performed. Running a control helps to ensure that the test kit is working properly.
4. Properly dispose of all equipment.	Proper disposal will help to eliminate cross-contamination.
5. Remove gloves and wash your hands.	Handwashing helps prevent cross-contamination.
6. Record the results in the laboratory log and also document the results in the patient's chart.	The results should be recorded in the log according to the facility's policies and also in the patient's chart so there will be a permanent record of the results.

DOCUMENTATION EXAMPLE:

10-10-XX 10:00 a.m.	Performed rapid mono test per Dr. Leonard, Result Positive, Manufacturer: Smith Diagnostics, Lot # 20937548900. Lillian Karnes, CMA (AAMA)----------

CHAPTER SUMMARY

- In a healthy body, specific mechanisms monitor and make adjustments to the internal environment to help maintain a constant state of balance known as homeostasis. Chemicals that help maintain homeostasis can be tested in different body fluids.
- Chemistry departments can test different chemicals in the blood to determine if there is a problem with homeostasis.
- Internal and external controls should be performed to make certain test kits and equipment are working properly.
- Serum is the liquid portion of the blood that remains after the blood has clotted. The usual color of serum is yellow but may be a different color in samples that are lipemic, icteric, or hemolyzed.
- In a lab setting, plasma is the liquid portion of the blood to which an anticoagulant has been added.
- Whole blood contains an anticoagulant and is not separated into components.
- Instead of ordering each chemistry test individually, the provider can order a group of tests known as a profile or panel.
- Instead of ordering each chemistry test individually, the provider can order a group of tests known as a profile or panel.
- Tests that check liver function include bilirubin, total protein, ALT, AST, LDH, GGT, and ALP.
- A renal panel tests kidney function. Tests that help to check kidney function include the following: Sodium, potassium, chloride, BUN, creatinine, and uric acid testing.
- Lipids are fats in the blood that contribute to coronary artery disease. A lipid panel may include the following: Total cholesterol, high-density lipoprotein (HDL), low-density lipoprotein (LDL), and triglycerides.
- Cardiac biomarkers include tests that help to determine if the patient has had a heart attack. Cardiac markers include the following: Troponin, creatinine kinase isoenzymes, and myoglobin.
- Glucose is the cell's preferred source of energy. High blood glucose is referred to as hyperglycemia. Low blood glucose is referred to as hypoglycemia.
- Type 1 diabetes was previously known as insulin-dependent diabetes mellitus (IDDM) and is frequently seen in patients under the age of 25. Type 2 diabetes was previously known as noninsulin-dependent diabetes (NIDDM) and is generally seen in patients over the age of 40.
- Tests that check blood glucose level include FBG, 2HPP, OGTT, and $HbA1_{c}$.
- Tests performed under the heading of serology and immunology evaluate antigen–antibody reactions and the body's immune response.
- Examples of rapid tests include a test to detect infectious mononucleosis and pregnancy.
- Human chorionic gonadotropin (hCG) is the hormone that helps to detect pregnancy.
- Common serology tests include VDRL, HIV CRP, and RA.
- Blood typing is a test that detects specific antigens present on the red blood cells. If you have A antigen, you have A blood type; if you have B antigen, you have B blood type; and if you have both A and B antigens present on the RBCs, you have AB blood type. If neither A nor B antigen is present on the red cell, you have O blood.
- Another factor to determine in blood typing is the Rh factor. Approximately 85% of North Americans are Rh positive. The Rh factor is very important to know during pregnancy.
- Chain of custody describes steps that must be taken to ensure the validity of a specimen for alcohol and drug testing.

CERTIFICATION REVIEW QUESTIONS

1. Which of the following tests screens for syphilis?
   a. VDRL
   b. HIV
   c. SYP
   d. STD

2. What is a blood glucose level of 50 mg/dL indicative of?
   a. Hyperglycemia
   b. Glycemia
   c. Glycogenemia
   d. Hypoglycemia

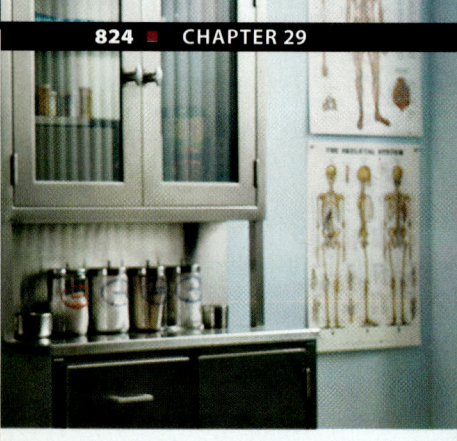

DEVELOPMENTAL OBJECTIVES

After completing this chapter, you should be able to:

1. Correctly spell and define essential terms.
2. Describe four patient positions used for radiographs.
3. Discuss the role of the medical assistant with regards to radiographic procedures.
4. List the risks associated with radiographs.
5. Explain safety precautions used by health care personnel and patients during X-rays.
6. Discuss patient preparation for various radiographic exams to include musculoskeletal, gastrointestinal, and urinary system exams.
7. Compare and contrast the different types of diagnostic radiographic procedures.
8. List the uses and side effects of radiation therapy.
9. Explain the advantages of sonography over radiograph (X-ray) during pregnancy.
10. Explain the role of molecular imaging and nuclear medicine in the diagnosis and management of disease.

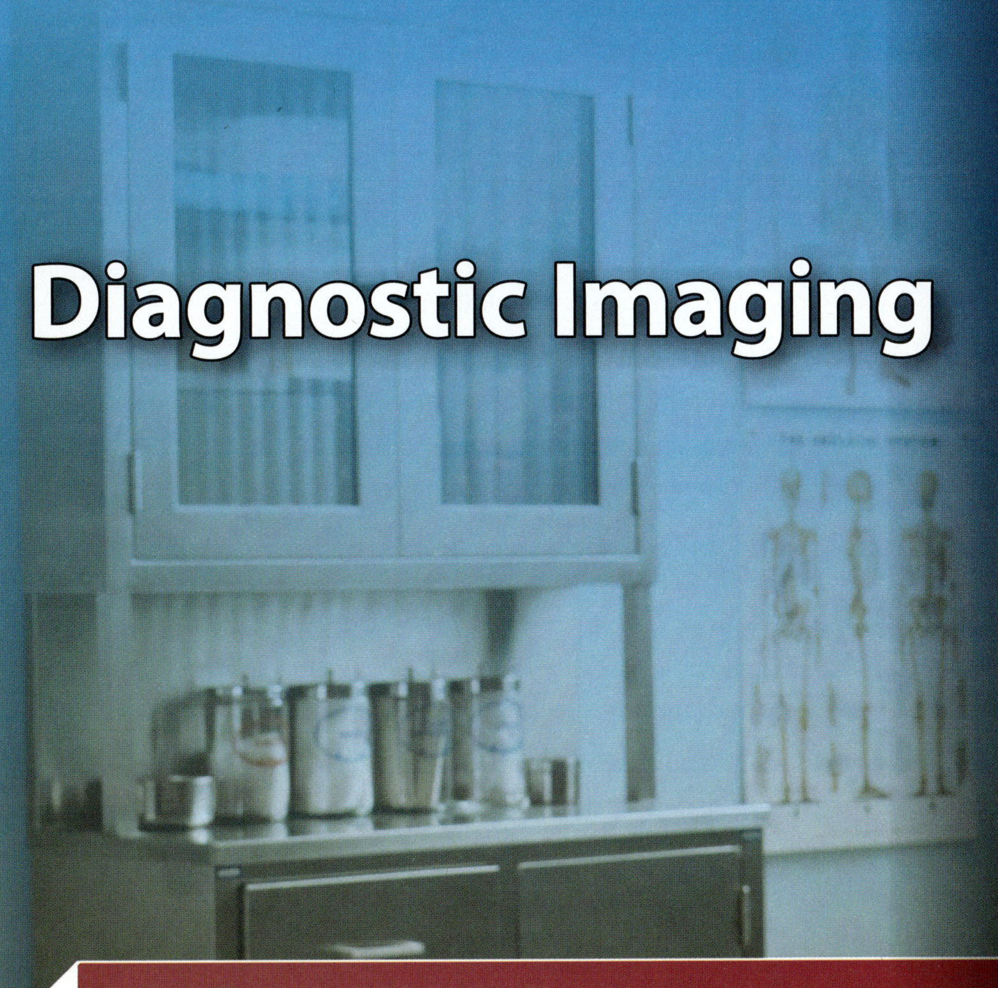

Diagnostic Imaging

29

ESSENTIAL TERMS

angiography
Bucky grid
cholangiography
collimator
computed tomography (CT)
contrast medium
endoscopic retrograde cholangiopancreatography (ERCP)
fluoroscopy
gray (Gy)
grid
magnetic resonance imaging (MRI)
molecular imaging
nuclear medicine
positron emission tomography (PET) scan
radiograph
radiologist
radiolucent
radiopaque
radiopharmaceuticals
scatter radiation
sievert (Sv)
sonogram
ultrasound
X-ray

CHAPTER OUTLINE

Radiology Overview

Legal Considerations for Diagnostic Imaging

Radiographic Equipment
- Digital Radiography

The Medical Assistant's Role in Radiographic Procedures
- Positioning the Patient

Common Types of Radiographs (X-rays) Performed in the Office

Processing and Displaying Radiographic Films

Storing and Disposing of Radiographic Films

Safety Precautions
- Personnel Safety Precautions
- Patient Safety Precautions

Scheduling Radiological Procedures Outside the Office
- Patient Preparation Instructions
- Explaining the Procedure

Radiological Procedures Commonly Performed Outside the Office

Other Diagnostic Imaging Procedures
- Computed Tomography (CT) Scan
- Magnetic Resonance Imaging (MRI)
- Ultrasound/Sonography

Molecular Imaging and Nuclear Medicine

Radiation Therapy

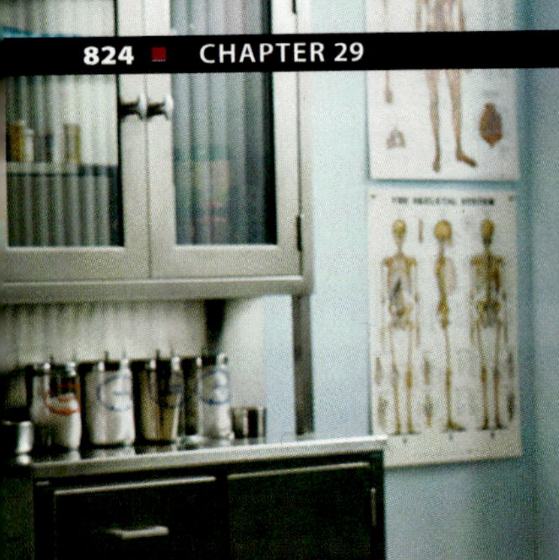

DEVELOPMENTAL OBJECTIVES

After completing this chapter, you should be able to:

1. Correctly spell and define essential terms.
2. Describe four patient positions used for radiographs.
3. Discuss the role of the medical assistant with regards to radiographic procedures.
4. List the risks associated with radiographs.
5. Explain safety precautions used by health care personnel and patients during X-rays.
6. Discuss patient preparation for various radiographic exams to include musculoskeletal, gastrointestinal, and urinary system exams.
7. Compare and contrast the different types of diagnostic radiographic procedures.
8. List the uses and side effects of radiation therapy.
9. Explain the advantages of sonography over radiograph (X-ray) during pregnancy.
10. Explain the role of molecular imaging and nuclear medicine in the diagnosis and management of disease.

CHAPTER SUMMARY

- In a healthy body, specific mechanisms monitor and make adjustments to the internal environment to help maintain a constant state of balance known as homeostasis. Chemicals that help maintain homeostasis can be tested in different body fluids.
- Chemistry departments can test different chemicals in the blood to determine if there is a problem with homeostasis.
- Internal and external controls should be performed to make certain test kits and equipment are working properly.
- Serum is the liquid portion of the blood that remains after the blood has clotted. The usual color of serum is yellow but may be a different color in samples that are lipemic, icteric, or hemolyzed.
- In a lab setting, plasma is the liquid portion of the blood to which an anticoagulant has been added.
- Whole blood contains an anticoagulant and is not separated into components.
- Instead of ordering each chemistry test individually, the provider can order a group of tests known as a profile or panel.
- Instead of ordering each chemistry test individually, the provider can order a group of tests known as a profile or panel.
- Tests that check liver function include bilirubin, total protein, ALT, AST, LDH, GGT, and ALP.
- A renal panel tests kidney function. Tests that help to check kidney function include the following: Sodium, potassium, chloride, BUN, creatinine, and uric acid testing.
- Lipids are fats in the blood that contribute to coronary artery disease. A lipid panel may include the following: Total cholesterol, high-density lipoprotein (HDL), low-density lipoprotein (LDL), and triglycerides.
- Cardiac biomarkers include tests that help to determine if the patient has had a heart attack. Cardiac markers include the following: Troponin, creatinine kinase isoenzymes, and myoglobin.
- Glucose is the cell's preferred source of energy. High blood glucose is referred to as hyperglycemia. Low blood glucose is referred to as hypoglycemia.
- Type 1 diabetes was previously known as insulin-dependent diabetes mellitus (IDDM) and is frequently seen in patients under the age of 25. Type 2 diabetes was previously known as noninsulin-dependent diabetes (NIDDM) and is generally seen in patients over the age of 40.
- Tests that check blood glucose level include FBG, 2HPP, OGTT, and $HbA1_c$.
- Tests performed under the heading of serology and immunology evaluate antigen–antibody reactions and the body's immune response.
- Examples of rapid tests include a test to detect infectious mononucleosis and pregnancy.
- Human chorionic gonadotropin (hCG) is the hormone that helps to detect pregnancy.
- Common serology tests include VDRL, HIV CRP, and RA.
- Blood typing is a test that detects specific antigens present on the red blood cells. If you have A antigen, you have A blood type; if you have B antigen, you have B blood type; and if you have both A and B antigens present on the RBCs, you have AB blood type. If neither A nor B antigen is present on the red cell, you have O blood.
- Another factor to determine in blood typing is the Rh factor. Approximately 85% of North Americans are Rh positive. The Rh factor is very important to know during pregnancy.
- Chain of custody describes steps that must be taken to ensure the validity of a specimen for alcohol and drug testing.

CERTIFICATION REVIEW QUESTIONS

1. Which of the following tests screens for syphilis?
   a. VDRL
   b. HIV
   c. SYP
   d. STD

2. What is a blood glucose level of 50 mg/dL indicative of?
   a. Hyperglycemia
   b. Glycemia
   c. Glycogenemia
   d. Hypoglycemia

3. The most likely way a patient contracts infectious mononucleosis is:
   a. sexual contact.
   b. contaminated food or water.
   c. vector.
   d. through contact with infected saliva.
4. A patient's blood tests negative with both Anti-A and Anti-B test serum, indicating which blood type?
   a. AB
   b. O
   c. A
   d. B
5. A pregnancy test determines the presence of:
   a. hCG.
   b. T3.
   c. TSH.
   d. FSH.
6. A high level of LDL cholesterol can put a patient at risk for developing:
   a. cancer.
   b. colitis.
   c. coronary artery disease.
   d. TIA.
7. Which of the following is a tumor marker for colorectal cancer?
   a. PSA
   b. ALP
   c. SGPT
   d. CEA
8. Which of the following tests is used as an indicator of blood glucose control?
   a. $HbA1_c$
   b. FBS
   c. OGTT
   d. 2HPP
9. Chemistry tests are usually performed on:
   a. serum.
   b. urine.
   c. stool.
   d. synovial fluid.
10. Blood specimens that are hemolyzed may be rejected by the lab. Hemolyzed specimens will have which of the following?
   a. Reddish tinge
   b. Whitish tinge
   c. Yellowish tinge
   d. Greenish tinge

STUDY RESOURCES

Resources to Test and Reinforce Your Knowledge:	
Certification Review Questions	Take this end-of-chapter quiz
Workbook	• Complete the activities for Chapter 28 • Perform the procedures for Chapter 28 using the Competency Checklists
Resources to Promote Critical Thinking:	
***Solve the Case* Activities**	• Consider these case studies and discuss your conclusions
Learning Lab	• Module 22: Laboratory Procedures
MindTap	• Complete Chapter 28 readings and activities

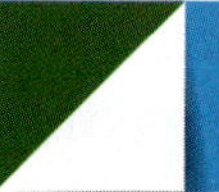

REFERENCES

American Diabetes Association. Standards of medical care in diabetes—2015. *Diabetes Care*. 2015; 38(suppl 1):S1-S93.

Association between Helicobacter pylori infection and duodenal ulcer. (n.d.). Retrieved August 12, 2015, from http://www.uptodate.com/contents/association-between-helicobacter-pylori-infection-and-duodenal-ulcer

Brain Natriuretic Peptide (BNP) Test. (n.d.). Retrieved August 12, 2015, from http://www.webmd.com/heart-disease/brain-natriuretic-peptide-bnp-test

Diabetes Mellitus (Type II). (n.d.). Retrieved August 12, 2015, from http://www.nmihi.com/d/niddm.htm

Peptic Ulcer Disease. (n.d.). Retrieved from http://www.niddk.nih.gov/health-information/health-topics/digestive-diseases/peptic-ulcer/Pages/overview.aspx

INTRODUCTION

Diagnostic imaging orders are often included in the "Plans" section of the progress note. Diagnostic imaging procedures may include radiography, sonography, CT scan, MRI scan, and nuclear medicine. The purpose of these procedures is to confirm a diagnosis or to rule out other possible causes related to the patient's symptoms. Radiological procedures may also be used for treatment purposes in particular types of malignancies. A **radiologist** is a physician who has received additional training in the use and interpretation of radiological examinations and is usually the medical specialist who oversees a hospital diagnostic imaging department or an outside imaging facility.

Some states allow medical assistants to perform certain radiographic procedures once they complete additional training and acquire a special X-ray license or certificate. Even if not permitted to perform X-rays, medical assistants should have a basic understanding of the different types of radiographic procedures that are commonly ordered and be familiar with preparation instructions for each one.

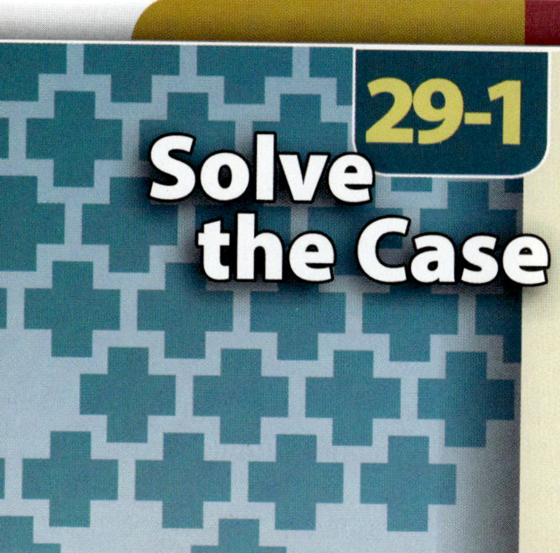

Enrique Monroy, a 46-year-old Hispanic male, comes to the family practice facility where you work. The patient has a productive cough of two weeks, a low-grade fever, and complains of chest pain when coughing. Sleep has been difficult. The English language is difficult for the patient. The provider has ordered a posterior-anterior (PA) and lateral chest radiograph on the patient.

1. **How will you describe the procedure to the patient?**
2. **What techniques can be used to enhance the communication process?**
3. **What must be considered when scheduling the patient's radiograph?**
4. **What might the radiograph show?**

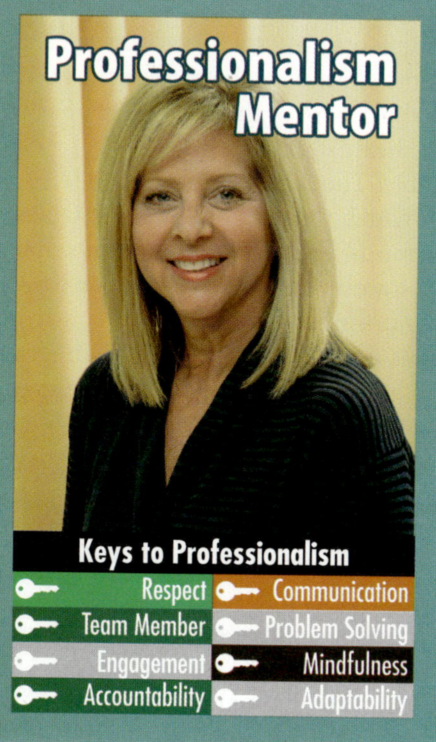

A new medical assistant in one of our surgical specialty clinics recently expressed that she never realized the variety of radiographic examinations available to patients. She admitted to feeling overwhelmed at times by all the specialized preparation required for each procedure. In addition to knowing general guidelines for these procedures, she also needed to be familiar with variances from one facility to another. I could see her frustration and offered to explain the different tests and why they are ordered. Diagnostic imaging is important for determining the presence of disease or injury. Providing the correct instructions for each test is vital to obtaining accurate results in an efficient time period. So, how do you become proficient in educating patients about these procedures? Start by learning all that you can while you are in school. Once you are in the field, collaborate with providers and staff members to build your knowledge. Make copies of each facility's preparation instructions and place them in a notebook for easy referencing at your workstation. Taking initiative to learn and share all you can about each procedure will result in greater compliance on the part of the patient and satisfaction in knowing that procedures won't have to be repeated due to poor preparation. ■

RADIOLOGY OVERVIEW

German physicist Wilhelm Roentgen (who received the Nobel Prize in 1901) is credited with discovering the **X-ray**. In 1895, while experimenting with electric current flow in a cathode-ray tube, he observed that a nearby piece of barium platinocyanide gave off light when the tube was in operation. He named his discovery "X-radiation," which has since been shortened to X-ray (commonly now referred to as radiograph). Further exploration found that the light could penetrate other materials, including human tissue, which permitted visualization of structures within the body without surgical intervention. The discovery of the X-ray proved to be a major step in the field of modern medicine.

In current medicine, X-rays (or **radiographs**) are the recorded image produced using X-radiation. Radiographic images represent various body parts in different shades of gray (black and white do not technically have shades), dependent on the mass of the tissue. Bones, being very dense, appear whiter on a radiograph. Muscles and organs take on gray hues, as they are less dense and can absorb more of the radiograph. If the beam passes through air, as occurs when passing through tissue within the lungs and parts of the colon, the rays appear as a darker shade of gray or black.

LEGAL CONSIDERATIONS FOR DIAGNOSTIC IMAGING

In many states, only a licensed radiologic technologist (or radiographer) may perform radiographs; however, some states allow individuals such as medical assistants the opportunity to obtain a limited license to perform certain radiographic procedures such as radiography of the chest, extremities, or spine. The individual will go through a short training class and sit for a special licensing exam that will allow the individual to take limited radiographs with particular types of equipment.

Many states allow individuals to obtain a limited radiography license (often referred to as a General X-ray Machine Operator [GXMO] license) to perform radiographs on the chest and extremities. Examples of states that presently allow limited radiography include California, Kentucky, Ohio, and Minnesota. Medical assistants interested in performing diagnostic imaging duties should check the licensing requirements in the states in which they work to determine if there is an opportunity to obtain a certificate or license. The American Registry of Radiologic Technologists is a resource that can aid in this process.

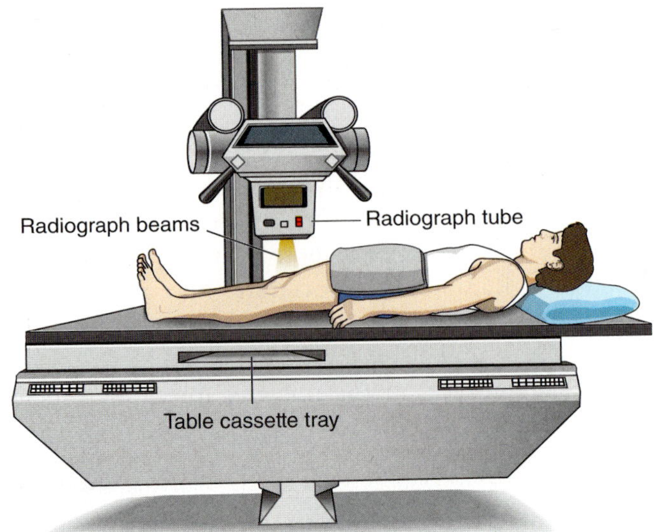

Figure 29-1 ■ An illustration of radiographic equipment used to take film radiographs.

RADIOGRAPHIC EQUIPMENT

Medical assistants who are licensed to perform radiography and work in offices that have radiographic equipment (Figure 29-1) should become familiar with the equipment and procedures that are used in each particular office. Radiographic equipment comprises the following components:

- Radiograph tube: The radiograph tube is the part of the equipment that emits radiation. The tube itself is encased in a protective covering in which different components are attached. These specialized components assist with the movement of the tube and the adjustment of the size and shape of the radiograph beam.
- Radiograph table: The table is the part of the equipment on which the patient lies. Most tables are adjustable for different positioning. The table may be raised, lowered, or tilted so that the patient is in a standing position.
- **Collimator**: This device, attached to the radiograph tube, controls the size and shape of the radiograph beam.
- Image Receptor: The image receptor is a frame that holds the film and two intensifying screens (Figure 29-2). The types in current use include: film/screen, computed radiography (CR), hardwired direct radiography (DR), tethered DR, and wireless DR.
- **Grid**: This component is placed below the radiograph table between the table and the image receptor to prevent the radiograph beam from scattering, which helps to produce a clearer image.

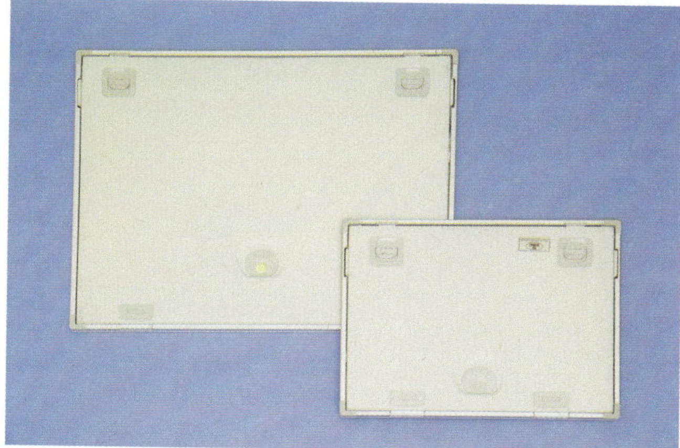

Figure 29-2 ■ The cassette, which houses the film, and the film together form the image receptor.

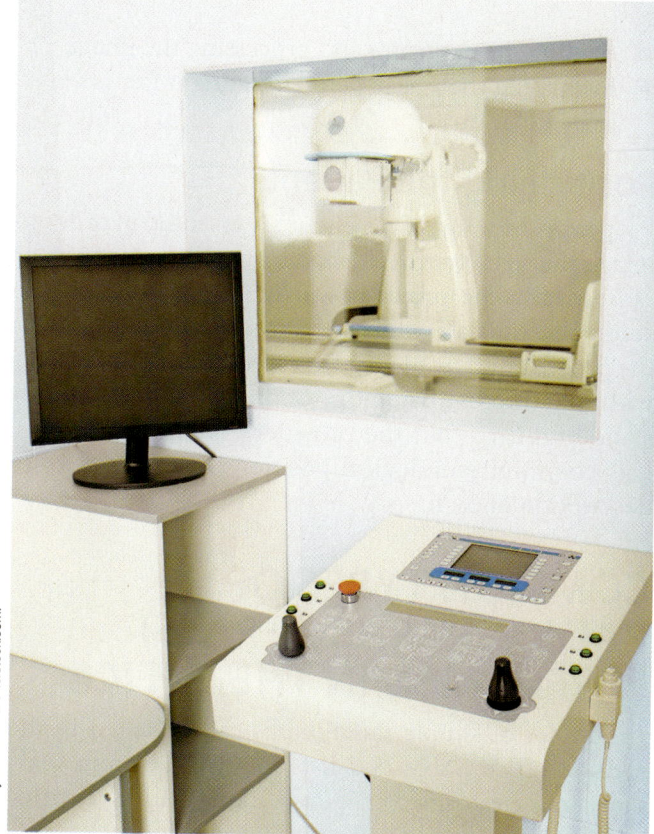

Figure 29-3 ■ The control panel of the radiograph unit is located in an enclosed area with lead walls to keep the medical assistant safe from scattering radiation.

- **Bucky**: The Bucky holds a cassette tray in which the Image Receptor is placed. During the radiograph, the Bucky moves the grid out of the way to prevent it from being visible on the Image Receptor.
- Control panel: The control panel is the part of the unit that controls the duration of the radiation being applied (Figure 29-3). When done appropriately, the image will be high quality and a low dose of radiation will be applied. The radiographer will determine the settings needed and stand either behind a lead shield or in an enclosed area with lead-lined walls while taking the radiograph (Figure 29-3).
- Radiograph processor: This unit develops the radiographic image.

Digital Radiography

As technology becomes more sophisticated, traditional film imaging is on the decline. Digital radiography provides better quality images and saves an enormous amount of space. There is no need for films and processors, and these images can be sent anywhere in the world in a matter of seconds, as long as the receiver has the technology to receive and view the images (Figure 29-4). The technology needed is simply a PC or tablet with Internet.

The advantages of digital images include the following:

- Reduced radiation exposure to the patient and operator due to fewer repeated images.
- Faster turnaround/processing/throughput.
- Ability to manipulate the image.
- Ability to copy, archive, and share the image with others for remote consultation using a Picture Archiving and Communication System (PACS).
- Minimal physical storage space. No longer need film processor, film processing darkroom, film storage, or film files.
- Reduced operating cost in terms of film purchase, processor chemistry, and maintenance.

Digital equipment is quite expensive for smaller clinics and provider's offices, but as prices continue to decline, more offices will move toward digital radiography.

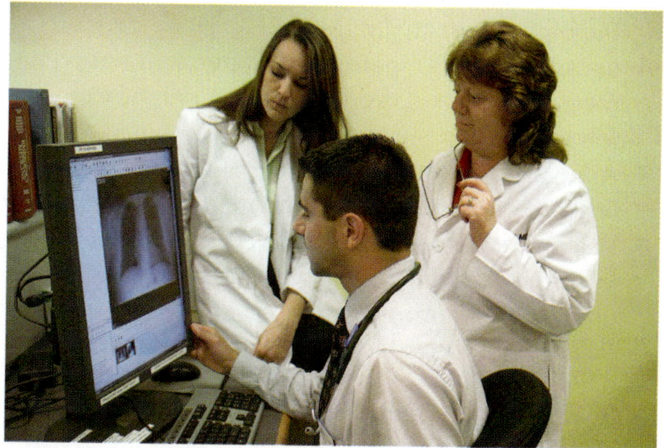

Figure 29-4 ■ The provider and other members of the health care team can view the very clear digital radiograph image by looking at the computer screen.

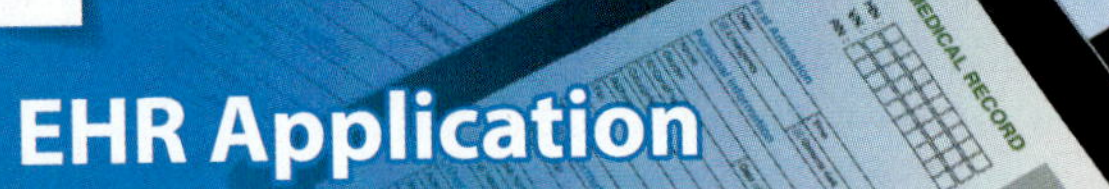

EHR Application

EHR makes viewing and storing digital radiographs very easy. When the radiograph is taken, the image is sent to the patient's EHR, where it is stored for future use. There is no longer a need for space to store the films. Images can be sent to other specialists at the click of a button. If the specialist doesn't have a compatible EHR, the medical assistant will make a CD of the image and send it with the patient.

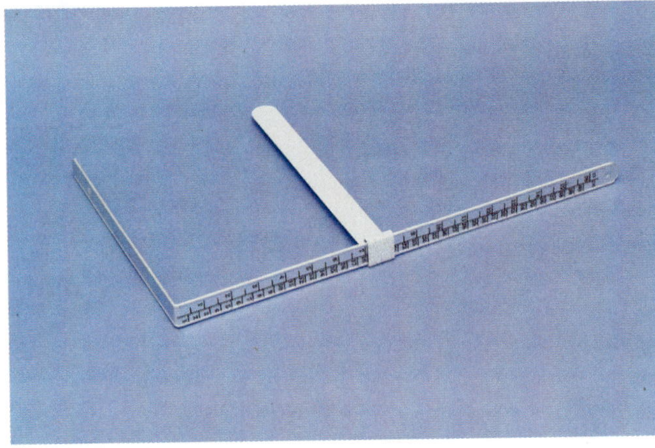

Figure 29-5 ■ A caliper that is used to measure parts of the body before taking a radiograph.

THE MEDICAL ASSISTANT'S ROLE IN RADIOGRAPHIC PROCEDURES

The medical assistant's role in taking radiographs will vary from office to office and from state to state. The following list explains the usual duties of the medical assistant who has been trained in performing radiographs and authorized to perform limited radiographic examinations:

- Explaining the procedure
- Ensuring that there is no risk of pregnancy for female patients before taking the radiograph
- Providing disrobing instructions for the patient and instructing the patient on what jewelry needs to be removed (any metals such as necklaces, earrings, rings, and so on, should be removed from the viewing area, or it will show up on the film)
- Preparing the Image Receptor: Ensure that the cassette has the patient's name, type of radiograph, date, and location of the radiograph, followed by positioning the film or image receptor to obtain the highest quality image
- Using a caliper (Figure 29-5) to perform body measurements on the surfaces that will be exposed to radiographs
- Adjusting the settings on the radiograph machine to match the patient's measurements
- Placing lead aprons or shields on the patient to limit the amount of radiograph exposure, especially to the reproductive organ area
- Positioning the patient so that the tube lines up with the cassette
- Adjusting the collimator so that the beam only includes the area to be viewed
- Instructing the patient regarding position and breathing during the exposure
- Making the exposure and processing the image
- Evaluating the image before sending it for interpretation

Positioning the Patient

Proper positioning of the patient is essential in order to image the right part of the body and to produce a clear radiograph. The provider will write an order for the study and indicate which position should be used for the procedure. The medical assistant should be familiar with the different patient positions in order to understand and carry out the provider's orders. Table 29-1 lists common radiological positions and gives a brief description of each.

COMMON TYPES OF RADIOGRAPHS (X-RAYS) PERFORMED IN THE OFFICE

A number of simple radiographs can be taken in the medical office. Table 29-2 lists some of the more common ones performed in-house, along with a description of the study and the positions used for each one.

CRITICAL THINKING CHALLENGE

A patient arrives for a radiograph of their forearm. On review of the order, the provider has requested PA, lateral, and oblique views of the right ulna and radius. The patient states that it is his left arm that hurts.

1. What should you do?

Table 29-1 Common Patient Positions for Radiographs

Position	Description
Anterioposterior (AP)	The radiograph beam is directed from the anterior surface to the posterior surface. If the patient is in a supine position, the radiograph tube will be directed toward the front of the patient's body and the patient's back will be positioned against the film. The radiograph beam travels from front to back. 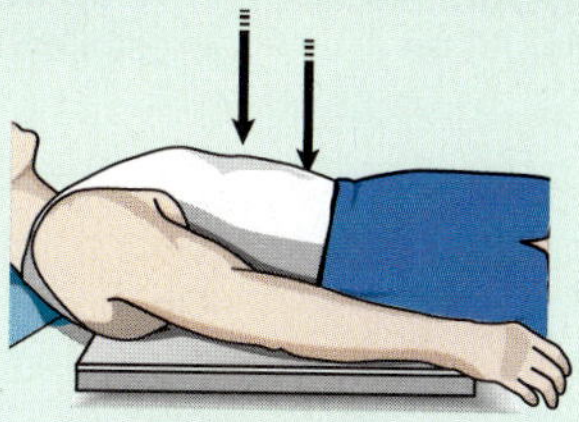
Posterioanterior (PA)	The radiograph beam is directed from the posterior surface to the anterior surface. If the patient is standing, the radiograph tube will be directed toward the patient's back and the front of the patient's body will be against the Image Receptor. The radiograph beam travels from back to front. In this image the beam is traveling from the back of the patient's hand to the front. 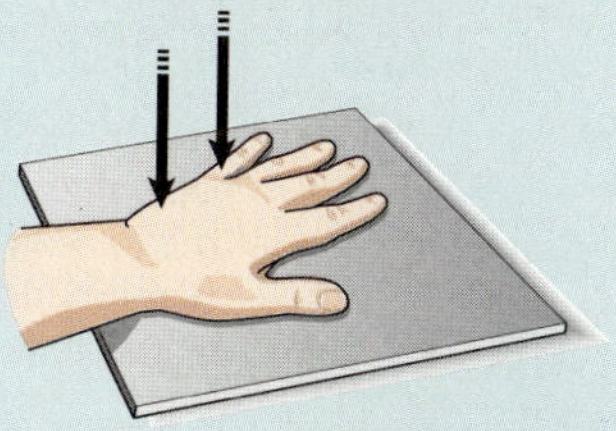
Lateral	This position can either be a right lateral or a left lateral. In a lateral position the direction (left or right) refers to the position of the patient in relation to the film, not the tube. The patient's right side is against the film in the right lateral position and the patient's left side is against the film in the left lateral position. 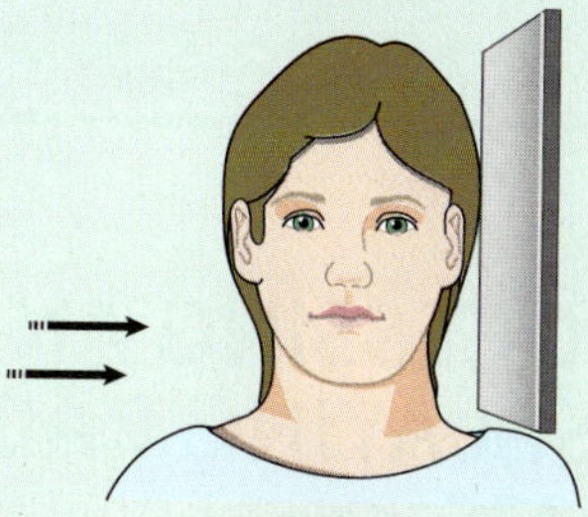
Oblique	The patient's body area is placed against the film at an angle. 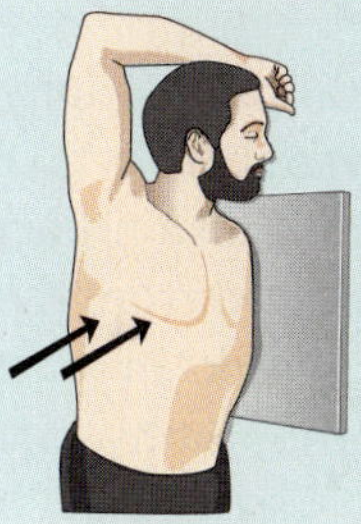
Erect	The patient is standing completely erect with the back surface of the body toward the film. 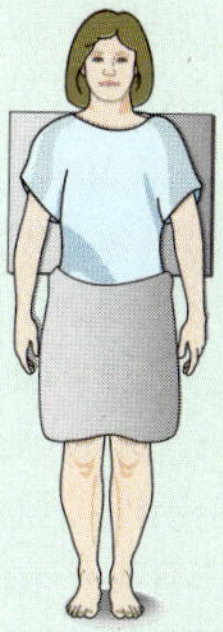
Supine	The patient lies flat on the back on the radiograph table. 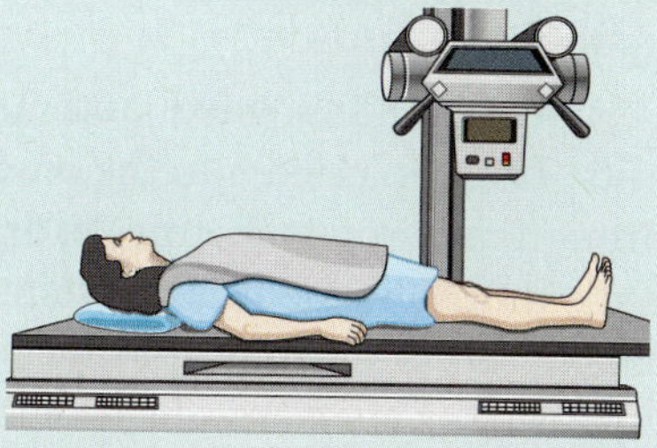

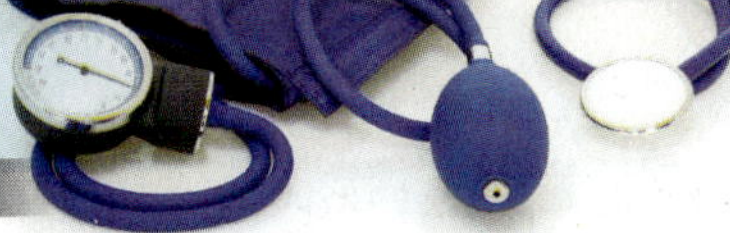

Table 29-2 Common Radiographs Performed in the Medical Office

Type of Radiograph	Routine Views	Description of the Procedure
Kidneys, ureters, and bladder (KUB)	AP (supine and erect view)	A supine film to view gas and stone patterns within the abdominal cavity. These patterns can assist in the diagnosis of kidney stones, gallstones, obstructed bowel, ileus, volvulus, and constipation.
Bone/skeletal	AP Lateral Oblique	Radiographs to view abnormalities or injuries associated with the bones (Figure 29-6). Spinal views are also part of this series and include: • Cervical views (neck region) • Thoracic views (middle back region) • Lumbar sacral (lower back region).
Chest	PA and Lateral Upright films allow the air fluid levels of infections to be visualized	Flat, upright films of the chest to view the lungs and heart for any abnormalities or lung disease such as pneumonia. This study can also detect an enlarged heart.
Sinus	PA The patient's face is against the film.	Radiograph of paranasal sinuses to detect signs of infection, inflammation, and other abnormalities.

Figure 29-6 ■ A radiographic image of a severe fracture of the femur.

PROCESSING AND DISPLAYING RADIOGRAPHIC FILMS

With digital radiography equipment, film is no longer necessary, so there is no need for darkrooms or processors. There is also no need for view boxes because the image is viewed from the computer screen.

If you work in a location that does not have digital radiography equipment, the following steps would be performed. Once the radiograph (term is interchangeable with X-ray) has been taken, the film must be developed to produce the image. Traditional radiographic films are developed in a darkroom, similar to those used to develop film from a camera. The medical assistant must avoid turning on overhead lighting or accidentally opening the door to the darkroom when working with radiograph film or it will become damaged. Radiograph film is very expensive, and because several films are contained in one case, the whole case may be ruined if light enters the room.

Many facilities have automated film-developing units. The film is fed into the processor, which moves it through the proper chemicals, dries it, and sends it out of the unit. The medical assistant should view the film and make certain that the image is clear, includes all regions requested, and that the identification information is correct before taking it out to the provider. Once the films are processed, the medical assistant will place the films in the view box.

STORING AND DISPOSING OF RADIOGRAPHIC FILMS

With digital radiography, films are no longer necessary. However, if the office you work in has not yet converted to digital equipment, proper storage and handling of radiograph film is crucial. Film can be damaged by light, moisture, heat, or exposure to chemicals. Unexposed films should be stored in a special metal drawer or cabinet located within a darkroom. Exposed films, such as patient radiographs, should be stored in envelopes made for that purpose (Figure 29-7) and should be filed in an appropriate area.

The length of time that patient radiographs have to be kept will vary according to individual state statutes

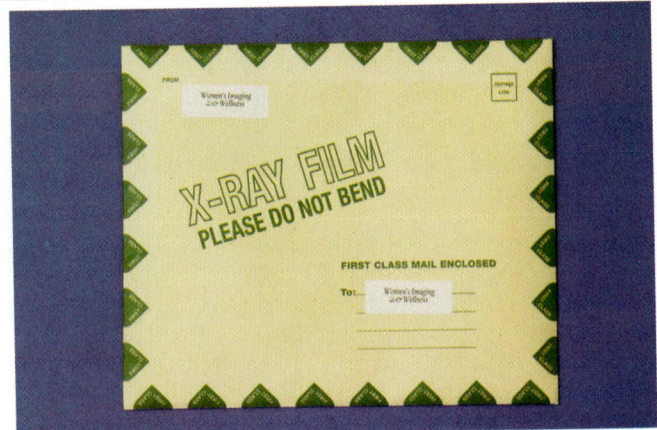

Figure 29-7 ■ Special envelopes designed for storage of radiographic films.

and provider preference, but will usually range from five to seven years. Once this time has passed, the radiographs can be disposed of using proper disposal techniques. Radiograph recycling companies will come to offices and remove outdated films, shred the films, and recycle the films for precious metals. The film is weighed, and the office may receive a fee for the silver extracted from the film.

SAFETY PRECAUTIONS

Individuals can be exposed to radiation when in close proximity to the area where radiographs are performed. Long-term exposure to low-level radiation can increase the risk of certain cancers later in life. There is also the risk of genetic effects that may affect future generations. Because these effects are subtle, it is imperative to practice ALARA—keep the radiation exposure "As Low As Reasonably Achievable." Safety Precautions should also include the following:

- No holding patients during an exposure.
- If in the room during an exposure, wear protective lead material.
- Stand behind the protective barrier when exposures are made.
- Make sure the equipment is in good working order, regularly inspected.
- Avoid any unnecessary radiation exposure and especially repeat radiographic exposures by making sure the first exposure is correct.

Exposure to high levels of radiation can lead to tissue damage, a lowered red blood and white blood cell count, bone marrow damage, damage to the ovaries and testes, fetal damage, cancer, and burns. Steps must be taken to protect both the health care worker and the patient from overexposure to radiation.

The amount of radiation emission is measured in several different ways. The **gray (Gy)** is a measurement of radiation energy per kilogram and is interchangeable with **sievert (Sv)**, as they both are International System of Units (SI). Radiation can also be found in the environment from facilities such as medical testing and treatment sites and nuclear weapons sites. Ionizing radiation can also come from the sun or radioactive natural sources such as radon. We often compare the dose of a chest radiograph to air travel from New York to California while a comparable dose of radiation from a chest CT would be the amount a commercial pilot receives in a year.

Personnel Safety Precautions

During a radiograph, the radiation that strikes the patient is known as "primary" radiation. **Scatter radiation** is emitted from the patient in all directions, which is considered "secondary" radiation. Another source of secondary radiation is leakage from the radiograph tube housing. It is the secondary radiation that health care workers must protect themselves from. When the patient becomes a source of scatter radiation, the barrier is only effective if placed between the operator and the patient. In other words, don't turn your back to the patient while wearing a lead apron that only covers the front. Barriers must be used to prevent absorption of the scatter radiation to other individuals outside of the room and to individuals undergoing a radiographic study.

An effective barrier to secondary radiation is lead. Lead aprons (Figure 29-8), thyroid guards, and gloves should be worn by the medical assistant if the medical

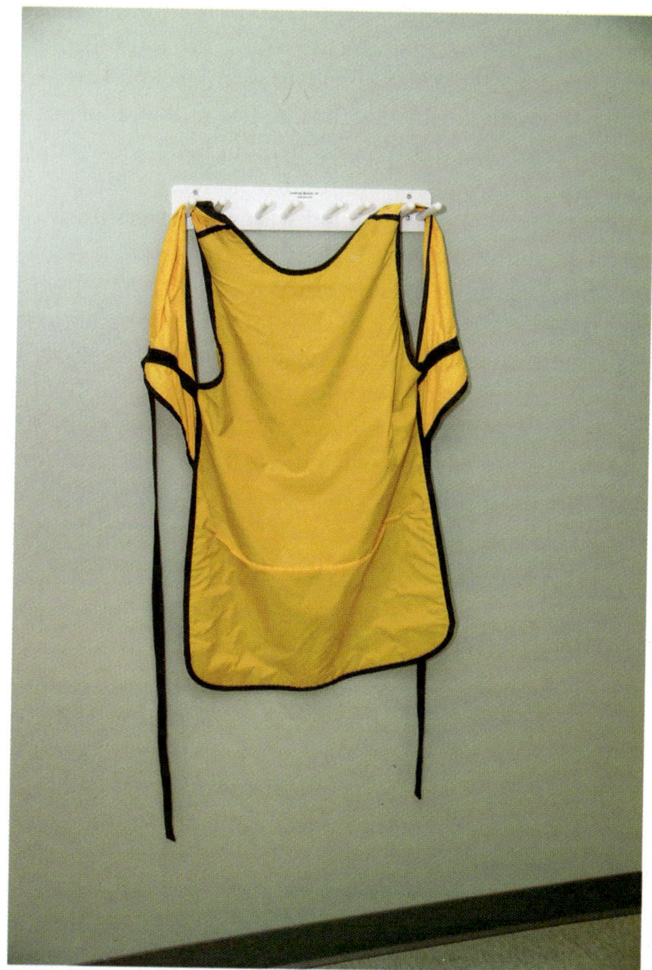

Figure 29-8 ■ An example of a lead apron.

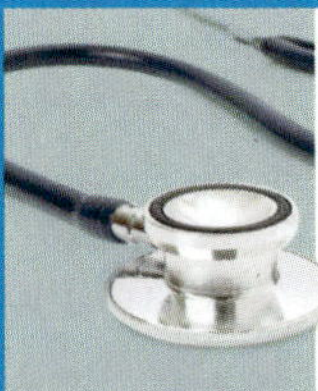

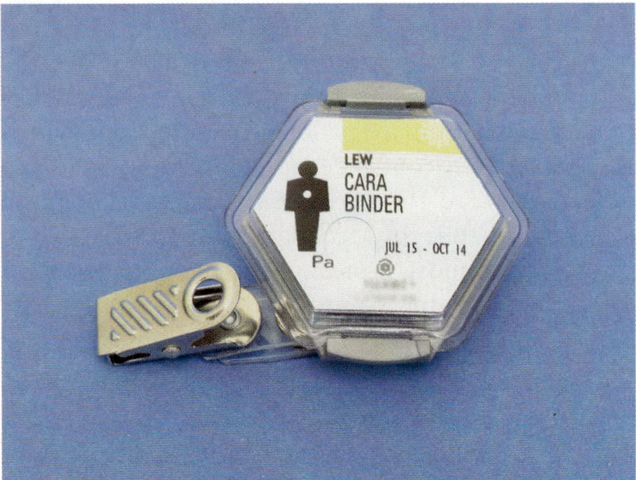

Figure 29-9 ■ A film badge worn by personnel working with radiographs or in the vicinity where radiographs are taken.

> **Field Smarts**
>
> All radioactive materials used in radiation therapy must be stored in containers made of lead and should never be handled with bare hands. Special equipment must be used when handling any of these radioactive materials to avoid contamination or radiation poisoning. Radiographic equipment that is used for radiographs and CT studies do not have ambient radiation and can be handled safely. Radiation is only produced when energy is applied to the system.

assistant must remain in the room while radiographs are taken. (This is sometimes necessary when a child is having a radiograph, or to hold a particular body part in place during a radiograph.) Since the radiographer does not usually remain in the room, the radiographer may stand behind a lead shield, or in an enclosed area in which the walls are lined with lead. The radiographer can then operate the control panel without being exposed to radiation. The walls of the room where the radiograph equipment is housed are lined with at least one inch of metal shielding material to prevent the scattered radiation from escaping outside of the room. Personnel who take radiographs or work in close proximity to radiologic equipment should wear a radiation monitor such as a film badge or optically stimulated luminescence (OSL) badge (Figure 29-9), known as a dosimeter, that contains a small piece of film that will indicate the level of radiation exposure based on color changes. The badge is checked at regular intervals to determine if radiation exposure has occurred and the level of radiation that was absorbed.

Patient Safety Precautions

When obtaining radiographs, the general rule of thumb is to use the smallest amount of radiation possible to achieve the best results. This will reduce the exposure to the patient as well. Female patients who may be pregnant should not receive radiographic studies unless it is deemed medically necessary by the provider. Many facilities require informed consent from the patient on risks and benefits of the study. Often in emergency situations, consent is considered to be implied.

A grid, which was discussed earlier in the chapter, is used to absorb the scatter radiation from the radiograph. A **Bucky grid** consists of alternating strips of lead—a **radiopaque** and a **radiolucent** (penetrable by radiographs) material. Both of these materials absorb some of the secondary radiation and allow the radiographs to penetrate the tissue at the same time. The radiation absorbed by the Bucky grid is to protect the Image Receptor, so alternate safety measures must be taken to protect the radiographer and the patient. Patients should be shielded with a lead apron that covers the thyroid gland, breasts, and gonad regions whenever possible.

SCHEDULING RADIOLOGICAL PROCEDURES OUTSIDE THE OFFICE

It is usually the medical assistant's responsibility to schedule radiological procedures performed outside the office. The following information should be provided to the outside facility when scheduling an appointment:

- The patient's full name and date of birth
- Insurance information, including precertification information, if needed
- Type of radiological study
- Diagnosis
- Provider information

Health Coach

Radiographic Procedures During Pregnancy

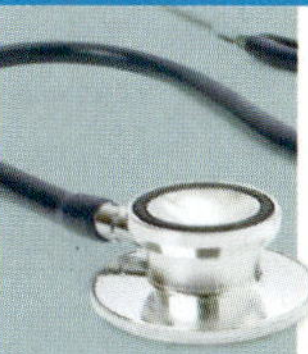

If a female patient is pregnant and a radiograph must be performed, the patient must be informed about the risks to the fetus before making the decision to have the radiograph. Many facilities will not take an radiograph if the patient is pregnant. They will look for alternative measures such as ultrasound or magnetic resonance imaging (MRI). When the patient is not certain about pregnancy, a pregnancy test should be performed prior to taking the radiograph. The provider will then decide how to proceed.

Patient Preparation Instructions

As mentioned earlier, it may be the medical assistant's responsibility to schedule and educate patients for outside radiograph examinations. Information provided to the patient should include the following:

- Date and time of procedure
- Facility where procedure is to be performed
- Paperwork to take to the facility
- Special preparation procedures
- Follow-up procedures

Explaining the Procedure

Many patients fear any type of medical exam, especially if it is a first-time procedure. Some diagnostic imaging equipment is large, noisy, and can be very intimidating to the patient; therefore, it is important to thoroughly explain all radiological procedures so the patient knows what to expect. Many radiographs are noninvasive and do not involve any pain or discomfort for the patient. Some, however, require the use of a **contrast medium**, which is a substance that is either ingested or injected to enhance internal structures for better visualization. A thorough explanation of the type of contrast medium to be used will help to alleviate patient anxiety.

Types of Contrast Media

As discussed earlier in the chapter, internal structures of the body appear as different shades of gray (which may appear white or black), depending on their density or thickness, when a radiograph is developed. Bone tissue is very dense and will appear lighter or white on the film because radiographs do not pass through as easily. In contrast, the lung tissue is less dense than the bone tissue and the radiographs will pass through, causing it to appear dark or blackened on the image.

Field Smarts

Several radiological studies may be ordered for the same day. Always check with the facility to be sure that all studies can be performed during the same visit. Some studies may require certain substances to be introduced into the patient's body that could interfere with subsequent studies, thus requiring the procedures to be scheduled on separate days. The typical recommendations for multiple radiography procedures the same day are the following:

- Non contrast procedures first (i.e., lumbar spine)
- Iodinated contrast procedures intravenous urography (IVU) or CT with contrast
- Barium contrast procedures upper gastrointestinal (UGI) series, also known as barium swallow or lower gastrointestinal (LGI) series, also known as a Barium enema (BE)

If an internal organ or structure is difficult to view on a radiograph, a contrast medium may be used. Contrast media are radiopaque, which means that the radiograph cannot penetrate the media. Therefore, if an internal structure, such as the intestines, is filled with a contrast medium, less rays will be absorbed, resulting in a lighter image that is easier to view. Contrast media are available in several forms:

- Liquid: Barium sulfate powder is mixed with water and the patient drinks the liquid to make the structures of the upper gastrointestinal tract more visible. Barium can also be administered as an enema for visualization of the lower GI tract.
- Iodine: Compounds containing iodine salts can be injected into the patient, usually intravenously, to visualize the kidneys, thyroid gland, heart, gallbladder, and blood vessels. It is important to determine if the patient has any allergies to iodine before scheduling the study. Shellfish allergy use to be considered the same as an iodine contrast allergy, but current research and guidelines no longer support this claim.
- Air or carbon dioxide: Air and other gases like carbon dioxide can be injected into the body to view the spinal cord and joints.

RADIOLOGICAL PROCEDURES COMMONLY PERFORMED OUTSIDE THE OFFICE

Clinical examinations may indicate the need for further diagnostic procedures to help identify a particular disorder or illness. A diagnosis often depends on exploration of the internal tissues of the body. Rather than relying on surgical intervention for visualization, radiograph and other radiological procedures provide a less invasive method for observation. There are presently many specialized radiological and diagnostic imaging procedures available, with new studies being developed all the time. Table 29-3 lists some of the more common radiological procedures performed outside the office as well as their purpose, the area(s) assessed, patient preparation instructions, and the route that the contrast medium is administered.

Table 29-3 Common Radiological Procedures Performed Outside of the Medical Office

Procedure Name	Purpose	Organs/Body Systems Assessed	Patient Preparation Instructions	Contrast Medium Routes
Angiography An angiogram of the coronary arteries after the injection of a contrast medium.	Visualization of the blood vessels to assess blood flow, clots, hemorrhaging, aneurysm	Heart Aorta Brain Lungs GI tract Kidneys	Nothing by mouth for six to eight hours prior to the exam	IV
Arthrography	Visualization of the inside of a joint to assess the tendons, ligaments, and cartilage	Knee Hip Shoulder	None prior to the procedure *Post-procedure:* Some swelling and discomfort in the joint area may be present for one to two days following the study	Injection
Barium Swallow/Upper GI Series GI Series with small bowel follow through A radiograph of the stomach after the ingestion of barium.	Visualization of the upper GI tract for assessment of ulcers, tumors, polyps, hiatal hernia, esophageal varices	Esophagus Stomach Small intestine	*Day before procedure:* Light evening meal and NPO (nothing by mouth) after midnight *Day of procedure:* NPO *During the procedure:* May have several images taken at specific time intervals. The test may take 3-5 hours. *Post-procedure:* Increased fluid intake and laxative, if prescribed	Oral contrast

Table 29-3 Common Radiological Procedures Performed Outside of the Medical Office *(continued)*

Procedure Name	Purpose	Organs/Body Systems Assessed	Patient Preparation Instructions	Contrast Medium Routes
Barium Enema/Lower GI Series	Visualization of the lower GI tract for assessment of polyps, tumors, or lesions	Colon	*Day before procedure:* Clear liquid diet, cleansing of the colon with laxative agents, light evening meal, NPO after evening meal *Day of procedure:* NPO and a cleansing enema Post-procedure: Increased fluid intake and if no bowel movement within 24 hours after the procedure, report to the provider	Administered by enema
Cholangiography	Visualization of the bile ducts for detection of possible stones or lesions (Generally used if **endoscopic retrograde cholangiopancreatogram (ERCP)** is not available or unsafe). ERCP is a procedure that combines upper gastrointestinal (GI) endoscopy and radiographs to treat problems of the bile and pancreatic ducts.	Bile ducts of liver	Possible cleansing enema prior to the procedure No meal before the exam	IV
Fluoroscopy	Visualization of moving body structures in real time, similar to a movie; often used during heart catheterizations	Heart Esophagus Stomach Blood vessels	NPO after midnight	Depending upon location of procedure: IV or oral contrast
Intravenous pyelogram (IVP)	Visualization of the urinary tract for stones, obstructions, cysts and tumors. (CT KUB and CT urography have generally replaced IVP as the study of choice.)	Kidneys Ureters Bladder	NPO prior to the procedure Laxatives the day prior to the procedure to cleanse the intestinal tract	IV

Health Coach

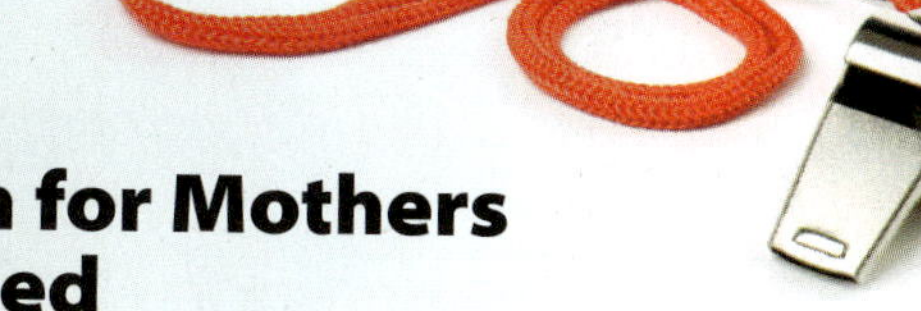

IV Contrast Information for Mothers who Breastfeed

Remind patients who are breastfeeding that there is a chance that the IV contrast media can be transferred to breast milk. Suggest that the patient use formula in place of breast milk for several days following a study in which an IV contrast medium is used. Barium contrast is not absorbed from the gastrointestinal tract and doesn't have the same risks to the infant or breastfeeding.

OTHER DIAGNOSTIC IMAGING PROCEDURES

Some diagnostic imaging procedures require the use of special equipment other than standard radiographic equipment. Many of these specialized procedures are performed in a hospital radiology department. However, some independent facilities have equipment that perform advanced imaging and more specialized procedures.

Computed Tomography (CT) Scan

The **computed tomography (CT)** scan combines radiograph along with a computer analysis of body tissues and organs and can be performed with or without a contrast medium. CT scans can supply the provider with more detailed information than a traditional radiograph and can eliminate the need for more invasive procedures. It is a valuable tool in detecting tumors and lesions in multiple areas of the body. CT scans can also be used to pinpoint the area where radiation should be administered to treat a tumor or mass.

During the scan, the patient lies on a table that moves into a doughnut-shaped scanner (Figure 29-10). The table advances in small increments while the scanner gathers separate images in the form of thin cross sections or slices of the tissue being studied (Figure 29-11). The scan does not usually require any special preparation and is both painless and noninvasive. If the scan requires the use of a contrast medium, the patient should be instructed not to eat or drink anything for four hours prior to the procedure.

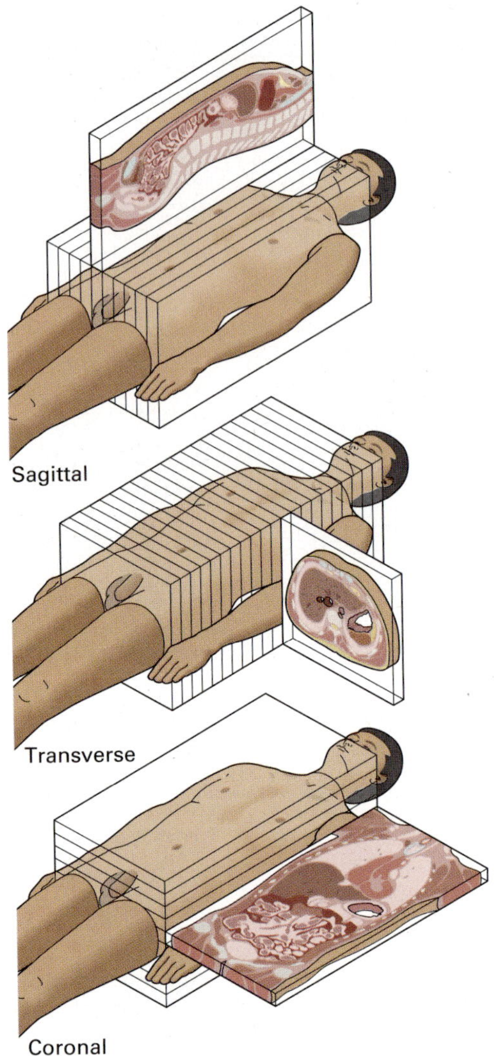

Figure 29-11 ■ Cross-sectional images produced by a CT scan.

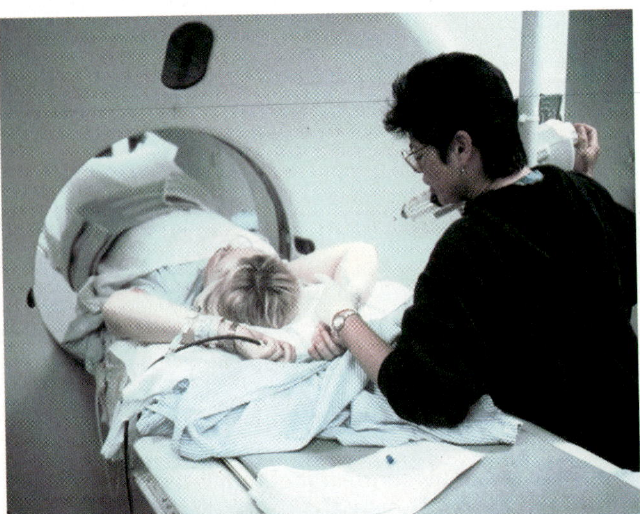

Figure 29-10 ■ The patient lies on the table ready to enter the CT scanner.

Magnetic Resonance Imaging (MRI)

Magnetic resonance imaging (MRI) has become the diagnostic imaging procedure of choice for many providers and hospitals. MRI uses no radiation and produces a high-quality, three-dimensional image that is much clearer than traditional radiographs (Figure 29-12). An MRI machine utilizes a powerful magnetic field, rather than radiation, to produce images of internal organs and soft tissue structures. Although any area of the body can be visualized by MRI, bone fractures are better visualized with a traditional radiography or CT scan.

During the MRI, the patient is placed in a cylindrical chamber and must remain inside and motionless for up to 60 minutes. Patients who suffer from claustrophobia may need to be sedated in order to undergo an MRI. Open MRIs are now available for patients who cannot

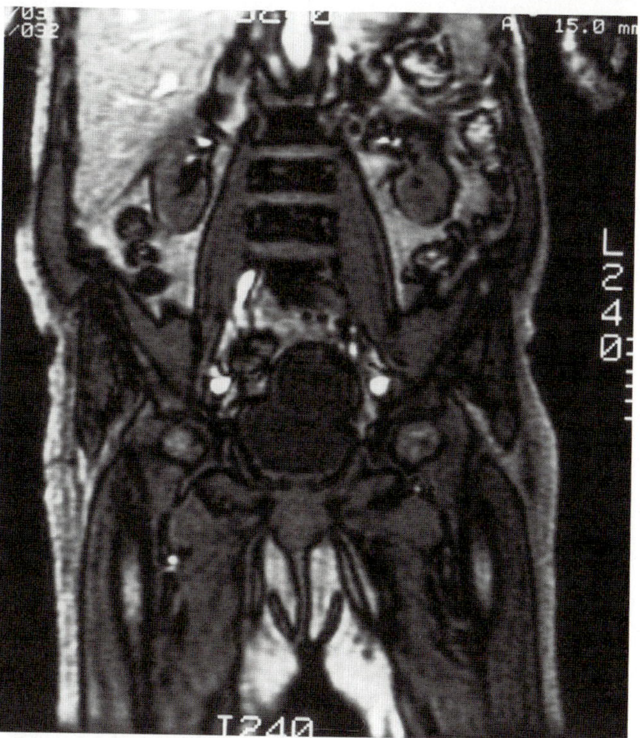

Figure 29-12 ■ An MRI image of the abdomen.

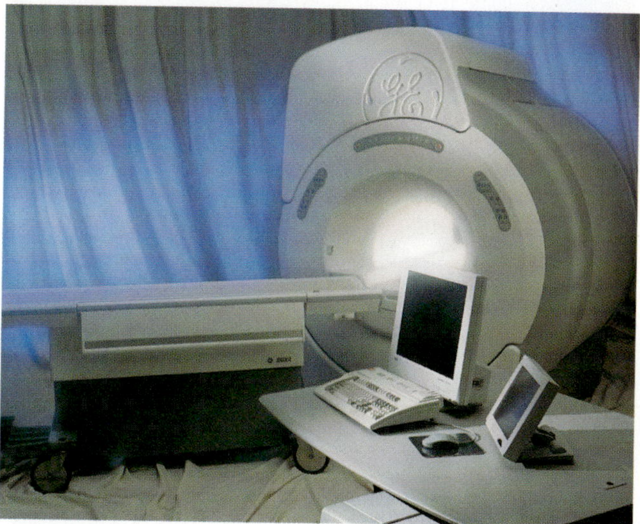

Courtesy of GE Medical Systems.

Figure 29-13a ■ A *closed* magnetic resonance imaging (MRI) system.

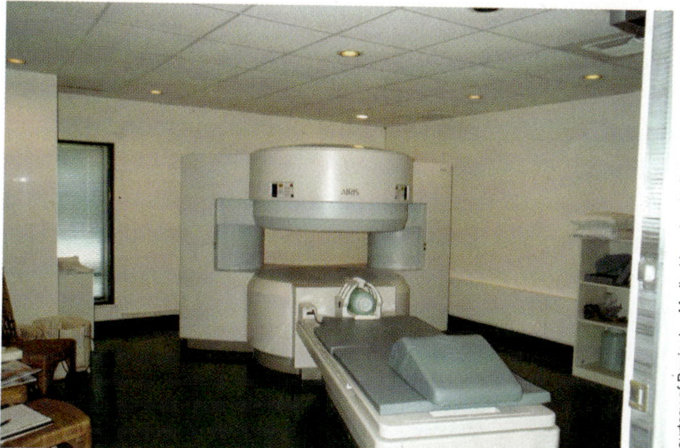

Courtesy of Barrington Medical Imaging, LLC, Cary, IL.

Figure 29-13b ■ Many patients are claustrophobic and cannot withstand a traditional MRI. For those patients, an *open* MRI can be used.

tolerate a traditional MRI, but depending on the open MRI machine used, the image quality is not as clear and accurate as those produced by a closed MRI. The machine makes loud knocking noises during the procedure and some patients prefer to wear ear plugs or headphones to listen to music during the procedure. Refer to Figures 29-13a and 29-13b for pictures of both a closed and open MRI machine.

While an MRI is a relatively easy procedure for the patient, there are some drawbacks, including the following:

- Patients with certain pacemakers or metal implants should not undergo an MRI, because the metal can interfere with the magnetic field. It is possible to burn the wires of the pacemaker unit and tissue surrounding the device. Many new devices and implants are MRI safe.
- Objects containing metal, such as jewelry, eyeglasses, belts, hairclips, watches, clothing with zippers, wire bras, clothes with metal studs, and even some forms of makeup (mascara) can interfere with the magnetic field and cause burns to the patients.
- Credit cards or hotel keys with metallic strips can interfere with the magnetic field and should not be taken into the room where the procedure is performed.
- Removable dental work (such as partial dentures) and hearing aids contain metal and may cause burns to the patient.

Ultrasound/Sonography

Ultrasound is a diagnostic imaging procedure that does not use radiation but instead bounces high-frequency sound waves off the internal structures of the body, creating a **sonogram** or picture (Figure 29-14) of the internal structure that is being scanned. Ultrasound is used to detect abnormalities within the internal organs, such as gallstones, tumors, and heart defects. Additionally, color Doppler ultrasound can show the velocity and direction of blood flow through vessels. Because ultrasound waves do not harm a developing fetus, ultrasonography is often used to monitor the baby's

Figure 29-14 ■ A sonogram image.

development during pregnancy. Ultrasound does not penetrate bone or any internal structures surrounded by bone, so it is not useful for assessing the brain, skeletal tissue, or the lungs. Other uses of ultrasound have been developed to include in physical therapy to warm soft tissues by increasing the duration, frequency, and intensity of the sound waves.

Ultrasound imaging is performed by specially trained personnel and can be performed in a medical office, hospital, or radiology facility. There is usually little to no preparation for an ultrasound procedure, but preparation instructions will vary depending on the structures being viewed. The patient should be instructed to wear loose-fitting, comfortable clothing because the procedure is conducted on bare skin. A conduction gel is placed on the patient's skin and the transducer (a wand-like part of the instrument) is moved over the area. As the sound waves bounce off the internal structure, an image is displayed on the screen or oscilloscope. A hard copy of the image can also be printed. Refer to Figure 17-17 in Chapter 17 for a picture of a patient having an ultrasound performed.

MOLECULAR IMAGING AND NUCLEAR MEDICINE

Molecular imaging provides detailed pictures that illustrate disease processes at the cellular or molecular level. This technology allows providers to study the function of organs rather than just the anatomy of organs. Providers are able to diagnose diseases like cancer at a much earlier stage and to treat diseases while they are still very manageable using this technology.

Nuclear medicine is included in molecular imaging and is a branch of medicine that uses radioactive material for the purpose of diagnosing and treating diseases. Substances known as **radiopharmaceuticals**, containing radioactive isotopes, are administered to the patient by mouth or by injection. Different areas of the body attract these isotopes, which can be detected on a special type of scan. Tumors and other types of abnormalities are detected as either "hot spots" where an unusually large amount of radiopharmaceuticals collect or "cold spots" where an unusually low amount of radiopharmaceuticals collect. A "hot spot" may indicate the presence of a particular type of tumor, or may be found in areas that are inflamed, infected, or where trauma is present. A "cold spot" may indicate a lack of blood supply to an area or some forms of cancer.

An example of a nuclear medicine study is a bone scan. Radioactive isotopes are injected into the patient and the patient is asked to return in two to four hours for the actual scan to be performed. The isotopes accumulate in areas of the body where increased bone turnover, such as arthritis or stress fracture, exists and appear as dark areas or spots on the image (Figure 29-15). Radio nuclides break down quickly, reducing unwanted side effects. In fact, the isotopes do not expose the patient to as much radiation as some traditional radiographic procedures. Table 29-4 lists and describes other types of nuclear medicine imaging studies.

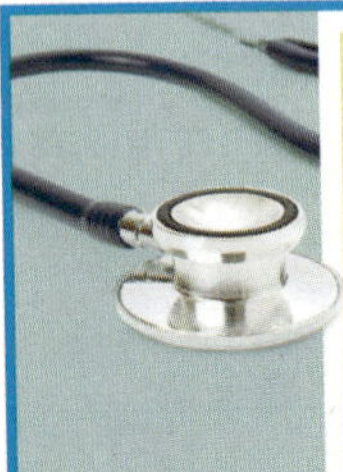

Field Smarts

In the past, patients with pacemakers and internal defibrillators were unable to have MRIs, creating a huge dilemma for these patients when an MRI study was necessary to diagnose other serious conditions. Because of the increase of patients with these types of devices, medical equipment manufacturers have come up with alternative solutions for these patients. One such device, referred to as an MRI-conditional pacemaker, received FDA approval for use in the United States in February 2011. There are some clinics that will perform MRIs on patients with traditional pace makers and implantable devices; however, these procedures are only performed if absolutely medically necessary and with the assistance of an MRI physicist and careful cardiac monitoring during the procedure. Many orthopedic plates and screws are also MRI safe, but may cause some distortions on the image.

Table 29-4 Nuclear Medicine Procedures

Procedure	Description
Positron emission tomography (PET) scan	This test uses a radioactive tracer to illustrate how tissues and organs are functioning. The test can diagnose cancer and check for metastasis, as well as check for heart problems and brain function. Types of PET scans include brain, breast, heart, lung, and PET/CT scans.
Single-photon emission tomography (SPECT)	This scan also analyzes function of different tissues and organs using a radioactive substance and special camera to create images in 3-D. This test can illustrate areas of the brain that are more or less active and illustrate how blood flows through the heart.
Targeted molecular ultrasound	This test combines ultrasound technology with special contrast micro bubbles to look for diseases such as atherosclerosis, tumor-related angiogenesis, and rejection of transplanted organs.
Magnetic resonance spectroscopy (MRS)	An MRI observes anatomical structures in the body but MRS looks at biochemical changes in the cell and is able to determine tumor type and aggressiveness and able to distinguish between tumor recurrence and radiation necrosis.

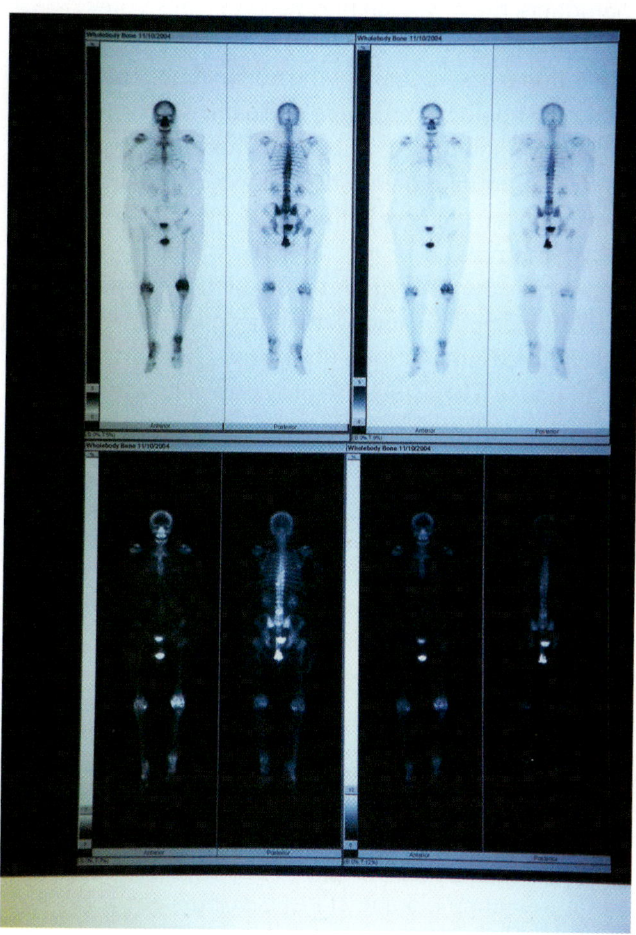

Figure 29-15 ■ An image produced by a nuclear medicine bone scan.

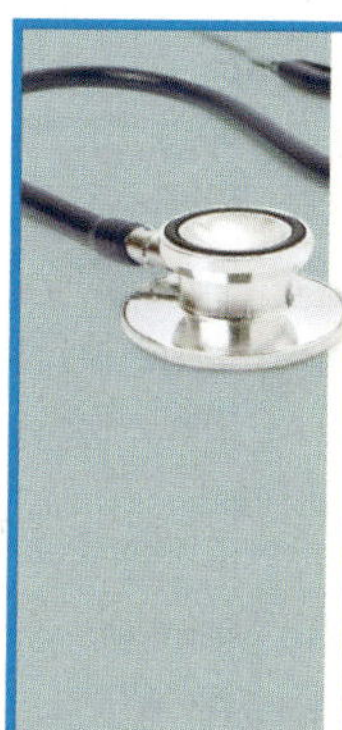

Field Smarts

Osteoporosis is usually only seen by radiograph when it has reached a very advanced stage. There are better tests for earlier detection of the disease, such as a dual-energy radiograph absorptiometry (DEXA), which is often referred to as a bone density scan.

RADIATION THERAPY

Radiation therapy is used to treat or reduce the burden of inoperable tumors. It is also used to destroy any cancer cells remaining after surgical tumor removal. The treatment causes damage to both normal and cancerous tissue alike, but with more sophisticated targeting methods, there is more damage to the cancer cells. Nonetheless, damage to the surrounding normal tissue is unavoidable at this time.

Radiation therapy can be administered through the skin to the target area in the body or by implanting radioactive "beads" or "seeds" inside the body and leaving them in place for a prescribed amount of time. This type of therapy interferes with the DNA of the malignant cells, which either destroys the cells or retards their growth.

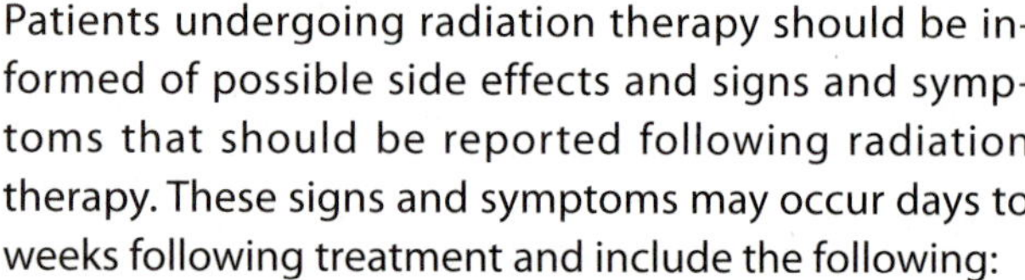

Radiation Therapy

Patients undergoing radiation therapy should be informed of possible side effects and signs and symptoms that should be reported following radiation therapy. These signs and symptoms may occur days to weeks following treatment and include the following:

- Redness of the skin that resembles a sunburn: Avoid using alcohol on the skin, avoid exposure to direct sunlight and other sources of heat, and do not lie on the reddened area.
- Hair loss: Some hair loss may occur if radiation burns are deep. Use mild shampoos and gently comb or brush the hair.
- Damage to the eyes: Signs of damage such as excessive tearing, dryness, injury to the lens, or conjunctivitis should be reported immediately. Artificial tears (eye drops) may be used along with antibiotics, if appropriate.
- Damage to the ears: The ears should be checked for blockage of the canal and bulging of the tympanic membrane (eardrum). Prevent falls due to dizziness and alert the office if there is any degree of hearing loss. Antibiotics may be administered if infection is present.
- Irritation of the mucosa of the mouth: If the mucosa is irritated, avoid spicy foods, smoking, and hot liquids. Sucking on ice chips may help to relieve some of the symptoms; however, frozen or cold foods and drinks may also be irritating. Try eating foods and drinking liquids that are room temperature.
- Irritation of the mucosa of the intestinal tract: Observe intake and output levels and report any diarrhea or vomiting. If diarrhea and vomiting are present, avoid dairy products and take over-the-counter (OTC) medications to help alleviate symptoms. If symptoms are not relieved with OTC products, the physician may need to write a prescription to treat the symptoms.
- Irritation of the mucosa of the urinary tract: Urine output should be measured and a urinalysis should be performed to determine if an infection is present. If so, antibiotics may be prescribed to treat the infection. An increase in fluids may help to decrease the symptoms.
- Bone marrow and lymph tissue damage: Report unusual bleeding, and watch for signs of anemia such as extreme fatigue, shortness of breath, and unusual bruising. The provider will perform blood counts on a regular basis and may start the patient on antibiotics to protect the patient from infection.
- Nervous system symptoms: Report any signs of pain, incontinence, slurred speech, cognitive dysfunction, dizziness, or weakness and tingling in the arms and legs.

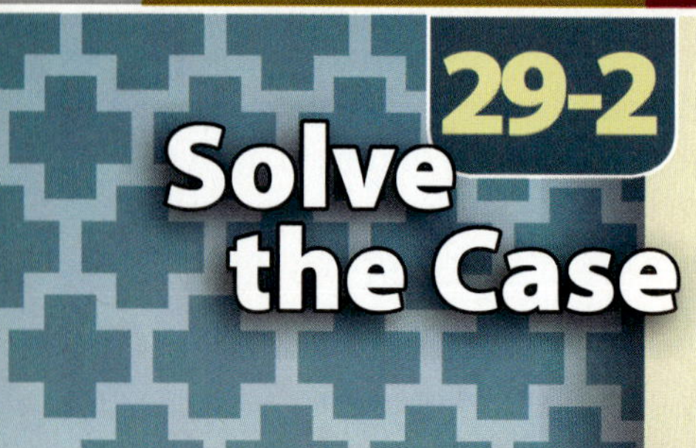

On completion of the chest radiograph of Mr. Monroy, the physician points to a white, triangular region within the lung field and states that the patient has pneumonia.

1. **Is the white region within the lung field radiolucent or radiopaque?**
2. **What shade should the lung fields be and why?**
3. **What shade is bone? What shade is fat?**

CHAPTER SUMMARY

- Diagnostic imaging, which includes radiology procedures, ultrasonography, and nuclear medicine, makes it possible for providers to view internal structures within the body.
- The medical assistant should be knowledgeable regarding the indications for radiograph procedures, including their uses for diagnosis and treatment.
- The ability of the medical assistant to provide accurate instructional information will be important for patient compliance and better results. When taking radiographs, medical assistants must institute safety measures to protect both the patient and themselves.
- Never take shortcuts, and avoid the need to retake radiographs because appropriate measures were not taken to get it right on the first try.

CERTIFICATION REVIEW QUESTIONS

1. Which of the following radiological procedures requires no patient preparation?
   a. Upper GI
   b. Lower GI
   c. Chest radiograph
   d. All of the above
2. Which of the following would be an example of a contrast medium?
   a. Barium cobalt
   b. Barium sulfate
   c. Barium sodium
   d. Barium citrate
3. In which of the following radiograph positions would the patient's chest be against the film?
   a. Lateral
   b. AP
   c. PA
   d. Oblique
4. Which of the following radiograph procedures would require a contrast medium?
   a. KUB
   b. IVP
   c. Foot
   d. Abdominal
5. All of the following can be side effects of radiation therapy *except*:
   a. hair loss.
   b. nausea.
   c. anemia.
   d. None of the above
6. Which part of the body is examined during an angiography?
   a. Joints
   b. Blood vessels
   c. Vertebrae
   d. Intestines
7. Which radiological procedure provides the radiologist with thin cross-sectional images of the body?
   a. CT scan
   b. Nuclear medicine scan
   c. MRI
   d. Both a and c
8. Which of the following items must be worn by health care workers who perform radiographs?
   a. Lab coat
   b. Dosimeter
   c. Oximeter
   d. Goggles
9. What does a cholangiography evaluate?
   a. Bile ducts
   b. Liver
   c. Gallbladder
   d. Both a and b
10. All of the following procedures require special patient preparation *except*:
    a. upper GI.
    b. lower GI.
    c. MRI.
    d. small bowel series.

STUDY RESOURCES

Resources to Test and Reinforce Your Knowledge:	
Certification Review Questions	Take this end-of-chapter quiz
Workbook	• Complete the activities for Chapter 29
Resources to Promote Critical Thinking:	
Solve the Case Activities	• Consider these case studies and discuss your conclusions
Learning Lab	• Module 29: Diagnostic Imaging
MindTap	• Complete Chapter 29 readings and activities

REFERENCES

"About Nuclear Medicine & Molecular Imaging." *SNMMI*. N.p., n.d. Web. August 24, 2015. http://www.snmmi.org/AboutSNMMI/Content.aspx?ItemNumber=6433

Kaneko, Osamu F., and Jürgen K. Willmann. "Ultrasound for Molecular Imaging and Therapy in Cancer." *Quantitative Imaging in Medicine and Surgery*. AME Publishing Company, n.d. Web. August 24, 2015. http://www.ncbi.nlm.nih.gov/pmc/articles/PMC3466813/

National Institutes of Health. (n.d.). What is ERCP? Retrieved June 15, 2015, from http://www.niddk.nih.gov/health-information/health-topics/diagnostic-tests/ercp/Pages/diagnostic-test.aspx

"Nuclear Exercise Stress Test." *Nuclear Exercise Stress Test*. N.p., n.d. Web. August 25, 2015. http://my.clevelandclinic.org/services/heart/diagnostics-testing/nuclear-imaging/nuclear-exercise-stress-test

"PET Scan: Medline Plus Medical Encyclopedia." *U.S. National Library of Medicine*. U.S. National Library of Medicine, n.d. Web. August 24, 2015. https://www.nlm.nih.gov/medlineplus/ency/article/003827.htm

"Positron Emission Tomography (PET) Scan."- *Mayo Clinic*. N.p., n.d. Web. August 24, 2015. http://www.mayoclinic.org/tests-procedures/pet-scan/basics/definition/prc-20014301

"SPECT Scan." *Mayo Clinic*. N.p., n.d. Web. August 24, 2015. http://www.mayoclinic.org/tests-procedures/spect-scan/basics/definition/prc-20020674

Wilhelm Conrad Röntgen. (2015). The Biography.com website. Retrieved July 1, 2015, from http://www.biography.com/people/wilhelm-conrad-röntgen-39707

30

Fundamentals of Pharmacology

CHAPTER OUTLINE

Pharmacology

Drug Origins
- Drug Sources

Medicinal Uses of Drugs

Drug Classifications

Pharmacodynamics
- Dose Response
- Drug Actions
- Drug Effects

Pharmacokinetics
- Variables that Affect a Drug's Blood Plasma Level
- Factors That Affect Drug Actions

Drug Names

Medication Tasks

Regulations and Legal Classifications of Drugs
- Controlled Substances

The Medication Order or Prescription Writing
- Prescription Abbreviations
- Rules for Creating Prescriptions for Controlled Substances
- Tamper-Resistant Prescription Pads

Drug Resources
- The Physicians' Desk Reference
- U.S. Pharmacopeia / National Formulary
- Drug Product Package Inserts
- Drug Resources on the Internet and E-versions of Drug References

Safe Drug Administration
- Seven Rights of Drug Administration
- Safety and Continuity during Medication Administration

Routes of Medication Administration
- Enteral Routes
- Parenteral Routes

ESSENTIAL TERMS

administer
adverse effects
affinity
agonist
anaphylaxis
antagonist
bioavailability
buccal
dispense
drug
drug ceiling
drug interaction
efficacy
enteral
local reaction
medicinal
parenteral
pharmacodynamics
pharmacokinetics
pharmacology
prescribe
prophylactic
receptor
side effect
sublingual
systemic reaction
therapeutic effect
therapeutic index
topical
transdermal patch

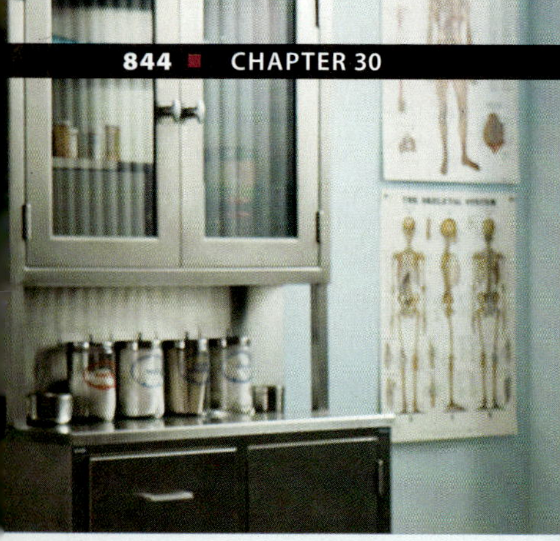

DEVELOPMENTAL OBJECTIVES

After completing this chapter, you should be able to:

1. Correctly spell and define the essential terms.
2. List and describe five different sources of drugs.
3. Compare and contrast five different uses of drugs.
4. Identify the drug classifications including their indications for use, desired effects, side effects, and adverse reactions.
5. Describe how drugs attach themselves to drug receptor sites and explain at what point the drug exerts its effect on the patient.
6. Describe dose-response curve and summarize factors that can affect a patient's response to particular medications.
7. Describe four processes that affect a drug's blood plasma levels.
8. Comply with federal, state, and local laws in regards to prescribing, delegating, administering, or dispensing medications.
9. Analyze the five schedules used to differentiate the various classifications of controlled substances and describe how prescriptions may be relayed to a pharmacist for each schedule.
10. Identify the parts of a prescription.
11. Properly utilize a Physicians' Desk Reference (PDR) and describe other resources available for referencing medications.
12. Verify the rules of medication administration including the seven rights.
13. List and describe the different routes of drug administration and properly administer oral, topical, and transdermal medications, and a rectal suppository.

INTRODUCTION

A **drug** is any substance that produces a change in the function of a living organism. **Pharmacology** is the study of drugs, including their origin, nature, properties, and effects upon living organisms. A drug's **efficacy** (effectiveness) and benefits have to be measured and compared to its risks in order to determine its viability.

Medical assistants must have a basic understanding of the fundamentals of pharmacology including drug uses, forms, classifications, and routes of administration. Becoming familiar with the effects that drugs have on the body and the physiological variables that can alter their performance will enable the medical assistant to properly administer drugs and provide appropriate education for patients.

In addition, the medical assistant must be familiar with (1) state and federal drug laws that dictate procedures that must be followed when working with special categories of drugs and (2) state delegation laws dictating who has authority to delegate pharmacological tasks to the medical assistant.

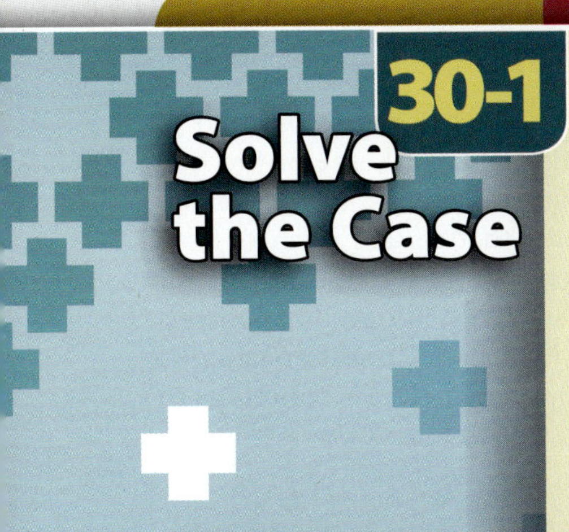

Twenty-year-old Isaac Kyeremateng comes into the office because of a lower back injury he received last week. He states that he felt a burning sensation after picking up a heavy box. He is complaining of some tingling in his legs and feet and horrible back pain in the tailbone area (pain is about a 10 on the pain scale). He is currently sitting on the exam table but appears very uncomfortable. His vitals are normal except for his blood pressure, which is 156/92, an unusually high reading for Isaac.

1. **Is there anything you can do to help Isaac get more comfortable while he waits for the provider?**
2. **What may be causing the unusual spike in Isaac's blood pressure?**
3. **What types of testing do you think the provider will order for Isaac?**

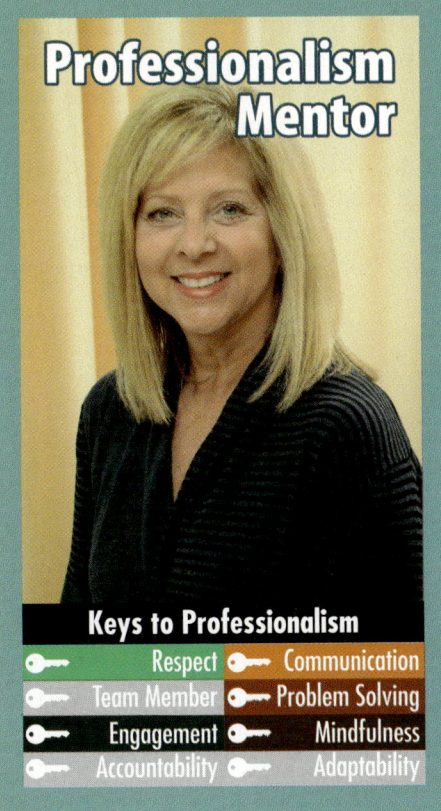

Most patients at some point in time will be placed on a medication. Some patients take a medication for a certain time period while others are placed on a medication for life. At a very busy cardiology practice, a patient called in for a medication refill but expressed concerns to the medical assistant taking his call that it might not be the right medication. He was feeling dizzy and had frequent headaches and felt like the medication might be the cause. Instead of just putting in a refill request, the medical assistant was actively listening to the patient and engaged with what he was saying to her. What she did next was what we call in health care a "good catch." She had the patient bring in his prescription, and she then looked up the medication that had been ordered in the patient's chart and contacted the pharmacy. The patient was right! The medication that he had been given by mistake was Lamictal, a seizure medication instead of his Labetalol, a blood pressure medicine. Two medications that sound alike yet have severe consequences if used improperly. Patients depend on members of the health care team to keep them safe and sometimes it takes really listening to a patient's concerns and hearing what they are trying to tell us. Kudos to that medical assistants and to all health care providers who take the time to make sure their patient's safety comes first! In your professional journal, explain how the professionalism keys in this feature box apply to the situation described. ■

PHARMACOLOGY

Pharmacology is a broad term that means the study of drugs. The field of pharmacology can be further broken down into five different subdivisions. The following bullets list those divisions with a *very basic* description of each subdivision:

- *Pharmacognosy*: Study of a drug's characteristics and its sources
- *Pharmacodynamics*: Study of the effects of drugs on living organisms, or what a drug does to the body
- *Pharmacokinetics*: Study of the movement of drugs throughout the body, or what the body does to a drug
- *Pharmacotherapeutics*: Study of the desired uses and effects of a drug
- *Toxicology*: Study of poisons, their effects, and antidotes

DRUG ORIGINS

One of the first historical records of drugs comes from Babylonia in the form of textbooks found on clay tablets tracing back to 2600 B.C. These tablets contained inscriptions describing symptoms of a disease, a drug formula that could be used as a remedy for the disease, compounding instructions, and a chant or spell that could be used to enhance the formula's effectiveness.

Throughout the early history of pharmacy, herbalists, physicians, and priests (whose roles often intertwined) all played active roles in apothecary (or pharmacological) functions. However, these individuals had very little training in apothecary studies, placing citizens seeking their guidance in harm's way. It wasn't until the Middle Ages that the roles of these practitioners diverged and the practice of pharmacy became a specialty.

The first college of pharmacy originated in 1821, and the American Pharmaceutical Association (APhA) was founded in 1852. During the early years of pharmacy, drugs didn't have to meet specific standards before being introduced to the public; hence, drug quackery was quite common. As a result of drug efficacy and safety concerns, drug laws were developed by the early 1900s to protect the public against drug scams and to promote overall drug safety.

Today, a drug must go through rigorous testing before being introduced to consumers. Scientists use a variety of sources to produce drugs including plants, minerals, animals, and synthetics.

Drug Sources

There are a variety of sources that can be used to manufacture drugs (Figure 30-1). Some of the first drug sources were plants, fruits, and vegetables. Further research revealed that certain extracts from animals were useful in alleviating patient symptoms or replacing missing chemicals. Today, bioengineering techniques allow chemists to modify particular genes within plants to perform certain functions or to alleviate particular side effects associated with their use.

Plant Sources

Medicinal use of plants for treating disease processes or disorders has been the foundation of pharmacological therapy for thousands of years. Studying the leaves, stems, roots, blossoms, or fruit of certain plants led to the discovery of their **medicinal** properties and functions. One example of a plant source used today is the genus *Digitalis*, which includes the perennial and Grecian foxglove plants, which are used to make digitalis and digoxin (drugs used to treat congestive heart failure). Other examples include ergot, a particular type of fungus that grows on grass and cereal grain, once

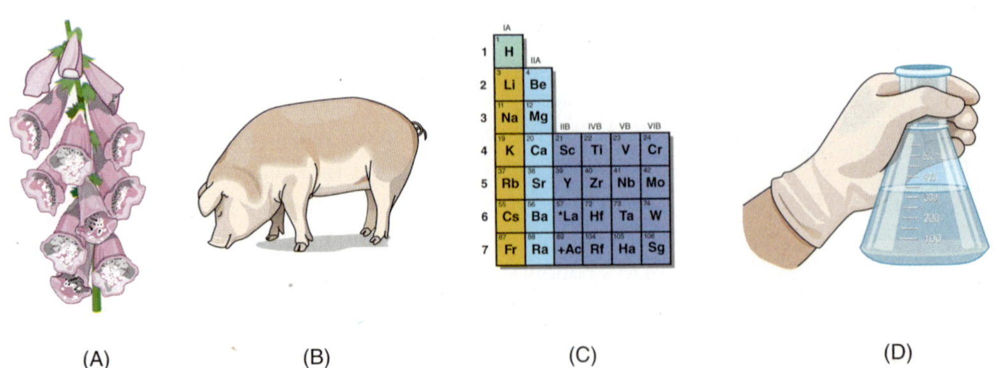

Figure 30-1 ■ Drugs are obtained from a variety of sources: (a) plant, (b) animal, (c) mineral, and (d) synthetic, as well as bioengineering (not shown).

used as a uterine stimulant and now used in the treatment of migraines, and opium, which originates from the poppy plant and is the key ingredient for all narcotics. Herbal medications come from a variety of plants as well and should be listed in a patient's drug history.

Animal Sources

Animals are sometimes used as sources for drugs. Drugs derived from animal sources include insulin, thyroid medications, cortisone, and adrenaline. These essential extracts are obtained from the tissues of the pancreas and adrenal glands of particular animals. Premarin, a conjugated estrogen, is made by extracting hormones from the urine of a pregnant mare and is used to treat menopausal symptoms. Even the eggs of a hen are used to develop certain vaccines. Animal sources are contraindicated when the patient has an allergy to any of the products or by-products used to develop the drug.

Mineral Sources

Minerals, such as silver nitrate and sulfur, are highly purified forms of elements that are used to treat specific diseases. A sulfonamide (a specific type of antibiotic) is an example of a drug that comes from a mineral source and is commonly used to treat bacterial infections of the urinary tract. The antipsychotic drug lithium carbonate is another example of a drug made from a mineral source and is used to treat bipolar disease. Due to the possibility of drug interactions, all minerals, including over-the-counter (OTC) products, should be included in the patient's drug history.

Synthetic Origins

Synthetic forms of drugs are created in pharmaceutical laboratories by experimenting with different chemicals. Scientists are able to create new drugs or compounds that are identical to natural drugs by altering and combining chemicals using a variety of different methods. One advantage of producing synthetic drugs is the ability to standardize the doses and to alter substances that may cause serious side effects. Synthetic drugs are usually more economical to manufacture than those coming from natural sources, resulting in less expense to the patient.

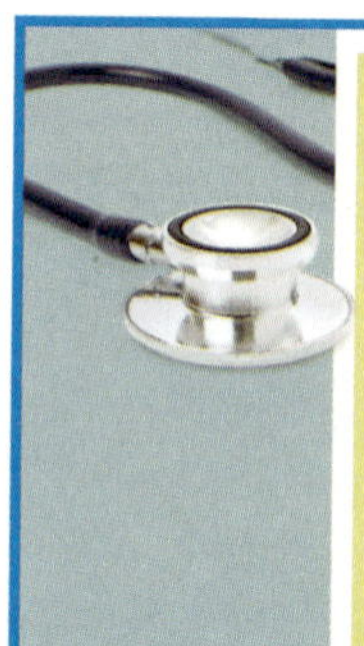

Field Smarts

Patients receiving flu vaccine should be thoroughly questioned about chicken egg allergies before administration. This is because the vaccine is developed using the eggs of hens. Administration of these products to a patient with an allergy could cause the patient to go into anaphylaxis, a severe life-threatening condition caused by the allergy.

Bioengineering

Genetic engineering is the latest process that is used to manufacture drugs. All living structures (plants, animals, and people) have the exact same DNA molecular structure consisting of six basic components—a phosphate, a sugar, and four bases. Recombinant technology takes genetic information from two different organisms and combines them together. These drugs are produced by utilizing the DNA within a bacterium or other microorganism and performing gene splicing to produce hybrid forms of drugs. By removing the bacterial walls of an *Escherichia coli* bacterium and combining it with an insulin gene, the drug Humulin (a form of human insulin) is made. The cells duplicate rapidly, making billions of new cells capable of producing insulin. Bioengineering has been practiced for many years in the agricultural and horticulture industry.

MEDICINAL USES OF DRUGS

Drugs are prescribed to patients for a variety of purposes. Listed below are the five medicinal uses of drugs:

- Therapeutic: A substance used in the treatment of a condition to relieve symptoms. An example is using aspirin to relieve symptoms of a headache.
- Diagnostic: A medicinal product used in combination with radiography and other imaging procedures to detect abnormalities, such as lesions and tumors, and to check how well a specific organ is functioning. An example of a diagnostic drug used to detect gastrointestinal (GI) abnormalities is barium sulfate. Radioactive iodine is a radionuclide used to check thyroid function.
- Curative: A medication that helps to remove an agent that causes disease. Antibiotic therapy is an example of a curative drug because of its ability to destroy bacteria.
- Replacement: These are agents used to replace chemicals that are deficient or missing in the

body, such as insulin and other hormones. Vitamins and minerals are examples of other substances that are commonly used in replacement therapy.

- Preventative (also termed **prophylactic**): These substances are used to prevent or lessen the severity of a disease. Examples include immunizing agents such as vaccines and antibiotics that are given prior to surgical procedures to reduce the risks of infection.

DRUG CLASSIFICATIONS

Drugs are categorized under different classifications and may be segregated by their actions upon the body, the change they produce in cellular activity, or by the body system they affect. Drugs that have multiple effects may be found under several classifications. Table 30-1 lists common drug classifications and their actions. Refer to Appendix E for a list of the top 50 drugs and their classifications.

Table 30-1 Drug Classifications and Their Actions

Classification	Indication for Use/ Desired Effect	Examples	Side Effects	Adverse Effects
Analgesic	Relieves pain	*Nonnarcotic examples*: Tylenol (acetaminophen) Bayer, Aspro, Dispril (aspirin) *Narcotic examples*: Hydrocodone	**Acetaminophen**—Nausea, rash, headache **Aspirin**—stomach ache, rash, tinnitus, dizziness, bleeding, diarrhea, constipation **Hydrocodone**—Constipation, nausea, pruritus, back pain, tremor	**Acetaminophen**—hypersensitivity, hepatotoxicity, anemia, thrombocytopenia **Aspirin**—GI ulcer, anaphylaxis, Nephrotoxicity **Hydrocodone**—Respiratory depression, apnea, hypotension, death, bradycardia, and dependency
Anesthetic	Produces a lack of feeling; may be local or general	*Local anesthetics:* Novacaine (procaine HCL) Xylocaine (lidocaine HCL) *General anesthetic*: Ultane (sevoflurane)	**Lidocaine**—pain, vasovagal reaction, tinnitus, euphoria, hallucinations, agitation **Sevoflurane**—nausea, vomiting, hypotension, shivering	**Lidocaine**—arrhythmia, respiratory depression or distress, coma, seizure **Sevoflurane**—malignant hyperthermia, cardiac arrest, apnea, airway spasm, and hepatotoxicity
Antacid	Neutralizes stomach acid	Mylanta, Maalox, Zantac, Prilosec	**Mylanta**—abdominal pain, constipation, dehydration, diarrhea, nausea, and vomiting.	**Mylanta**—aluminum intoxication, encephalopathy, osteomalacia
Antiacne	Treats acne	Accutane (Isotretinoin) Differin Gel (adapalene gel) Benzoyl peroxide Cleocin gel (clindamycin)	**Accutane**—dry skin, hypertriglyceridemia, headache, lab abnormalities, palpitations **Benzoyl peroxide**—dermatitis, dry skin	**Accutane** -osteopenia, hepatotoxicity, pancreatitis, vasculitis, **Benzoyl peroxide**—hypersensitivity
Antianginal	Relieves the symptoms of angina	Imdur (isosorbide mononitrate), Isordil (isosorbide), Nitrostat (nitroglycerin)	Nitroglycerin—headache, lightheadedness, hypotension, tachycardia	Nitroglycerin—severe hypotension, paradoxical bradycardia
Antianxiety	Relieves anxiety and muscle tension	Librium (chlordiazepoxide HCL), Valium (diazepam), Xanax (alprazolam)	**Valium**—drowsiness, confusion, depression, urinary retention, nausea	**Valium**—Lab abnormalities, respiratory depression, dependency, bradycardia, and hypotension
Antiarrhythmic	Controls cardiac arrhythmias	Norpace (disopyramide) Procan SR (procainamide) Cardioquin (quinidine), metoprolol, amiodarone	**Amiodarone**—bradycardia, nausea, vomiting, low blood pressure, fatigue **Quinidine**—diarrhea, nausea, rash, fatigue	**Amiodarone**—heart failure, shock, death **Quinidine**—thrombocytopenia, respiratory arrest, death

Table 30-1 Drug Classifications and Their Actions *(continued)*

Classification	Indication for Use/ Desired Effect	Examples	Side Effects	Adverse Effects
Antibiotic	Inhibits or destroys bacteria	Ceftin (cefuroxime), Cleocin HCl (clindamycin HCL), Levaquin (levofloxacin), Amoxil (amoxicillin), azithromycin	**Ceftin**—diarrhea, nausea, vomiting, vaginitis **Azithromycin**—diarrhea, nausea, vomiting, vaginitis, rash, anorexia	**Ceftin**—toxic-epidermal necrolysis, anaphylaxis, and seizures **Azithromycin**—toxic-epidermal necrolysis, anaphylaxis, pancreatitis
Anticholinergic	Reduces muscle spasms in the bladder, lungs, intestines, and eye muscles (also known as an antispasmotic)	AtroPen (atropine sulfate) Ditropan (oxybutynin) Donnatal (scopolamine sulfate)	**Atropine**—Dry skin, dry mouth, nausea, headache, rash, blurred vision, ataxia, palpitations	**Atropine**—Anaphylaxis, severe bradycardia, heat stroke, death
Anticoagulant	Prevents or delays blood clotting	Coumadin (warfarin sodium) Dicumarol (heparin sodium) Lovenox (enoxaparin sodium)	**Heparin**—bleeding, thrombocytopenia, urticaria **Warfarin**—bleeding, abdominal complaints, fatigue, rash, cold intolerance, alopecia	**Heparin**—heparin induced thrombocytopenia and hemorrhage **Warfarin**—hemorrhage, gangrene, tissue necrosis, hypersensitivity, and anaphylaxis
Anticonvulsant	Prevents or relieves convulsions	Klonopin (clonazepam) Neurontin (gabapentin) Tegretol (carbamazepine)	**Carbamazepine**—dizziness, nausea, vomiting, hypertension, tremor, dry skin	**Carbamazepine**—Suicidality, toxic epidermal necrolysis, arrhythmia, pancytopenia
Antidepressant	Prevents or relieves symptoms of depression	Celexa (citalopram) Effexor XR (venlafaxine) Wellbutrin-SR (bupropion)	**Citalopram**—nausea, ejaculatory dysfunction, diaphoresis, tremor, insomnia	**Citalopram**—suicidality, mania, serotonin syndrome, hyponatremia
Antidiabetic	Helps to lower blood glucose levels	*Oral hypoglycemics*: Actos (pioglitazone), Glucophage (metformin), Micronase (glyburide) *Forms of insulin*: Humulin R (short acting) Humulin N (long acting)	**Metformin**—diarrhea, nausea, vomiting, flatus, ovulation, rash **Pioglitazone**—URI, headache, weight gain, fluid retention Injection site reaction, lipodystrophy, myalgia, pruritus, peripheral edema	**Metformin**—lactic acidosis, megaloblastic anemia **Pioglitazone**—hypoglycemia, heart failure, bladder cancer Severe hypoglycemia, hypokalemia, anaphylaxis
Antidiarrheal	Counteracts diarrhea	Kaopectate (kaolin/pectin) Pepto-Bismol (bismuth subsalicylate) Lomotil (diphenoxylate/atropine)	**Kaopectate**—black stool, black tongue, tinnitus **Lomotil**—nausea, vomiting, anorexia, euphoria, confusion, gingival hyperplasia	**Kaopectate**—Reye's syndrome **Lomotil**—respiratory depression, ileus, pancreatitis, toxic megacolon, angioedema
Antiemetic	Counteracts nausea and vomiting	Compazine (prochlorperazine) Dramamine (dimenhydrinate) Phenergan (promethazine) Zofran (ondansetron)	**Compazine**—drowsiness, galactorrhea, abnormal glucose, ejaculatory dysfunction **Zofran**—headache, constipation, fatigue, dizziness, pruritus	**Compazine**—blood dyscrasias, thrombocytopenic purpura **Zofran**—urinary retention, hypersensitivity
Antiflatulant	Relieves gas and bloating in the GI tract	Gas-X (simethicone) Mylicon—infant drops	**Gas-X**—Diarrhea, nausea	None reported

continues

Table 30-1 Drug Classifications and Their Actions *(continued)*

Classification	Indication for Use/ Desired Effect	Examples	Side Effects	Adverse Effects
Antifungal	Kills or prevents the growth of fungi and yeast	Diflucan (fluconazole) Monistat (miconazole) Nizoral (ketoconazole)	**Diflucan**—abdominal complaints, rash, taste changes **Nizoral**—abdominal complaints, rash, pruritus, headache, fatigue	**Diflucan**—hepatotoxicity, seizures and anaphylaxis **Nizoral**—hepatotoxicity, adrenal insufficiency, anaphylaxis, leukopenia, thrombocytopenia
Antigout agent	Prevents or lessens the occurrence of gout attacks	Benemid (probenecid) Zyloprim (allopurinol) Colcrys (colchicine) Uloric (febuxostat)	**allopurinol**—rash, abdominal complaints and gout exacerbation **Uloric**—LFT elevation, gout exacerbation	**allopurinol**—hypersensitivity, toxic epidermal necrolysis, alopecia **Uloric**—stroke, myocardial infarction, and hepatotoxicity
Antihistamine	Counteracts the effects of histamine in the body; helps to relieve symptoms of allergic reactions	Allegra (fexofenadine) Benadryl (diphenhydramine) Claritin (loratidine) Zyrtec (centirizine)	**Benadryl**—CNS stimulation, urinary retention, double vision, blurred vision **Zyrtec**—drowsiness, appetite stimulation, diarrhea, dizziness, dry mucous membranes	**Benadryl**—anaphylaxis, toxic psychosis, labryinthitis, and seizures **Zyrtec**—bronchospasm, hepatotoxicity, syncope, and hypotension, thrombocytopenia
Antihyperlipidemic or cholesterol-lowering agent	Helps to decrease cholesterol or lipid levels	*Statin* Crestor (rosuvastatin Lipitor (atorvastatin calcium) Zocor (simvastatin) *Other* Zetia (ezetimibe) Niaspan (niacin)	**Crestor**—headache, myalgia, abdominal complaints, proteinuria, diabetes mellitus	**Crestor**—myopathy, hepatotoxicity, pancreatitis, angioedema
Antihypertensive	Reduces high blood pressure	*ACE Inhibitors* Accupril (quinapril) Altace (ramipril) Vasotec (enalapril) *Angiotensin receptor blockers (ARB)* telmisartan valsartan Cozaar (losartan) *Calcium Channel Blockers* Norvasc (amlodipine) Calan (verapamil) *Thiazides* chlorthalidone hydrochlorothiazide	**Lisinopril**—hypotension, cough, fatigue, dizziness, headache, hyperkalemia, **Amlodipine**—fatigue, flushing, abdominal complaints, swelling **Chlorthalidone**—hypokalemia, hyponatremia, hypotension	**Lisinopril**—anaphylaxis, arrhythmia, toxic epidermal necrolysis, angioedema, pancreatitis, fetal malformations **Amlodipine**—angina exacerbation, hepatitis, myocardial infarction **Chlorthalidone**—arrhythmia, necrotizing angiitis, and agranulocytosis
Antimanic	Treats manic disorders	Eskalith (lithium) Depakene (valproic acid) Depakote (divalproex) Abilify (aripiprazole) Geodon (ziprasidone)	**Valproic Acid**—Severe drowsiness, worsening seizures, unusual bleeding, and many others **Lithium**—muscle weakness, tremor, edema, anorexia, weight gain	**Valproic Acid**—Liver or pancreas problems, upper stomach pain, jaundice, and many others **Lithium**—coma, hyperparathyroidism, diabetes insipidus
Antimigraine	Relieves migraines	Imitrex (sumatriptan) Zomig (zolmitriptan)	**Zomig**—dizziness, abdominal complaints, dry mouth, chest discomfort, vertigo	**Zomig**—coronary vasospasm, myocardial infarction, severe hypertension, and stroke

Table 30-1 Drug Classifications and Their Actions *(continued)*

Classification	Indication for Use/ Desired Effect	Examples	Side Effects	Adverse Effects
Antineoplastic	Destroys or inhibits the growth of malignant cells	Cytoxan (cyclophosphamide) Myleran (busuflan) Taxol Onxol (paclitaxel) Paraplatin (carboplatin)	**General**—Pancytopenia, alopecia, abdominal complaints, joint pain, infection	**General**—Can shut down any organ system, arrhythmia, myocardial infarction, anaphylaxis, ischemic colitis, GI bleed, or obstruction
Antiparkinson's agent	Treats symptoms associated with Parkinson's disease	Sinemet (carbidopa/ levodopa) Requip (ropinirole) Mirapex (pramipexole) Zelapar, Eldepryl (selegiline)	**Sinemet**—UTI, dizziness, headache, dry mouth, hypotension, hallucinations, confusion, compulsive behaviors, depression	**Sinemet**—sudden sleep episodes, psychosis, GI bleed, melanoma, blood, arrhythmias, syncope, myocardial infarction
Antiprotozoal	Treats protozoal infections	Flagyl (metronidazole)	Abdominal complaints, metallic taste, dark red-brown urine	Seizures, aseptic meningitis, peripheral neuropathy, encephalopathy
Antipsychotic	Treats schizophrenia and other associated brain disorders	Haldol (haloperdol) Seroquel (quetiapine) Zyprexa (olanzapine)	**Haldol**—insomnia, weight changes, gynecomastia	**Haldol**—retinopathy, pneumonia, heat stroke, dystonia, hyperprexia
Antiretrovial	Treats HIV infections	Retrovir (zidovudine) Truvada (emtricitabine / tenofovir)	**Truvada**—gastrointestinal complaints, fatigue, abnormal dreams, depression, hypercholesterolemia	**Truvada**—hepatomegaly, hepatotoxicity, renal failure, osteomalacia, pancreatitis, autoimmune disorders
Antispasmotic	Relieves cramps or spasms of the stomach, intestines, and bladder	Bentyl (dicyclomine) Levsin (hyoscyamine) Donnatal (phenobarbital / hyoscyamine / atropine / scopolamine)	**Bentyl**—dry mouth, dry eye, dizziness, nausea, constipation, muscle weakness, palpitations	**Bentyl**—psychosis, hallucinations, delirium, anaphylaxis, heat stroke
Antitussive	Prevents or relieves cough	Benylin (cough syrup with codeine) Tessalon (benzonatate)	**Tessalon**—sedation, headache, itchy rash, abdominal complaints, rigors	**Tessalon**—hallucinations, hypersensitivity reaction
Antiulcer	Treats ulcers of the stomach and upper intestine	*Proton Pump Inhibitor (PPI)* Prevacid (lansoprazole) Priolsec (omeprazole) Protonix (pantoprazole) *Binds border* Carafate (sucralfate)	**Prilosec**—abdominal complaints, headache, B12 deficiency **Carafate**—constipation	**Prilosec**—anaphylaxis, hepatic impairment, renal failure, fractures **Carafate**—anaphylaxis, hyperglycemia
Antiviral	Works against a viral infection	Symmetrel (amantadine) Zovirax (acyclovir) Tamiflu (oseltamivir)	**Tamiflu**—abdominal complaints, nosebleed, ear complaints	**Tamiflu**—delirium, anaphylaxis, toxic epidermal necrolysis
Bone resorption inhibitor	Prevents and treats osteoporosis	Evista (raloxifene) Fosamax (alenfronate)	**Evista**—hot flashes, flu like symptoms, peripheral edema, depression, cough, insomnia **Fosamax**—abdominal and musculoskeletal complaints	**Evista**—DVT, PE, stroke **Fosamax**—dysphagia, GI ulcer or bleed, hypocalcemia, jaw osteonecrosis
Bronchodilator	Eases breathing by dilating the bronchial tubes	Atrovent (ipratropium) Combivent (ipratropium, albuterol) Proventil (albuterol)	**Proventil**—nervousness, tremor, tachycardia, headache, nausea	**Proventil**—hypersensitivity, hypertension, angina, cardiac arrest, arrhythmia

continues

Table 30-1 Drug Classifications and Their Actions *(continued)*

Classification	Indication for Use/ Desired Effect	Examples	Side Effects	Adverse Effects
Cardiac glycoside	Strengthens the heart muscle; treats congestive heart failure	Digitek (digitoxin) Lanoxin (digoxin)	**Lanoxin**—dizziness, abdominal complaints, visual changes, gynecomastia	**Lanoxin**—AV block, ventricular arrhythmia, hallucinations, intestinal ischemia, and necrosis
Central nervous stimulant	Treats attention-deficit/ hyperactivity disorder	Adderall (amphetamine-dextroamphetamine) Strattera (atomoxetine HCl)	Anorexia, dry skin, insomnia, abdominal complaints, libido changes, taste change, elevated BP	Dependency, depression, psychosis, Tourette syndrome, hypertension, myocardial infarction
Contraceptive	Prevents conception	*Injectable*: Depo Provera (medroxyprogesterone) *Oral*: Yasmin (ethinyl estradiol/ drospirenone)	**Depo Provera**—abnormal cycles, abdominal complaints, weight gain, hirsutism **Yasmin**—abdominal complaints, breast tenderness, elevated BP	**Depo Provera**—thromboembolism, hypertension, stroke, breast and ovarian cancer **Yasmin**—thromboembolism, stroke, hypertension, anaphylaxis
Corticosteroid	Treats inflammation	Cortone (cortisone) Flovent (fluticasone) Kenalog (triamcinolone)	**Cortone**—fluid retention, hypokalemia, hyperglycemia, BP elevation, abdominal complaints, skin atrophy, weight gain	**Cortone**—anaphylaxis, adrenal insufficiency, psychosis, Cushing syndrome, diabetes mellitus, GI bleed, tendon rupture
Cough expectorant	Liquefies mucus and promotes its removal	Robitussin (guaifenesin)	**Robitussin**—rash, vomiting, nausea	**Robitussin**—nephrolithiasis
Decongestant	Reduces nasal congestion and swelling	Afrin (oxymetazoline) Sudafed (pseudoephedrine)	**Sudafed**—insomnia, abdominal complaints, CNS stimulation, tachycardia, tremor	**Sudafed**—urinary retention, hypertension, arrhythmias
Diuretic	Increases the output of urine	Dyrenium (triamterene) Lasix (furosemide) Bumex (bumetanide)	**Lasix**—urinary frequency, dizziness, hypotension, electrolyte abnormalities	**Lasix**—severe electrolyte abnormalities, arrhythmia, ototoxicity, renal failure
Hemostatic	Assists in blood coagulation or clotting	vitamin K thrombin Lysteda Cyklokapron (tranexamic acid) DDAVP (desmopressin)	**Lysteda**—headache, URI, abdominal complaints, vision changes **DDAVP**—flushing, headache, rhinitis, abdominal complaints, cough, hypertension	**Lysteda**—anaphylaxis, thromboembolism, cerebral edema, seizures **DDAVP**—anaphylaxis, respiratory arrest, hyponatremia, water intoxication, seizures
Histamine (H2) receptor antagonist	Blocks all phases of gastric acid secretion	Tagamet (cimetidine) Zantac (ranitidine)	**Zantac**—headache, abdominal complaints, malaise, myalgia, dry skin and mouth, dizziness	**Zantac**—thrombocytopenia, hepatotoxicity, pneumonia
Hormone replacement	Replaces hormones that are diminished (menopausal symptoms, thyroid disorder, etc.)	Premarin (conjugated estrogen) Prempro (conjugated estrogen/progesterone)	**Prempro**—vaginal bleeding and spotting, abdominal complaints, libido changes, blood pressure elevation	**Prempro**—stroke, thromboembolism, anaphylaxis, erythema, ischemic colitis
Immunosuppressant	Suppresses the immune system (RA and transplant patients)	Neoral Dandimmune (cyclosporine) Prograf Hecoria FK506 (tacrolimus)	**Tacrolimus**—tremor, diarrhea, headache, infection, abdominal complaints, electrolyte disorders	**Tacrolimus**—immunosuppression, malignancy, toxic epidermal necrolysis, nephrotoxicity, diabetes mellitus

Table 30-1 Drug Classifications and Their Actions *(continued)*

Classification	Indication for Use/ Desired Effect	Examples	Side Effects	Adverse Effects
Laxative	Loosens stools and promotes normal bowel elimination	Metamucil (psyllium) Miralax (polyethylene glycol 3350) Dulcolax (disacodyl)	**Metamucil**—GI obstruction, diarrhea, constipation, bronchospasm **Dulcolax**—nausea, abdominal cramps, vomiting, diarrhea	**Metamucil**—none **Dulcolax**—electrolyte disturbances, cathartic colon
Miotic	Contracts pupils of the eyes	Miostat (carbachol intraocular) Pilopine HS (pilocarpine ophthalmic)	**Pilopine HS**—blurred vision, ciliary spasm, myopia	**Pilopine HS**—retinal detachment, lens opacification
Mydriatic	Dilates pupils of the eyes	AK-Dilate Neo-Synephrine (phenylephrine) Isopto Atropine (atropine ophthalmic)	**Isopto Atropine**—blurred vision, photophobia, IOP increased	**Isopto Atropine**—psychosis, seizures, arrhythmias, hypotension, respiratory depression, hallucinations
Muscle relaxant	Aids in relaxation of skeletal muscles	Flexeril (cyclobenzaprine) Robaxin (methocarbamol) Soma (carisoprodol)	**Flexeril**—drowsiness, dry mouth, dizziness, blurred vision, confusion	**Flexeril**—seizures, arrhthymia, myocardial infarction, heat stroke, anaphylaxis, psychosis
Nonsteroidal anti-inflammatory drug (NSAID)	Relieves mild to moderate fever, pain, and inflammation	Advil Motrin (ibuprofen) Bextra Naprosyn (naproxen) Celebrex (celecoxib)	Abdominal complaints, rash, LFT elevations, fluid retention	Renal failure, GI bleeding, myocardial infarction, stroke, hypertension, bronchospasm
Sedative, hypnotic, tranquilizer	Produces a calming effect; used to treat insomnia	Ambien (zolpidem) Lunesta (eszopiclone)	**Lunesta**—unpleasant taste, headache, somnolence	**Lunesta**—depression, suicidality, aggression, hallucinations, angioedema, dependency
Thrombolytic agents	Aids in dissolving blood clots that already exist	Activase (alteplase) Streptase (streptokinase)	**Activase**—bleeding	**Activase**—intracranial hemorrhage, stroke, arrhythmia, anaphylaxis
Vasodilator	Produces relaxation of blood vessels; lowers blood pressure	Natrecor (nesiritide) Nitrostat (nitroglycerin) Nesiritide	**Nitrostat**—headache, lightheadedness, dizziness, flushing, rash, hypotension	**Nitrostat**—syncope, paradoxical bradycardia, exfoliative dermatitis
Vasopressor	Produces constriction of blood vessels; elevates blood pressure and cardiac output	Intropin (dopamine) Levophed (norepinephrine)	**Levophed**—headache, anxiety, bradycardia, dyspnea	**Levophed**—severe hypertension, arrhythmia, asthma exacerbation, extravasation necrosis

Note: Drugs in the "Example" column that are capitalized indicate brand names. Drugs in parentheses and/or in lower case letters indicate generic names.

PHARMACODYNAMICS

The term **pharmacodynamics** refers to the study of the effects of drugs on living organisms. Drugs exert a forceful and specific action in the body by forming a bond to protein molecules or chemical groups found within a cell or on its surface. These bonding proteins or sites are referred to as **receptors**, each having a unique structural design. Receptors are normally activated by neurotransmitters or hormones (Figure 30-2a).

To bind correctly with cell receptors, drugs must have a similar or complementary chemical structure to that of its receptor. **Affinity** is a measurement of how tightly a drug attaches or binds to a receptor. This binding creates a signal for the cell to function or respond in a particular manner; the tighter the binding, the better the result.

Drugs that bind to receptors and affect cell response are referred to as **agonists** (Figure 30-2b), while drugs that prevent cell response are called **antagonists**

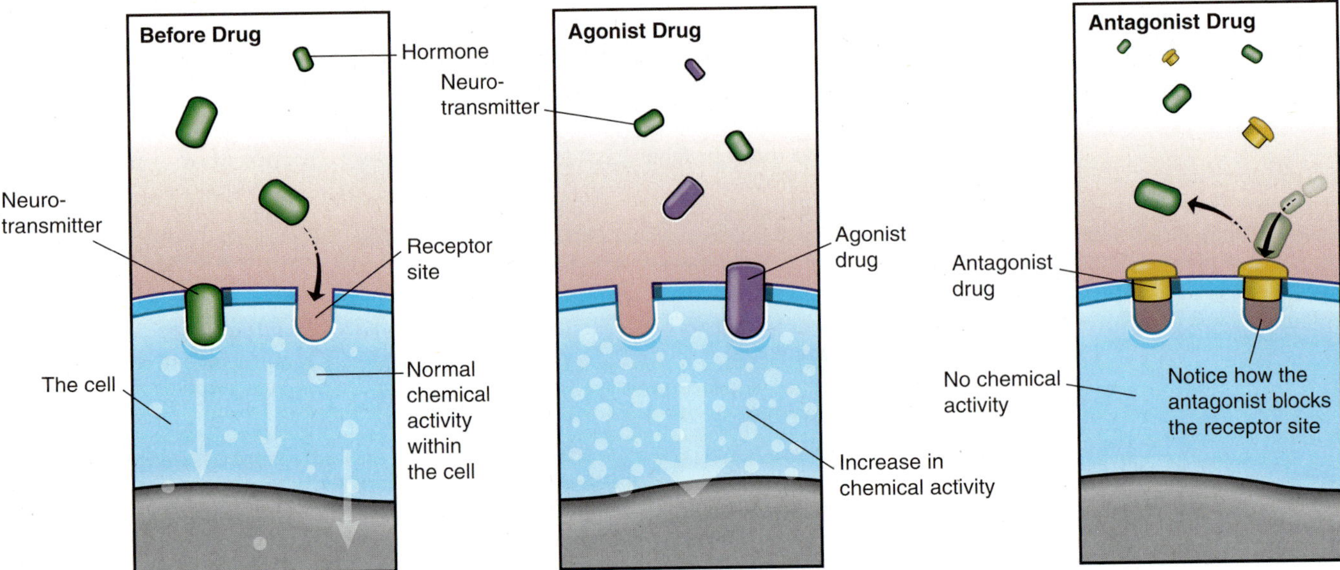

Figure 30-2a ■ The body's natural chemicals or neurotransmitters are specially designed to lock into the cell's receptor site, stimulating the cell to take a specific action.

Figure 30-2b ■ An agonist drug works with the body's natural chemicals by enhancing cellular activity.

Figure 30-2c ■ An antagonist drug works against the body's natural chemicals by blocking the cell's receptor site so that the neurotransmitters cannot get through.

(Figure 30-2c). Agonists mimic or enhance the action of the receptor, whereas antagonists block or inhibit the action of a receptor.

Albuterol is an example of a short-acting beta$_2$-agonist used in the treatment of acute asthma. Albuterol acts on the beta$_2$-adrenergic receptors, resulting in relaxation of muscles lining the airway, stimulating the bronchial tubes to dilate.

Zofran is an example of a serotonin antagonist. It works by blocking the effects of serotonin produced in the brain and stomach and helps to prevent nausea and vomiting in patients with nausea.

Dose Response

Drug manufacturers perform a proliferation of testing prior to a drug's distribution to determine its risk-to-benefit ratio. The manufacturer must also determine the drug's **therapeutic index**, or the range between the therapeutic dose of a drug and the dose at which the drug becomes toxic (Figure 30-3). Some drugs, such as non-opioid pain relievers, have what is referred to as a **drug ceiling**. A drug's ceiling is the maximum dose at which the drug will provide its greatest effect. Taking higher doses than those listed as the maximum dose on the drug's label will provide no further therapeutic value and in some cases may cause harm to organs such as the kidneys and liver. Opioid drugs such as morphine do not have a ceiling effect and are used in patients that are terminally ill or to manage patients who are in excruciating pain.

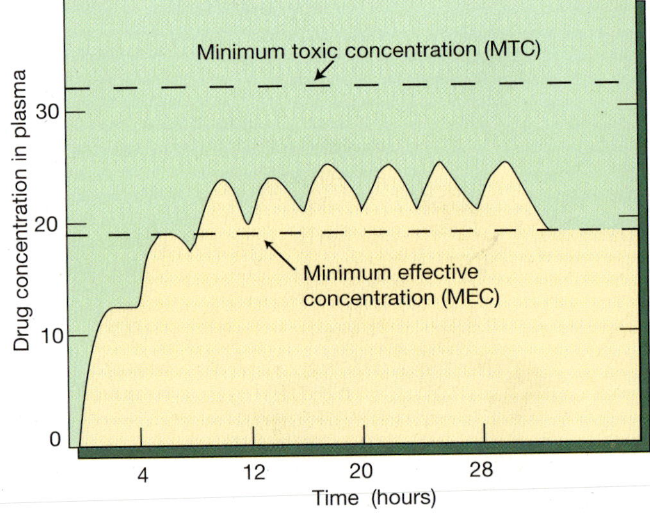

Figure 30-3 ■ Notice the separation between the therapeutic dose (minimum effective concentration) and the concentration of the drug at which the drug becomes toxic.

The effect that a drug will have at the site of action is directly related to the amount of the drug received and how it is administered. The **bioavailability** of a drug refers to the extent to and the rate at which the drug enters the blood plasma and is made available at the site of action. Figure 30-4a is an example of a dose–response curve, illustrating the bioavailability of a hypothetical drug (taken in oral form) and the point that the drug should reach its peak plasma level, or level of highest concentration. This example illustrates that the drug should start being released within minutes of consumption and should peak in concentration approximately 1.6 hours following consumption. All intravenous drugs have 100 percent bioavailability, meaning that the entire drug is automatically released into the bloodstream upon injecting into the vein and available at the site of action (Figure 30-4b). Notice how the drug's peak concentration occurs immediately following IV administration.

The bioavailability of oral medications may be influenced by acids and enzymes in the stomach, foods in the stomach, and any pathological conditions associated with organs of digestion. This process may take anywhere from several minutes to days depending on the drug's consistency when the drug is given by mouth. Generally speaking, the order in which drugs are absorbed within the digestive tract are as follows: solutions, suspensions, capsules, tablets, and coated tablets.

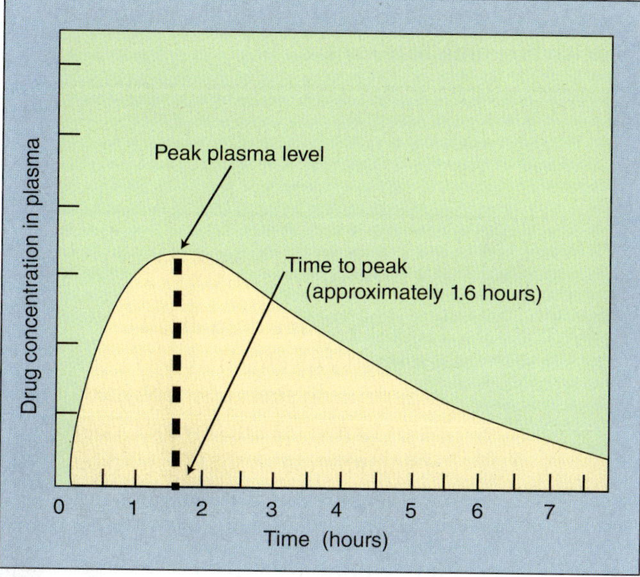

Figure 30-4a ■ The time it takes for the drug to reach its peak plasma level following oral ingestion of the drug.

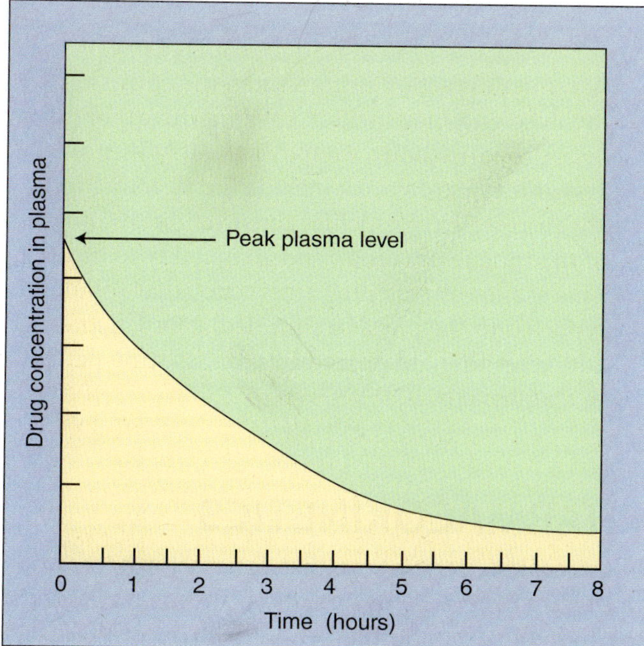

Figure 30-4b ■ The time it takes for the drug to reach its peak plasma level following single-bolus intravenous administration.

Once a drug reaches its therapeutic level within the blood plasma, the patient is able to reap its full benefits. To jump-start this process, the physician may choose to give the patient a loading or priming dose of the medication. In this scenario, the patient is initially given higher doses of medication than the usual maintenance dose. This practice assists in getting the drug to a therapeutic level in a quicker time frame. Once the drug reaches the therapeutic level in the blood plasma, the dose is tapered off to a standard maintenance dose.

Drug Actions

Drugs may be grouped by the type of action they produce in the body. Drug actions include the following:

- Local action: The drug acts on the area of tissue in which it is administered. Examples include topical medications applied to a joint to relieve pain or a local anesthetic injected into an area where a surgical procedure is going to be performed for numbing purposes.
- Remote action: The drug has an effect in a different location of the body than where it was administered, such as a nerve block (for instance, injecting analgesics and narcotics along the spine to block the pain of labor).
- Systemic action: The drug is absorbed into the bloodstream and carried to other parts of the body as with oral medications, injections, and suppositories. A large percentage of the drugs that are administered in ambulatory settings are systemic medications.

CRITICAL THINKING CHALLENGE

A patient calls and states that her headache is not subsiding after taking the maximum dose of Tylenol. The patient asks if it would be okay to take one more capsule.

1. Do drugs like Tylenol have a drug ceiling?
2. What are potential risks of taking a dose beyond the recommended maximum dose?
3. What might be an appropriate response to give to the patient?

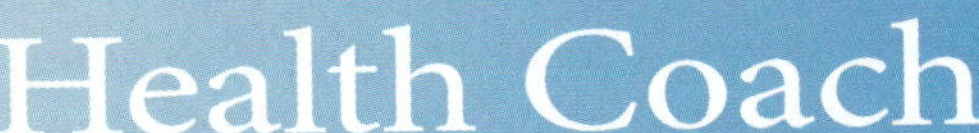

Health Coach

Therapeutic Index of Drugs

Patients taking drugs with a narrow therapeutic index must be continually monitored to make certain that the drug plasma levels are within the therapeutic range. Patients should receive education on the importance of taking drugs as directed and should be advised of the importance of routine drug monitoring. Drug blood plasma levels below the therapeutic range will prevent the patient from experiencing the drug's full benefits. Levels higher than the therapeutic range may cause significant organ damage. Examples of drugs that should be routinely monitored include: Digoxin, Phenobarbital, Theophylline, Lithium, Cyclosporin, and Ritonavir. Any critical lab values should be given to the physician for immediate review.

Drug Effects

While the primary effects of therapeutic drugs may be beneficial, other effects from particular drugs can be detrimental. The combination of various drugs, chemicals, or foods can change the effect that a drug has on the body.

Different effects that a drug may have in the body include the following:

- **Therapeutic effect**: The desired effect that a drug has on the body.
- **Side effect**: A secondary effect in addition to the therapeutic effect. Some side effects are therapeutic and end up becoming another use for the drug. However, most side effects are unpleasant and may even be harmful (these are often referred to as **adverse effects**). Harmful or even deadly side effects may be the result of an incorrect dosage and often occur at the beginning of treatment, when changes are made to the dose, or when the drug is discontinued.
- **Drug interaction**: This occurs when one drug diminishes or increases the effects of another drug. Many electronic health record (EHR) programs have drug interaction tools that flag the provider when there is a drug interaction between two or more drugs.
- Drug allergy: An allergy to a drug occurs when the body forms antibodies against specific chemicals in a drug, stimulating an allergic response. A less severe allergic reaction is referred to as a **local reaction**, such as occurs when the patient experiences pruritus (itching), edema (swelling), and erythema (redness) at the site at which the medication was administered.

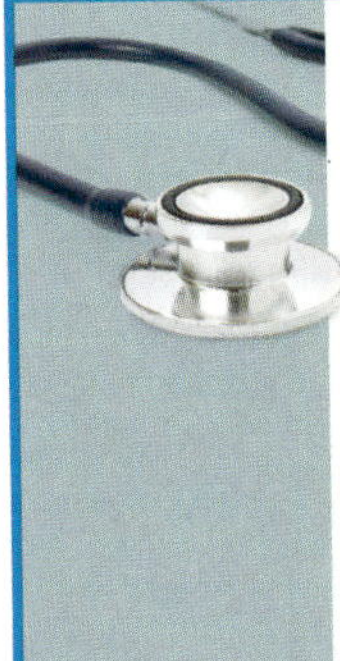

Field Smarts

Epinephrine is a drug that is commonly given to patients experiencing signs of anaphylaxis. It helps to reverse anaphylaxis. Epi-Pens or Epinephrine should be stocked in every room where medications are administered. Remember never to give a drug without an order from the physician. You can, however, draw up the medication.

A **systemic reaction** occurs when the entire body is involved and may include urticara (hives) or a rash over the entire body. **Anaphylaxis**, an advanced systemic reaction, may include the systemic signs above as well as bronchial constriction, swelling of the tongue or throat, and an inability to breathe. This is a life-threatening emergency that should be reported to the physician immediately. Chapter 33 addresses first aid procedures for assisting patients in anaphylaxis.

PHARMACOKINETICS

Pharmacokinetics is a term that describes how the body reacts to a drug, which depends on specific variables of the individual taking the drug, the form of the drug, the chemical composition of the drug, and the route or mode of administration.

Variables That Affect a Drug's Blood Plasma Level

Four processes that drugs go through after being administered into the body include the following:

1. Absorption: This is the process by which the drug passes into the body tissues or body fluids. This process depends on how the drug was administered, gastrointestinal function (when the drug is taken orally), and the chemical makeup of the drug.
2. Distribution: The process by which the drug is transported from the blood to the intended site of action.
3. Biotransformation: This is the process in which the drug is chemically altered and undergoes changes in order to be utilized as intended by the body. This process occurs in the liver for most drugs.
4. Elimination: The process by which the drug is excreted from the body. Numerous drugs are eliminated through the kidneys. Elimination can also occur through the gastrointestinal tract, the respiratory tract, the skin, the mucous membranes, or even the mammary glands.

The concentration of a single dose of an oral medication increases until the drug plasma level reaches its peak. As the drug is broken down and eliminated from the body, the drug plasma level declines, thus weakening its effects.

Factors That Affect Drug Actions

There are other factors that can affect the anticipated response that each patient may have to a drug. Table 30-2 lists and describes these factors.

DRUG NAMES

A single drug may have up to three names—chemical, generic, or brand:

- Chemical name: This is the name assigned to a drug that comes from its chemical formula. The chemical formula includes letters and numbers that illustrate the molecular structure of the compound. For example, $C_9H_8O_4N$ is the chemical formula for aspirin. The chemical name for aspirin is acetylsalicylic acid.
- Generic name: This is the drug's official name, which is assigned by the United States Adopted Names (USAN) Council. A generic drug contains the same ingredients as the trade drug but is

Table 30-2 Factors That Affect Drug Actions

Age	Newborns have immature body systems, whereas an elderly person's organs are diminishing in function. As drugs are metabolized differently in these special populations, patients and caregivers of patients should be educated on the importance of taking or administering medication as prescribed and symptoms or signs that could be an indicator for alarm in these special populations.
Body weight	Adult medications are calculated based on the average adult weight of 150 pounds. Pediatric medications are calculated based on body surface area or the child's weight. The physician will need to make adjustments in dosages to match the patient's specifications.
Compliance	If the patient does not take the drug in the manner in which it is intended, the patient will not receive the maximum benefits. Education is essential to promote compliance.
Disease	Patients may experience an adverse response to certain drugs if a disease has complicated their ability to absorb or excrete the drug properly. For example, patients with renal or liver disease may be unable to metabolize or excrete the medication properly. Chronic use of acetaminophen, ibuprofen, aspirin, antibiotics, steroids, and statin (anticholesterol) drugs may lead to kidney or liver failure.
Gender	Drugs may affect men and women differently due to muscle–fat ratios and the presence of certain hormones. Pregnant women have to be extremely cautious when taking medication to avoid damage to the developing fetus.
Idiosyncrasy	Some patients may react to a drug in an unusual manner; for example, a patient takes a tranquilizer to rest and feel less anxious but instead the opposite occurs.
Interactions from other drugs or foods	Sometimes interactions from other drugs or food can change the desired outcome of drug therapy. For example, the effects of oral hypoglycemics may be diminished when the patient takes both an oral hypoglycemic and specific types of diuretics. Female patients taking certain antibiotics or antifungals in combination with oral contraceptives may be at risk of becoming pregnant due to an interaction between the two.
Timing	The time of day that the drug is taken may have an impact on its effect. Gastric activity can affect the absorption of some drugs, so labels are placed on the medication bottle to instruct the patient when to take the drug (such as before or after meals). Drugs affecting the body's diurnal rhythms (day/night processes) should be given at times to match the body's natural responses. For instance, sedatives should be taken in the evening and stimulants should be taken at the beginning of the day.
Tolerance	Tolerance to a drug occurs when the body becomes overly adapted to the drug and fails to respond to the drug at the cellular level. Acquired tolerance occurs after taking a particular drug for an extended period of time.

usually much less expensive. The generic name of a drug will start with a lowercase letter, whereas the brand name will begin with a capital letter—for example, aspirin is the generic name for Bufferin, Ascriptin, and Ecotrin, and acetaminophen is the generic name for Tylenol. Generic drugs may be manufactured by more than one drug company, though each company produces the drug under its own unique brand or brand name (while keeping the generic name the same).

- Brand Name (AKA Proprietary Name): The exclusive name of a drug substance or drug product owned by a company under trademark law. Brand names of drugs include the following: Celebrex (celecoxib), Keflex (cephalexin), and Lasix (furosemide).

MEDICATION TASKS

In order to perform medication tasks, health care workers must be familiar with common terms used in medication tasking:

- **Prescribe**: To order a medication from the pharmacy, usually by prescription.
- **Dispense**: To personally hand the patient a medication to take later; in ambulatory care, drug samples and stock samples are commonly dispensed to patients.
- **Administer**: To prepare and personally give the patient a medication through any method, at the point of care.

Physicians are licensed to prescribe, dispense, and administer medications for their patients. Depending on the state, midlevel practitioners such as nurse practitioners and physician assistants may also participate in these tasks. The medical assistant cannot prescribe or order medications but *may be* able to dispense or administer certain types of medications or create or call in prescriptions with a direct order from the physician.

REGULATIONS AND LEGAL CLASSIFICATIONS OF DRUGS

For the safety of the consumer, the U.S. Food and Drug Administration (FDA) establishes standards for pharmaceutical companies to follow in the development and sale of prescribed and OTC medications.

Drug companies must gain FDA approval before their drugs can be sold to consumers. This process is lengthy and very costly. The approval process incorporates a variety of testing measures to ensure the quality and safety of the drug, including laboratory testing, animal testing, and human testing performed on volunteers. Upon FDA approval, exclusive production can be granted for seven years for orphan drugs, or five years for new chemicals of an existing drug class. The total length of the patent is 20 years after filing for the patent. After the initial copyright period has elapsed, the drug patent is released and other manufacturers may produce the drug under a different brand name.

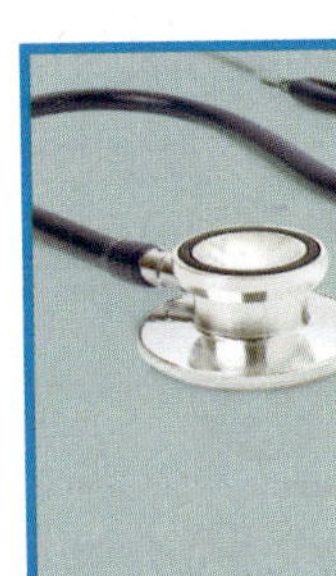

Field Smarts

Medication delegation rules will vary from one state to another. Always check the rules in the state in which you are employed before accepting medication orders from a midlevel practitioner.

Supplemental mineral products and other herbal supplements are not required to go through the same rigorous testing as other drugs. In many cases, the labeling information and packaging does not accurately depict the supplement's contents. To help ease the mind of consumers, some manufacturers voluntarily have these products tested at their own expense. The U.S. Pharmacopeia (USP) verified mark (Figure 30-5)

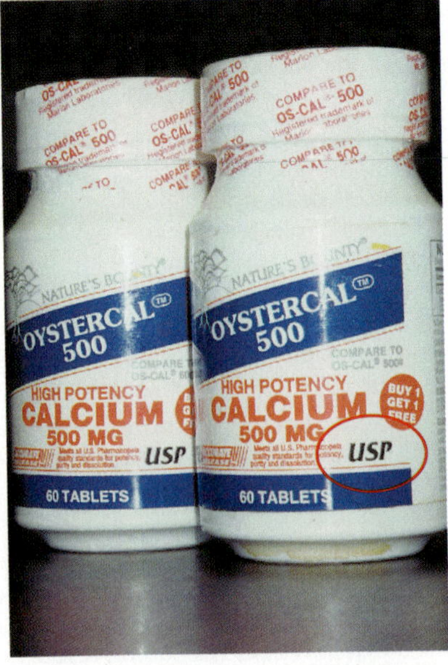

Figure 30-5 ■ The USP symbol assures consumers that products have been properly tested and that the contents on the inside of the container match the label information on the outside.

assures consumers that these products have been properly tested and that the products are safe. Encourage patients to look for this label when purchasing these products.

Controlled Substances

Providers that prescribe, dispense, or administer controlled substances must be registered with the U.S. Drug Enforcement Administration (DEA), a part of the Department of Justice. The DEA, established in 1973, is responsible for enforcing U.S. controlled substance laws and regulations.

The Controlled Substances Act (CSA) defines drugs or substances that may have the potential for illegal use or abuse. Based on CSA guidelines, controlled substances are divided into five schedules according to their addictive properties and degree of abuse. It is important to stay up to date with this schedule, as it is updated frequently. Table 30-3 lists each of the schedules, the drug's potential for abuse in that schedule, accepted medical uses of each of the drugs, and examples of drugs in each schedule.

To apply for a DEA number, the physician must complete and submit DEA Form 224, Application for Registration either online or by mail. This certificate is renewable every three years. Each DEA number is site specific so if the physician practices at more than one location, most likely he or she will need a separate DEA number for each location (this may vary when practicing at more than one location in the same area—check with the local DEA office). A physician's DEA number must be included on any prescription for a controlled substance.

Storage of Controlled Substances

Controlled substance labels include a large "C" followed by the Schedule classification (Figure 30-6). All controlled substances should be kept separate from other drugs and must be stored in a secure cabinet or drawer. Medical facilities that house large amounts of Schedule II drugs, or that are located in high crime areas, usually have more stringent storage specifications, such as storing the drugs in a floor safe or a steel container affixed to a cabinet or wall (Figure 30-7). Further security measures may include an alarm system, security cameras, and the appointment of a security manager. All prescription pads and order blanks for controlled substances should also be securely locked away. Only a minimal number of staff members (usually the physician and/or supervisor) should have keys to cabinets containing these items.

Recordkeeping Requirements of Controlled Substances

The DEA requires that a full inventory of all controlled substances be completed every two years. Records

Table 30-3 Controlled Substances Schedule

Schedule and Classification Listing on Label	Potential for Abuse	Accepted Medical Uses	Examples
Schedule I C-I on label	High potential for abuse; there is a lack of accepted safety for use under medical supervision	Not accepted for medical use within the United States; may be used for research under certain conditions	acetorphine, etorphine, heroin, myophine
Schedule II C-II on label	High potential for abuse; abuse may lead to severe psychological or physical dependence	Accepted medical use within the United States but with severe restrictions	codeine, Dilaudid, methadone, morphine, nembutal, oxycodone, percodan, Ritalin
Schedule III C-III on label	Potential for abuse but less than first two schedules; may lead to low to moderate physical dependence, or moderate to high psychological dependence	Accepted medical use within the United States	barbituric acid, Codeine with aspirin, dronabinol in sesame oil, ketamine, Talbutal, Testosterone
Schedule IV C-IV on label	Low potential for abuse compared to drugs in schedule III; may lead to limited physical or psychological dependence	Accepted medical use within the United States	Buspar, Chloral hydrate, Darvon, diazepam, Librium, Valium, Xanax
Schedule V C-V on label	Low potential for abuse compared to drugs in schedule IV; may lead to limited physical or psychological dependence	Accepted medical use within the United States	Motofen, Kapectolin PG, Robitussin A-C (with Codeine)

Note: Tradenames are capitalized; generic names are lowercased. Prescription refill information for drugs in each schedule can be found in Table 30-4.

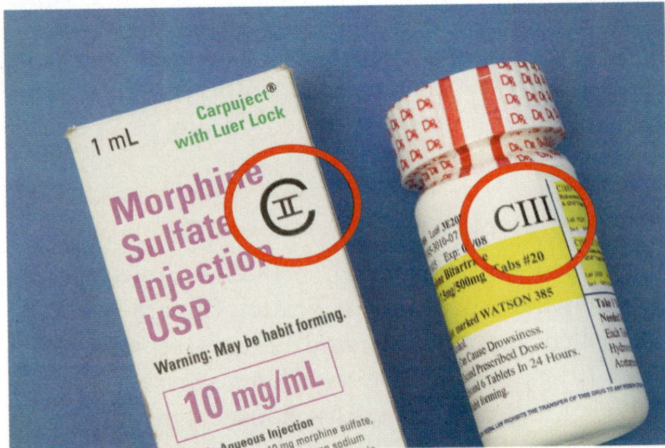

Figure 30-6 ■ Notice the Roman numeral beside the C. This indicates that the medication is a controlled drug.

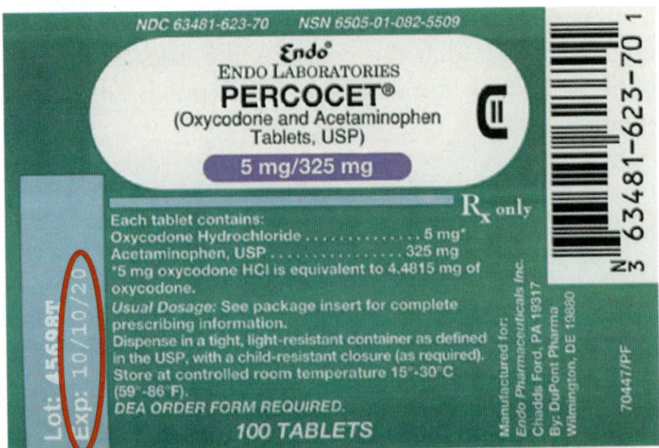

Figure 30-8 ■ Notice the location of the expiration date.

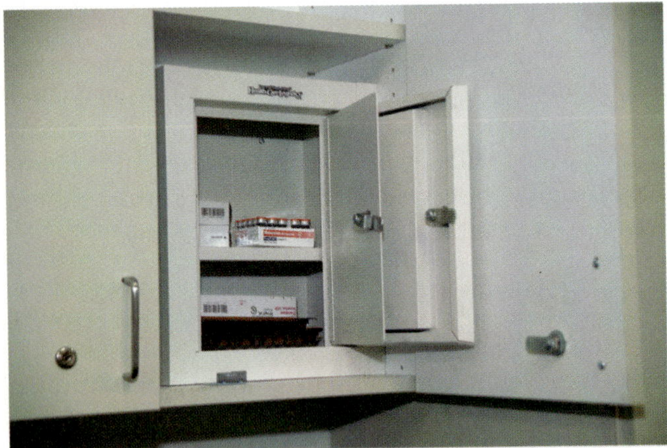

Figure 30-7 ■ Controlled substances should be double-locked for extra protection.

from that inventory must be kept for a minimum of two years. A minimum of monthly inventories should be performed with additional inventories every shift in which staff has access, and witnesses should be present.

Any time controlled substances are received, dispensed, or administered, they should be recorded in a special log. New shipments should be witnessed by at least two other persons. Inventory records of controlled substances should be stored securely in a safe or locked cabinet.

Proper Disposal of Both Controlled and Noncontrolled Drugs

Drugs should never be used past their expiration date. When the expiration date (Figure 30-8) has been reached, the medications must be removed from the current drug inventory and disposed of in a proper manner. Drugs should always be removed from their original containers prior to disposal to keep others from using them. Solids, such as tablets and capsules, should be placed in sealable plastic bags with a little water to assist in dissolving. The bags should be sealed and discarded in regular trash. Liquid substances should be mixed in plastic sealable bags with items such as coffee grounds, cat litter, or absorbent paper towels and sealed closed before discarding in the trash. Drugs should not be flushed down a drain or toilet unless instructions on the label advise to do so. Some offices place expired medications in the biohazardous trash or take them to a pharmaceutical take-back location that disposes of expired medications in an appropriate manner.

Before disposing of controlled substances, the registrant (physician) or agent for the registrant (office supervisor) should complete and submit DEA Form 41, Registrants Inventory of Drugs Surrendered, and wait for instructions from the DEA to proceed. The DEA will send the form back with instructions on what to do. Once the office has disposed of the drug per the DEA instructions, the original and two copies of the DEA form should be sent back to the DEA office and a copy should be kept for the office. There are a variety of responses that the DEA may send, such as disposing of the substance in front of two other witnesses, mailing the substance to the DEA office, or having a DEA agent present during the disposal. Disposal records should be kept for a minimum of two years. The practice may use the services of a reverse distributor (a company authorized to accept and destroy all types of expired drugs for a fee) to dispose of these drugs.

If a controlled substance spills or breaks in the container in which it is stored and is not recoverable, the registrant must document the incident in the inventory record. When possible, two individuals who witnessed the breakage should sign the inventory records indicating what they witnessed.

EHR Application

Many EHR programs house medication logs within the EHR software (Figure 30-9). Individual patients should have a medication log stored within their personal electronic chart. The software may also include a global log that tracks vaccines and narcotics given to the entire patient population. Global logs provide tracking information that is useful when there is a problem with a particular lot number of medication. These logs can also provide statistical data that identifies the prescribing activities of individual physicians.

THE MEDICATION ORDER OR PRESCRIPTION WRITING

The prescription is a written legal document that lists compounding, dispensing, and administering instructions for particular medications. The prescription can be broken down into nine different sections. Figure 30-10 shows an example of a prescription and lists and defines the different parts of a prescription.

Written prescriptions must be written in permanent black ink. Prescriptions may be given directly to the patient, sent to the pharmacy in digital format, faxed to the pharmacy, or called into the pharmacy. All handwritten prescriptions must be signed by the physician. Electronic prescriptions must include the physician's digital signature to verify that the prescription is authentic. Providers participating in governmental

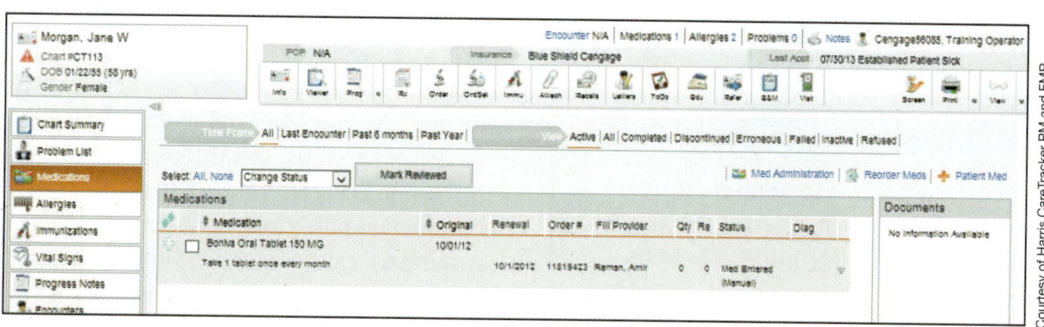

Courtesy of Harris CareTracker PM and EMR

Figure 30-9 ■ An example of a medication log in Harris CareTracker.

Parts of a Prescription

1. The physician's name, address, telephone number, and DEA number.
2. The patient's name, address, and the date on which the prescription is written.
3. The *superscription* that includes the symbol Rx ("take thou").
4. The *inscription* that states the names and quantities of ingredients to be included in the medication.
5. The *subscription* that gives directions to the pharmacist for filling the prescription.
6. The *signature* (Sig) that gives the directions for the patient.
7. The physician's signature blanks. Where signed, indicates if a generic substitute is allowed or if the medication is to be dispensed as written.
8. REPETATUR 0 1 2 3 PRN. This is where the physician indicates whether or not the prescription can be refilled.
9. LABEL. Direction to the pharmacist to label the medication appropriately.

L&K **LEWIS & KING**
2501 CENTER STREET
NORTHBOROUGH, OH 12345
(614) 555-1124

Name *Juanita Hansen*
Address *143 Gregory Lane, Apt. 43* Date *4/7/XX*
℞ *Northborough, OH 12345*
Furadantin 50 mg Tabs
#56
Sig 1 tab p.o. q.i.d X14 days

Generic Substitution Allowed *Susan Rice* M.D.
Dispense As Written ______ M.D.
REPETATUR (0) 1 2 3 PRN
☑ LABEL

Figure 30-10 ■ All prescriptions should have a minimum of the nine sections shown here.

reimbursement programs like Medicare are required to create prescriptions electronically or receive penalties in reimbursement.

The role of the medical assistant regarding prescription tasks will vary according to state law and office policy, but may include the following:

- Writing prescriptions under the direction of the physician for medications that are nonscheduled or that are listed in Schedules III–V
- Calling in prescriptions to pharmacies under the direction of the physician for medications that are nonscheduled or listed in Schedules III–V
- Faxing prescriptions under the direction of the physician to the pharmacy
- Creating prescriptions in the EHR under the direction of the physician
- Providing patients with instruction on how to properly take their medications and what side effects to look for

EHR Application

In order for medical assistants to enter medication orders into the electronic health record, they must be credentialed. This meets the Stage 2 Meaningful Use Computerized Provider Order Entry (CPOE) requirements. To learn more about CPOE requirements refer to Chapter 3.

Prescription Abbreviations

The use of standard medical abbreviations is greatly discouraged when performing clinical documentation. This is especially true when writing orders in a patient's chart. A vast number of injuries and deaths have been associated with the use of abbreviations. As a result, some health care organizations are banning the use of all abbreviations in regards to clinical documentation, while other organizations are only banning abbreviations that are considered dangerous.

The Joint Commission's 2004 "Do Not Use" list of abbreviations was part of a larger initiative, National Patient Safety Goals, designed to keep patients safe. This list features several abbreviations that are considered dangerous and are not permitted when performing clinical documentation in organizations accredited by the Joint Commission, such as hospitals, clinics, and skilled nursing centers. Many other health care accrediting organizations are instituting the "Do Not Use" list as part of their standards as well.

Appendix A provides a listing of common abbreviations that are still used in many medical organizations. Refer to the Joint Commission's website for a full listing of the "Do Not Use" list of abbreviations.

Procedure 30-1 lists steps for writing a prescription; however, keep in mind that the majority of offices are completely paperless, meaning that all prescriptions are generated electronically. When creating prescriptions in the EHR, the medical assistant will just click on the prescription writer and follow the prompts. Refer to Figure 30-11 for a sample of a medication order management screen from Harris CareTracker. Information

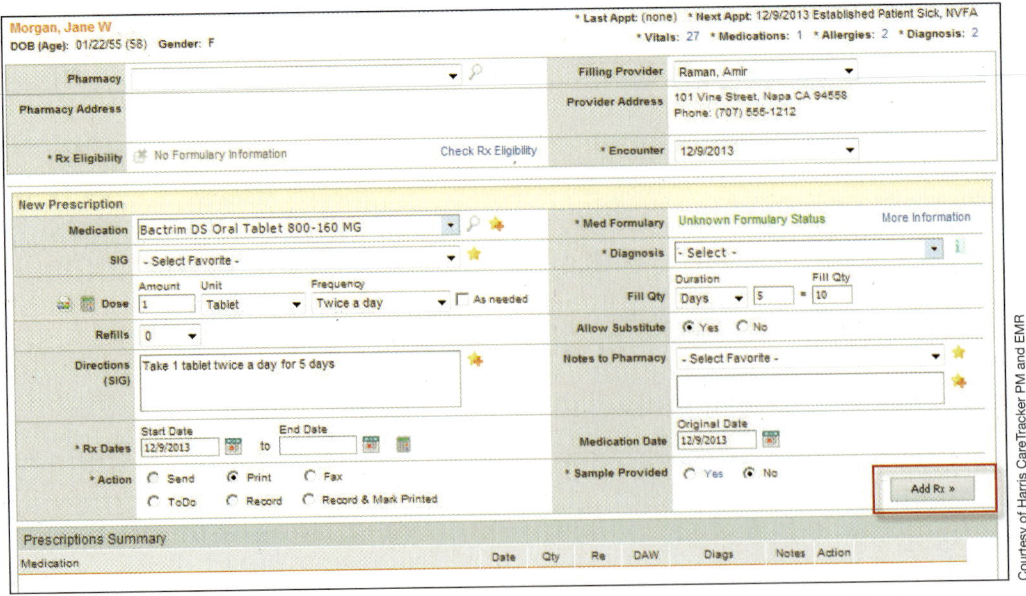

Courtesy of Harris CareTracker PM and EMR

Figure 30-11 ■ An example of a medication order management screen in Harris CareTracker.

for documenting prescriptions within the patient's chart can be found in Chapter 4.

Rules for Creating Prescriptions for Controlled Substances

Medical assistants must be familiar with rules and guidelines associated with their particular state and office when it comes to creating or calling in prescriptions for controlled substances. Information that should be included when writing or calling in prescriptions for controlled substances is similar to those for noncontrolled substances but with a few inclusions. Table 30-4 lists rules for prescriptions for controlled substances.

Tamper-Resistant Prescription Pads

Federal law requires prescriptions for controlled substances (Schedule II) to be written on specialized tamper-resistant prescription pads and signed in ink on the day issued. Examples of required tamper-resistant

Table 30-4 Rules for Prescriptions for Controlled Substances

All controlled substances	The form must include the physician's DEA number. The amount must be written out (six rather than 6) or combined [six (6)]. The amount prescribed is usually limited to smaller quantities than noncontrolled substances. Many states require controlled substance orders to be written on a special security tamper-resistant prescription pad.
Schedule II	Except in emergencies, drugs in this schedule must be both handwritten and signed by the physician in permanent ink (many states also require prescription orders to be written on a special tamper-resistant pad). The physician may call in an order for schedule II drugs for emergency purposes, but only for the amount of the drugs necessary to get through the emergency. The pharmacy must receive a written prescription within seven days following a phone order from this schedule. Some states require the diagnosis to appear on the prescription for certain categories of drugs within this schedule. Currently, *no refills are permissible in any state;* however, some states allow physicians to write one prescription for a 60- or 90-day supply under special circumstances. Medical assistants may not create or call in a prescription for drugs in this schedule under any circumstance.
Schedules III–V	Orders may be computer generated, handwritten, or given over the phone. The required use of tamper-resistant prescription pads varies according to state and federal guidelines. May be refilled up to five times within a six-month period. There may be some variances with Schedule V drugs depending on the state. Some Schedule V drugs can be dispensed by a pharmacy without a prescription. Orders may be written in 30-, 60-, or 90-day increments. Many states will allow the medical assistant to call in these drugs, but the state's pharmacy statutes should be checked.

Health Coach

Prescription Medications

Patients should receive the following instructions regarding prescription medications:

- Take medication as directed by the physician.
- Take all of the medication for the length of time prescribed.
- Do not stop taking the medication(s) without consulting the physician first.
- Inform the physician of any unusual or adverse effects from taking the medications.
- Do not combine OTC medications or herbal supplements without notifying the physician.
- Do not take someone else's medication or give the medication to someone else.
- Store all medications away from children.
- Properly discard unused medications.
- Follow all warning labels on the medication container.
- Check the medication storage area at home regularly for expired or unused drugs and properly dispose of them.

CRITICAL THINKING CHALLENGE

A busy physician leaves an order for you to write prescriptions for two separate patients. One of the patients' needs a prescription for Valium and the other patient needs a prescription for Percodan. Using a drug reference book, check to see which schedule these drugs fall under.

1. **Is the medical assistant able to write prescriptions for these two drugs?**
2. **If not, explain why. Does a special prescription pad need to be used for either of these prescriptions?**

features in the state of California include the following: (i) the prescription paper must be both heat and chemically sensitive, (ii) the paper must have anti-copy features that cause the word "void" to appear if someone tries to make a copy of the prescription, (iii) the opaque Rx symbol must disappear if someone tries to lighten the form, and (iv) a warning band describing the form's security features must be printed on the prescription. California also requires a statement, "Prescription is void if the number of drugs prescribed is not noted," with a line allowing physicians to write in the number. These prescription pads can only be ordered from state-approved vendors that use security printers to create the pads. Other states also require tamper-resistant pads, but most states do not yet require all of the features that California requires.

DRUG RESOURCES

There are a number of resources and reference books available that provide helpful information about particular drugs. These resources and reference books are updated periodically to provide the most current drug listings and information. Common resources include the *Physicians' Desk Reference*, the *U.S. Pharmacopeia/National Formulary*, drug package inserts, nursing drug books, and drug-related websites.

The Physicians' Desk Reference

The *Physicians' Desk Reference* (*PDR*) is published every year by PDR, LLC. This reference is one of the most popular drug reference guides and is commonly found in physicians' offices, hospitals, and specialty clinics. Many providers now have access to the most current information via mobile PDR (downloadable on moble devices) and PDR.net. The *PDR* is divided into color-coded sections. Table 30-5 lists each of those sections and includes a description of each.

There are additional reference tables in the PDR, including poison antidotes, drugs that should not be crushed, and drugs excreted in breast milk.

Table 30-5 *PDR* Sections

Section	Page Color	Section Title	Content Description
1	White	Manufacturers' Index	This section lists pharmaceutical manufacturers in alphabetical order along with the name and address of each manufacturer. A list of drugs supplied by each manufacturer and page numbers that elaborate on each drug are also included in this section.
2	Pink	Brand and Generic Name Index	This section lists drugs in alphabetical order by both generic and brand name, followed by two sets of page numbers. The first number indicates the page on which a picture of the drug can be found, and the second number indicates the page on which product information can be found. This is a great starting place when looking up drug information.
3	Blue	Product Category Index	This section divides drugs alphabetically into categories by classification. This section gives the reader an opportunity to compare similar drugs made by different manufacturers.
4	Gray	Product Identification Guide	This section provides full-color (*actual size*) photographs of the tablets and capsules of those included in the *PDR* and is arranged alphabetically by manufacturer. This section can be used when the patient knows what the pill looks like, but doesn't know the name of the drug.
5	White	Product Information	This is the main section of the book. It includes product information arranged alphabetically by manufacturer. The information in this section comes directly from the package insert and includes the following information about the drug: description, clinical pharmacology, indications, contraindications, warnings, precautions, adverse reactions, dosage and administration, and how the drug is supplied.
6	White	Dietary Supplement Information	This section presents information on herbal preparations and nutritional supplements. Listings are arranged alphabetically by manufacturer.

U.S. Pharmacopeia/National Formulary

The *U.S. Pharmacopeia/National Formulary (USP/NF)* is considered the official book of drug standards. It contains standards for all medications, dietary supplements, and medical devices. It also contains a national formulary of all drugs that have been approved for use in the United States. The *USP/NF* is published every five years and includes drugs that have been tested and certified that meet specific standards of quality, purity, and potency. It is used most often by pharmaceutical companies, research laboratories, and companies that manufacture medical devices. It is occasionally used by providers.

Drug Product Package Inserts

Drug product inserts are included in every packaged medication. This insert describes all significant aspects of the drug, such as the chemical name, generic name, recommended dosage, and dosage intervals. The information provided may also include findings of clinical studies and possible side effects of the drug throughout the drug studies.

Drug Resources on the Internet and E-versions of Drug References

Many health care professionals have come to rely on the Internet for reviewing drug listings and finding the most current drug information available. Pharmaceutical company websites provide product information, and a variety of other websites developed for health advocacy have wonderful resources as well. Many health care professionals prefer to download drug reference books to their phones and other mobile devices. There is usually a fee associated with this download, while others are free.

SAFE DRUG ADMINISTRATION

Medication preparation and administration should take place in a well-lit area. The medical assistant should avoid becoming distracted while preparing medications to reduce the risks of medication errors. Drugs should always be checked to make certain that they have not yet reached their expiration date and that they have been stored correctly to ensure drug effectiveness. Many drugs can be stored at room temperature; however, some drugs must be stored in a refrigerator or freezer.

Seven Rights of Drug Administration

The medical assistant should have a complete understanding regarding a drug's use, dosage, how it is to be given, and common side effects. Patient safety is further promoted by following the *Seven Rights of Drug Administration:*

1. The *Right Patient*: Verify the patient's name with the chart and confirm it is the right patient by using another identifier such as the patient's date of birth or last four digits of the patient's social security number (the National Patient Safety Goals requires the use of two identifiers).
2. The *Right Drug*: Check the label a minimum of three times to confirm that it is the right drug and the right strength by comparing the physician's written order against the drug label. Read the drug label when:
   - Removing the medication from the storage area
   - Preparing the medication
   - Placing the medication back into the storage area or before discarding the used container
3. The *Right Dose*: If necessary, perform the proper calculations to determine the correct dosage to be given. Refer to Chapter 32 for examples of dosage calculations.
4. The *Right Route*: Check the drug order to ensure that the route of administration is the correct route for the drug being given and for the patient receiving the drug.
5. The *Right Time*: This is usually not a factor in ambulatory health centers because drugs are normally administered at the time they are ordered, but always read the order for clarification.
6. The *Right Technique*: Learning the procedures for proper drug administration will assist the medical assistant in knowing how to administer the medications. When in doubt, check the drug insert or ask the physician for clarification.
7. The *Right Documentation*: Giving the medication is only half of the procedure; the other half is documentation.

Most EHR programs include templates that can be used for entering drug information. Items such as expiration dates, route, manufacturer's name, etc. automatically populate once you enter the medication's lot number. Reports for any lot number can easily be generated which eliminates the need for separate logs. Figure 30-12 shows an example of an electronic medication entry screen within an EHR. Refer to Chapter 4 for information that must be documented in medication entries.

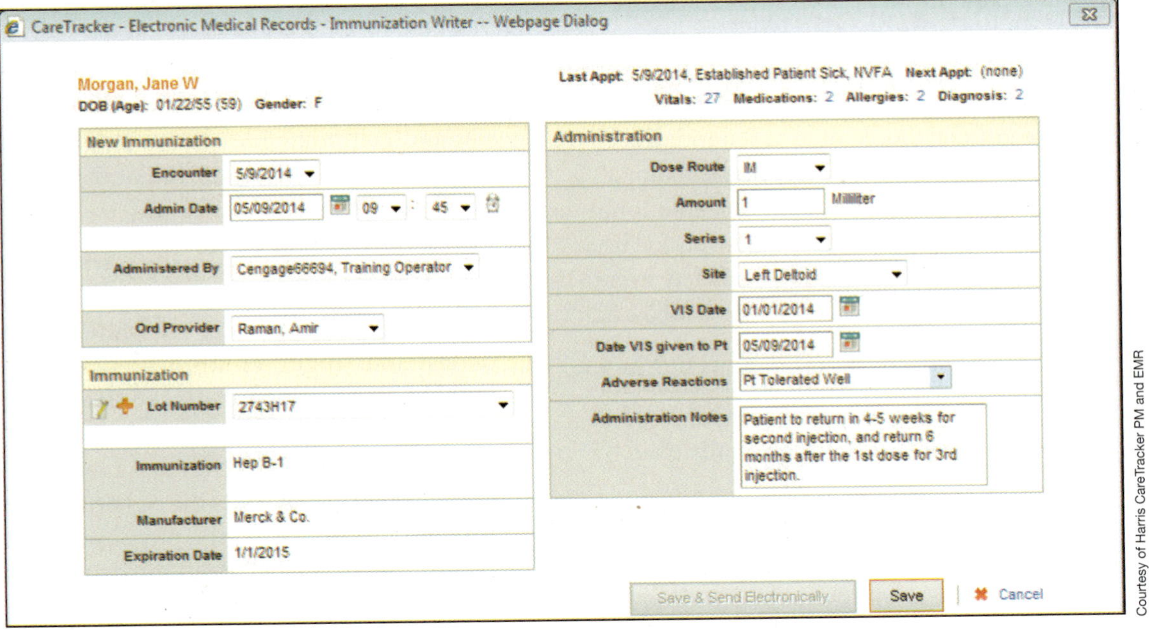

Courtesy of Harris CareTracker PM and EMR

Figure 30-12 ■ An example of a medication entry screen in Harris CareTracker.

Always have the patient wait 20 to 30 minutes following drug administration. This is the usual time period in which anaphylactic reactions occur. Signs of anaphylaxis and treatment steps for treating anaphylaxis can be found in Chapter 33.

Safety and Continuity during Medication Administration

"PAD" is an acronym that can be used during the drug administration process. It stands for "Preparation, Administration, and Documentation," which is the chain of events that should be performed by only *one person* during medication administration. Errors during any step of the process can lead to serious consequences for the patient.

- Preparation: Never allow another person to prepare a medication that you are going to administer. You cannot guarantee that the medication was prepared properly.
- Administration: Never allow another person to administer a medication that you prepare. If an error occurs during administration, you may be held accountable should an adverse event occur.
- Documentation: Following preparation and administration, you need to make certain that documentation is correct and complete. Never have someone else document for you. Remember the adage, "If you didn't document it, you didn't do it!"

Field Smarts

The latest National Patient Safety Goals state that drugs that look-alike/sound-alike (LASA) should be stored separately from one another. Drug alert stickers can be purchased to place on shelves that store LASA products. Health care personnel may also consider highlighting the part of the drug that is different, such as hydr-OXY-zine and hydr-ALA-zine.

Reporting Medication Errors

Medication errors can occur at any time and the medical assistant must know how to respond in the event an error should occur. It is important to understand the reasons why the medication error occurred and to thoroughly evaluate the incident to ensure that the error is not repeated. Some of the most common reasons medication errors occur are the following:

- Not reading the label carefully.
- Confusing a drug with another that is spelled almost the same or sounds almost the same.

- Not calculating the dosage correctly.
- Trying to multitask while preparing a medication.

If a medication error occurs, there are specific steps that must be followed:

- Recognize that an error has occurred: *Never* try to conceal a drug error. It could be fatal for a patient.
- Remain calm: Panic may delay the appropriate treatment.
- Notify the physician *stat:* Calmly and discretely provide the necessary details.
- Assess the patient for any reaction to the medication: Review the patient's vital signs and look for any other signs of distress.
- Respond appropriately to the physician's orders.
- Document the error in the patient's medical chart and complete an incident report.

ROUTES OF MEDICATION ADMINISTRATION

There are two major routes by which drugs can be administered: enteral and parenteral. The term **enteral** means pertaining to the alimentary canal or intestines. Medications that pass through any structures within the alimentary canal may be considered enteral medications and include the following specific routes: oral, buccal, sublingual, and rectal. (Buccal, rectal, and sublingual routes *may also* be considered submucosal routes because they pass through a mucus membrane within the alimentary canal to get into the blood stream.) Nasogastric tubes (NG) and gastric tubes may be used to deliver enteral medications in patients unable to take medications orally.

Parenteral means pertaining to beside or outside of the intestines. Parenteral medications include any drugs delivered by a method other than through the digestive tract, including topical, transdermal, mucosal, inhalation, injectable, and intravenous. The most common parenteral medications are administered by injection. See Chapter 32 for procedures relating to administering injections and intravenous medications.

The route that is used to deliver the medication is determined by several factors, including the manufacturer's recommendations, the physician's preference, and special requests from the patient. Some drugs can only be given through one route due to the chemical composition of the drug or because the drug can be caustic or toxic when given through other routes.

Enteral Routes

Again, enteral medications pertain to medications that pass through any organs of digestion. Enteral routes used in ambulatory care are usually limited to the oral and rectal routes.

Oral Medications

Oral medications come in a variety of different forms and should only be given to conscious patients who can swallow without difficulty. Table 30-6 lists information regarding oral medications that are in solid forms.

Oral medications commonly travel through the digestive tract, where they are digested and absorbed in the stomach or intestines. Other medications are taken into the oral cavity but do not travel through the digestive tract. **Buccal** medications are placed between the gums of the upper molars and the inside cheek (Figure 30-13) where they are rapidly absorbed through vasculature within the mucus membranes. **Sublingual** medications are placed under the tongue (Figure 30-14) and also provide rapid absorption into the bloodstream. Nitroglycerine is an example of a drug that is given sublingually. Buccal and sublingual medications should not be swallowed and medications that are meant for absorption in the intestines should not be given bucally or sublingually.

Liquid Medications

Liquids are often used as a vehicle to deliver medication (Table 30-7). Whenever possible, children should be given liquids until they can safely swallow pills. Adults that have great difficulty swallowing pills may also be offered liquids. The medical assistant should read the entire label for clarification. Liquid medications for pediatric patients are frequently packaged with a medicine cup (Figure 30-15), oral syringe, medicine spoon (Figure 30-16), or a calibrated medicine dropper (Figure 30-17). Patients should not be allowed to consume any liquids after drinking a liquid medication until confirming with instructions on the medication label.

Refer to Procedure 30-2 for steps on how to administer oral and liquid medications.

Administering Medications through Feeding Tubes

Some enteral medications may be delivered through a patient's feeding tube. Medical assistants do not typically administer drugs using this route. Patients who have neuromuscular disorders, are unconscious, or are in a vegetative state are often fed through a feeding tube.

Table 30-6 Solid Oral Medications

Type	Explanation
Tablets	A medication that is usually mixed with a special binding powder and pressed and molded into a particular shape, most often a round disc. Most tablets are designed to be absorbed high in the gastrointestinal tract but may be *enteric coated*, designed to break down and be absorbed in the intestines. Some tablets are *buffered* to help decrease acidity in the stomach. Coated tablets should never be altered by smashing into a powder and mixing with a liquid because it prevents the drug from being absorbed properly. Tablets may be *scored (*lined*)* for cutting in half.
Caplet	A smooth, oval, coated tablet designed for easier swallowing.
Capsules	A dose of oral medication housed in a special soluble container, usually gelatin. Capsules usually dissolve in the stomach but may be enteric coated (designed to dissolve in the intestines). May be sustained release (SR) or time released, meaning that the different granules within the capsule are designed to be released at different times.
Gel caps	An oil-based medication that is encased in a gelatin shell.
Lozenge or troche	Medication that is encased in round or oval candy coating. Designed to be dissolved in the mouth and assists with soothing irritated tissue of the throat.

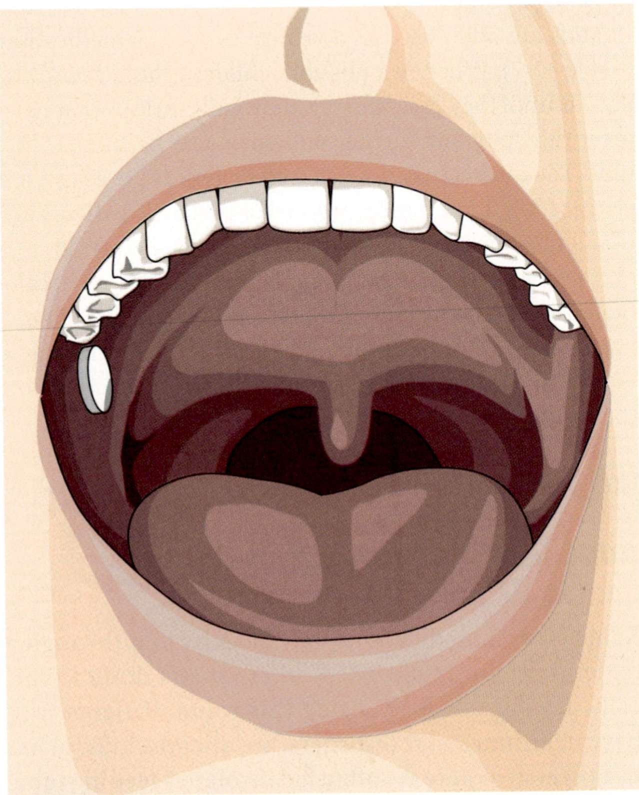

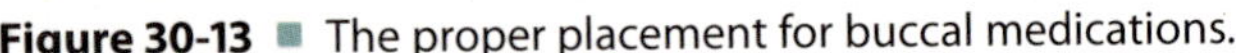

Figure 30-13 ■ The proper placement for buccal medications.

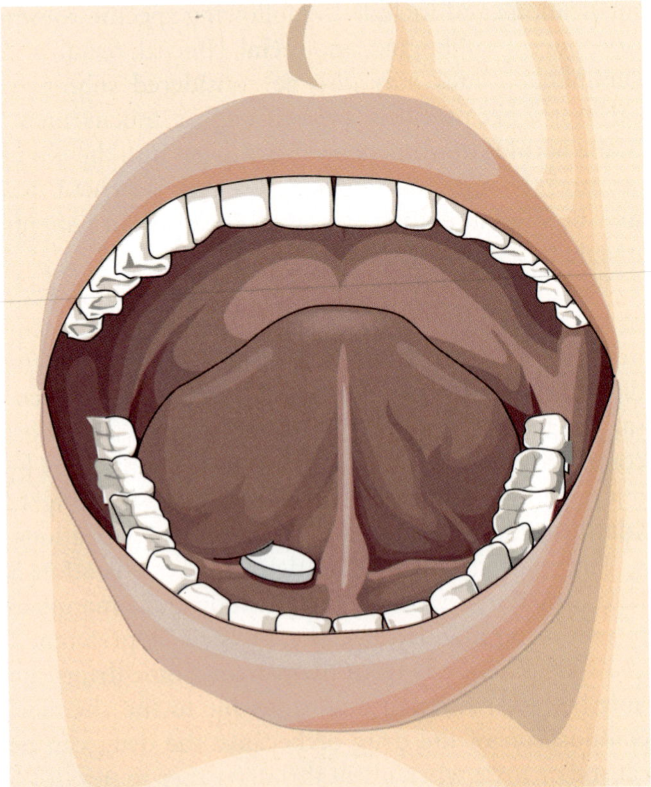

Figure 30-14 ■ The proper placement for sublingual medications.

Table 30-7 Types of Liquid Medications

Type	Examples	Description
Syrups	Cough syrup	A concentration of medicine mixed with sugar water. Used as a vehicle to transport distasteful medications.
Extracts	Allergy extracts	A highly concentrated form of medicine made by mixing the leaves of a plant with alcohol. The solid matter is removed (extracted), leaving just the plant oils mixed with alcohol. This produces a much more concentrated form of the drug than its original form.
Elixirs	Cough or cold medications	A medication sustained in a sweetened liquid usually containing alcohol. It may be used for its flavoring or medicinal properties.
Tinctures	St. John's wort, tincture of iodine	A chemical or soluble drug prepared in an alcoholic solvent.
Magmas	Milk of magnesia	Minerals suspended in water. These should be well mixed before use.
Suspension	Ear and eye medications (such as Zithromax)	Medication particles that are dissolved in a liquid. Must be mixed well before administering.
Sprays	Throat and nasal sprays	Sprays may be used to anesthetize the back of the throat to relieve pain. Some nasal sprays are delivered into the nasal mucosa for relief of allergy symptoms.
Washes	Oral rinses	Frequently used for oral health. These are rinses that are gargled and spit back out.

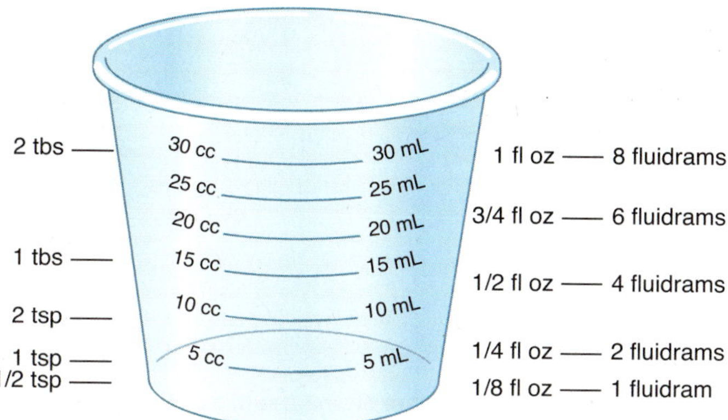

Figure 30-15 ■ A medication cup with measurement markings for proper dosage.

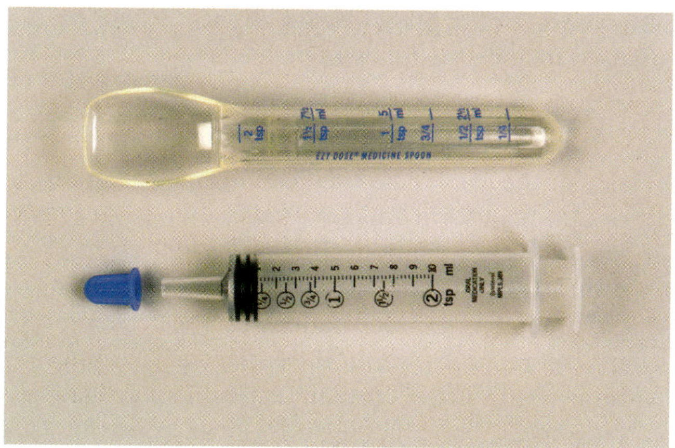

Figure 30-16 ■ Oral syringes and medication spoons are great for administering liquids to young children.

A feeding tube may extend from the nasal cavity into the stomach or intestines, or may be directly attached to the stomach or intestines through an opening in the skin.

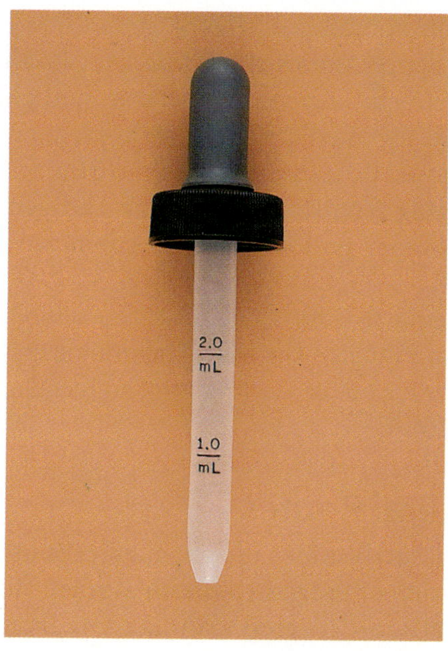

Figure 30-17 ■ Droppers are good for instilling eye or ear drops and for administering oral medications to infants.

Rectal Medications

Rectal medications are often given to patients who cannot keep medication down due to gastrointestinal disturbances, are unconscious, or have problems with swallowing. This method of drug absorption minimizes the changes or alterations of drugs that, if given orally, may lose their effectiveness due to gastrointestinal secretions.

Rectal medications such as suppositories are often coated with gelatin or cocoa butter (Figure 30-18), which easily melts due to the warm temperatures within the cavity. This promotes rapid absorption of

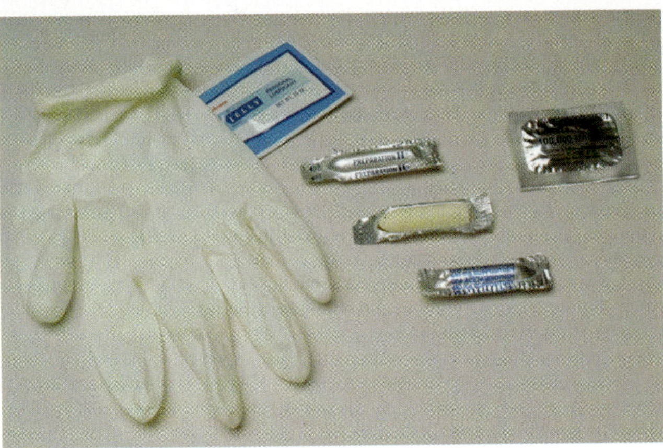

Figure 30-18 ■ Rectal suppositories are often coated with gelatin or cocoa butter to assist with absorption.

the medication through the vasculature located within the rectal mucosa. These medications are often used to soften the stool, stimulate bowel movements, or relieve nausea and vomiting when the stomach is especially irritated. Suppositories should be kept in a cool area and not directly exposed to heat or sunlight, as this may cause the medication to melt prematurely. The patient should be instructed to remove the foil wrapper or packaging from the suppository and gently insert the suppository past the internal sphincter along the rectal wall.

An enema (Figure 30-19) is a procedure that may be used to evacuate the bowel before a suppository is inserted or for better viewing prior to rectal exams (see Chapter 16).

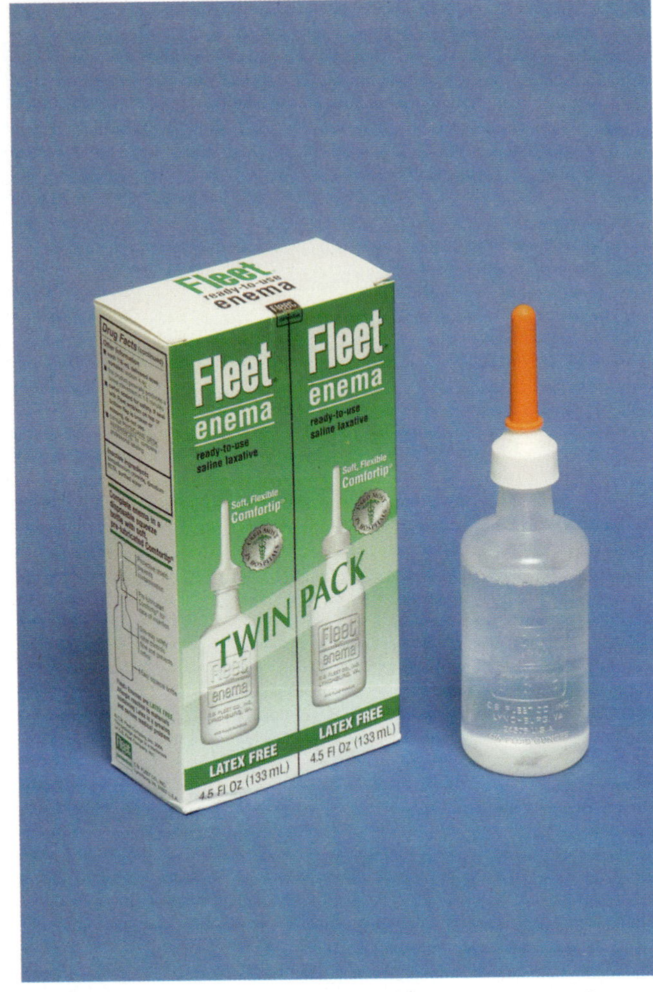

Figure 30-19 ■ Enemas are often used to assist in bowel evacuation.

Parenteral Routes

Parenteral medications are any medications administered outside of the gastrointestinal tract. Advantages of medications delivered via this route include rapid absorption (resulting in a faster response time) and absence of the common side effects often associated with medication taken through the gastrointestinal tract. Disadvantages include rapid onset of allergy symptoms or anaphylaxis and possible injuries to soft tissue or bone tissue during the injection process. Chapter 32 expands on injections and infusion therapy, while other parenteral routes are described in this chapter.

Mucosal Membrane Medications

The mucous membranes can be used for administering particular types of medications to produce a systemic effect. Mucous membranes used within the alimentary canal to deliver medications include those membranes used for buccal, sublingual, and rectal medications. Other parts of the body in which mucous membranes are used include the following:

- Ophthalmic membranes: Medications can be delivered within the upper or lower conjunctival sacs of the eye. These medications may be in drop or ointment form and are usually used to treat eye infections or irritation. Chapter 13 includes a procedure for instilling eye ointments and drops.
- Otic membranes: Medications can be delivered into membranes within the ear to treat ear infections or to soften cerumen (earwax) for irrigation purposes. Chapter 13 includes a procedure for instilling ear drops.
- Nasal membranes: Medications can be administered through mucus membranes of the nose. These medications may help to relieve rhinitis or to relieve nasal congestion. They may be local or systemic, and may be in the form of drops or sprays. *Inhalation therapy* may be delivered

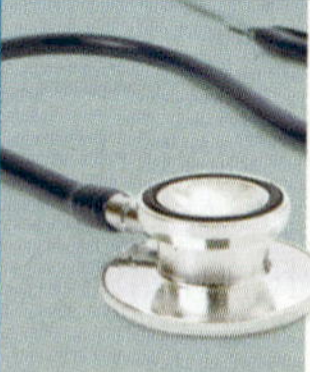

Field Smarts

Any time you apply a topical product to the patient's skin for medicinal purposes, you should wear gloves to avoid penetration of the product into your skin and to avoid possible disease transmission whenever there is a risk of infection. A new disposable spatula or tongue blade may be used when removing these products from their original containers and an applicator such as a tongue blade or cotton-tip applicator should be used when applying liniments or ointments to the skin. Sterile products and supplies should be used when applying topical products to a wound site.

through oral or nasal passages in the form of an aerosol or liquid that is vaporized with warm steam or administered by a metered dose inhaler. Medications that are inhaled can produce a local effect by opening air passages within the cavity or a systemic effect by supplying medication to the lungs to be absorbed into the bloodstream. Examples of inhalation drugs include bronchodilators, mucolytic agents, and steroids. Chapter 15 includes a procedure for administering nebulizer treatments and provides tips for using an inhaler.

- Vaginal membranes: Medications administered vaginally include sprays, tablets, suppositories, creams, and foams. Hormone creams, contraceptives, and antifungal creams are all examples of the types of medications delivered by this route. Creams are usually administered using an applicator. Patients should be instructed to wear a pad following the administration of vaginal medications to prevent drainage onto the patient's underwear.

Topical Applications

Topical agents are medications applied to the skin. They generally provide a localized action. Such medication forms include the following:

- Lotion: A medication that comes in liquid form and is applied externally to the skin. Lotions are often used as a topical cleanser to stop pruritus (itching) or to help relieve pain. Lotions may be applied using a soft cloth, cotton ball, or gauze squares and are typically rubbed into the skin. Gold Bond medicated lotion is an example.
- Liniment: A medical preparation that is rubbed into the skin. It is usually mixed with a quick drying solvent such as alcohol or acetone. Aromatic chemical compounds are often included to create a pleasant scent. Liniments are often applied to the skin for the relief of stiff joints and pain and may be applied during therapeutic or relaxation massages.
- Ointments: These medications are usually oil-based and used for a variety of purposes. Examples include Vicks Vaporub ointment, which is used to help relieve chest congestion, and burn ointments, which are used to stimulate healing and to stop the pain.

Transdermal Patches

Transdermal patches (Figure 30-20) are adhesive patches applied to the skin that are impregnated with medication for slow release into the bloodstream. The different layers within the patch (Figure 30-21) allow

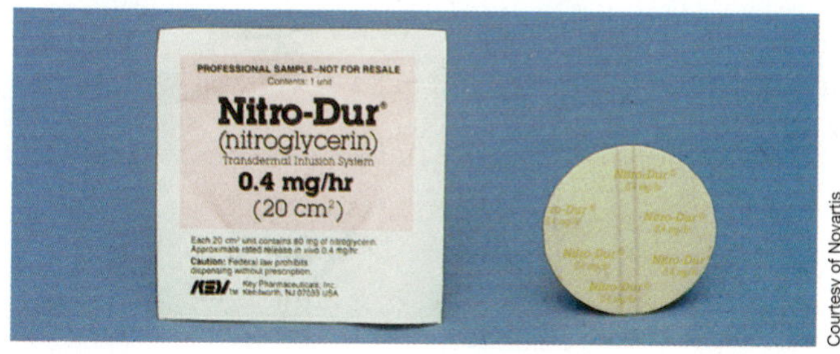

Figure 30-20 ■ Nitro-Dur is an example of a transdermal patch that delivers nitroglycerine into the bloodstream.

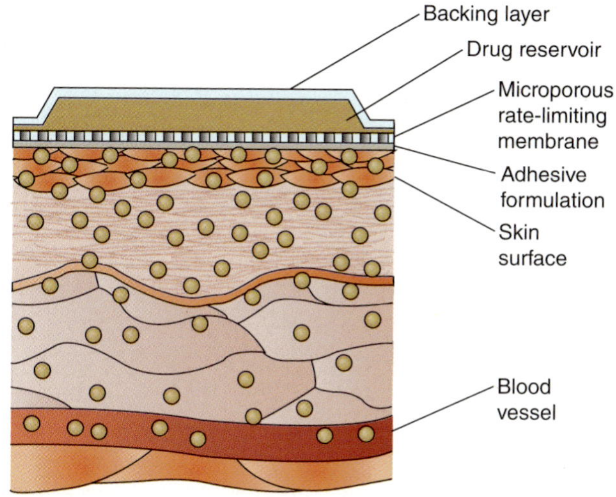

Figure 30-21 ■ The Nitro-Dur patch is a multilayered unit. It consists of a blocking layer, a reservoir of nitroglycerin, a rate controlling membrane, and an adhesive layer that has a priming dose of nitroglycerine.

the medicine to be released at varying time intervals. The date and time that the patch was applied should be written on the patch so that the patient knows when it needs to be changed. The medical assistant should always wear gloves when applying these patches to avoid penetration of the medication into the medical assistant's skin. Examples of transdermal medications include nicotine patches for smoking cessation, estrogen patches for hormone replacement therapy, morphine patches for management of chronic and debilitating pain, and nitroglycerin for treatment of angina or chest pain.

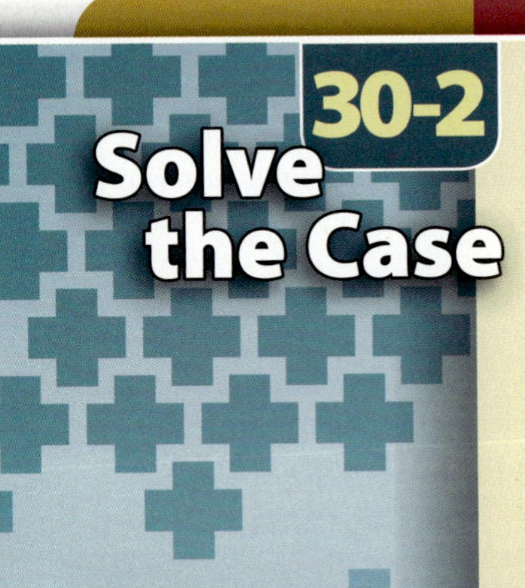

The doctor decides he wants to refer Isaac to an orthopedist. He also wants you to give Isaac Demerol (100 mg), IM.

1. **Look up Demerol on the Internet and see what schedule it is.**
2. **According to medication delegation rules in your state, are you allowed to give this medication?**
3. **Isaac came by himself today. Should he be allowed to drive home by himself?**
4. **If you are not allowed to administer controlled substances, how will you respond to the doctor when he asks you to give Isaac the Demerol injection?**

PROCEDURE 30-1

Write a Prescription

Objective:

To correctly write a prescription onto a paper prescription blank.

Equipment/Supplies:

- Medication order from physician
- Patient's chart/EHR
- Prescription blank
- Writing instrument

PROCEDURAL STEPS	DETAILS AND/OR RATIONALE
1. Assemble the chart, order for medication, and prescription pad.	You will need all of these resources to write the prescription.
2. Read the order and ask any questions if you do not understand the order.	Guessing what the physician wants could result in serious complications or even death to the patient.
3. Write in the patient's name, address, and age or date of birth.	The pharmacy will need this information to process the prescription.
4. If not already on the form, write the superscription, or Rx symbol.	This symbol is usually preprinted on the prescription form.
5. Fill in the information included in the inscription (name of the drug, form of the drug, and strength of the medication).	Being specific will help to prevent potential errors.
6. Fill in the information that should be included in the subscription. This usually refers to the dispense amount. (The dispense amount should include the number itself followed by the written amount in parentheses.)	Writing the amount both numerically and in writing helps to prevent someone from changing the amount later.
7. Fill in the information included in the signature (instructions for taking).	These are special instructions that allow the patient to know how to take the medication and how often.
8. If applicable, check the box that states: Do Not Substitute or Dispense as Written.	If the physician does not want the pharmacist to change to a generic drug, this box should be checked.
9. Circle or write the amount of refills.	If refills are ordered, it needs to be documented.
10. Insert the DEA number if applicable.	This may vary from state and practice.
11. Give the prescription to the physician to read and sign.	All prescriptions must be signed by the physician in order to be legal.
12. Document the order in the patient's record.	Illustrates that the prescription was written and what was included in the order.

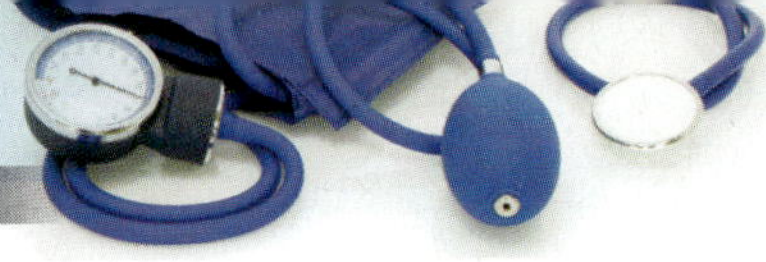

DOCUMENTATION EXAMPLE:

DOUGLASVILLE MEDICINE ASSOCIATES
5076 BRAND BLVD
DOUGLASVILLE, NY 01234
(123) 456-7890

Patient's Name: *Sydney Heller* DOB: *02-04-XX*

Address: *1234 Hickory Hills, Polaris, NY, 01298* Date: *12-14-XX*

Rx

Amoxicillin Capsules, 250 mg
Dispense: # 90 (Ninety)
Sig: 1 cap. PO tid x 10 days

__*X*__ Dispense as Written ______ Do Not Substitute

Signature: *Trent Valentine, M.D.*

DEA # ____________________ Number of Refills: *0*

PROCEDURE 30-2

Administer an Oral Medication

Objective:

To properly administer an oral medication to a patient as ordered by the physician.

Equipment/Supplies:

- Written medication order
- Proper medication
- Plastic medication cup
- Medication transport tray
- Water
- Gloves (optional)
- Patient's chart/EHR

PROCEDURAL STEPS	DETAILS AND/OR RATIONALE
1. Working in a well-lit area, verify the physician's order. Be certain to follow the Seven Rights of Drug Administration.	Understanding the physician's order and following the seven rights will help to prevent errors.
2. Wash your hands and apply gloves (gloves are optional). Assemble the medication and supplies. Check the label on the medication bottle as you retrieve it from the cabinet **(Medication check #1)**.	Washing hands and gloving helps to reduce the number of microorganisms on your hands and protects you from becoming contaminated when retrieving the cup and medication container back from the patient. Checking the label helps to confirm that you have the correct medication.
3. Compare the written drug order with the drug label before preparing the drug. Make certain that you have the right drug and the right dose **(Medication check #2)**. Perform dosage calculation if necessary.	Checking the drug once again helps to verify that you have the correct drug.

continues

PROCEDURE 30-2 continued

PROCEDURAL STEPS	DETAILS AND/OR RATIONALE
4. Check the expiration date of the drug.	Outdated drugs may be altered or have deteriorated in their effectiveness and should not be used.
5. Loosen the lid and remove it from the bottle. Place the lid on the counter so that the inside of the lid is pointing upward. Pour the correct amount of pills into the cap of the medication vial without contaminating the inside of the cap (Figure 30-22), and then into the medicine cup. (When measuring a liquid form of medication, palm the label before pouring and hold the medication cup at eye level, as in Figure 30-23. Read the volume at the lowest point of the curve in the liquid, or at the meniscus.)	Placing the lid in a downward position onto a counter surface will contaminate the inside of the lid. Pouring the pills into the cap first allows you to pour any extra pills that fell into the lid during pouring right back into the pill bottle, keeping them as clean or sterile as possible. Palming the label of a liquid medication prevents the label from becoming damaged in the event that the liquid runs onto the label. **Figure 30-22** ■ The medical assistant pours the pills into the cap before pouring into the medicine cup. **Figure 30-23** ■ Liquid medications should be read at eye level.
6. Replace the medication in its proper storage area. Read the label once again before returning it to verify that it is the correct drug and dosage **(Medication check #3)**.	Checking the drug against the order three times before administering will confirm that you have the correct drug and correct dose.
7. Properly transport the medication to the patient. Be careful not to touch the medication or the inside of the container.	Touching the inner part of the medicine cup will contaminate the container holding the medication, thus contaminating the medication.
8. Identify the patient, using a minimum of two identifiers.	Patient verification is important before administering any drugs to prevent error in administering the wrong drug to the wrong patient. This also complies with the Joint Commission rules for patient safety.
9. Identify yourself, and ***explain the rationale for the performance of the procedure to the patient, showing awareness of the patient's concerns related to the procedure being performed***.	Explaining to the patient what drug(s) the patient is taking and why will encourage compliance.

continues

PROCEDURE 30-2 continued

PROCEDURAL STEPS	DETAILS AND/OR RATIONALE
10. Give the patient the medication to swallow (Figure 30-24) and observe the patient to make sure there is no difficulty in taking the medication. With a pill, allow the patient to have plenty of water to ensure the medication has passed from the esophagus into the stomach. Do not give the patient water when giving a liquid medication unless you have confirmed with the package insert and the physician that it is okay to do so.	Drinking water after a liquid medicine can dilute the medication, minimizing its effects.
11. Properly dispose of the medication cup and other disposable equipment into the garbage and remove gloves and wash hands.	
12. Provide the patient with any relevant educational materials and ask the patient to repeat back any instructions to confirm that the patient comprehends the information.	Education is important to encourage patient compliance.
13. Document the procedure in the patient's record.	Documentation proves that the procedure was performed.

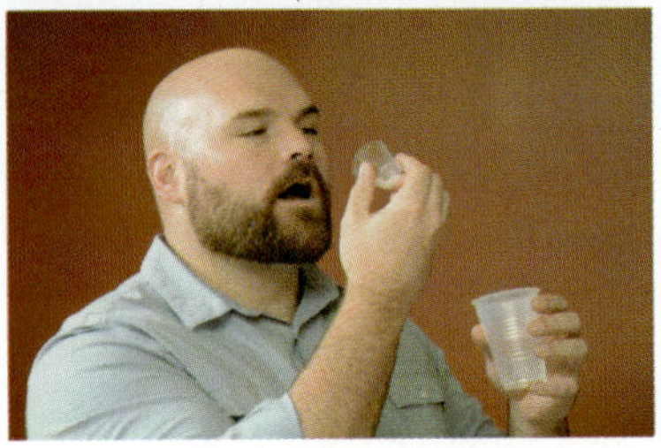

Figure 30-24 ■ The medical assistant should make certain that the patient swallows the medication.

DOCUMENTATION EXAMPLE:

07-12-XX 10:15 A. M.	Tylenol, 500 mg po per Dr. Legg. Observed pt. swallow med. Gave pt. both verbal and written home care. instructions for taking medication at home. Jane Barnes, CMA (AAMA)--

CHAPTER SUMMARY

- Pharmacology is the study of drugs, including their origin nature, properties, and effect upon living organisms.
- Throughout the early history of pharmacy, herbalists, physicians, and priests (whose roles often intertwined), all played active roles in apothecary functions; however, that has all changed now with formal training and mandated licensure.
- Sources of drugs include: plants, animal, mineral, synthetic, and drugs that are genetically engineered.
- Medicinal uses of drugs include, therapeutic, diagnostic, curative, replacement, and preventative.
- Reference Table 30-1 for common drug classifications.
- Pharmacodynamics refers to the study of the effects of drugs on living organisms.
- Drugs may be grouped by the type of action they produce in the body. Three different actions of drugs include, *local reaction* (the drug acts on the area of tissue in which it is administered), *remote action* (the drug has an effect in a different location of the body than where it was administered, such as a nerve block), and *systemic action* (the drug is absorbed into the bloodstream and carried to other parts of the body).

- Pharmacokinetics is a term that describes how the body reacts to a drug, which depends on specific variables of the individual taking the drug.
- Different effects that a drug may have in the body include: therapeutic effect, side effect, drug interaction, or a drug allergy.
- Factors that affect drug actions include: age, body weight, compliance, disease, gender, idiosyncrasy, interactions from other drugs or foods, timing, and tolerance.
- A single drug may have three names, chemical name (chemical structure of the drug), generic name (the drug's official name), and brand name (the words, names, slogans, pictures, or symbols that are used to identify a company).
- Three medication tasks include to prescribe (to order a medication), dispense (to give to the patient to take home), and to administer (to prepare and give to the patient at the point of care).
- The U.S. Food and Drug Administration (FDA) establishes standards for pharmaceutical companies to follow in the development and sale of prescribed and OTC medications.
- Providers that prescribe, dispense, or administer controlled substances must be registered with the U.S. Drug Enforcement Administration (DEA), a part of the Department of Justice.
- The Controlled Substances Act (CSA) defines drugs or substances that may have the potential for illegal use or abuse.
- Controlled substances are divided into five schedules, according to their addictive properties and degree of abuse.
- The DEA requires that a full inventory of all controlled substances be completed every two years. Records from that inventory must be kept for a minimum of two years. A minimum of monthly inventories should be performed with additional inventories every shift in which staff has access, and witnesses should be present.
- The prescription is a written legal document that lists compounding, dispensing, and administering instructions for particular medications.
- The Physicians' Desk Reference (PDR) is one of the most commonly used drug reference guides and is used in a variety of healthcare settings. It is divided into six different sections including: manufacturers' index, brand and generic index, product category index, product identification guide, product information section, and dietary supplements section.

CERTIFICATION REVIEW QUESTIONS

1. An example of a type of drug that is developed from a mineral source is:
   a. digoxin.
   b. insulin.
   c. sulfonamide.
   d. hormones.
2. A drug may have up to three names. The generic name is the drug name based on which of the following?
   a. The chemical formula that states the molecular structure
   b. The drug brand name
   c. The official name of the drug
   d. Where it falls in the Controlled Substance Drug Schedule
3. Which of the following is a Controlled Substance Drug Schedule II?
   a. Cough syrup with codeine
   b. Morphine
   c. Darvocet
   d. Heroin
4. If a provider asks you to administer a controlled substance that you aren't allowed to under state delegation laws, how should you respond?
   a. Respect the provider's order and do it anyway.
   b. Tell the provider that you need additional training before administering the medication.
   c. Tell the provider to give it himself.
   d. Explain that according to state law, you are unable to administer a controlled substance but that you would be happy to ask the nurse to assist him with the request.
5. What is the minimum number of times a medical assistant must read the medication label when administering the Seven Rights of proper drug administration?
   a. One
   b. Two
   c. Three
   d. Four

6. A patient has a surgery and wakes up unable to swallow. After lots of testing, the staff concludes that the patient has paralysis of the throat muscles and is unable to eat or drink food or swallow medications. Which of the following would be the best method of administering the patient's medications?
   a. Through a G-tube
   b. Through injection
   c. Transdermally
   d. Both a and b

7. Mr. Adkins is a diabetic who takes insulin. Which medicinal method describes how insulin is used?
   a. Curative
   b. Diagnostic
   c. Therapeutic
   d. Replacement

8. Mr. Muhammad was diagnosed with congestive heart failure. His heart isn't working with the force it once was. He has pitting edema in his feet and legs. What class or classes of medication(s) would be best for Mr. Muhammad's symptoms?
   a. Antiarrhythmic
   b. Diuretic
   c. Cardiotonic
   d. Both b and c

9. A patient complains that she doubled the maximum dose of acetaminophen for her headache but two hours later she still hasn't received any relief. What is the most likely problem?
   a. She has reached the drug's ceiling.
   b. She hasn't taken enough medication to get the maximum results.
   c. She doesn't have any drug receptors.
   d. She hasn't reached the therapeutic index.

10. A patient is experiencing urticaria after receiving a penicillin injection. She has no other symptoms. She most likely is experiencing a(n):
   a. anaphylactic reaction.
   b. systemic reaction.
   c. local reaction.
   d. side effect.

STUDY RESOURCES

Resources to Test and Reinforce Your Knowledge:	
Certification Review Questions	Take this end-of-chapter quiz
Workbook	• Complete the activities for Chapter 30 • Perform the procedures for Chapter 30 using the Competency Checklists
Resources to Promote Critical Thinking:	
***Solve the Case* Activities**	• Consider these case studies and discuss your conclusions
Learning Lab	• Module 25: Pharmacology and Medication Administration
MindTap	• Complete Chapter 30 readings and activities

REFERENCES

Blesi, M. (2017). *Medical assisting: Administrative and clinical competencies.* (8th ed.). Clifton Park, NY: Cengage Learning.

Lindh, W. Q., Pooler, M. S., Tamparo, C. D., Dahl, B. B., & Morris, J. A. (2014). *Delmar's comprehensive medical assisting.* (5th ed). Clifton Park, NY: Cengage Learning.

Rice, J. (2011). *Principles of pharmacology for medical assisting.* (5th ed). Clifton Park, NY: Cengage Learning.

U.S. Food and Drug Administration. (n.d.). Retrieved September 9, 2015, from http://www.fda.gov/Drugs/DevelopmentApprovalProcess/ucm079031.htm#How many years is a patent granted for?

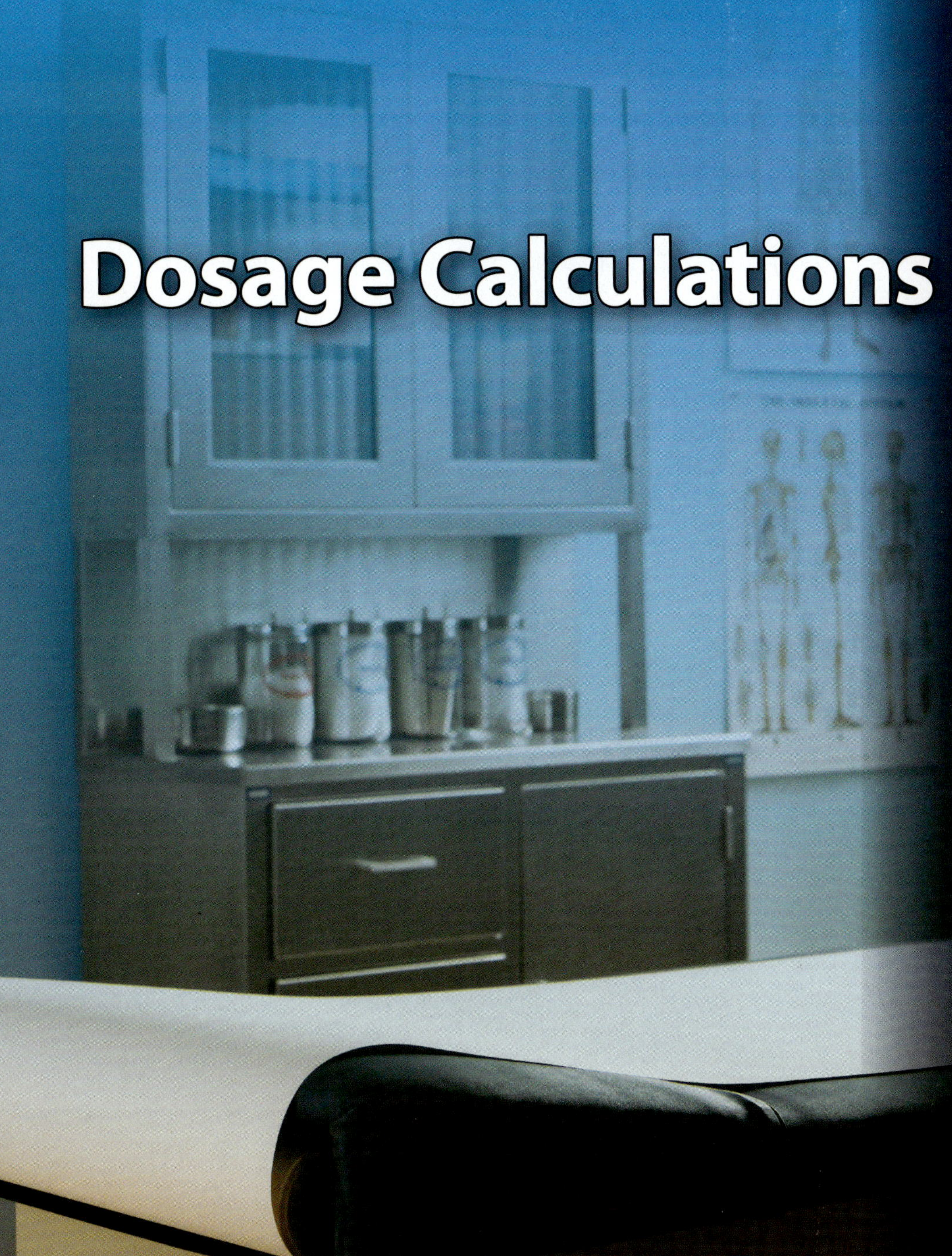

31 Dosage Calculations

ESSENTIAL TERMS

apothecary
apothecary system
body surface area (BSA)
conversion
drug dosage
expiration date
generic name
gram (g, gm)
liter (L)
lot control
medication label
meter (m)
metric system
National Drug Code (NDC)
nomogram
prescription
product name

CHAPTER OUTLINE

Medication Order

Medication Math Fundamentals
- The Apothecary System
- The Metric System
- Household Measurements

Calculating Drug Dosages for Administration
- Rounding Equations
- Proportional Method
- Formula Method
- Calculating Pediatric Dosages

Calculating Insulin Dosages
- Types of Insulin

Reading Medication Labels
- Warning Labels

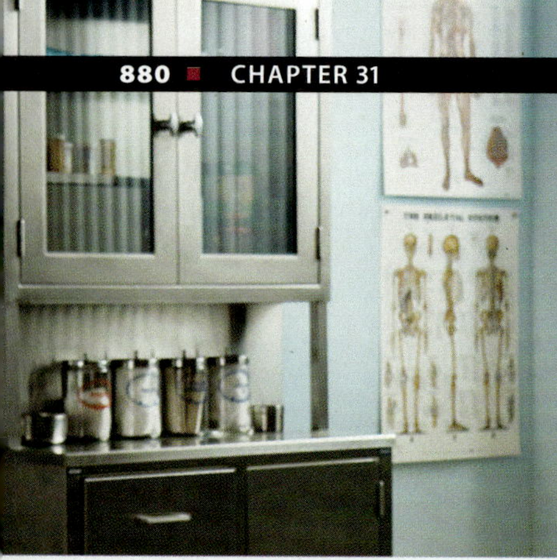

DEVELOPMENTAL OBJECTIVES

After completing this chapter, you should be able to:

1. Correctly spell and define the essential terms.
2. Demonstrate and perform conversions between the various systems of measurements.
3. Correctly calculate an adult dose of medication based on the order given and the label.
4. Calculate children's dosages according to body surface area (BSA) and according to kilograms of body weight.
5. Describe how insulin is measured and what type of syringe is used.
6. List and describe the types of insulin that are available.
7. List the important parts of a medication label and describe what should be checked every time a medication is administered.

INTRODUCTION

Medical assistants are often called upon to prepare medications. In order to properly prepare a medication, the medical assistant must be able to read and comprehend the physician's order, read and comprehend the medical label, and calculate the appropriate dose.

The medical assistant should be able to educate patients on how to take medication and assist the patient with understanding the different types of warning labels that appear on medication bottles.

This chapter will provide a review of fundamental math principles and will introduce math formulas that are necessary for calculating medication dosages. Learning the information in this chapter is vital to patient safety and the patient's overall well-being.

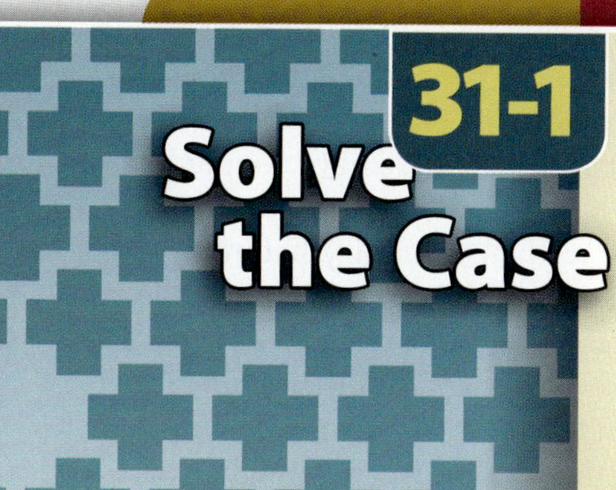

Sixty-year-old Sarah Hamilton comes into the office today because of flu-like symptoms. When you go to retrieve another patient from the reception room, you notice that Mrs. Hamilton is barely able to keep her head up and is forcefully coughing. The reception room is packed.

1. **What concerns immediately come up as you observe Mrs. Hamilton?**
2. **What types of actions may help to minimize danger to other patients?**
3. **How will you take these steps without offending Mrs. Hamilton?**

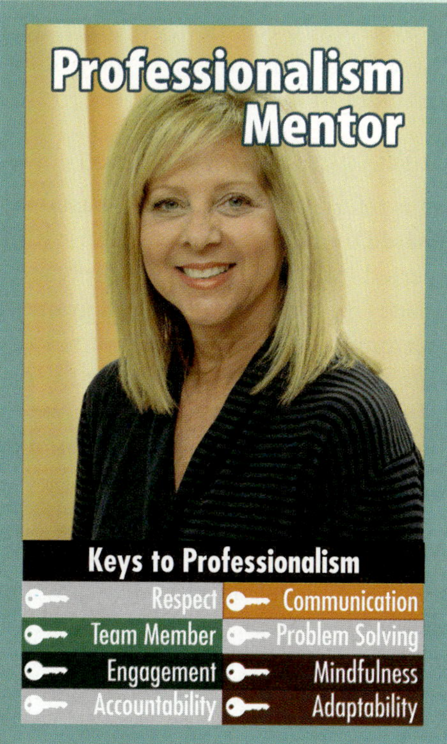

One of the most frequently requested classes for the medical assistant in our ambulatory areas is the class on medication administration and dosage calculations. Medication errors can happen in any practice and that's why we stress that everyone attend this class. In one instance, a medical assistant was questioning why she had to come to the class. She had been a medical assistant for several years and wasn't sure she needed a refresher course on medication and vaccination administration. To be honest, I was baffled by her resistance to ensuring she was administering medications and vaccinations correctly. Medication errors can be devastating, and once given incorrectly, cannot be undone. I reminded her that being in the health care field requires continuing education. It also requires a good attitude and realizing that there will always be changes in best practice in the health care field. How will you feel about continuing to learn after you have been out of school for a while? Continuing to maintain proficiency in medication administration and dosage calculation is critical to your success as a medical assistant who delivers safe and effective patient care. ■

MEDICATION ORDER

Medical assistants are often assigned the task of administering medications to patients while they are in the office. They may also be responsible for dispensing medications and creating or calling in prescriptions for patients. In order to perform these tasks, the medical assistant must be familiar with the information included in a medication order.

A medication order is an order that includes the following:

- Name of the drug to be administered, dispensed, or prescribed
- Drug form
- **Drug dosage**
- Frequency of administration
- Special instructions for taking the medication

The physician is usually the health care team member responsible for creating medication orders; however, other providers in the practice—including nurse practitioners and physician's assistants—may also create medication orders. Because medical assistants are not licensed, they must be familiar with delegation laws for administering medications in the states in which they work. Many medical practice statutes dictate that only a physician can delegate the administration of parenteral medications to an unlicensed individual, which would include the medical assistant. It is important to check these laws before proceeding with such tasks.

MEDICATION MATH FUNDAMENTALS

In order to calculate medication dosages, medical assistants must have an understanding of basic math principles. Some math skills that are necessary for calculating dosages include the ability to perform metric conversions and set up and solve equations (formulas). There are two major systems used to calculate medication dosages: the apothecary system and the metric system. The **apothecary system** was the original primary method used for calculating and measuring medication dosages; however, the metric system is now considered the primary method.

The Apothecary System

A pharmacist or chemist was formerly known as an **apothecary**. The traditional math system that was used to determine medication dosages in English-speaking countries was known as the "apothecary system of mass." This system was replaced by the metric system during the first half of the twentieth century. Since this system is not commonly used in today's medical office, we will not elaborate on this system.

The Metric System

Prior to the early 1800s, there was no standardization between countries in regard to units of measurement. Each country had its own units for measuring, which made it very difficult when trading, buying, or selling.

In the late 1700s, the French National Assembly called upon the Academy of Science to create a simple, decimal-based system of units that could be used by people in all countries. Members of the academy went to work and carefully reviewed proposals submitted by scientists throughout France.

In 1801, the French National Assembly adopted a decimal-based system based on the circumference of the earth submitted more than a century before by a French scientist by the name of Gabriel Mouton. The system that Mouton created is today referred to as the **metric system**. It took several years for other countries to adopt the system, but the metric system is now considered the primary method for measuring weight, volume, and length (area) throughout the world.

In the United States, scientific measures and formulations are based on the metric system, though other systems of measurement, such as apothecary measurements and the household system, may be used as well. The metric system has evolved into the modern system known as Le Système International d'Unités (SI), or International System of Units, which is the primary method of measurement in medicine.

Metric System Weights and Measures

The metric system is referred to as a decimal-based system because it is based on multiples of 10. Metric units can easily be converted into other units by simply moving the decimal place (milliliters to liters and grams to micrograms, for example). There are 14 prefixes that are used within the metric system to describe the size of a metric unit; however, only a portion of those are used in health care. Table 31-1 lists the most common prefixes and their standard values.

Units of the Metric System

The three fundamental units used in the metric system are liters, meters, and grams. **Meter (m)**, the fundamental unit of length, is used when measuring distance. It was the initial unit of the metric system and set the foundation for the remainder of the system. Centimeters (cm) are often used when measuring lesions, nodules, moles, wheals, and the diameter of burns and lacerations.

Table 31-1 Common Prefixes and Their Values

Unit	Pronunciation	Unit Value	Decimal Value/Whole Number
micro-	mi´kro	1/1000,000 of a unit	0.000001
milli-	mil´i	1/1000 of a unit	0.001
centi-	sen´ti	1/100 of a unit	0.01
deci-	des´i	1/10 of a unit	0.1
deka-	dek´a	10 units	10
hecto-	hek´to	100 units	100
kilo-	kil´o	1000 units	1000

Liter (L) is the fundamental unit of volume and is used when measuring liquids. One milliliter (mL) is equivalent to one cubic centimeter (cc). This is because the amount of space that is needed to occupy a milliliter is equivalent to one cubic centimeter; hence, these terms may be used interchangeably. However, cc is on the Joint Commission's list for possible future inclusion in the Do Not Use List, and therefore mL, not cc, should be used. Injectables and liquid medications are measured in liters (specifically, milliliters) when using the metric system.

Gram (g, gm) is the metric unit that is used when measuring anything that has mass or weight. One gram weighs approximately 1 cubic centimeter. Solid medications are often recorded in subunits of grams (mg or mcg) and the patient's weight is recorded in kilograms (kg).

Table 31-2 illustrates common metric units that are used in medicine and gives examples of how they are used.

Metric System Guidelines

The following guidelines have been provided to assist in learning how to use the metric system correctly:

1. For all units except liters (L), use lowercase letters: mg, g, mm, mL.
2. Always leave a full space between the number and unit: 2 mL, 5,250 km.
3. Avoid mixing symbols with names that are spelled out in the same expression:

Correct	Incorrect
8 kg/L	8 kg/liter
5 kg/L	5 kg per L
10 kilograms per liter	10 kilograms/liter

4. Arabic numbers are used to denote whole numbers: 1, 10, 100, 1,000.
5. Fractions are converted to their decimal equivalents for quantities less than 1: 0.1, 0.05, 0.005.
6. A zero should always be placed before a decimal point for numbers less than 1 to avoid confusion: 0.1, 0.05, 0.001.
7. Metric units do not have a singular or plural form: 5 mL, 2 mL, 60 mg (no "s" at the end).
8. The Arabic number always precedes the metric unit of measurement: 10 grams, 2 milliliters, 5 liters.
9. Gram is abbreviated by writing gm or g. The preferred abbreviation is g.
10. When a measurement/symbol is named after a person, capitalize the measurement and symbol: Celsius (C).

By combining prefixes with the roots, you get multiples or submultiples of the metric system. For example, milli (prefix) and liter (root) are combined to form milliliter (refer to Table 31-3).

Table 31-2 Common Metric Units Used in Health Care

Medication Dosages Are Usually Measured In	Medication Volumes Are Usually Measured In	Laboratory Results Are Usually Measured In	Miscellaneous
Grams (gm, g) Milligrams (mg) Micrograms (mcg) Units (U) ("U" is an error-prone abbreviation; write out "units" instead)	Milliliters (mL) Cubic centimeter (cc) ("cc" is an error-prone abbreviation; use mL instead)	Milligrams (mg) Micrograms (mcg) Grams per deciliter (g/dL) Units per liter (U/L)	Blood pressure is measured in millimeters of mercury (mmHg) Wounds and lesions are usually measured in centimeters (cm) Organs are usually measured in grams (g)

Table 31-3 Common Units Used in the Metric System

Length: Meter	Volume: Liter
0.001 of a meter = 1 millimeter (mm)	0.001 of a liter = 1 milliliter (mL)
0.01 of a meter = 1 centimeter (cm)	0.01 of a liter = 1 centiliter (cL)
0.1 of a meter = 1 decimeter (dm)	0.1 liter = 1 deciliter (dL)
1 meter = 1 meter (m)	1 liter = 1 liter (L)
10 meters = 1 dekameter (dam)	10 liters = 1 dekaliter (daL)
100 meters = 1 hectometer (hm)	100 liters = 1 hectoliter (hL)
1000 meters = 1 kilometer (km)	1000 liters = 1 kiloliter (kL)
Mass and/or Weight: Gram	**Frequently Used Metric Equivalents**
0.000001 gram = 1 microgram (mcg)	2.54 centimeters (cm) = 1 inch (in)
0.001 of a gram = 1 milligram (mg)	1000 millimeters (mL) = 1 liter (L)
0.01 of a gram = 1 centigram (cg)	1,000 cubic centimeters (cc) = 1 liter (L)
0.1 of a gram = 1 decigram (dg)	1,000 micrograms (mcg) = 1 milligrams (mg)
1 gram = 1 gram (g)	1,000 milligrams (mg) = 1 gram (g)
10 grams = 1 dekagram (dag)	1,000 grams (g) = 1 kilograms (kg)
100 grams = 1 hectogram (hg)	1 kilogram (kg) = 2.2 pounds (lb)
1000 grams = 1 kilogram (kg)	

Metric Conversions

The term **conversion** means to switch from one unit to another. Conversion may be necessary when the physician orders a medication in a unit that is not available, such as when the physician orders a drug in milligrams and the measurements on the drug label measure the drug in grams. There are a number of different methods that can be used to perform conversions—two are presented here.

Conversion Factor Method

The conversion factor method can be used both for performing conversions within the metric system and for performing conversions between two different systems.

To perform conversions using the conversion factor method, a factor equivalent table will need to be available to use when setting up problems. Table 31-3 is a factor equivalent table for the most common metric system units. (Be very careful when using a factor equivalent table. Pay attention to detail to avoid setting the problem up the wrong way.)

Example: 5 g = ___ mg

Step 1. Write down the initial measurement and place it over the number 1 (you are creating a fraction—the initial measurement becomes the numerator, and the number 1 is the denominator). Next to this, create a second fraction. Place the number 1 beside the units you want to convert to (in this case, mg). This will be the numerator in the second fraction. Proceed to Step 2 to add the denominator to the second fraction.

$$\frac{5\text{ g}}{1}\ \frac{1\text{ mg}}{} = \underline{\qquad}\text{ mg}$$

Step 2. The denominator of the second fraction is the converting factor from the appropriate factor equivalent table, the factor that matches the unit of the initial measurement to the units necessary for the final measurement. Referring to Table 31-3, the factor equivalent for this problem is 0.001 g = 1 mg. Place 0.001 g as the denominator of the second fraction. Note that the units you want to eliminate (in this case, grams) must be in opposite positions (numerator and denominator) so they cancel out; otherwise, you have set the problem up incorrectly.

$$\frac{5\text{ }\cancel{g}}{1}\ \frac{1\text{ mg}}{0.001\text{ }\cancel{g}} = \underline{\qquad}\text{ mg}$$

Step 3. Multiply the two numerators and the two denominators. Note that the grams are in opposite position and therefore cancel each other out.

$$\frac{5\text{ }\cancel{g}}{1} \times \frac{1\text{ mg}}{0.001\text{ }\cancel{g}} = \frac{5\text{ mg}}{0.001}$$

Step 4. Divide the numerator by the denominator.

$$\frac{5\text{ mg}}{0.001} = 5{,}000\text{ mg}$$

The answer is 5 g = 5,000 mg.

Shortcut or Counting Method

Another method that can be used when performing conversions within the metric system is the shortcut or counting method. Since the metric system uses multiples of 10, it is relatively easy to perform conversions within the metric system, because all you are doing is moving the decimal point a specific number of places to the right or to the left.

Table 31-4 is a metric conversion table that can be used when performing metric conversions. It illustrates the common metric units used in health care and their values in descending order. The bottom row of the table has a counting section with arrows. The arrows point to the metric unit that each arrow represents. This is the section used to determine how many places and in which direction to move the decimal. To illustrate how to use this table, use the following metric conversion problem:

Example: 1 g = ___ mg

1. Start by placing your finger in the box of the arrow that represents the unit of the known value. (For this problem, place your finger in the box above the arrow for the standard unit, gram.)
2. Next, move your finger the number of places that it takes to get from the known value to the unknown value. (In this case, move from grams to milligrams, which is three places to the right.)
3. Next, move the decimal in the number of the known value the number of places that it took to get from the known value to the unknown value. The decimal in any whole number is immediately to the right of the whole number. (For this problem, add three zeros, since you moved three places to the right.)

The answer is 1 gram = 1,000 mg.

It gets a little trickier when you move the decimal from the right to the left. Convert the following unit:

Example: 5 mg = ___ g

1. Place your finger on the arrow that represents the prefix milli-.
2. Next, move your finger the number of spaces that it takes to get from milli to grams. (You should have moved your finger three places to the left to move from milli to grams.)
3. Next, move the decimal in the number of the known value the number of places that it takes to get from the known value to the unknown value. (So move your decimal point three places to the left.) Since the decimal point immediately follows the whole number, moving the decimal one place would represent 0.5 g, moving the decimal two places would represent 0.05 g, and moving the decimal three places represents 0.005 g.

The answer is 5 mg or 0.005 g.

Household Measurements

The imperial system (also known as the household system) of measuring volume and weight can be found in any kitchen in the United States. This system is important to the patient who has no prior experience working

Table 31-4 Metric Conversion Table

Whole Numbers				Fractions or Decimals					
Increasing Value				←	→				Decreasing Value
1000	100	10	1	1/10	1/100	1/1000	—	—	1/1,000,000
				0.1	0.01	0.001			0.000001
kilo	hecto	deka	Standard Unit (*gram, liter* and *meter*)	deci	centi	milli	PH*	PH*	micro
							—	—	
↑	↑	↑	↑	↑	↑	↑	↑	↑	↑
PLACE HOLDER COUNTING SECTION									

*The letters PH stand for "place holder." The majority of metric units are separated by one unit of 10; however, the separation between milli and micro jumps from 10 to 1,000. So that you don't get confused, place holders between milli and micro are there as a reminder to move the decimal place three places between the two units.

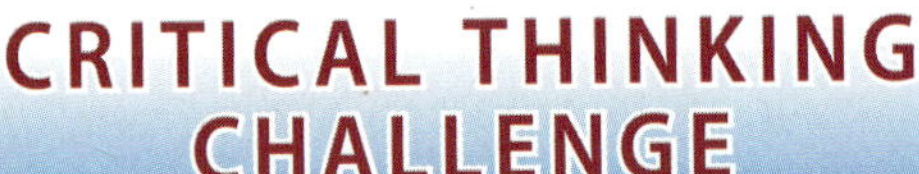

CRITICAL THINKING CHALLENGE

Using either the conversion factor method or the shortcut method, convert the following measurements:

1. **0.25 grams = ___ milligrams**
2. **750 micrograms = ___ milligrams**
3. **1 kilometer = ___ meters**
4. **1 liter = ___ microliters**

with the metric system. Most Americans will be familiar with this system because they use it in their everyday lives. Household measurements may be used as reference points during patient education. The medical assistant should always keep in mind that household measurements are not exact and should not be used in a clinical setting.

The household system measures weight in increments called pounds, and volume is measured in drops (gtt). Pounds are still the standard unit for patient weight in the United States.

Liquid oral medications can be easily measured and are sometimes prescribed in household units such as teaspoon, tablespoon, drops, and ounces. (Keep in mind that many pharmaceutical manufacturers are now packaging their liquid medications with droppers or medication cups that feature both household and metric units.) Table 31-5 lists some of the most common household measurements.

Some common conversions between the household system and the metric system can be found in Table 31-6.

Table 31-5 Common Household Measurements

60 drops = 1 teaspoon (tsp)
1 dash = less than 1/8 tsp
3 teaspoons = 1 tablespoon (tbsp)
2 tbsp = 1 ounce (oz)
4 oz = 1 juice glass
6 oz = 1 teacup
8 oz = 1 glass or cup
16 tbsp or 8 oz = 1 measuring cup
2 cups = 1 pint
2 pints = 1 quart
4 quarts = 1 gallon

CRITICAL THINKING CHALLENGE

Using Table 31-6 as a reference, read and respond to the following:

A patient is concerned because her mammogram stated that she had a 0.6 cm lesion in her right breast. There is no indication that the lesion is cancerous. The patient appears to be more upset about the size of the lesion than anything else and keeps referring to the size as 0.6 inches.

1. **How might you comfort the patient based on the conversion in Table 31-6?**
2. **Should this patient be referred to the physician?**

Table 31-6 Common Conversions between Household Measurements and Metric Measurements

Household Measurement	Metric Measurement
1 teaspoon (tsp)	5 mL
1 tablespoon (tbsp)	15 mL
1 ounce (oz)	30 mL
16 oz cup (c)	180 mL
1 glass or 8 ounces (oz)	240 mL
2.2 pounds (lb)	1 kilogram (kg)
1 inch (in)	2.5 centimeter (cm)

CALCULATING DRUG DOSAGES FOR ADMINISTRATION

It is important for the medical assistant to be able to properly calculate medication dosages. An error in medication dosage can cause great harm to the patient. There are two major methods used for calculating adult dosages: the proportional method and the formula method. The method you will use will be the one that is most comfortable for you.

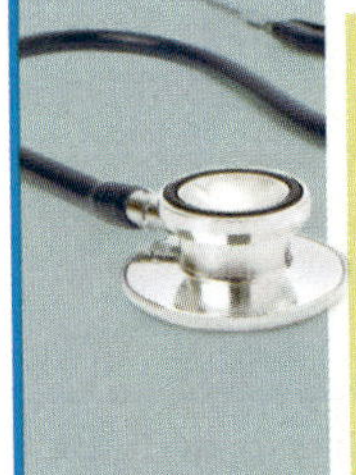

Field Smarts

Cutting tablets that are not scored is highly inadvisable; it is very difficult to cut the pills into two even halves. Always use a pill splitter for the most accurate measurement.

Table 31-7 Guidelines for Rounding Adult Dosages

Liquids	Solids
1. Round to the nearest tenth when giving more than 1 mL of medication. (Use a 3 mL syringe, marked in tenths.) 2. Round to the nearest hundredth when giving less than 1 mL. (Use a TB syringe marked in hundredths.) 3. For digits 1 through 4, round down. For digits 5 through 9, round up. For example, 1.42 mL would be rounded to 1.4 mL, and 1.78 mL would be rounded to 1.8 mL.	1. When working with tablets that are not scored, round to the nearest whole number of what is available. If your calculation comes out to 1.8 tablets, you will round up and give the patient 2 tablets. (Always check with the physician for clarification, however.) 2. If you are working with tablets that are scored (grooved), round to the nearest half or whole tablet. For example, if your answer is 1.5 tablets and the tablets are scored, you will give the patient 1½ tablets.

Note: When performing multiple step problems, wait until the last step to round. If two separate problems are necessary to obtain an answer, round the last step of each problem. All weights should be rounded to the nearest hundredth. For example, 25.256 kg = 25.26 kg.

Rounding Equations

There will be some occasions when it will be necessary to round your answers to obtain the correct dosage. Table 31-7 illustrates guidelines for rounding adult dosages.

Because young children are so small, rounding becomes much more complicated. Always check the physician's preference when rounding for children.

Proportional Method

Some people prefer to use the proportional method when calculating dosages. The steps are listed below:

Example: The physician orders 0.75 g of Luvox. The medication on hand is 500 mg tablets.

Step 1. Determine if the ordered dose is in the same units as the dose on hand. If not, convert so that the two are in the same units before calculating the dosage.

Change 0.75 g to mg using the conversion factor formula. (Hint: 0.001 g = 1 mg.)

$$\frac{0.75\ \not{g}}{1} \times \frac{1\text{ mg}}{0.001\ \not{g}} = \frac{0.75\text{ mg}}{0.001}$$

$$0.75\text{ g} = 750\text{ mg}$$

Step 2. Next, set up a proportion to calculate the dosage.

Unit on hand : Medication form =
Dosage ordered : Unknown amount to be given

500 mg: 1 tab = 750 mg : x tab

Step 3. Remember that a proportion is the same as a fraction, so this can be written as:

$$\frac{500\text{ mg}}{1\text{ tab}} = \frac{750\text{ mg}}{x\text{ tab}}$$

Step 4. Cross multiply the numbers. This means to multiply the numerator from the left fraction with the denominator of the right fraction, and vice versa.

$$500x = 750$$

Step 5. Solve for x. To solve for x, divide both sides of this equation by 500. This leaves just "x" on the left side of the equation.

$$\frac{500x}{500} = \frac{750}{500}$$

$$x = \frac{750}{500}$$

$$x = 1.5$$

The answer is 1.5 tablets should be given.

Step 6. To check whether your answer is correct, insert your answer into the original formula in place of x and cross multiply.

500 mg : 1 tablet = 750 mg : 1.5 tablets

$$\frac{500\text{ mg}}{1\text{ tab}} = \frac{750\text{ mg}}{1.5\text{ tab}}$$

$$500 \times 1.5 = 750 \times 1$$

$$750 = 750$$

Formula Method

The formula method of calculating adult dosages requires the use of the following mathematical formula:

$$\frac{\text{Amount Desired}}{\text{Amount Available}} \times \text{Quantity (how it comes stocked, for example: 1 mL, 1 cap)}$$

The following steps can be used to calculate dosages using the formula method:

1. Determine if the dose desired is in the same units as the dose available or on hand. If not, convert so that they are in the same units.
2. Next, use the formula listed above to calculate the dosage.
3. Round the calculation using the criteria listed in Table 31-7.

Example: The physician orders 50 mg of Demerol. It comes stocked as 25 mg/mL, which means that there are 25 mg of Demerol in 1 mL of medication.

Step 1. The desired amount is already in the same units as the available amount, so no conversion is necessary.

Step 2. Set up the equation:

$$\frac{50 \text{ mg (Desired)}}{25 \text{ mg (Available)}} \times 1 \text{ mL} =$$

$$\frac{50}{25} \times 1 \text{ mL} =$$

$$2 \times 1 \text{ mL} = 2 \text{ mL}$$

(The unit mg cancels out.)

The answer is the patient should receive 2 mL of Demerol. (There is no need to round this answer.)

Refer to Procedure 31-1 for a procedure on calculating dosages for drug administration.

Calculating Pediatric Dosages

Because children are continuously growing, their size and weight must be considered when calculating pediatric dosages. The two common methods used to calculate the proper drug dosages for a pediatric patient are based on body surface area (BSA) and by kilograms of weight.

Calculating Pediatric Dosage by Body Surface Area (BSA)

The medical industry considers the **body surface area (BSA)** the most accurate method of calculating drug dosages for infants and children up to 12 years of age. In order to use this method, the child's height and weight must be known. A **nomogram** (Figure 31-1) is a graph that illustrates a relationship between two known values. The BSA is figured by drawing a straight line from the patient's height to the patient's weight. Where the numbers intersect on the surface area (SA) line is the figure that is used for the BSA. The BSA is then placed in the formula (equation) below to determine the proper dosage for the child.

$$\frac{\text{BSA of Child in m}^2}{1.7 \text{ (m}^2\text{)}} \times \text{Adult Dose} = \text{Child's Dose}$$

This formula is based on the average adult who weighs 140 lb and has a body surface area of 1.7 square meters (1.7 m^2).

Example: Michelle Turner is a five-year-old child who is 40 inches tall and weighs 38 lb. Find her BSA on the nomogram (BSA 0.7). The physician has ordered Demerol for extreme pain due to a fractured leg. The average adult dose of Demerol is 50 mg/mL. What dosage would be correct for Michelle according to the BSA method?

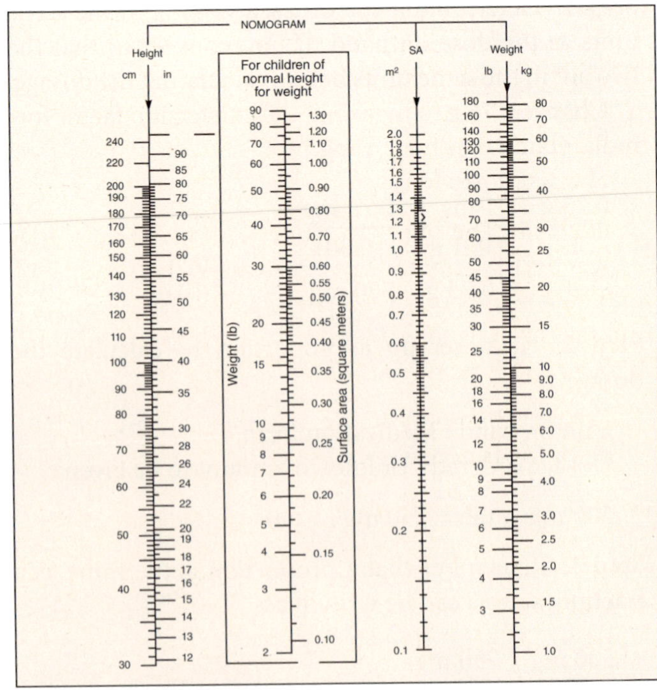

Figure 31-1 Information provided by the nomogram can help with dosage calculations.

CRITICAL THINKING CHALLENGE

Calculate the following dosage problems using either the proportional or formula method:

1. Order: 500 mg of Cipro (ciproflaxin HCL). Available: 250 mg tablets. Amount to be given?
2. Order: 50 mg of Thorazine. Available: 25 mg/mL. Amount to be given?
3. Order: 100 mg of Terramycin (oxytetracycline) IM. Available: 50 mg/mL. Amount to be given?

$$\frac{0.7\text{ m}^2}{1.7\text{ m}^2} \times 50\text{ mg} = \text{Child's Dose (round dose to the nearest whole number)}$$

$$\frac{0.7\text{ m}^2}{1.7\text{ m}^2} \times 50\text{ mg} = \frac{35}{1.7} = \text{20.5 mg (rounded = 21 mg)}$$

Once it has been determined that the pediatric patient is to get a 21 mg dosage of medication, it can be plugged into the formula used for calculating adult doses. For example, if the label reads that there is 50 mg/mL of medication, convert mg to mL using the following formula:

$$\frac{\text{Amount Desired}}{\text{Amount Available}} \times \text{Quantity}$$

Example:

$$\frac{21\text{ mg}}{50\text{ mg}} \times 1\text{ mL} = \frac{21}{50} = 0.42\text{ mL}$$

(Remember that anything less than 1 mL when rounding liquids is rounded to the nearest hundredth.)

Calculating Pediatric Dosage by Kilogram of Body Weight

Another way to calculate pediatric medication dosages is based on kilograms of body weight. Refer to the steps below:

1. Convert pounds into kilograms by dividing the number of pounds by 2.2. (Round the answer to the nearest hundredth.)
2. Multiply the dose ordered by kilogram of body weight.
3. If applicable, divide the child's dose by the number of equal doses to be given in a 24-hour period.

Example: The physician orders ceftriaxone sodium (Rocephin) 50 mg/kg. The medication should divided into equal doses every 12 hours (not to exceed 2 g) for Emma Porter, who weighs 66 pounds. How many milligrams will Emma receive?

1. Convert the pounds to kilograms. (In this case, no rounding is necessary.)

$$\frac{66\text{ lb}}{2.2} = 30\text{ kg}$$

2. Multiply the dose ordered by the weight in kilograms. (Cancel out like units.)

$$\frac{50\text{ mg}}{\text{kg}} \times 30\text{ kg} = 1{,}500\text{ mg} = 1.5\text{ g}$$

CRITICAL THINKING CHALLENGE

1. A child has a BSA of 0.5. The adult dose is 250 mg. How many mg of medication should the child receive? The label on the bottle states that there is 100 mg/mL of medication. How many mL should the child receive?
2. A child has a BSA of 0.8. The adult dose is 500 mg. What would be the correct dosage for this child? The label reads that there is 500 mg/2 mL of medication. How many mL of medication should the patient receive?

EHR Application

Some EHR programs feature an electronic dosage calculator within the software, which calculates the dosage after you enter the required information into the appropriate fields. There are also electronic dosage calculators available on the Internet (search for "online dosage calculators"). However, do not rely on the answer you receive from an electronic calculator. Always work the problem out first manually, and use the electronic calculator to check your work. This will help ensure you have the correct dose.

3. If applicable, divide the child's dose by the number of equal doses to be given in a 24-hour period.

   Divide 1,500 mg by 2 to obtain the divided dose = 750 mg

The answer is Emma will receive 750 mg of Rocephin every 12 hours, as ordered. (Note that this does not exceed 2 grams.)

CALCULATING INSULIN DOSAGES

Insulin is measured in units and should be administered with a U-100 syringe. U-100 means that there are 100 units in one milliliter or cubic centimeter of medication. Never use a standard mL syringe when administering insulin. The physician will determine the exact number of units to be given to the patient. Because of the role that insulin plays in the body, an error in dosage can lead to serious complications or even death. Because there are so many types of insulin, make certain that you have the correct type by reading the label thoroughly. When mixing insulin, make certain that the two are compatible. Start with clear and move to cloudy.

Types of Insulin

As you learned in Chapter 7, there are two types of diabetes: type 1 and type 2. Type 1 diabetics need insulin to control their blood sugar, however, type 2 diabetics may or may not need insulin.

There are three different types of human insulin available.

- Regular (Short acting, starts working 30–60 minutes after administration and lasts 3 to 6 hours).
- Intermediate-acting (Starts to work 2 to 4 hours post administration and lasts anywhere from 10 to 16 hours).
- Premixed (A mixture of both).

Analogs are insulin medicines that have been altered to help in faster absorption or last longer in the body. They include the following:

- Rapid-acting insulin: This means that its action is very quick (15–60 minutes following administration) and is usually taken shortly before or after meals. Examples of rapid-acting insulins include: Humulin R, Crystalline Zink, Humalog, Semilente, Velosulin, and Novolin.
- Long-acting insulin: This type of insulin takes the longest to exert its effects, usually 4 to 24 hours. It helps to control blood sugar between meals and when patients sleep. It is usually taken once to twice a day at the same time/s every day. Examples include: Ultralente, PZI or Protomaine Zink Insulin, and Insulin Glargine.
- Premixed: This insulin provides both intermediate and fast acting effects and is manufactured in different combinations. NovoLog 70/30 FlexPen is an example of a pre-mixed medication.

READING MEDICATION LABELS

The **medication label** is the product label that gives vital information about the medication. Medications normally come with an insert that has additional information that may be helpful in administering the medication. Medical assistants must be able to read and understand medication labels so that they can properly administer medications. Figure 31-2 shows an example

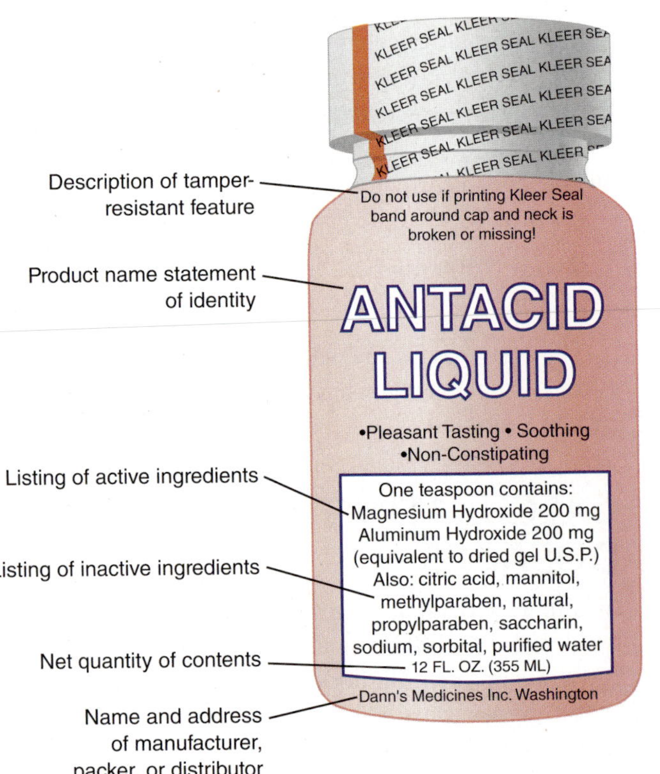

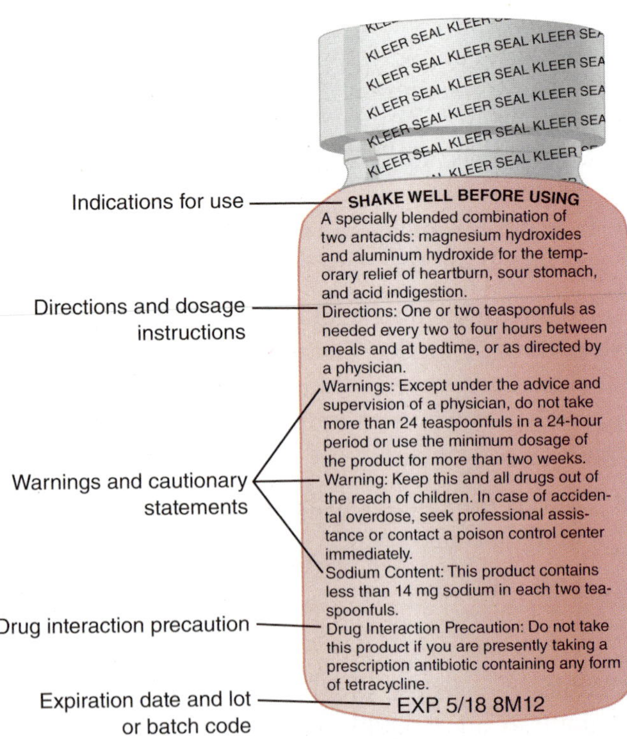

Figure 31-2 ■ Information found on a nonprescription label.

of a nonprescription product label that contains the following:

- A description of the tamper-resistant feature.
- The product name and dosage amount (if applicable).
- The active and inactive ingredients. Sometimes, this information appears on the medication insert.
- The quantity of the solution.
- The name and address of the manufacturer, packer, or distributor.
- The back of the label lists indications for use, dosage instructions, warnings, interaction problems, lot number, and expiration date.

Prescription medication labels are a little different than nonprescription labels. A **prescription** is an order for a prescribed drug. Prescription labels include vital information for the person dispensing the medication (Figure 31-3). Some specific parts of a prescription medication label include the following:

- **Product name** (Vistaril): Refers to the brand name of the medication.
- **Generic name** (if applicable) (hydroxyzine hydrochloride): This is the drug's official name; it can also be a listing of active and nonactive ingredients within the medication. Generic drugs are usually more affordable then brand name drugs.
- **National Drug Code (NDC)** (0049-5460-74): These are the numbers used to identify the manufacturer, the product, and the size of the container.
- Dosage strength (50 mg): This is the dosage strength for each unit.
- The drug form (liquid): This is the form in which the drug is supplied.
- The number of units (10 mL), or total volume: The number of units, capsules, mL, or tablets in the entire bottle.
- Usual dose and frequency (25 to 100 mg every four to six hours): The usual dosage administered to the patient in one dose and how often the dose is administered.
- Route of administration (intramuscular): This information indicates how the medication is to be given: IM, Sub-q, topically, rectally, and so on.
- Manufacturer's name (Pfizer Roerig).
- **Expiration date** (shown on Figure 31-4: 8/2020): The manufacturer only guarantees the effectiveness and safe use of the medication up to the expiration date posted on the drug package or container. If a drug is expired, it should be disposed of properly.
- **Lot control** or batch number (shown on Figure 31-4: 401803c): The manufacturer places a lot control or batch number on the label in order to track medications in the event that a bulk production of the drug is recalled due to numerous reports of severe adverse reactions or product contamination.
- Other information (refer again to Figure 31-3): Drug storage information (store below 86°F [30°C]; do not freeze), photosensitivity information, and so on.

FOR INTRAMUSCULAR USE ONLY.
USUAL ADULT DOSE: Intramuscularly: 25 - 100 mg stat; repeat every 4 to 6 hours, as needed.
See accompanying prescribing information.
Each mL contains 50 mg of hydroxyzine hydrochloride, 0.9% benzyl alcohol and sodium hydroxide to adjust to optimum pH.
To avoid discoloration, protect from prolonged exposure to light.
Rx only
10 mL
NDC 0049-5460-74
Vistaril®
(hydroxyzine hydrochloride)
Intramuscular Solution
50 mg/mL
Pfizer Roerig
Division of Pfizer Inc, NY, NY 10017
Store below 86°F (30°C).
PROTECT FROM FREEZING.
PATIENT: ____________
ROOM NO.: ____________
05-1111-32-4
MADE IN USA
9249

Figure 31-3 ■ Prescription drug labels contain vital information regarding the medication. Labels reproduced with permission of Pfizer Inc.

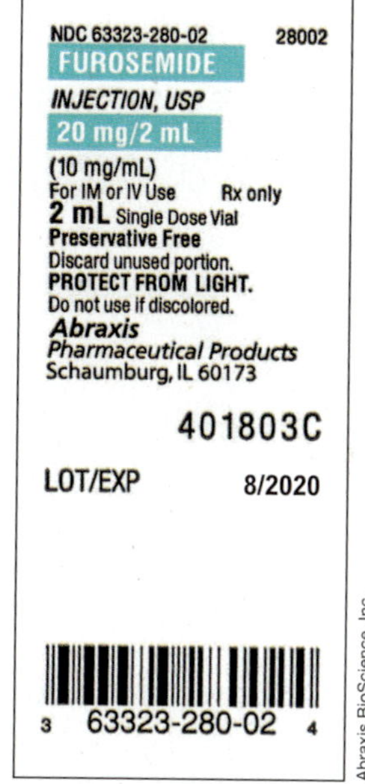

Figure 31-4 ■ Furosemide injection.

CRITICAL THINKING CHALLENGE

Using the product label in Figure 31-4, answer the following questions:

1. What is the product name?
2. What is the expiration date on the bottle?
3. What form does the medication come in?
4. What is the dosage amount for the medication?
5. Who is the manufacturer?

Warning Labels

Warning labels are placed on medications indicating special instructions for proper and effective usage of the drug. Patients must be informed of medication side effects, such as drowsiness or dizziness, which could make driving or operating machinery dangerous. Other warning labels may include instructions on how or when to take the medication. Examples include instructions to take the medication with food to lessen gastric distress or to take on an empty stomach due to interference with the drug's absorption or effectiveness. Additionally, warning labels may instruct patients to take their drugs with lots of water, to refrigerate the medication between doses, and even to shake the bottle well to resuspend the particles of some medications. Figure 31-5 illustrates a variety of instructions and warning labels for prescription medications.

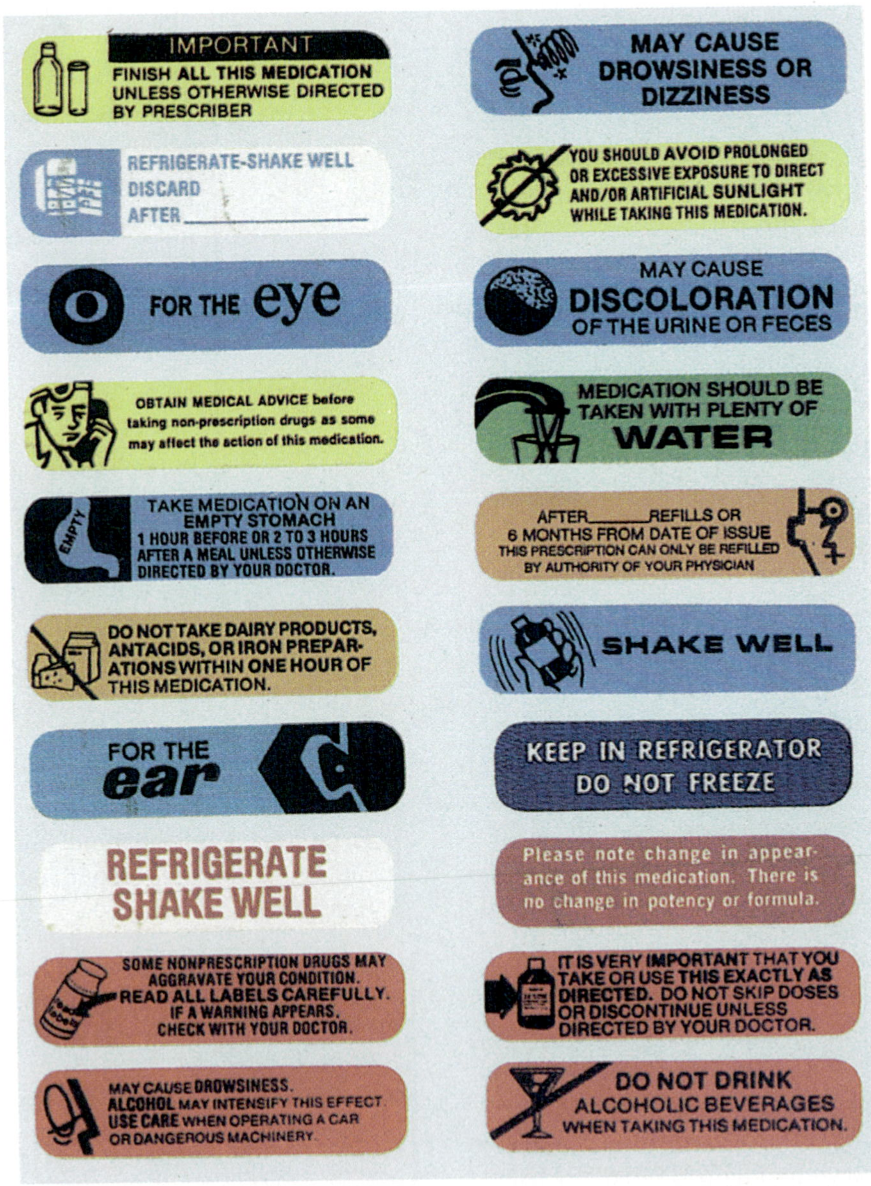

Figure 31-5 ■ Warning labels and instruction labels used on prescription medications.

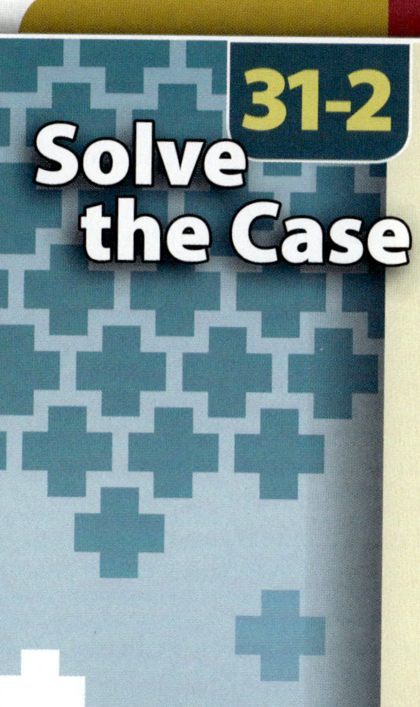

Mrs. Hamilton's chief complaint and vitals signs: Pt. c/o a productive cough and fever × three days. "My body aches from the tip of my head down to my feet." Temperature: 102.8 degrees Fahrenheit; pulse: 104; respiration: 26; and blood pressure: 146/88. The doctor ordered both a rapid influenza test and chest X-ray. The patient is positive for Type B influenza and the chest X-ray revealed that she has bilateral pneumonia. Dr. Bumgardner orders 1 G of Rocephin to be given IM and a breathing treatment. She also orders educational materials for influenza and pneumonia. The patient is to return in five days for a follow-up exam.

The label on the Rocephin reads as follows: 500 mg/2 mL.

1. **How many mL of Rocephin will you give the patient?**

Look up educational materials for pneumonia and influenza type B. Also look up common side effects of Rocephin.

2. **On a sheet of paper, write down the common side effects of Rocephin.**
3. **Using the educational materials you obtained, practice discharging the patient with another student.**

Procedure 31-1

Calculate a Medication Dosage for Administration

Objective:

To properly calculate a medication dosage for administration.

Equipment/Supplies:

- Patient's chart/EHR with the provider's order
- Medication vial
- Pencil/scrap paper
- Calculator

PROCEDURAL STEPS	DETAILS AND/OR RATIONALE
1. Obtain medication order, medication vial or bottle, pencil, a piece of scrap paper, and calculator.	Having all equipment and supplies together will make the process flow much better when calculating the dosage.
2. Compare the order with the medication label a minimum of three times to make certain you have the correct medication. (Check the name of the medication, the strength, and the expiration date.)	Checking the medication label a minimum of three times helps to confirm that you have the correct medication for the correct patient.
3. Compare the order with the medication label to make certain the prescribed units match the available units. (If not, do a metric conversion to get both into like units.)	If the order and available medication are not in like units, the dosage calculation will not be correct.
4. Calculate the correct dosage by applying the appropriate formula. ***Incorporate critical thinking skills when performing patient care.***	You must use the appropriate formula based on the size and age of the patient.
5. Write down the amount of medication to administer on the piece of scrap paper.	This will assist you in not forgetting the exact amount to give.

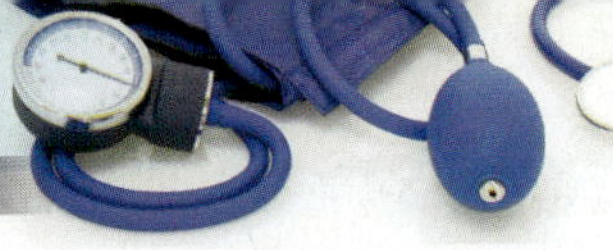

CHAPTER SUMMARY

- The medication order is an order that includes the name of the drug, the drug form, drug dosage, frequency of administration, and special instructions for taking the medication.
- Medical assistants must be familiar with delegation laws associated with medication administration.
- The apothecary system was the original primary method used for calculating and measuring medication dosages; however, the metric system is now considered the primary method.
- The metric system has evolved into the modern system known as Le Système International d'Unités (SI), or International System of Units, which is the primary method of measurement in medicine.
- The metric system is referred to as a decimal-based system because it is based on multiples of 10.
- There are 14 prefixes that are used within the metric system to describe the size of a metric unit; however, only a portion of those are used in health care.
- The three fundamental units used in the metric system are liters, meters, and grams. Meter (m), the fundamental unit of length, is used when measuring distance. Liter (L) is the fundamental unit of volume and is used when measuring liquids. Gram (g, gm) is the metric unit that is used when measuring anything that has mass or weight.
- Common metric prefixes and units can be are found in Tables 31-1 through 31-3.
- The term *conversion* means to switch from one unit to another. Conversion may be necessary when the physician orders a medication in a unit that is not available.
- The imperial system (also known as the household system) of measuring volume and weight can be found in any kitchen in the United States.
- Common household units and conversions between household measurements and metric measurements can be found in Tables 33-5 and 33-6.
- There are two major methods used for calculating adult dosages: the proportional method and the formula method.
- The two common methods used to calculate the proper drug dosages for a pediatric patient are based on body surface area (BSA) and by kilograms of weight.
- Table 33-7 lists guidelines for rounding adult dosages.
- Insulin is measured in units and should be administered with a U-100 syringe. U-100 means that there are 100 units in one milliliter or cubic centimeter of medication.
- There are three different types of insulin: rapid-acting, intermediate-acting, and long-acting.

CERTIFICATION REVIEW QUESTIONS

1. The fundamental units of the metric system include all of the following except:
   a. meters.
   b. liters.
   c. pounds.
   d. grams.
2. A physician orders Amoxicillin 500 mg by mouth (p.o.) *stat*. On hand you have 250 mg/1 tab. How much medication is to be administered to the patient?
   a. ½ tablet
   b. 1 tablet
   c. 1½ tablets
   d. 2 tablets
3. What is the decimal form that represents one/one hundredth?
   a. 1/100
   b. 0.01
   c. 0.1
   d. 1/10
4. When should household measurements be used?
   a. In a clinical setting
   b. When you can't do the conversion calculation
   c. When you want an exact dosage calculated
   d. When assisting patients with medication that they will administer at home

5. What chart is used to calculate dosages using the BSA method for pediatric patients?
   a. Metric chart
   b. Nomogram chart
   c. Household measurement chart
   d. No chart is necessary

6. Components of a medication label include all of the following except:
   a. the generic name of the medication.
   b. the price of the medication.
   c. the manufacturer of the medication.
   d. the listing of active ingredients.

7. The drug's official name is referred to as the:
   a. product name
   b. generic name
   c. NDC
   d. both a and c

8. When working with patients who have a very limited income, which type of drug would be more affordable?
   a. Brand drug
   b. Generic drug
   c. NDC
   d. Both a and c

9. Insulin is measured in:
   a. mL.
   b. units.
   c. mg.
   d. mEq.

10. When mixing insulins, you always move from:
   a. cloudy to clear.
   b. clear to cloudy.
   c. thin to thick.
   d. thick to thin.

STUDY RESOURCES

Resources to Test and Reinforce Your Knowledge:	
Certification Review Questions	Take this end-of-chapter quiz
Workbook	• Complete the activities for Chapter 31 • Perform the procedure for Chapter 31 using the Competency Checklist
Resources to Promote Critical Thinking:	
***Solve the Case* Activities**	• Consider these case studies and discuss your conclusions
Learning Lab	• Module 25: Pharmacology and Medication Administration
MindTap	• Complete Chapter 31 readings and activities

REFERENCES

Blesi, M. (2017). *Medical assisting: Administrative and clinical competencies*. (8th ed.). Clifton Park, NY: Cengage Learning.

Lindh, W. Q., Pooler, M. S., Tamparo, C. D., Dahl, B. B., Morris, J. A. (2014). *Delmar's comprehensive medical assisting*. (5th ed.). Clifton Park, NY: Cengage Learning.

Rice, J. (2011). *Principles of pharmacology for medical assisting*. (5th ed.). Clifton Park, NY: Cengage Learning.

"Your Insulin Options." *Cornerstones4Care*. Novo Nordisk Inc. May 2015. https://www.cornerstones4care.com/medicine/what-to-know/your-insulin-options.html

32

Administration of Parenteral Medications

ESSENTIAL TERMS

ampule
aqueous
aspirate
bolus
cannula
cartridge unit
cubic centimeter (cc)
diluent
extravasation
gauge
hypodermic
infiltration
intra-articular
intradermal
intramuscular (IM)
Luer-Lok
occlusion
parenteral
patency
phlebitis
precipitate
primary drug
secondary drug
subcutaneous (Sub-Q)
taut
thrombosis
trocar
vial
viscosity
wheal

CHAPTER OUTLINE

Administration of Parenteral Medications
- Parenteral Equipment and Supplies
- Preparing Medications
- General Guidelines for Parenteral Medications

Routes of Administration
- Intradermal Injections
- Subcutaneous Injections
- Intramuscular Injections

Parenteral Complications

Immunizations
- Contraindications and Precautions in Vaccine Administrations

Basics of Intravenous (IV) Therapy
- Equipment and Supplies Employed in Intravenous Therapy
- Documentation of IV Therapy
- Risks, Complications, and Adverse Reactions of IV Therapy
- Discontinuation of Intravenous Infusion Therapy

Intra-Articular Injections

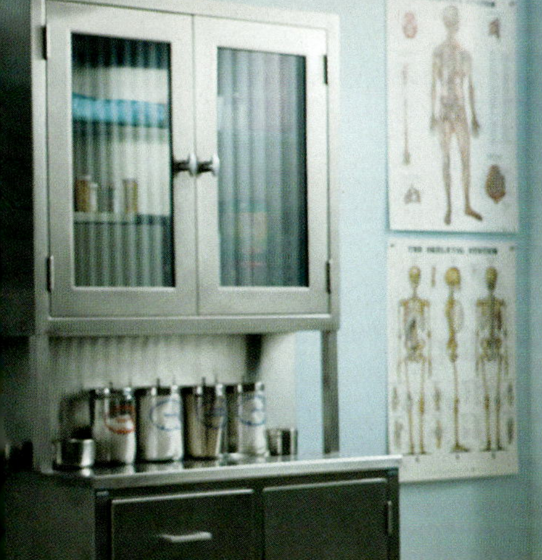

DEVELOPMENTAL OBJECTIVES

After completing this chapter, you should be able to:

1. Correctly spell and define the essential terms.
2. List six separate routes used for delivering parenteral medications.
3. List four common parenteral routes by injection and list which ones are routinely performed by the medical assistant.
4. Name and describe the components of a hypodermic needle and syringe.
5. Describe various designs of needle safety devices, and discuss the importance of using these devices.
6. Describe the importance of needle safety when administering injections.
7. Describe factors that help determine the size of the syringe, the length of needle, and the gauge of needle to be used.
8. List complications that may occur when incorrect equipment is used or the medication is administered using the wrong route.
9. Describe the role of the medical assistant in the administration of intravenous (IV) medications.
10. List several complications that may occur when administering IV medications.
11. List instances in which IV therapy should be discontinued.

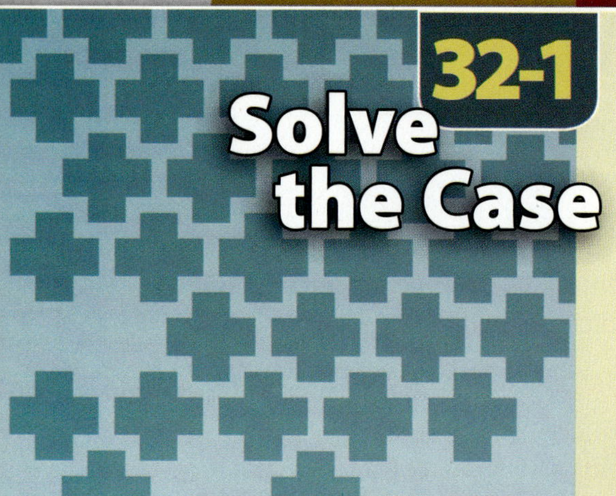

A 35-year-old female with prior history of menstrual migraines presents to clinic with a headache rated as a constant 8/10 throbbing pain over her right eye. The pain is identical to her prior migraines but more severe, associated with photophobia (sensitivity to light) and nausea. Vital signs are all within normal ranges. Based on your current level of understanding, answer the following questions.

1. **What can be done now to help relieve some of the patient's current symptoms?**
2. **Do you think that everyone that comes into a medical clinic with pain is actually in pain?**
3. **How do you keep from being judgmental toward patients in pain?**

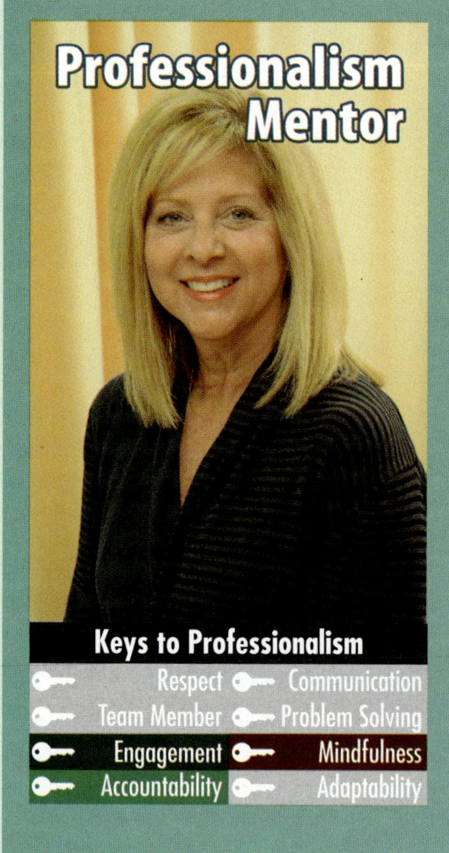

One thing I know for sure after many years in the medical field, is that patients do not like getting injections. I'm fairly certain I have never heard a patient say "Oh good, I'm getting a shot today!" Once in a while, following an injection, a patient will say, "that didn't hurt too bad." However, when it does hurt, you always hear about it. Knowing how to administer an injection requires both knowledge and skill. You cannot be a successful medical assistant by only having one of those attributes. You will get better at giving injections over time with practice. However, many of the medical assistants I work with don't always follow the seven rights of administration or forget to aspirate or check expiration dates. In other words, they get careless in their practice and sooner or later one of their patients gets hurt. It can be a painful stick, wrong site, or needle size, or even inadvertent contamination of the insertion site that leads to infection. The list is long and it's easy to fall into noncompliant behaviors. To be successful as a medical assistant you must gain the trust of the health care providers you work with and the patients you serve. You must pay attention to detail and demonstrate excellence in work ethic by always following the correct protocol for administering any medication you give. A true professional will never take short cuts. How will you practice? Will you take short cuts when you get busy or behind in your work? It happens! In your journal, describe how the keys listed in this feature apply to this scenario. Then write a pledge to yourself to always be vigilant when giving medications. Read your pledge often; it will help you to always make the right call. ■

INTRODUCTION

Medical assistants are often responsible for the administration of parenteral medications. The most common form of parenteral medication is injectables. In order to successfully perform this task, the medical assistant must be able to select the appropriate equipment, properly prepare the medication, select a suitable site, and administer the medication using the correct technique. Both providers and patients want to know that they can depend on the medical assistant to institute safety checks along the way to ensure that the entire procedure is performed with absolute accuracy.

Failure to institute safety measures can result in serious consequences for the patient and possible litigation for the office. This chapter will address the many duties associated with parenteral drug administration and provide useful tips that will aid in decreasing patient discomfort and anxiety.

ADMINISTRATION OF PARENTERAL MEDICATIONS

The term **parenteral** means pertaining to outside the intestines. When referring to parenteral medication, it means to deliver medication via a route other than through the digestive tract. The most common route used to deliver parenteral medications is through injection; however, other parenteral routes include intravenous (within the vein), transdermal (through the skin), transmucosal (through the mucus membrane), topical (on the skin), and inhalation (through the respiratory tract). This chapter addresses parenteral medications delivered through the injection and intravenous routes; refer to Chapter 30 for all enteral and other forms of parenteral routes. Common parenteral routes by injection include intradermal, subcutaneous, intramuscular, and intra-articular. Of those routes, only three are routinely used by the medical assistant: intradermal, subcutaneous, and intramuscular. Some medical assistants are also responsible for administering intravenous medications; however, this will vary according to the state's medical practice act and office policy.

Parenteral medications are delivered into the bloodstream much more rapidly than oral medications, usually within minutes. The following list provides information regarding the amount of time it takes for a medication to enter the bloodstream through selected parenteral routes:

- Intravenous: Instantly to seconds
- Intramuscular: 5 to 15 minutes, depending on the drug
- Subcutaneous: Several minutes

Table 32-1 lists both the advantages and disadvantages of parenteral administration.

Parenteral Equipment and Supplies

There is a multitude of equipment and supplies available for the delivery of parenteral medications. Syringes and needles come in many sizes and are selected according to the route the medication is to be given, the patient's body size, the **viscosity** (or thickness) of the medication, and the amount of medication to be given.

Syringes

Syringes (Figure 32-1) used today are primarily made of plastic and are completely disposable. Typical syringe sizes range from 1 to 5 mL. Larger syringes (10–60 mL) are used for irrigating wounds or body cavities, drawing large amounts of blood, and for aspirating fluid from a patient's joint or body cavity. Syringe selection is primarily based on the amount of medication to be administered.

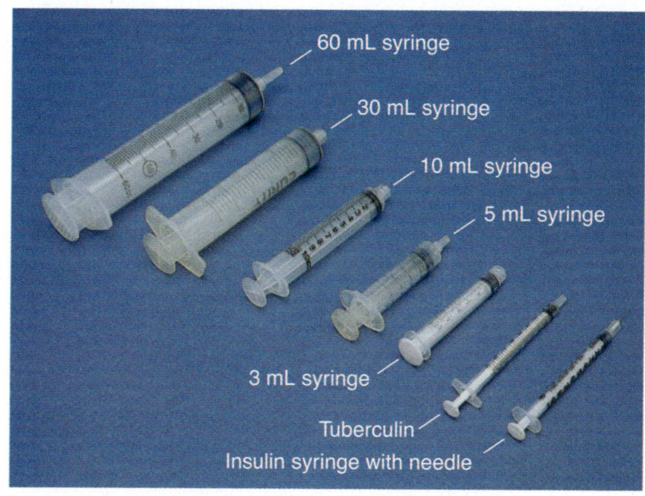

Figure 32-1 ■ Syringes come in a variety of sizes.

Table 32-1 Advantages and Disadvantages of the Parenteral Route of Administration

Advantages	Disadvantages
Effective route when other routes would be difficult to use. For example, if the patient is unconscious or unresponsive.	Unsanitary equipment or mishandling of the equipment could cause microorganisms to be introduced into the patient.
Medications administered by injection do not cause irritation to the patient's digestive system, nor are they altered by gastric acids.	An allergic reaction to a parenteral drug may occur more rapidly and may be more severe than an allergic reaction to an oral medication because of how quickly it is absorbed into the bloodstream and the amount that is given in one dose.
An exact dose can be administered to a direct site by injection.	Improper injection procedures could cause damage to the patient's nerves, tissue, veins, and other vessels.
Effects of the medication take place much more rapidly than the oral route, so a patient who is in excessive pain would receive faster relief from a parenteral pain reliever than an oral pain reliever.	Veins could be traumatized by an intravenous injection.

Syringes are packaged in hard plastic containers or peel-apart packages and are sealed to ensure sterility. If a syringe package appears to have already been opened, the syringe should not be used and should be disposed of properly.

The components of a syringe include the calibrated barrel, plunger, flange, and tip (Figure 32-2). Table 32-2 explains each component of a syringe.

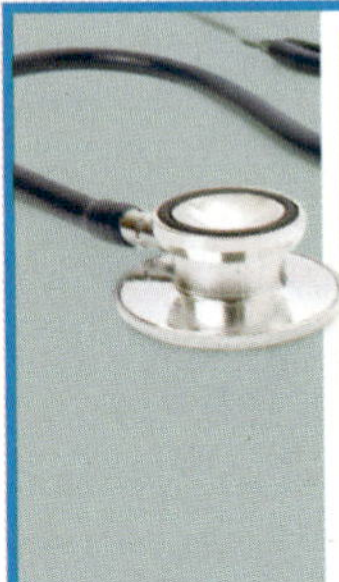

Field Smarts

In order to prevent the medication from becoming contaminated, you must never touch the inside of the barrel of the syringe, the rubber stopper on the plunger, or the tip of the syringe that connects to the needle.

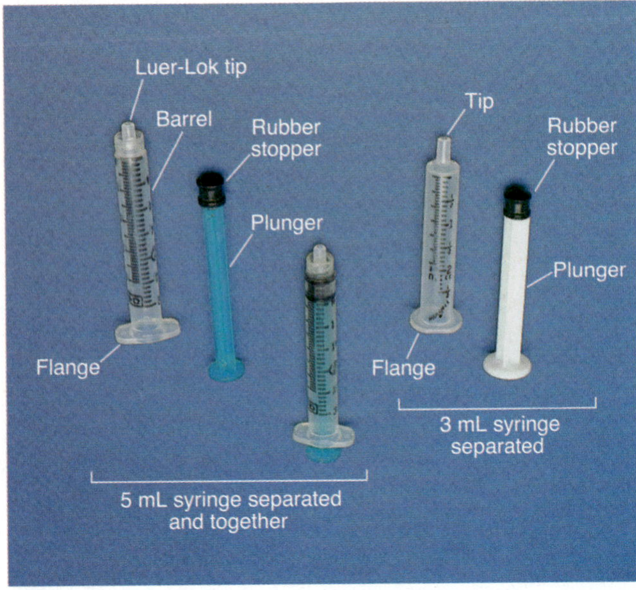

Figure 32-2 ■ The parts of a syringe.

Needles

Needles are available in various sizes and lengths and come in disposable and non-disposable forms. Needle selection is determined by the type of medication to be administered, the route of administration, and the size of the patient. Disposable needles are more commonly used and are prepackaged in sterile plastic or paper wrappers. Disposable safety needles are the standard of care in most facilities as there is reduced risk of accidental needle sticks and blood contamination.

A needle's **gauge** (G) refers to the diameter of the needle. Gauge selection is determined by the viscosity or thickness of the medication. Gauge sizes that are typically used in ambulatory care range from 18 to 27 G. The larger the gauge, the smaller the diameter of the needle (for example, a 22 G needle would be smaller in diameter than a 20 G needle). Figure 32-5 illustrates a variety of different needle gauges and lengths available.

Table 32-3 provides specific details for selecting the appropriate gauge based on the route and the viscosity of the medication. *Note*: The general guidelines for needle gauges are provided later in the chapter under "Routes of Administration" and should be used as guidelines for certification and registration testing.

The length of the needle is determined by the route of administration, the site of the injection, and the amount of adipose tissue over the injection site. Intramuscular (IM) injections will require a longer needle than a subcutaneous or intradermal injection because muscles are deeper than the other two types of tissue. The location of the injection also plays a role in the selection of needle length. The deltoid and ventrogluteal muscle are two common muscles that are used for intramuscular

Table 32-2 Description of the Components of a Syringe

Barrel	The cylinder that holds the medication and contains calibrations for precise measuring. The barrel is typically calibrated or marked in milliliters (mL) or **cubic centimeters (cc)**; however, manufacturers are phasing out syringes labeled in cubic centimeters (cc). Some specialty syringes contain other calibrations such as the insulin syringe, which is calibrated in Units.
Plunger	A plastic rod with a *rubber stopper* on one end that seals the medication within the syringe and flared edges on the other end for maneuvering the plunger. This apparatus either draws medication in or pushes medication out of the barrel.
Flange	The flared plastic rim on the syringe used for guiding the plunger.
Tip	The part of the syringe in which the needle is attached. Different types of syringe tips include: the *Slip-tip* (Figure 32-3), a smooth tip in which the needle is attached just by slipping it onto the syringe; and the **Luer-Lok** tip (Figure 32-4), which has a threaded end in which the needle can be locked by twisting. The tip of the syringe must remain sterile throughout the entire procedure.

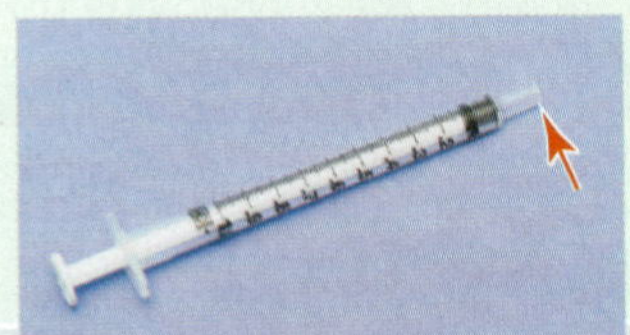

Figure 32-3 ■ An example of a syringe with a slip-tip.

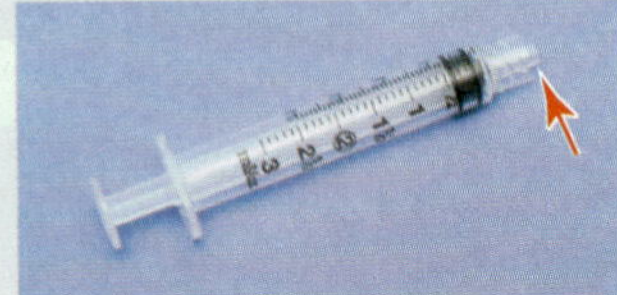

Figure 32-4 ■ An example of a syringe with a Luer-Lok tip.

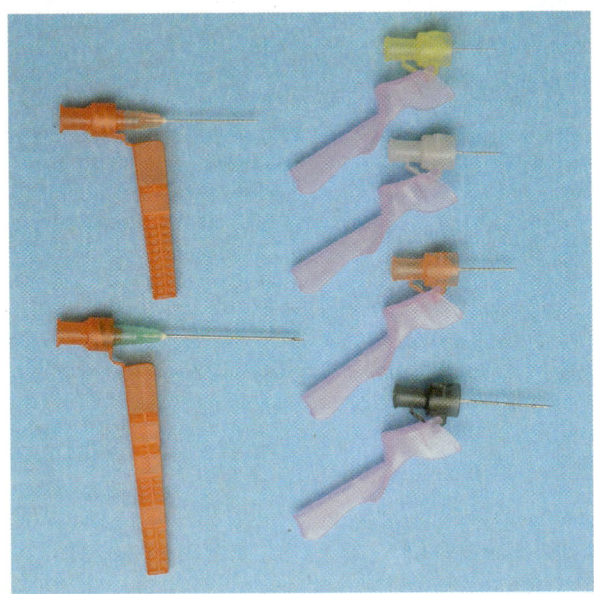

Figure 32-5 ■ A variety of needles with different lengths and gauges.

injections, but each muscle is a different size and at a different depth. The deltoid is smaller and more superficial than the ventrogluteal muscle and, therefore, would take a shorter needle. Finally, the amount of adipose tissue that the patient has in the area in which the injection is being administered will also play a role in the length of the needle that is used. Patients with larger amounts of adipose tissue will require a longer needle to penetrate through the extra layers than patients with little adipose tissue.

Table 32-4 provides specific needle lengths based upon the route of administration, the location of the injection, and the size of the patient. *Note:* The general guidelines for needle lengths are provided later in the chapter under "Routes of Administration" and should be used as guidelines for certification and registration testing.

Table 32-3 Gauge Sizes Based upon the Route of Administration and Viscosity of the Medication

Gauge of Needle	Viscosity of Medication	Route	Examples
18–20	Thicker or oil-based medications	IM	Hormones, steroids, penicillin, and certain vitamin preparations
21–23	**Aqueous** or water-based medications	IM	Immunizations and other water-based medications
23–25	Aqueous-based medications	Sub-Q	Immunizations, allergy medications, etc.
26–27	Aqueous-based medications	ID	Allergy testing extracts and PPD extract
30 (usually ultra-fine point)	Aqueous-based medications	Sub-Q	Used when repeated injections are given, such as insulin

Table 32-4 Needle Lengths Based upon the Route of Administration, Location of the Injection, and Size of the Patient (Adult Chart)

Intradermal Injections	
Patients of all sizes	⅜″ to ½″
Subcutaneous Injections	
Patients with little adipose tissue (muscular patients)	⅜″ to ½″
Patients with an average to large amount of adipose tissue	½″ to ⅝″
Intramuscular Injections	
Deltoid: Adult with an underdeveloped or atrophied deltoid muscle and very little adipose tissue (i.e., frail adult)	⅝″
Deltoid: Adult with a well-developed deltoid muscle and an average amount of adipose tissue	1″
Deltoid: Adult with a well-developed deltoid and a large amount of adipose tissue	1″
Ventrogluteal: Adult with very little adipose tissue	1″
Ventrogluteal: Adult with an average amount of adipose tissue	1″ to 1½″
Ventrogluteal: Adult with a large amount of adipose tissue	1½″ to 2″
Vastus lateralis (thigh): Adult with very little adipose tissue	1″
Vastus lateralis (thigh): Adult with an average amount of adipose tissue	1″ to 1½″
Vastus lateralis (thigh): Adult with a large amount of adipose tissue	1½″ to 2″

Little adipose tissue: Can only pull up very little adipose tissue when lightly pinching the skin in the area in which you are administering the injection (typically females or males less than 130 lb).

Average amount of adipose tissue: Can pull up an average amount of adipose tissue when lightly pinching the skin in the area in which you are administering the injection (typically females 130 to 200 lb or males 130 to 260 lb).

Large amount of adipose tissue: Can pull up a large amount of adipose tissue when lightly pinching the skin in the area in which you are administering the injection (typically females 200+ lb or males 260+ lb).

Parts of the Needle

Even though needles come in disposable and non-disposable forms, they all have similar components. Figure 32-6 illustrates different needles that are used for various routes and Figure 32-7 illustrates the different parts of a needle.

The parts of a needle include the following:

- Point: The sharpened end of the needle, cut in a slanted edge called the bevel.
- Lumen: The bore of a hollow needle.
- Bevel: The flat, slanted edge of the needle that helps to ease the insertion of the needle into the tissue; there are finer cuts and different lengths of bevels, such as a fine tip bevel, which is used for insulin syringe needles. The finer the cut of the bevel, the less pain felt by the patient and the less trauma to the patient's tissue.
- Shaft: The hollow steel tube of the needle through which the medication passes into the patient.
- Hub: The component that facilitates the attachment of the needle to the syringe; the hub is color-coded for easy recognition of the size and must remain sterile when assembling the needle and syringe.
- Hilt: The part of the needle in which the shaft attaches to the hub.
- Safety device: A mechanism to shield the needle after use (also see Figure 32-8).

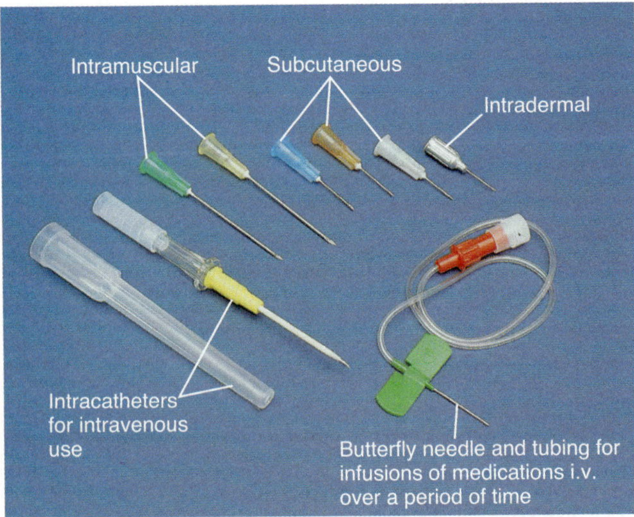

Figure 32-6 ■ Different needles used for various routes of administration. (Safety devices not shown so that all parts of the needle are visible.)

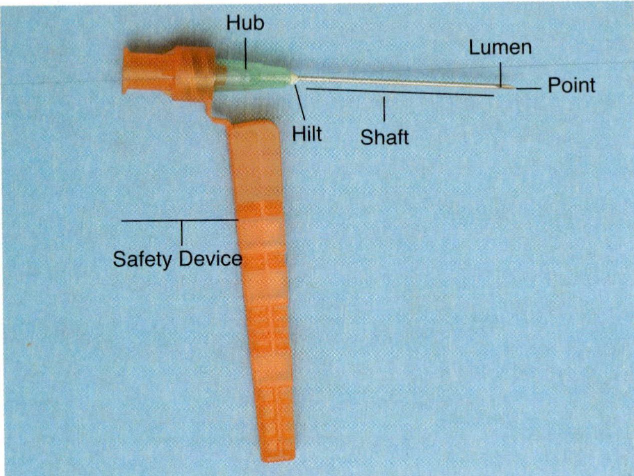

Figure 32-7 ■ The parts of a needle.

Needle Safety when Using Parenteral Equipment

Needle safety is very important when working with parenteral equipment. Each office should use safety devices to help prevent accidental needle sticks from

CRITICAL THINKING CHALLENGE

An elderly, frail patient comes into the practice to obtain a flu vaccine, which is an aqueous or water-based solution. The patient's deltoid muscle is not very prominent and the patient has very little fat over the deltoid. The needles available are 23 G ⅝″, 22 G 1″, and 20 G 1½″.

1. **What needle would work best for this particular medication and patient? Give the reason for your selection.**

CRITICAL THINKING CHALLENGE

Mrs. Sims in room 2 is waiting for an ACTH injection. ACTH is a very thick, oily hormone. Mrs. Sims has a large amount of adipose tissue around her hips and buttocks region and weighs 253 pounds. The needle sizes available include 27 G ⅜″, 25 G ⅝″, 22 G 1″, 21 G 1½″, and 20 G 2″.

1. **Which needle would work best under these conditions? List your reasons.**

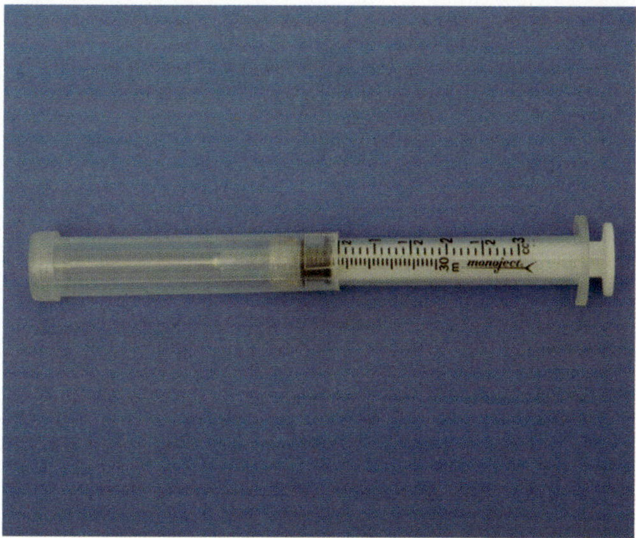

Figure 32-8 ■ Syringe with safety shield that pulls over the needle.

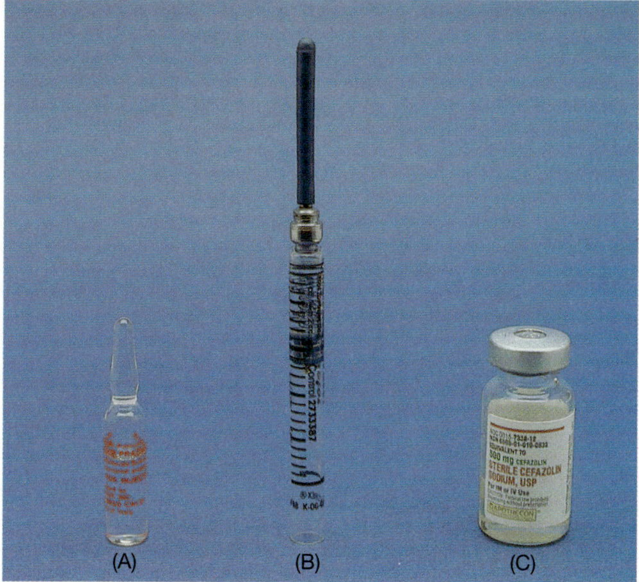

Figure 32-9 ■ Various medication containers: (a) ampule; (b) cartridge unit; (c) vial.

contaminated needles. There are a variety of different types of safety devices, including retractable needles and plastic sheaths that slide down over the needle. Figure 32-8 shows another type of safety device.

If the medical assistant is accidentally stuck by a contaminated needle during or following an injection she should wash the area immediately with soap and water and report the incident to a supervisor. An incident report should be completed and the employee should receive counseling regarding what lab testing should be performed and possible treatment options. Depending upon the risk, bloodwork from the patient and the employee will be necessary for immediate testing, and the employee may require repeated testing over several months. Refer to Chapter 10 for a review of needle safety guidelines and procedures to follow in the event of a needle stick.

Preparing Medications

Medications for parenteral administration are stored in a variety of different containers. Medications may be stored in a(n):

- **Ampule** (Figure 32-9a): A glass container with a stem that holds a single dose of medication
- **Cartridge unit** (Figure 32-9b): A disposable, prefilled, single-dose cartridge of medication that slips into a nondisposable injection device
- **Vial** (Figure 32-9c): A glass or plastic container that may contain either a single dose or multiple doses of medication

Measuring Medication in a Syringe

The type of syringe used will be based on the amount of medication to be administered and sometimes on the type of medication (e.g., insulin). Syringes are normally calibrated in mL. To draw up the correct amount of medication, the medical assistant must be able to properly read the calibrations on the outside of the syringe. The shorter lines (Figure 32-10a) on a 1 mL tuberculin syringe are measured in increments of hundredths. Each small line represents 0.01 mL, or 1/100 of a milliliter. The longer lines (Figure 32-10b) are measured in tenths—each line represents 0.1 mL, or 1/10 of an mL, and range from 0.1 to 1.0 mL. On a 3 mL syringe, the smaller calibrations (Figure 32-10c) are measured in tenths and represent 0.1, or 1/10 of an mL. The larger lines (Figure 32-10d) represent increments of ½, 1, 1½, 2, 2½, and 3 mL. On a 5 mL syringe, the smaller calibrations (Figure 32-10e) are measured on a scale of 0.2, or 2/10 of an mL, with the longer calibration (Figure 32-10f) lines representing 1, 2, 3, 4, and 5 mL.

Some specialty syringes are measured in units. A unit is the amount of a substance necessary to stimulate a biological effect. The biological effect that one unit of medication has upon body tissue is decided upon by the International Conference for the Unification of Formulas. Unit increments are commonly used for substances such as insulin and particular vitamins and are specific to the individual substance or medication being administered;

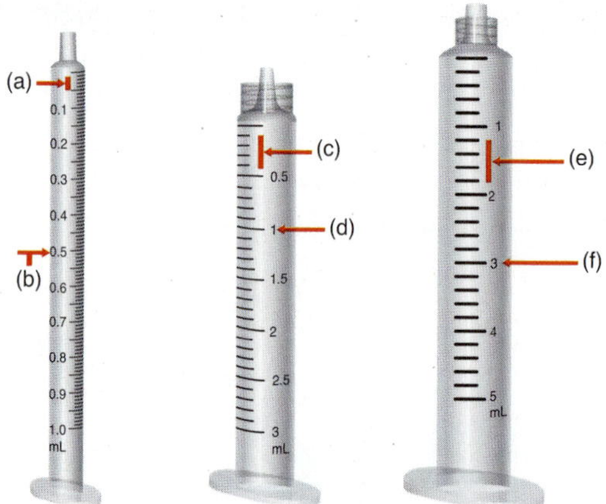

Figure 32-10 ■ The markings on 1, 3, and 5 mL syringes. (a) The shorter lines on a 1 mL syringe are measured in hundredths. (b) The longer lines on a 1 mL syringe are measured in tenths. (c) The shorter lines on a 3 mL syringe are measured in tenths. (d) The longer lines on a 3 mL syringe are measured in wholes or halves. (e) The shorter lines on a 5 mL syringe are measured in 2/10 of an mL or 0.2 mL increments. (f) The longer lines on a 5 mL syringe are measured in whole numbers.

therefore, insulin syringes may not be interchanged with other types of syringes.

To correctly fill a syringe, the plunger should be pulled back so that the top ring on the plunger is even with the calibration line on the outside of the syringe, matching the amount of medication ordered by the physician (Figure 32-11), which in this case is 70 units.

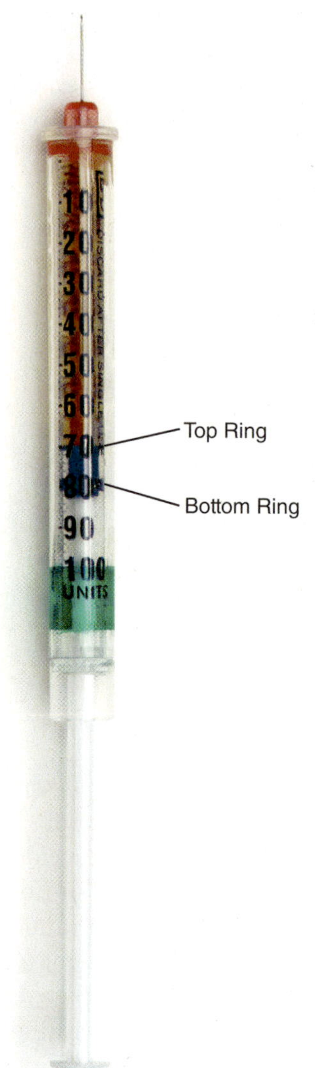

Figure 32-11 ■ Use the top ring of the plunger for measuring medication volumes.

Withdrawing Medication from a Vial

When medication is stored in a vial, it may be in a single -dose vial (containing an individual dose of medication) or a multiple-dose vial (containing several doses). The name and strength of the drug should be checked on the medication label a minimum of three times and verified with the physician's order. Always check the expiration date on the vial as well. This information is usually checked:

- When removing the medication vial from the shelf
- Right before preparing the medication
- Right after preparing the medication

A vial is packaged with a sterile cap that protects the rubber stopper. Remove the metal or sterile cap and cleanse the rubber stopper with an alcohol swab.

Medication in a multi-dose vial must be aspirated, or pulled into the syringe through a needle, by pulling back on the plunger of the syringe.

To prepare the syringe for use, remove it from the wrapper and assemble the needle. Pull the plunger within the barrel back to the calibration line that matches the amount of medication to be removed. For example, for removing 1½ mL of medication from the vial, 1½ mL of air must be inserted into the vial before withdrawing the medication.

There is an air pressure vacuum inside the vial that makes it easier to pull up the medication. The purpose of forcing air into the vial is to equalize the pressure within the vial after the medication has been removed. If the proper amount of air is not inserted within the vial, the pressure within the vial will drop, making it very difficult to pull back on the plunger when filling subsequent syringes. On the other hand, if too much air is inserted within the vial, the pressure within the vial will become very powerful, causing the medication to be involuntarily forced out through the stopper and out into the syringe.

Once the vial is prepared and the plunger is pulled back to the amount of medication being withdrawn, insert the needle into the vial (Figure 32-13), in the space above the solution. With the vial still in an upright position, push the plunger forward to expel the air within the syringe into the vial. Pick up the vial and invert it with the needle in it. Make certain that the needle is below the liquid line before pulling back on the plunger (Figure 32-14).

Carefully pull back on the plunger until reaching the desired amount of medication to be withdrawn. Gently pull the needle out of the vial and carefully place the

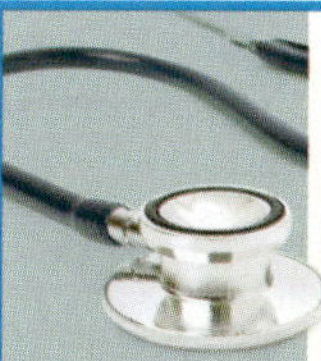

Field Smarts

Always inspect the rubber stopper of the vial to make certain that the rubber is completely intact. Check the medication in the vial to make sure the there is no **precipitate** (pieces of solid material or crystals) or unusual cloudiness. If anything unusual does appear, do not use the medication and check with a supervisor to see if it should be discarded. If at all possible, you should only use single-dose vials; however, if it is not possible, place an expiration date on the vial once the vial is opened. Typically, the medication is only good for 28 days, but always check the manufacturer's instructions. Always clean the rubber stopper off with alcohol before filling syringes.

CRITICAL THINKING CHALLENGE

Review Figure 32-12 and write down the amount of medication in each of the syringes shown.

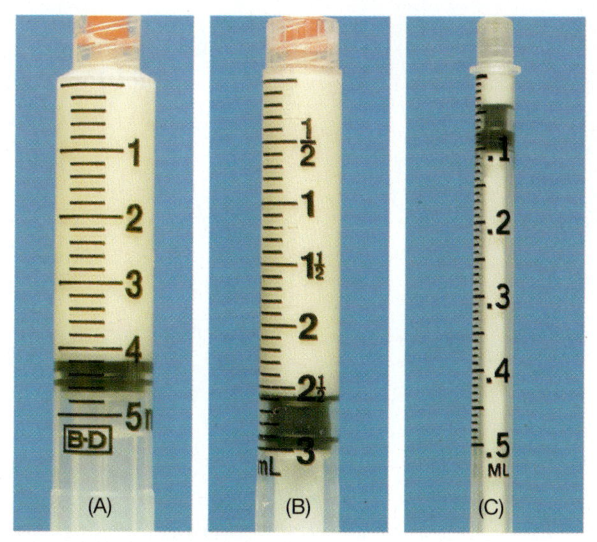

Figure 32-12 ■ What is the volume of medication in each of the following syringes?

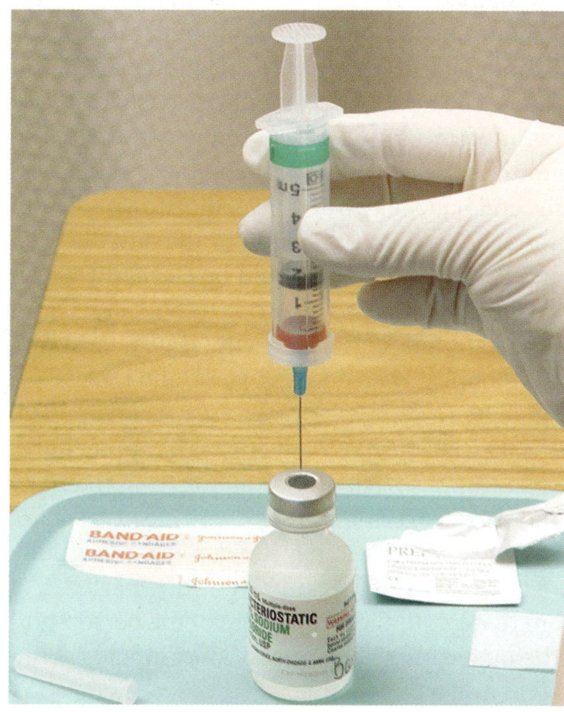

Figure 32-13 ■ Expel an amount of air into the vial that is equal to amount of medication to be withdrawn.

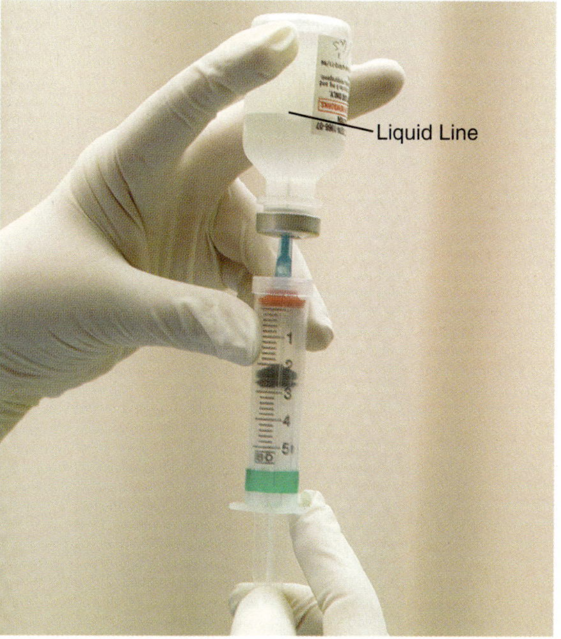

Figure 32-14 ■ The needle must be below the liquid line in the vial before withdrawing the medication.

cap on the needle following institutional policy. (Tiny air bubbles in the syringe may need to be removed by gently flicking the syringe prior to withdrawing the needle from the vial.) Procedure 32-1 lists the proper steps for performing this procedure.

Withdrawing Medication from an Ampule

An ampule is made of sterile glass and contains one single dose of medication premeasured to the exact volume or amount needed. Examples of single-dose medications contained in an ampule include heparin and sterile saline. The neck of the ampule is constricted and may cause medication to become trapped at the top of the ampule (Figure 32-15). By flicking the ampule with your wrist and hand, any trapped medication in the top will be forced down into the body of the ampule. The outer surface of the ampule should be cleaned with an alcohol pad or other antiseptic prior to opening.

The glass ampule is hermetically sealed, meaning the dose is completely enclosed in glass, and the neck is scored (indented), so it will break easily when opened. The medical assistant should practice safety procedures when separating the neck of the ampule from the body of the ampule by covering the neck with a gauze square or safety device and breaking it away from the body (Figure 32-16). This will help prevent tiny particles of glass from flying into the face or eyes of the person preparing the medication. The neck of the ampule should be placed in a sharps container.

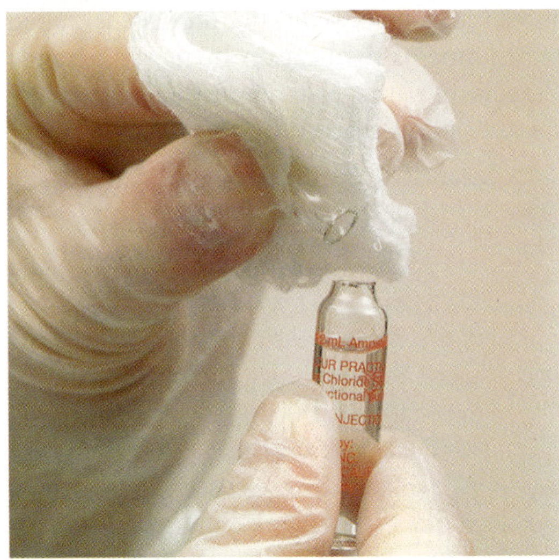

Figure 32-16 ■ Cover the neck of the ampule with gauze and snap the neck off away from you.

A special needle that contains a small filter within the lumen should be used to remove any glass particles that may have mixed with the medication when the top was snapped from the body of the ampule. A membrane filter (Figure 32-17) may also be attached to the syringe before attaching the needle to keep glass contaminants out of the syringe. The filter needle is then removed and replaced with a **hypodermic** needle before injecting the patient. Refer to Procedure 32-2 for the proper steps to follow when withdrawing medication from an ampule.

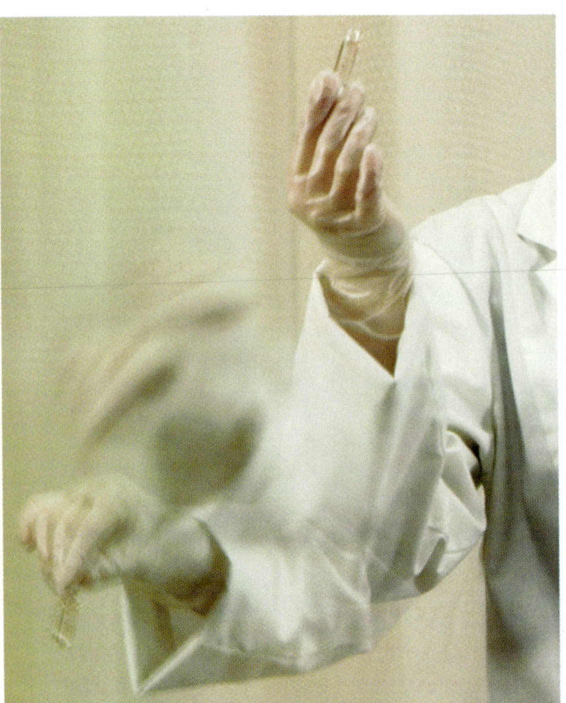

Figure 32-15 ■ Force medication from the neck of the ampule by a quick snap of the wrist.

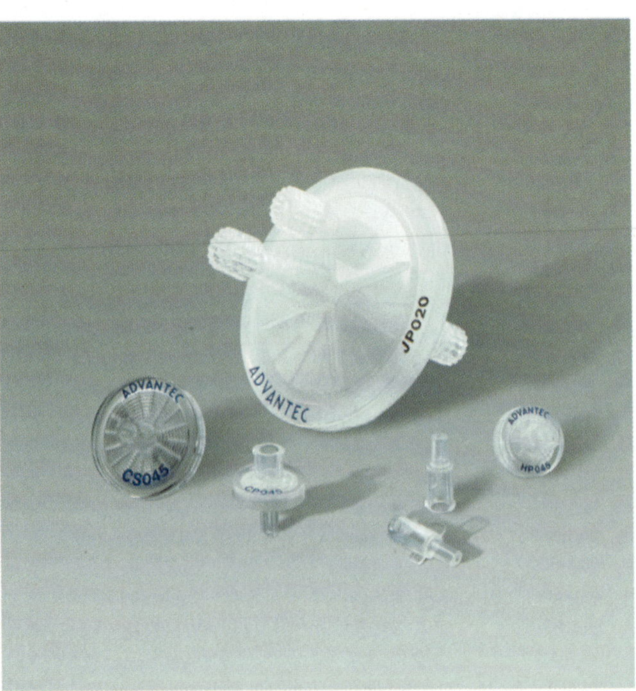

Figure 32-17 ■ Various membrane filters that can be attached to syringes of all sizes, in place of using a standard filter needle.

Reconstituting Medications for Injection

Certain medications are packaged in powdered (dry) form and must be reconstituted with a liquid in order to be injected. Powder forms of medication have a longer shelf-life than liquid forms. A **diluent** (liquid) is used to reconstitute the powder. Normally this solution is sterile saline (NaCl), sterile water (H_2O), or lidocaine. The diluent may be supplied with the medication or may need to be drawn up separately. The medical assistant must always follow the manufacturer's instructions when reconstituting a medication.

Once the diluent is removed from its original container, it is injected into the powdered drug vial and gently mixed by rolling the solution between both hands until the all of the powder particles are dissolved.

Once the particles are completely dissolved, the medical assistant will draw up the freshly made dilution (medication) following the physician's orders. Procedure 32-3 provides detailed instructions on the steps required for reconstituting powdered drugs.

Mixing Two Medications in a Single Syringe

When a physician orders two medications, it is sometimes possible to combine the two drugs into one syringe, thus making it possible to give one injection instead of two separate injections. It is most important to check with the physician or pharmacist to clarify if the two medications can be combined. Some medications are incompatible and may cause problems when combined.

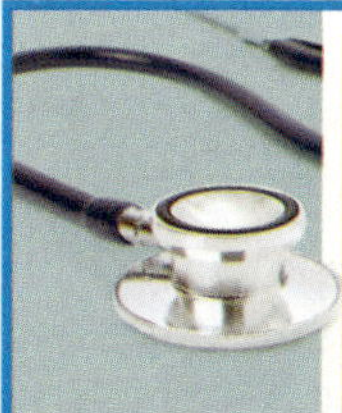

Field Smarts

Changing the needle between the vial and patient reduces complications during and following the injection. Each time the needle is pushed through the stopper of a vial, it becomes dulled, making it difficult to puncture the skin and creating more pain for the patient. In addition, irritating substances such as allergy extracts may adhere to the needle upon aspiration from the vial. As the needle penetrates the skin, a small amount of the medication may adhere to the skin, causing a painful local reaction at the site of the injection.

When combining two medications, the medical assistant must determine which medication is the **primary drug** and which is the **secondary drug**. The primary drug is the first drug to be drawn up into the syringe. When administering insulin, the primary drug is the clear insulin and the secondary drug is the cloudier insulin. Always check with the physician when in doubt. Procedure 32-4 lists step-by-step instructions for mixing two medications in a single syringe.

Using a Medication Cartridge or an Injector Device

Some medications come in sealed, prefilled disposable glass cartridges that hold a single dose of medication. Depo-Provera, penicillin G benzathine, Phenergan, and interferon are examples of medications that are available in cartridges. The prefilled cartridge–needle units require no mixing, no special calculations, and are easily administered to the patient.

The cartridge–needle units are designed to fit into a cartridge unit holder, referred to as an injector device (Figure 32-18). Injector devices, such as Tubex® and Carpuject® syringes, are usually nondisposable, made of nonchrome-plated brass or plastic, and are interchangeable with many brands of cartridges. Procedure 32-5 lists steps that are performed when using a cartridge injector device.

Prefilled Syringes

Many manufacturers are turning to disposable prefilled syringes (Figure 32-19). These syringes contain unit doses of medications and may be either glass or plastic. They are even easier to use than a cartridge set because

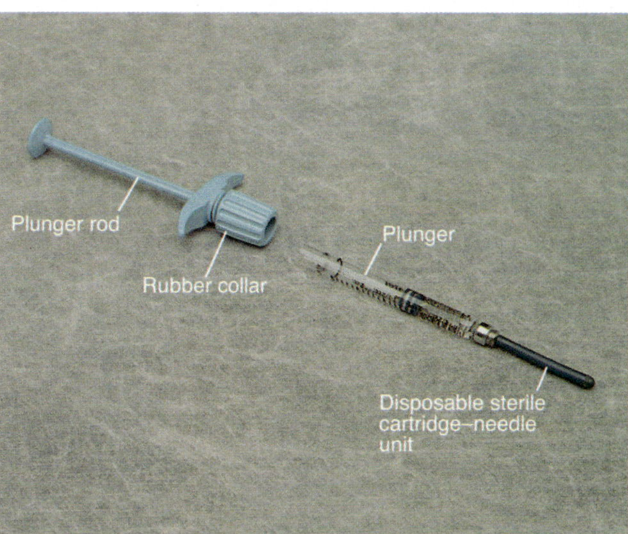

Figure 32-18 ■ A cartridge–needle unit and a reusable injector device.

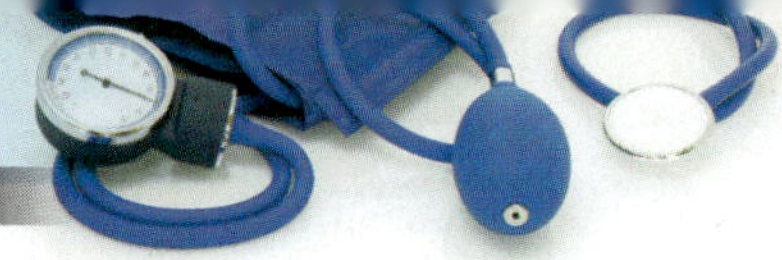

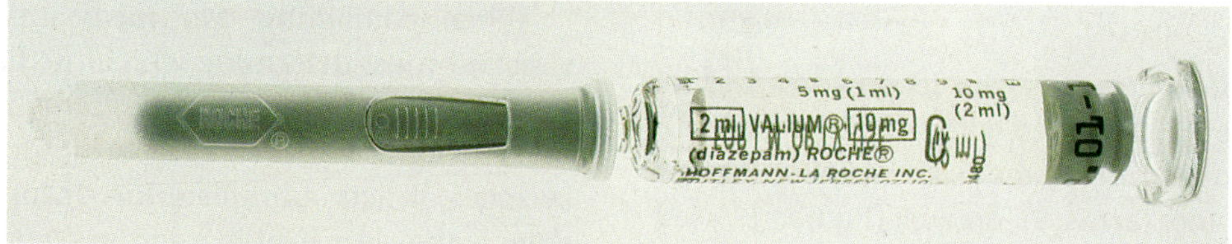

Figure 32-19 ■ Practices can now choose between a vial or pre-packaged syringe that is ready to go. Courtesy of Roche Laboratories, Inc.

they are ready to go. Once you have identified the medication and dosage, you just remove the cap, apply the needle (if applicable), and administer the medication.

General Guidelines for Parenteral Medications

In most medical facilities, the medication is prepared in a different room than the examination room and transferred to the exam room prior to injecting. Below are guidelines to follow when preparing and administering all types of injections:

- Prepare only one order of medication at a time and for one patient at a time. If the patient is to be given multiple injections, prepare each one separately and label syringes or syringe wrappers with a marking pen so that you can identify which syringe holds what medication.
- Follow standard safety precautions when dealing with needles and syringes.
- Ensure that contamination does not occur to the equipment during preparation or transport.
- Never allow another health care worker to prepare a medication that you will administer, nor should you prepare a medication for someone else. The responsibility for a medication error falls on the person who administers the medication.
- Follow the seven rights of medication administration (as described in Chapter 30) when administering all medications.
- Use two patient identifiers before administering any medications (part of the Patient Safety Act).
- Check the patient's drug allergy status, latex allergy status, and adhesive allergy status prior to administering any medication.
- Wash your hands and wear gloves just prior to administering any parenteral medications. The gloves are to protect you against possible bleeding from the site.
- Never allow a patient to stand while receiving an injection. The patient's blood pressure may drop and the patient may faint.
- Sites should be free of scar tissue, wounds, lesions, rashes, moles, or any other disturbance in tissue growth.
- Cleanse all sites with an approved skin antiseptic using a circular motion working from the inside out, prior to the injection.
- Stabilize your hand when holding the needle and syringe. Hand movement may cause the needle to move, nicking a blood vessel or nearby nerve.
- Follow the same track coming out of a site that you use going in. This will decrease injury to the surrounding tissue.
- Engage the needle sheath or safety device on the syringe immediately following the injection and dispose of the unit in the sharps container.

Patients should wait a minimum of 20 to 30 minutes following the injection to monitor for anaphylaxis.

Angles of Insertion

The angle used when administering medications is based on the route of the injection (Figure 32-20). When administering intradermal injections you should use a 10- to 15-degree angle, when administering a subcutaneous injection use a 45-degree angle, and when administering an intramuscular injection use a 90-degree angle. The angle helps to keep you in the correct layer of tissue or muscle.

Guidelines for Aspiration

Aspiration has been a common practice when administering medications for several decades; however, this philosophy is changing. The term **aspirate** means to pull back slightly on the plunger to look for blood in the tip of the syringe to see if you are in a blood vessel. The thought behind aspiration is that depositing drugs that are meant for slower absorption directly into the bloodstream could result in complications to the patient. The latest studies, however, state that there is no reported evidence that aspiration with or without blood return confirms needle placement.

As a matter of fact, the following organizations now state that aspiration is not necessary when administering vaccines (subcutaneous or IM) and include:

- Centers for Disease Control and Prevention (CDC)
- Advisory Committee on Immunization Practices (ACIP)

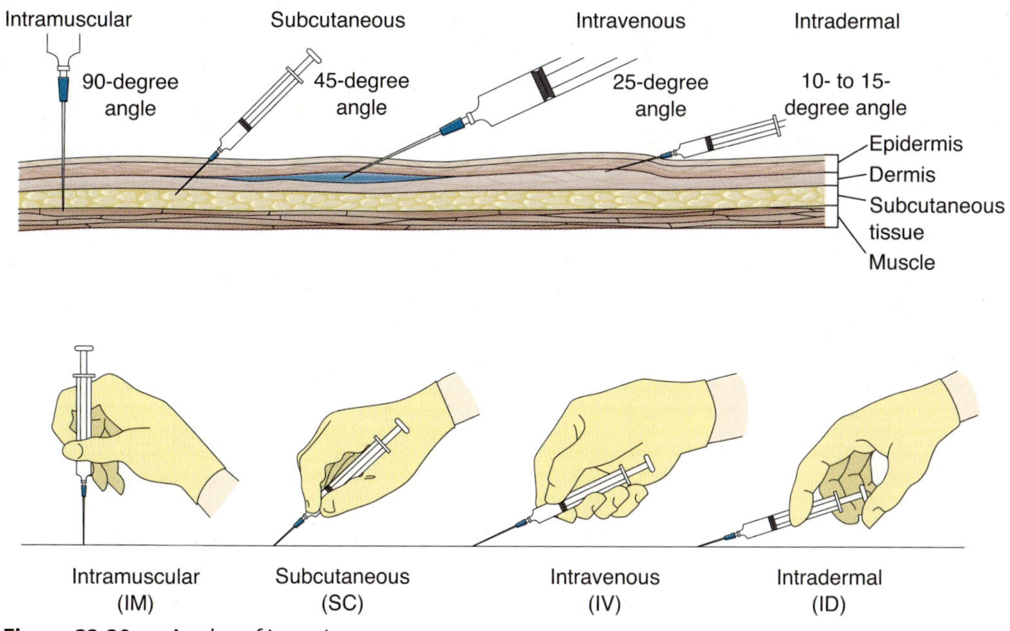

Figure 32-20 ■ Angles of insertion.

- Department of Health and Human Services (HHS)
- American Academy of Family Physicians (AAFP)

There is nothing conclusive regarding the practice of aspiration during allergy injections. The American Academy of Allergy, Asthma & Immunology leaves the practice of aspiration up to the individual provider. The practice of not aspirating during insulin injections has been accepted for many years now.

Based on the latest research, the following aspiration practices are recommended based on the types of medications administered in ambulatory care settings; however, always check the manufacturer's instructions and with the provider for specifics:

- No aspiration for intradermal injections
- No aspiration for subcutaneous injections; however, check with provider regarding aspiration for allergy injections
- Aspirate on intramuscular injections except for immunizations

Guidelines for Massaging the Site Following the Injection

At the conclusion of subcutaneous and intramuscular injections, gently massage the site with a gauze pad to assist with the disbursement of the medication. Massaging is contraindicated with particular types of medications, especially those that may be irritating to the tissue or those that can stain the skin. Examples of medications in which massage is contraindicated include heparin, insulin, Fragmin, and Lovenox. Massaging after these injections can damage tissue at the site or cause the medication to be absorbed incorrectly.

Massaging is contraindicated when performing all intradermal injections due to the disbursement of the extract into deeper tissue and when administering all Z-track injections.

Following the Procedure

Patients should be monitored for anaphylaxis (life-threatening allergic reaction) for 20 to 30 minutes following the injection. Most anaphylactic reactions will occur during this time period. Check the patient at the end of the monitoring period to make certain there are no concerns. Observe the site where the injection was administered and look for any local reactions including redness, wheals, or swelling. Ask if the patient is experiencing any breathing difficulties or any other unusual symptoms. If the patient experiences anything out of the ordinary, check with the provider before dismissing the patient. Provide the patient with education on how to manage the injection site and what to expect over the next few days. Document the procedure and the follow-up observations in the patient's chart. Refer to Chapter 4 for a complete procedure on documenting medications. Medications such as immunizations and narcotics should also be documented in designated log. Figure 32-21 shows a hospital medication log. In practices using EHR, manual logs are no longer necessary because they can be generated electronically.

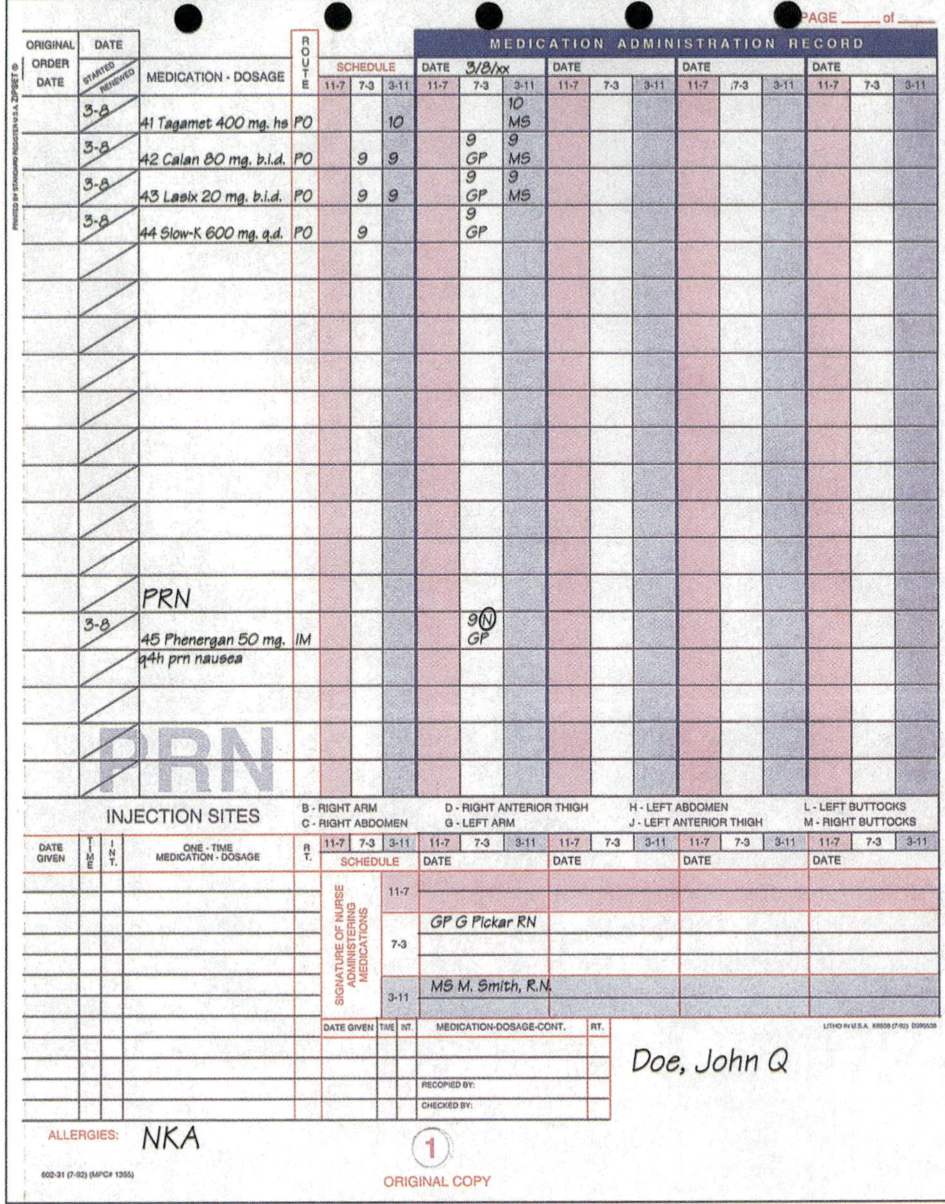

PAGE ____ of ____

MEDICATION ADMINISTRATION RECORD

ORIGINAL ORDER DATE	DATE STARTED RENEWED	MEDICATION - DOSAGE	ROUTE	SCHEDULE 11-7	SCHEDULE 7-3	SCHEDULE 3-11	DATE 3/8/xx 11-7	7-3	3-11	DATE 11-7	7-3	3-11	DATE 11-7	7-3	3-11	DATE 11-7	7-3	3-11
	3-8	41 Tagamet 400 mg. hs	PO			10			10 MS									
	3-8	42 Calan 80 mg. b.i.d.	PO		9	9		9 GP	9 MS									
	3-8	43 Lasix 20 mg. b.i.d.	PO		9	9		9 GP	9 MS									
	3-8	44 Slow-K 600 mg. q.d.	PO		9			9 GP										
		PRN																
	3-8	45 Phenergan 50 mg. q4h prn nausea	IM					9Ⓝ GP										

PRN

INJECTION SITES: B - RIGHT ARM; C - RIGHT ABDOMEN; D - RIGHT ANTERIOR THIGH; G - LEFT ARM; H - LEFT ABDOMEN; J - LEFT ANTERIOR THIGH; L - LEFT BUTTOCKS; M - RIGHT BUTTOCKS

DATE GIVEN	TIME	INT.	ONE - TIME MEDICATION - DOSAGE	RT.

SIGNATURE OF NURSE ADMINISTERING MEDICATIONS

SCHEDULE	DATE	DATE	DATE	DATE
11-7				
7-3	GP G Pickar RN			
3-11	MS M. Smith, R.N.			

DATE GIVEN	TIME	INT.	MEDICATION-DOSAGE-CONT.	RT.

RECOPIED BY:

CHECKED BY:

Doe, John Q

ALLERGIES: NKA

1 ORIGINAL COPY

Figure 32-21 ■ An example of a hospital medication log used to document all medications for a specific patient.

ROUTES OF ADMINISTRATION

The route that is selected for parenteral delivery will be primarily based on the manufacturer's recommendation and the intended use of the drug. Routes selected by the manufacturer are based on absorption properties of the drug and possible irritants or dyes in the drug that may make it harmful to surrounding tissue. Altering any drug routes could cause harmful side effects for the patient, such as tissue abscess and degeneration, tissue staining, and shock.

Intradermal Injections

The term **intradermal** means pertaining to within the skin. The epidermis (outer layer of the skin) is the layer of skin that is used for intradermal injections. In order for the needle to stay within this layer, the needle should be positioned at a 10° to 15° angle (Figure 32-22). When the medication is slowly injected at this angle, a bubble of fluid called a **wheal** (Figure 32-23) should appear on the outer surface of the skin.

The standard sites used for intradermal (ID) injections are the inner lower forearm and the middle of the back (Figure 32-24). These sites are used due to the lack of hair found in these areas and the thinness of the skin. Because of the location of the injection, aspiration is not necessary when performing intradermal injections.

Common types of injections administered through this route include allergy extract for testing purposes

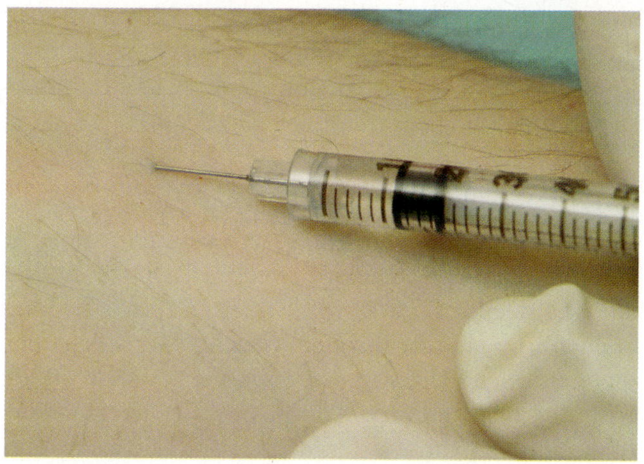

Figure 32-22 ■ The needle is inserted at a 10° to 15° angle for an intradermal injection.

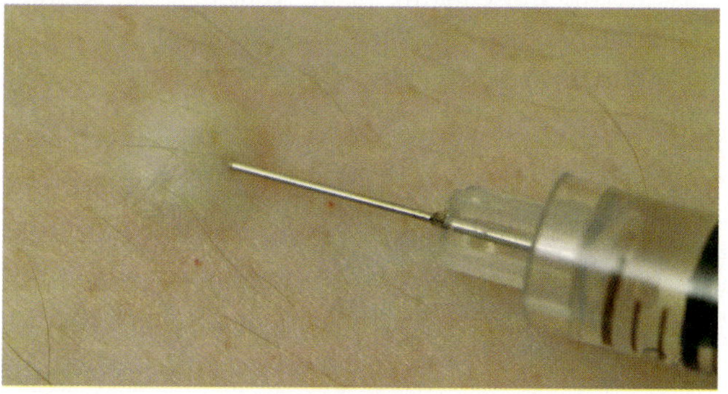

Figure 32-23 ■ A wheal should appear on the surface of the arm following an intradermal injection.

and the purified protein derivative (PPD) or tuberculin (TB) skin test. Intradermal injections should never be massaged because it will force the liquid to be dispersed in deeper tissues, causing the wheal to disappear.

Patients receiving intradermal injections will need to have the site evaluated within a prescribed time frame. The provider will measure the site where the wheal was induced. If the wheal extends over a specific parameter, it means that the test is positive. Table 32-5 is a summary chart for key information regarding intradermal injections. Refer to Procedure 32-6 for a complete procedure on administering intradermal injections.

Table 32-5 **Intradermal Injection Summary Chart**

Needle size	26–27 G, ⅜″–½″
Syringe size	1 mL
Angle of insertion	10°–15°
Aspirate	No
Common medications or extracts given this route	Allergy extract, TB extract
Maximum amount of mL per location	0.1 mL
Massage	No

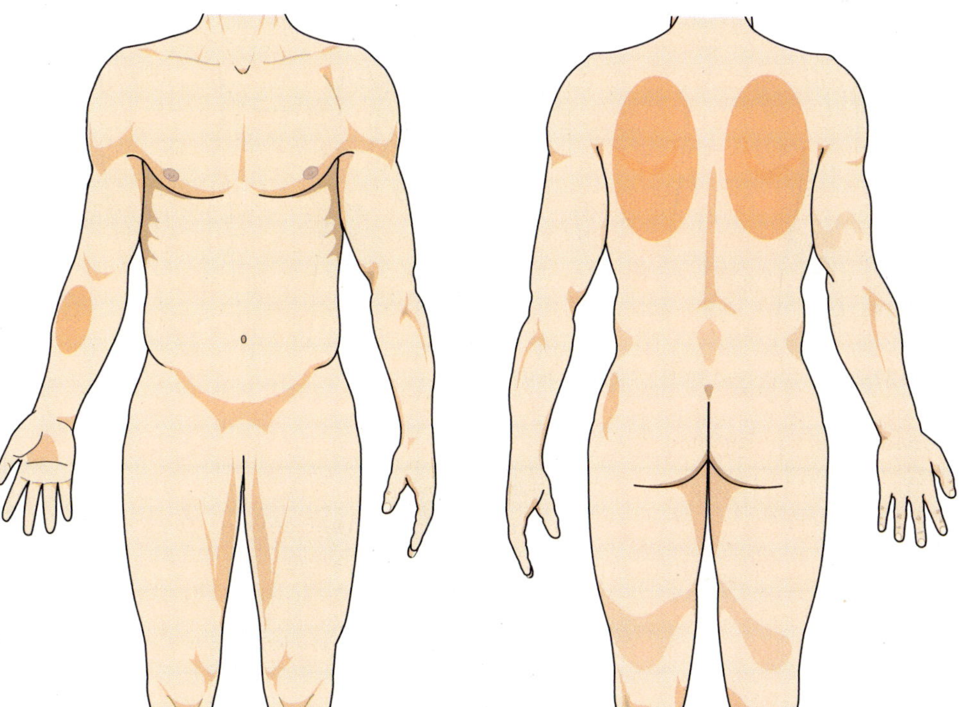

Figure 32-24 ■ Sites for an intradermal injection include the inner forearm and the upper portion of the back.

Subcutaneous Injections

The term **subcutaneous** (Sub-Q) is a medical term that means pertaining to under the dermis (or true layer of the skin). Subcutaneous tissue is made up of fatty and connective tissue. When administering a subcutaneous injection, the adipose tissue should be slightly pinched between the finger and thumb to help differentiate the adipose tissue from the muscle. The injection is placed in the fatty tissue of the body, not the muscle. In order to reach this tissue, the medical assistant should position the needle at a 45° angle; however, a 90° angle may be appropriate for patients with lots of adipose tissue or when using a shorter needle.

Aspiration is no longer recommended for the majority of medications given subcutaneously. Always check with the provider for specifics. Sites commonly used for this route include the fatty outer portion of the upper arms, the lower abdomen, the middle and lower back, and the thigh region (Figure 32-25). Table 32-6 lists important facts about subcutaneous injections. Refer to Procedure 32-7 for instructions on how to administer subcutaneous injections.

Intramuscular Injections

The term **intramuscular (IM)** means within the muscle. Intramuscular injections are given with a longer needle and at a steeper angle of 90°. The needle must be long enough to penetrate through the skin and subcutaneous tissues and deep into the muscular tissue; otherwise, the medication will seep into the subcutaneous tissue and may cause a sterile abscess or malabsorption of the medication.

Body areas normally used for intramuscular injection sites are the musculature of the ventrogluteal regions, vastus lateralis, and the deltoid. When administering an intramuscular injection, the tissue overlying the muscle

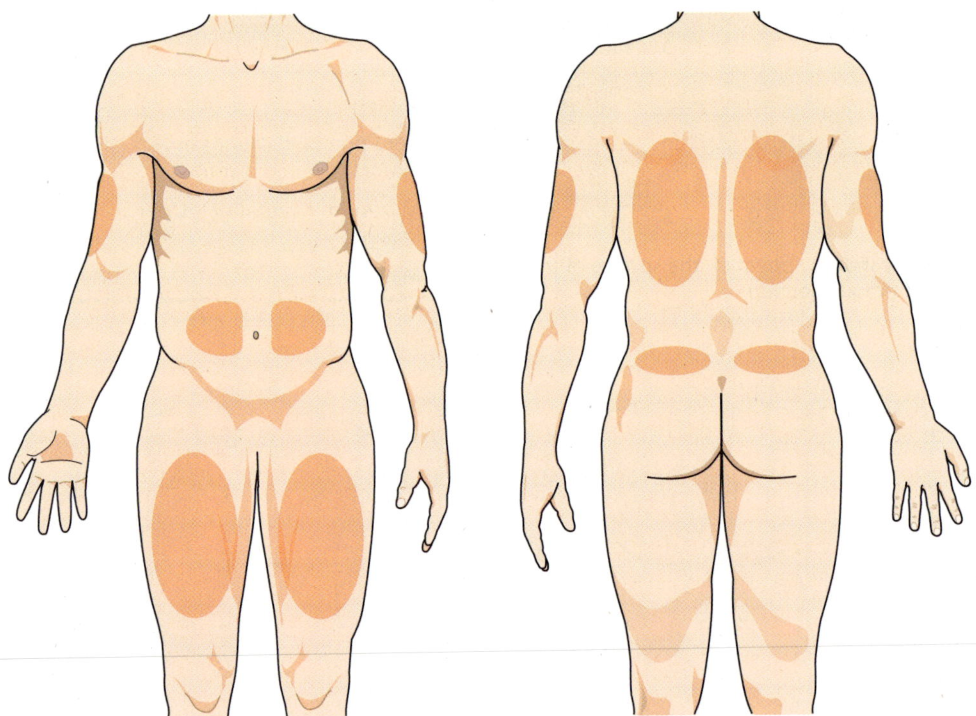

Figure 32-25 ■ Common sites for a subcutaneous injection.

Table 32-6 Subcutaneous Injection Summary Chart

Needle size	23–25 G, ½″–⅝″
Syringe size	1–3 mL (use an insulin syringe when giving insulin)
Angle of insertion	45°–90°
Aspirate	No
Common medications or extracts given this route	Allergy injections, insulin injections, heparin, Lovenox, MMR vaccine, small pox vaccine, IPV vaccine, VAR vaccine
Maximum amount of mL per location	1 mL
Massage	Yes, except in a select few medications (read manufacturer's instructions)

Table 32-7 Intramuscular Injection Summary Chart

Needle size	20–23 G, 1–2"
Syringe size	3–6 mL
Angle of insertion	90°
Aspirate	Yes, except for vaccines
Common medications or extracts given this route	Most vaccines, analgesics, antibiotics, steroids, hormones
Maximum amount of mL per location	Deltoid: I mL; large muscles such as the vastus lateralis: 3 mL
Massage	Generally: yes; Z-Track: no

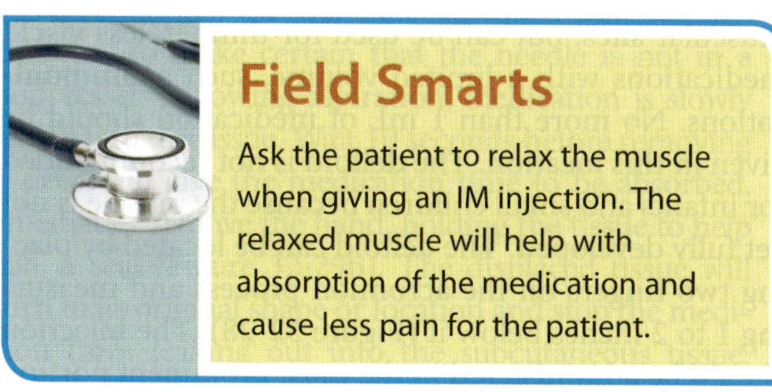

Field Smarts

Ask the patient to relax the muscle when giving an IM injection. The relaxed muscle will help with absorption of the medication and cause less pain for the patient.

should be held **taut** (a term that means to pull or draw tight) to ascertain that the medicine is deposited into the muscle and not the subcutaneous tissue. Table 32-7 provides facts regarding IM injections. Procedure 32-8 lists specific steps for administering IM injections.

Dorsogluteal

The dorsogluteal site was previously used to administer medications; however, this site is no longer recommended because of the danger of nicking the sciatic nerve. Therefore, we will not be covering it in this text.

Ventrogluteal

The ventrogluteal muscle can accommodate many of the same medications injected into the dorsogluteal muscle and may be used for patients of all ages. The ventrogluteal area is free of major nerves and vessels so it is considered safer than the dorsogluteal site.

To locate the ventrogluteal site, the medical assistant should be positioned to face the lateral side of the patient's hip. Center the top of the hand or fingers over the patient's gluteal medial muscle, just below the iliac crest. If facing the patient's right side, place the left lower palm over the greater trochanter of the femur, place the index finger of the left hand on the anterior superior iliac spine, and spread the middle finger posteriorly as far as it will reach along the iliac crest. This should create a "V." Within the "V" is where the injection will be administered (Figure 32-26).

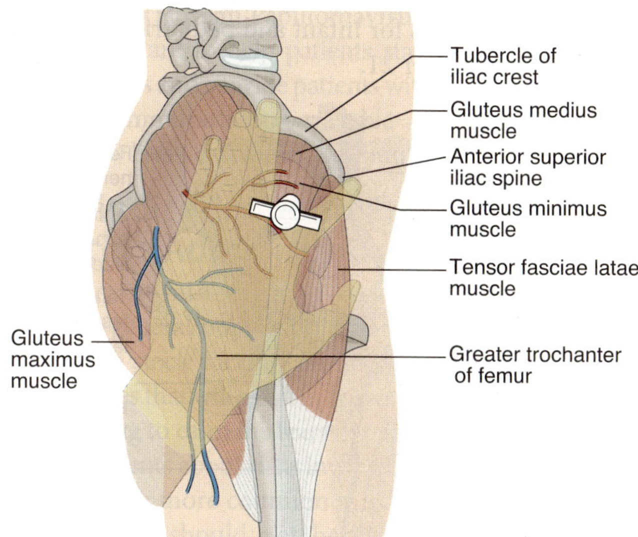

Figure 32-26a ■ Landmarks for ventrogluteal site.

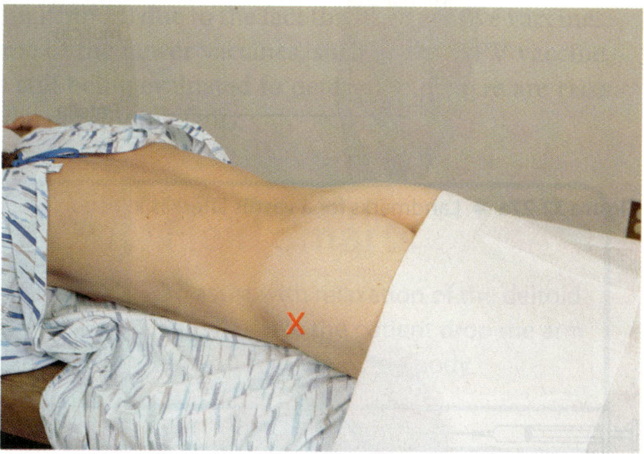

Figure 32-26b ■ Where to administer a ventrogluteal injection.

Vastus Lateralis

The vastus lateralis is part of the quadriceps group of the thigh and is the preferred site for administering injections on infants and young children. This is because it is larger and more developed than any of the

Table 32-8 Possible Parenteral Complications

Incorrect Technique	Consequences	Effects
Failure to change the needle between the vial and patient	Tissue irritation or discoloration. Excess pain to the patient.	Local reaction to the skin or muscle; discoloration of the skin increased amount of pain because of the needle's dullness.
Using a needle that is too short	Medication will be deposited into incorrect tissue	Medication will not be absorbed the way the manufacturer intended it to be absorbed, thus changing the desired effects of the medication; abscess tissue degeneration.
Using a needle that is too long	Medication will be deposited into incorrect tissue	Medication will not be absorbed the way the manufacturer intended it to be absorbed, thus changing the desired effects of the medication; could cause damage to the periosteum, resulting in infection and bone retardation; needle could break off into the bone.
Failing to aspirate on medications that should be aspirated	Depositing medication directly into a vein or artery	Shock: Medication was not intended to go directly into the bloodstream. May cause patient's heart to beat faster, respiration rate to increase, blood pressure to drop. Patient may become unconscious.
Break in sterile technique	The introduction of microorganisms into the muscle, subcutaneous tissue, or blood stream	Blood infection; an abscess in the subcutaneous tissue, muscle tissue, or surrounding tissue; tissue degeneration.
Choosing a muscle that is underdeveloped	May cause injury to the nearby nerves	Tingling; excruciating pain; paralysis.
Injecting a patient with a small-gauge needle when administering a viscid solution	May cause injury to the surrounding tissue	Burning; tissue degeneration; increased pain to the patient.

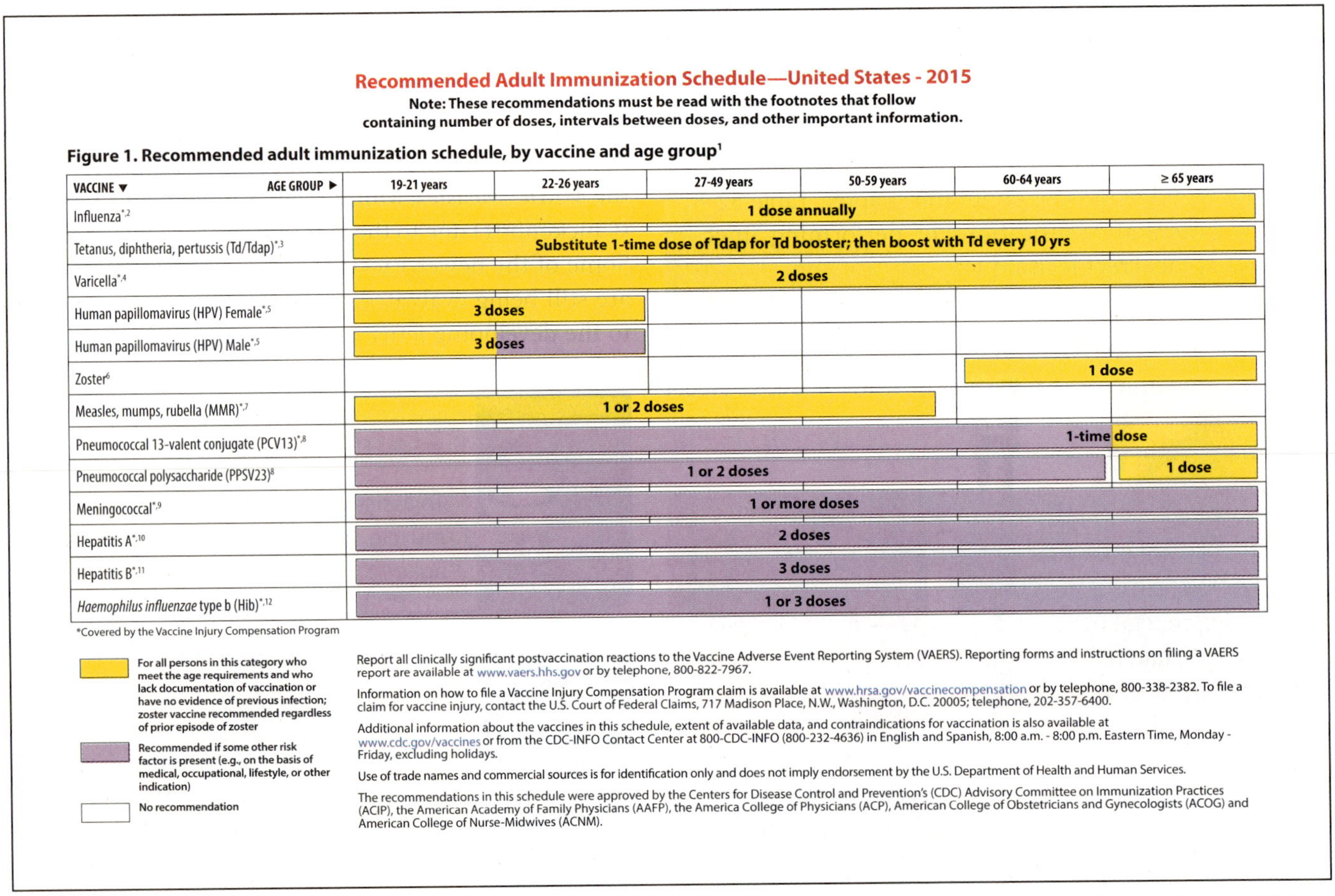

Recommended Adult Immunization Schedule—United States - 2015

Note: These recommendations must be read with the footnotes that follow containing number of doses, intervals between doses, and other important information.

Figure 1. Recommended adult immunization schedule, by vaccine and age group[1]

<table>
<tr><th>VACCINE ▼ AGE GROUP ▶</th><th>19-21 years</th><th>22-26 years</th><th>27-49 years</th><th>50-59 years</th><th>60-64 years</th><th>≥ 65 years</th></tr>
<tr><td>Influenza*,2</td><td colspan="6">1 dose annually</td></tr>
<tr><td>Tetanus, diphtheria, pertussis (Td/Tdap)*,3</td><td colspan="6">Substitute 1-time dose of Tdap for Td booster; then boost with Td every 10 yrs</td></tr>
<tr><td>Varicella*,4</td><td colspan="6">2 doses</td></tr>
<tr><td>Human papillomavirus (HPV) Female*,5</td><td colspan="2">3 doses</td><td></td><td></td><td></td><td></td></tr>
<tr><td>Human papillomavirus (HPV) Male*,5</td><td colspan="2">3 doses</td><td></td><td></td><td></td><td></td></tr>
<tr><td>Zoster6</td><td></td><td></td><td></td><td></td><td colspan="2">1 dose</td></tr>
<tr><td>Measles, mumps, rubella (MMR)*,7</td><td colspan="4">1 or 2 doses</td><td></td><td></td></tr>
<tr><td>Pneumococcal 13-valent conjugate (PCV13)*,8</td><td colspan="6">1-time dose</td></tr>
<tr><td>Pneumococcal polysaccharide (PPSV23)8</td><td colspan="5">1 or 2 doses</td><td>1 dose</td></tr>
<tr><td>Meningococcal*,9</td><td colspan="6">1 or more doses</td></tr>
<tr><td>Hepatitis A*,10</td><td colspan="6">2 doses</td></tr>
<tr><td>Hepatitis B*,11</td><td colspan="6">3 doses</td></tr>
<tr><td>Haemophilus influenzae type b (Hib)*,12</td><td colspan="6">1 or 3 doses</td></tr>
</table>

*Covered by the Vaccine Injury Compensation Program

[Yellow] For all persons in this category who meet the age requirements and who lack documentation of vaccination or have no evidence of previous infection; zoster vaccine recommended regardless of prior episode of zoster

[Purple] Recommended if some other risk factor is present (e.g., on the basis of medical, occupational, lifestyle, or other indication)

[White] No recommendation

Report all clinically significant postvaccination reactions to the Vaccine Adverse Event Reporting System (VAERS). Reporting forms and instructions on filing a VAERS report are available at www.vaers.hhs.gov or by telephone, 800-822-7967.

Information on how to file a Vaccine Injury Compensation Program claim is available at www.hrsa.gov/vaccinecompensation or by telephone, 800-338-2382. To file a claim for vaccine injury, contact the U.S. Court of Federal Claims, 717 Madison Place, N.W., Washington, D.C. 20005; telephone, 202-357-6400.

Additional information about the vaccines in this schedule, extent of available data, and contraindications for vaccination is also available at www.cdc.gov/vaccines or from the CDC-INFO Contact Center at 800-CDC-INFO (800-232-4636) in English and Spanish, 8:00 a.m. - 8:00 p.m. Eastern Time, Monday - Friday, excluding holidays.

Use of trade names and commercial sources is for identification only and does not imply endorsement by the U.S. Department of Health and Human Services.

The recommendations in this schedule were approved by the Centers for Disease Control and Prevention's (CDC) Advisory Committee on Immunization Practices (ACIP), the American Academy of Family Physicians (AAFP), the America College of Physicians (ACP), American College of Obstetricians and Gynecologists (ACOG) and American College of Nurse-Midwives (ACNM).

Figure 32-30 ■ Recommended adult immunization schedule by vaccine and age group, updated annually, and posted on the CDC's website, www.cdc.gov.

Z-Track Method of Injection

The Z-track method is used when the medication may cause irritation to the skin or cause discoloration of the tissues. This method seals the medication deeply within the muscle and allows no exit path back into the subcutaneous tissue and skin. The skin and subcutaneous tissue over the ventrogluteal tissue are displaced or pulled laterally before the needle is inserted by placing the palm of the nondominant hand on the surface of skin, and pulling it several inches to the side (Figure 32-29a). This hand should not move until the end of the procedure. The needle is inserted and the syringe is aspirated (one-handed technique) to make certain that the needle is not in a blood vessel. Following aspiration, medication is slowly injected into the tissue. Wait 10 seconds before removing the needle to give the medication time to be absorbed. Immediately remove the hand, holding the tissue to help create a seal (Figure 32-29b). The displaced tissue will return to its original shape or location and stop the medication from leaking out into the subcutaneous tissue. The pathway of the needle is interrupted when using this technique and is quite effective in preventing the loss of medication. Common medications given by the Z-track method include iron preparations and medications that are irritating to superficial tissue, such as Vistaril®.

PARENTERAL COMPLICATIONS

To reduce the risks of parenteral complications, follow the guidelines listed throughout the chapter. Table 32-8 lists the potential ramifications of performing injections using incorrect techniques.

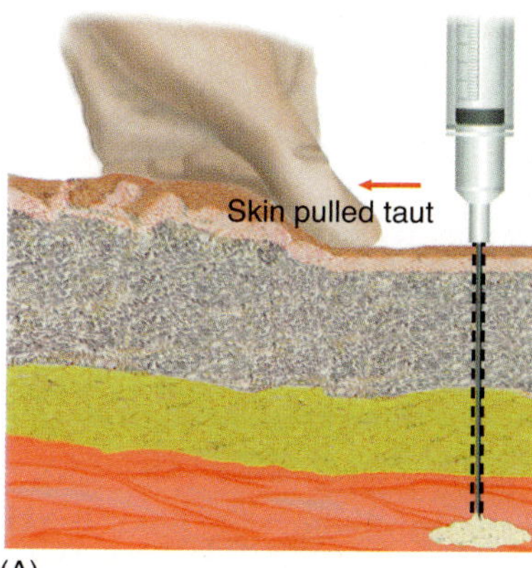

Figure 32-29a ▪ Pull the skin laterally before inserting the needle into the muscle.

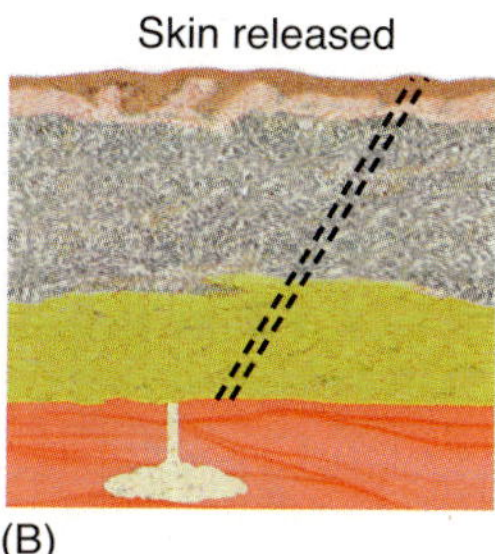

Figure 32-29b ▪ Removing the hand that held the skin back will create a seal and prevent the medication from leaking into the subcutaneous tissue.

IMMUNIZATIONS

When most people think about immunizations, often they just think about children (refer to Chapter 21 for information about immunizations in children), but adults are encouraged to maintain immunity through booster shots every 3–5 years. Immunizations such as the hepatitis B series, DTaP, influenza, and pneumonia vaccinations are just a few of the common immunizations that are listed on the adult immunization schedule. There have been a few new immunizations introduced in recent years, including the shingles (Zoster) vaccine and the HPV (Human Papillomavirus) vaccine.

It is important to help patients stay up to date with immunizations and provide patients with education about the newest immunizations available and their benefits. Figure 32-30 lists the standard immunizations for adults.

Contraindications and Precautions in Vaccine Administrations

There are many misconceptions regarding immunizations among the general population. It is important for medical offices to stock vaccination information sheets (VIS) and brochures that will assist in answering these questions and in helping to calm the fears of patients and parents of pediatric patients about risks involved with immunizing.

Some of the more common misconceptions are that immunizations should not be given to women who are pregnant or breastfeeding. The only two vaccines known to actually cause harm to a developing fetus are the *MMR* (Measles, Mumps, and Rubella) and *Varicella* (Chickenpox) due to the fact that they are live vaccines. Some of the newer vaccines, such as the HPV vaccine, are still being evaluated to determine if there are risks to the developing fetus.

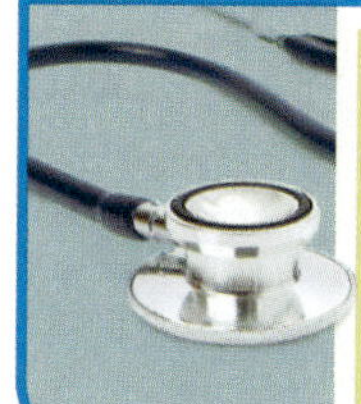

Field Smarts

To assist with relaxation of the deltoid muscle, have the patient drop the arm against the side of the body.

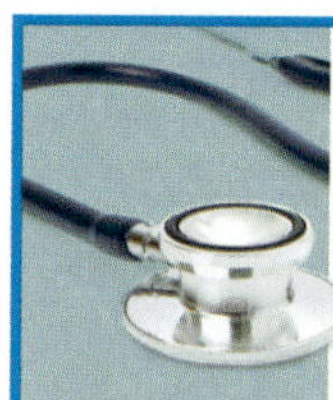

Field Smarts

When administering an immunization in the deltoid muscle, use the patient's dominant arm. Increased muscle use will promote better circulation and will help to work out the soreness from the injection much faster.

Table 32-8 Possible Parenteral Complications

Incorrect Technique	Consequences	Effects
Failure to change the needle between the vial and patient	Tissue irritation or discoloration. Excess pain to the patient.	Local reaction to the skin or muscle; discoloration of the skin increased amount of pain because of the needle's dullness.
Using a needle that is too short	Medication will be deposited into incorrect tissue	Medication will not be absorbed the way the manufacturer intended it to be absorbed, thus changing the desired effects of the medication; abscess tissue degeneration.
Using a needle that is too long	Medication will be deposited into incorrect tissue	Medication will not be absorbed the way the manufacturer intended it to be absorbed, thus changing the desired effects of the medication; could cause damage to the periosteum, resulting in infection and bone retardation; needle could break off into the bone.
Failing to aspirate on medications that should be aspirated	Depositing medication directly into a vein or artery	Shock: Medication was not intended to go directly into the bloodstream. May cause patient's heart to beat faster, respiration rate to increase, blood pressure to drop. Patient may become unconscious.
Break in sterile technique	The introduction of microorganisms into the muscle, subcutaneous tissue, or blood stream	Blood infection; an abscess in the subcutaneous tissue, muscle tissue, or surrounding tissue; tissue degeneration.
Choosing a muscle that is underdeveloped	May cause injury to the nearby nerves	Tingling; excruciating pain; paralysis.
Injecting a patient with a small-gauge needle when administering a viscid solution	May cause injury to the surrounding tissue	Burning; tissue degeneration; increased pain to the patient.

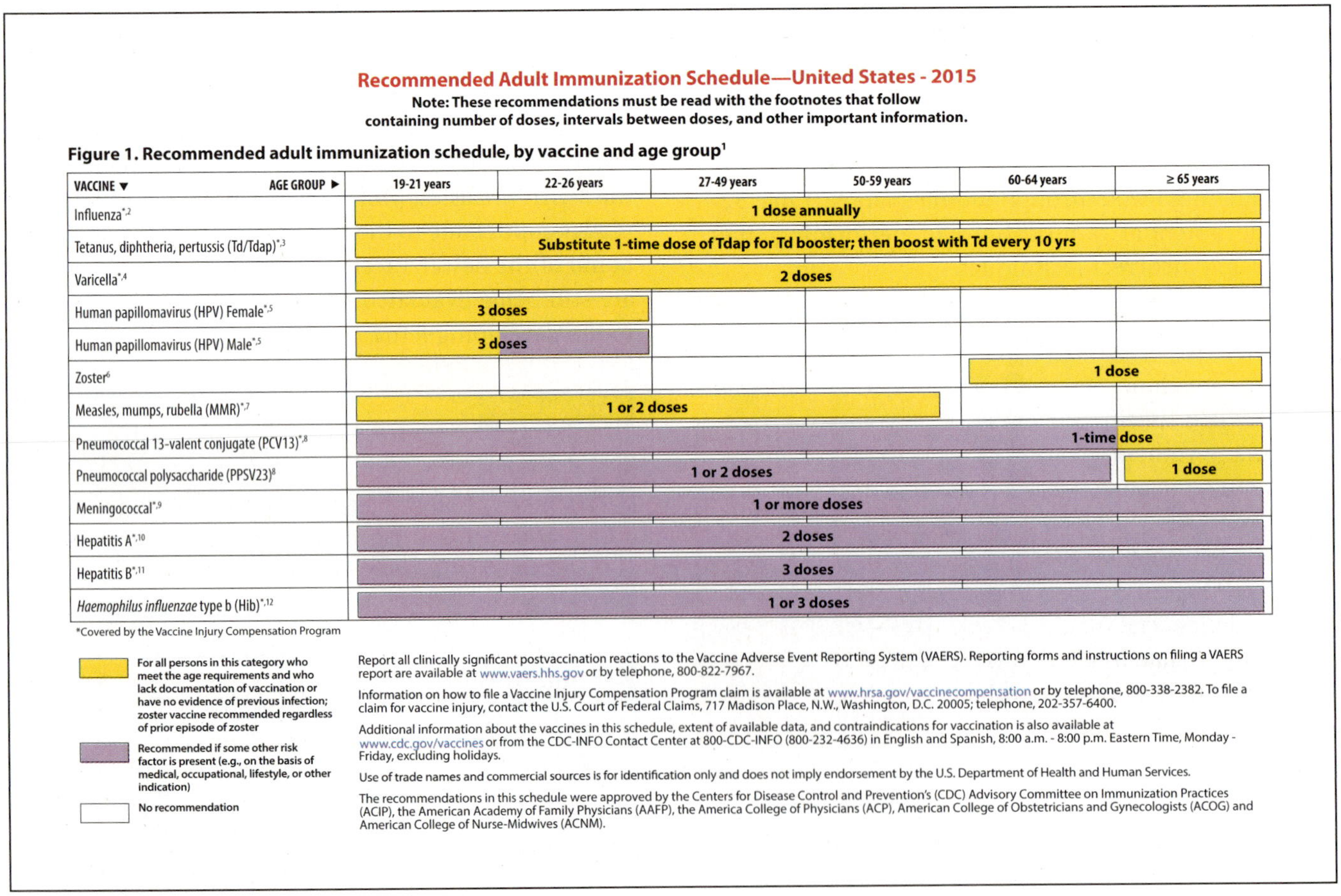

Recommended Adult Immunization Schedule—United States - 2015

Note: These recommendations must be read with the footnotes that follow containing number of doses, intervals between doses, and other important information.

Figure 1. Recommended adult immunization schedule, by vaccine and age group[1]

<table>
<tr><th>VACCINE ▼ AGE GROUP ▶</th><th>19-21 years</th><th>22-26 years</th><th>27-49 years</th><th>50-59 years</th><th>60-64 years</th><th>≥ 65 years</th></tr>
<tr><td>Influenza[*,2]</td><td colspan="6">1 dose annually</td></tr>
<tr><td>Tetanus, diphtheria, pertussis (Td/Tdap)[*,3]</td><td colspan="6">Substitute 1-time dose of Tdap for Td booster; then boost with Td every 10 yrs</td></tr>
<tr><td>Varicella[*,4]</td><td colspan="6">2 doses</td></tr>
<tr><td>Human papillomavirus (HPV) Female[*,5]</td><td colspan="2">3 doses</td><td></td><td></td><td></td><td></td></tr>
<tr><td>Human papillomavirus (HPV) Male[*,5]</td><td colspan="2">3 doses</td><td></td><td></td><td></td><td></td></tr>
<tr><td>Zoster[6]</td><td></td><td></td><td></td><td></td><td colspan="2">1 dose</td></tr>
<tr><td>Measles, mumps, rubella (MMR)[*,7]</td><td colspan="4">1 or 2 doses</td><td></td><td></td></tr>
<tr><td>Pneumococcal 13-valent conjugate (PCV13)[*,8]</td><td colspan="6">1-time dose</td></tr>
<tr><td>Pneumococcal polysaccharide (PPSV23)[8]</td><td colspan="5">1 or 2 doses</td><td>1 dose</td></tr>
<tr><td>Meningococcal[*,9]</td><td colspan="6">1 or more doses</td></tr>
<tr><td>Hepatitis A[*,10]</td><td colspan="6">2 doses</td></tr>
<tr><td>Hepatitis B[*,11]</td><td colspan="6">3 doses</td></tr>
<tr><td>Haemophilus influenzae type b (Hib)[*,12]</td><td colspan="6">1 or 3 doses</td></tr>
</table>

*Covered by the Vaccine Injury Compensation Program

For all persons in this category who meet the age requirements and who lack documentation of vaccination or have no evidence of previous infection; zoster vaccine recommended regardless of prior episode of zoster

Recommended if some other risk factor is present (e.g., on the basis of medical, occupational, lifestyle, or other indication)

No recommendation

Report all clinically significant postvaccination reactions to the Vaccine Adverse Event Reporting System (VAERS). Reporting forms and instructions on filing a VAERS report are available at www.vaers.hhs.gov or by telephone, 800-822-7967.

Information on how to file a Vaccine Injury Compensation Program claim is available at www.hrsa.gov/vaccinecompensation or by telephone, 800-338-2382. To file a claim for vaccine injury, contact the U.S. Court of Federal Claims, 717 Madison Place, N.W., Washington, D.C. 20005; telephone, 202-357-6400.

Additional information about the vaccines in this schedule, extent of available data, and contraindications for vaccination is also available at www.cdc.gov/vaccines or from the CDC-INFO Contact Center at 800-CDC-INFO (800-232-4636) in English and Spanish, 8:00 a.m. - 8:00 p.m. Eastern Time, Monday - Friday, excluding holidays.

Use of trade names and commercial sources is for identification only and does not imply endorsement by the U.S. Department of Health and Human Services.

The recommendations in this schedule were approved by the Centers for Disease Control and Prevention's (CDC) Advisory Committee on Immunization Practices (ACIP), the American Academy of Family Physicians (AAFP), the America College of Physicians (ACP), American College of Obstetricians and Gynecologists (ACOG) and American College of Nurse-Midwives (ACNM).

Figure 32-30 ■ Recommended adult immunization schedule by vaccine and age group, updated annually, and posted on the CDC's website, www.cdc.gov.

Table 32-7 Intramuscular Injection Summary Chart

Needle size	20–23 G, 1–2″
Syringe size	3–6 mL
Angle of insertion	90°
Aspirate	Yes, except for vaccines
Common medications or extracts given this route	Most vaccines, analgesics, antibiotics, steroids, hormones
Maximum amount of mL per location	Deltoid: l mL; large muscles such as the vastus lateralis: 3 mL
Massage	Generally: yes; Z-Track: no

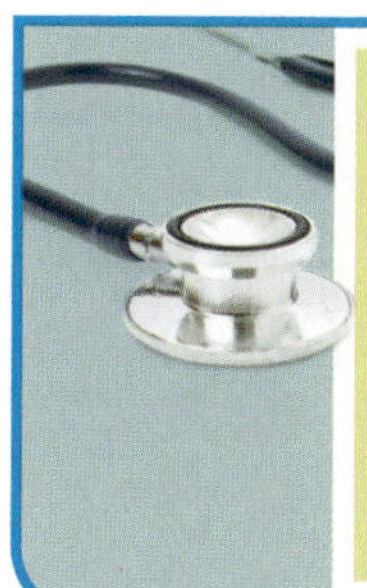

Field Smarts

Ask the patient to relax the muscle when giving an IM injection. The relaxed muscle will help with absorption of the medication and cause less pain for the patient.

should be held **taut** (a term that means to pull or draw tight) to ascertain that the medicine is deposited into the muscle and not the subcutaneous tissue. Table 32-7 provides facts regarding IM injections. Procedure 32-8 lists specific steps for administering IM injections.

Dorsogluteal

The dorsogluteal site was previously used to administer medications; however, this site is no longer recommended because of the danger of nicking the sciatic nerve. Therefore, we will not be covering it in this text.

Ventrogluteal

The ventrogluteal muscle can accommodate many of the same medications injected into the dorsogluteal muscle and may be used for patients of all ages. The ventrogluteal area is free of major nerves and vessels so it is considered safer than the dorsogluteal site.

To locate the ventrogluteal site, the medical assistant should be positioned to face the lateral side of the patient's hip. Center the top of the hand or fingers over the patient's gluteal medial muscle, just below the iliac crest. If facing the patient's right side, place the left lower palm over the greater trochanter of the femur, place the index finger of the left hand on the anterior superior iliac spine, and spread the middle finger posteriorly as far as it will reach along the iliac crest. This should create a "V." Within the "V" is where the injection will be administered (Figure 32-26).

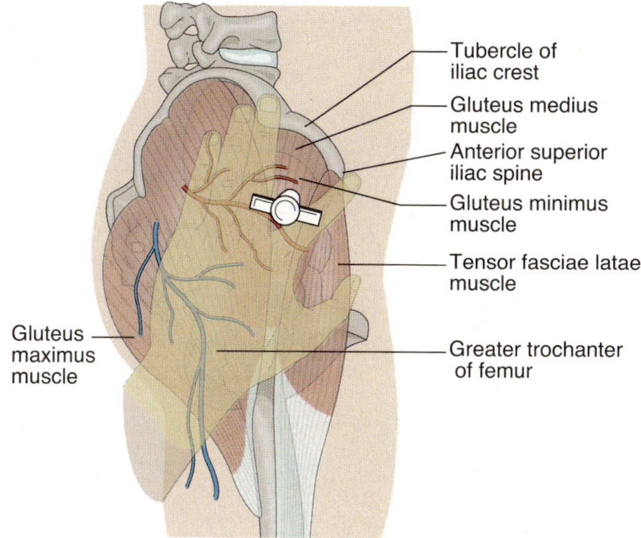

Figure 32-26a ■ Landmarks for ventrogluteal site.

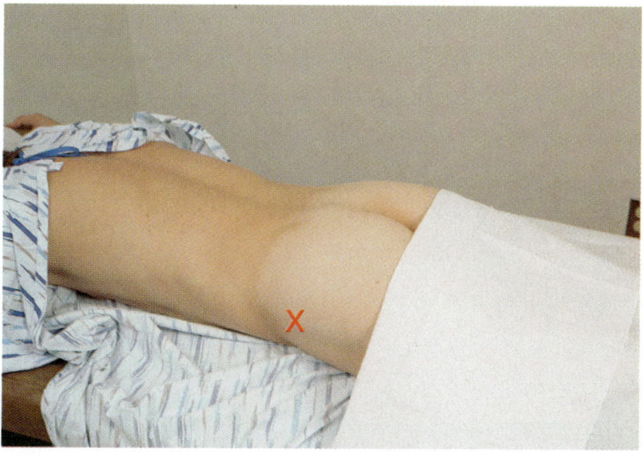

Figure 32-26b ■ Where to administer a ventrogluteal injection.

Vastus Lateralis

The vastus lateralis is part of the quadriceps group of the thigh and is the preferred site for administering injections on infants and young children. This is because it is larger and more developed than any of the other large muscle groups at birth. The vastus lateralis can also be used to administer IM injections to adults and is relatively free of large vessels and major nerves. Some adults may find it more painful to use this site than the ventrogluteal site. To find the correct location of the vastus lateralis in adults, the medical assistant should position the hand so that it is at least one hand's width below the proximal end of the greater trochanter of the femur. Place the other hand so that it is at least one hand's width above the kneecap. The injection may be placed anywhere between those two landmarks along the lateral or outer portion of the thigh (Figure 32-27). Sites for infant and pediatric injections are found in Chapter 21.

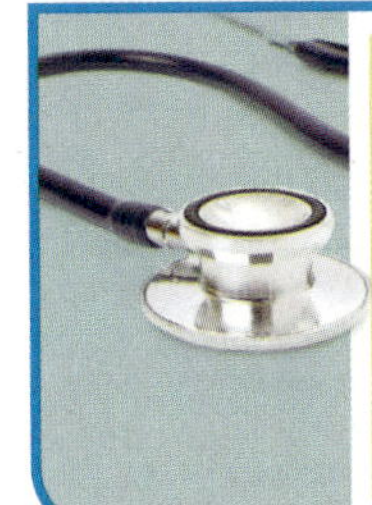

Field Smarts

To assist with relaxing the vastus lateralis, have the patient sit at the edge of the table with legs dangling over the edge of the table.

Deltoid

The deltoid is a smaller muscle than the other intramuscular sites, but can be used for thinner, less viscid medications with a limited volume, such as immunizations. No more than 1 mL of medication should be given in this location. The deltoid is not recommended for infants and small children because the muscle is not yet fully developed. The deltoid can be located by placing two fingers on the acromion process and measuring 1 to 2 inches below it (Figure 32-28). The injection should be administered in the most prominent portion of the muscle.

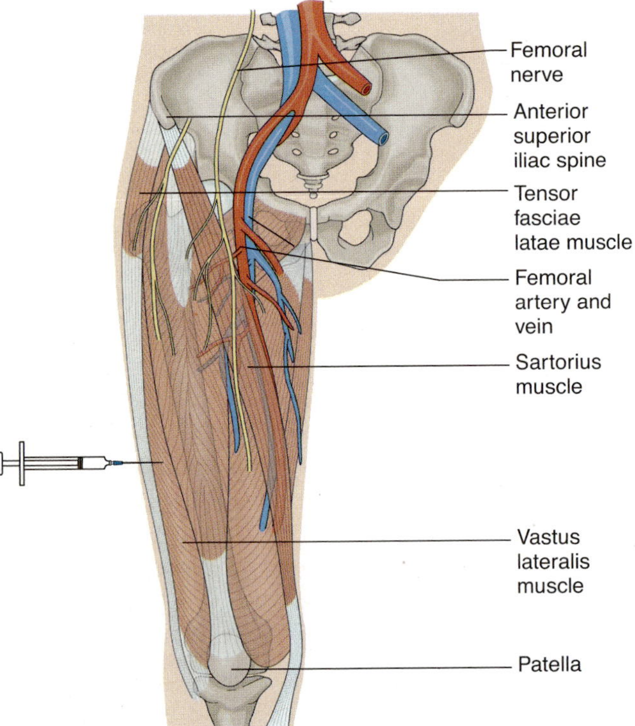

Figure 32-27a ■ Landmarks for a vastus lateralis injection.

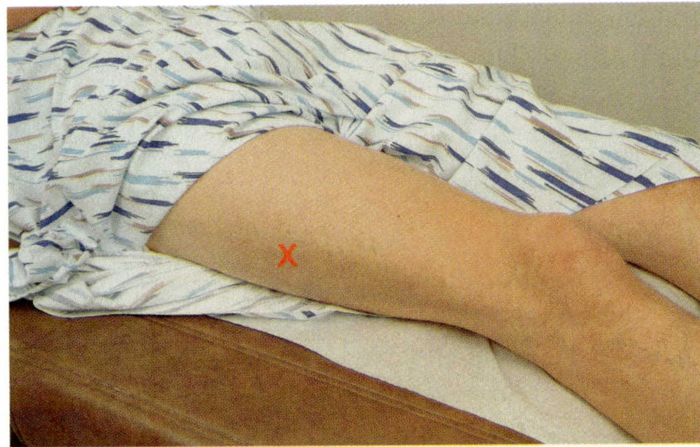

Figure 32-27b ■ Where to administer a vastus lateralis injection.

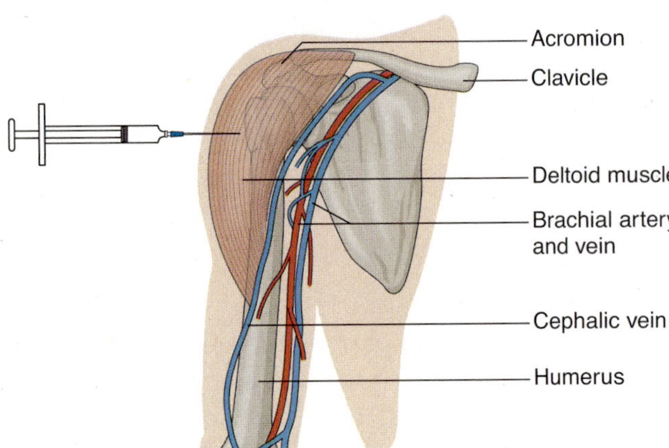

Figure 32-28a ■ Landmarks for a deltoid injection.

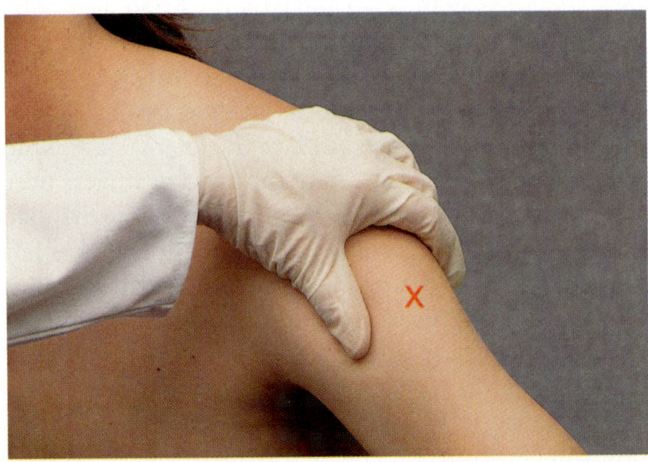

Figure 32-28b ■ Where to administer a deltoid injection.

Immunocompromised patients should explore the benefits and risks of immunization and make an informed decision on what is best for their particular situation.

Some contraindications to vaccines include the addition of preservatives or stabilizers that may be the cause of allergy sensitivity such as gelatin, eggs, or other types of plant derivatives used in processing the vaccines. Read the package inserts very carefully and screen the patient before administering the immunizing agents to verify prior history of sensitivity or allergic reaction. The CDC has a great deal more information regarding immunization contraindications on their website at www.cdc.gov.

BASICS OF INTRAVENOUS (IV) THERAPY

Intravenous (IV) therapy is the administration of fluids or medications directly into a vein. The purpose of administering fluids intravenously may be to replace lost fluids or to introduce medication, solutions, or nutrients to a patient. IV injections are usually administered directly into the vein (**bolus**) or injected into an access port on the IV line. Intravenous therapy is preferred when the patient requires fast absorption and can bring quick results because fluids enter the bloodstream immediately. IV therapy is drug specific, meaning only certain drugs are administered by this route. It is important to understand the difference between intravenous injections and intravenous infusion. IV injections consist of a relatively small amount of fluid being introduced into the veins, while IV infusion is the process of infusing fluid volumes of 50 to 500 mL or more into the body.

Laws vary from state to state as to whether medical assistants can perform procedures directly related to intravenous therapy. Health care facilities such as ambulatory care clinics and urgent care centers have started to delegate specific job duties to the medical assistant including gathering the supplies, starting the IV, monitoring the patient for adverse reactions, and discontinuing the IV. A licensed physician is the one who prescribes IV therapy. Whether or not the medical assistant will be able to start IVs will be determined by state law and office policy. The medical assistant must be aware of the laws in the state in which she practices so that the medical assistant does not go beyond the scope of practice.

Equipment and Supplies Employed in Intravenous Therapy

Equipment and supplies available for use in IV therapy are continually being updated to comply with federal and state laws regarding safe work practices and for patient comfort. Containers for IV fluids have changed from glass containers to pliable plastic bags (Figure 32-31) that are lightweight and not at risk of becoming broken or damaged. IV fluid bags range in size from 50 to 2000 mL, with the smaller bags often referred to as "piggyback" bags. When prescribed, the pharmacy will open the bag to add additional medications to the fluids and label the bag with the specific prescription the physician has ordered. If a bag is found with the opaque outer bag removed, do not use the solution because sterility and viability of the product may be compromised.

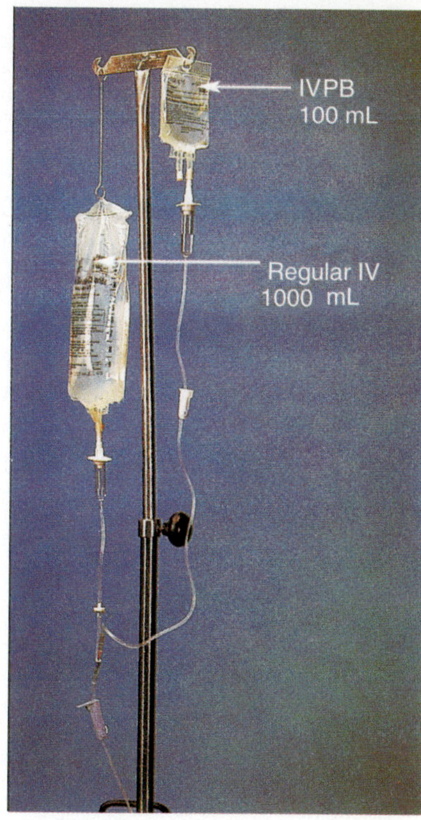

Figure 32-31 ■ Standard intravenous line with piggyback (PB IV).

The tamper-proof additive caps are removed when additive drugs are mixed within the IV bag. Piggyback containers are used for reduced volume of fluid infusion and are filled with ready-to-use medications at the time of manufacturing. The pharmacy will add additional medications if prescribed, such as antibiotics.

The commonly used fluids contained within an IV bag for infusion are normal saline (NaCl) or dextrose in water. Infusions are given to replace lost body fluids, restore fluid balance of cellular tonicity, or to provide medications or nutrients to the body. Homeostasis of the body and its functions is the primary reason for infusion of fluids. The fluid choice is based on the electrolyte balance and the patient's needs at the time. While there are numerous types of fluids used during IV administration, some common products are included in Table 32-9.

Table 32-9 Common Fluids Used for IV Therapy

Infusion	Indications
5% Dextrose in water (D5W)	Fluid replacement for rehydration
Normal saline (0.9% NaCl)	Used to replace sodium losses
Dextrose in saline solutions	Fluid replacement for burns, rehydration, maintenance infusion, circulatory insufficiency, and in cases of shock
Ringer's Solution (Na 147 mEq/L, K 4 mEq/L, Cl 155 mEq/L)	Restores fluid and electrolyte balance, used when patients have lactose intolerance, may be used as a blood replacement for a short time

Infused fluids are introduced to the body through administration sets, which is tubing that connects the IV bags to the IV cannula in the patient. Administration sets come in a variety of styles, from the very basic solution set to multiple administration tubing. All IV tubing sets have common components including clamps, a piercing pin, a drip chamber, and a cannula adapter.

Basic IV Administration Sets

Each IV administration set has similar components, including the following:

- Piercing pin (Figure 32-32): A hollow spike that is inserted into the administration port of the IV bag. It is important this remains sterile when inserted.
- Drip chamber (Figure 32-32): This is where the solution flows prior to its entry into the tubing; it acts as a pressurizing chamber for nonvented bags.
- Slide clamp (Figure 32-32): This is used to restrict fluid flow and act as a quick on/off control for the IV tubing. The tubing ends in a sterile-capped adapter, which is attached to the cannula.
- Roller clamp (Figure 32-33): This is used to regulate the flow of fluids through the IV tubing.
- IV **cannula** or catheter (Figure 32-34): A flexible tube that is used to insert medication within a body cavity or blood vessel. It has a **trocar** (Figure 32-34) (a sharp-pointed needle) attached to it that punctures the skin to get the catheter within the vein.

Because of the legal issues involved with IV administration, the medical assistant's responsibilities for IV therapy are usually to collect the equipment and supplies and to assist with taping the IV in place. The provider or nurse will usually be responsible for starting the IV.

The infusion of fluids can be achieved by either an infusion pump or by gravity flow (Figure 32-35). The gravity method is controlled by a roller clamp on the IV tubing. The tighter the clamp, the less fluid that flows through the tube. The drip chamber is used in calculating the drops per minute that flow into the IV tubing.

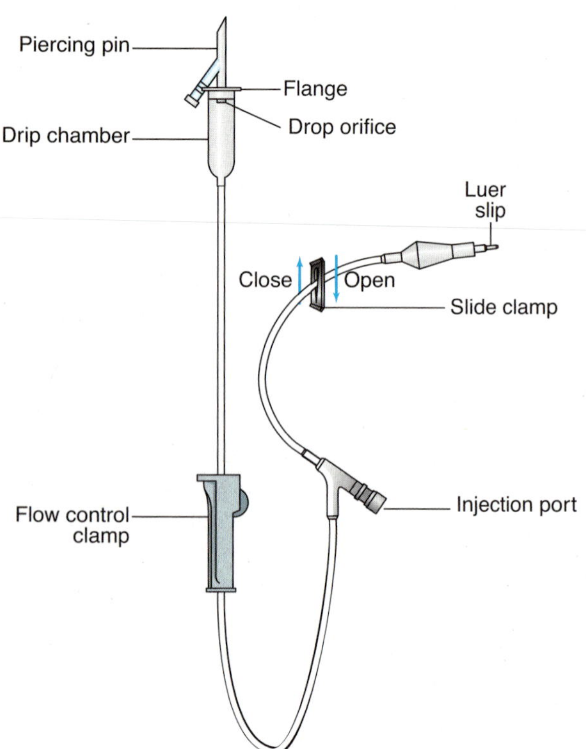

Figure 32-32 ■ An IV administration tubing set.

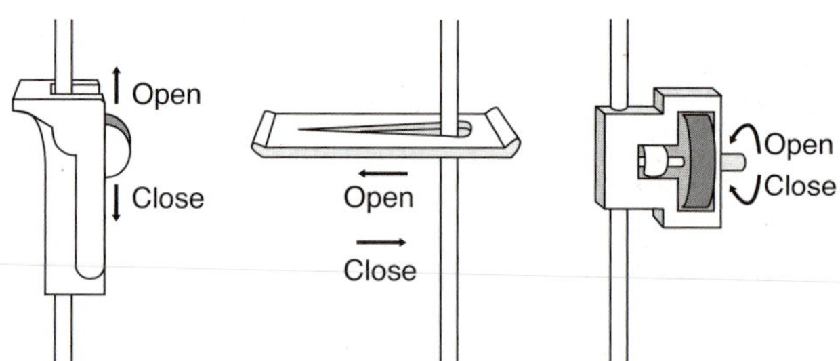

Figure 32-33 ■ Parts of the tubing clamp.

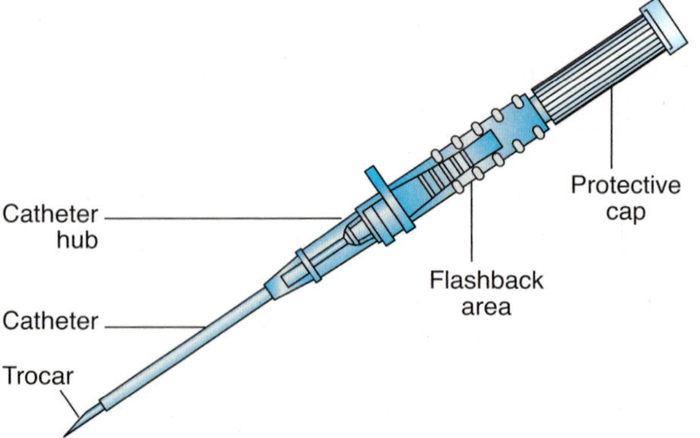

Figure 32-34 ■ A catheter and needle.

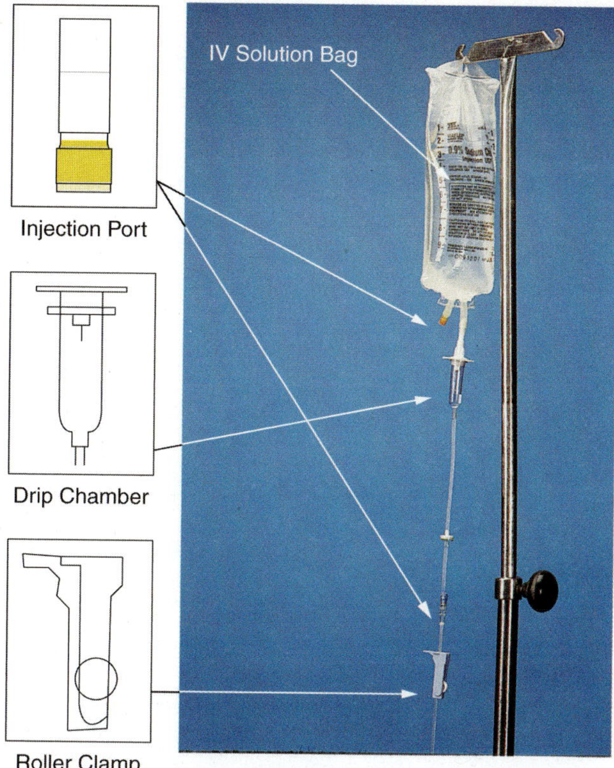

Figure 32-35 ■ Standard gravity flow intravenous system.

The IV pumps are more precise in delivery and more practical and safe for the patient. Constant monitoring of the IV set for occlusions is not necessary with the IV pumps. The pump will sound an alarm if an **occlusion** (blockage or closure) is detected or if the timing of the flow rate indicates the bag is almost empty. With the pump, the fluid is forced with light pressure into the veins and lessens reflux, which is the backing up of fluids into the veins and tissues. The pump can be set for different lengths of time and rates of infusion. Some pumps can run multiple IV lines on the same patient.

Documentation of IV Therapy

The health care professional that inserts and starts the IV will be responsible for documenting the procedure. Documentation in the patient's chart should include the IV site location, number of attempts of insertion, any complications of the procedure, the date and time of insertions, the needle gauge and length, and the person's initials that inserted the catheter. Any adverse reactions to the procedure such as redness, pain, swelling, bruising, and other essential findings that are not problematic at this point but could lead to complications at a later date and time should also be documented.

Risks, Complications, and Adverse Reactions of IV Therapy

Intravenous therapy can have numerous inherent risks and complications associated with this type of medication administration procedure. The medical assistant must be knowledgeable in recognizing the complications, signs, and symptoms that may arise from the IV infusion. The different complications can be classified as local, systemic, or be a combination of the two.

Local complications may consist of pain and irritation at the insertion site, cannula dislodgement, catheter or needle occlusion, and **phlebitis** (inflammation of the vein). Other complications may involve hematoma formation, venous spasm, vessel collapse, **thrombosis** (blood clot), and nerve, tendon, or ligament damage.

It is essential to communicate with the patient to assess complications of IV therapy or patient intolerance of the IV catheter. The medical assistant may be the health care professional that monitors the patient for complications and should know when the provider or nurse should be alerted. Table 32-10 explains some questions to ask a patient to clearly define the effectiveness of the therapy and patient tolerance.

Once the medical assistant has determined the patient's pain level, it is important to relay this information to the provider so the provider can determine the most appropriate intervention. Depending on the findings, the actions may include discontinuation of the therapy, changing position of the extremity, adjusting the flow rate of infusion, re-taping the site, or applying a warm or cool compress. Table 32-11 explains in further detail more of the complications and risks of IV therapy.

Systemic complications are much more dangerous and can be life-threatening. The medical assistant should become familiar with symptoms that may indicate a

Table 32-10 **Guideline Questions for Patient Pain Assessment**

1. Tell me about the pain you are having.
2. Where does it hurt?
3. When did it start?
4. Is the pain in one spot, or does it radiate to other places?
5. What kind of pain is it? Aching? Gnawing? Burning? Stabbing or piercing? Dull? Throbbing?
6. Are there any other symptoms of discomfort?
7. Rate the pain on a scale of 0 to 10, with 10 being the worst pain.

Table 32-11 Complications and Risks of Intravenous Therapy

Complications and Risks	Description	Symptoms
Infiltration or **extravasation**	Medication fluid leaks from the cannula or from the vein into the tissues surrounding the site	Redness, severe swelling, hardness at the site, pain, and edema.
Catheter and needle displacement	Self-explanatory.	Redness.
Occlusion	The cannula becomes blocked and allows blood to back up into the IV tubing.	Blood in IV tubing or loss of flow.
Loss of **patency** (the openness of the vein)	Occurs when the vein wall has been damaged.	Blood in IV tubing or loss of flow.
Phlebitis (inflammation of the vein wall)	Bacteria can form as a normal immune response due to the death of leukocytes and other tissue cells.	Vein may be hard, red streak along vein, inflammation, and swelling.
Thrombosis	Blood clots form, causing slow or stopped infusion	Slow or stopped infusion. Fever and malaise may be present.
Hematoma	Blood infiltrates into the tissues	Discoloration of the skin, discomfort, and swelling.
Cellulitis	A bacterial infection that can spread to surrounding tissues.	Redness, red streak at the site of the needle or nearby.

Table 32-12 Signs and Symptoms of Systemic Complications

Systems Affected by Systemic Complications	Signs and Symptoms
Cardiovascular system	Facial edema, generalized edema, erythema along veins, palpitations, hypotension, cardiac arrest
Gastrointestinal system	Dysphagia, gastric cramping, intestinal cramping, nausea, vomiting
Integumentary system	Flushing, red flare, rash, IV site edema, pruritus (itching), urticaria (hives)
Nervous system	Agitation, anxiety, confusion, disorientation, headache, loss of sensation or numbness, vertigo
Respiratory system	Nasal congestion, runny nose, cough, sensation of tightness in throat, mucous membrane edema, bronchospasm, respiratory arrest
Special senses	Pruritus, watery eyes, scratchy throat, tinnitus (ringing in ears), buzzing sound in ears, tingling or numbness in fingers or toes, vertigo

systemic reaction. Table 32-12 provides details of systemic complications that may occur during IV infusion therapy. If the medical assistant notices any of the signs as noted in Table 32-12, immediately alert the provider.

Discontinuation of Intravenous Infusion Therapy

When the physician determines the patient no longer needs IV infusion, the IV must be discontinued. The first step in discontinuing IV infusion is proper aseptic technique and the application of gloves. Then the IV tubing is clamped off and removed from the adapter or extension set. Take care to not remove the adapter—this will cause blood to leak profusely out of the cannula hub. Remove the transparent dressing by rubbing the patient's skin with an alcohol pad, which will loosen the adhesive in the dressing. This helps patients who have a lot of hair on their arm or in cases in which the adhesive dressing has adhered to the skin and is difficult to remove.

Once the transparent dressing is removed, the tape securing the cannula hub should be removed. Take care not to accidentally dislodge the hub from the site during this process. When the tape is completely removed, prepare a gauze pad and place above the cannula site. Inform the patient to take a deep breath and when the patient breathes in, remove the cannula in one smooth continuous movement without pressing down on the cannula. Place the gauze over the site and apply pressure for five minutes. Be sure to inspect the cannula (Figure 32-36) to make sure it is in one piece and has not broken off within the vein. Document in the patient's chart the state of the cannula for its "intact" form (e.g., "Cannula removed from right anterior forearm. Cannula intact. Patient tolerated procedure well. No swelling, no bruising, or other complications noted.").

Intravenous therapy is a concise procedure and should be performed only by specially trained individuals. If medical assistants are asked to perform duties that exceed their training, a life-threatening event may occur to the patient. If unsure of what exactly is detailed in the procedure, verify with the ordering physician to ensure complete understanding of the expectations of

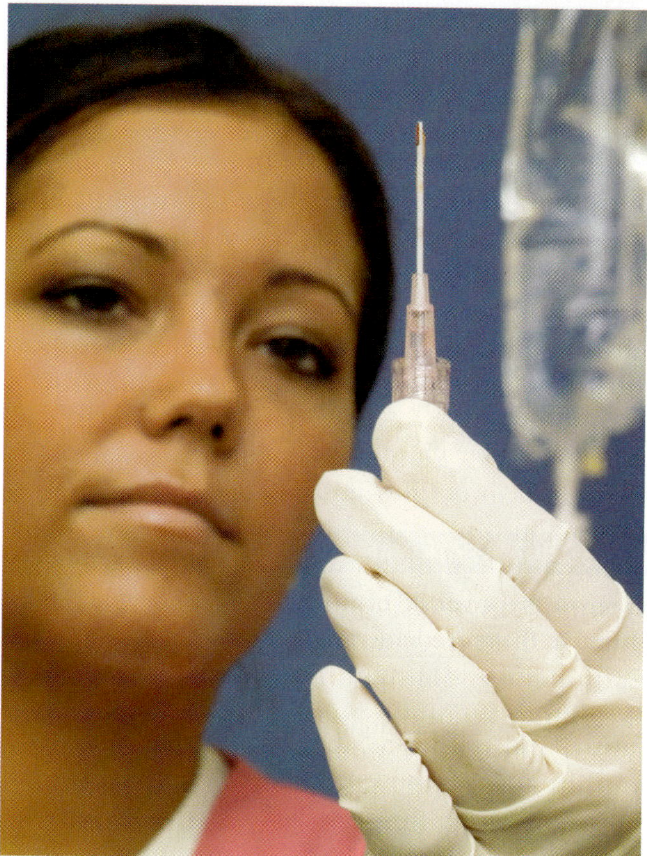

Figure 32-36 ■ Inspect the cannula following withdrawal from the patient's vein.

performance and completion of the administration of intravenous therapy. If medical assistants are allowed to perform IVs in their state but feel uncomfortable performing the procedure, they should get assistance from their superior or the provider.

INTRA-ARTICULAR INJECTIONS

The term **intra-articular** means within a joint. Some injections are given within a joint to help reduce inflammation and pain. Patients that suffer with osteoarthritis are usually good candidates for these types of injections. The knee is the most common joint in which these injections are given but other joints can be injected as well. Viscosupplementation, ketorolac, and steroids to reduce inflammation are the common drugs used to treat osteoarthritis.

The medical assistant's duty for these injections would be to prepare the patient for the injection and to have all of the equipment ready for the physician. The medical assistant may need to help hold the joint still during the injection procedure.

CRITICAL THINKING CHALLENGE

You work in an urgent care center and the physician instructs you to start an IV on a specific patient. You know that the Medical Practice Act in the state in which you work requires a licensed health care provider or registered nurse to perform this procedure. All of the rest of the medical assistants in the facility start IVs. One of the medical assistants tells you that she will assist you with your first IV.

1. How will you respond to the physician?

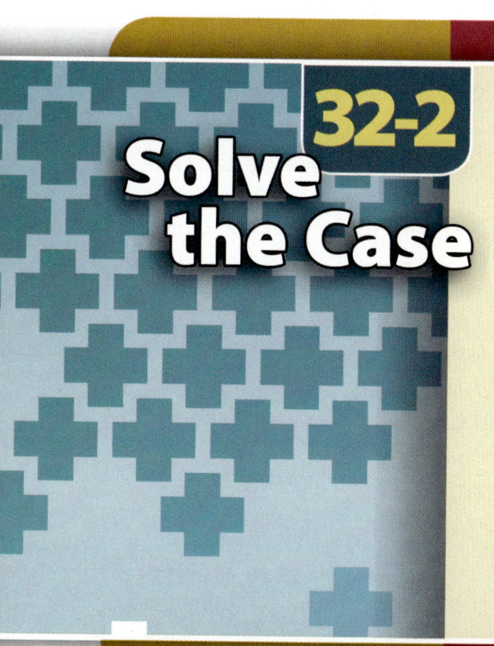

The same 35 year-old patient presented in the first case has been diagnosed with an acute migraine exacerbation by the provider. After you placed the patient in a cool, dark, quiet room she reports immediate improvement in her pain to 5/10. The provider orders ketorolac 60 mg intramuscularly now, promethazine 25 mg IV.

1. **Look up the ketorolac and see if you can administer it. How will you know if you can administer it? Refer back to Chapter 30 regarding scheduled medications.**
2. **If you are allowed to administer this drug, state how many mL you will give the patient if the label on the bottle reads 100 mg/mL. (Refer back to Chapter 31 if you don't remember how to calculate a dosage.)**
3. **Using the information that you obtained on ketorolac, role-play with a fellow student and practice providing patient education for this drug.**

PROCEDURE 32-1

Withdraw Medication from a Vial

Objective:

To prepare medication from a vial for administration.

Equipment/Supplies:

- Provider's order
- Vial of medication
- Antiseptic wipe
- Needle and syringe appropriate for procedure
- Gauze 2 × 2 sponges
- Sharps container
- Medication tray

PROCEDURAL STEPS	DETAILS AND/OR RATIONALE
1. Wash your hands and apply gloves.	This prevents the spread of infection and contamination during the procedure.
2. Assemble the equipment.	
3. Work in a quiet and well-lit area.	Distractions and poor lighting may lead to medication errors.
4. Select the correct medication from the storage area and check the drug label **(Medication Check #1).**	This assists in making certain you have the correct medication.
5. Check the expiration date.	Using a medication beyond the expiration date may decrease the effectiveness of the drug.
6. Compare the medication with the physician's order **(Medication Check #2).**	This alleviates the mistakes and wasting of valuable medication.
7. Calculate the correct dose to be given, if needed. ***Incorporate critical thinking skills when performing patient care***. Verify the correct calculations with the physician if necessary.	Giving the correct dose helps to obtain the desired effects and avoid complications.
8. Open the syringe and attach the needle to the syringe.	
9. Open the antiseptic wipe and clean the vial stopper (Figure 32-37).	This prevents contamination of the vial and the needle when preparing the injection.
10. Holding the syringe at eye level, pull back on the plunger of syringe to draw an amount of air into the syringe equal to the amount of medication to be withdrawn from the vial.	This keeps the pressure in the vial at atmospheric pressure.
11. Check to make sure the needle is firmly attached to the syringe and remove the cap from the needle.	If the needle is not firmly attached to the syringe, it may become disconnected and cause an injury to the person preparing the medication or to the patient during the procedure.
12. Insert the needle through the rubber stopper (Figure 32-38) until it reaches the empty space between the stopper and the fluid level.	

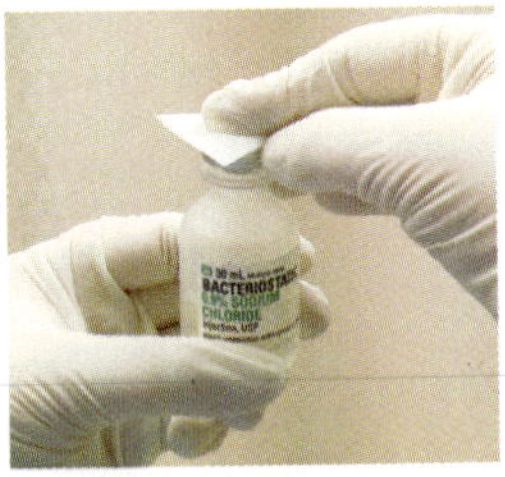

Figure 32-37 ■ Cleanse the stopper of the vial.

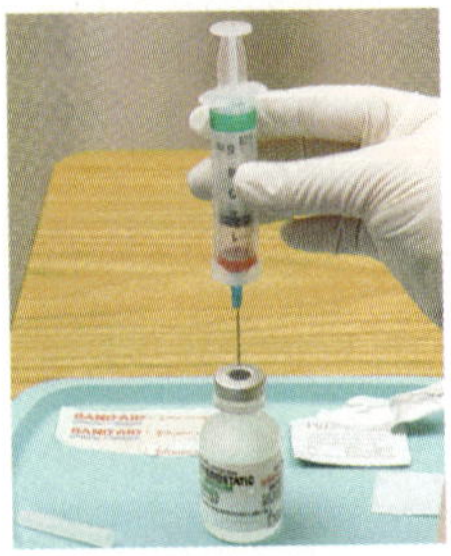

Figure 32-38 ■ Insert the needle through the rubber stopper.

continues

PROCEDURE 32-1 continued

PROCEDURAL STEPS	DETAILS AND/OR RATIONALE
13. Push forward on the plunger to inject air into the vial. Keep the needle above the fluid level.	Forcing air into the medication can cause the fluid to break down or bubble, thus creating more bubbles in the medication vial.
14. Invert the vial while holding onto the syringe and plunger. Hold the vial and syringe without contaminating the needle or hub of the syringe. These parts of the syringe must remain sterile.	This helps prevent microorganisms from entering the vial and the patient from obtaining an infection.
15. Hold the syringe at eye level and withdraw the proper amount of medication (Figure 32-39).	This ensures that you are reading the calibration lines correctly.
16. Keep the tip of needle below the fluid level.	This helps to prevent air from forming in the syringe.
17. Remove any air bubbles in the syringe by tapping or flicking the side of the syringe where the bubbles are located (Figure 32-40).	If there are air bubbles in the syringe, you may not have the correct amount of medication. Air bubbles can take up extra space. Air bubbles may also cause pain to the patient.
18. Remove any air remaining in the tip of the syringe. Check to make certain that you still have the correct amount of medication. If you do not, make the appropriate adjustments to confirm you have the correct amount before removing the needle from the vial.	Removing air bubbles and expelling any air could change the volume of medication in the syringe.
19. Remove the needle from the rubber stopper of the vial.	
20. Replace the needle cap on the syringe (Figure 32-41) or replace with a new needle and cap setup.	Replacing the needle unit reduces the risk of a local reaction if the needle used to withdraw the medication is changed between the vial and patient. Pushing the needle through the rubber stopper dulls the needle; a new needle pierces the skin much easier.
21. Read the medication label, record the date the vial was opened, and place your initials on the vial. Replace the medication vial in the correct storage cabinet (**Medication Check #3**).	Three checks help to ensure you have the correct medication and prevents errors from occurring.
22. Place the syringe on to a clean tray with other items necessary for the injection, including an alcohol wipe, a gauze pad, and an adhesive bandage.	

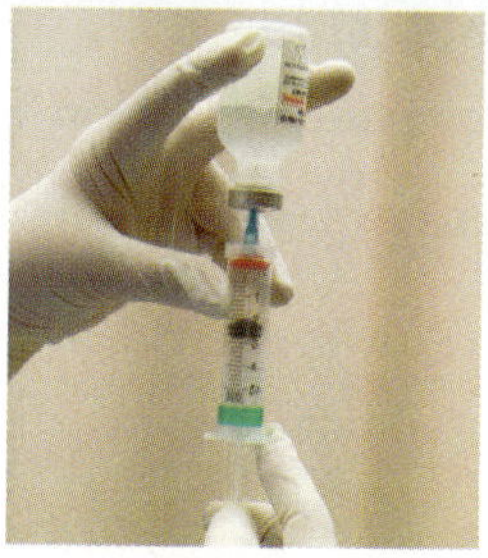

Figure 32-39 ■ Hold the vial at eye level during withdrawal of the medication.

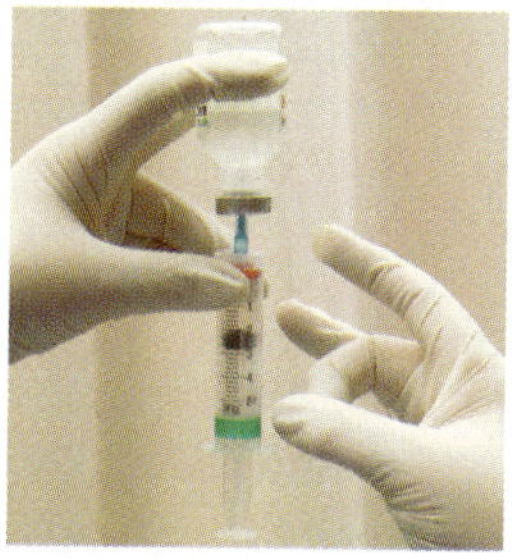

Figure 32-40 ■ Flick the syringe to remove any air bubbles.

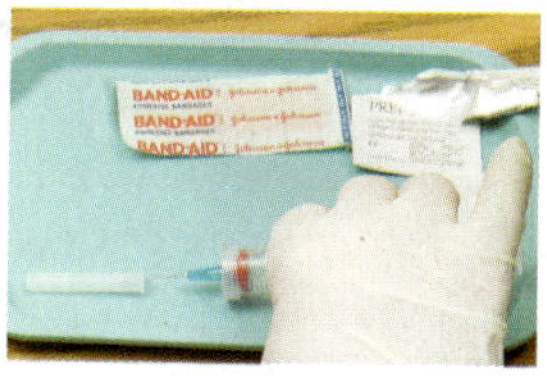

Figure 32-41 ■ Replace the needle cap.

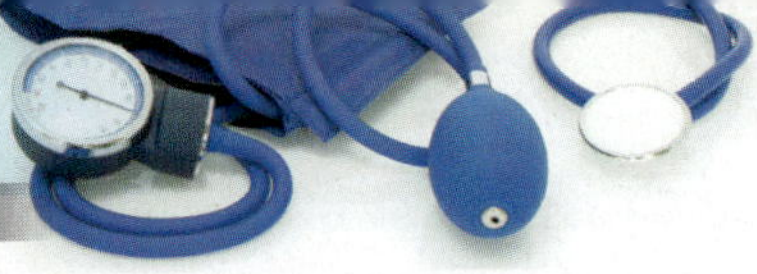

PROCEDURE 32-2

Withdraw Medication from an Ampule

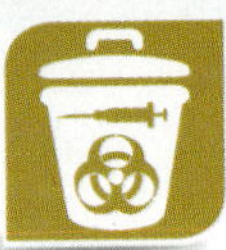

Objective:

To prepare medication from an ampule for administration.

Equipment/Supplies:

- Provider's order
- Ampule of medication
- Antiseptic wipes (2)
- Needle and syringe appropriate for procedure
- Filter needle
- Gauze 2 × 2 sponges
- Sharps container
- Medication tray

PROCEDURAL STEPS	DETAILS AND/OR RATIONALE
1. Wash your hands and apply gloves.	This prevents the spread of infection and contamination during the procedure.
2. Assemble the equipment.	
3. Work in a quiet and well-lit area.	Distractions and poor lighting may lead to medication errors.
4. Select the correct medication from the storage area and check the drug label **(Medication Check #1).**	This helps to confirm you have the correct medication and prevents error from occurring.
5. Check the expiration date.	No medication should be given if the drug has reached the expiration date, as it may not be effective.
6. Compare the medication with the physician's order **(Medication Check #2).**	This alleviates the possibility of mistakes and wasting of valuable medication.
7. Calculate the correct dose to be given, if needed. ***Incorporate critical thinking skills when performing patient care.***	An incorrect dose could cause great harm to the patient.
8. Open the syringe and filter needle and assemble, if necessary.	A filter needle filters out possible glass fragments that may be present from snapping the stem from the body of the ampule.
9. Tap the stem of the ampule lightly, or snap the wrist of the arm holding the ampule, to remove any medication in the neck of the ampule.	This forces the medication into the base of the ampule container.
10. Open the antiseptic wipe and clean the ampule container. Allow the ampule to dry completely.	This prevents contamination of the needle when preparing the injection.
11. Place a piece of gauze around the neck of the ampule. Hold the ampule firmly between the fingers and the thumbs of both hands.	This protects the fingers when breaking open the neck of the vial.
12. Break off the stem by snapping it quickly and firmly away from the body. Discard the top in a sharps container and carefully set the ampule down on a flat, firm surface.	This keeps glass fragments from flying into the medical assistant's eyes or face.

continues

PROCEDURE 32-2 continued

PROCEDURAL STEPS	DETAILS AND/OR RATIONALE
13. Check to make sure the filter needle is firmly attached to the syringe and remove the cap from the needle.	If the needle is not firmly attached it may cause injury to the person preparing the medication.
14. Insert the needle into the ampule below the fluid level. Hold the ampule at a slight angle while advancing the needle within the glass body. Completely draw up all the medication into the syringe (Figure 32-42).	Tilting the ampule facilitates emptying the entire ampule.
15. Remove the needle from the ampule without allowing the needle to touch the edges of the ampule.	This prevents contamination of the needle.
16. Dispose of the ampule into the sharps container. Check the medication label before discarding the ampule **(Medication Check #3).**	Immediately disposing of the ampule prevents injury to the person preparing the medication for injection.
17. Remove any bubbles in the syringe.	This helps to prevent any air bubbles from entering the patient.
18. Pull back slightly on the plunger to draw the medication from the needle into the syringe, engage the safety device, and remove the filter needle.	This removes any medication that remains within the filter needle. Medication cannot be administered to the patient with the filter needle.
19. Open a new needle for administering medication to the patient and attach it correctly to the syringe.	The filter needle may have glass fragments inside, so it is not used.
20. Remove the cap from the needle and push slightly forward on the plunger to remove air that is within the tip of the syringe and shaft of the needle.	This expels any air that is within the syringe tip and shaft of the new needle to ensure that air is not being injected into the patient's tissues.
21. Replace the needle cap on the syringe following institutional policy.	
22. Prepare the medication tray. Place a bandage, a gauze pad, an antiseptic wipe, and the syringe on a medication tray for transporting to the exam room to administer the injection to the patient.	

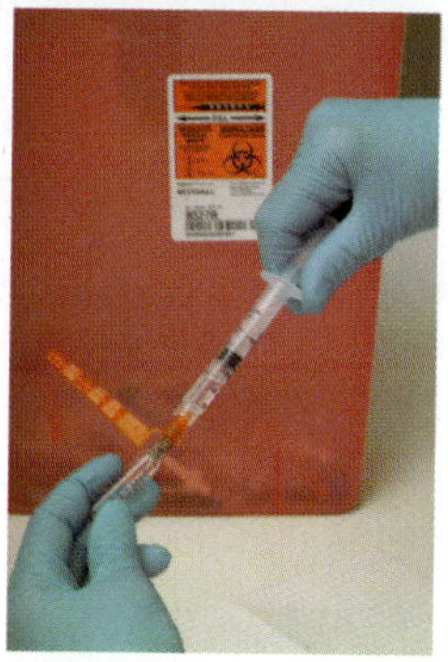

Figure 32-42 ■ Hold the ampule at a slight angle when withdrawing medication.

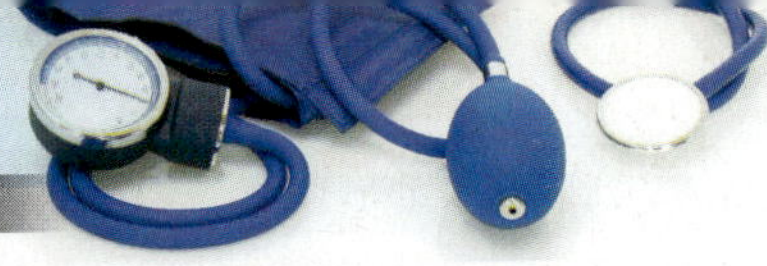

PROCEDURE 32-3

Reconstitute a Powdered-Base Medication with a Diluent

Objective:

To reconstitute a powdered-base medication for preparation of administering an injection to a patient.

Equipment/Supplies:

- Provider's order
- Vial of powdered medication
- Vial of diluent
- Antiseptic wipe
- Two needles and a syringe appropriate for procedure
- Gauze 2 × 2 sponges
- Sharps container
- Medication tray

PROCEDURAL STEPS	DETAILS AND/OR RATIONALE
1. Wash your hands and apply gloves.	This prevents the spread of infection and contamination during the procedure.
2. Assemble the equipment.	
3. Work in a quiet and well-lit area.	Distractions and poor lighting may lead to medication errors.
4. Select the correct medication and diluent from the storage area, and check both drug labels (**Medication Check #1).**	Having the wrong medication or diluent could cause harm to the patient.
5. Check the expiration date on both labels.	Medication should not be given if the drug has reached the expiration date, because it may not be effective.
6. Compare the medication with the physician's order **(Medication Check #2).**	This reduces the chances of making a medication error and the wasting of valuable medication.
7. Calculate the correct dose to be given, if needed. ***Incorporate critical thinking skills when performing patient care***. Verify the correct calculations with the provider if necessary.	Giving the wrong dose could cause great harm to the patient.
8. Open the syringe and needle and assemble, if necessary.	
9. Clean both the powder vial and the reconstituting fluid vial stopper with alcohol before use (Figure 32-43).	This prevents possible contamination to the medication vials or the patient.
10. Pull back on the plunger to fill the syringe with the amount of air equal to the amount of diluting liquid required for reconstitution from the vial containing the diluent.	This equalizes the pressure within the vial.
11. Check to make sure the needle is firmly attached to the syringe and remove the needle cap.	If the needle is not firmly attached to the syringe, it may become disconnected and cause an injury to the person preparing the medication.
12. Insert the needle into the diluent vial.	

Figure 32-43 ■ Cleanse the rubber stopper of both vials.

continues

PROCEDURE 32-3 continued

PROCEDURAL STEPS	DETAILS AND/OR RATIONALE
13. Push in the plunger, forcing the air from the syringe into the vial of diluent (Figure 32-44).	This equalizes the amount of air in the vial.
14. Invert the vial in the dominant hand, holding between the thumb and index finger.	
15. Keep the needle immersed in the solution while drawing the solution into the barrel of the syringe.	If the needle tip is not inserted in the fluid, air will be drawn into the syringe.
16. Check for air bubbles and determine that the exact amount of diluent is withdrawn from the vial before removing the needle from the vial.	
17. Carefully remove the needle from the vial.	
18. Insert the needle into the vial containing the powdered medication (Figure 32-45).	
19. Add the appropriate amount of reconstituting liquid to the powdered drug, slowly rotating vial while injecting fluid into it.	This allows the powder to be flushed with the fluids and helps to minimize the formation of clumps within the powder.
20. Replace the needle cap on the syringe following institutional policy.	
21. Roll the vial between the hands to thoroughly mix the medication (Figure 32-46).	This allows all of the particles to be suspended appropriately.
22. Record the new date of expiration on the label of the medication vial.	Once the medication has been prepared, it is only good for a certain amount of time.
23. Recheck the medication label before returning the vial to the proper storage area **(Medication Check #3).**	A third check helps in confirming you have the correct medication.
24. Prepare to administer the medication to the patient. Place a bandage, a gauze pad, an antiseptic wipe, and the syringe on a medication tray for transporting to the exam room to administer the injection to the patient.	

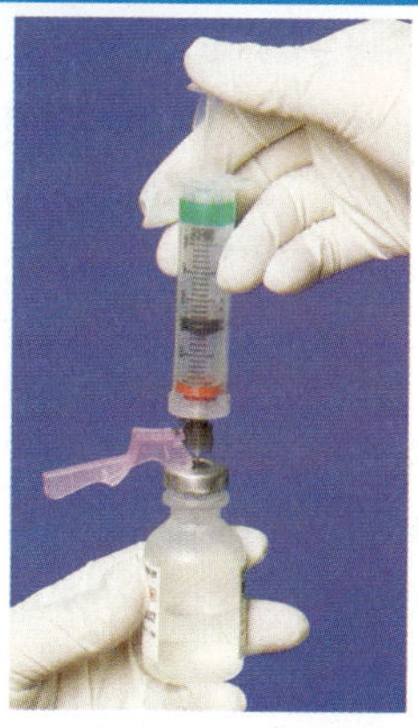

Figure 32-44 ■ Inject air into the diluent vial.

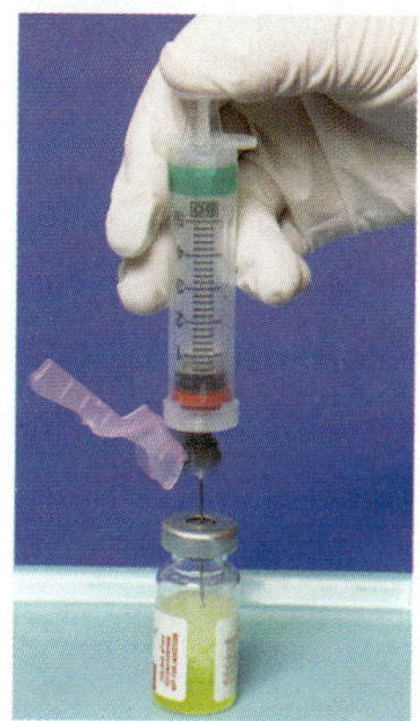

Figure 32-45 ■ Inject the diluent into powdered medication vial.

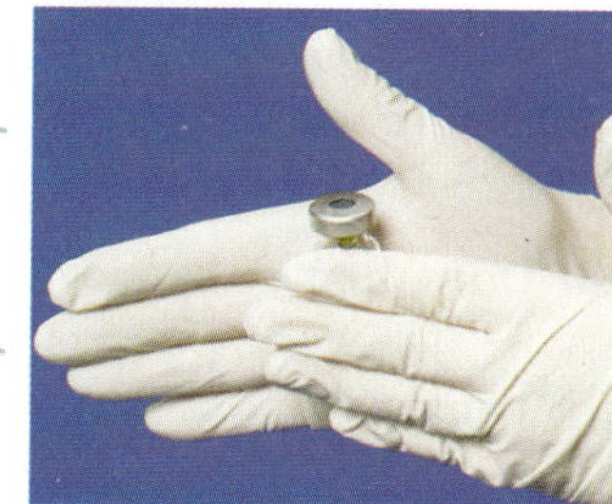

Figure 32-46 ■ Gently roll the vial between the hands to mix well.

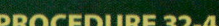

PROCEDURE 32-4

Mix Two Medications into One Syringe

Objective:

To draw two medications into one single syringe for injection administration to a patient.

Equipment/Supplies:

- Provider's order
- Two vials of medication
- Antiseptic wipe
- Two needles and a syringe appropriate for procedure
- Gauze 2 × 2 sponges
- Medication tray
- Sharps container

PROCEDURAL STEPS	DETAILS AND/OR RATIONALE
1. Wash your hands and apply gloves.	This prevents the spread of infection and contamination during the procedure.
2. Assemble the equipment.	
3. Work in a quiet and well-lit area.	Distractions and poor lighting may lead to medication errors.
4. Select the correct medications from the storage area and check their drug labels (**Medication Check #1**).	Reading the label helps to be certain you have the correct medication.
5. Check the expiration dates on both vials.	No medication should be given if the drug has reached the expiration date, as the medication may not be as effective.
6. Compare the medications with the physician's order (**Medication Check #2**).	This alleviates the possibility of mistakes and wasting of valuable medication.
7. Calculate the correct doses to be given, if needed. ***Incorporate critical thinking skills when performing patient care***. Verify the correct calculations with the provider if necessary.	Giving an incorrect dose could cause great harm to the patient.
8. Open the syringe and needle and remove them from their packaging. Attach the needle to the syringe.	
9. Clean the rubber stopper of both vials with an alcohol wipe.	This removes microbes that may be on the stoppers.
10. Determine which medication is the primary medication vial. Do not do anything with the primary medicine at this point.	The primary medication is the first medication to be drawn up.
11. Draw up an amount of air into the syringe that is equal to the amount of medication required from the second vial.	Air is injected into the second vial at this point because once the syringe is filled with medication from the first vial, it will no longer be possible to inject air into the vial.
12. Check to make sure the needle is firmly attached to the syringe and remove the needle cap.	If the needle is not firmly attached it may become detached from the syringe, causing harm to the preparer.

continues

PROCEDURE 32-4 continued

PROCEDURAL STEPS	DETAILS AND/OR RATIONALE
13. Insert the needle into the second vial and push the air from the syringe into the vial to replace the medication that will be taken out later. Do not allow the needle to touch the liquid.	Pushing the needle into the medication will contaminate the needle, affecting the next vial.
14. Carefully remove the needle from the vial.	
15. Draw up an amount of air into the syringe that is equal to the amount of medication required to be taken from the primary vial.	This equalizes the pressure due to the fluid being removed from the vial.
16. Insert the needle into the primary vial. Push forward on the plunger, forcing air from the syringe into the primary vial without contacting the medication.	Pushing air into the liquid could create bubbles in the syringe and vial.
17. Invert the vial in the dominant hand, holding it between the thumb and index finger.	
18. Keep the needle immersed in the solution while drawing the solution into the barrel of the syringe.	If the needle tip is not inserted in fluid, air will be drawn into the syringe.
19. Remove any air remaining in the tip of the syringe. If there is medication lacking in the syringe, pull back on the plunger so that the correct amount of medication is drawn into the syringe.	This expels any remaining air within the syringe and the needle and confirms you have the correct amount of medication.
20. Remove the needle from the stopper of the first vial, engage the safety device, and discard into a sharps container. Replace the needle with a new needle.	This reduces the risk of medication from the first vial carrying over to the second vial.
21. Smoothly insert the needle into the secondary vial.	
22. Invert the vial and slowly withdraw the medication required from the vial. Do not allow any medication from the first vial to be inadvertently injected into the second vial. Pulling slowly to avoid creating air bubbles, pull the plunger back to the correct calibration mark on the syringe.	If medication from the primary vial mixes with the secondary vial it will contaminate the contents of the second vial.
23. Remove the needle from the second vial.	
24. Check for air bubbles and remove them from the syringe.	
25. Check again that the total amount of medication in the syringe is the correct total to be administered.	If the incorrect dosage is in the syringe, the patient may not obtain the full effects of the medication.
26. Replace the needle cap on the syringe following institutional policy.	Some facilities will allow recapping of clean needles, while other facilities prefer the scoop method.
27. Recheck the medication labels of both vials before returning the vials to the proper storage area (**Medication Check #3**).	Checking the label three times helps to confirm you have the correct medication and prevents errors from occurring.

continues

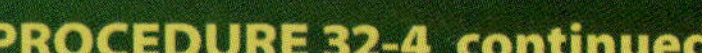

PROCEDURE 32-4 continued

PROCEDURAL STEPS	DETAILS AND/OR RATIONALE
28. Prepare to administer the medication to the patient. Place a bandage, a gauze pad, an antiseptic wipe, and the syringe on a medication tray for transporting to the exam room to administer the injection to the patient.	

PROCEDURE 32-5

Load a Cartridge into an Injector Device

Objective:

To prepare medication from a prefilled cartridge for administration.

Equipment/Supplies:

- Provider's order
- Prefilled cartridge of medication
- Cartridge holder
- Antiseptic wipe
- Gauze 2 × 2 sponges
- Sharps container
- Injection tray

PROCEDURAL STEPS	DETAILS AND/OR RATIONALE
1. Wash your hands and apply gloves.	This prevents the spread of infection and contamination during the procedure.
2. Assemble the equipment.	
3. Work in a quiet and well-lit area.	Distractions and poor lighting may lead to medication errors.
4. Select the correct medication from the storage area and check the drug label (**Medication Check #1**).	This confirms that you have the correct medication.
5. Check the expiration date.	No medication should be given if the drug has reached the expiration date, as it may not be effective.
6. Compare the medication with the physician's instructions (**Medication Check #2**).	This lessens the possibility of mistakes and wasting of valuable medication.
7. Calculate the correct dose to be given, if needed. ***Incorporate critical thinking skills when performing patient care.***	There may be instances in which a patient does not need the entire dose within the cartridge.
8. Pick up the cartridge unit holder (the injector).	
9. Turn the ribbed collar toward the open position until it stops (Figure 32-47).	This allows for the insertion of the cartridge into the holder.

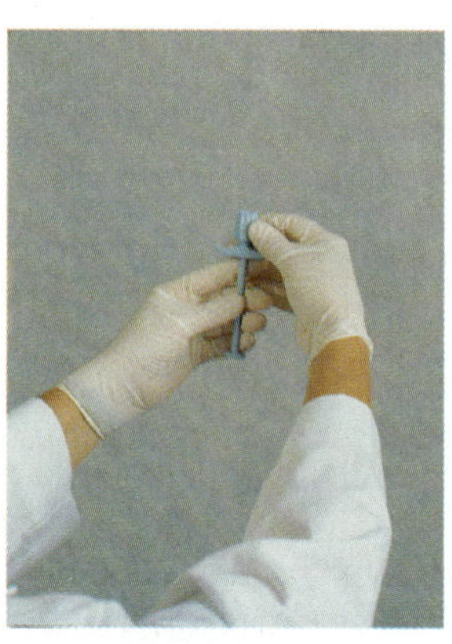

Figure 32-47 ■ Turn the ribbed collar to the open position.

continues

PROCEDURE 32-5 continued

PROCEDURAL STEPS	DETAILS AND/OR RATIONALE
10. Hold the injector with the open end up and fully insert the sterile cartridge–needle unit.	
11. Firmly tighten the ribbed collar of the unit at the syringe base by turning the ribbed collar toward the "close" arrow. (Hold the cartridge to prevent it from swiveling inside the holder while tightening.)	
12. Thread the rod of the plunger into the cartridge unit until a slight resistance is felt (Figure 32-48).	If the cartridge is not tightened securely onto the holder, the needle unit may move during the injection procedure.
13. Prepare the medication for injection into the patient at this time. Place a bandage, a gauze pad, an antiseptic wipe, and the syringe on a medication tray for transporting to the exam room. Check the medication label one last time (**Medication Check #3**).	Checking the label three times confirms you have the correct medication and prevents errors from occurring.
14. After use, do not recap the needle.	
15. Disengage the plunger rod from the cartridge unit holder while holding the needle down and away from the fingers or hands over a sharps unit (Figure 32-49).	This prevents the fingers from being in front of the needle.
16. Unscrew the ribbed collar of the cartridge unit holder.	
17. Allow the needle cartridge unit to drop into the sharps container (Figure 32-50).	This helps to prevent an accidental needlestick.
18. Cleanse the cartridge holder with an antiseptic cleanser and allow to dry.	This prevents cross-contamination from occurring to the next patient receiving medication from a prefilled cartridge.
19. Cleanse the work area and remove gloves and wash your hands.	

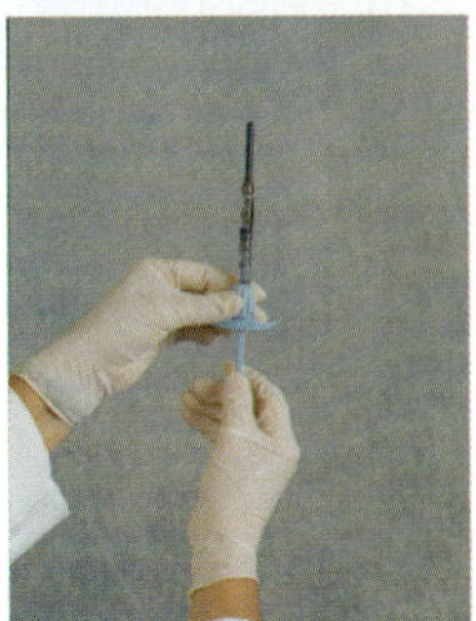

Figure 32-48 ■ Thread the plunger onto the cartridge unit.

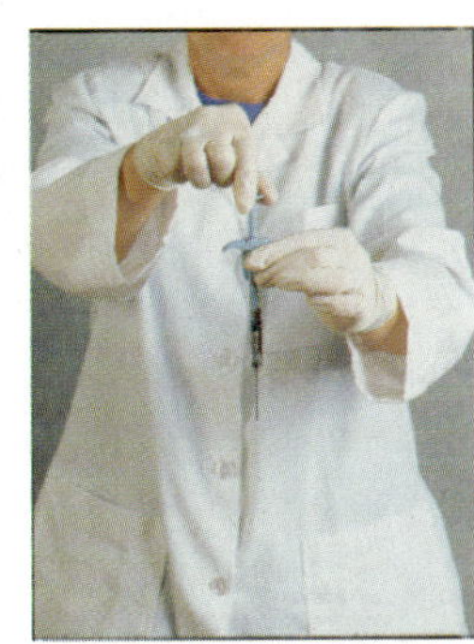

Figure 32-49 ■ After the injection is given, disengage the plunger from the cartridge unit.

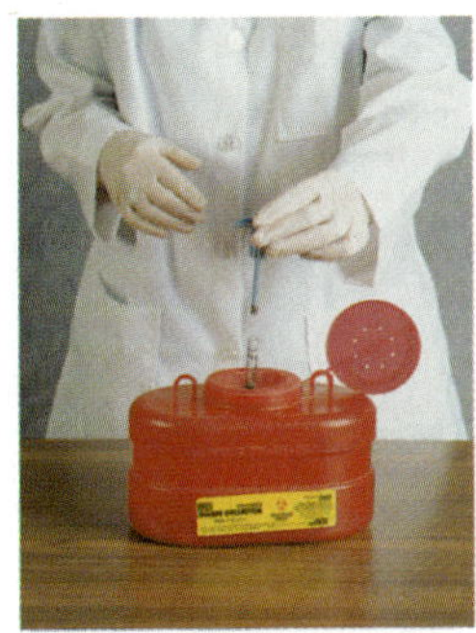

Figure 32-50 ■ Allow the cartridge to drop freely into the sharps container.

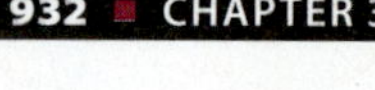

PROCEDURE 32-6

Administer an Intradermal Injection

Objective:

To administer an intradermal injection into a patient.

Equipment/Supplies:

- Appropriate sized needle and syringe unit with correct medication
- Antiseptic wipe
- Gauze 2 × 2 sponges
- Sharps container
- Disposable gloves
- Medication tray
- Patient's chart/EHR

PROCEDURAL STEPS	DETAILS AND/OR RATIONALE
1. Wash your hands.	This prevents the spread of infection and contamination during the procedure.
2. Assemble the equipment. Follow the Seven Rights of Drug Administration.	Following the seven rights helps to alleviate errors.
3. Identify the patient using two identifiers, identify yourself, and ***explain the rationale for performance of the procedure, showing awareness of the patient's concerns related to the procedure being performed***.	Giving the medication to the wrong patient can cause serious problems for the patient.
4. Ask patient about drug allergies or latex allergies.	Giving the patient a drug or using products that the patient is allergic to can cause an anaphylactic reaction.
5. Select the proper injection site (anterior forearm or middle of back).	
6. Cleanse the site with antiseptic and allow to air dry completely. (Cleanse in a circular motion working outward to an area of 2 to 3 inches.)	This prevents the possible contamination of the injection site and ensures the removal of microorganisms from the injection site area. Wet alcohol may cause the site to burn when you inject the medication.
7. Prepare the equipment and apply gloves.	Wearing gloves prevents contamination from bloodborne pathogens during the procedure.
8. Remove the needle cap. Pull the cap straight off, never twist.	Twisting may loosen the needle attached to the syringe.
9. Stretch the skin taut at the site of administration.	This allows the needle to be inserted easier and keeps the tissue from moving during insertion.
10. Insert the needle at a 10° to 15° angle with the bevel upward just under the skin (Figure 32-51).	

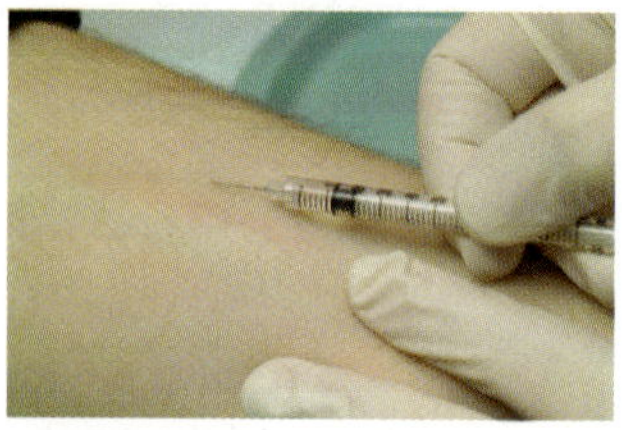

Figure 32-51 ■ Insert the needle bevel up just below the surface of the skin.

continues

PROCEDURE 32-6 continued

PROCEDURAL STEPS	DETAILS AND/OR RATIONALE
11. Inject the medication slowly and steadily. A wheal should form (Figure 32-52).	This allows the tissue to slowly displace and provides space for the fluid. If the needle is too deep, a wheal will not form and the injection will have to be repeated.
12. Remove the needle quickly at the same angle of insertion.	This prevents injury to the tissue.
13. Do not press on or massage the injection site. Do not apply a bandage to the site.	The medication will be dispersed into deeper tissue if pressure is applied to the area. A bandage will absorb the medication.
14. Properly engage the safety device on the needle and dispose of the needle-syringe unit in the sharps container.	Engaging the safety device will help to prevent an accidental needlestick.
15. Remove gloves and wash your hands.	This prevents contamination and the spread of infection.
16. Give proper patient education for caring for the site and inform the patient to wait 20 to 30 minutes.	The 20- to 30-minute wait is to observe the patient for anaphylaxis.
17. Perform postinjection observation and document the procedure in the patient's chart and the appropriate logs.	Documentation illustrates that the procedure was performed.

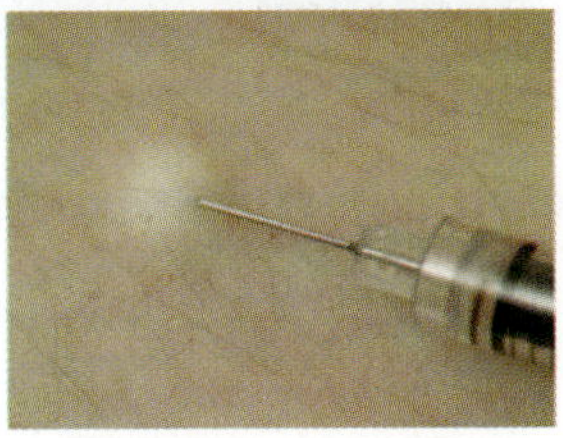

Figure 32-52 ■ A wheal will form if the procedure was performed correctly.

DOCUMENTATION EXAMPLE:

05-22-XX 3:15 p.m.	Tubersol, 0.1 mL, ID, right lower forearm, per Dr. Jones. Manf—Kline Beecham, Lot number—K449, exp. date—12/XX. Pt. tolerated well, instructions given to return to clinic 48–72 hours for PPD reading. Negative complications during post-injection observation. Sherri Jones, CMA (AAMA)--

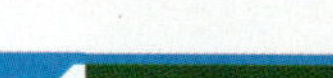

PROCEDURE 32-7

Administer a Subcutaneous Injection

Objective:

To administer an injection through the subcutaneous tissue.

Equipment/Supplies:

- Appropriate sized needle and syringe unit with correct medication
- Antiseptic wipe
- Gauze 2 × 2 sponges
- Sharps container
- Disposable gloves
- Medication tray
- Adhesive bandage
- Patient's chart/EHR

PROCEDURAL STEPS	DETAILS AND/OR RATIONALE
1. Wash your hands.	This prevents the spread of infection and contamination during the procedure.
2. Assemble the equipment. Follow the Seven Rights of Drug Administration.	Following the seven rights will help prevent errors from occurring.
3. Identify the patient using two identifiers, identify yourself, and ***explain the rationale for performance of the procedure, showing awareness of the patient's concerns related to the procedure being performed.***	Giving the medication to the wrong patient can cause serious problems for the patient.
4. Ask the patient about drug allergies, latex allergies, or adhesive allergies.	Giving the patient a drug or using products that the patient is allergic to can cause an anaphylactic reaction.
5. Select the proper injection site (fatty tissue of the arms, thighs, or stomach).	
6. Cleanse the site with antiseptic and allow to air dry completely. (Cleanse in a circular motion working outward to an area of 2 to 3 inches.)	This prevents the possible contamination of the injection site and ensures the removal of microorganisms from the injection site area. Wet alcohol may cause the site to burn when you inject the medication.
7. Prepare the equipment and apply gloves.	This prevents contamination from bloodborne pathogens during the procedure.
8. Remove the needle cap. Pull the cap straight off, never twist.	Twisting may loosen the needle attached to the syringe.
9. Grasp or pinch the tissue lightly with one hand.	This helps to determine the subcutaneous layer of tissue and helps with the needle insertion.
10. Insert the needle at a 45° angle with the other hand, using a quick and smooth motion (Figure 32-53).	A 90° angle may be appropriate for patients with lots of adipose tissue or when using a shorter needle.
11. Stabilize the needle within the tissue. Check the guidelines of your office in regard to aspiration.	Unnecessary movement of the syringe can cause tissue damage and pain to the patient.

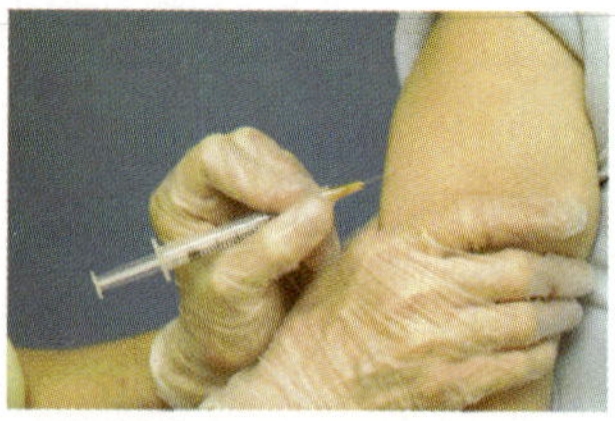

Figure 32-53 ■ The proper angle of insertion for a subcutaneous injection.

continues

PROCEDURE 32-7 continued

PROCEDURAL STEPS	DETAILS AND/OR RATIONALE
12. Inject the medication slowly and steadily.	Injecting the medication too quickly can cause discomfort to the patient and not allow the medication to be absorbed properly.
13. Remove the needle quickly at the same angle of insertion.	This helps to prevent trauma to the tissue.
14. Place a gauze sponge over the injection site and gently massage the area, if applicable.	This helps ease the discomfort caused from the injection and accelerates absorption of the medication (unless massaging is contraindicated).
15. Properly engage the needle's safety device and dispose of the needle and syringe into the sharps container. Apply a bandage to the site to prevent the patient's clothes from becoming contaminated with blood.	Engaging the safety device helps to reduce the possibility of a needlestick.
16. Remove gloves and wash your hands.	This prevents contamination and the spread of infection.
17. Give proper patient educational materials and waiting instructions.	
18. Perform post-check of the patient and site 20 to 30 minutes following the procedure.	Allergic reactions usually occur within 20 to 30 minutes of the procedure.
19. Chart the procedure correctly on the progress note and appropriate logs.	Documentation illustrates that the procedure was performed.

DOCUMENTATION EXAMPLE:

05-22-XX 3:15 p.m.	Varivax #1, 0.5 mL, sub-q, right arm per Dr. Sullivan. Manf.–Kline Beecham, Lot number–K449, exp. date – 12/XX. Pt. tolerated well, instructions given to pt. for site care and VIS (12/XXXX) provided—consent form signed and filed in chart. Post injection follow-up, negative complications. Sherri Jones, CMA (AAMA)--

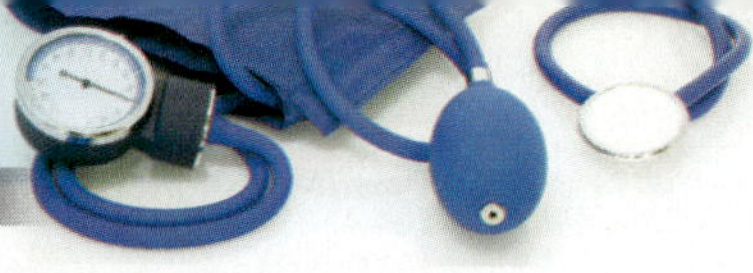

PROCEDURE 32-8

Administer an Intramuscular Injection

Objective:

To administer an injection within the muscular tissue.

Equipment/Supplies:

- Appropriate sized needle and syringe unit with correct medication
- Antiseptic wipe
- Gauze 2 × 2 sponges
- Medication tray
- Sharps container
- Disposable gloves
- Adhesive bandage
- Patient's chart/EHR

PROCEDURAL STEPS	DETAILS AND/OR RATIONALE
1. Wash your hands.	This prevents the spread of infection and contamination during the procedure.
2. Assemble the equipment. Follow the Seven Rights of Drug Administration.	Following the seven rights will help prevent errors from occurring.
3. Identify the patient using two identifiers, identify yourself, and ***explain the rationale for performance of the procedure, showing awareness of the patient's concerns related to the procedure being performed.***	This prevents the wrong patient from receiving the medication.
4. Ask the patient about drug allergies, latex allergies, or adhesive allergies.	Giving the patient a drug or using products that the patient is allergic to can cause an anaphylactic reaction.
5. Locate the proper injection site (deltoid, ventrogluteal, or vastus lateralis).	The right site must be selected in order for the drug to be absorbed properly.
6. Cleanse the site with antiseptic and allow to air dry completely. (Cleanse in a circular motion working outward to an area of 2 to 3 inches.)	This prevents the possible contamination of the injection site and ensures the removal of microorganisms from the injection site area. Wet alcohol may cause the site to burn when you inject the medication.
7. Prepare the equipment and apply gloves.	This prevents contamination from bloodborne pathogens during the procedure.
8. Remove the needle cap. Pull the cap straight off, never twist.	Twisting may loosen the needle attached to the syringe.
9. Stretch the tissue to hold the skin taut with your nondominant hand.	
10. Using your dominant hand, insert the needle at a 90° angle using a quick and smooth motion (Figure 32-54).	This helps with the needle insertion.
11. Stabilize the needle within the tissue.	Unnecessary movement of the hand holding the syringe can cause tissue damage and pain to the patient.

Figure 32-54 ■ The proper angle of insertion for an intramuscular injection.

continues

PROCEDURE 32-8 continued

PROCEDURAL STEPS	DETAILS AND/OR RATIONALE
12. Aspirate if instructed to do so to ensure the needle is not in a blood vessel. If blood enters the syringe, do not inject, but remove the needle immediately. If there is no bloody return into the needle, proceed with the injection process.	Depositing the medication into the bloodstream could cause great harm to the patient. (Aspiration while giving IM medications is under review; however, some nursing boards are eliminating aspiration during immunization procedures. Check the policy of your office.)
13. Inject the medication slowly and steadily.	Injecting the medication too quickly can cause discomfort to the patient and not allow the medication to be absorbed appropriately.
14. Remove the needle quickly at the same angle of insertion.	This helps to prevent trauma to the tissue.
15. Place a gauze sponge over the injection site and gently massage the area, if applicable.	Massaging the area helps to disburse the medication, unless contraindicated.
16. Engage the safety device on the needle, and dispose of the needle-syringe unit in the sharps container.	This protects you from an accidental needlestick from a contaminated needle.
17. Place an adhesive bandage over the site and remove gloves and wash your hands.	This prevents contamination and the spread of infection.
18. Give related patient educational materials and proper waiting instructions.	
19. Perform post-check of the patient and site 20 to 30 minutes following the procedure.	Allergic reactions usually occur within 20 to 30 minutes of the procedure.
20. Chart the procedure correctly on the progress note and appropriate logs.	Documentation illustrates that the procedure was performed.

DOCUMENTATION EXAMPLE:

05-22-XX 3:15 p.m.	Hepivax 0.5 mL, IM, R. Deltoid per Dr. Jones. Manf.—Kline Beecham, Lot number–K449, exp. date—12/XX. Pt. tolerated well, instructions given to pt. for site care and VIS (02/XXXX) provided and consent form signed and filed. No problems during post check. Sherri Jones, CMA (AAMA)--

CHAPTER SUMMARY

- The term *parenteral* means outside of the intestines and the most common route to deliver parenteral medications is through the injection route.
- Other parenteral routes include intravenous, transdermal, transmucosal, topical, and inhalation.
- Common parenteral routes by injection include intradermal, subcutaneous, intramuscular, and intra-articular; however, the medical assistant will routinely only be performing the first three routes of injections.

- The speed at which injectables and IV medications are delivered into the body is as follows: intravenous (instantly), intramuscular (5 to 15 minutes), and subcutaneous (several minutes).
- The part of a syringe include the barrel, plunger, flange, and tip.
- A needle's gauge refers to the diameter of the needle and the gauge that you will use is determined by the viscosity of medication you are administering.
- The length of the needle is determined by the specific route of administration and the size of the patient.
- The parts of a needle include the point, lumen, bevel, shaft, hub, and safety device.
- Injectable medications may be stored in ampules, vials, cartridge units, or prefilled syringes.
- 1 mL syringes are measured in tenths/hundredths, 3 mL syringes are measured in 1/2 or whole mL/tenths, and 5 mL are measured in full mL/2/10 mL.
- Vials of medications come in unit doses or multiple doses.
- An ampule is made of sterile glass and contains one single dose of medication. Filtered needles should be used with ampules.
- When combining two medications, you must determine the primary drug and the secondary drug.
- Medication cartridges hold a single dose of medication. The cartridge fits into an injector device.
- Prefilled syringes are single doses of medications stocked with specific medications.
- Aspiration is pulling back on the plunger to make certain you are not in a blood vessel.
- Intradermal injections are given in the outer layer of the skin, using a 10°–15° angle. The goal is to obtain a wheal. Accepted needle sizes for intradermal injections are 26–27 G, ⅜″–⅝″. The common solutions given this route include allergy testing extract and tuberculosis (TB) skin testing solution.
- Subcutaneous injections are administered under the dermis or in the fatty connective tissue. These are typically given at a 45° angle. The average size needle for subcutaneous injection is 23–25 G, ½″–⅝″. The common medications for this route include allergy injections, MMR, polio (IPV), and varicella vaccines.
- Intramuscular means within a muscle. These injections are given at a 90° angle. The average size needles include the following: 20–23 G, 1″–2″. Types of medications given this route include: many vaccines, analgesics, antibiotics, steroids, and hormones.
- Intravenous medications are medication administered through a vein. Medical assistants should check legislation in their state before administering these medications. The majority of states require licensure in order to perform this task.
- Solutions commonly used for IV therapy is 5 percent dextrose, normal saline, dextrose in saline, and Ringer's solution.
- A basic IV administration set includes the following: piercing pin, drip chamber, roller clamp, cannula, and side clamp.
- Complications that may occur during IV therapy includes infiltration, needle or catheter displacement, occlusion, loss of patency of the vein, phlebitis, hematoma, and cellulitis.
- Intra-articular medications are administered in a joint.

CERTIFICATION REVIEW QUESTIONS

1. Tuberculin syringes come in what syringe size?
   a. 1 mL syringes
   b. 3 mL syringes
   c. 5 mL syringes
   d. 10 mL syringes
2. The gauge of the needle indicates:
   a. the diameter of the needle.
   b. the length of the needle.
   c. the length of the hub.
   d. the size of the syringe.
3. A subcutaneous injection is usually given at what degree in regards to angle of insertion?
   a. 10°
   b. 15°
   c. 45°
   d. 90°
4. The two vaccines that are contraindicated for pregnant women are:
   a. hepatitis B and tetanus.
   b. Varicella and MMR.
   c. PPD and hepatitis B.
   d. small pox and hepatitis A.

5. The gauge used for an injection is determined by:
   a. the viscosity of the medication.
   b. the site of the injection.
   c. the amount of fat the patient has.
   d. All of the above
6. Which of the following gauges are considered the largest diameter?
   a. 23 G
   b. 22 G
   c. 21 G
   d. 20 G
7. Aspiration is encouraged in which of the following?
   a. During intradermal injections
   b. During most subcutaneous injections
   c. During all intramuscular injections
   d. During all intramuscular injections with the exception of immunizations
8. Other parenteral routes include which of the following?
   a. Buccal
   b. Sublingual
   c. Transdermal
   d. Both a and b
9. When drawing up two medications you inject air into which of the vials first?
   a. Primary medication
   b. Secondary medication
   c. You don't inject air into any vial
   d. None of the above
10. The part of the syringe that prevents the syringe from rolling off the table is the:
   a. barrel.
   b. plunger.
   c. flange.
   d. tip.

STUDY RESOURCES

Resources to Test and Reinforce Your Knowledge:	
Certification Review Questions	Take this end-of-chapter quiz
Workbook	• Complete the activities for Chapter 32 • Perform the procedures for Chapter 32 using the Competency Checklists
Resources to Promote Critical Thinking:	
***Solve the Case* Activities**	• Consider these case studies and discuss your conclusions
Learning Lab	• Module 25: Pharmacology and Medication Administration
MindTap	• Complete Chapter 32 readings and activities

REFERENCES

Antipuesto, Dausy Jane. *Z-Track Method.* Nursing Crib. n.d. Web. July 11, 2015.

"Are Techniques Used for Intramuscular Injection Based on Research Evidence?" *Are Techniques Used for Intramuscular Injection Based on Research Evidence?* N.p., n.d. Web. September 15, 2015, from http://www.nursingtimes.net/nursing-practice/specialisms/prescribing/are-techniques-used-for-intramuscular-injection-based-on-research-evidence/1952004.article

"Aspiration in Injections: Should We Continue or Abandon the Practice? - F1000Research." *Aspiration in Injections: Should We Continue or Abandon the Practice? - F1000Research.* N.p., n.d. Web. September 15, 2015, from http://f1000research.com/articles/3-157/v1

Crawford, Cecelia. "To Aspirate or Not to Aspirate, That Is the Question." N.p., n.d. Web. September 15, 2015, from www.stti.iupui.edu/pp07/vancouver09/41810.Crawford

"How to Give a Subcutaneous Injection - Care Guide." *How to Give A Subcutaneous Injection - Care Guide.* N.p., n.d. Web. September 15, 2015, from http://www.drugs.com/cg/how-to-give-a-subcutaneous-injection.html

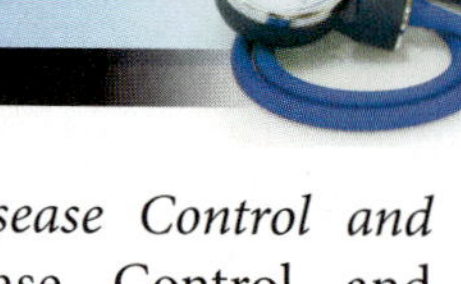

"Injection Safety." *Centers for Disease Control and Prevention*. Centers for Disease Control and Prevention, 01 Apr. 2015. Web. September 15, 2015, from http://www.cdc.gov/injectionsafety/

"Is It Necessary to Aspirate When Giving an Allergy Injection." *Is It Necessary to Aspirate When Giving an Allergy Injection*. N.p., n.d. Web. September 15, 2015, from http://www.aaaai.org/ask-the-expert/aspirate-allergy-injection.aspx

Rheuminfo. *Performing an Injection Using a Pre-Filled Syringe*. n.d. Web. July 11, 2015.

Adkins, Janice et al. *A Grown Preference for Ready-to-Administer Vaccines: New Guidelines, Evidence, and Trends*. Pharmaceutical Commerce. August 27, 2013. Web. July 11, 2015.

33

Responding to Medical Office Emergencies

CHAPTER OUTLINE

Preparing Personnel for Emergencies

The Medical Assistant's Role in Office Emergencies

Assessment and Screening in the Ambulatory Health Care Setting

Identification and Response to Emergencies

Acute Abdominal Emergencies

Anaphylaxis

Breathing Emergencies

Cardiac Arrest

Cerebrovascular Accident (CVA)

Bleeding/Pressure Points

Burns

Diabetic Ketoacidosis and Insulin Shock

Poisoning

Seizures

Shock

Syncope

Vertigo

Thermal Emergencies

Wounds

Musculoskeletal Injuries

Animal Bite

Insect Bites and Stings

Concussion and Other Head and Neck Injuries

Mentally or Emotionally Distressed Patients

ESSENTIAL TERMS

abrasions
acute abdomen
algorithm
anaphylaxis
asthma
automated external defibrillator (AED)
cardiopulmonary resuscitation (CPR)
cerebrovascular accident (CVA)
concussion
crash cart
defibrillation
diabetic coma
diabetic ketoacidosis
diaphoresis
embolus
frostbite
heat cramp
heat exhaustion
heat stroke
hemorrhaging
hypothermia
incision
insulin shock
ischemia
laceration
myocardial infarction (MI)
orthostatic hypotension
puncture
seizure
shock
syncope
thrombus
transient ischemic attack (TIA)
traumatic brain injury
triage
ventricular fibrillation

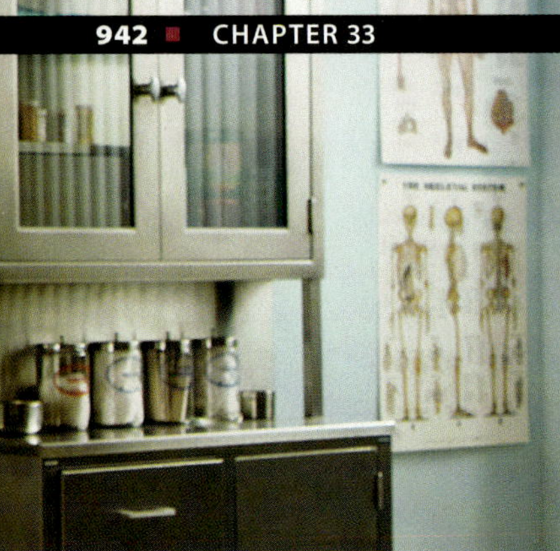

DEVELOPMENTAL OBJECTIVES

After completing this chapter, you should be able to:

1. Correctly spell and define the essential terms.
2. Discuss the role of the medical assistant in screening emergencies in the ambulatory health care setting.
3. Identify and respond to emergencies.
4. Understand the use and purpose of triage and treatment algorithms or flowcharts in an emergency.
5. List diseases and conditions that may be considered life-threatening and describe the proper steps that should be taken with each one.
6. List patient conditions that are not considered life-threatening and describe what factors should be considered in determining the order in which these patients are seen.
7. Define cardiopulmonary resuscitation and explain its purpose.
8. Describe the purpose of an automated external defibrillator (AED) and the medical assistant's role in using an AED.
9. List common medications and supplies found on a crash cart and explain each of their uses.
10. Demonstrate the different bandaging techniques and explain when to use each method.
11. Perform basic first aid procedures.

INTRODUCTION

Most people think of emergency medicine as something that only occurs at the scene of an accident or in a hospital trauma center; however, ambulatory health care centers also get their fair share of smaller-scale emergencies. This is especially true with the rapid expansion of urgent care centers. Medical assistants need to know not only how to respond at the scene of an emergency, but also how to properly assist patients upon their arrival at the office. The contents of this chapter will provide the medical assistant with the knowledge that is necessary to respond to emergencies in the ambulatory health care setting.

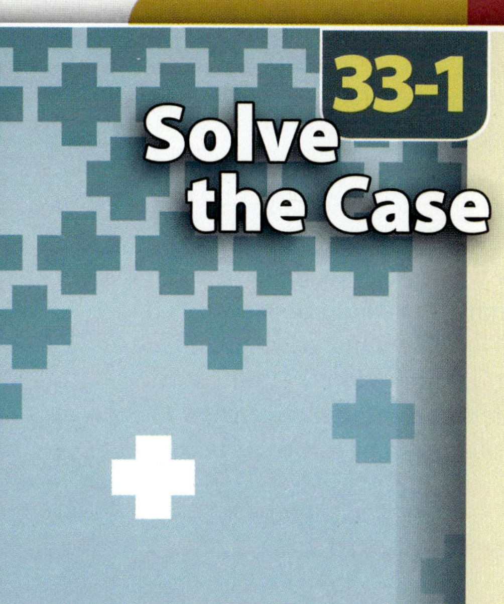

The ambulatory care center is really busy this afternoon. In addition to the regularly scheduled patients, five patients just entered the reception room within five minutes of each other. All the regular examination rooms are full. One patient burned her arm on a hot pot and appears to be in quite a bit of discomfort. One patient is complaining of intense abdominal pain that came on very quickly, another patient cut his foot on a piece of broken glass and is bleeding through the towel, one patient is in the middle of an asthma attack, and the last patient fainted while at school today but is conscious now and his mother wants to have him evaluated. Given your present level of knowledge:

1. **How would you determine in what order to see the patients?**
2. **What types of resources or special equipment may be necessary based on each patient's complaints?**
3. **One of the patients who had a minor injury is upset because you took back a more seriously ill patient first, even though that patient had arrived after her. How will you respond?**

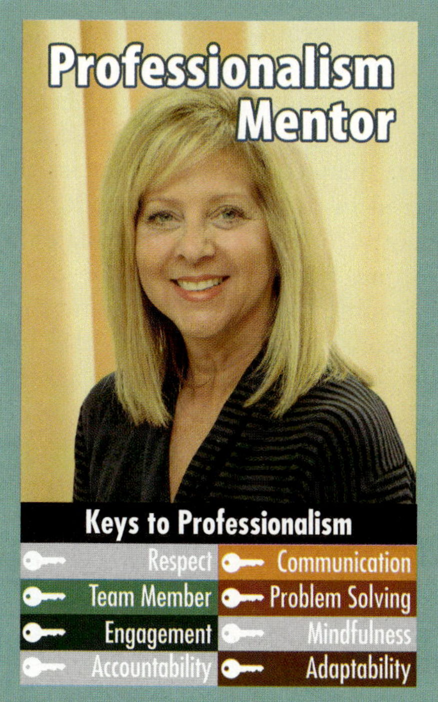

When you work in health care, sooner or later you will encounter an emergency. It is during these times that the true nature of your professionalism and competency will be tested. Situations can go from bad to worse very quickly. Consider the following scenario involving a patient being seen with a complaint of shortness of breath: The patient had a history of asthma and the harder it was for her to breath, the more panicked she became. The medical assistant who just happened to be in the reception room to call back another patient, saw the woman struggling to breathe. Using *critical thinking* skills to recognize the potential for a serious event, the medical assistant told the front desk to get the provider immediately, while the medical assistant stayed with the patient to keep her calm and to prevent a possible fall should the patient pass out. This *attention to detail* and *teamwork* were the keys to success in this instance. The patient received a breathing treatment to help open her airways and then was taken to the emergency room (ER) by squad for further evaluation. After reading this chapter, consider whether you would have done anything different than the medical assistant in this scenario? Should the receptionist have noticed there was a problem? ■

PREPARING PERSONNEL FOR EMERGENCIES

All medical facilities should provide employees with emergency and disaster training. To learn more about disaster training and emergency preparedness refer to the Emergency Preparedness section of *MindTap for Clinical Medical Assisting*. Occasionally, patients who aren't aware they are in the middle of a life-threatening emergency will visit an urgent care center or doctor's office. The most common life-threatening emergencies that occur in the doctor's office are patients with chest pain and breathing emergencies such as patients experiencing an asthma attack. When assessing the order in which patients are seen, life-threatening emergencies always take priority over patients with non-life-threatening disorders. The majority of patients seen in a doctor's office or urgent care facility are seen for non-life-threatening disorders; however, careful screening is still very important for determining levels of priority. The medical assistant will need to consider the following factors when working with patients with non-life-threatening disorders:

1. The possible complications or damages that may incur from a delay in treatment
2. The patient's discomfort level (both physical and emotional)
3. The environment and atmosphere of the reception area

The Medical Assistant's Role in Office Emergencies

The role of the medical assistant in medical office emergencies will vary from one office to another and in some instances, from one state to another. In some states, medical assistants are permitted to administer oxygen and start IVs under the provider's direction, while other states require licensure. All medical assisting students should have formal first aid and cardiopulmonary resuscitation (CPR) training prior to going into their externship program, including the ability to use the automated external defibrillator (AED). CPR stands for **cardiopulmonary resuscitation** and means to restore heart and lung function. An AED is a defibrillator that is completely automated and easy to use. The AED is designed to shock the heart into a normal rhythm during periods of ventricular fibrillation and is discussed in more detail later in this chapter. *Important note:* For more information on CPR, log onto the AHA website (www.heart.org) or the Red Cross website (www.redcross.org) and search "CPR" and "AED."

Assessment and Screening in the Ambulatory Health Care Setting

Triage is a French term coined in 1794 by Baron Dominique Jean Larrey, a French military surgeon. It was designed to assist those delivering emergency care on the battlefield and refers to a process in which things are ranked in terms of importance or priority. Hospital ER departments have triage stations where specially trained nurses and medics take the patient's complaint and vital signs and determine the severity of the patient's symptoms. Once the patient has been assessed, the patient is either immediately placed in a room or sent back to the waiting area.

Medical offices rarely see patients with life-threatening disorders, so the triaging or screening process is not nearly as intense as the hospital ER. However, there may still be situations when prioritizing is necessary. Patient order is determined by the seriousness of the patient's symptoms. Thus, patients with potentially life-threatening conditions should be examined prior to patients with non-life-threatening emergencies. This is where the use of an algorithm or flowchart becomes important.

Triage and Treatment Algorithms or Flowcharts

To better assess and screen for emergency management and basic first aid, use of an algorithm or flowchart helps to identify the appropriate steps to follow. An **algorithm** outlines a detailed sequence of actions to perform in order to accomplish a task. Figure 33-1 illustrates an emergency algorithm for providers to use in the treatment of syncope. Many medical offices, however, will use protocol charts or tables to determine steps that should be taken during an emergency. Table 33-1 represents an example of a protocol chart that separates emergencies that may be encountered in the ambulatory health care setting into categories of first tier (life-threatening emergencies), second tier (emergencies or conditions that could become life-threatening), and third tier (emergencies considered non-life-threatening). Of course, steps will vary from one office to another so always check the protocol of the office in which you work.

IDENTIFICATION AND RESPONSE TO EMERGENCIES

The following section provides information about different types of emergencies that occur in the medical office. Even though medical assistants do not diagnose patients, they must have the ability to identify conditions that are considered emergencies and be able to respond appropriately until the provider is available.

Acute Abdominal Emergencies

Acute abdomen is a term that refers to the *sudden or abrupt onset of intense abdominal pain* and related symptoms, which may include fever, vomiting, diarrhea, dyspnea (difficult breathing), and shock. Sudden abdominal

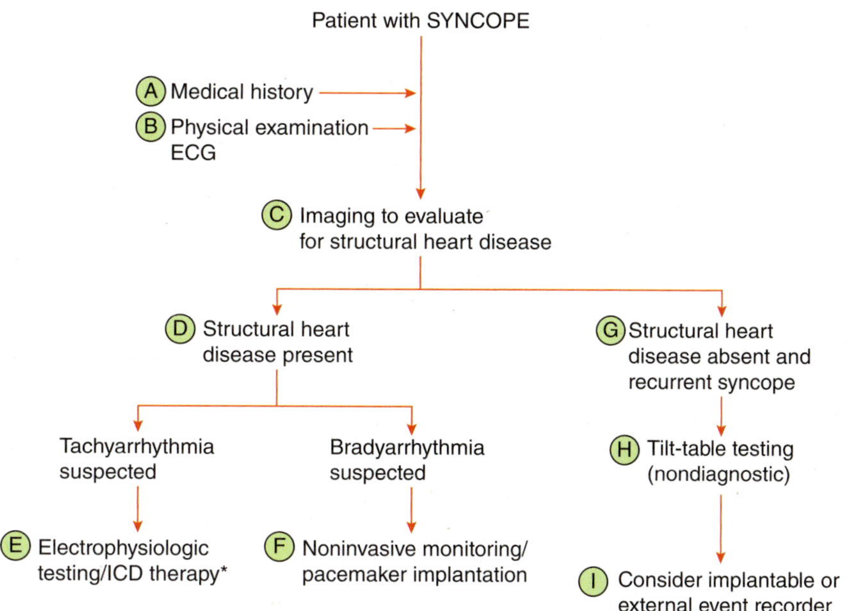

Figure 33-1 ■ Illustration of emergency algorithm for providers on how to treat patients with syncope.

Table 33-1 Medical Office Emergencies Triage and Treatment Chart

First Tier: Life-Threatening Emergencies Actions to Take				
Cardiac Emergencies	**Breathing Emergencies**	**Severe Bleeding Emergencies/Shock**	**Anaphylaxis**	**CVA**
Notify provider stat Put patient on heart monitor or run an ECG Take vital signs including oxygen saturation Have administrative staff call 911, if applicable Be prepared to provide CPR or assist in code if applicable Have nitroglycerin, aspirin, oxygen, and IV equipment ready for the provider's order	Notify provider stat Get vital signs including oxygen saturation level Provider may order oxygen to be delivered if saturation falls below 95% (the medical assistant may be asked to administer if legal in the state she works) Have nebulizer, IV equipment, and breathing medications available in the event the provider gives an order Be prepared to provide CPR or assist in code if applicable	Notify provider stat Immediately apply direct pressure to wound using several gauze pads and elevate limb if applicable If bleeding continues, apply pressure to the proximal limb or artery, have tourniquet accessible for the provider Monitor patient for shock (if applicable, lower head or elevate feet) Have administrative staff call 911 if applicable	Notify provider stat Immediately take vital signs including oxygen saturation Have epinephrine, diphenhydramine, cimetidine, steroids, and oxygen ready, and be prepared to administer once order is received Have administrative staff call 911 if applicable If breathing or heart stops, provide CPR	Notify provider stat Get vital signs and perform CVA assessment questions Have administrative staff call 911 if applicable If breathing or heart stops, provide CPR

continues

Table 33-1 Medical Office Emergencies Triage and Treatment Chart *(continued)*

Second-Tier: Emergencies that Could Become Life-Threatening if Left Untreated Actions to Take				
Diabetic Emergencies	**Convulsions/Seizures/ Syncope**	**Thermal Emergencies**	**Concussions**	**Abdominal Emergencies**
Notify provider stat ***Diabetic*** Immediately take patient's blood sugar and vital signs ***Insulin shock—hypoglycemia*** If glucose is below 80 mg/dL, provide a diabetic snack such as peanut butter and orange juice If glucose is below 50 mg/dL, be prepared to administer glucagon ***Diabetic ketoacidosis*** If glucose is above 200 mg/dL and patient has acetone smell, have insulin ready If glucose is above 400 mg/dL and patient is unresponsive, be prepared to administer insulin and call 911	Notify provider stat Break patient's fall if possible and remove anything that could cause more harm to the patient If having a seizure, try to place patient on side and clear the area to avoid any further injury to the patient. Have lorazepam IM available in case the seizure persists If syncope episode, lower head or elevate feet and obtain vital signs every 5 minutes. Have water and a snack available for the patient.	Notify provider stat If a thermal injury is suspected, obtain rectal temperature If heat emergency (temperature above 104°F or 40°C), emersion bath in ice water is best, but evaporative cooling with cold saline bags, wet towels, and fans may be helpful if that is all that is available. Goal temperature is 98.6°F or 37°C, the faster this is obtained, the less damage to internal organs such as the brain. If cold emergency (temperatures at or below 95°F or 35°C), remove any damp clothing, place in a dry and warm area, and provide full body insulation with warm sleeping bag. If the patient's temperature falls below 91°F or 32.8°C, call 911 and be prepared to conduct CPR.	Notify provider stat If a patient has sustained a blow to the head, look for clues of a concussion (loss of consciousness, slow to recover, balance issues, or disorientation) Assess for red flags such as neck pain, worsening confusion, or headache, repeated vomiting, seizures, weakness, or tingling suggesting nerve injury, or double vision. Patients with these symptoms should be prepared for transport, and 911 should be called.	Notify provider stat Patients complaining of severe abdominal pain with an associated fever, anorexia, or constipation, should be considered emergencies until proven otherwise Providers will need vital signs The provider should decide if a patient needs to be transported
Third-Tier Emergencies (Non-Life-Threatening) Actions to Take				
Possible Fractures, Strains, or Dislocations	**Animal Bites**	**Burns**	**Vertigo**	**Wounds**
Notify provider stat Immobilize joint and elevate. If swelling is present, apply ice to area. Identify any skin wounds, address bleeding issues Be ready for a possible X-ray, splinting or casting	Notify provider stat Find out what animal bit patient Control bleeding with direct pressure with gauze If bleeding is controlled, wash bite area with antiseptic soap and water. Remove any debris. Have sterile gloves, a basin, large volume of water, a splash guard and 50 mL syringe, sterile gauze, scissors, and hemostats (thumb or tissue) available for the provider	Notify provider stat Obtain vital signs Identify what caused the burn (electricity, heat, chemical, freeze) If there are signs of inhalation injury (burns of the face and mouth) or third degree/full thickness burns, provider may want to have patient transported to ER If surface area is limited to one portion of the body, prepare sterile gloves, sterile saline, and topical antibiotics for care of the wounds	Notify provider stat Obtain vital signs Place the patient in a position of least symptoms If patient wants to lie down, make certain that one side of exam table is pushed against wall. The medical assistant will need to stay with patient guarding the open side to prevent a fall.	Notify provider stat Control active bleeding with gloved hand, gauze, and direct pressure Obtain vital signs Have sterile gloves, a basin, 500 mL water, a splash guard and 50 mL syringe, sterile gauze, and suture kit ready for the provider

[Patients that have breathing emergencies, cardiac symptoms, or ambulatory problems should be wheeled back to the appropriate room (Cardiac bay, procedure room or exam room) in a wheelchair. If the patient collapses in the reception room, the patient should not be moved. The doctor should be notified immediately and the emergency medical services (EMS) should be summoned. No medications should be administered unless ordered by provider.]

pain should be treated as a life-threatening emergency until a diagnosis can be made. Chronic abdominal pain is usually not classified as a life-threatening emergency. Organs that may be involved in acute abdomen emergencies include the appendix, gall bladder, intestines, and spleen. Related conditions include appendicitis, the rupture of any of the above organs, and hemorrhage.

Anaphylaxis

Anaphylaxis is a severe allergic reaction to an allergen usually in the form of a food, medication, chemical, or insect sting or bite. It is a systemic reaction (meaning that it affects the entire body) and typically occurs within minutes to two hours following contact with the allergen, but may be delayed as much as four hours. Refer to Table 33-2 for a more detailed listing of the timeline for the onset of symptoms related to the source of the allergen.

After an initial exposure to the allergen, the person's immune system may become sensitized to the offending agent. During subsequent exposures, a severe allergic reaction may occur, leading to the release of histamine throughout the body's tissues. Histamine affects various systems of the body in different ways. The following is a list of the effects of histamine on different body systems during an anaphylactic crisis.

The effects of histamines and symptoms of anaphylaxis can vary by body system:

- *Respiratory system.* Histamine may cause the bronchial tubes to constrict, resulting in bronchospasms.
- *GI tract.* Histamine can cause cramping, bowel swelling, vomiting, and diarrhea.
- *Circulatory system.* Histamine may cause vasodilation, which in turn promotes hypotension, or a dip in blood pressure, and a leaking of fluid from the blood vessels into the body's tissues. The leaking of the blood vessels causes blood volume to diminish, resulting in shock.
- *Integumentary system.* Histamine can cause hives to occur throughout the body but may be more prevalent on the lips, tongue, and throat, blocking critical air passages.

The symptoms of anaphylaxis include a rapid or weak pulse, confusion, slurred speech, reddish skin, rash, or hives on the body with severe itching, swollen throat, hoarseness, swelling in other parts of the body, syncope, breathing problems, cyanosis, abdominal cramping, diarrhea, vomiting, heart palpitations, and chest tightness. Eventually, if left untreated, the anaphylactic patient will go into cardiac arrest and die.

Table 33-2 Timelines for Symptoms of Anaphylaxis Based on the Source

Source	Timeline for Anaphylaxis to Kick in	Interesting Facts
Food	Minutes to two hours.	Peanuts, tree nuts (walnuts, cashews, etc.), shellfish, fish, milk, and eggs are examples of foods that are commonly seen as causes of anaphylactic reactions. It may only take a trace amount of the food product to stimulate a reaction. Individuals who are allergic to foods and have asthma are believed to be at a higher risk for developing an anaphylactic reaction.
Medications	Typically occur within one hour, but may be several hours later in rare cases.	According to literature from the American Academy of Allergy, Asthma and Immunology, a patient is more likely to develop an allergy when taking a medication frequently. Taking a medication by rubbing it on the skin or by injection is also more likely to lead to an allergy than taking the medication by mouth. Examples of drugs that may be more likely to provoke a reaction include antibiotics such as penicillin and tetracycline and certain pain relievers such as morphine and codeine. Patients receiving allergy injections are always in danger of anaphylaxis.
Insect stings or bites	Usually occurs within minutes, but may also be delayed.	Honeybees, bumblebees, yellow jackets, hornets, wasps, fire ants, and harvester ants are the most common causes of insect stings and allergic reactions in the United States.
Latex	Anaphylaxis may be immediate, but delayed sensitivity reaction may occur 12 to 36 hours later, usually in the form of redness and blistering.	Those who wear latex frequently have an increased risk of becoming sensitized to latex. Patients with spina bifida and patients who have had multiple urinary surgeries seem to be at a higher risk than others of developing a latex allergy.

Breathing Emergencies

Breathing emergencies often can become life-threatening and medical assistants need to know their role during breathing emergencies. Breathing emergencies in the office often include asthma attacks, hyperventilation, and choking emergencies. Refer to Table 33-1 to learn how to respond to patients with breathing emergencies.

Asthmatic Attack

Asthma is a chronic lung disease that causes the bronchial tubes to constrict and blocks the flow of air to and from the lungs. It quite often is the result of allergens, but may be exacerbated by physical activity and stress. Other conditions that may provoke breathing emergencies include foreign bodies in the respiratory tract, emphysema, sudden infant death syndrome (SIDS), and chronic obstructive pulmonary disease (COPD). Breathing emergencies will eventually lead to cardiac failure; therefore, prompt treatment is essential. The symptoms may include blueness of the lips and nail beds, a wheezing sound coming from the lungs, and an inability to breathe.

Hyperventilation

Hyperventilation is the rapid or deep breathing that often occurs with panic or anxiety. In the normal breathing process, you breathe in oxygen and exhale carbon dioxide. Excessive breathing creates low levels of carbon dioxide in the blood and causes many of the symptoms of hyperventilation. In addition to fast breathing, common symptoms of hyperventilation include belching, bloating, and chest pain from swallowing air; confusion; dizziness; light-headedness; numbness and tingling in extremities and mouth; shortness of breath from the abnormal blood gas levels and pH; and muscle spasms, sleep disturbances, and palpitations from the electrolyte shifts.

The provider will perform a physical exam and ask the patient detailed questions about his symptoms. In addition, further tests may be ordered such as a blood test to determine the oxygen and carbon dioxide levels in the blood, ECG, chest X-ray, chest CT scan, and/or nuclear scans to measure breathing (ventilation) and circulation (perfusion).

Foreign Body Airway Obstruction and Choking Emergencies

Foreign body airway obstruction (FBOA) causes asphyxia and can be terrifying to the patient. It can result in rapid loss of consciousness and death if the symptoms are not immediately detected and treated. Choking is the physiological response to airways obstruction. Inhaling a foreign body usually occurs while eating. In order to have a successful outcome, immediately ask the victim if she is choking. If the victim is unable to speak, but still conscious, she can at least respond by nodding.

Choking Emergencies

Choking is a common cause of breathing emergencies, especially in children. Patients should be educated on how to prevent choking emergencies.

The universal distress signal for a choking victim is the placement of the victim's hands around the throat. If an adult or child appears to be choking while in the office, the medical assistant should ask if the patient can speak (victims with a truly blocked airway will be unable to speak). Once the medical assistant has established that the patient is choking, the medical assistant should get positioned behind the patient, placing the dominant leg between the patient's legs (this is to support the patient in the event that the patient collapses). Next, the medical assistant should perform the Heimlich maneuver by wrapping his arms around the patient's waist and making a fist, placing it in between the patient's naval and sternum (Figure 33-2). The medical assistant should then give the patient

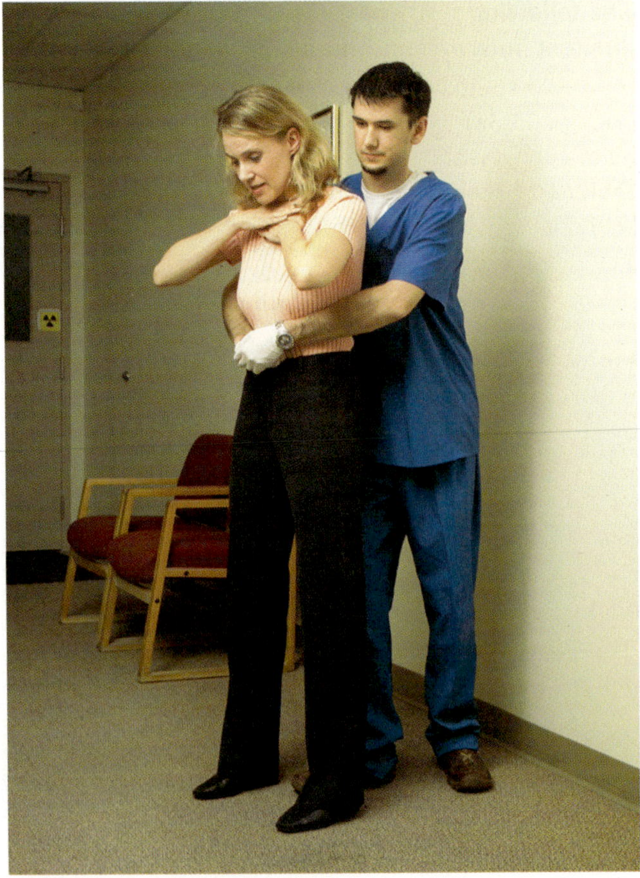

Figure 33-2 ■ The proper placement of the rescuer's hands when giving abdominal thrusts to relieve an obstructed airway.

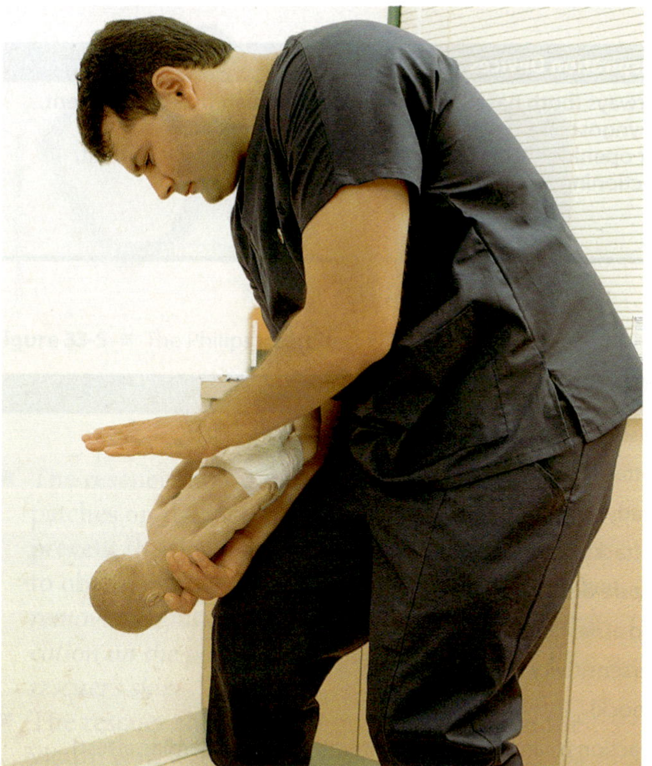

Figure 33-3a ■ When infants have an obstructed airway, the rescuer starts by administering back blows to the infant.

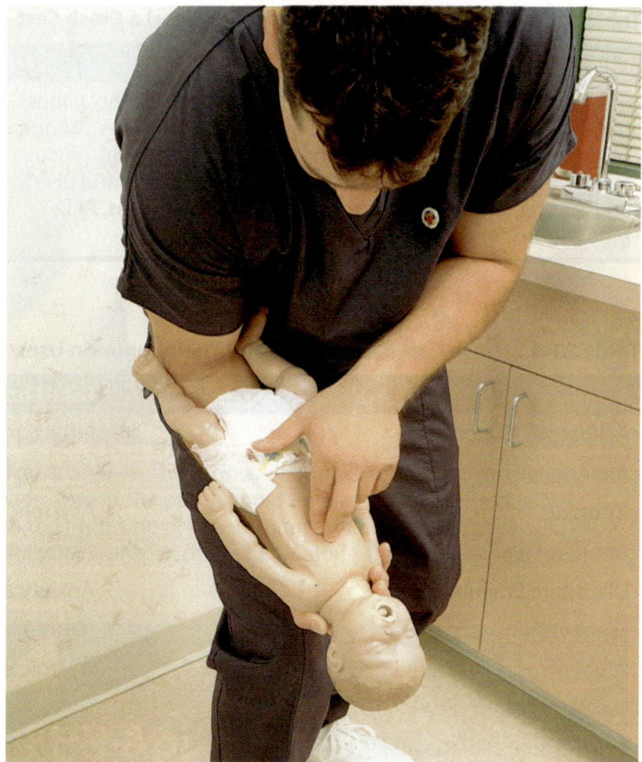

Figure 33-3b ■ The rescuer then gives the infant chest compressions to assist in expelling the object from the infant's airway.

several upward abdominal thrusts until the object is dispelled or the patient becomes unconscious.

Infants should receive a combination of back blows (Figure 33-3a) and chest thrusts (Figure 33-3b) to relieve airway obstructions. For more information on choking and the Heimlich maneuver, log on to the National Library of Medicine website (www.nlm.nih.gov) and search the topic "Heimlich maneuver."

Cardiac Arrest

The medical term for heart attack is **myocardial infarction (MI)**. A myocardial infarction may be the result of atherosclerosis or a buildup of plaque in the coronary arteries.

The symptoms and signs of a heart attack include uncomfortable tightness or squeezing in the chest that may radiate to the arm, neck, or jaw (especially on the left side), shortness of breath, nausea and vomiting, ashened appearance, **diaphoresis** (excessive sweating), and dizziness. Refer to Table 33-1 for instructions on responding to patients with chest pain. Refer to Chapter 14 for more information relating to cardiology.

Crash Cart Supplies

A **crash cart** is a cart that stocks all of the medications and supplies used in an emergency (Figure 33-4).

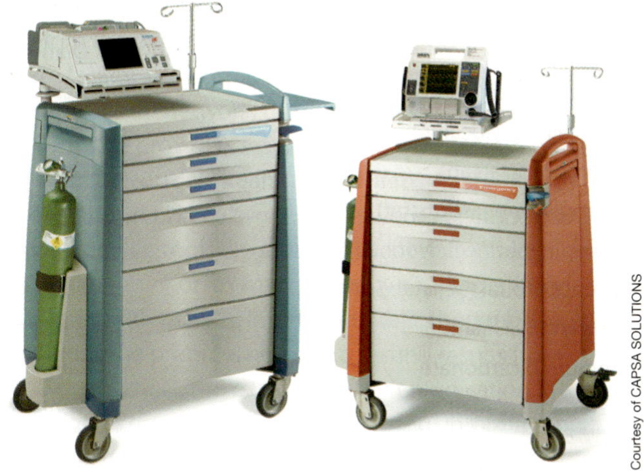

Figure 33-4 ■ A crash cart.

Table 33-3 outlines common items stocked in a crash cart. Table 33-4 describes the various medications stocked in the crash cart and their intended use.

The crash cart should be inspected at regular intervals established by office policy. Check that all items are present and no dated material has passed its expiration date. The best practice is to include a chart or file attached to the cart that provides an inventory of the materials and check-off date to use during inspection and use of the cart in an emergency. Restock the cart after any use.

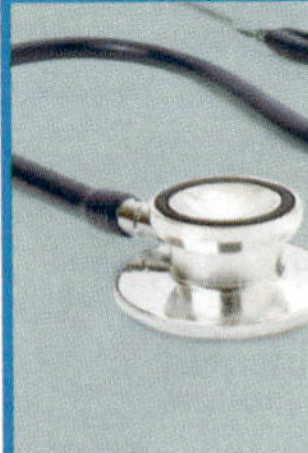

Field Smarts

Today, aspirin is commonly prescribed to help prevent heart attack and stroke. Studies indicate that aspirin, a blood thinner, may also reduce the severity of heart attack if taken immediately when symptoms first occur, and that survival rates are better as a result. If an aspirin is taken during a heart emergency, it should be chewed up and then swallowed with water so that it gets into the bloodstream quicker. Never give aspirin without a directive from a provider.

and symptoms of stroke usually come on rapidly and include facial asymmetry, one-sided paralysis, severe headache, slurred speech, dilated pupils, loss of bladder or bowel control, weakness or a lack of coordination, blurred vision, and dizziness (Figure 33-7). Patients who are at a higher risk for a CVA include African Americans, males, patients with hypertension, heart disease, or diabetes, patients with a history of **transient ischemic attacks (TIA)** or ministrokes, and patients who smoke. The symptoms of TIAs include headache, confusion, tinnitus, and personality changes. TIAs usually only last a few minutes and may be a predecessor to a stroke.

Acting "F.A.S.T." can help stroke patients get the treatments they desperately need. The most effective stroke treatments are only available if the stroke is recognized and diagnosed within three hours of

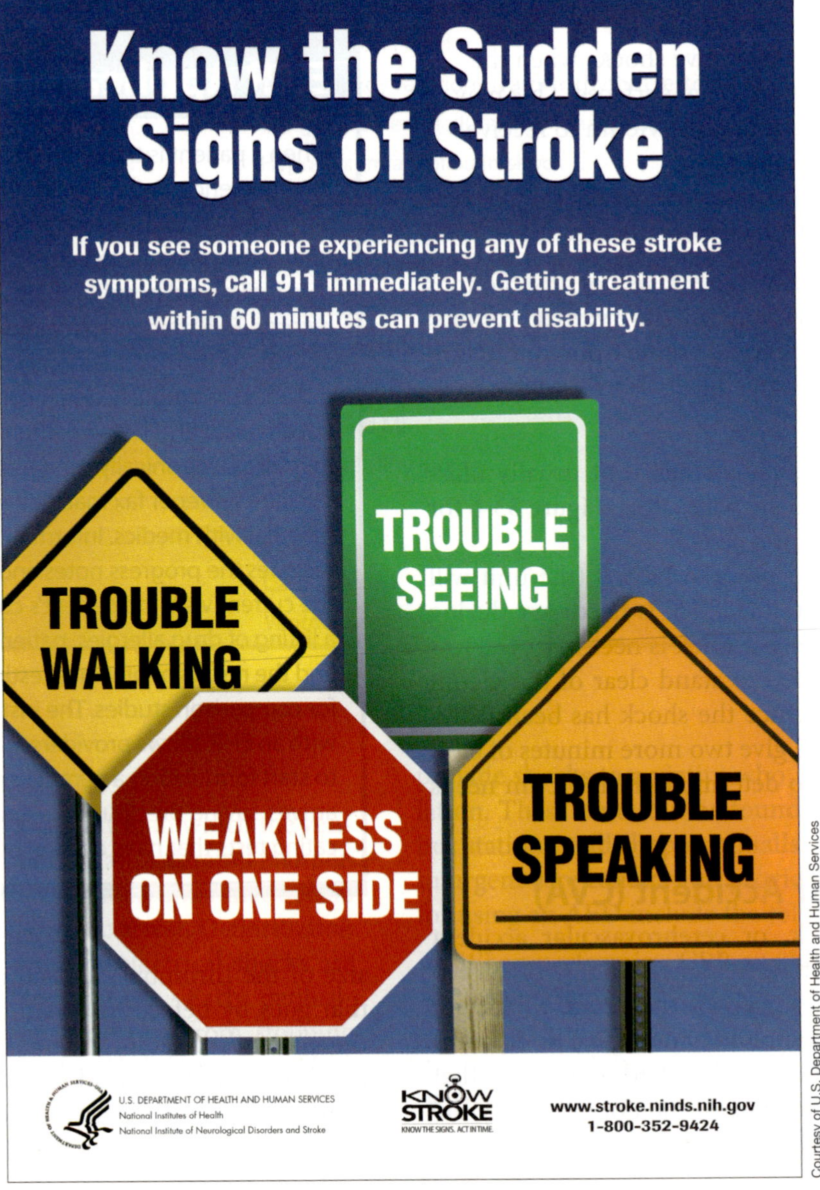

Courtesy of U.S. Department of Health and Human Services

Figure 33-7 ■ Know the sudden signs of stroke.

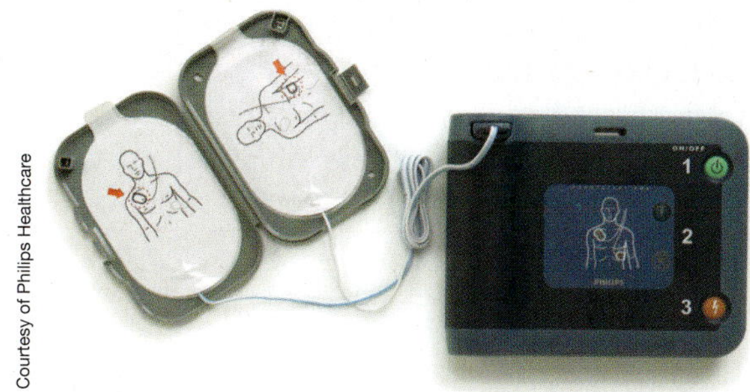

Courtesy of Philips Healthcare

Figure 33-5 ■ The Philips HeartStart FR2+ ECG/EKG.

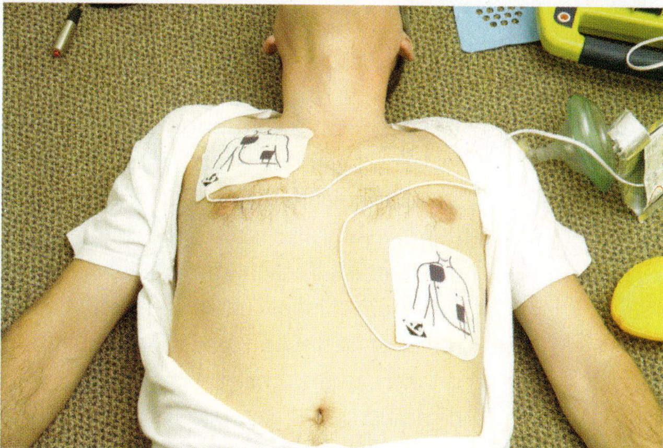

Figure 33-6 ■ The proper electrode placement for the AED pads: One of the pads should be placed under the clavicle on the right side of the sternum and the other pad should be placed at the apex of the heart along the lower left rib cage.

- The rescuer should remove any transdermal patches on the victim's chest. These patches may prevent the flow of electricity or cause the patient to obtain a burn. *Rescuers should wear gloves when removing transdermal patches to prevent the medication on the patch from being absorbed into the rescuer's skin.*
- The rescuer should never give shocks when the victim is in water or on metal surfaces. This may cause both the rescuer and the victim to receive burns.
- If the victim has a pacemaker, the rescuer should place electrode pads about 1 inch from the pacemaker.

The AED will usually have a list of instructions secured to the unit and many will have verbal prompts; however, the major steps are the same from unit to unit and include the following:

1. Turn the power on.
2. Attach the electrode pads (each unit usually illustrates where to place the pads). (See Figure 33-6 for proper placement of the pads.)
3. Clear the victim and press "Analyze" (the unit will be able to determine if a shock is necessary during the analyzing cycle). If a shock is necessary, the rescuer will be instructed to stand clear of the victim and press "Shock." Once the shock has been delivered, the rescuer will give two more minutes of CPR before reanalyzing to determine if the victim needs another shock.

EHR Application

When a patient is transported to the hospital due to an emergency, important information can be sent electronically to the emergency department (ED) before the patient even arrives. When the ambulatory care facility and hospital share an electronic health records (EHR) network, the information will be available to the providers instantly simply by accessing the patient's electronic health record. If the hospital does not share an EHR network then it would be important to either electronically send pertinent data through a secure server or fax machine or by sending printed material with medics. Information that should be sent includes the progress notes and testing results from the current visit, the patient's current medication list, a listing of drug allergies, patient history information, and the results of previous testing that can be used for comparison studies. The instant access provided with an EHR allows providers in the ED an opportunity to start formulating a game plan before the patient arrives, saving precious time and money by not duplicating tests that have already been performed.

Cerebrovascular Accident (CVA)

A stroke, brain attack, or **cerebrovascular accident (CVA)**, are terms that refer to a blockage or bleeding within the blood vessels of the brain. Blockages may be caused by a **thrombus** (blood clot) or **embolus** (air bubble, foreign body, or detached blood clot) that makes its way from one part of the body (usually the heart) to the vessels within the brain. The location and size of the thrombus, as well as the amount of time that goes by before intervention, will greatly impact the patient's disability status and recovery process. Blocked vessels can lead to **ischemia** (a loss of blood supply to the affected area), eventually resulting in an infarct (death of the involved brain tissue). The signs

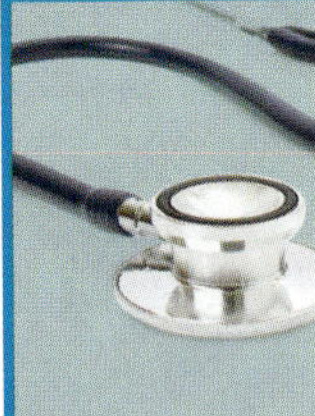

Field Smarts

Today, aspirin is commonly prescribed to help prevent heart attack and stroke. Studies indicate that aspirin, a blood thinner, may also reduce the severity of heart attack if taken immediately when symptoms first occur, and that survival rates are better as a result. If an aspirin is taken during a heart emergency, it should be chewed up and then swallowed with water so that it gets into the bloodstream quicker. Never give aspirin without a directive from a provider.

and symptoms of stroke usually come on rapidly and include facial asymmetry, one-sided paralysis, severe headache, slurred speech, dilated pupils, loss of bladder or bowel control, weakness or a lack of coordination, blurred vision, and dizziness (Figure 33-7). Patients who are at a higher risk for a CVA include African Americans, males, patients with hypertension, heart disease, or diabetes, patients with a history of **transient ischemic attacks (TIA)** or ministrokes, and patients who smoke. The symptoms of TIAs include headache, confusion, tinnitus, and personality changes. TIAs usually only last a few minutes and may be a predecessor to a stroke.

Acting "F.A.S.T." can help stroke patients get the treatments they desperately need. The most effective stroke treatments are only available if the stroke is recognized and diagnosed within three hours of

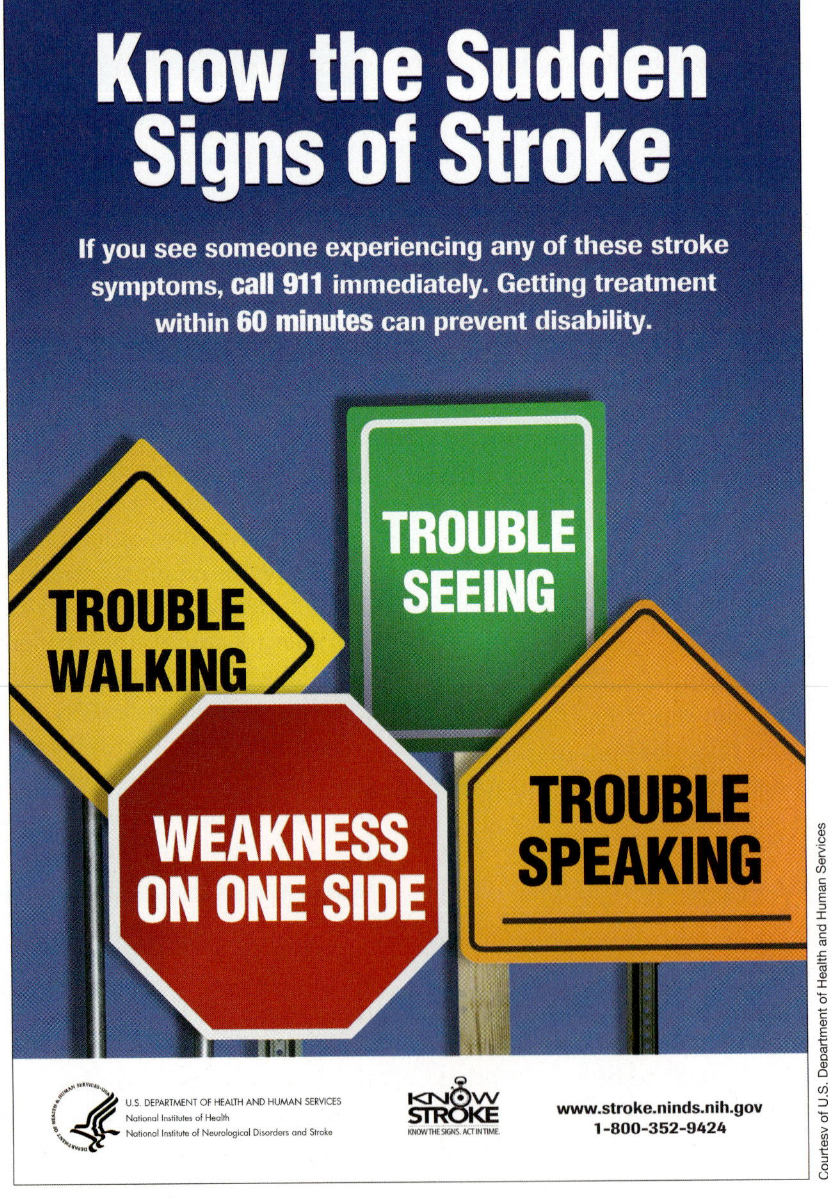

Figure 33-7 ■ Know the sudden signs of stroke.

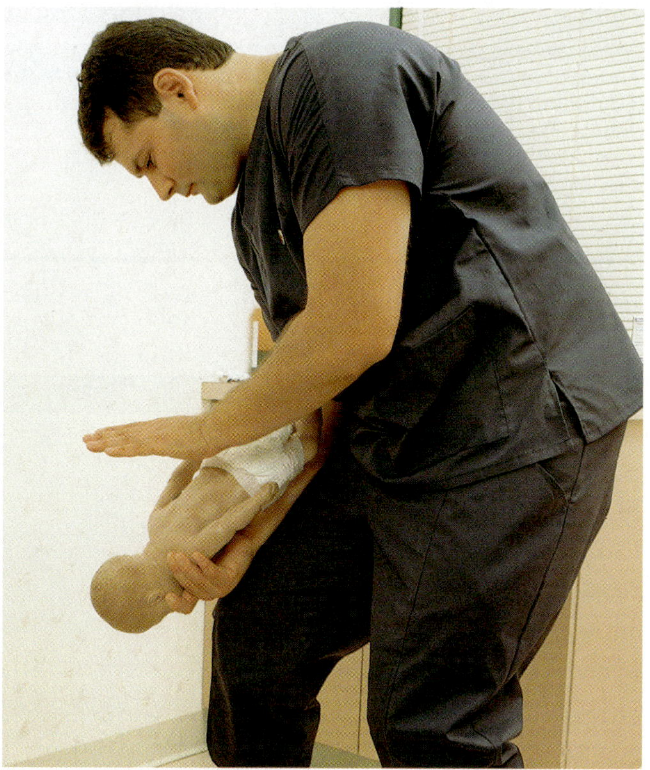

Figure 33-3a ■ When infants have an obstructed airway, the rescuer starts by administering back blows to the infant.

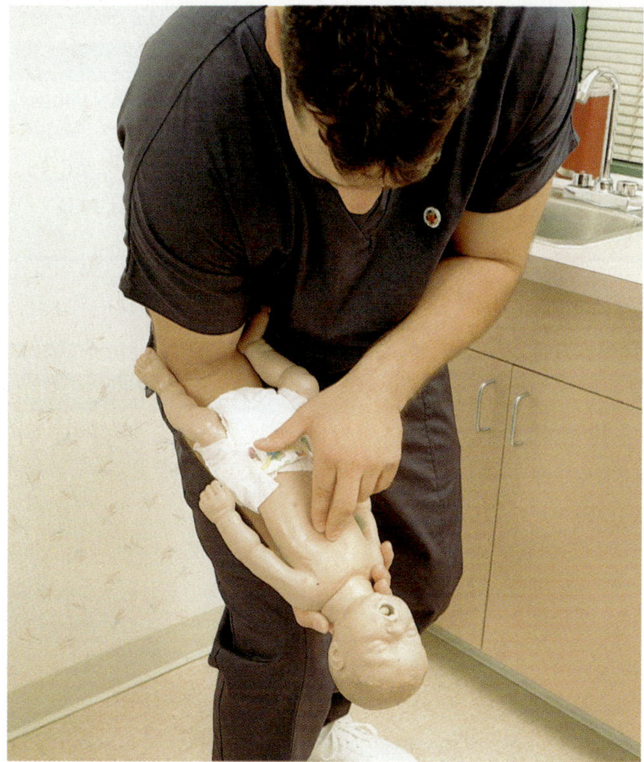

Figure 33-3b ■ The rescuer then gives the infant chest compressions to assist in expelling the object from the infant's airway.

several upward abdominal thrusts until the object is dispelled or the patient becomes unconscious.

Infants should receive a combination of back blows (Figure 33-3a) and chest thrusts (Figure 33-3b) to relieve airway obstructions. For more information on choking and the Heimlich maneuver, log on to the National Library of Medicine website (www.nlm.nih.gov) and search the topic "Heimlich maneuver."

Cardiac Arrest

The medical term for heart attack is **myocardial infarction (MI)**. A myocardial infarction may be the result of atherosclerosis or a buildup of plaque in the coronary arteries.

The symptoms and signs of a heart attack include uncomfortable tightness or squeezing in the chest that may radiate to the arm, neck, or jaw (especially on the left side), shortness of breath, nausea and vomiting, ashened appearance, **diaphoresis** (excessive sweating), and dizziness. Refer to Table 33-1 for instructions on responding to patients with chest pain. Refer to Chapter 14 for more information relating to cardiology.

Crash Cart Supplies

A **crash cart** is a cart that stocks all of the medications and supplies used in an emergency (Figure 33-4).

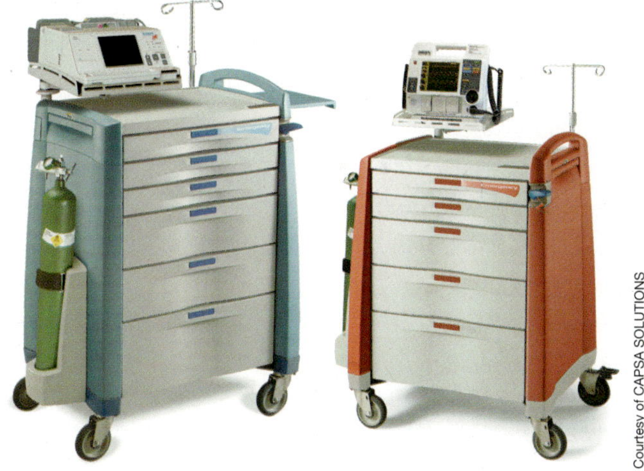

Courtesy of CAPSA SOLUTIONS

Figure 33-4 ■ A crash cart.

Table 33-3 outlines common items stocked in a crash cart. Table 33-4 describes the various medications stocked in the crash cart and their intended use.

The crash cart should be inspected at regular intervals established by office policy. Check that all items are present and no dated material has passed its expiration date. The best practice is to include a chart or file attached to the cart that provides an inventory of the materials and check-off date to use during inspection and use of the cart in an emergency. Restock the cart after any use.

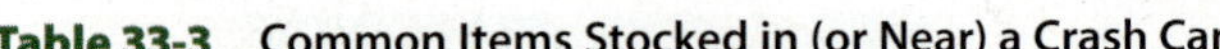

Table 33-3 Common Items Stocked in (or Near) a Crash Cart

Equipment and Supplies	Respiration Devices
Stethoscope, blood pressure cuff, adhesive tape, alcohol wipes, bandage supplies, scissors, iodine swabs, alcohol wipes, tongue blades, tourniquets, gloves (both sterile and nonsterile), glucose supplements, hot and cold packs, IV supplies (tubing and needles, and fluids), penlight, PPE, disposable syringes, needles, AED, medications for emergency use	Airways (both nasal and oral in all sizes), bag-mask equipment, laryngoscope, oxygen tank with flow meter and wrench for opening the tank, oxygen mask/tubing and equipment, suctioning equipment

Table 33-4 Crash Cart Medications and Their Common Uses

Name	Used For
Activated charcoal	Ingestion of poisons
Aminophylline	Acute asthma attacks or bronchial spasms
Atropine	Asystole and bradycardia
Albuterol (Proventil)	Acute asthma attacks or bronchial spasms
Diazepam (Valium)	Anxiety and seizure disorders
Digoxin (Lanoxin)	Heart failure and atrial fibrillation
Diphenhydramine (Benadryl)	Allergic or hypersensitivity reactions
Dopamine (Intropin)	Hypotension (shock)
Epinephrine (Adrenaline)	Acute allergy reactions (cardiac rhythm restoration during cardiac arrest)
Furosemide (Lasix)	Congestive heart failure, pulmonary edema
Glucagon or glucose	Hypoglycemia or insulin shock
Intravenous solutions (Dextrose [5%], normal saline, and Ringer's lactate solution)	Rehydration
Insulin	Diabetic hyperglycemia or hyperkalemia
Isoproterenol (Isuprel)	Acute conditions of bradycardia
Lidocaine (Xylocaine)	Ventricular arrhythmias
Naloxone (Narcan)	Drug overdoses, shock, alcoholic coma
Nitroglycerine (Nitrostat)	Angina and MI
Norepinephrine (Levophed)	Acute hypotension
Phenobarbital (Bellatal; Solfoton)	Seizures
Phenytoin (Dilantin)	Seizures
Sodium bicarbonate	Cardiac arrest
Verapamil (Calan)	Ventricular tachycardia

Providing Defibrillation

Ventricular fibrillation is a condition in which the ventricle of the heart beats in a disorganized, rapid manner. This is one of the most common rhythms that occurs in adult victims of sudden cardiac arrest. **Defibrillation** is a procedure in which drugs or electrical shocks are used to restore normal contractions. Early defibrillation is necessary to keep the heart from stopping altogether. An **automated external defibrillator (AED)** (shown in Figure 33-5) is a type of defibrillator that allows persons with very little training the ability to provide shocks to a victim who is in ventricular fibrillation. These units can be found in factories, airports, bus stations, and shopping malls. AEDs are also found in urgent care centers and providers' offices. Some tips for using an AED include the following:

- When performing CPR on children (ages 1-8 or under 55 pounds), use a pediatric dose attenuator system and pads.
- Only use adult pads on adult victims.
- The rescuer should make certain that the skin is clean and dry before placing the pads on the chest.

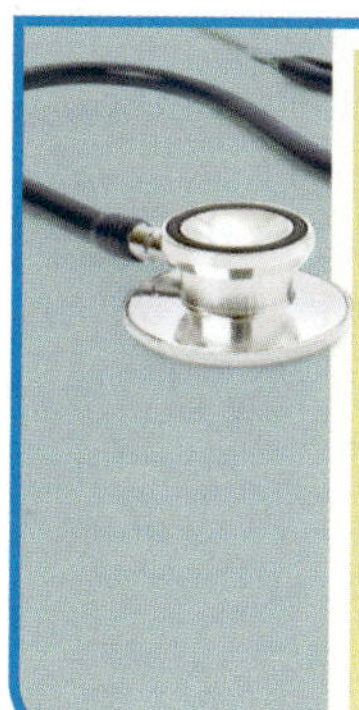

Field Smarts

In order to have the best chances of a full recovery, clot-busting drugs such as tissue plasminogen activator (tPA) should be administered within three hours from the onset of stroke symptoms, making early transport to the hospital critical.

the first symptoms. If they don't arrive at the hospital in time, patients may not be eligible for the most effective treatments for stroke. The American Stroke Association (www.stroke association.org) developed F.A.S.T. to recognize the warning signs and symptoms of a stroke:

F—Face: Ask the person to smile. Does one side of the face droop?
A—Arms: Ask the person to raise both arms. Does one arm drift downward?
S—Speech: Ask the person to repeat a simple phrase. Is their speech slurred or strange?
T—Time: If you observe any of these signs, call 911 immediately.

Bleeding/Pressure Points

Hemorrhaging is a term that means uncontrollable bleeding. It is usually the result of a traumatic injury. Any time a patient severs a major blood vessel, it can lead to hemorrhage and shock. Most patients who are truly hemorrhaging will go directly to the ER; however, occasionally patients will show up at the urgent care center with a bleeding crisis that should be managed in an ER. Refer to Table 33-5 for examples of blood vessels that may be involved during a bleeding emergency. Figure 33-8 depicts a medical assistant applying direct pressure and elevating the patient's arm to control bleeding. Figure 33-9 represents common arteries that can be used to control bleeding. Refer to Procedure 33-1 for a complete procedure on controlling bleeding.

Internal Bleeding

Internal bleeding is very difficult to recognize because it is not something that can be observed with the naked eye. It may be the result of a traumatic injury such as a fractured pelvis or gunshot or knife wound, or may be the result of an aneurysm. Post-surgical patients may experience internal bleeding following a procedure so pay close attention to any symptoms that may point to internal bleeding. The symptoms include rapid and weak pulse, shallow breathing, hypotension, dizziness, cold and

Table 33-5 Blood Vessels That May Be Involved during a Bleeding Emergency

Possible Location	Symptoms	Severity
Artery	Bright red blood that spurts from the open artery every time the heart beats	Very severe, hard to control, and could lead to death if it is a major artery
Vein	Dark red blood due to low oxygen levels. Does not usually spurt out, but will flow steadily.	May cause great blood loss, but is not as severe as an arterial injury because of the lower pressure in the vein
Capillary (located between veins and arteries)	Usually dark red blood that just gently oozes. May be accompanied by clots.	Not considered life-threatening or severe. Easy to control with direct pressure.

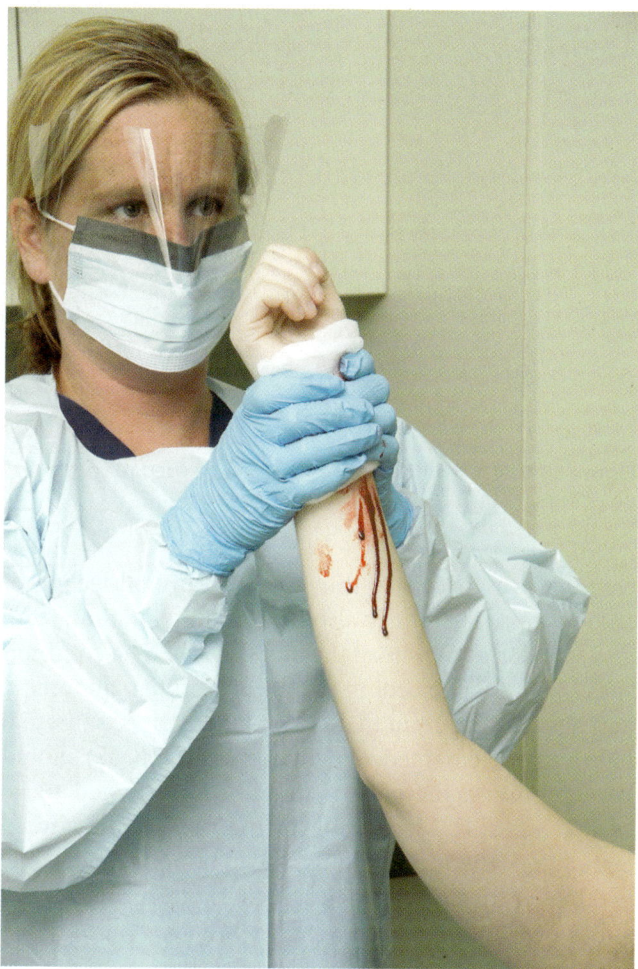

Figure 33-8 ■ The medical assistant is applying direct pressure and elevating the patient's arm to control the patient's bleeding.

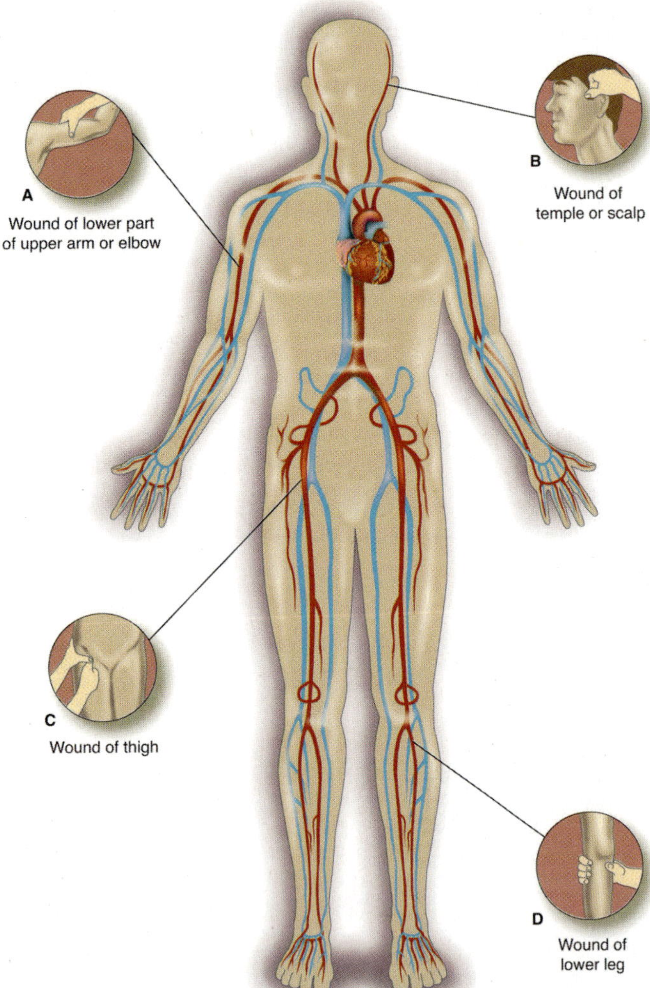

Figure 33-9 ■ Common arteries that can be used to control bleeding.

clammy skin, excessive thirst, and an overall feeling of anxiousness. There may also be skin discoloration, pain, and swelling at the site of the hemorrhage. The common sites for internal bleeding are the extremities, abdomen, and head. In the event that the provider suspects internal bleeding, the emergency medical services (EMS) should be alerted and the patient should be instructed to lie completely still. Monitoring of the patient's breathing, circulation, and mental status should be performed while waiting for the EMS, and the patient should be treated for shock by elevating his feet and keeping him warm.

Bleeding Emergencies (Non-Life-Threatening)

The majority of bleeding emergencies in the office will be on a smaller scale and include lacerations and other open wounds. Even though these patients may not be in danger of hemorrhaging to death, a smaller bleeding emergency can be quite distressful to the patient, the patient's family, and other families sitting in the reception area. The medical assistant should also consider the sanitary conditions of the reception area. If the patient is dripping blood on the floor or on the furniture in the reception room, the environment of the room is now unsanitary and unsafe. Patients who are bleeding through bandages and towels should be escorted back to the triage area immediately following patients with life-threatening conditions.

Nosebleeds

Patients may lose large volumes of blood during a nosebleed. There are two types of nosebleeds:

- *Anterior nosebleed.* These occur in the lower part of the septum, which is highly vascular. Anterior nosebleeds usually just involve one side. They may occur as the result of a minor injury or dry climate.
- *Posterior nosebleed.* These are rarer and more dangerous than anterior nosebleeds, usually occurring higher and deeper in the nasal cavity. These types of nosebleeds occur more often in older patients, patients with facial or nasal injuries, and in patients with hypertension.

Burns

Burns are of high concern because of complications that may arise.

The following criteria may be used to assess the seriousness of a burn. Patients who exhibit any of the signs or symptoms listed or match the following criteria are usually sent on to the emergency room.

1. Patients with breathing problems (be prepared to assist with the breathing emergency)
2. Patients with burns located on the head, neck, hands, feet, and genitals (these are considered severe)
3. Patients with multiple burns or burns that cover a large surface area

CRITICAL THINKING CHALLENGE

You take a phone call from a patient who just had surgery. The patient states that he just does not feel right and that his heart is racing.

1. What other questions should you ask the patient to obtain a better grasp of the patient's condition?
2. What piece of information did the patient provide that should send up an automatic red flag?
3. What could be wrong with the patient and what should be your next course of action?

4. Patients of certain ages (the pediatric patient and older adults are more susceptible to complications from burns)
5. All full thickness burns are considered critical burns

Table 33-6 describes how various types of burns are classified.

Another factor that helps to assess the severity of a burn is the percentage of body surface area that is

Health Coach

Nosebleeds

To help prevent nosebleeds, use a dehumidifier during the winter months, and lubricate the interior of the nose with an ointment or cream. Avoid picking the nose or blowing really hard. Sleep with the head elevated.

When a nosebleed occurs, remain calm and avoid tilting the head back, as this will cause the blood to run down the back of the throat. Try pinching the soft tissue of the nose with the thumb on one side and the index finger on the opposite side, pressing against the bones of the face. Pinch close for five minutes (you may breathe through your mouth). The head should always remain elevated; do not lay flat. Place an ice bag filled with crushed ice above the area in which you are pinching. This will constrict blood vessels in the area, thus decreasing the amount of blood loss. If bleeding does not slow down or stop, activate the EMS.

Table 33-6 Types of Burns

Types of Burns	Degrees of Burns	Example
Thermal burn: Caused by heat, such as a hot surface or flames. *General first aid for all thermal burns*: Cool the burn by pouring cool sterile saline or water over the site to provide comfort for the patient. If the burn is minor and does not cover a large area, cover the burn with a sterile dressing.	***Superficial burns*** (formally known as first degree burns): Involves the first layer of the skin. *Symptoms:* Reddening of the skin, warmth and pain; skin remains intact.	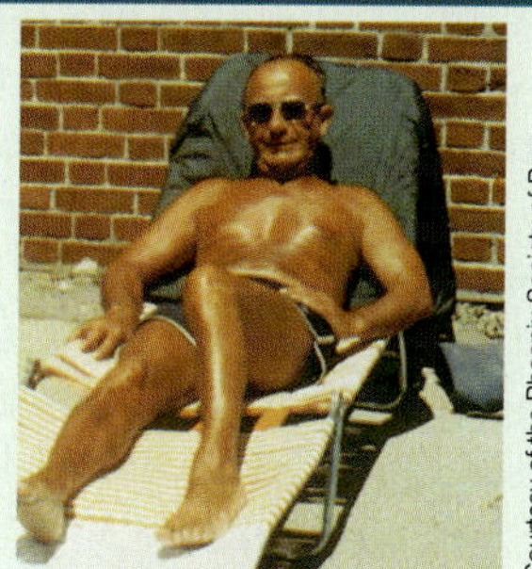 Courtesy of the Phoenix Society of Burn Survivors, Inc. A superficial burn.
Chemical burn: Caused by contact with acids or alkalis. *General first aid*: Clothes should be removed and the area should be flooded with water for a minimum of 15 minutes. Dry chemicals should be brushed off before flushing the patient's skin. Some dry chemicals are activated by water. Cover the burn with a sterile dressing. The burn should be assessed by a provider. *Chemical burn to the eye:* Should be flushed with water from the inside to the outside for 10–15 minutes.	***Partial thickness burns*** (formally known as second degree burns): Burns that extend into the dermis or second layer of the skin. *Symptoms:* Skin may appear white to pink; may have some fluid loss and blisters; mild to moderate pain.	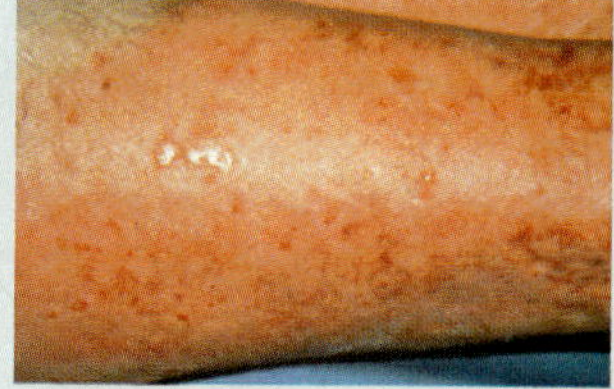 A partial thickness burn. Courtesy of the Phoenix Society of Burn Survivors, Inc.
Electrical burn: Occurs after contact with electrical wiring (can also be caused by a lightning strike); hard to assess outwardly; could be internal injuries that are not visible to the naked eye. *General first aid*: Make sure the electrical source has been shut down prior to applying first aid (never touch an electrical wire!); administer CPR if necessary and call the EMS.	***Full thickness burns*** (formally known as third and fourth degree burns): Involves all three layers of the skin including fat and muscle tissue, which may decrease the motility and function of the affected area. Nerve endings are usually destroyed, so the patient may have no pain. *Symptoms:* The surface of the burn may have a hardened appearance that appears pearly white and leathery. Greatly damaged tissue has a charcoal appearance and underlying tissue is usually visible.	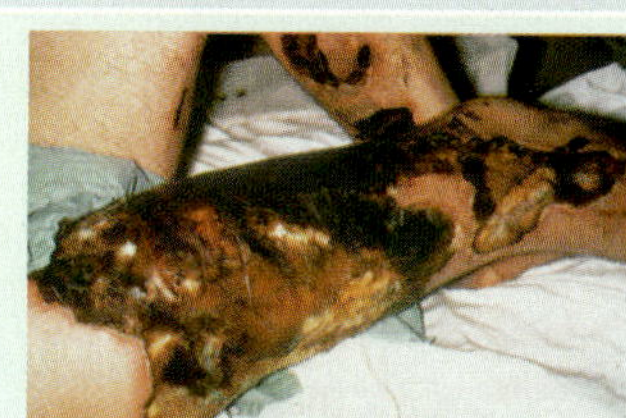 A full thickness burn. Courtesy of the Phoenix Society of Burn Survivors, Inc.

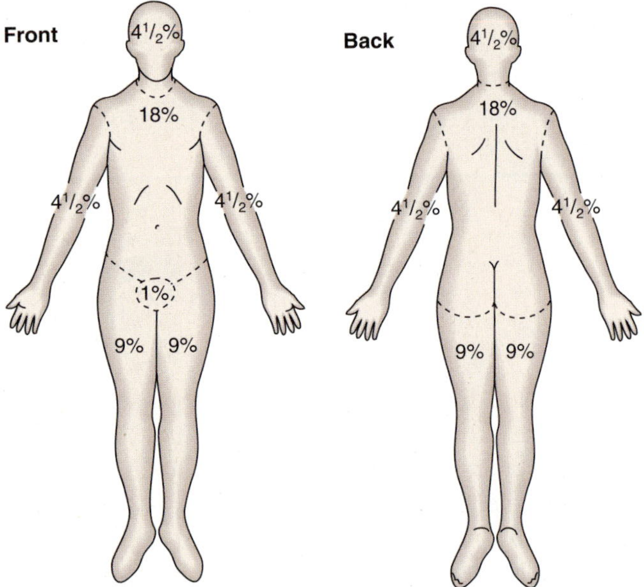

Figure 33-10 ■ The *Rule of Nines* is used to estimate the percentage of body surface area burned (adult example).

involved in the burn. The *Rule of Nines* formula is used most often in the field by medics who need to determine very quickly how much of the body is affected.

Figure 33-10 illustrates *the Rule of Nines* by assigning a skin surface percentage to 11 different body parts. When the major surface areas are tallied together, it totals 99 percent. The remaining 1 percent is assigned to the genitals. The *Rule of Nines* does not apply to infants and children because of differences in head and body proportions; however, there are charts that can assist in tallying affected areas in their age groups as well. Refer to Figure 33-11 for a breakdown of body surface percentages in babies and children. Infection is a big concern for patients who sustain burns.

Eye Injuries Related to Burns

Severe eye injuries or chemical burns to the eyes are usually considered emergencies because damage to the eye can occur very quickly and a delay in treatment may lead to serious eye damage or blindness.

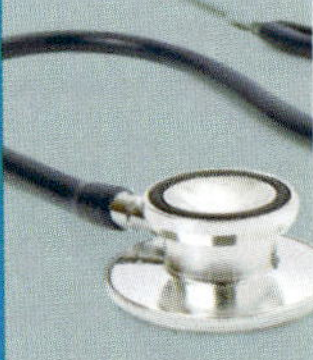

Field Smarts

Patients with severe eye injuries, such as chemical burns or foreign bodies in the eye, should be assessed right away. Chemical burns are normally irrigated with tepid water or saline for several minutes to help remove the chemicals. If the eye has been injured and it will be a few minutes before the provider is available, the provider may want the medical assistant to cover both of the patient's eyes to prevent further damage to the affected eye. Obtain the eye tray, numbing drops, dye, ultraviolet light, and ophthalmoscope. Some practices may have the medical assistant perform a visual acuity test to screen for vision damage.

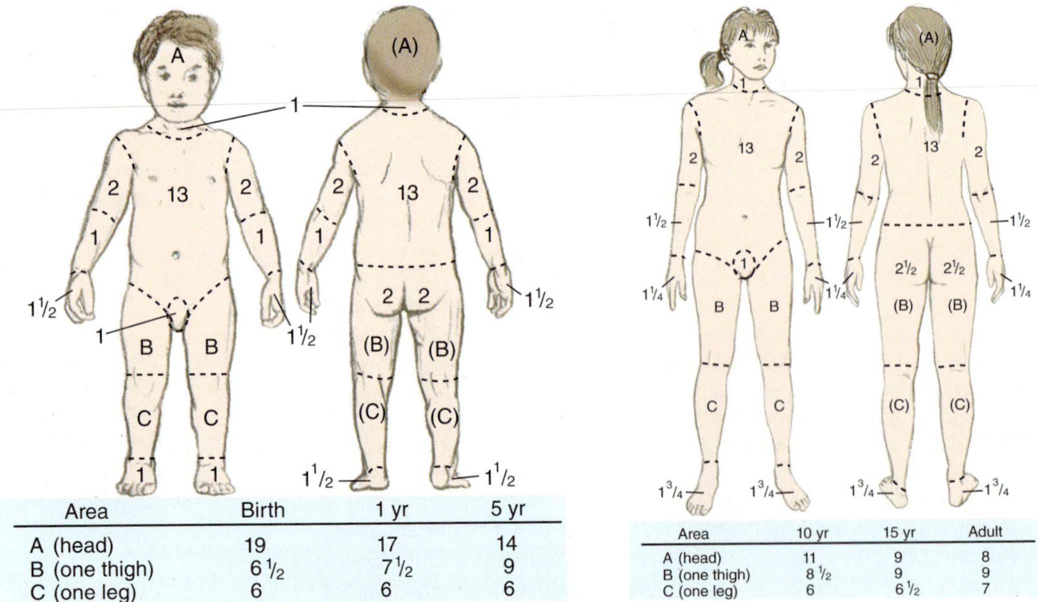

Area	Birth	1 yr	5 yr
A (head)	19	17	14
B (one thigh)	6 1/2	7 1/2	9
C (one leg)	6	6	6

Area	10 yr	15 yr	Adult
A (head)	11	9	8
B (one thigh)	8 1/2	9	9
C (one leg)	6	6 1/2	7

Figure 33-11 ■ The Lund and Browder chart is used for estimating the extent of burns in infants and children.

Diabetic Ketoacidosis and Insulin Shock

Diabetic emergencies can be very serious and even life-threatening. **Diabetic ketoacidosis** is a serious complication of diabetes that occurs when the body produces high levels of blood acids called ketones, and develops when the body is unable to produce enough insulin. Medical assistants should become familiar with the signs of both diabetic coma and insulin shock. **Diabetic coma** is a life-threatening condition in which the patient's blood sugar is dangerously high, causing the patient to go into a coma. **Insulin shock** is a life-threatening condition in which the patient's blood sugar drops to a dangerously low level, causing the patient to go into shock. Medical assistants should know how to properly respond in the event of a diabetic crisis. The following is a list of questions that should be asked when you suspect a diabetic emergency.

1. Are you a diabetic? If yes, type 1 or 2? (The patient's chart can help answer this question.)
2. What type of medication do you take for your diabetes? (The patient's chart can help answer this question.)
3. When was your last dose of medication, and how much did you take?
4. When did you eat last? (Especially important for patients with hypoglycemia.)
5. Have you recently exercised? (Exercise lowers blood sugar.)
6. Have you been sick to your stomach or vomiting? (Especially important for patients with hypoglycemia.)
7. Do you feel confused? (Often seen in hypoglycemia patients.)
8. Have you had a recent infection? (Could be related to hyperglycemia.)

Table 33-7 depicts the differences between insulin shock and diabetic ketoacidosis, which can lead to diabetic coma.

If unsure whether the victim is suffering from hyperglycemia or hypoglycemia, treat for hypoglycemia. Hypoglycemia is usually more serious than hyperglycemia, due to how quickly the patient deteriorates. If you as the medical assistant suspect any diabetic emergency, alert the provider immediately to obtain order for stat glucose testing.

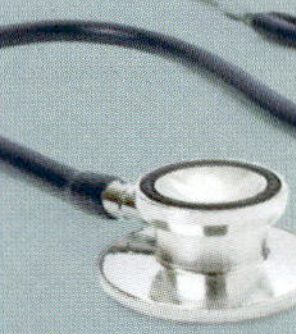

Field Smarts

Ambulatory and urgent care centers usually stock emergency supplies of glucose that may be in the form of pastes, gels, or tablets and may be given sublingually (under the tongue) or bucally (between the gums and cheek) for rapid absorption. Patients with diabetes should keep these supplies as well. If you are at the scene of an emergency and these items are unavailable, you may want to try giving the patient a sugary liquid such as orange juice, apple juice, or a sugary cola. Liquid forms of glucose are best when emergency items are unavailable because they are absorbed at a faster rate into the bloodstream than solids.

Table 33-7 Differences between Insulin Shock and Diabetic Ketoacidosis

Insulin Shock	Diabetic Ketoacidosis or Coma
Low blood sugar: Causes include an overdose of insulin or hypoglycemic medications, vomiting/diarrhea, lack of food/dieting, or excessive exercising.	High blood sugar: Causes include excessive eating, not taking insulin or oral hypoglycemic, fever or infections, and stress.
Immediate onset	Gradual onset
Pulse is full and pounding	Pulse is weak and thready
Respiration is normal to shallow	Respiration is rapid and deep
Skin is pale, cool, and clammy	Skin is red, hot, and dry
Feeling lightheaded or shaky (poor coordination)	May have a fruity odor coming from the mouth
Headache is normally present	Drowsiness
Confused and disoriented	Intense thirst
May be angry and in a rage	Eventual stupor or unconsciousness
Eventual stupor or unconsciousness	

continues

Table 33-7 Differences between Insulin Shock and Diabetic Ketoacidosis *(continued)*

Insulin Shock	Diabetic Ketoacidosis or Coma
Field Smarts Tip: Ask diabetic assessment questions if the patient is conscious. Notify the provider stat. Obtain vitals and be prepared to perform blood glucose testing. Wait for the provider's instructions. The provider may order a sugary substance (see the Field Smarts box) to help stabilize the patient's blood sugar. Retest blood sugar according to the provider's instructions. If unable to regulate, the patient may need to be transported to the ER.	*Field Smarts Tip:* If the patient is conscious, ask appropriate diabetic screening questions and alert the provider. Be prepared to perform blood glucose testing. If the patient is unconscious, notify the provider stat. Be prepared to administer insulin via injection or IV according to the provider's instructions (as long as it is allowed under your state's scope of practice for medical assistants).

Table 33-8 Information on Poisons

Route	Definition	Symptoms	Types	First Aid
Ingestion (Figure 33-12a)	Poison is taken in through the mouth, where it will eventually enter the digestive system.	Burning or swelling of the lips, mouth, tongue, and throat. May have discoloration of mouth. Nausea, vomiting, and diarrhea may also be present.	Household products such as bleach, cleaners, and alcohol. Garage products may include radiator fluid and oil or gasoline.	If at the scene, examine the mouth and remove any foreign bodies, powders, or tablets. Wipe the mouth out with a cloth. Do not induce vomiting and do not give any liquids without instructions from poison control. Call EMS if directed.
Inhalation (Figure 33-12b)	Poison is inhaled through the nose and/or mouth.	Coughing, breathing difficulties, nausea/vomiting, headache, and loss of consciousness.	Dangerous fumes from household cleaners, carbon monoxide, and cyanide.	If at the scene, minimize your risk and move the patient to fresh air. Start artificial breathing if the patient stops breathing.
Injected (Figure 33-12c)	Poison is delivered into the circulatory system by needle or insect.	Edema, erythema, and pain at the injection site. The patient may go into an anaphylactic reaction.	IV drugs, bites and stings from snakes and insects.	If at the scene, remove the object if you can do so without causing greater harm. Get the patient to a hospital stat.
Absorption (Figure 33-12d)	Poison is absorbed through the skin.	Itching, burning, erythema, and rash on the skin. Nausea and vomiting may be present. The patient may go into shock.	Insecticides and poisons from plants.	If at the scene, remove contaminated clothing, rinse for a minimum of 10 minutes. Shower with soap and water. Throw away contaminated clothes.

Poisoning

Poisonings can be very serious and may progress into a respiratory or cardiac emergency. More than 90 percent of poisonings occur in the home and over 50 percent of poisonings occur among children under the age of six. Poisons can enter the body through one of four routes. Refer to Table 33-8 and Figure 33-12 for an in-depth look at poisons.

Seizures

Seizures are sudden attacks that result from a malfunction of the brain. Seizures are normally not life-threatening but may become life-threatening if patients choke on vomit or injures themselves during the seizure. There are two major types of seizures: petite mal seizures and grand mal seizures.

Petite Mal Seizure

Petite mal seizures are also known as absence seizures. They are usually seen in children between the ages of 6 and 12. The symptoms include staring, blinking, and tasting movements made by the mouth. They usually only last 10–20 seconds and the patient rarely remembers anything about the seizure. First aid is usually not necessary for this type of seizure.

Grand Mal Seizure

Typically, a grand mal seizure starts with a loss of consciousness. The patient usually has a history of epilepsy or another brain disorder. The patient may initially become stiff and then start violently shaking. The skin may turn gray and the patient may lose both bladder and bowel control or even vomit during the episode.

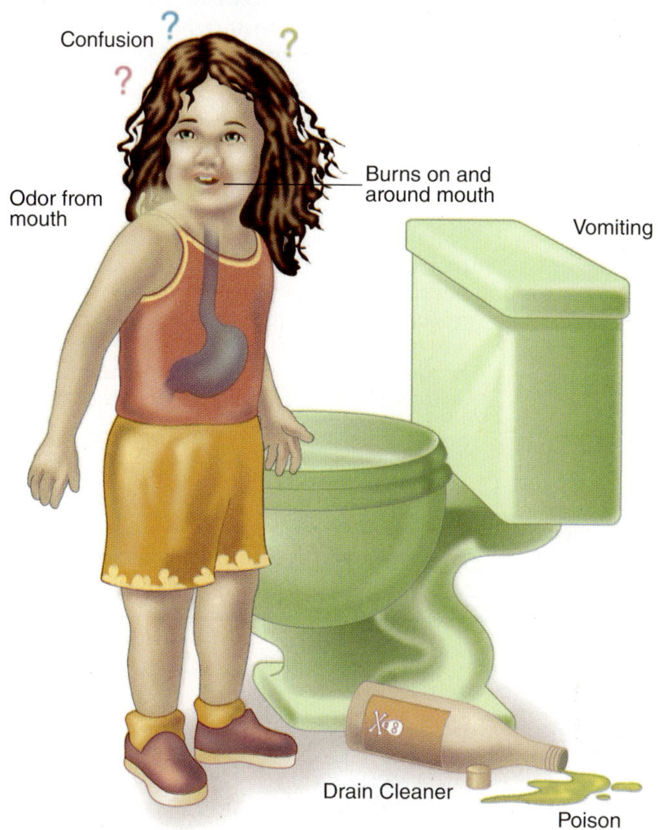

Figure 33-12a ■ Poisoning through ingestion.

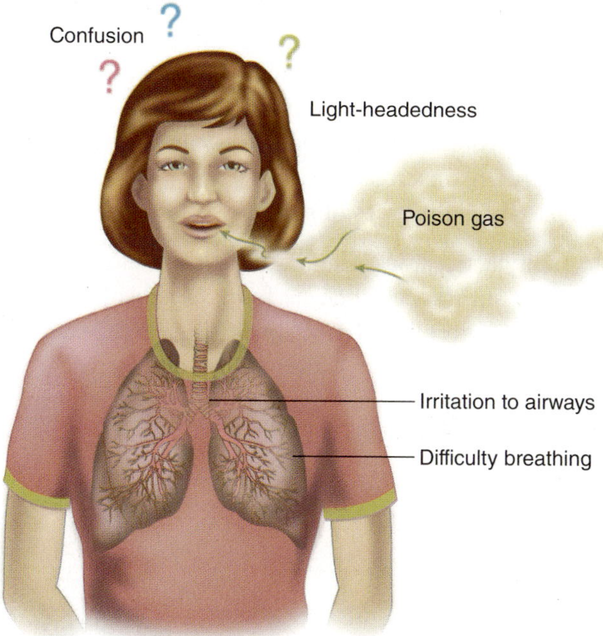

Figure 33-12b ■ Poisoning through inhalation.

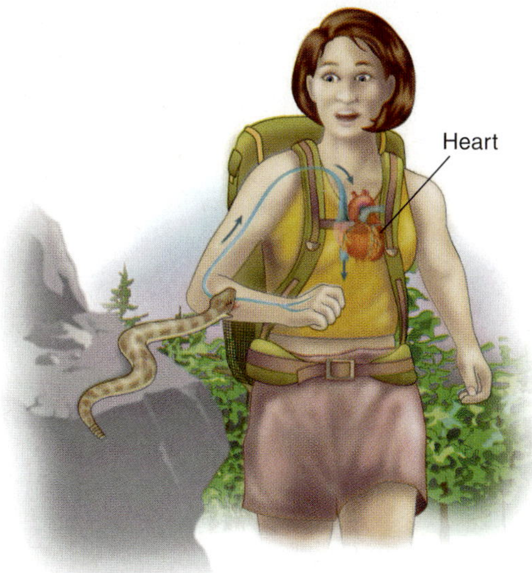

Figure 33-12c ■ Poisoning through injection.

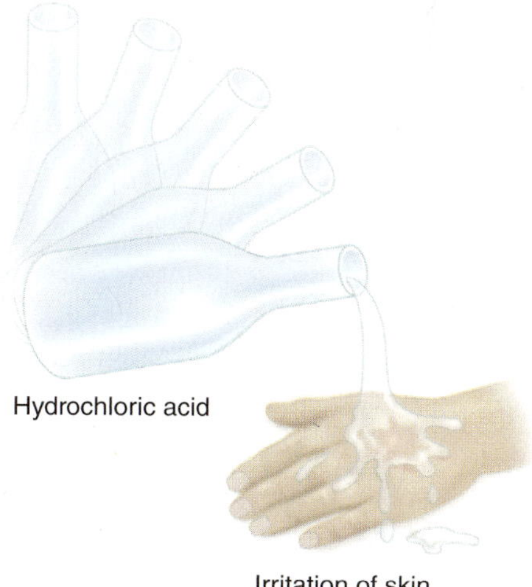

Figure 33-12d ■ Poisoning through absorption.

The episode may last 30 seconds to five minutes. Following the seizure, the patient may have a headache, appear confused, and generally feel very tired. Refer to Table 33-1 on how to respond to a patient having a seizure.

Shock

Shock is a potentially fatal condition that can be brought on by disease, injury, decrease in circulation, and fluid loss. During shock, organs and tissues of the body receive an inadequate flow of blood, depriving the organs and tissues of oxygen. Various systems within the body react to the lack of perfusion and try to preserve the blood for the major organs. Table 33-9 illustrates what happens to various systems when shock occurs.

If blood flow to the organs becomes compromised, the body will sacrifice blood flow to specific organs to help maintain blood supply to the organs most affected by hypoperfusion. Figure 33-13 illustrates perfusion order during cases of shock.

Early symptoms of shock include a rapid, weak pulse and clammy skin. As shock progresses, symptoms progress to include confusion, chest pain, dyspnea, and eventually unconsciousness.

There are eight types of shock:

1. Anaphylactic shock: Caused by a severe allergic reaction to substances such as foods, medications, and insect stings or bites (described earlier in the chapter)
2. Cardiogenic shock: Caused by acute myocardial ischemia or cardiac dysfunction resulting in a decrease of oxygen to cells

Table 33-9 The Effects of Shock on Various Body Systems

Body System	What Occurs
Circulatory	The blood vessels constrict, heart rate increases, and blood pressure drops.
Intestinal	The bowel becomes anoxic causing tissue to become necrotic, which releases bacteria into the abdominal cavity. The patient becomes nauseated and vomiting starts.
Kidneys	Initially the kidneys are fine, but as the blood pressure starts to fall, the body tries to preserve its water volume by sending out hormones that cause the patient to retain fluid. The patient has scanty urination and excessive thirst as a result. The kidneys become unable to properly regulate the acid–base balance and other electrolytes.
Respiratory	Because the cells are starved for oxygen, the body will begin to hyperventilate, resulting in respiratory alkalosis.
Nervous system	The patient becomes very nervous, possibly combative, and eventually unconscious.
Skin	The skin becomes cold and clammy.

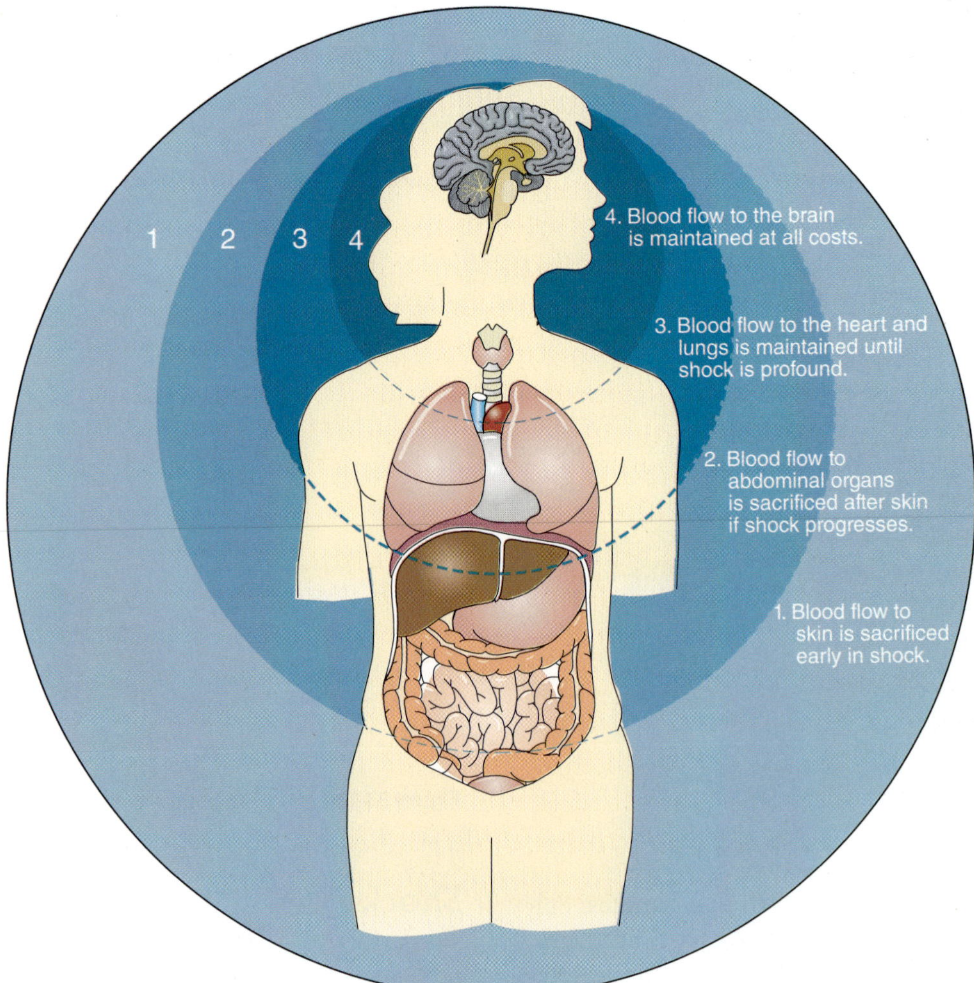
1
2
3
4
4. Blood flow to the brain is maintained at all costs.
3. Blood flow to the heart and lungs is maintained until shock is profound.
2. Blood flow to abdominal organs is sacrificed after skin if shock progresses.
1. Blood flow to skin is sacrificed early in shock.

Figure 33-13 ■ When blood volume diminishes, as in cases of shock, the body tries to compromise by sacrificing blood supply to the less-significant organs in order to preserve blood for the vital organs such as the heart and brain.

3. Hypovolemic shock: Caused by excessive blood volume loss brought on by internal bleeding, external bleeding, severe burns, and severe dehydration
4. Metabolic shock: Caused by an impairment in homeostatis such as acid–base balance changes during a diabetic emergency
5. Neurogenic shock: Caused by dilation of blood vessels that may be secondary to brain injury or excessive deep spinal anesthesia
6. Psychogenic shock: Caused by traumatic emotional factors such as grief and fear; usually not fatal
7. Respiratory shock: Caused by a traumatic injury to the respiratory tract; there is an inadequate exchange of oxygen and CO_2
8. Septic shock: Caused by a toxic substance accumulating in the bloodstream, as in toxic shock syndrome

When to Anticipate Shock

Shock is most likely to occur following surgical procedures, during certain metabolic disorders, during severe infections, and following severely traumatic physical or emotional events. Table 33-1 lists steps that should be taken when a patient is in shock. In Procedure 33-1 you will appropriately detect the signs of shock and respond accordingly.

Syncope

Syncope is a brief episode of unconsciousness or fainting. Fainting is not a disease but rather a symptom of an underlying condition or disease. It may be triggered by a variety of factors, including emotional stress, pain, pooling of the blood due to poor positioning of extremities, severe coughing episodes, and **orthostatic hypotension** (blood pressure that drops upon standing). It may also be related to heart and lung disorders, brain or neurological disorders, and certain medications such as antihypertensives, antidepressants, and diuretics.

Cause for elevated concern if:

- Syncope is in conjunction with a heart irregularity.
- There is a family history connected with sudden death following a syncope episode.
- The syncope episode occurs in combination with exercise.

Refer to Table 33-1 to learn steps for responding to syncope episodes.

Vertigo

Vertigo is a "spinning" sensation or feeling "dizzy" that is most frequently caused by an inner ear problem. The symptoms described by people with vertigo include the following: spinning, tilting, swaying, feeling unbalanced, and being pulled to one direction.

The symptoms can last as little as a few minutes, or up to a few hours or more, and can come and go. Treatment is determined based on the cause. Much of the time vertigo goes away without treatment.

Thermal Emergencies

Because certain temperature-related emergencies can be life-threatening, they are listed under life-threatening emergencies. Table 33-10 provides a list of symptoms for each type of heat-related emergency. Refer to Table 33-1 for instructions on how to respond to heat-related emergencies.

Cold-Related Emergencies

Frostbite is a local injury of the skin due to freezing or subfreezing conditions. Factors that can increase the risk of frostbite include wet gloves and socks, high wind conditions, and prolonged exposure to cold temperatures. The nose, toes, fingers, face, and ears are the most vulnerable sites to frostbite. Frostbite is not

Table 33-10 Symptoms for Heat-Related Emergencies

Condition	Symptoms
Heat cramps are usually confined to the abdomen and legs and result from a combination of factors, including elevated temperature, loss of fluids, and a loss of salt from the body.	Abdominal and leg cramps, general weakness or fatigue, heavy sweating, possible dizziness, or fainting. *Heat cramps occur when the body becomes overheated and are the least serious of all of the heat-related emergencies.*
Heat exhaustion most commonly occurs as the result of exposure to excessive heat while working or exercising. The victim sweats and loses large volumes of water and salts. The blood capillaries rise to the surface of the skin, where the blood pools to assist in the cooling process.	General weakness, rapid and shallow respirations, weak pulse, cool clammy skin, diaphoresis, and may be unresponsive. *This whole process creates a mild form of shock, which may lead to heat stroke if not remedied.*
Heat stroke occurs when the body is either unable to cool itself down due to dehydration, physiological conditions, or a progression of heat exhaustion factors that go untreated.	A temperature of 104°F (40°C) or higher, general weakness, initial deep respirations that change to shallow respirations, pulse may start out as rapid and strong but may change to rapid and weak, dry hot skin, very little or no sweating, dilated pupils, muscle twitching, convulsions or unconsciousness. *Heat stroke is a life-threatening emergency and the EMS should be activated right away.*

a life-threatening condition itself but is associated with life-threatening conditions because it is categorized with hypothermia.

The symptoms of frostbite include skin that feels frozen or hard, a white, waxy appearance, swelling, and blisters. The skin may be red, purple, or mottled. Proper treatment includes removal of the victim from the cold environment, removal of cold, wet clothing, and warming the affected part by natural means such as body-to-body contact and blankets. Avoid rubbing, massaging, or quick heat treatments with hot water or heating pads, as this may cause further injury.

Hypothermia is another type of cold-related emergency that affects the body's core temperature. Normal body temperature is around 98.6°F (37°C). Hypothermia victims usually have body temperatures that fall below 95°F (35°C) and may be at a serious risk of dying without medical intervention, which is why hypothermia is listed under life-threatening conditions. Factors that make persons more susceptible to hypothermia include age (the very old and very young), prolonged exposure to cold and wet environments, various medications, and alcohol and drug use. The symptoms include cold skin, shivering, dizziness, mental impairment, a decrease in motor function, and a very rigid posture. Respiration and pulse rates will slow down and eventually stop, so victims should be monitored for the CABs (which consists of checking circulation and providing compressions if necessary, opening the airway, and breathing for the patient) of CPR. Other treatment measures for hypothermia are similar to the management of frostbite. Do not give hypothermic victims anything by mouth. Activate EMS as soon as possible.

Wounds

The majority of wounds that are seen in an ambulatory or urgent care center are not the type of life-threatening wounds that are seen in an emergency room, but may involve bleeding and a great deal of pain. There are two major types of wounds: opened and closed.

Open Wounds

Open wounds are wounds that break the skin and may include abrasions, incisions, lacerations, and punctures. The following are examples of open wounds.

Abrasions

Abrasions (Figure 33-14) are superficial scrapes that may be very painful. These types of injuries are usually not serious and can be treated at home unless gravel and dirt are embedded within the wound. Usual home care involves gentle cleansing of the area, application of an over-the-counter antibiotic cream, and a dressing to keep the

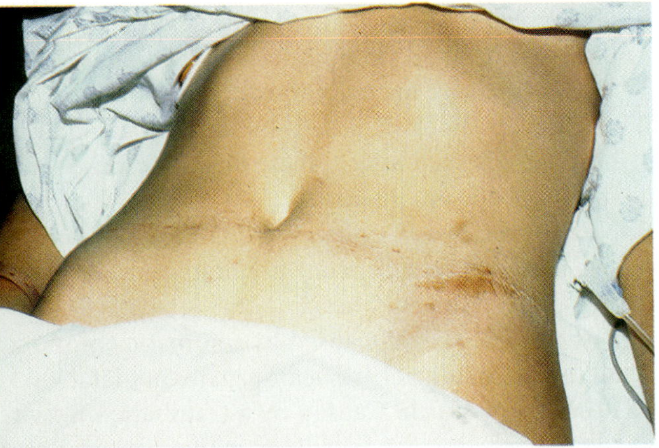

Figure 33-14 ■ An example of an abrasion.

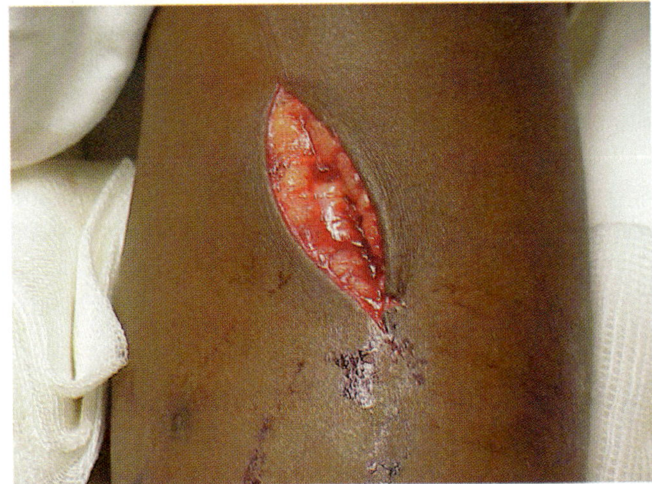

Figure 33-15 ■ An example of an incision.

site clean. Reinjury, which occurs quite often with young children, creates an increased risk of infection.

Incisions

Incisions (Figure 33-15) are cuts in the skin made from items such as sharp instruments or glass. Deeper incisions may involve a great deal of bleeding and can become easily infected. These types of incisions should be closed within six hours of the injury by one of the following methods: adhesive skin closures, suturing, or surgical adhesives. Treatment for minor incisions includes gentle cleansing to the area and the application of a dressing. Check to see when the patient's last tetanus shot was performed. If it was more than 10 years prior, the patient will probably need to have a tetanus booster.

Lacerations

Lacerations (Figure 33-16) are different from incisions because they are usually irregularly shaped cuts with jagged edges. They may also appear as tears. Bleeding is usually very heavy and the patient often needs sutures. If bleeding is minimal, this may create an increased

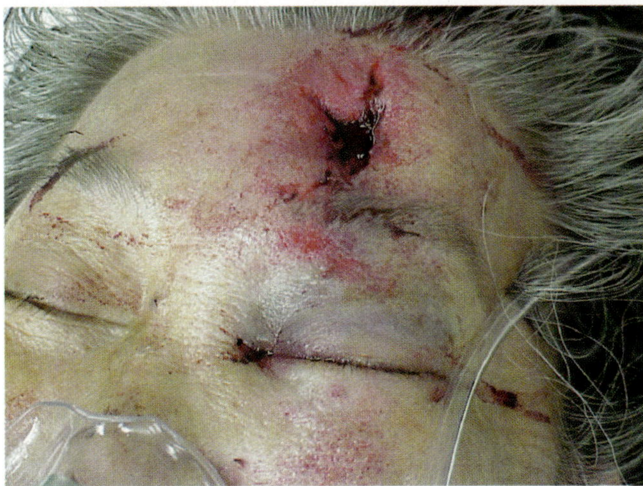

Figure 33-16 ■ An example of a laceration.

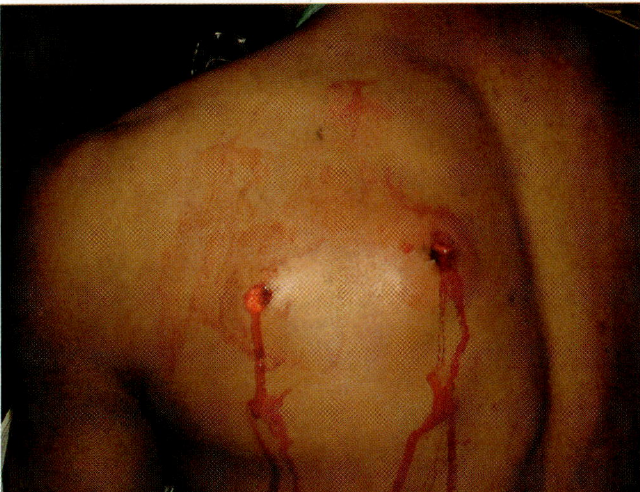

Figure 33-17 ■ An example of a puncture.

risk of infection because bleeding promotes cleansing. Treatment usually involves cleansing of the wound and possible wound closure. Check to see when the patient's last tetanus shot was performed.

Punctures

Punctures (Figure 33-17) are usually caused by objects such as sticks, pins, nails, or pieces of glass that penetrate the skin, leaving a hole in the skin. They may be superficial or deep. There is usually little bleeding with superficial punctures, so these kinds of wounds are also very susceptible to infection. Superficial wounds should be cleansed and bandaged and the patient should be encouraged to watch for signs of infection. Deeper wounds should be professionally examined, cleaned, and X-rayed. The patient's tetanus status should be checked.

Closed Wounds

Closed wounds include bruises, hematomas, strains, and sprains. Wound care for hematomas and bruises are usually very minor. Ice may be applied to area to decrease pain, local blood flow, and bruising. Coverings are usually not necessary for these types of wounds. Strains and sprains are addressed in detail in Chapter 22.

Musculoskeletal Injuries

Fractures and other limb injuries are commonly seen in patients who use urgent care services. These types of injuries are often non-life-threatening but patients are usually in a great deal of pain and discomfort. It is difficult to determine the seriousness of the injury without the aid of radiographs (X-rays). Types of musculoskeletal injuries include bone fractures, strains, sprains, and dislocations.

Bone Fracture

A fracture is another term for a broken bone (partial or complete), usually the result of major trauma or injury, and requires medical attention. Fractures often involve injury to surrounding tissue such as the tendons, ligaments, and nerves and involve a great deal of pain and swelling. Refer to Chapter 22 for a listing of different fractures and treatments.

Strain

A strain results from overuse or exertion of the affected muscle. There usually is no swelling, but the patient may have significant pain upon movement.

Sprain

A sprain results from a twisting or wrenching of a joint, which causes the attached ligament to stretch or tear, resulting in bleeding within the tissue. The bone is usually not affected, but the patient may experience a great deal of pain and swelling.

Treatment for Strains and Sprains

In general, the treatment for soft tissue injuries such as sprains and strains is the same. Refer to the mnemonics RICE and MICE in Table 33-11 for a description of both. The focus for the first 24 hours following an injury is to reduce swelling and inflammation; therefore, the RICE treatment is usually followed. Some providers now encourage following the MICE mnemonic, which incorporates movements with ice.

Table 33-11 RICE and MICE Descriptions

Rice	Mice
R = Rest	M = Movement or motion
I = Ice	I = Ice, heat, or both
C = Compression (ace bandage)	C = Compression (ace bandage)
E = Elevation	E = Elevation

The second 24 hours may involve changes that are designed to promote circulation and healing and may exchange cold therapy with heat therapy or may combine the two. The provider will give instruction. The exact steps for applying heat and cold therapy are outlined in Chapter 22.

Dislocation

This is a separation of a bone from its normal place of attachment or position within a joint, most common in the shoulders and fingers, but can occur in the elbows, hips, and knees. The joint may be visibly out of place or deformed or immovable. The patient is usually in a great deal of pain and discomfort and there may be damage to surrounding structures such as the ligaments, blood vessels, nerves, and soft tissue. Radiographs (X-rays) are often ordered and treatment may include reduction, immobilization, surgery, or rehabilitation. Reduction and splinting may take place in the medical office. Providers may try to give the patient a local anesthetic prior to reducing, but sometimes patients need a general anesthetic because of the pain involved and therefore will need to be transported to the hospital.

Splinting

Prior to diagnosis, all musculoskeletal injuries should be treated as possible fractures. Patients with lower musculoskeletal injuries should be transported to the clinical area by wheelchair and placed in a special procedure room that has casting and splinting supplies. The affected limb should be immobilized and elevated and a cold pack should be placed over the site of the injury to help reduce swelling. Musculoskeletal injuries will usually require radiographs, and the medical assistant may be responsible for assisting the provider with splinting or casting.

The Purpose of Splinting

Splinting is a procedure that is performed to prevent further damage or injury to the affected extremity. Refer to Chapter 22 for a full procedure on splinting.

Bandaging Techniques

Different types of bandaging techniques may be used for both open and closed wounds. Wounds that are open usually require the application of sterile dressings prior to bandaging. To learn more about the proper application of sterile dressings, refer to Chapter 10. Figure 33-18 illustrates different bandaging techniques that can be used for different types of injuries.

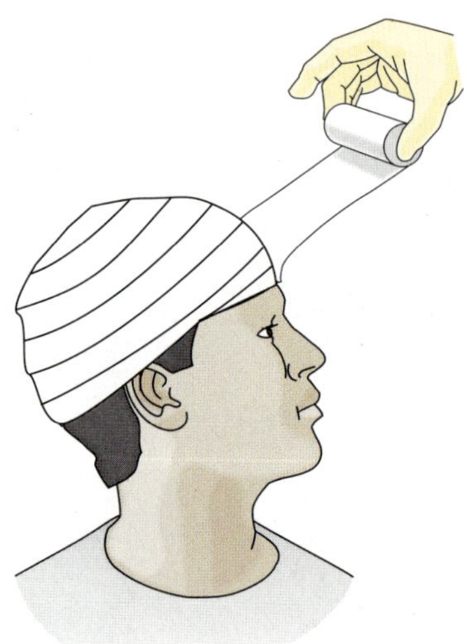

Figure 33-18a ■ A recurrent bandage may be used on the head.

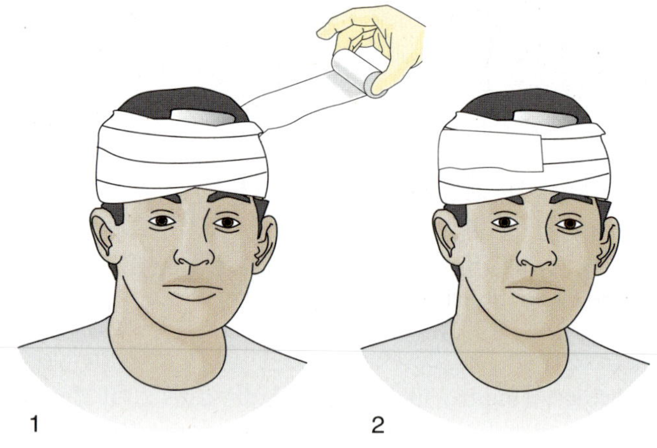

Figure 33-18b ■ A roller bandage may be used to cover a head wound.

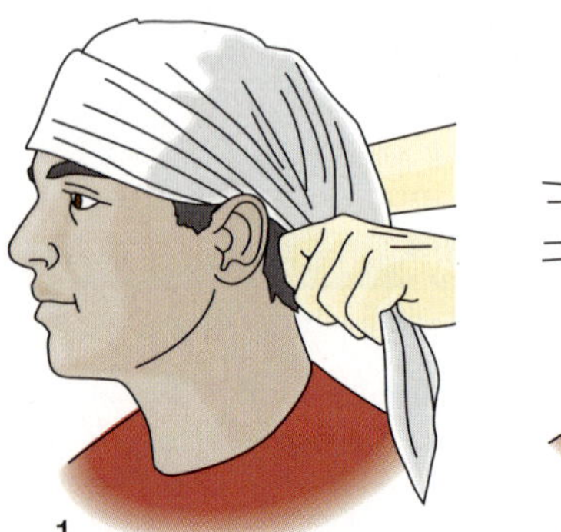

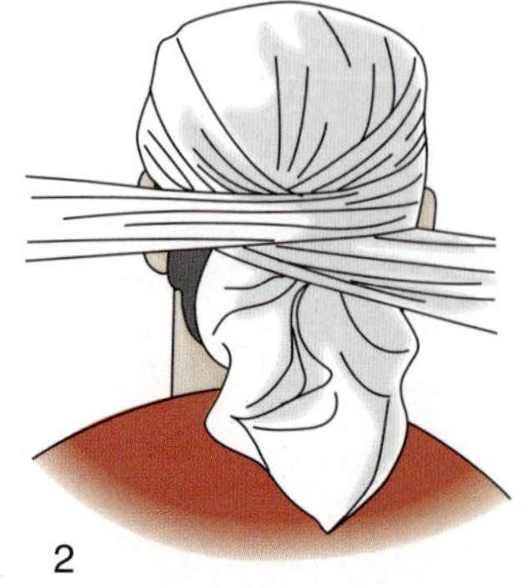

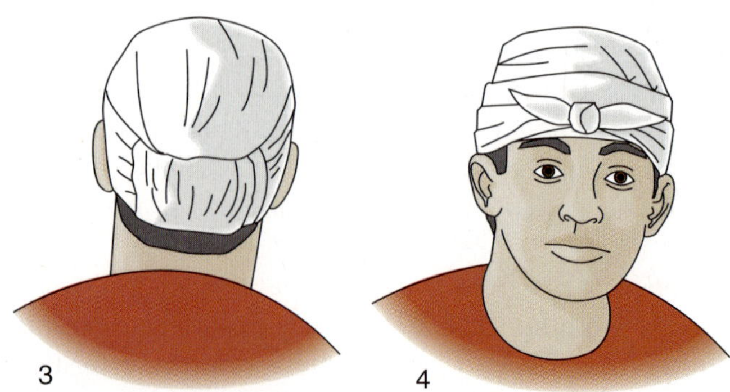

Figure 33-18c ■ A triangular bandage may also be used to cover a head wound.

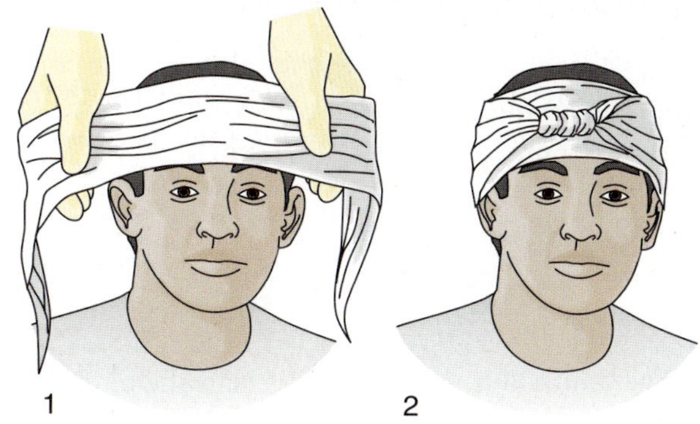

Figure 33-18d ■ A cravat may be used to hold a dressing in place on the head.

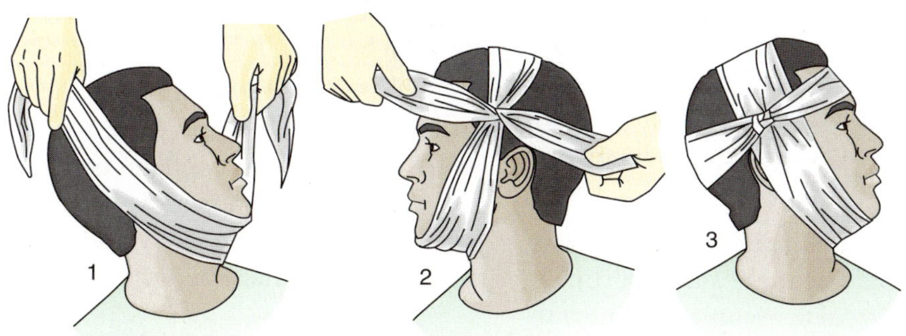

Figure 33-18e ■ A double cravat may be used to cover and secure an ear injury.

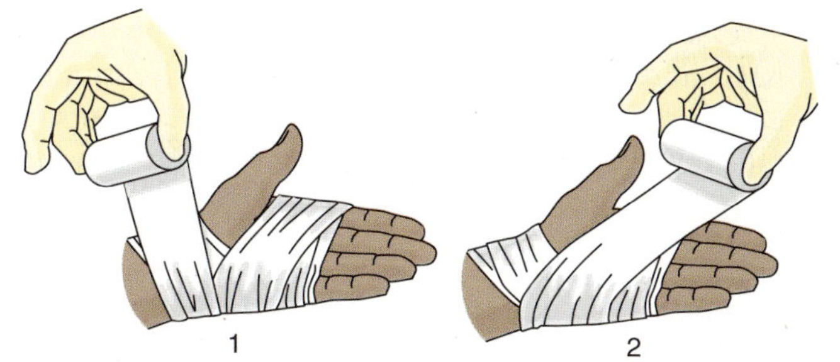

Figure 33-18f ■ A figure eight bandage is used to immobilize a joint.

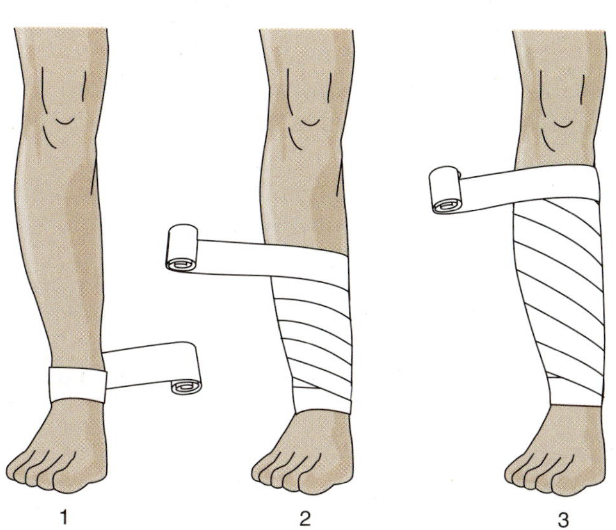

Figure 33-18g ■ A spiral bandage may be used to cover an extremity.

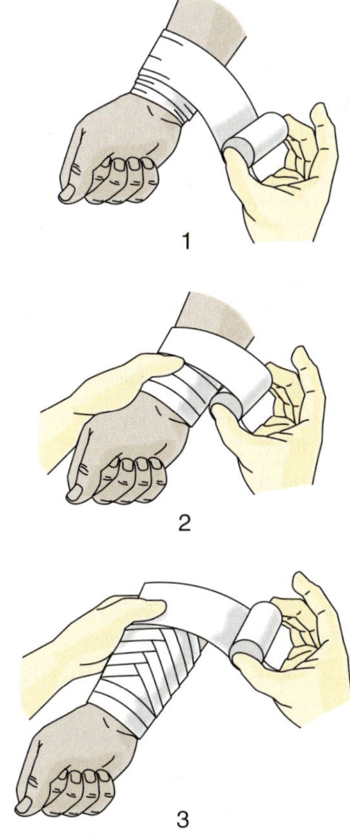

Figure 33-18h ■ A reverse spiral turn may be used when extra padding is essential.

Animal Bite

Typically wild animals avoid people, but if they are sick, feel threatened, or are protecting their young, they might attack. Attacks by domestic pets are more common. Typically animal bites are not life-threatening, but they can become infected, resulting in serious medical issues. The ways to prevent bites and complications include the following:

- Never pet, handle, or feed unknown animals
- Leave snakes alone
- Keep a close watch on children around animals
- If you are a pet owner, vaccinate your cats, ferrets, and dogs against rabies (also called hydrophobia)
- If you are a pet owner, spay or neuter your dog to make it less aggressive
- Get a tetanus booster if you have not had one recently
- Wear boots and long pants when you are in areas with venomous snakes

Animal bite reporting requirements vary by state. Medical assistants should refer to the health department for the state they are working in to become familiar with reporting requirements. Patients who have been bitten should wash the bite wound with soap and water, seek attention from a medical provider to determine care based on the situation, and report the bite as required. Medical assistants should follow state, local, and office policy in regards to reporting animal bites.

Insect Bites and Stings

Most insect bites (also called bug bites) are harmless, though they sometimes cause discomfort. Bites that hurt include the bee, wasp, and hornet stings, and the fire ant bites. Bites that usually itch come from the mosquito, flea, and mite. Disease can also spread through insect bites. For example, in the United States, some mosquitoes spread West Nile virus, and travelers outside the United States may be at risk for malaria and other infections. Ticks can carry Lyme disease, Rocky Mountain spotted fever, and other tick-borne infections. Some tips to prevent insect bites and complications are the following:

- Don't bother insects
- Use insect repellant
- Wear protective clothing
- Be careful eating outside because food attracts insects
- If you know you have severe allergic reactions to insect bites, carry an emergency epinephrine kit
- Avoid wooded and brushy areas where ticks are known to be present; use repellents that contain 20–30% *N*, *N*-diethyl-meta-toluamide (DEET); bathe or shower as soon as possible after coming in contact with ticks; conduct a full-body check. If a tick is attached to your skin, use fine-tipped tweezers to grasp the tick as close to the skin's surface as possible, then pull upward with steady even pressure. Do not twist or jerk the tick as this may cause the tick to break off and parts to remain in the skin. After removal of the tick, thoroughly clean the bite area and your hands with rubbing alcohol, iodine scrub, or soap and water. Properly dispose of the tick (never crush a tick with your fingers). If a rash or fever develops within several weeks of removing a tick, see your provider and tell her about the recent bite, when and where the bite occurred.

As a medical assistant, you will need to remember that a patient who suffers an allergic reaction to an insect bite or sting could go into anaphylactic shock if untreated. Immediately contact your provider, and reference the triage/algorithm instructions.

Concussion and Other Head and Neck Injuries

Head and neck injuries are very serious due to the risk of paralysis and possible death and should be assessed and treated immediately. The majority of head and neck injuries are the result of automobile accidents, sports injuries, motorcycle accidents, and falls. Any injury to the brain caused by trauma is termed a **traumatic brain injury**. Typical head injuries include the following:

- ***Concussion***. An injury in which the brain is jarred.
- *Brain contusion*. A bruising of the brain that may cause some internal bleeding and swelling. Often caused by a skull fracture, but may also be caused by a severe jarring sensation, such as in shaken baby syndrome, or when a car stops abruptly.
- *Skull fracture*. An injury in which the skull cracks; may cause the edges of the skull to cut into the brain.
- *Hematoma*. Bleeding in the brain that eventually clots. The symptoms are not always immediate and may be delayed for several weeks.

Head and cervical neck symptoms will vary depending on the severity and location of the injury, but may include severe head, neck, and back pain that radiates down to the shoulders, arms, or legs, tingling in or slight paralysis of the extremities, confusion, listlessness, and dilation of one or both pupils. The symptoms of head injuries may also include drainage coming from the eyes, ears, mouth, or nose. Lower injuries involving the spinal cord may cause paralysis, breathing difficulties, and a loss of bowel or bladder control.

CRITICAL THINKING CHALLENGE

The receptionist calls you to tell you that a patient has just collapsed in the reception area. The provider just ran downstairs to consult with a specialist and there are no other clinical team members available. When you get to the reception area, several other patients are surrounding the victim.

1. What should you do first?

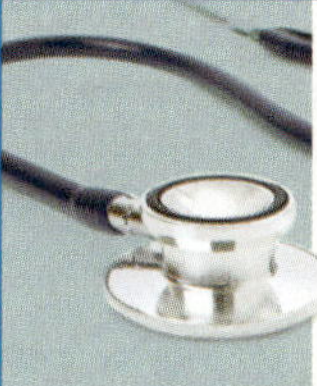

Field Smarts

Alert the provider STAT with any head or neck injuries. Do not allow the patient to move. Obtain a cervical collar and be prepared to assist the provider with head and neck immobilization (Figure 33-19). If the provider feels the injury is critical, the medical assistant may need to notify the EMS so that the patient can be transported to the nearest emergency facility.

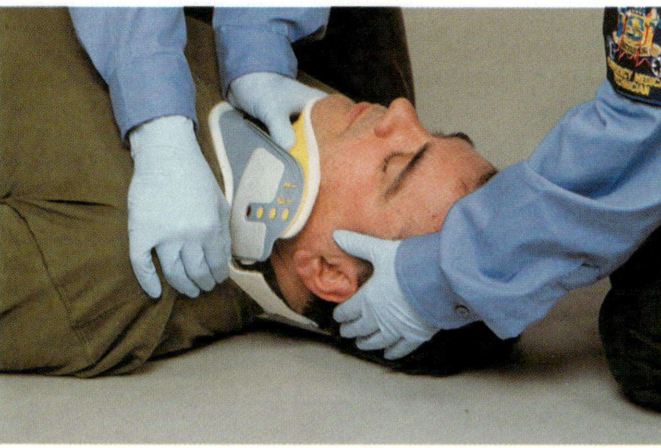

Figure 33-19 ■ A cervical collar is carefully applied when neck injuries are suspected.

Spinal cord injuries (SCI) are very serious because any additional movement can cause significant damage to the already injured vertebrae and spinal cord. Patients who sustain traumatic head and spinal injuries are usually transported by the EMS to the nearest trauma center. There are those occasions in which the patient has few or no symptoms at the time of the injury but may have an exacerbation of symptoms days following the injury. The patient may not realize the seriousness of the injury and may seek the services of a family practitioner or urgent care center rather than a hospital.

Mentally or Emotionally Distressed Patients

One final category of possible emergencies involves considerations of dealing with the emotional or mental state of the patient or others. If the person appears highly agitated and is very vocal in the reception area, this can be quite distressing to others in the waiting area. Safety is also a concern in these cases because mentally or emotionally unstable persons may pose a physical threat to themselves, office personnel, or other patients sitting in the reception area. Consider the recent attacks and shootings at various medical centers, including the Veteran's Administration clinics or hospitals. Raise your awareness, practice emergency drills, and openly discuss potential situations, and how to handle with your provider and practice manager.

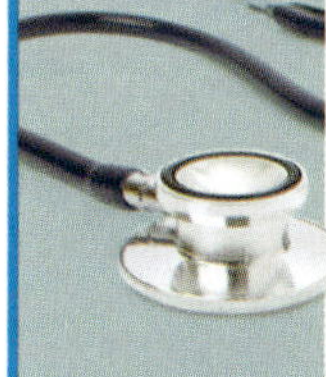

Field Smarts

Alert the provider of the patient's mental or emotional state and be prepared to give the provider a list of local mental health centers. Assist the patient to an examination room as soon as possible and encourage the patient to discuss fears or concerns until the provider takes over. If the patient starts making threats to the provider or other staff members, be prepared to call both the police and EMS for professional intervention.

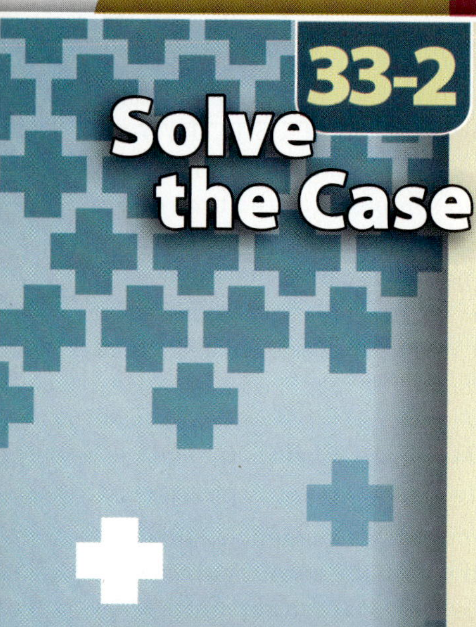

Of the five patients who entered the clinic on the really busy afternoon as described in "Solve the Case 33-1," determine the correct order that the patients should be seen now that you have received emergency training. Describe your emergency response to each medical emergency scenario:

1. **Patient burned her arm on a hot pot and appears to be in quite a bit of discomfort.**
2. **Patient is complaining of intense abdominal pain that came on very quickly.**
3. **Patient cut his foot on a piece of broken glass and is bleeding through the towel.**
4. **Patient comes into the office in the middle of an asthma attack.**
5. **Patient fainted while at school today but is conscious now; his mother wants to have him evaluated.**

PROCEDURE 33-1

Performing Basic First Aid in the Medical Office Setting

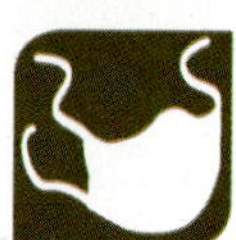

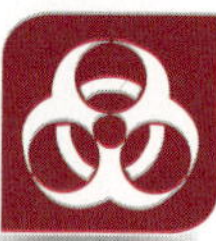

Objective:

To properly apply basic first aid steps for each of the conditions below: Bleeding emergencies, shock, fractures, seizures, syncope, and diabetic emergencies.

Equipment/Supplies:

- Patient's chart/EHR

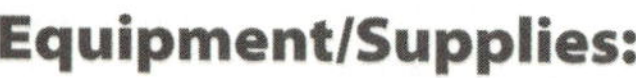

For Bleeding Emergencies:

- Sterile 4 × 4s
- Gauze
- Laceration tray
- Tetanus vaccine

To Treat Shock:

- Pillows
- Sheets/blanket

For Possible Fractures:

- Ice
- Casting Supplies

For Syncope Episodes:

- Blankets
- Pillows

For Seizures or Convulsions:

- Blankets
- Pillows
- Lorazepam (IV Supplies; or Syringe and Needle)

For a Diabetic Emergency:

- Glucose Testing Meter and Supplies
- Sugary Snacks (Hypoglycemic patients)
- Insulin (IV Supplies or Sterile Needle and Syringe [Hyperglycemic patients])

continues

PROCEDURE 33-1 continued

PROCEDURAL STEPS	DETAILS AND/OR RATIONALE
1. ***Demonstrate self-awareness in responding to an emergency situation.*** Identify the patient using two identifiers, identify yourself, and observe the area ***recognizing the physical and emotional effects on persons involved in an emergency situation.***	
2. Wash hands and apply PPE. Assemble equipment and supplies. ***Show awareness of a patient's concerns related to the procedure being performed***.	
3. ***Incorporate critical thinking skills when performing patient assessment and care. Explain to a patient the rationale for performance of a procedure.***	Explaining the procedure to the patient will help alleviate stress and encourage patient cooperation.
4. *For Bleeding Emergencies:* **a.** If the area is already bandaged and blood is seeping through the bandage, apply 4 × 4s over the top of the existing bandage. If no bandage is present, apply sterile/clean 4 × 4s over the bleeding wound and apply pressure (Figure 33-20).	Removing the existing bandage before the blood is clotted could interrupt the clotting process.
b. While still applying direct pressure to the site, elevate the arm above the level of the heart (Figure 33-21).	Elevating the arm decreases the amount of blood flowing to the area.
c. Apply direct pressure to the artery between the point of attachment and the site of the injury (Figure 33-22). Compress the artery against the bony surface of the limb. (Use the brachial artery for the upper limbs and the femoral artery for the lower limbs.) Continue to apply direct pressure and elevate the extremity.	Applying direct pressure to the artery above the site of injury slows down the bleeding process due to constriction of the artery.
d. If bleeding is still uncontrolled, a tourniquet should be applied. The provider should apply the tourniquet just above the affected area. Once applied, the tourniquet should not be loosened. Attach a note to the patient's clothes, close to the tourniquet, stating when the tourniquet was applied.	Tying a tourniquet just above the affected area will stop the bleeding, but may also promote major tissue damage to all the tissue located inferior to the site where the tourniquet is attached. This is why the provider should apply it. Indicating the time will alert hospital personnel to how long the tourniquet has been on so that they may act accordingly.

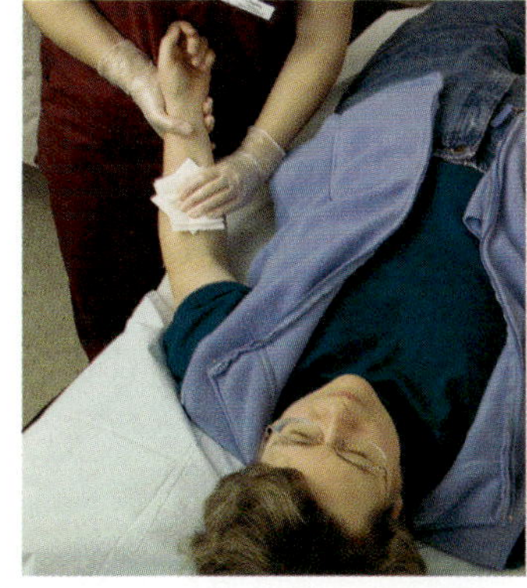

Figure 33-20 ■ Apply direct pressure using a sterile bandage whenever possible.

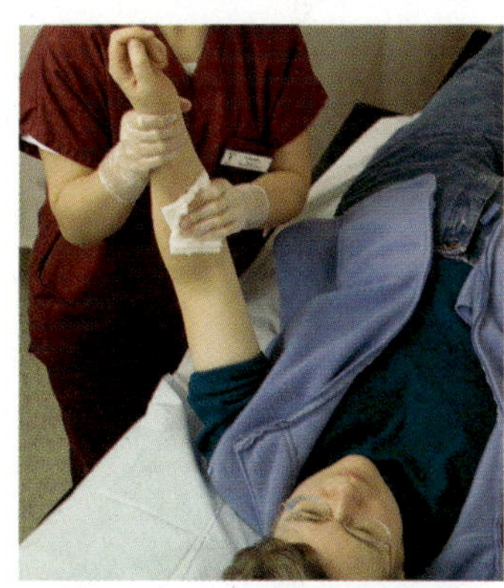

Figure 33-21 ■ Elevate the arm above the level of the heart.

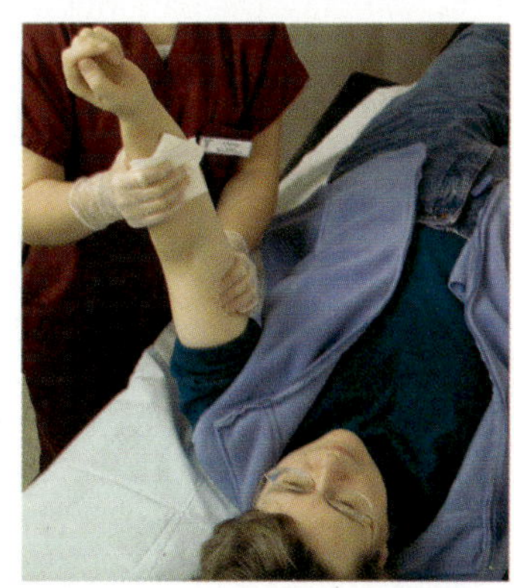

Figure 33-22 ■ Apply pressure to the nearest pressure point.

continues

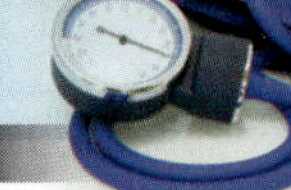

PROCEDURE 33-1 continued

PROCEDURAL STEPS	DETAILS AND/OR RATIONALE
e. Treat the patient for shock and help the patient to remain calm while waiting for the EMS.	Patients that lose large amounts of blood are candidates for shock.
f. Continue to monitor the patient for breathing and heart function.	Critical bleeding emergencies may advance to cardiac arrest.
g. Document the incident.	Documentation is necessary for legal purposes.
h. Dispose of soiled bandages in the biohazarous trash and clean and disinfect the area.	
5. *To Treat Shock:* ***a.*** Recognize that the patient may be going into shock and take the patient's vital signs. The symptoms of shock include an increase in pulse and respiration; pale, cool, clammy skin; and restlessness.	The heart rate and respiration rate increases because of the lack of blood flow throughout the body.
b. Alert the provider or activate the EMS.	The more quickly the patient can get help the better the chances are for a full recovery.
c. Elevate the patient's legs. You may use pillows or blankets if the exam table does not have a mechanism to elevate the legs (Figure 33-23).	Elevating the legs will help the blood to circulate back toward the brain.
d. Place a sheet or blanket over the patient to keep the patient warm.	Patients in shock are usually cold due to the decrease of blood supply.
e. Monitor the patient's airway, breathing, and circulation, ***demonstrating critical thinking when performing patient assessment***.	Patients experiencing shock symptoms may slip into respiratory or circulatory arrest. It is important to monitor the patient until help arrives.
f. Keep the patient calm and reassure the patient that help is on the way.	This may help delay unconsciousness.
6. *For Possible Fractures:* **a.** Recognize possible fracture. If open fracture, control bleeding and treat for shock. If closed, elevate limb and apply ice.	Elevating the limb and applying ice will reduce swelling.
b. Notify provider and get ready to send patient for radiographs (X-rays).	The medical assistant cannot obtain an X-ray without order from provider.
c. Obtain casting supplies and assist provider with casting if applicable.	If fracture is confirmed, casting will help the bone to heal properly.

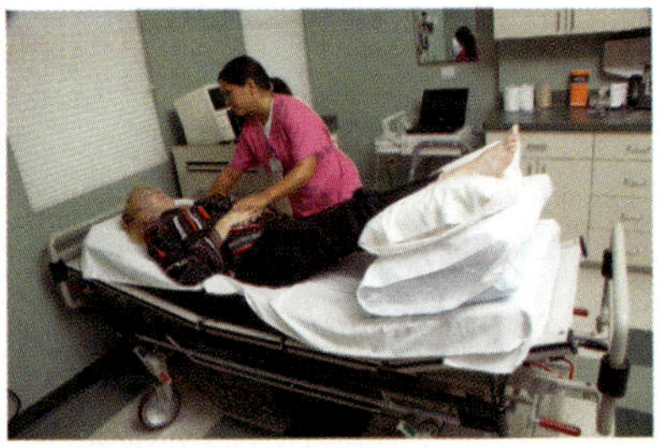

Figure 33-23 ■ Elevating the patient's legs will help the blood to flow back down toward the brain.

continues

PROCEDURE 33-1 continued

PROCEDURAL STEPS	DETAILS AND/OR RATIONALE
7. *For Syncope Episodes:* **a.** Recognize symptoms of syncope and immediately have patient lay down elevating feet above the head. (If possible, place patient in Trendelenburg position.)	Placing patient in Trendelenburg position will help get blood flow back to the brain.
b. Apply cold compresses to patient's forehead and neck.	The cooling compress will help patient feel better.
c. Place a blanket or sheet over patient if the patient is cold.	Patients are often cold following a syncope episode; blankets will help keep them warm.
d. Monitor patient's vital signs and have them evaluated by provider before releasing.	Patient's blood pressure usually drops during a syncope episode. Releasing the patient too early may evoke another syncope episode.
e. If patient actually faints, break fall if possible. Check for injuries and place patient in Trendelenburg position. Notify provider as soon as possible. Monitor vital signs.	Breaking the patient's fall will help to prevent injury.
8. *For Seizures or Convulsions:* **a.** Recognize that patient is having a seizure. (Wash hands and apply gloves when possible.)	The gloves are applied in the event the patient is bleeding or vomits.
b. Notify provider as soon as possible.	
c. Clear area of items that may cause injury to patient.	
d. Try to keep patient on side, if possible.	Keeping the patient on his side will keep the patient from aspirating vomit in lungs if patient is nauseated.
e. Once seizing subsides, place pillow underneath patient's head and a blanket over patient.	Patient is often cold following a seizure so placing a blanket over patient will help keep him warm.
f. Allow patient time to rest. Have provider assess patient for release.	Patients are often very tired following a seizure. Allowing them to rest will help them feel better before leaving.

continues

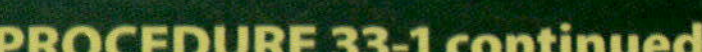

PROCEDURE 33-1 continued

PROCEDURAL STEPS	DETAILS AND/OR RATIONALE
9. *For a Diabetic Emergency:* **a.** Recognize signs of a diabetic emergency. Ask assessment questions as described in this chapter. Signs of insulin shock include bounding pulse; shallow respiration; pale, cool, and clammy skin; shaking; headache; possibly anger. Signs of diabetic ketoacidosis or coma include thread pulse; deep and rapid respirations; red, hot, and dry skin; possible fruity odor coming from mouth; drowsiness; and intense thirst.	Asking assessment questions will help you determine what is going on before blood glucose testing so that you gather the correct supplies.
b. Notify provider right away and obtain order for blood glucose testing.	Provider needs to be informed right away so that testing and treatment can begin.
c. Test patient's blood glucose and obtain vital signs.	Testing the blood glucose will allow the provider to know the type and severity of diabetic crisis.
d. If patient's blood glucose is low, offer sugary liquid or sugary snack. If patient's blood glucose is high, prepare insulin and wait for order to administer.	Sugary liquids will get into the blood stream faster than sugary snacks. Insulin will lower the patient's blood sugar, helping to prevent patient from going into a coma.
e. Have provider assess patient for release.	
f. Be prepared to call EMS if applicable.	
10. Provide patient education.	The patient needs to know how to prevent emergencies from happening in the future and how to manage problems that may incur from current episode.
11. Clean exam table, floor, and so on with disinfectant and dispose of trash in proper receptacles.	
12. Document procedure in the patient's chart.	

DOCUMENTATION EXAMPLE:

02-16-XX 6:00 P.M.	Pt. entered the urgent care after being in a car accident. While taking pt.'s vitals the pt. started sweating profusely. Skin was clammy and cool. Vitals: BP: 88/40, P 106, R 28. Alerted provider. Treated pt. for shock by elevating pt.'s legs and placing a blanket over pt. Dr. Legg had EMS dispatched. Pt. transported to hospital. Rosa Garcia, RMA (AMT)--

CHAPTER SUMMARY

- The medical assistant must have a thorough knowledge of emergency procedures before working in a provider's office or urgent care center. Emergencies can occur at any time and office personnel must be ready to respond in an appropriate manner.
- You must be familiar with the use of various emergency equipment in the office, including the crash cart and related supplies, the AED, and obtain CPR certification.
- Acute abdomen is a term that refers to the *sudden or abrupt onset of intense abdominal pain* and related symptoms, which may include fever, vomiting, diarrhea, dyspnea (difficult breathing), and shock.
- Anaphylaxis is a severe allergic reaction to an allergen usually in the form of a food, medication, chemical, or insect sting or bite.
- Hemorrhaging is a term that means uncontrollable bleeding. It is usually the result of a traumatic injury. Any time a patient severs a major blood vessel, it can lead to hemorrhage and shock.
- Internal bleeding is very difficult to recognize because it is not something that can be observed with the naked eye. It may be the result of a traumatic injury such as a fractured pelvis or gunshot or knife wound, or may occur following a surgical procedure.
- Burns are very concerning because of the complications that may arise as a result of a burn. Severe eye injuries or chemical burns to the eyes are usually considered emergencies as well, because damage to the eye can occur very quickly and a delay in treatment may lead to serious eye damage or blindness.
- An automated external defibrillator (AED) is a type of defibrillator that allows persons with very little training the ability to provide shocks to a victim who is in ventricular fibrillation.
- Foreign body airway obstruction (FBOA) causes asphyxia and can be terrifying to the patient. It can result in rapid loss of consciousness and death if the symptoms are not immediately detected and treated. Choking is the physiological response to airways obstruction.
- Diabetic emergencies can be very serious and even life-threatening. Diabetic coma is a life-threatening condition in which the patient's blood sugar is dangerously high, causing the patient to go into a coma. Insulin shock is a life-threatening condition in which the patient's blood sugar drops to a dangerously low level, causing the patient to go into shock.
- A fracture is a broken bone (partial or complete), usually the result of major trauma or injury, and requires medical attention.
- Poisonings can be very serious and may progress into a respiratory or cardiac emergency. More than 90 percent of poisonings occur in the home and over 50 percent of poisonings occur among children under the age of six.
- Seizures are sudden attacks that result from a malfunction of the brain. There are two major types of seizures: petite mal seizures and grand mal seizures.
- Shock is a potentially fatal condition that can be brought on by disease, injury, decrease in circulation, and fluid loss. During shock, organs and tissues of the body receive an inadequate flow of blood, depriving the organs and tissues of oxygen.
- Early symptoms of shock include a rapid, weak pulse and clammy skin. As shock progresses, symptoms progress to include confusion, chest pain, dyspnea, and eventually unconsciousness.
- A stroke, brain attack, or cerebrovascular accident (CVA), are terms that refer to a blockage or bleeding within the blood vessels of the brain.
- Acting "F.A.S.T." can help stroke patients get the treatments they desperately need. The most effective stroke treatments are only available if the stroke is recognized and diagnosed within three hours of the first symptoms.
- Syncope is a brief episode of unconsciousness or fainting. Fainting is not a disease but rather a symptom of an underlying condition or disease.
- Vertigo is a "spinning" sensation or feeling "dizzy" that is most frequently caused by an inner ear problem.
- Closed wounds include bruises, hematomas, strains, and sprains; in general, soft tissue injuries.
- Open wounds and abrasions are superficial scrapes that may be very painful.
- Because certain temperature-related emergencies can be life-threatening, they are listed under life-threatening emergencies.
- There are three heat-related emergencies or conditions that are brought on by heat exposure: (1) heat cramps, (2) heat exhaustion, and (3) heat stroke.

- Cold-related emergencies include frostbite and hypothermia.
- Fractures, strains, sprains, and dislocations (musculoskeletal injuries) are common emergencies seen in an outpatient or urgent care clinic.
- Asthma is a chronic lung disease that causes the bronchial tubes to constrict and blocks the flow of air to and from the lungs.
- Hyperventilation is the rapid or deep breathing that often occurs with panic or anxiety.
- Animal bite reporting requirements vary by state. Medical assistants should refer to the health department for the state they are working in to become familiar with reporting requirements.
- As a medical assistant, you will need to remember that a patient who suffers an allergic reaction to an insect bite or sting could go into anaphylactic shock if untreated. Immediately contact your provider, and reference the triage/algorithm instructions.
- Head and neck injuries are very serious due to the risk of paralysis and possibly death and should be assessed and treated immediately. Spinal cord injuries (SCI) are very serious because any additional movement can cause significant damage to the already injured vertebrae and spinal cord. Patients that sustain traumatic head and spinal injuries are usually transported by EMS to the nearest trauma center.

CERTIFICATION REVIEW QUESTIONS

1. _________ is a brief episode of unconsciousness or fainting.
   a. Stroke
   b. Syncope
   c. TIA
   d. Mini-stroke
2. Defibrillation is performed on:
   a. adults.
   b. children older than 8.
   c. infants.
   d. Both a and b
3. Which of the following would indicate the proper triage order for the conditions listed below?
   a. Sore throat, asthma attack, non-life-threatening bleeding emergency, emotional crisis
   b. Asthma attack, emotional crisis, non-life-threatening bleeding emergency, sore throat
   c. Asthma attack, non-life-threatening bleeding emergency, emotional crisis, sore throat
   d. Emotional crisis, asthma attack, non-life-threatening bleeding emergency, sore throat
4. Which of the following symptoms are not associated with diabetic coma?
   a. Rapid and pounding pulse
   b. Skin which is red, hot, and dry
   c. A fruity odor coming from the mouth
   d. Drowsiness
5. _____________________ is the rapid or deep breathing that often occurs with panic or anxiety.
   a. Hyperventilation
   b. Hypotension
   c. Hypertension
   d. Hypothyroidism
6. Acting "F.A.S.T." can help stroke patients get the treatments they desperately need. The acronym F.A.S.T. stands for:
   a. Fast—Action—Speed—Trauma.
   b. Fast—Action—Speech—Time.
   c. Face—Arms—Speech—Time.
   d. Face—Action—Speed—Trauma.
7. Heat-related symptoms of a temperature of 104°F (40°C) or higher, general weakness, initial deep respirations that change to shallow respirations, is referred to as:
   a. heat cramps.
   b. heat exhaustion.
   c. heat stroke.
   d. overheating.
8. Which blood vessel(s) involved in a bleeding emergency display the symptoms of dark red blood due to low oxygen levels and does not usually spurt out, but will flow steadily?
   a. Artery
   b. Vein
   c. Capillary
   d. All of the above

9. Diabetic ketoacidosis is presents as which of the following?
   a. Low blood sugar; causes include an overdose of insulin or hypoglycemic medications, vomiting/diarrhea, lack of food/dieting, or excessive exercising.
   b. Immediate onset.
   c. Pulse is full and pounding.
   d. High blood sugar; causes include excessive eating, not taking insulin or oral hypoglycemic, fever/infections, and stress.

10. ________________________ is a severe allergic reaction to an allergen usually in the form of a food, medication, chemical, or insect sting or bite.
    a. Anaphylaxis
    b. Ketoacidosis
    c. Hyperallergenic reaction
    d. All of the above

STUDY RESOURCES

Resources to Test and Reinforce Your Knowledge:	
Certification Review Questions	Take this end-of-chapter quiz
Workbook	• Complete the activities for Chapter 33 • Perform the procedure for Chapter 33 using the Competency Checklist
Resources to Promote Critical Thinking:	
***Solve the Case* Activities**	• Consider these case studies and discuss your conclusions
Learning Lab	• Module 26: Emergencies and First Aid
MindTap	• Complete Chapter 33 readings and activities

REFERENCES

American Academy of Allergy Asthma & Immunology (n.d.). Drug allergy overview. Retrieved April 13, 2015, from http://www.aaaai.org/conditions-and-treatments/allergies/drug-allergy.aspx

American Stroke Association (n.d.). Spot a Stroke. Retrieved January 14, 2015, from http://www.strokeassociation.org/STROKEORG/WarningSigns/Stroke-Warning-Signs-and-Symptoms_UCM_308528_SubHomePage.jsp

Anonymous (n.d.). Choking and Foreign Body Airway Obstruction (FBAO). Retrieved January 14, 2015, from http://www.patient.co.uk/doctor/choking-and-foreign-body-airway-obstruction-fbao

Blesi, M. (2017). *Medical assisting: Administrative & clinical competencies* (8th ed.). Clifton Park, NY: Cengage Learning.

Brigham and Women's Hospital (n.d.). Types of Fractures. Retrieved January 14, 2015 from http://healthlibrary.brighamandwomens.org/RelatedItems/89,P07392

Centers for Disease Control and Prevention (n.d.). Ticks. Retrieved January 14, 2015, from http://www.cdc.gov/ticks/

Food Allergy Research & Education (n.d.). About Food Allergies. Retrieved April 10, 2015, from www.foodallergy.org/allergens

Lindh, W. et al. (2014). *Delmar's comprehensive medical assisting: Administrative and clinical competencies* (5th ed.). Clifton Park, NY: Cengage Learning.

Mayo Clinic (n.d.). Diabetic Ketoacidosis. Retrieved January 14, 2015, from http://www.mayoclinic.org/diseases-conditions/diabetic-ketoacidosis/basics/definition/CON-20026470?p=1

Purdue University (n.d.). Biological Waste. Retrieved January 14, 2015, from http://www.purdue.edu/ehps/rem/eh/biowaste.htm

U.S. Department of Labor Occupational Safety and Health Administration (n.d.). (Lack of) Personal Protective Equipment. Retrieved January 12, 2015, from https://www.osha.gov/SLTC/etools/hospital/hazards/ppe/ppe.html

U.S. Department of Labor Occupational Safety and Health Administration (n.d.). Needlestick/Sharps Injuries. Retrieved January 12, 2015, from https://www.osha.gov/SLTC/etools/hospital/hazards/sharps/sharps.html#needlestick_injuries

U.S. Environmental Protection Agency (n.d.). Medical Waste. Retrieved January 14, 2015 from http://www.epa.gov/osw/nonhaz/industrial/medical/index.htm

U.S. National Library of Medicine National Institutes of Health (n.d.). Animal Bites. Retrieved January 14, 2015, from http://www.nlm.nih.gov/medlineplus/animalbites.html

U.S. National Library of Medicine National Institutes of Health (n.d.). Heimlich maneuver. Retrieved January 14, 2015, from http://www.nlm.nih.gov/medlineplus/ency/article/000047.htm

U.S. National Library of Medicine National Institutes of Health (n.d.). Hyperventilation. Retrieved January 14, 2015, from http://www.nlm.nih.gov/medlineplus/ency/article/003071.htm

WebMD (n.d.). Brain & Nervous System Health Center (Vertigo). Retrieved January 14, 2015, from http://www.webmd.com/brain/vertigo-symptoms-causes-treatment

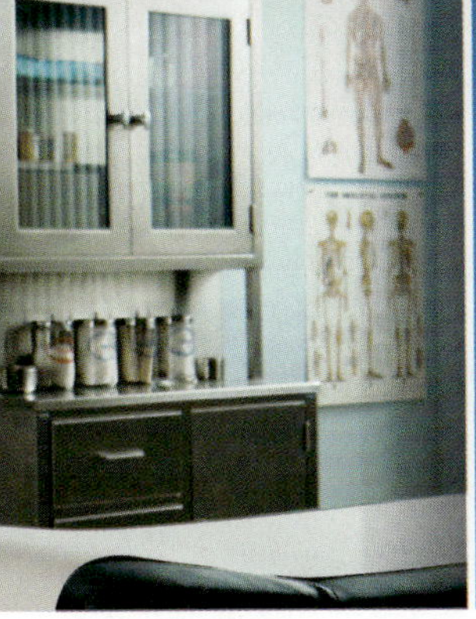

Appendix A

Medical Abbreviations

Common Charting Abbreviations

ADL; ADLs	activities of daily living
ADM	admit; admission; admitted
AM	before noon; morning
ant.	anterior
AP	anterior/posterior
ax	axillary
BCP	birth control pills
BM	bowel movement; bone marrow; breast milk
BMI	body mass index
BP	blood pressure
BSE	breast self-examination
c̄; c; W	with
CC	chief complaint
c/o	complains of
CPE	complete physical exam
def	deficiency
DNS/NS	did not show/no show
DOB	date of birth
Dx	diagnosis
EDC	expected date of confinement
EDD	expected date of delivery
EMS	emergency medical services
Ex	exam
FB	foreign body
FH	family history
FHS/FHT	fetal heart sounds/fetal heart tones
FTT	failure to thrive
HA	headache; hearing aid
H/O	history of
H & P	history and physical
HPI	history of present illness
Hx; hx	history
LMP	last menstrual period
Lt or Ⓛ	left
neg	negative
NKA	no known allergies
NKDA	no known drug allergies
N/V	nausea and vomiting
OV	office visit
PA	posterior-anterior
PH	past history
PX or PE	physical exam
PM	afternoon, evening, or night
Post-op	postoperative
Pt.	patient
R/O	rule out
ROM	range of motion
Rt or Ⓡ	right
Rx	prescription drug
s̄	without
SH	social history
Spec	specimen
SOAP	subjective, objective, assessment(s), plan(s)
SOB	shortness of breath
S & S	signs and symptoms
STAT; stat	immediately
Sx	symptom
UCHD	usual childhood diseases
VO	verbal order
w̄	with
w/o	without
WNL	within normal limits
yr	year

Common Laboratory Abbreviations

ABG	arterial blood gases
ACTH	adrenocorticotropic hormone
ADH	antidiuretic hormone
ALB; Alb	albumin
ALP	alkaline phosphatase
ALT	alanine aminotransferase
ANA	antinuclear antibody
aPTT	activated partial thromboplastin time
Bx	biopsy
BUN	blood, urea, nitrogen
C & S	culture and sensitivity
Ca or Ca^{2+}	calcium
CBC	complete blood count
CEA	carcinoembryonic antigen
CK	creatinine kinase
CMV	cytomegalovirus
CO	carbon monoxide
CO_2	carbon dioxide
CPK	creatine phosphokinase
CRP	c reactive protein
CR	creatinine
CSF	cerebrospinal fluid
DIFF	differential
EBV	Epstein Barr virus
ELISA	enzyme-linked immunosorbent assay
ETOH; EtOH	ethyl alcohol
ESR	erythrocyte sedimentation rate
FBS	fasting blood sugar
FPG	fasting plasma glucose
Fe or Fe^{2+}	iron
FSH	follicle-stimulating hormone
GC	gonorrhea culture or gonorrhea/chlamydia
GTT	glucose tolerance test
Hgb, hb, or hgb	hemoglobin
$HbA1_c$ or $HgA1_c$ or $A1_c$	hemoglobin $A1_c$
HCG; hCG	human chorionic gonadotropin hormone
HCT; Hct	hematocrit
HDL	high-density lipoprotein
HGH	human growth hormone
HIV	human immunodeficiency virus
H Pylori	*Helicobacter pylori* bacterium
INR	international normalized ratio
K or K^+	potassium
Lab	laboratory
LDH	lactate dehydrogenase
LDL	low-density lipoprotein
LFT	liver function test
Mag or Mg	magnesium
MCH	mean corpuscular hemoglobin
MCHC	mean corpuscular hemoglobin concentration
MCV	mean corpuscular volume
Na	sodium
OGTT	oral glucose tolerance test
P	phosphorus
Pap	Papanicolaou test
PAT	preadmission testing
PBI	protein-bound iodine
PKU	phenylketonuria
POL	physician's office laboratory
PPE	personal protective equipment
PSA	prostate-specific antigen
PT	prothrombin time
PTT	partial thromboplastin time
QA	quality assurance
QC	quality control
qns	quantity nonsufficient
qs	quantity sufficient
RA	rheumatoid arthritis
RBC or rbc	red blood cell
RBS	random blood sugar
RF	rheumatoid factor
RPR	rapid plasma regain test
Sed rate	sedimentation rate
sp gr	specific gravity
Staph	staphylococcus
Strep	streptococcus
STS	serological test for syphilis
TC	throat culture
TP	total protein
TSH	thyroid stimulating hormone
T3	triiodothyronine
T4	thyroxine
UA	urinalysis; uric acid
UC	urine culture
VDRL	venereal disease reference lab
WBC or wbc	white blood cell
WNL	within normal limits

Common In-Office Procedure Abbreviations

AP	apical pulse
BP	blood pressure
Drg or Drsg	dressing
DVA	distance visual acuity
ECG or EKG	electrocardiogram
HC	head circumference
Ht	height
NVA	near visual acuity
P	pulse
PFT	pulmonary function testing
R	respiration(s)
SaO_2	oxygen saturation
T	temperature
TPR	temperature, pulse, and respiration
VA	visual acuity
VC	vital capacity
VS	vital signs
Wt	weight

Common Medication Abbreviations

a	before
ac	before meals
amp	ampule
bid	twice a day
$\bar{c}$	with
cap(s)	capsule(s)
DAW	dispense as written
DS	double strength
D/W	distilled water
elix	elixir
emul	emulsion
fl.	fluid
fl. oz.	fluid ounce
hs	hours of sleep or bedtime
ID	intradermal
IM	intramuscular
Inj	injection
IT	inhalation therapy
IV	intravenous
IVP	intravenous push
IVPB	intravenous piggyback
NKDA	no known drug allergies
NPO	nothing by mouth
p	after
pc	after meals
PDR	*Physicians' Desk Reference*
PO or po	by mouth
PR	per rectum
PRN or prn	as needed
q	every
qAM	every morning
qhr	every hour
qid	four times a day
qnoc	every night
Rx	prescription
$\bar{s}$	without
sig	let it be labeled
sol	solution
STAT	immediately
Subcut, Sub-Q, or SQ	subcutaneous
supp	suppository
syr	syrup
tab(s)	tablet(s)
tid	three times daily
tinc	tincture
TPN	total parenteral nutrition
Ung	ointment
W/O	without

Common Measurement Abbreviations

g	gram
gt	drop
gtt	drops
kg	kilogram
IU (Do not use abbreviation)	international units
lb	pounds
L	liter
mcg	microgram
mEq	milliequivalent
mg	milligram
mL	milliliter
ng	nanogram

Common Symbols

△	change
↓	decrease
'	foot
○ or ♀	female
"	inch
↑	increase
Ⓛ	left
□ or ♂	male
⊖	negative
∅	none or negative
#	number
○	pint
⊕	positive
Ⓡ	right

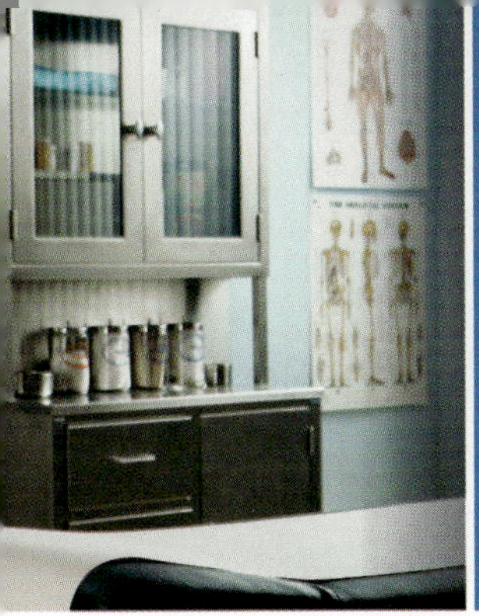

Appendix B

ISMP's List of *Error-Prone Abbreviations, Symbols,* and *Dose Designations*

The abbreviations, symbols, and dose designations found in this table have been reported to ISMP through the ISMP National Medication Errors Reporting Program (ISMPMERP) as being frequently misinterpreted and involved in harmful medication errors. They should **NEVER** be used when communicating medical information. This includes internal communications, telephone/verbal prescriptions, computer-generated labels, labels for drug storage bins, medication administration records, as well as pharmacy and prescriber computer order entry screens.

Abbreviations	Intended Meaning	Misinterpretation	Correction
μg	Microgram	Mistaken as "mg"	Use "mcg"
AD, AS, AU	Right ear, left ear, each ear	Mistaken as OD, OS, OU (right eye, left eye, each eye)	Use "right ear," "left ear," or "each ear"
OD, OS, OU	Right eye, left eye, each eye	Mistaken as AD, AS, AU (right ear, left ear, each ear)	Use "right eye," "left eye," or "each eye"
BT	Bedtime	Mistaken as "BID" (twice daily)	Use "bedtime"
cc	Cubic centimeters	Mistaken as "u" (units)	Use "mL"
D/C	Discharge or discontinue	Premature discontinuation of medications if D/C (intended to mean "discharge") has been misinterpreted as "discontinued" when followed by a list of discharge medications	Use "discharge" and "discontinue"
IJ	Injection	Mistaken as "IV" or "intrajugular"	Use "injection"
IN	Intranasal	Mistaken as "IM" or "IV"	Use "intranasal" or "NAS"
HS **hs**	Half-strength At bedtime, hours of sleep	Mistaken as bedtime Mistaken as half-strength	Use "half-strength" or "bedtime"
IU**	International unit	Mistaken as IV (intravenous) or 10 (ten)	Use "units"
o.d. or OD	Once daily	Mistaken as "right eye" (OD-oculus dexter), leading to oral liquid medications administered in the eye	Use "daily"
OJ	Orange juice	Mistaken as OD or OS (right or left eye); drugs meant to be diluted in orange juice may be given in the eye	Use "orange juice"
Per os	By mouth, orally	The "os" can be mistaken as "left eye" (OS-oculus sinister)	Use "PO," "by mouth," or "orally"
q.d. or QD**	Every day	Mistaken as q.i.d., especially if the period after the "q" or the tail of the "q" is misunderstood as an "i"	Use "daily"
qhs	Nightly at bedtime	Mistaken as "qhr" or every hour	Use "nightly"
qn	Nightly or at bedtime	Mistaken as "qh" (every hour)	Use "nightly" or "at bedtime"
q.o.d. or QOD**	Every other day	Mistaken as "q.d." (daily) or "q.i.d. (four times daily) if the "o" is poorly written	Use "every other day"
q1d	Daily	Mistaken as q.i.d. (four times daily)	Use "daily"
q6PM, etc.	Every evening at 6 PM	Mistaken as every 6 hours	Use "daily at 6 PM" or "6 PM daily"
SC, SQ, sub q	Subcutaneous	SC mistaken as SL (sublingual); SQ mistaken as "5 every;" the "q" in "sub q" has been mistaken as "every" (e.g., a heparin dose ordered "sub q 2 hours before surgery" misunderstood as every 2 hours before surgery)	Use "subcut" or "subcutaneously"
ss	Sliding scale (insulin) or ½ (apothecary)	Mistaken as "55"	Spell out "sliding scale;" use "one-half" or "½"
SSRI **SSI**	Sliding scale regular insulin Sliding scale insulin	Mistaken as selective-serotonin reuptake inhibitor Mistaken as Strong Solution of Iodine (Lugol's)	Spell out "sliding scale (insulin)"
i/d	One daily	Mistaken as "tid"	Use "1 daily"
TIW or tiw	3 times a week	Mistaken as "3 times a day" or "twice in a week"	Use "3 times weekly"
U or u**	Unit	Mistaken as the number 0 or 4, causing a 10-fold overdose or greater (e.g., 4U seen as "40" or 4u seen as "44"); mistaken as "cc" so dose given in volume instead of units (e.g., 4u seen as 4cc)	Use "unit"
UD	As directed ("ut dictum")	Mistaken as unit dose (e.g., diltiazem 125 mg IV infusion "UD" misinterpreted as meaning to give the entire infusion as a unit [bolus] dose)	Use "as directed"
Dose Designations and Other Information	**Intended Meaning**	**Misinterpretation**	**Correction**
Trailing zero after decimal point (e.g., 1.0 mg)**	1 mg	Mistaken as 10 mg if the decimal point is not seen	Do not use trailing zeros for doses expressed in whole numbers
"Naked" decimal point (e.g., .5 mg)**	0.5 mg	Mistaken as 5 mg if the decimal point is not seen	Use zero before a decimal point when the dose is less than a whole unit
Abbreviations such as mg. or mL. with a period following the abbreviation	mg mL	The period is unnecessary and could be mistaken as the number 1 if written poorly	Use mg, mL, etc. without a terminal period

Dose Designations and Other Information	Intended Meaning	Misinterpretation	Correction
Drug name and dose run together (especially problematic for drug names that end in "l" such as Inderal40 mg; Tegretol300 mg)	Inderal 40 mg Tegretol 300 mg	Mistaken as Inderal 140 mg Mistaken as Tegretol 1300 mg	Place adequate space between the drug name, dose, and unit of measure
Numerical dose and unit of measure run together (e.g., 10mg, 100mL)	10 mg 100 mL	The "m" is sometimes mistaken as a zero or two zeros, risking a 10- to 100-fold overdose	Place adequate space between the dose and unit of measure
Large doses without properly placed commas (e.g., 100000 units; 1000000 units)	100,000 units 1,000,000 units	100000 has been mistaken as 10,000 or 1,000,000; 1000000 has been mistaken as 100,000	Use commas for dosing units at or above 1,000, or use words such as 100 "thousand" or 1 "million" to improve readability
Drug Name Abbreviations	**Intended Meaning**	**Misinterpretation**	**Correction**
To avoid confusion, do not abbreviate drug names when communicating medical information. Examples of drug name abbreviations involved in medication errors include:			
APAP	acetaminophen	Not recognized as acetaminophen	Use complete drug name
ARA A	vidarabine	Mistaken as cytarabine (ARA C)	Use complete drug name
AZT	zidovudine (Retrovir)	Mistaken as azathioprine or aztreonam	Use complete drug name
CPZ	Compazine (prochlorperazine)	Mistaken as chlorpromazine	Use complete drug name
DPT	Demerol-Phenergan-Thorazine	Mistaken as diphtheria-pertussis-tetanus (vaccine)	Use complete drug name
DTO	Diluted tincture of opium, or deodorized tincture of opium (Paregoric)	Mistaken as tincture of opium	Use complete drug name
HCl	hydrochloric acid or hydrochloride	Mistaken as potassium chloride (The "H" is misinterpreted as "K")	Use complete drug name unless expressed as a salt of a drug
HCT	hydrocortisone	Mistaken as hydrochlorothiazide	Use complete drug name
HCTZ	hydrochlorothiazide	Mistaken as hydrocortisone (seen as HCT250 mg)	Use complete drug name
MgSO4**	magnesium sulfate	Mistaken as morphine sulfate	Use complete drug name
MS, MSO4**	morphine sulfate	Mistaken as magnesium sulfate	Use complete drug name
MTX	methotrexate	Mistaken as mitoxantrone	Use complete drug name
PCA	procainamide	Mistaken as patient controlled analgesia	Use complete drug name
PTU	propylthiouracil	Mistaken as mercaptopurine	Use complete drug name
T3	Tylenol with codeine No. 3	Mistaken as liothyronine	Use complete drug name
TAC	triamcinolone	Mistaken as tetracaine, Adrenalin, cocaine	Use complete drug name
TNK	TNKase	Mistaken as "TPA"	Use complete drug name
ZnSO4	zinc sulfate	Mistaken as morphine sulfate	Use complete drug name
Stemmed Drug Names	**Intended Meaning**	**Misinterpretation**	**Correction**
"Nitro" drip	nitroglycerin infusion	Mistaken as sodium nitroprusside infusion	Use complete drug name
"Norflox"	norfloxacin	Mistaken as Norflex	Use complete drug name
"IV Vanc"	intravenous vancomycin	Mistaken as Invanz	Use complete drug name
Symbols	**Intended Meaning**	**Misinterpretation**	**Correction**
ʒ ♏	Dram Minim	Symbol for dram mistaken as "3" Symbol for minim mistaken as "mL"	Use the metric system
x3d	For three days	Mistaken as "3 doses"	Use "for three days"
> and <	Greater than and less than	Mistaken as opposite of intended; mistakenly use incorrect symbol; "< 10" mistaken as "40"	Use "greater than" or "less than"
/ (slash mark)	Separates two doses or indicates "per"	Mistaken as the number 1 (e.g., "25 units/10 units" misread as "25 units and 110" units)	Use "per" rather than a slash mark to separate doses
@	At	Mistaken as "2"	Use "at"
&	And	Mistaken as "2"	Use "and"
+	Plus or and	Mistaken as "4"	Use "and"
°	Hour	Mistaken as a zero (e.g., q2° seen as q 20)	Use "hr," "h," or "hour"
Φ or ⊘	zero, null sign	Mistaken as numerals 4, 6, 8, and 9	Use 0 or zero, or describe intent using whole words

**These abbreviations are included on The Joint Commission's "minimum list" of dangerous abbreviations, acronyms, and symbols that must be included on an organization's "Do Not Use" list, effective January 1, 2004. Visit www.jointcommission.org for more information about this Joint Commission requirement.

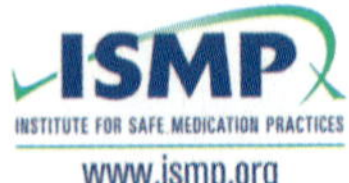

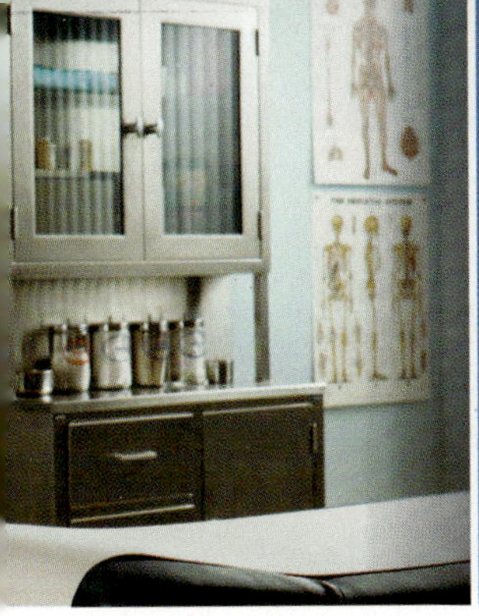

Appendix C

Top 50 Drugs (based on number of prescriptions)

DRUG NAME	OTHER NAME	CLASSIFICATION	SCHEDULE	USUAL DOSE
Adalimumab	Humira	DMARD: Tumor necrosis factor inhibitor	None	40 mg injected subcutaneously every 2 weeks
Albuterol HFA	Proair HFA; Proventil HFA; Ventolin HFA	Short-acting beta-2 agonist	None	90 mcg/spray 1–2 puffs inhaled every 4–6 hours
Amphetamine / dextroamphetamine	Adderall; Adderall XR	Stimulant	Schedule II	5–30 mg immediate release by mouth divided one to three times daily; 20–60 mg extended release tabs by mouth daily
Aripiprazole	Abilify	Second generation antipsychotic	None	2–30 mg by mouth daily 9.75–15 mg intramuscularly once
Aspart	Novolog	Short-acting insulin	None	0.5–1 Unit/kg/day divided based on individual need
Budesonide	Uceris (oral, foam); Pulmicort (inhaled)	Corticosteroid	None	9 mg oral daily; 2 mg foam rectally twice daily; 180–720 mcg inhaled twice daily
Budesonide / formoterol	Symbicort	Corticosteroid / Long-acting beta-2 agonist	None	80–160/4.5 mcg spray two puffs inhaled twice daily
Buprenorphine / Naloxone	Suboxone; Bunavail; Zubsolv	Opioid agonist / opioid antagonist	Schedule III	4–24 mg/1–6 ml tablet sublingually daily
Celecoxib	Celebrex	NSAID: Selectively inhibits cyclooxygenase-2 prostaglandin synthesis	None	50–400 mg by mouth daily
Cyclosporine ophthalmic	Restasis	Immunomodulator	None	0.05% Suspension 1 drop in each eye every 12 hours
Dabigatran etexilate	Pradaxa	Thrombin inhibitor	None	150 mg by mouth twice daily
Detemir	Levemir	Long-acting insulin	None	0.1–0.2 units/kg divided 1–2 times daily; individualized dosing
Dexlansoprazole	Dexilant; Kapidex	Proton pump inhibitor	None	30–60 mg by mouth daily
Doxycycline	Acticlate; Adoxa; Avidoxy; Doryx; Monodox; Oracea; Periostat; Vibramycin	Antibiotics: Tetracycline	None	20–200 mg by mouth 1–2 times daily; 100 mg by mouth twice daily

continues

DRUG NAME	OTHER NAME	CLASSIFICATION	SCHEDULE	USUAL DOSE
Duloxetine	Cymbalta	Serotonin Norepinephrine reuptake inhibitor	None	60–120 mg by mouth daily
Enoxaparin	Lovenox	Anticoagulant; long-acting heparin	None	30 mg subcutaneously every 12 hours; 40 mg subcutaneously daily; 0.75–1 mg/kg subcutaneously daily
Esomeprazole	Nexium	Proton pump inhibitor	None	20–40 mg by mouth 1 hour prior to meal once daily
Etanercept	Enbrel	DMARD: Tumor necrosis factor inhibitor	None	50 mg injected subcutaneously weekly
Ezetimibe	Zetia	Inhibits the absorption of cholesterol in small intestine	None	10 mg by mouth daily
Ezetimibe / simvastatin	Vytorin	Cholesterol combination medication	None	10/10–80 mg by mouth at night
Fenofibrate	Fenoglide; Lipofen; Lofibra; Tricor; Triglide	Inhibits triglyceride synthesis	None	48–160 mg by mouth daily
Fluticasone propionate	1. Flovent HFA 2. Flovent Diskus	Corticosteroid	None	1. 44–220 mcg/spray 2 puffs inhaled twice daily 2. 100–250 mcg/actuation DPI 1–2 puffs inhaled twice daily
Fluticasone propionate / Salmeterol	Advair Diskus	Corticosteroid / Long-acting beta-2 agonist	None	100–500 mcg/50 mg 1 puff inhaled twice daily
Hydrocodone / Acetaminophen	Hycet, Lorcet, Lortab, Norco, Vicodin, Zamicet, Zydone	Opioid combination	Schedule II	2.5–10/300–325 mg; 7.5–10/ 325 mg/15 ml
Infliximab	Remicade	Immunomodulary : Inhibits tumor necrosis factor alpha	None	3–10 mg/kg intravenously at variable intervals
Insulin glargine	Lantus ; Toujeo	Long-acting insulin	None	10–50 units injected subcutaneously once to twice daily
Ipratropium bromide / albuterol	Combivent; Duoneb	Anticholinergic / Short-acting beta-2 agonist	None	0.5/2.5 mg/3 ml nebulized treatment inhaled every 6 hours; 20/100 mcg/spray 1 puff inhaled every 6 hours
Levothyroxine	Levothroid; Levoxyl; Synthroid; Tirosint; Unithroid	Hormone	None	25–300 mcg pills by mouth daily
Lidocaine	Xylocaine	Local anesthetic: Inhibits sodium ion channels in nerve cells		Depends on formulation. Viscous lidocaine 1 ml swish, gargle, spit up to 4 times daily
Lisdexamfetamine	Vyvanse	ADD/ADHD: Stimulant	Schedule II	10–70 mg by mouth daily
Lispro	Humalog	Short-acting insulin	None	0.5–1 Unit/kg/day divided based on individual need
1. Metoprolol succinate 2. Metoprolol tartrate	1. Toprol XL 2. Lopressor	Beta-blocker: cardiac specific	None	1. 25–400 mg by mouth daily 2. 50–225 mg by mouth twice daily

continues

DRUG NAME	OTHER NAME	CLASSIFICATION	SCHEDULE	USUAL DOSE
Memantine	Namenda	*N*-methyl-D-aspartate receptor blocker	None	5–20 mg by mouth daily
Methylphenidate	Concerta; Metadate; Methylin; Quillivant; Ritalin	ADD/ADHD: Stimulant	Schedule II	5–15 mg immediate release tabs by mouth twice to three times daily; 10–60 mg extended release tabs by mouth one to two times daily
Mometasone nasal	Nasonex	Corticosteroid	None	0.05% suspension (50 mcg/spray) 2 spray in each nostril daily
Olmesartan medoxomil	Benicar	Angiotensin II receptor blocker	None	5–40 mg by mouth daily
Omega-3-acid ethyl esters	Lovaza	Reduces triglyceride synthesis	None	4 grams by mouth daily
Oseltamivir	Tamiflu	Influenza neuraminidase inhibitor	None	30–75 mg by mouth daily to twice daily
Oxycodone extended release	OxyContin	Opioid	Schedule II	Individualized dosing
Pregabalin	Lyrica	Antiepileptic	Schedule V	25–300 mg by mouth 2–3 times daily (max of 600mg daily)
Raloxifene	Evista	Osteoporosis: Estrogen receptor modulator	None	60 mg by mouth daily
Rivaroxaban	Xarelto	Anticoagulant: Factor Xa blocker	None	10–20 mg by mouth daily
Rosuvastatin	Crestor	Statin: HMG-CoA reductase inhibitor	None	5, 10, 20, 40 mg by mouth at night
Sitagliptin	Januvia	DPP-4 inhibitor : Diabetes	None	100 mg by mouth daily (comes in 25, 50, and 100 mg pills)
Sitagliptin / metformin	Janumet	Diabetes: DPP-4 inhibitor / Biguanides	None	50/500–1000 mg 1 tab by mouth twice daily
Solifenacin	Vesicare	Antispasmodic: Muscarinic receptor antagonist	None	5–10 mg by mouth daily
Tadalafil	Cialis; Adcirca	Phosphodiesterase type 5 inhibitor	None	2.5–20 mg tab by mouth prior to sex; 5 mg by mouth daily for BPH; 40 mg by mouth daily for pulmonary hypertension
Testosterone	AndroGel; Axiron; Fortesta; Testim; Vogelxo	Testosterone hormone	Schedule III	1% gel 4–8 pumps applied to skin; 1.62% gel 1–4 pumps applied to skin
Valsartan	Diovan	Angiotensin II receptor blocker	None	40–320 mg by mouth daily

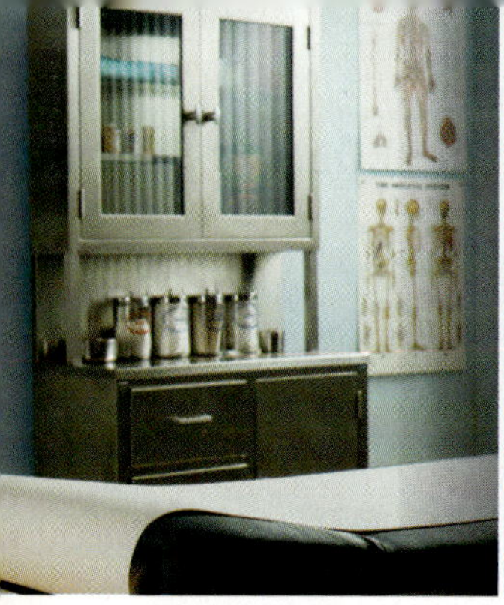

Glossary

A

abnormal uterine bleeding (AUB): AUB has replaced the terms *menorrhagia* (excessive menses) and *merorrhagia* (abnormal timing). AUB is categorized as structural (PALM: Polyps, Adenomyosis, Leiomyoma, and Malignancy) and nonstructural (COEIN: Coagulopathy, Ovulatory dysfunction, Endometrial, Iatrogenic, and Not yet classified)

abortion: termination of pregnancy prior to the fetus becoming viable; may be induced or spontaneous, as in the case of a miscarriage

abrasion: superficial scrape that may be very painful

accountable care organization: organizations made up of a variety of health care providers including doctors, nurse practitioners, social workers, and hospitals that work collaboratively to provide coordinated health care to their patients

accountability: honesty, self-confidence, integrity, and dependability; taking responsibility for one's own actions

Accrediting Bureau of Health Education Schools (ABHES): accrediting organization that oversees accreditation standards for various certifying bodies, such as the American Medical Technologists

Achilles tendonitis: inflammation of the Achilles tendon

activated partial thromboplastin time (aPTT): common coagulation test that measures clotting time in seconds

active listening: listening to focus on the information at hand

activities of daily living (ADLs): activities that are performed on a daily basis such as bathing, dressing, grooming, eating, and walking

acupressure: a method used to stimulate acupoints, using firm pressure to massage the acupoints

acupuncture: a form of traditional Chinese medicine that can be traced back at least 2,500 years and is widely practiced in the United States. Thin needles are placed at specific points in the body to release the flow of the body's vital energy (of "chi") by stimulating points along 14 energy pathways

acupuncturist: a provider who inserts very thin needles through a patient's skin in varying depths at specific points on the body. Licensure varies from state to state

acute abdomen: sudden or abrupt onset of intense abdominal pain

adaptability: an effective change in response to an altered situation

ADA Standards for Accessible Design: federal standards that mandate construction companies to design buildings that are accessible to all persons, including those who have dexterity and limited mobility problems

addendum: an addition or supplement to a previous chart (or progress) note

additive: substance such as a clot activator, separator gel, anticoagulant, or cell preservative that helps to maintain the integrity or function of the specimen

administer: to prepare and personally give the patient a medication through any method at the point of care

adolescent: age classification that is related to the onset of puberty and development of secondary sex characteristics

advance directive: legal documents, such as the living will, durable power of attorney, and health care proxy, that allow people to convey their decisions about end-of-life care ahead of time

aerobic: class of bacteria that require oxygen to grow

afebrile: without fever

affinity: measurement of how tightly a drug attaches or binds to a receptor

agar: gelatin-like substance containing additives and nutrients that support the growth and multiplication of microorganisms

agglutination: antigen–antibody reaction that involves clumping of cells due to the antibody attaching itself to the antigen

aggressive: behavior that means to stand up for your rights, but in a way that violates the rights of others

agonist: drugs that bind to cell receptors and affect or enhance the cell's natural response

algorithm: outlines a detailed sequence of actions to perform in order to accomplish a task; also referred to as a flowsheet

aliquot: portion of the whole specimen used for testing

allergen: defined as a substance that causes an allergic reaction

allergist: a provider who is specially trained to diagnose, treat, and manage allergies, including specialty training to identify factors that trigger allergies or asthma

allograft: tissue grafted from a donor

alternative medicine: refers to using a nonmainstream approach in place of conventional medicine

alternative therapy: using a method (of medicine) other than conventional medicine

Alzheimer's disease: occurs when certain areas of the brain that control thinking, communication, and behavior deteriorate. Some of the deterioration may be caused by a decrease of the neurotransmitter acetylcholine

amenorrhea: absence of menstrual flow

American Association of Medical Assistants (AAMA): professional organization that promotes and certifies medical assistants

American Medical Technologists (AMT): nonprofit certification agency and professional membership association that certifies medical assistants and other health care professionals

American Sign Language (ASL): distinct language for the deaf; considered the native language of the deaf

Americans with Disabilities Act (ADA): act that requires businesses to extend civil rights to people with disabilities similar to those now available on the basis of race, color, sex, national origin, and religion; businesses may not discriminate against persons with disabilities and must provide an environment that accommodates the individual's disability

Americans with Disabilities Act Amendments Act (ADAAA): The act, which became effective January 1, 2009, emphasizes that the definition of disability should be construed in favor of broad coverage of individuals to the maximum extent permitted by the terms of the ADA and generally shall not require extensive analysis. The act made important changes to the definition of the term "disability" by rejecting the holdings in several Supreme Court decisions and portions of EEOC's ADA regulations

amniocentesis: procedure in which a needle is introduced into the amniotic sac through the mother's abdominal wall to withdraw fluid for various lab tests

amplitude: when referring to an ECG, amplitude is the measure of the height of the cardiac deflection or the strength of the contraction

ampule: glass container with a stem that holds a single dose of medication

anaerobic: class of bacteria that do not require oxygen or that cannot grow when oxygen is present

analyte: any substance that is being chemically analyzed

anaphylaxis: advanced systemic or allergic reaction to a chemical, drug, food, or insect sting or bite; symptoms may include bronchial constriction, swelling of the tongue or throat, and an inability to breathe

anastomosis: a surgical connection between two hollow, or tubular structures

anesthetic: medication used to produce a lack of feeling in patients undergoing a surgical procedure

angioedema: swelling under the skin

angiography: visualization of blood vessels after a radiopaque contrast medium has been injected to assess blood flow, blood clots, hemorrhaging and aneurysms

anisocytosis: marked difference in the size of cells, especially red blood cells

anorexia of aging: the loss of appetite for food in the later years of life

anorexia nervosa: eating disorder in which the individual limits its food intake or does not eat at all to the point of starvation

anoscope: type of speculum used to visualize the anus and lower portion of the rectum

antagonist: drugs that prevent or block a cell response

antecubital space: front of the arm (or inside) at the bend of the elbow; site commonly used for venipuncture

anterior cruciate ligament (ACL): the ligament that stabilizes the knee

antibody: protein particle produced by B-lymphocytes of the immune system; attaches to a specific antigen to neutralize or control it

anticoagulant: substance that keeps blood from coagulating or clotting

antigen: invading organism such as a bacterium or virus that stimulates antibody production within the body

antiserum: serum that contains antibodies to a specific antigen, used to perform blood typing

anuria: no urine is being formed by the kidneys

apothecary: term formerly used for a pharmacist or chemist

apothecary system: the original or primary system used for calculating and measuring medication dosages

appearance: the outward or visible portion of a person

aqueous: water-based solution

arrhythmia: an irregular heart rhythm

arthrectomy: a procedure to remove fatty plaque from a coronary artery

arthritis: inflammation of a joint or multiple joints with pain, swelling, stiffness, or deformity

arthroscopy: visualization of a joint and joint capsule through a lighted instrument

artifact: unwanted interference on an ECG tracing

ascites: the abnormal accumulation of serous fluid in the peritoneal cavity

asepsis: free of germs

aspirate: pulling back on the plunger of a syringe to make certain that the needle is not in a blood vessel

aspiration: removal of excess fluid from a body cavity or structure

assertive: being able to articulate and express your ideas, needs, and feelings in a way that is honest and direct; assertive behavior is described as standing up to express your feelings, rights, and thoughts honestly and directly in a way that respects the feelings of other people

assessment: evaluation of the patient through medical questioning, physical examination, diagnostic and other lab testing; when referring to the "SOAP" format, assessment is an interpretation of subjective and objective findings

Assessment Based Recognition in Order Entry (ABR-OE): a program offered by the AAMA that allows noncredentialed medical assistants to gain a credential following successful completion of the program. This allows the medical assistant to enter orders into the electronic health record.

assistive device: device such as a cane, crutches, walker, or wheelchair that helps a patient to walk or move about freely

asthma: chronic lung disease causing the bronchial tubes to constrict and block the flow of air to and from the lungs
astigmatism: abnormal curvature of the cornea causing blurred vision
asymptomatic: without symptoms
atherosclerosis: a buildup of cholesterol, calcium, and other substances in the coronary arteries
atraumatic needle: needle that is packaged with suture material fused to an eyeless needle
atrophy: lack of nutrition causing shrinkage of a muscle
attitude: the way one feels about someone or something
atypical: not normal; nonconforming
audiologist: health care professional trained to identify and treat hearing or balance problems
audiometer: device used to measure hearing acuity at different sound frequencies
augmented lead: a lead on an ECG in which a single positive electrode is referenced against "null point" (a point with little or no significant electronic variation) between the remaining limb electrodes.(aVR, aVL, and aVF)
auricle: external ear
auscultatory gap: an occurrence in which Korotkoff sounds diminish and become inaudible (a period of silence) during phase two or phase three of the blood pressure measurement
auscultation: the act of listening to body sounds with the aid of a stethoscope
autoclave: instrument that sterilizes items by displacing air with steam within its chamber and exposing items to large amounts of heat over a specified time period
autograft: tissue grafted from the patient's own body
automated external defibrillator (AED): defibrillator that is completely automated and easy to use; designed to shock the heart into a normal rhythm during periods of ventricular fibrillation
auxiliary services: aids that assist in the communication process for patients with special needs, especially those with hearing disabilities, such as qualified interpreters, telephone handset amplifiers, assistive listening devices, telephones compatible with hearing aids, closed caption decoders, open and closed captioning, telecommunications devices for deaf persons (TDD), and videotext displays
Ayurveda: the traditional medicine of India that emphasizes reestablishing balance in the body through diet, lifestyle, exercise, cleansing of the body, and on the health of the mind, body, and spirit

B

bacilli: rod-shaped bacteria; may contain spores
bacteria: single-celled microorganisms lacking a nucleus that can cause infections
bandage: wrapping material placed over a dressing or a closed wound
bariatrics: medical practice directed at the prevention and control of obesity as well as associated diseases
baseline: the flat, horizontal line separating two ECG cycles, or the point on an ECG in which there is no electrical activity; also known as the isoelectric line
baseline value: initial results established for the purpose of comparing future results
basophil: type of white blood cell, known as a granulocyte, that contains dark, purplish-black granules in the cytoplasm
benign prostatic hyperplasia (BPH): benign condition in which the prostrate is enlarged
bile: a digestive juice, secreted by the liver for the digestion of fats
bilirubin: orange-yellow pigment found in bile that is formed when RBCs are broken down; found in urine of patients with certain liver diseases
binge: eating behavior where huge amounts of food are consumed
bioavailability: the extent to and the rate at which a drug enters the blood plasma and is made available at the site of action
biofeedback: a therapy used to enable a person to learn to control otherwise involuntary bodily functions, usually with the help of electronic equipment
biohazard: any substance contaminated with blood or body fluids that could transmit disease
bipolar leads: leads on an ECG that record the electrical activity from two limb electrode at the same time (Leads I, II, and III)
bisphosphonates: a class of drugs to prevent loss of bone mass, most often prescribed to treat osteoporosis
bloodborne pathogen: disease-causing microbe found in blood and blood components
blood urea nitrogen (BUN): kidney function indicator test that measures the amount of nitrogen in the blood
body language: gestures, postures, and facial expressions by which a person manifests various physical, mental, or emotional states and communicates nonverbally with others
body mass index (BMI): numerical correlation between a patient's height and weight used to calculate the patient's body fat percentage
body surface area (BSA): most accurate method of calculating drug dosages for infants and children up to 12 years of age
bolus: loading dose of medication that is introduced directly through the vein as opposed to through an access port or IV line
box lock: hinged part of the instrument found on ring handled instruments that contain ratchets
bradycardia: heart rate below 60 beats per minute
bradypnea: abnormally slow breathing
Braxton–Hicks contractions: periodic and painless irregular uterine contractions; not true labor
bronchoscopy: procedure that utilizes a lighted scope to view the lungs
buccal: medication placed between the gums of the upper molars and the inside cheek for rapid absorption into the blood stream

Bucky grid: special film holder that contains a moveable grid that helps to reduce the scatter of secondary radiation during an X-ray

bulimia nervosa: eating disorder in which the individual develops a pattern of consuming large amounts of food (binging) followed by eliminating the food from the body by vomiting, using laxatives, or diuretics (purging)

bursitis: the inflammation of the bursa

business associate agreement: document signed by all business partners that defines how PHI is to be handled

butterfly: small winged needle attached to tubing and an adapter to be used with a syringe or vacuum tube system for venipuncture

C

caesarian section (C-section): delivery of a fetus through a surgical incision into the uterus

calcitonin: a hormone that decreases blood calcium

calipers: instrument used for measuring different parts of the body; body fat calipers are devices that measure skin folds on different parts of the patient's body

campylobacter: a type of bacteria. The most common cause of diarrhea worldwide

cannula: flexible tube that is used to insert medication within a body cavity or blood vessel

capillary puncture: skin puncture method used to obtain small amounts of blood for testing; usually performed on fingertips or great toe

carbohydrates: a primary nutrient essential for cellular function, providing the main source of energy for the body. When carbohydrates are consumed in excess of energy needs, they are converted to fat and stored in the body's fat cells

carcinogen: cancer-causing agent

cardiac ablation: a procedure that destroys electrical tissue in the heart that causes an abnormal rhythm

cardiac catheterization: a procedure in which a long catheter is threaded either from the groin region (femoral artery) or arm region (brachial artery) with the assistance of an X-ray camera (fluoroscopy) to look for occlusions in the blood vessels or heart

cardiac cycle: the time between ventricular contraction and relaxation

cardiac pacemaker: a small device placed in the chest or abdomen to help control arrhythmias

cardiologist: medical doctor who specializes in treating diseases and disorders of the heart and related structures

cardiopulmonary resuscitation (CPR): technique that is used to restore the victim's breathing and heart action when they fail

cardiothoracic surgeon: performs procedures on the heart and great vessels of the heart

cardiovascular surgeon: physician who specializes in performing surgical procedures on the heart and related structures

cardioversion: to restore normal sinus rhythm through the use of medications or electrical current

carpal tunnel syndrome: a syndrome of numbness and pain in the hand and fingers, caused by compression of the median nerve in the wrist

cartilage: connective tissue located between the articular surfaces of the bones, joints, and vertebrae, which acts as a shock absorber

cartridge unit: disposable, prefilled cartridge of medication that slips into a nondisposable injection device

case manager: usually a registered nurse (RN) who can manage and consolidate the information acquired through multiple modalities

cast: (1) device made of plaster or fiberglass used to immobilize a fracture or dislocation; (2) structure sometimes found in the urine due to the accumulation of protein in the renal tubules

catheterization: insertion of a sterile tube directly into the bladder through the urethra to obtain a sterile urine specimen

cell-mediated immunity: type of immunity involving T-lymphocytes, which directly attack cancer cells, fungi, and viruses to make them powerless in the body

Celsius (C): the official scientific measurement of temperature; also called the centigrade scale

Centers for Disease Control and Prevention (CDC): one of the major operating components of the Department of Health and Human Services; responsible for the development of standard precautions and universal precautions

centrifuge: instrument that spins test tubes containing specimens at high speeds to separate and concentrate the components

cerebrovascular accident (CVA): blockage or bleeding within the blood vessels of the brain; also known as a stroke

certification: fulfillment of the necessary requirements of a specific organization to perform specific tasks, usually acquired through an assessment tool such as a test

Certification Commission for Healthcare Information Technology (CCHIT): commission appointed by the U.S. Department of Health and Human Services (HHS) to develop and evaluate the certification criteria and inspection process for EHRs; this commission certifies a vendor's EHR software. In November 2014, CCHIT® ceased testing and certification of EHRs. The reason given by CCHIT® was that it had become difficult to plan new services due to the slowing of the pace of ONC 2014 Edition certification, delays to subsequent meaningful use implementation, and the unreliable timing of future federal health IT requirements

Certified Medical Assistant (AAMA) [CMA (AAMA)]: medical assistant who has passed the medical assisting exam through the American Association of Medical Assistants

cerumen: ear wax

chelation: therapy used to remove excess or toxic metals or minerals from the body using a chemical substance to bind molecules, such as metal or minerals, and hold them tightly so they can be removed from the body

chest circumference: measurement of the chest at the nipple level to screen for physiological abnormalities of the heart and lungs

chief complaint: the reason that the patient is being seen. It is a listing of the patient's symptoms and should be written using the patient's own words whenever possible

child: age classification that correlates with school attendance

chiropractor: providers who practice a drug-free, hands-on health care approach that focuses on the musculoskeletal and nervous systems. The most common procedure performed is "spinal manipulation," also referred to as "chiropractic adjustment." The purpose of chiropractic manipulation is to restore joint mobility

cholangiography: visualization of the bile ducts for detection of possible stones or lesions

cholesterol: type of lipid found in the blood; it is made in the liver and is the major component of bile

choroid layer: the middle layer of the eye; contains blood supply and connective tissue

circumcision: procedure in which the prepuce or foreskin of the penis is cut away; usually performed on newborns

Civil Rights Act: act designed to protect individuals from being discriminated against because of race, color, sex, national origin, or religion

clean-catch midstream (CCMS) specimen: urine specimen collected in a sterile container after cleansing the urinary meatus using only the middle stream of the specimen

clinical diagnosis: identification of a disease or condition from facts obtained through the medical history, physical exam, lab testing, and radiological testing

Clinical Laboratory Improvement Amendment (CLIA '88): legislation enacted to protect the public by regulating all laboratory tests performed on human specimens

clinician: health practitioner such as a physician, physician assistant, or nurse practitioner; can also refer to an individual that works in a clinical setting

closed wound: wound that does not break the skin, such as contusions, hematomas, strains, and sprains

coagulation cascade: a series of steps that occur during the coagulation or clotting process; one step triggers another

cocci: round or spherical shaped bacteria

collaboration: the action of working with someone to accomplish a task or project, or to produce or create something

Colles (fracture): fracture of the distal end of the radius bone in the wrist

collimator: device attached to the X-ray tube that controls the size and shape of the X-ray beam

colonoscopy: examination of the colon with a lighted scope

colostomy: the surgical creation of an artificial excretory opening between the colon and the body surface

colposcopy: visualization of the cervix and vagina through a lighted scope

comminuted (fracture): bone is broken or splintered into fragments

Commission on Accreditation of Allied Health Education Programs (CAAHEP): commission that oversees accreditation standards for various certifying bodies, such as the AAMA

Commission on Office Laboratory Accreditation (COLA): established in 1988 as a private alternative to assist clinical laboratories in complying with the CLIA '88 standards

communication: the exchange of thoughts, messages, or information by speech, signals, writing, or behavior

compassion: to show concern or empathy for another individual

complementary and alternative medicine (CAM): CAM refers to a broad set of health care practices that are not part of that country's own tradition and are not integrated into the dominant health care system

complete blood count (CBC): group of blood tests that includes hemoglobin, hematocrit, red and white blood cell counts, differential count, and red blood cell indices

comprehensive medical history: history covering the patient's personal, social, and family history from the time of birth until the time that the history is developed

compression (fracture): a bone fragment driven inward; seen in skull fractures

computed tomography (CT): radiographic procedure that produces cross-sectional images of the body

computer physician order entry (CPOE): CPOE is an application used by physicians and other health care providers to enter patient care information. Using CPOE for medication and orders will allow results, to be automatically checked for potential errors or problems. CPOE entails the provider's use of computer assistance to directly enter medication orders from a computer or mobile device. The order is also documented or captured in a digital, structured, and computable format for use in improving safety and organization. EHRs with the CPOE feature also provide support tools that result in improved care and patient outcomes. Use of CPOE supports Measure 1 of 13, Stage 1 of Meaningful Use

concentric circle: technique that is used to apply antiseptic; the medical assistant paints the antiseptic directly over the site starting in the center and working to the outer periphery

conceptually accurate signed English (CASE): type of sign language that uses ASL conceptual signs but in English word order

concussion: injury in which the brain is jarred

cones: specialized cells in the eye that are used in bright light and help to process color

confidentiality: to keep secret or private

conjunctiva: the lining over the sclera (the white part of the eye) and the inner eyelids

constipation: defined as having a bowel movement fewer than three times per week

constrict: narrowing of a blood vessel

consumer-mediated exchange: the safest way to communicate with patients via electronic means. The patient portal is an example of a consumer mediated exchange

contact dermatitis: a reaction that appears when the skin comes in contact with an irritant or an allergen

contrast medium: substance that is either injected or ingested prior to X-ray studies that enhances internal structures for better visibility

conversion: to change from one unit to another

coronary artery bypass graft: an artery or vein from another part of the body is connected or graphed to a blocked coronary artery/arteries so that blood can flow around it

coronary artery disease: a condition in which the coronary arteries become sclerotic (hardened) and narrow due to a condition known as atherosclerosis; a buildup of cholesterol, calcium and other substances

cosmetic dermatologist: in addition to those conditions treated by a dermatologist, treatments that fall in to the category of cosmetic dermatology include surgery to diminish acne scars, injecting fillers and botulinum toxins (Botox) to give an aging face a more youthful appearance, chemical peels, and laser surgery to diminish or remove small veins, age spots, and wrinkles

courtesy: showing respect for others and having polished manners

craniosacral therapy: a therapy developed by osteopath physician John Upledger in the 1970s (cranio meaning the head and sacral referring to the area at the base of the spine). Therapists (usually D.O.s) sense the pulse and look for any subtle restrictions in the flow of craniosacral fluid

crash cart: cart that stocks all of the medications and supplies used in an emergency

credentialing: documentation that validates that an individual has been successful in attaining the educational components necessary to perform a specific job title

cryotherapy: therapeutic use of cold modalities to treat an injury or other physical condition

cubic centimeter (cc): metric unit used to measure medications; mL is the preferred measurement

cultural diversity: unique differences in various cultures

culture: to grow and identify microorganisms in a laboratory from a patient sample

culture and sensitivity (C&S) test: test involving bacteria grown on a plate to which antibiotic disks have been added, to determine which drugs the bacteria is sensitive or resistant to

culture medium: material (liquid or solid) containing nutrients that help bacteria to grow

cystitis: inflammation of the bladder

cystoscopy: insertion of a lighted scope into the urethra, which is then directed into the bladder for visual inspection

cytologic: the examination of material for the purposes of cytology

cytology: (1) branch of science dealing with the configuration, structure, and function of cells; (2) laboratory department that performs microscopic examinations of cells, such as pap tests

D

DASH (Dietary Approaches to Stop Hypertension): a diet that can reduce hypertension by limiting sodium, sugars, and red meats

debridement: to remove dead tissue

defibrillation: procedure in which drugs or electrical shock is used to restore normal contractions

dementia: ongoing and irreversible decrease in mental functioning affecting memory, reasoning, and judgment

dentist: a provider who diagnoses and treats the teeth, oral cavity, and associated structures, and treats related diseases including prevention and the restoration of defective and missing tissue (e.g., cosmetic dentistry). Many dentists are now providing anti-aging procedures such as Botox and fillers, such as Juvéderm

dependability: to be reliable, dependable, or trustworthy

depolarization: in reference to the heart, a discharge of electricity that commences the heart to beat

dermatologist: a provider who specializes in assisting patients with itchy skin associated with allergies

diabetic coma: life-threatening condition in which the patient's blood sugar is dangerously high, causing the patient to go into a coma

diabetic ketoacidosis: a serious complication of diabetes that occurs when the body produces high levels of blood acids called ketones, and develops when the body is unable to produce enough insulin

dialysis: procedure in which the patient's blood is passed through a machine that filters out waste products and returns the blood back to the patient's body

diaphoresis: profuse sweating

diastole: phase when the cardiac ventricles relax

diastolic pressure: period of least pressure in the arterial vascular system; the bottom reading of a blood pressure

dietetic technician: a person with an associate degree in foods and nutrition

dietitian: a professional who counsels patients on the special diets that are required for specific diseases

differential count: count of 100 white blood cells on a stained blood smear for the purpose of determining the approximate percentage of each type of white blood cell; red blood cell morphology is also observed

differential diagnosis: identification of a disease or condition by comparing similar symptoms and performing diagnostic and lab tests to identify the unknowns, leading to a final diagnosis

digital rectal exam (DRE): procedure in which the provider inserts his or her gloved finger into the patient's rectum to check the size of the prostate

dignity: showing respect and assurance

dilatation: expansion of a body opening

dilation: expansion of the cervix during labor to facilitate passage of the fetus

diluent: solution used to reconstitute powder

diplomacy: tact or tactfulness; the art or skill of handling negotiations or relations

directed exchange: used by providers to easily and securely send patient information—such as laboratory orders and results, patient referrals, or discharges summaries—directly to another health care professional

disinfection: process of using special liquids or pasteurization techniques on inanimate objects to destroy or inhibit the growth of microorganisms

dislocation: temporary displacement of a bone from its usual position in the joint

dispense: to personally hand the patient a medication to take later; in ambulatory care, drug samples and stock samples are commonly dispensed to patients

dissect: to cut open or cut apart

diurnal rhythms: biological processes or activities, such as hormone secretion, sleeping, feeding, and so on that must be in sync with the day and night cycle

diversity: the condition of having or being composed of differing elements; especially the inclusion of different types of people (as people of different races or cultures) in a group

"Do Not Use" abbreviations list: a list of abbreviations created by the Joint Commission that are commonly misinterpreted and should no longer be used when documenting medication orders within the patient's medical record

dobutamine stress test: for patients who are unable to exercise on a treadmill due to physical limitations or age

doctor of osteopathy (D.O.): both D.O.s and M.D.s are fully qualified physicians licensed to prescribe medication and perform surgery. Osteopathic medicine is a parallel branch of American medicine with a distinct philosophy and approach to patient care, practicing a "whole person" approach. D.O.s focus on preventive health care and have received extra training in the musculoskeletal system. A D.O. incorporates osteopathic manipulative treatment into his or her practice, using their hands to diagnose illness and injury and to encourage the body's natural tendency toward good health

dressing: piece of bandage material placed over an open wound

drug: any substance that produces a change in the function of a living organism; often used in the diagnosis, treatment, or prevention of a disease

drug ceiling: maximum dose at which the drug will provide its greatest effect

drug dosage: strength of the drug or amount to be given

drug interaction: occurs when one drug diminishes or increases the effects of another drug

dynamics: the unconscious, psychological forces that influence the direction of a team's behavior and performance

dysmenorrhea: difficult or painful menstruation

dyspnea: difficult or labored breathing

dysrhythmia: irregularities in heart rhythm

dysuria: painful urination

E

***Escherichia coli*:** a bacteria which is transmitted through contaminated foods that have not been properly cooked

echocardiography: a noninvasive diagnostic test that uses ultrasound to visualize internal cardiac structures

eclampsia: progressed form of preeclampsia that may also include seizures and coma

ectopic: abnormal position; tubal pregnancy

effacement: thinning and shortening of the cervix to permit the fetus to pass through

efficacy: effectiveness of a drug

elder abuse: any abuse and neglect of persons age 60 and older by a caregiver or another person in a relationship involving an expectation of trust

electrocardiogram (ECG or EKG): recording or tracing of the electrical activity of the heart

electrocardiograph: instrument or machine used to record the ECG

electrode: sensors attached to the patient's skin during electrocardiography; designed to detect the electrical activity coming from the heart

electrolyte: solution, gel, or cream that helps to conduct electrical current during an ECG

electron beam CT scan: a scan that takes images of the heart between beats detecting calcium deposits associated with atherosclerosis

electronic health record (EHR): refers to the interoperability of electronic medical records, or the ability to share medical records with other health care facilities; an EHR also integrates the administrative functions (known as practice management) and the clinical functions, typically referred to as EMR; in this textbook we use the term EMR to refer to clinical duties, PM for administrative duties, and EHR for the combined PM/EHR electronic application that is interoperable

electronic medical record (EMR): patient records in a digital format

embolus: air bubble, foreign body, or detached blood clot that makes its way from one part of the body (usually the heart) to the vessels within the brain

emergency preparedness: preparing for potential disasters, including infectious, occupational, environmental, or terrorist threats; may also be referred to as disaster preparedness, emergency management, or disaster management

empathy: to identify with another's feelings and respond with understanding

endocrine: the endocrine system produces hormones through which the body maintains a constant internal environment

endocrinologist: a physician who diagnoses and treats diseases of the endocrine system, which includes the pancreas and the treatment of diabetes

endoscopes: illuminated flexible or sometimes rigid tubes used to view body structures or organs

endoscopic retrograde cholangiopancreatogram (ERCP): a procedure that combines upper gastrointestinal (GI) endoscopy and X-rays to treat problems of the bile and pancreatic ducts

endoscopy: the visual examination of the interior of a body cavity

endospore: inner layer of the wall of a spore found in particular types of bacteria

engagement: encompasses enthusiasm, excellence, work ethic, initiative, and education/credentialing; the emotional commitment an employee has to the organization and its goals

enteral: pertaining to the alimentary canal or intestines; enteral medications are medications that go through the digestive tract

eosinophil: type of white blood cell, known as a granulocyte, that contains orange-red granules in the cytoplasm

epidemiology: the study of infectious diseases and their origin, cause, and patterns of occurrence

epidermis: the outer layer of skin

epinephrine: the only medication that can reverse the symptoms of anaphylaxis

erectile dysfunction (ED): the inability of a man to achieve and maintain an erection during sexual intercourse; also known as impotence

erosion: the wearing away of a surface

erythrocyte: red blood cell; transports oxygen to the cells of the body and carbon dioxide to the lungs

erythrocyte sedimentation rate (ESR): measurement of how far red cells fall in a given amount of blood in one hour

ethics: intangible elements of life we deal with on a daily basis; represents the innate knowledge of right and wrong; an ethical dilemma is where two moral principles are in conflict, such as when there is no clear-cut right or wrong on any matter; it might also be true when the right behavior leads to the wrong outcome

etiology: the study of the causes of disease

evacuated tube: collection tube that contains a vacuum that facilitates the collection of blood during venipuncture

examination: the process of inspecting the body and its systems to determine the presence or absence of disease

exhalation: the exhaling of waste products; breathing out

exocrine: secreting through a duct; related to the exocrine system

expiration: see exhalation

expiration date: date that guarantees the effectiveness and safe use of the medication up to the date posted on the package or container

exploitation: the unauthorized or improper use of the resources of an elder for monetary or personal benefit, profit, or gain

exposure control: plan developed by the employer as part of infection control to protect at risk employees from exposure to blood and OPIM

external controls: evaluates the entire testing process and that the control results are in the expected ranges

extracorporeal: outside the body

extracorporeal shock wave lithotripsy (ESWL): shock waves that break kidney stones down into small particles so that they can pass through the urinary tract with more ease

extravasation: infiltration or leaking of fluid into the tissue around the vein

exudate: fluid secreted by tissue that may include blood, pus, dead cells, and tissue fluid as a result of disease or injury

F

Fahrenheit (F): the standard grade of measurement generally used for temperatures in the United States

familial stature: height or body type that occurs within a family

family medical history: detailed information about the present and past health of the patient's family members

febrile: feverish

fee for service: a delivery model in which the provider is reimbursed according to the type and amount of services provided with no emphasis on patient outcomes

fenestrated: to have one or more openings

fever: abnormal elevation of the body temperature

fiber: that part of plant foods that is not digested

fibrin: fiber-like; forms a network of fibers to help form the needed blood clot

fissure: linear ulcer located on the edge of the anus

fistula: a crack-like sore of the skin surface

flow sheet: log sheet found in the patient's chart that assists the physician in monitoring repetitive information

fluoroscopy: X-ray of moving body structures in real time, similar to a movie

Foley catheter: type of urinary catheter that has a balloon that inflates to keep the catheter in place

fomites: inanimate objects, such as equipment, contaminated with infectious material and capable of transmitting disease

fovea centralis: an area of the retina that allows for the sharpest vision. Contains only cones, no rods

fracture: break in a bone

frostbite: local injury of the skin due to freezing or subfreezing conditions

fungi: group of microorganisms that includes yeasts and molds

G

gastritis: inflammation of the stomach lining

gastroenteritis: inflammation of the mucous membrane lining the stomach and intestines

gastroenterologist: medical doctor that specializes in treating diseases and disorders of the digestive tract and accessory glands

gastroesophageal reflux disease (GERD): a backflow of stomach contents into the esophagus because of a weak sphincter muscle; also known as acid reflux

gauge: diameter of the lumen of a needle

generic name: official name of a drug

genogram: medical family tree

gestation: period of time from conception to birth

gesture: sign, signal, or cue used to communicate in combination with or apart from words

glaucoma: eye disease characterized by an increase in intraocular pressure resulting in possible blindness

gluten: a class of proteins found in grains such as wheat, rye, and barley

glycemic index (GI): measures how quickly carbohydrate foods raise the blood glucose level

gram (g, gm): unit used when measuring anything that has mass or weight

Gram negative: bacteria that stain pink/red during the Gram staining process

Gram positive: bacteria that stain purple during the Gram staining process

Gram stain: special testing method that differentiates bacteria based on their color reactions to various stains

gravida: the number of pregnancies a woman has had, including the current pregnancy

gray (Gy): a measurement of radiation energy per kilogram

greenstick (fracture): bone is bent/partially broken; seen in children

grid: structure located inside the bucky made up of alternating strips of radiolucent and radiopaque material

guide dogs: specially trained dogs that guide their visually impaired or blind owners

H

handle: the part of the instrument that the surgeon uses to hold the instrument

head circumference: measurement that traces the growth of the cranium and the brain

health coach: a person who provides individualized evaluation and subsequent management and encouragement to achieve superior patient health outcomes

health information technology (HIT): the exchange of health information between providers, payers, and consumers in a secure electronic environment

Health Insurance Portability and Accountability Act of 1996 (HIPAA): another name for privacy act; act that governs and protects the handling of protected health information

heat cramp: cramps caused by the body becoming overheated; the least serious of all of the heat emergencies

heat exhaustion: condition in which a victim becomes overheated, causing the victim to sweat and lose large volumes of water and salts

heat stroke: occurs when the body is either unable to cool itself down due to dehydration, physiological conditions, or a progression of heat exhaustion factors that go untreated; may lead to death if untreated

hematochezia: bright red blood in the stool. Usually indicating that the blood is coming from the lower part of the gastrointestinal tract

hematocrit: percentage of packed red blood cells in a given volume of blood

hematoma: swelling or accumulation of blood due to leakage from a blood vessel during or following venipuncture

hematuria: presence of blood in the urine; intact red cells present in the urine upon microscopic examination

hemoconcentration: pooling of blood at the venipuncture site caused by leaving the tourniquet in place too long; may lead to inaccurate test results

hemodialysis: dialysis in which the patient is hooked up to a dialysis unit through tubes that connect to the patient's blood vessels

hemoglobin: pigment in the red blood cells that carries iron and oxygen

hemoglobinuria: blood found in the urine without the presence of intact red blood cells

hemolysis: rupturing of the red blood cells during venipuncture, which releases hemoglobin into the serum or plasma, giving it a reddish appearance

hemorrhaging: uncontrollable bleeding

hemorrhoids: painful, swollen, and bleeding veins in the anal region

hemostasis: stopping the flow of blood

hepatologist: medical doctor that specializes in treating diseases and disorders of the liver

herniation: the protrusion of a structure from its normal position in the body

high-complexity testing: similar to moderate-complexity testing with respect to not being available for home use. In addition, regulations require detailed record keeping, proficiency testing, and biannual inspections

high-density lipoprotein (HDL): lipoprotein that removes cholesterol from the body by taking it to the liver, where it is excreted in bile; "good cholesterol"

history of present illness (HPI): series of symptoms or signs that are related to the patient's complaint

Holter monitor: portable ambulatory ECG worn by the patient for 24 hours to detect cardiac arrhythmias

homeopathy: A 200-year-old system of medicine based on the law of similars: If a dose of a substance can cause a symptom, that same substance in minuscule amounts can cure the symptom

homeostasis: state of equilibrium within the body when systems are functioning normally; state in which the body's internal conditions are able to remain constant in the midst of changing environments

honesty: truthful and sincere

human chorionic gonadotropin (hCG): hormone produced by the fertilized egg that is present in the blood and urine of pregnant females

humoral immunity: type of immunity that involves antibody production by B cells

hyperbaric oxygen (HBO_2) therapy: therapy involving placing the patient into a hyperbaric chamber to treat difficult wounds; elevated level of oxygen under decreased pressure helps to increase oxygen stores in the blood stream and at the wound site, resulting in faster healing

hyperglycemia: increased levels of glucose in the blood

hyperopia: farsightedness

hyperpnea: increase in respiratory rate or breathing that is rapid and deeper than normal

hypertension: high blood pressure

hyperthermia: state in which the body temperature is elevated above the normal range
hypertrophy: increase in organ size from an increase in the size of the cells
hyperventilation: rapid and deep respirations that result in higher blood oxygen levels and lowered carbon dioxide levels
hypodermic: pertaining to under the skin; when referring to syringes, it is a syringe that punctures the skin
hypoglycemia: decreased levels of glucose in the blood
hypotension: low blood pressure
hypothermia: condition in which the victim's core body temperature falls below 95°F; may lead to death if left untreated
hypoxic: decreased oxygen level

I

idiopathic: an illness without a known cause
ileostomy: the surgical creation of an artificial excretory opening between the ileum, at the end of the small intestine, and the outside of the abdominal wall
immunizations: the process of stimulating an antibody reaction through the delivery of a vaccine in order to generate an immune response
immunoglobulin: antibody produced by cells of the immune system that protects the body from pathogens
immunosuppressed: patient whose immune system has been weakened by disease, chemotherapy, medications, and so on, making the patient more susceptible to infection
immunotherapy: the prevention or treatment of disease that stimulates the immune response (allergy shots)
incision: cuts in the skin usually made from items such as sharp instruments or glass
incubation: the act of incubating; placing a culture in an environment that provides optimal temperature, humidity, and darkness for the purpose of growth and multiplication of microorganisms
individually identifiable health information (IIPI): see protected health information (PHI)
induration: degree of hardening of normally soft tissue
infant: refers to the first year of life
infectious waste: objects contaminated with blood, body fluids, or OPIM
infertility specialist: a provider who specializes in assisting patients who are experiencing problems with conception or carrying pregnancies to term delivery
infiltration: see extravasation
inflammatory response: the body's attempt to protect itself from microorganisms that enter the body and to heal and replace injured tissue
informed consent: a legal doctrine that requires practitioners to provide patients with a complete set of facts prior to surgical procedures or medical experiments. Information must include the nature of the treatment, possible benefits, possible risks, and possible alternative treatments
inhalation: the act of breathing in
inhalers: handheld portable devices that deliver medication directly to the lungs
initiative: to take the lead or to work independently
inoculation: to apply microorganisms onto a culture medium
inspection: visual examination of the surface of the body as well as the body's posture and movement to detect disease and other conditions
inspiration: see inhalation
instillation: to instill liquid, such as medication, into a body orifice or cavity like the eye or ear
Institute for Safe Medication Practices (ISMP): a governmental organization that specifically seeks ways to promote medication safety
insulin: a hormone secreted by the pancreas in response to high levels of glucose in the bloodstream
insulin shock: life-threatening condition in which the patient's blood sugar drops to a dangerously low level, causing the patient to go into shock
integrative health care: a growing trend where providers and health care systems are integrating various practices into treatment and health promotion
integrity: (1) to have character; (2) normal structure without damage, guaranteeing the purity of the specimen
internal controls: these evaluate whether or not the test is working as it was designed, the correct amount of sample was added, the sample moving through the test correctly or whether the instrument is in good working order
international normalized ratio (INR): a standardized ratio used by all labs for blood coagulation testing
intervals: in a lab setting, timelines in which particular lab tests should be performed; testing intervals may be based on age, health history, race, and a variety of other factors
intra-articular: medication that is administered directly into a joint
intradermal: within the skin
intramuscular (IM): within the muscle
intravenous pyelogram/pyelography (IVP): radiographic procedure that views the kidneys, ureters, and bladder after a contrast medium has been injected through an IV
irrigation: to flush a body canal, such as the eye or ear, with a flowing solution for the purposes of cleansing and removing debris and other unwanted objects
ischemia: temporary lack of blood flow to an organ such as the heart

J

Jaeger chart: assessment chart for near vision acuity consisting of a series of readings with the type ranging in size from newspaper headline print to the small print commonly found in telephone directories
jaws: tips of certain instruments used to grasp or clamp items
Joint Commission (JC): a national organization that focuses on improving the quality and safety of services provided by health care organizations

K

kcalorie: a measurement of energy when a food is burned

ketone: normal products of fat metabolism found in the urine of patients with uncontrolled diabetes; can also be found due to starvation and vomiting

kinesiology: the study of the principles of mechanics and anatomy in relation to human movement

Korotkoff sounds: sounds heard during auscultation of the blood pressure

kyphosis: abnormal forward curvature of the spine

L

lab requisition form: an order form that is used to request laboratory testing

laboratory report form: a form that provides patient results for specific lab tests

laceration: jagged wound or cut that may be the result of a traumatic injury; may also appear as a tear

lactose: a protein found in milk products

lancet: sterile, disposable, sharp-pointed blade used to puncture the skin for the purpose of collecting a blood sample

language development: stage of development that begins with noises and progress into words, phrases, and sentences

leads: (1) a recording of the electrical impulses coming from the heart at different angles; (2) sensors or electrode conductors attached to the patient's skin during an ECG

lens: transparent crystalline structure behind the iris of the eye. Works along with the cornea to focus light on the retina

leukocyte: white blood cell; main function is to fight infection and tissue damage

licensing: legal document that permits or authorizes a person to perform a specific task or tasks. Examples of professionals who must be licensed to practice medicine include doctors, dentists, and nurse practitioners; currently, no state offers licensing opportunities for medical assistants

ligature: (1) the act of tying or binding; (2) suture material used to tie off tubular structures such as the fallopian tubes or vas deferens following a surgical procedure

limited English proficiency (LEP): persons with a primary language other than English or those who have a difficult time, reading, speaking, or comprehending English

lipemia: abnormal amount of fat in the blood causing the serum or plasma to appear cloudy or milky

lipoprotein: simple protein bound to fat (cholesterol) that carries lipids in the blood

liter (L): fundamental unit of volume when measuring liquids

lithotomy: a position of the patient lying on the back, face up, with the feet and legs raised and supported in stirrups

lithotripsy: the crushing of stones by the application of sound waves

local reaction: allergic reaction to a drug that involves only the local tissue such as hives, swelling, and tenderness

lochia: discharge of blood, mucous, and tissue from the uterus following delivery

lot control: identifying number that allows the medication to be tracked in the event of a recall

low-density lipoprotein (LDL): lipoprotein deposited as fat in the tissues of the body and in the walls of the blood vessels, which increases the risk of coronary artery disease; "bad cholesterol"

Luer-Lok: special tip on a syringe that allows the needle to be screwed onto the syringe for a snug fit

lymphocyte: type of white blood cell with no granules in the cytoplasm; responsible for a major portion of the body's immune response

M

macrocephaly: abnormally large head that may indicate a pathologic disorder

macrocyte: larger than normal red blood cell

magnetic resonance imaging (MRI): diagnostic imaging procedure that uses a magnetic field to produce images of the body

malabsorption syndrome: the inability of the GI tract to absorb some nutrients

manipulation: applying passive movement to a joint while using force

Mantoux skin test: common screening test for tuberculosis

massage: the use of pressure, friction, and kneading to promote muscle relaxation

massage therapist: A massage therapist is a CAM provider who has a background and history of massage and its various techniques (e.g., soft-tissue, deep tissue myoskeletal alignment), and has studied anatomy, physiology, kinesiology, pathology, and theory. Many massage therapists today have 500 or more classroom hours, including assessment, practice, and student clinic

meaningful use: the set of standards defined by Centers for Medicare and Medicaid Services (CMS) incentive programs that governs the use of EHRs and allows eligible providers and hospitals to earn incentive payments by meeting specific criteria

meconium: earliest stools of the newborn

medical asepsis: cleansing methods used to destroy microorganisms found in blood and other body fluids once they leave the body

medication label: product label that gives vital information about the medication

medicinal: relating to or having the properties of a medication

melena: black, tarry and foul-smelling stools; the appearance of the stools is caused by the presence of digested blood and often indicates a disorder in the upper part of the gastrointestinal tract

melanocytes: pigment-containing cells

menarche: woman's first menstrual cycle

menopause: permanent cessation of menstruation

menses: bloody discharge of the endometrial lining; occurs monthly during a woman's fertile years if fertilization is not achieved

menstruation: see menses

mensuration: the act of measuring, including height and weight measurements

mental health: person's state of mind; how people look at themselves, their lives, and the other people in their lives, evaluate their challenges and problems, and explore choices

mental illness: condition or illness that impairs the mind's ability to process information in a "normal" fashion

mental impairment: see mental illness

mentally challenged: individual whose brain functions at a subnormal intellectual level

metabolic syndrome: a combination of medical disorders, primarily caused by obesity, including high blood pressure, high blood sugar levels, abnormal cholesterol levels and the accumulation of body fat around the waist

metabolism: sum of all chemical and physical changes that take place within an organism

meter (m): fundamental unit of length when measuring distance

metered-dose inhalers (MDI): inhalers that use a chemical propellant to push the medication out of the inhaler and deliver it to the patient's lungs by direct inhalation or by squeezing the canister

metric system: primary system for measuring weight, volume, and length (area)

microbiology: (1) the study of microorganisms, especially as they relate to infectious diseases; (2) the laboratory department that grows and identifies microorganisms

microcephaly: abnormally small head that may indicate a chromosomal disorder

microcyte: smaller than normal red blood cell

microscope: utilized to view objects like blood cells, microorganisms, and urine components that cannot be seen with the naked eye

midwife (midwives): can be either a Certified Nurse Midwives (CNM) or Certified Professional Midwives (CPM), both have specialty training in the care of the pregnant female as well as labor, delivery, and the postpartum periods

milestones: set of activities that indicate acceptable growth and development patterns

mindfulness: to be aware, alert, and attentive

minerals: inorganic elements that are essential for normal body function and include elements such as sodium, potassium, and magnesium

minimum effective concentration (MEC): the concentration of a high-level disinfectant that is necessary to kill bacterial spores; MEC concentration changes after repeated use of a chemical disinfectant

minimum necessary: part of the HIPAA rule; must release only the Protected Health Information (PHI) in the minimum necessary amount to accomplish the purpose for which use or disclosure is sought; does not apply when patients provide a valid, signed authorization for release of PHI, de-identify information—meaning PHI with all HIPAA identifiers removed

miscarriage: loss of a fetus before viability; also known as spontaneous abortion

modality: physical agent such as, heat, cold, water, and electricity used in physical therapy to improve or restore lost function to musculoskeletal tissue

moderate-complexity tests: require an understanding of test methodology, quality control, and instrument calibration. Unlike waived tests, tests for moderate-complexity are not available for home use. Detailed record keeping, proficiency testing, and biannual inspections are required

monocyte: type of white blood cell with no granules in the cytoplasm containing a large, irregularly shaped nucleus

morals: cultural and religious-based distinctions of right and wrong

morphology: study of structure and form; when referring to red blood cell morphology, it is a study of the cells' size, shape, and the amount or lack of color

motor development: area of development that includes reflexes, gross motor, and fine motor skills

mucosa: the membranes that secrete mucus to protect and lubricate tissues in the body

multiple allergosorbent test system (MAST): a method for measuring total and allergen-specific IgE levels

muscularis: the muscular layer of the gastrointestinal tract

myopia: nearsightedness

N

National Drug Code (NDC): numbers used to identify the drug manufacturer, the product, and the size of the container

National Committee for Quality Assurance: a nonprofit organization that strives to improve the quality of health care. The NCQA certifies a wide range of health care organizations including health plans, disease management programs, and physician organizations

National Healthcareer Association (NHA): a medical assisting certifying organization

nebulizer: instrument used for the treatment of asthma and other lung conditions that changes liquid medications into an aerosol mist so that they can be inhaled through a mouthpiece or facemask

neglect: the failure or refusal of a caregiver or other responsible person to provide for an elder's basic physical, emotional, or social needs, or failure to protect them from harm

neonate: refers to the first month of life

nephrologist: kidney specialist

neurologist: physician who specializes in diagnosing and treating diseases and disorders of the nervous system, including the brain, spinal cord, and nerves

neutrophil: most common type of granulocytic white blood cell that contains light purple granules in the cytoplasm

newborn: refers to the initial period following birth

nocturia: frequent urination during the night

nomogram: graph that illustrates a relationship between two known values

noninvasive heart scan: a test to evaluate and measure plaque in the coronary arteries by determining the amount of calcium present

nonsteroidal anti-inflammatory drug (NSAID): a drug that reduces inflammation and is not a steroid medication

nonverbal: communication using perception, body language, facial expression, eye contact, gestures, distance, silence, therapeutic touch, and active listening

normal flora: microorganisms normally present in different parts of the body that are nonpathogenic and pose no health threat to the host under ordinary circumstances; may provide protection to the host

normal sinus rhythm: the heart's rhythm within normal limits

normal value: values or ranges that are expected in certain populations; each lab has its own set of normal values based on test methodology and the testing population

normocyte: normal sized cell

notice of privacy practices: notice given to and signed by patients explaining how their PHI will be used

nuclear medicine: branch of medicine that uses radioactive isotopes for the purpose of diagnosing and treating diseases

nutrition: the process by which organisms take in and utilize food materials

nutritionist: a person trained in food and nutrition, who is not registered

O

obesity: condition present when a person is 20% to 30% over the normal weight for their age, size, and gender

objective impressions: information provided by the clinician or provider that includes a list of measurable or reproducible data

observation: the process of watching or visualizing

occlusion: lockage or closure that may occur during IV therapy, which blocks the medication from going into the vein

occult: medical term for "hidden"

Occupational Safety and Health Administration (OSHA): government agency that sets forth regulations for a safe and healthy workplace

occupational therapist (OT): medical professional who is responsible for assisting patients with basic motor function, reasoning, and activities of daily living

oliguria: a scant amount of urine that can be caused by renal failure or dehydration

oncologist: a physician who diagnoses and treats cancers

opened-container life: amount of time a disinfecting solution may be used once the bottle has been opened

open wound: wound that breaks the skin, including abrasions, incisions, lacerations, and punctures

ophthalmic: pertaining to the eye

ophthalmologist: medical doctor who specializes in the diagnosis and treatment (including surgery) of diseases and disorders of the eye

ophthalmoscope: instrument used to visualize the interior of the eye

opportunistic infections: infections that normally do not occur unless the infected individual has an impaired or weakened immune system

optician: eye professional (technician) who fills prescriptions for eye glasses

optometrist: doctor of optometry licensed to perform visual acuity testing and able to prescribe corrective lenses to patients with refractive errors

organizational ethics: represent the values by which the organization conducts its business; organizations frequently include a values statement as part of their mission and vision statements

orthomolecular medicine: the administration of vitamins, minerals, amino acids, hormones, and metabolic intermediates for the prevention and treatment of disease

orthopedist: physician who specializes in the treatment of diseases and disorders of the bones and muscles

orthopnea: breathing that is easiest while in a sitting or standing position

orthostatic hypotension: blood pressure that drops upon standing

ossicles: the three small bones of the middle ear: the malleus, incus, and stapes

osteopathic manipulative therapy (OMT): a hands-on treatment where DOs use their hands to examine the back and other parts of the body such as joints, tendons, ligaments, and muscles, for pain and restriction during motion that could signal an injury or impaired function

osteoporosis: condition in which the bones become brittle and porous due to a lack of calcium storage in the bone

other potentially infectious material (OPIM): body fluids other than blood that could be infectious

otic: pertaining to the ear

otolaryngologist: a provider who specializes in assisting patients who are experiencing sinus problems, including those associated with allergies

otorhinolaryngologist: the medical name for an ear, nose and throat doctor, or ENT

otoscope: instrument used to visualize the external ear canal and tympanic membrane

oval window: an oval-shaped membrane set within the cochlea. The stapes rests against the oval window and transmits its vibrations into the cochlea. The oval window serves as the division between the middle ear and the inner ear

oxygen saturation: the amount of oxygen in the hemoglobin of red blood cells (RBC)

P

pain management specialist: a medical doctor (MD) or doctor of osteopathy (DO) who has undergone specialized training in managing pain. Many pain management specialists also have specialty training as an anesthesiologist

palpate: method of examination that uses touch to locate veins for venipuncture

palpation: examination by application of the hands and fingers to the body to evaluate size and function of the body and to determine abnormality in size or texture

pancreatitis: the inflammation of the pancreas

para: number of live births

parasite: organism that lives within, upon, or at the expense of the host

parenteral: pertaining to outside of the intestines; any drugs delivered by a method other than through the digestive tract

paresthesia: tingling or burning sensation associated with nerve injury or damage

parietal pain: pain in the abdominal wall caused by inflammation and aggravated by movement

participating provider: a facility that contracts with the insurance company to provide laboratory or diagnostic services

parturition: another term for labor

passive: behavior characteristic is to typically avoid situations

past history (PH) or past health history (PHH): record of usual childhood diseases and other diseases, conditions, injuries, and hospitalizations that the patient has endured in the past

patency: the openness of a structure in the case of an IV; usually referring to veins

pathogen: disease-causing microorganism

pathogenic: disease-producing

patient advocate: an impartial party who listens to the patient's concerns and provides them access to the systems in place that would resolve their conflict

patient-centered: a model of care that emphasizes care coordination places the needs and preferences of the patient at the core of health care

patient-centered medical home (PCMH): a health care delivery model that emphasizes coordination of care and facilitates partnerships between patients and their health care team; may be part of an accountable care organization

patient navigator: the person who is able to assist a patient navigating the health system

Patients' Bill of Rights: a way to communicate the legal rights patients have while under the care of a provider or facility, from a government standpoint. The regulations proposed include a set of protections that apply to health coverage

pay for coordination: a type of health care delivery model that is often used in medical home environments and involves payment for specified care coordination services. In this environment, the provider, usually a primary care physician, leads a team of professionals to oversee and coordinate the patient's overall health

pay for performance organization: a health care delivery model in which providers are paid for how well patients are progressing in particular populations. Providers are rewarded for such things as better glucose control in their diabetic population, lower blood pressures in their hypertensive patients, and an increase in preventative screenings in other patient populations

peak expiratory flow (PEF): test that measures the speed of exhalation with the greatest effort

pediatric: specialty with a focus on working with patients from birth through young adulthood

pediatrician: medical specialist who treats the patient population from birth through young adulthood (usually age 18)

percentiles: group of percentages that compare measurements such as height and weight to other children of the same age

percussion: to use the fingertips to tap the body slightly but sharply to determine position, size, and consistency of an underlying structure or cavity

percutaneous transluminal coronary angioplasty (PTCA): a procedure similar to heart catheterization in which a balloon is guided through the coronary arteries and inflated to widen the artery

perimenopause: phase 1 of menopause; the beginning of menopause, characterized by irregular menses and amenorrhea

peristalsis: a series of wave-like contractions of the smooth muscles in a single direction that moves the food forward into the digestive system

peritoneum: a multilayered membrane that protects and holds the organs in place within the abdominal cavity

personal health record (PHR): copy of the patient's own medical record that may be in paper or digital format

personal medical history: history of the patient's current and previous health concerns

personal protective equipment (PPE): items that place a barrier between the employee and blood or OPIM, such as gloves, goggles, and gowns

pH: measure of the acidity or alkalinity of a substance

pharmacodynamics: the study of the effects of drugs on living organisms

pharmacokinetics: describes how the body reacts to a drug

pharmacology: the study of drugs, including their origin, nature, properties, and effects upon living organisms

phenylketonuria (PKU): congenital and familial disease in which the patient is deficient in the enzyme phenylalanine hydroxylase, which prevents the patient from converting phenylalanine to a protein needed for metabolism

phlebitis: inflammation of the vein

phlebotomist: health care employee who performs phlebotomy or blood drawing procedures

phlebotomy: act of drawing blood

physiatrist: physical medicine doctor who diagnoses and treats neuromuscular and bone diseases and injuries; works closely with the physical therapist

physical disability: impairment restricting or preventing normal functioning of a particular limb or group of limbs

physical therapist (PT): medical professional who is responsible for the management of a patient's rehabilitation through the use of different physical means or modalities

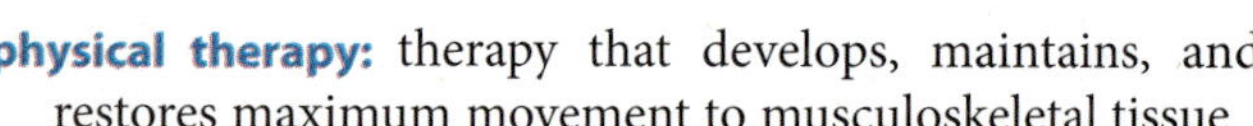

physical therapy: therapy that develops, maintains, and restores maximum movement to musculoskeletal tissue

physician's office laboratory (POL): laboratory located in physicians' offices to provide clinicians with faster turn-around times in relation to test results; tests may be waived or moderately-complex

placebo effect: refers to the fact that some people respond favorably to a known ineffective treatment because they believe it is working; occurs in about 30 to 40% of the patients

plan: part of the SOAP note that includes plans for testing, treatment, and education for each problem for which the patient is seen

plantar fasciitis: inflammation of the fascia in the foot

plasma: liquid portion of whole blood; obtained when the blood is centrifuged in a blood drawing tube containing an anticoagulant and separated from the cells

plastic surgeon: a surgical specialist who deals with the repair, reconstruction, or replacement of physical defects of form or function involving the skin, musculoskeletal system, craniomaxillofacial structures, extremities, breast and trunk, and external genitalia

pleural effusion: excessive amount of fluid in the pleural space

podiatrist: a physician specializing in the diagnosis and treatment of foot conditions

poikilocytosis: marked difference in the shape of the red blood cells

point-of-care testing (POCT): testing performed at the point of care (the patient's bedside, in the exam room, and so on)

polyps: a mushroom-like growth from the surface of a mucous membrane

polyuria: excessive urination

postlingual: individuals who became deaf after they started speaking

postpartum: time period between the delivery of the baby to the time of the mother's six-week check-up following delivery

posture: the position of the body whether standing, sitting, or lying down

Potts (fracture): a fracture that occurs at the distal end of tibia or fibula, just above the ankle

management: the administrative functions in an EHR

precipitate: pieces of solid materials or crystals that may form from a chemical reaction in a medication vial

precordial leads: the six chest leads of a standard 12-lead ECG

preeclampsia: complication of pregnancy marked by an increase in blood pressure, protein in the urine, and edema; may progress rapidly to eclampsia; another name for toxemia

prelingual: individuals who were deaf before they started speaking

prenatal: before birth

presbyopia: farsightedness due to aging and the loss of elasticity of the lens

prescribe: to order a medication from the pharmacy, usually by prescription

prescription: order for a prescribed drug or treatment

primary container: original container in which the specimen was collected

primary dressing: dressing that lies directly over the wound

primary drug: drug that should be drawn first when combining two drugs in the same syringe

problem list: list of specific problems identified by the patient history that is placed at the front of the patient chart for easy referencing

problem-oriented medical record (POMR): medical record documentation format developed by Lawrence L. Weed in the early 1970s that incorporates organized structure within the medical chart

problem-solving: the process of working through the details of a problem to reach a solution

proctologist: medical doctor who specializes in treating diseases and disorders of the lower bowel, rectum, and anus

procurement station: satellite locations where samples are collected

product name: trade name or brand name of the medication

professionalism: conduct, aims, or qualities that characterize or mark a professional or a professional person

proficiency testing: a program designed to evaluate the quality of a laboratory's performance; a form of external quality control

profile: related lab tests grouped by body system or function

progress note: note that tracks a patient's progress; the heart of the patient record; includes physician notes about current problems and is a chronological listing of the patient's overall health status

prophylactic: substances used to prevent or lessen the severity of a disease

prosthesis: artificial joint or body part; device that augments natural function, like a hearing aid or an artificial limb

protected health information (PHI): the patient's private health information

proteins: proteins are essential for the structure, function, and regulation of the body's cells

prothrombin time (PT): common coagulation test that measures clotting time in seconds

provider-performed microscopy (PPM) procedures: microscopic examinations that are part of CLIA's moderately-complex category of tests; these examinations require the expertise of a physician or second-level provider qualified in microscopic procedures

puberty: age at which both males and females are able to reproduce

puerperium: another name for the postpartum period

pulmonary function testing: noninvasive test that detects the lung's ability to function

pulmonologist: physician who specializes in respiratory care

pulse pressure: the difference between systolic and diastolic pressures

pulse rate: the number of pulse beats per minute that can be counted and are assessed for regularity
pulse rhythm: regularity of the pulse beats
pulse volume: strength of the pressure felt when palpating a pulse for characteristics, such as strong or weak, bounding or thready
puncture: wound that is usually caused by an object such as sticks, pins, nails, or pieces of glass that penetrate the skin, leaving a hole
pure culture: culture that contains only one organism
purulent: discharge containing pus
pyelonephritis: inflammation of the kidney and kidney pelvis

Q

qualitative: these results usually identify the presence or absence of a substance and are interpreted as positive or negative
quality assurance (QA): inclusive term for all policies, procedures, and practices that ensure reliable and accurate documentation, calibration, and maintenance of equipment, quality control, proficiency testing, and staff training
quality control (QC): procedures that monitor the processing of laboratory specimens; includes test control samples, documentation, and analyzing statistics for diagnostic tests
quantitative: these results provide an actual measurement of the substance in specific units. Always write out the result and unit when documenting the value
quantity not sufficient (QNS): describes a specimen received by the lab whose volume is not sufficient to perform the required test

R

radiate: to send out or to spread to another location
radiograph: see X-ray
radioallergosorbent test (RAST): a blood test to detect specific IgE antibodies to allergens used to determine the substance(s) a patient is allergic to
radiologist: medical specialist who uses radioactive substances for visualization of internal body structures and diagnosis and treatment
radiolucent: penetrable by X-rays
radionuclide: radioactive substance, such as iodine or cobalt, that is administered to patients prior to a nuclear medicine study
radiopaque: unable to be penetrated by the X-ray beam; allows visualization of tissue
radiopharmaceuticals: a radioactive drug used in the treatment of disease
random collection: urine specimen collected at any time with no special preparation
range of motion (ROM): exercise designed to move a joint through its full range of motion
ratchet: the part of a ring-handled instrument centered between the two rings; the locking mechanism that tightens or locks the tips of the instrument at varying degrees
reagent test strip: narrow plastic strip with reagent pads that have been treated with specific chemicals to test urine for the presence of substances such as glucose, blood, bacteria, WBCs, bilirubin, urobilinogen, protein, and ketones
receptor: bonding proteins or sites on cells to which drugs attach to stimulate or block a cell response
red blood cell indices: a group of tests that provides complete information about the red blood cells
reduction: realignment of a bone back into to its original position following a break
reference ranges: also known as normal values, expected values, or reference intervals
reflexes: involuntary or automatic response to a stimulus
reflux: a backward or return flow of fluid
refractive disorder: conditions in which the lens and cornea do not bend light correctly, resulting in visual defects
refractometer: handheld device that consists of a lens and a prism; used in POLs to measure the specific gravity of urine
Registered Medical Assistant (RMA): the medical assisting credential offered by the American Medical Technologists
registration: to enroll a person's name in a register, based on their successful completion of a specific program and/or their ability to pass an examination designed specifically for that particular specialty
rehabilitation: in regards to musculoskeletal rehabilitation, the act of restoring function and mobility to injured or diseased musculoskeletal tissue
renal threshold: point at which a substance reaches a blood concentration high enough for the kidneys to start removing it and it is detected in the urine
repolarization: period of relaxation of the heart
respect: treat a person with a positive feeling and appreciation, and to treat others the way you would want them to treat you
respiration: the act of breathing; one complete inhalation and exhalation
responsibility: a duty or obligation
reticulocyte: an immature red blood cell
retina: the inner-most layer at the back of the eye; light-sensitive
reuse life: amount of time a solution may be used once it has been prepared or activated
reverse chronological order: referring to medical records, meaning the most recent (in order of date and time) note or item is on top
rhythm strip: separate 12-inch recording of a particular lead (generally lead II) to observe heart rhythm variances
rods: specialized cells in the eye that are useful in dim light

S

salmonella: a bacteria that is transmitted through feces, either through direct contact with animals, or by eating contaminated raw/ undercooked meats or eggs or drinking unpasteurized milk or eating unpasteurized cheese products

sanguineous: discharge or exudate that contains blood

sanitization: cleaning process to remove tissue, blood, or body fluids from instruments or fomites, usually by scrubbing the items with a special soap

scatter radiation: emitted from the patient in all directions, which is considered "secondary" radiation

sclera: the white of the eye

scoliosis: abnormal lateral curvature of the spine

scope of practice: working under a physician's direct supervision, and consistent with his or her education, training, and experience; there is no uniform, national definition of a medical assistant's scope of practice, and duties will vary according to state law; a medical assistant's duties shall not constitute the practice of medicine

scrub: when the PM side of an EHR captures a patient encounter with CPT and ICD codes, then scrubs (verifies procedure(s) are supported with appropriate diagnoses and meet the approval of the insurance carrier) the claim(s)

secondary dressing: dressing that is placed over a primary dressing and assists with absorption of excess wound fluid or exudates from the inside, while keeping outside moisture from entering the wound

secondary drug: drug that should be drawn second when combining two drugs in the same syringe

secondary sex characteristics: visual changes seen in males and females as they reach puberty

sediment: solid material found in urine after centrifugation that is examined microscopically

segment: this is the space between two waves

seizure: sudden attack that is usually the result of a malfunction in the brain

sensitivity testing: technique that evaluates which antibiotics will destroy a particular microorganism

sensory development: development of the senses, such as vision and hearing, which continue to promote further motor development

serosanguineous: discharge or exudate that contains both serum and blood

serous: discharge or exudate that contains serum

serrations: markings etched into the tips of certain surgical instruments to help improve gripping power when working with tissue that is slippery

serum: liquid portion of the blood that remains after the blood has clotted; obtained from a blood drawing tube that does not contain an anticoagulant

service: to extend help to others

sexually transmitted disease (STD): also referred to as sexually transmitted infections; infections that are transmitted through sexual contact; examples include chlamydia, gonorrhea, and syphilis

sexually transmitted infections (STIs): infections that are transmitted through sexual contact, such as chlamydia, gonorrhea, and syphilis

shank: connects the handle to the working end of the instrument and extends the instrument to work in deeper tissue

sharps: sharp objects that could cause puncture wounds when handled, including needles, sharp instruments, scalpels, glass slides, glass tubes, and pipettes; these items should be placed in a sharps container to avoid injury

shelf life: amount of time a solution may be stored unopened before losing its potency

shelter-in-place: the process of moving vertically or horizontally to the safest area in the building, based on the type of emergency encountered

shingling: filing system commonly used for lab reports that are not on standard-size paper; reports are shingled in reverse chronological order about a half inch above each other in paper charts

shock: potentially fatal condition that can be brought on by disease, injury, decrease in circulation, and fluid loss; during shock, the blood may pool, preventing vital organs from receiving blood

side effect: secondary effect in addition to the therapeutic effect; some side effects are therapeutic and end up becoming another use for the drug; however, most side effects are unpleasant and may even be harmful

sievert (Sv): interchangeable with gray (Gy)

sighted guide assistance: to act as a guide for a person who is blind

signed English: type of sign language similar to Signed Exact English (SEE), though it often borrows vocabulary terms from American Sign Language (ASL); more similar to ASL than SEE

signed exact English (SEE): form of sign language that codes English words into a visual form

sleep apnea: periods of breathing cessation during hours of sleep

Snellen chart: chart used to test distance visual acuity

social history: lifestyle questions such as amount of alcohol consumed in a regular week, number of packs of cigarettes smoked per day, and so on

sonogram: a picture of the internal structure that is being scanned during an ultrasound

source-oriented medical record (SOMR): more traditional format used for entering data in the medical record; data is usually entered in narrative format in a related section of the chart; there is no systematic cross-referencing for this documentation format

specific gravity: measure of the amount of dissolved substances found in the urine; measure of the concentration of the urine

sphygmomanometer: instrument used to determine arterial blood pressure

spirometer: device that is used during spirometry testing to measure breathing capacity

splint: stiff device used to support and immobilize a part of the body that has been injured or fractured
sprain: trauma to ligaments, tendons, or muscles
sputum: fluid that is produced in the lungs and bronchi
standard of care: the diagnostic and treatment process that is reasonable and prudent that a clinician should follow for a certain type of patient, illness, or clinical circumstance
Standard Precautions: set of precautions developed by the CDC that take universal precautions to the next level by treating all body fluids except sweat as though they are potentially infectious
standardization: mark that is made at the beginning of each lead or group of leads when performing an ECG to make certain the unit is functioning properly
sterile conscience: continual mindset of sterility; making certain that nothing happens that compromises the patient's safety before, during, or following the surgical procedure
sterilization: the complete destruction of all microorganisms
sterilization indicators: devices that help in determining whether or not a package has been exposed to the high heat and whether the items inside are sterile
strain: injury to a body part caused by overuse or exertion
stress echocardiography: ultrasonic pictures of the heart taken at rest and during high levels of stress
stylus: heated wire on the ECG machine that produces the graphic tracing on the ECG paper
subatmospheric pressure device: device that uses negative pressure to help close wounds
subcutaneous: under the dermis or true layer of skin
subjective impressions: information provided by the patient
subjective information: information supplied by the patient
subjective, objective, assessment, plan (SOAP): charting format used in the POMR; each letter represents a different section of the documentation
sublingual: medication placed under the tongue for rapid absorption of the medication into the blood stream
sudden infant death syndrome (SIDS): death of an infant usually under one year of age with no known cause
supernatant: liquid portion of urine that is discarded after centrifugation
supplements: a product containing a dietary ingredient that when consumed is intended to provide additional nutritional value to the diet
surgical adhesive: surgical glue containing sealants to hold a wound closed; used in place of staples or sutures
surgical asepsis: procedures and practices used to destroy and eliminate all microorganisms from instruments and other objects in order to protect patients having surgical procedures from developing infections; maintaining sterile conditions during any invasive procedure
surgical wick: device that is used to introduce medications into a body cavity such as the ear and eye or to act as a drainage conduit for wound management
suture: (1) the process of sewing; (2) the type of strand or fiber used to sew; purpose of a suture is to hold the edges of a wound together until the natural healing process joins the tissue permanently
symptom: signal or sign experienced by the patient indicative of a specific disease or condition; may include, pain, fever, itching, and so on
syncope: brief episode of unconsciousness or fainting
systemic reaction: reaction that affects the entire body
systole: period in which the cardiac ventricles contract
systolic pressure: the highest amount of pressure within the arteries during ventricular contraction

T

tachycardia: heart rate greater than 100 beats per minute
tachypnea: rapid respirations in combination with normal or shallow breathing; respiration rate is usually above 40 breaths per minute
tact: sensitivity for knowing what to say and when to say it; sometimes referred to as diplomacy; the presentation or the way you deliver the message to the receiver involves the tone of your voice as well as the body language you use
taut: to pull or draw tight, as when you pull the skin tight when administering an intramuscular injection
taxonomy: classification of living organisms into the proper category
telecommunications device for the deaf (TDD): device that allows deaf persons to type messages over phone lines
Telecommunications Relay Services (TRS): service for deaf persons when they are calling a party or business that does not have a TDD or TTY in which a relay operator relays information between the two parties
teletypewriter (TTY): type of TDD; typewriter that transmits messages between a deaf person and a hearing person via telephone lines
testicular self-examination (TSE): procedure in which the patient examines his testicles monthly for any changes such as lumps or enlargement
therapeutic communication: exchange of information between the health care worker and the patient that leads to the advancement of the patient's physical and emotional well-being
therapeutic effect: desired effect that a drug has on the body
therapeutic index: range between the therapeutic dose of a drug and the dose at which the drug becomes toxic
thermotherapy: applying dry or moist heat to a body part to promote healing and restore function
thixotropic separator gel: gel contained in some vacuum tubes that forms a barrier between the cellular portion and the serum or plasma after centrifugation
thoracentesis: medical procedure performed to withdraw fluids from the pleural space
thrombocyte: blood platelet
thrombosis: blood clot
thrombus: blood clot
tinnitus: ringing in the ears

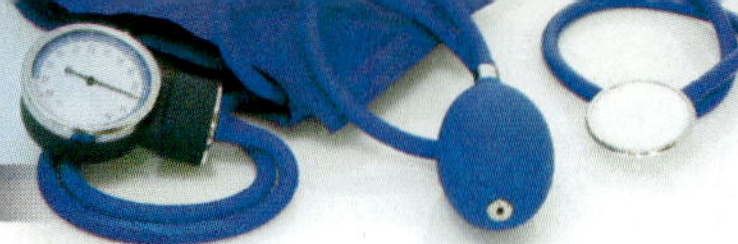

toddler: age classification referring to late in the first year of life continuing until the preschool years

tonometer: instrument that checks intraocular pressure

topical: medication applied to the skin

tourniquet: device used to distend veins to assist with venipuncture

toxemia: see preeclampsia

transdermal patch: adhesive patch applied to the skin, impregnated with medication that is slowly released into the blood stream

transfats: an unhealthy substance made through the chemical process of hydrogenation of oils, which turn liquid fats into fats that are solid at room temperature

transient flora: bacteria on the hands that is picked up throughout the day through direct contact with items that are contaminated

transient ischemic attack (TIA): also known as mini-stroke; symptoms include headache, confusion, tinnitus, and personality changes; TIAs usually only last a few minutes and may be a predecessor to a stroke

transmission-based precautions: precautions in addition to standard precautions that should be followed when working with patients with known highly infectious diseases

transrectal ultrasound (TRUS): procedure in which an ultrasound probe is inserted into the rectum to produce images of the prostrate

transurethral resection of the prostate (TURP): procedure performed on males with BPH, which cuts away overgrown tissue of the prostate to facilitate urination

traumatic brain injury: injury to the brain caused by trauma

traumatic needle: eyed needles are packaged so that the needle is separate from the suture material requiring the person performing the suturing to thread the needle

treadmill stress test: a noninvasive procedure during which the patient walks on a treadmill while connected to an ECG machine

triage: sorting patients according to the extent of their injuries or illnesses; process in which things are ranked in terms of importance or priority

triglyceride: neutral fat found in the blood stream that transports the fat to body tissues to be used as a source of energy

trimester: time period of three months; pregnancy is divided into three trimesters

Triple Aim Initiative: a movement by the Institute for Healthcare Improvement developed to address three dimensions: patient experience of care, improving health populations, and to reduce the per capita cost of health care

trocar: sharp, pointed needle

tuberculosis (TB): infection caused by Mycobacterium, a slow-advancing bacterium that commonly affects the lungs but can affect other tissue as well

turbid: opaque appearance of urine

tympanic membrane: thin membrane separating the external ear canal from the middle ear; eardrum

tympanometer: electronic device with an attached probe that is placed snugly in the patient's ear to determine if the middle ear is sending sound waves

tympany: drum-like sound upon percussion that indicates air or gas within the related region

U

ultrasonic cleaner: device that cleans instruments by transmitting sound waves through a cleaning fluid

ultrasound: (1) diagnostic procedure that uses high-frequency sound waves to produce an image of an internal body structure; (2) sound waves used to generate heat in deep tissues of the body as a method of treatment for an injury or other condition of the muscles

Universal Precautions: set of guidelines developed by the CDC to protect health care workers from infectious diseases by treating all human blood and OPIM products as if they were known to be infected with bloodborne pathogens

urea: nitrogenous end product of protein metabolism cleared from the blood by the kidneys into the urine

urethritis: the inflammation of the urethra

urochrome: pigment that gives urine its color

urology: medical specialty that involves the study of the structure, physiology, and diseases of the urinary system in both males and females and the reproductive system of males

urticaria: also known as hives

usual childhood diseases (UCD or UCHD): list of routine childhood diseases experienced by most children during the time frame that the patient was a child, such as chickenpox, mumps, measles, and so on; these are decreasing due to the immunization process

V

vaccinations: introduction of a vaccine or toxoid to provide protection from a specific disease

vacuum tube: test tube that contains a vacuum, forcing blood from the vein into the tube through aspiration

vasectomy: sterilization procedure in which the vas deferens is cut, clamped, or sealed to prevent sperm from entering the ejaculate

vasoconstriction: decrease in the diameter of the blood vessels

vasodilation: increase in the diameter of the blood vessels

vasography: radiological procedure that is used to evaluate patency (openness) of the vas deferens and ejaculatory ducts

vector: carriers such as insects or rodents that can serve as a reservoir in the chain of infection

vegan: a diet that excludes meats, fish, dairy, eggs or any other products which come from animals

vegetarian: a diet that excludes meat, but includes eggs and dairy products

venipuncture: to pierce a vein with a needle to obtain a blood specimen

ventricular fibrillation (VF or V-fib): condition in which the ventricles of the heart twitch or flutter with no organized movement; very common in adult victims of sudden cardiac arrest

verbal: written or oral

vertigo: disturbance in the equilibrium of the body and balance that causes the patient to be dizzy

vial: a small, prefilled glass or plastic bottle that contains either a single dose or multiple doses of medication

virus: submicroscopic parasites of plants, animals, and bacteria that often cause disease and require a living host in order to grow and multiply

viscosity: thickness of a substance

viscosupplementation: injection of hyaluronic acid into an arthritic knee joint

visual acuity: clearness or sharpness of vision

vital capacity (VC): the maximum amount of air the patient is able to inhale and exhale

vital signs: traditional signs of life such as blood pressure, pulse rate, respiration, and body temperature; also referred to as cardinal signs

vitamins: organic substances in the diet which are found in plants and animals and are necessary for normal growth and development

voiding: to evacuate the bladder

W

waived tests: low-complexity tests that are simple to perform, require a minimum of quality control and documentation, and a minimum of judgment and interpretation

wheal: bubble of fluid under the skin that develops from an intradermal injection

winged infusion: butterfly set used to collect blood from small or difficult veins

X

X-ray: high-energy beam capable of penetrating the body to produce images on film; radiographs

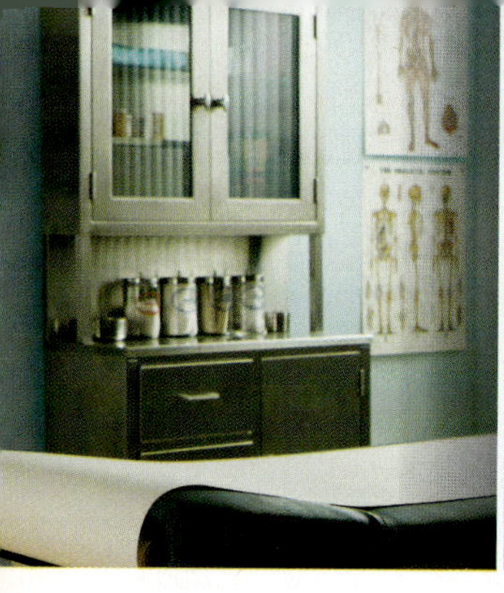

Index

A

AAMA (American Association of Medical Assistants), 3, 4, 5
ABHES (Accrediting Bureau of Health Education Schools), 13
Abnormal Uterine Bleeding (AUB), 473
ABO blood typing, 811
Abortions, 489
Abrasions, 962
ABR-OE (Assessment Based Recognition in Order Entry), 654
Abscess, 253
Accountability, professionalism, 15–16
Accountable care organizations (ACOs), 31–32, 154
Accrediting Bureau of Health Education Schools (ABHES), 13
ACL (Anterior cruciate ligament), 617
ACOs (Accountable care organizations), 31–32, 154
Activated partial thromboplastin time(APTT), 754
Active listening, 103, 155
Active listening, professional communication, 9
Activities of daily living (ADLs), 136
Acupressure, 541
Acupuncture, 541
Acupuncturist, 540
Acute abdomen, 945
Acute stage, 185
ADA (Americans with Disabilities Act), 123
ADAAA (Americans with Disabilities Act Amendments Act), 123
ADAMS (Aging, Demographics, and Memory Study), 137
Adaptability, professionalism, 17–18
ADA Standards for Accessible Design, 125
Addendum, 44, 92
Additives, 678
ADLs (Activities of daily living), 136
Administer, 858
Administer cold therapy treatments, 635–636
Administer heat therapy treatments, 632–635
Adolescent, 574
Adolescent care, 587–588
Advance directives, 59
adverse effects, 856
AED (Automated external defibrillator), 950
Aerobic, 772
Afebrile, 295
Affinity, 853
Agar, 776
Agency for Healthcare Research and Quality (AHRQ), 33
Agglutination, 810
Aging, Demographics, and Memory Study (ADAMS), 137
Agonists, 853
AHRQ (Agency for Healthcare Research and Quality), 33
Alcohol-based hand rub, 203
Algorithm, 944
Aliquot, 690
Alkaline phosphatases (ALPs), chemistry tests, 807
Allergen, 532
Allergist, 534
Allergy specialty
- antiaging procedures, 537–539
- complementary and alternative medicine (CAM), 539–542
- diagnostic tests, 534–537
- types and causes of, 530–533

Allergy testing, 534–535
Allograft, 621
Alternative therapy, 539
Alzheimer's disease, 137
Ambulation, 613
Amenorrhea, 472
American Association of Medical Assistants (AAMA), 3, 4, 5
American Medical Technologists (AMT), 3, 4–5
American Recovery and Reinvestment Act (ARRA), 62
American Sign Language (ASL), 133
Americans with Disabilities Act (ADA), 123
Americans with Disabilities Act Amendments Act (ADAAA), 123
Amniocentesis, 493
Amplitude, 395
Ampule, 903
AMT (American Medical Technologists), 3, 4–5
Amylase, chemistry tests, 807
Anaerobic, 772
Analytes, 799
Anaphylaxis, 532, 856, 947
Anastomosis, 451
Anesthetics, in minor surgery, 232
Angioedema, 531
Angiography, 834
Animal bite, 966
Anisocytosis, 748
Anorexia nervosa, 564, 589
Anorexia of aging, 452
Anoscope, 453
Antagonists, 853
Antecubital space, 683
Anterior cruciate ligament (ACL), 617
Antibodies, 186
Antibody, 807
Anticoagulant, 678
Anticoagulation teaching, 162
Antidote, 163
Antigen, 186, 532, 810
Antiserum, 810
Anuria, 512
Apical pulse rate, 317–318
Apical-radial pulse, 302
Apothecary, 882
Apothecary system, 882
Appearance, professionalism, 17–19
aPTT (Activated partial thromboplastin time), 754
Aqueous, 901
Aroma therapy, 542
ARRA (American Recovery and Reinvestment Act), 62
Arrhythmias, 301, 386
Art and/or Music Therapy, 542

Arterial blood, 799
Arthritis, 605, 610
Arthroscopy, 617
Artifacts, 399
Ascites, 450
Asepsis, 187, 213
Aseptic technique, 187
ASL (American Sign Language), 133
Aspirate, 908
Aspiration, 253
Aspiration pneumonia, 452
Assessment, 47
Assessment Based Recognition in Order Entry (ABR-OE), 654
Assistive device, 618
Asthma, 948
Astigmatism, 356
Asymptomatic, 643
Atherosclerosis, 388
Atraumatic needles, 234
Atrophy, 611
Attitude, professionalism, 10–11
Atypical, 483
AUB (Abnormal Uterine Bleeding), 473
Audiometer, 349, 362
Augmented leads, 397
Auricle, 350
Auscultation, 334
Auscultatory gap, 308
Autoclave, 217
Autoclaving, 217
  labeling, 219
  maintaining, 219–220
  operate, 241
  proper loading of, 219
  shelf life, 219
  sterilization indicators, 218–219
  wrapping items, 217–218, 239–240
Autograft, 621
Automated external defibrillator (AED), 950
Automated hematology analyzers, 753
Auxiliary services, 123
Axillary crutches, 628–629
Ayurveda, 542

B

Bacilli, 771
Bacitracin testing, 778
Bacteria, 769
  bacilli, 771
  binomial nomenclature system for, 769
  characteristics of, 770
  cocci, 770–771
  identification of, 775
  morphology of, 770
  spirilla, 771
Bandage, 267
Bariatrics, 562
Bariatric surgery, 563
Baseline, 295, 392
Baseline values, 643
Basic first aid, 968–972
Basophils, 743
Benign prostatic hypertrophy, 512
Bilirubin, 713, 802
Bimanual pelvic exam, 485
Binge, 564
Bioavailability, 854
Biofeedback, 542
Biohazard, 190
Biohazard label, 190–191
Bipolar leads, 396
Bisphosphonates, 623
Bleeding/pressure points, 953
Bloodborne diseases
  hepatitis, 194
  HIV/AIDS, 193–194
Bloodborne Pathogens, 197
Blood collection techniques
  blood collection tray, 681–682
  the syringe method, 684–685
  vacuum tube system, 677
  venipuncture, 674–677, 683–684
  winged infusion (butterfly) system, 680–681
Blood glucose, 817–818
Blood pressure monitoring, 164
Blood typing, 810–811
Blood urea nitrogen (BUN), 803
Blood vessels, 383
BMI (body mass index), 562
Body fluid precautions, 189–190
Body language, 103, 129
Body language, professional communication, 8
Body mass index (BMI), 293
Body's natural defenses
  immune response, 186
  immune system, 186
  immunizations, 187
  inflammation process, 186
  types of immunity, 186–187
  vaccines type, 187
Body substance isolation (BSI), 189
Body surface area (BSA), 888
Bolus, 917
Bone density scan, 164
Botox, 539
Box lock, 221
BP measurement, 319–320
Bradycardia, 301
Bradypnea, 304
Braxton-Hicks contractions, 494
Breast exam, 480–481
Breast self-examination (BSE), 480–481, 498–500
Bronchoscopy, 429
BSA (Body surface area), 888
BSI (Body substance isolation), 189
Buccal, 867
Bucky grid, 832
Bulimia nervosa, 564, 589
BUN (Blood urea nitrogen), 803
Burns, 954–956
Bursitis, 610
Business associate agreement, 67
Butterfly, 674

C

CAAHEP (Commission on Accreditation of Allied Health Education Programs), 13
Calcitonin, 623
Calcium (Ca), chemistry tests, 807
Calipers, 294
CAM (Complementary and alternative medicine), 530
Campylobacter, 565
Cane, 626–627
Cannula, 918
Capillary puncture, 688
Capillary puncture and microhematocrit test, 755–757
Carbohydrates, 553
Carcinoembryonic antigen (CEA), chemistry tests, 807
Carcinogen, 421
Cardiac arrhythmias, 386–387
Cardiac biomarker, 804
Cardiac catheterization, 403
Cardiac conduction system, 384
Cardiac cycle, 391
Cardiopulmonary resuscitation, 944
Cardiovascular exams and procedures
  abbreviation review, 385
  cardiovascular diseases, 385–390
  common lab tests, 403–405
  in-office and telephone screening tips, 385
  system snapshot, 382–385
  treatments and medications, 403
Cardiovascular physiology, 384
Cardioversion, 387

Carpal tunnel syndrome, 606, 610
Cartilage, 611
Cartridge unit, 903
CASE (Conceptually Accurate Signed English), 133
Case manager, 166
Cast, 612, 713
Cataracts, 352
Catheterization, 517
Catheterized, 709
CBC (complete blood count), 744
CCMS (Clean-catch midstream specimen), 709
CDC (Centers for Disease Control and Prevention), 179
Cell-mediated immunity, 186
Celsius (C), 296
Centers for Disease Control and Prevention (CDC), 179
Centers for Medicare & Medicaid Services (CMS), 31
Centrifuge, 659
Cerebrovascular accident (CVA), 951
Certification, 13
Certification Commission for Healthcare Information Technology (CCHIT®), 44
Certified Medical Assistant (CMA), 13, 14
Cerumen, 356
Cerumen impaction, 356
Cesarean section (C-section), 496
Chelation, 541
Chemical sterilizing agents, 217
Chemistry abbreviation review, 799
Chest CT, 429
Chief complaint, 79
Child, 574
Childhood obesity, 587
Chiropractic, 542
Chiropractor, 540, 605
Cholangiography, 835
Cholesterol, 803
Choroid layer, 350
Circumcision, 521, 586
Cirrhosis, 449, 450
Civil Rights Act, 123
Clean-catch midstream specimen (CCMS), 709
Clean-catch midstream urine collection, 725–727
Clia '88 for medical assistant, 646
CLIA-waived mono test, 820
Clinical chemistry tests, 799
Clinical diagnosis, 643
Clinical information
  drug allergies, 49
  electronic patient history form, 50
  immunizations, 49
  medical history, 49
  medication records, 50–51
  medications, 49
  physical exam, 50
  preventive screenings, 49
  progress notes, 50
Clinical Laboratory Improvement Amendments of 1988 (CLIA '88), 643
Clinically asymptomatic stage, 193–194
Clinically symptomatic stage, 194
Clinical medical assistant, 3–7
  credentialing/certification opportunities, 14–15
  errors, 6
  high degree of, 5
  legal scope of practice, 21–22
  nature of work, 6
  proximity factor, 5–6
  time factor, 6
  visibility factor, 5
Closed wounds, 264
CMA (Certified Medical Assistant), 13, 14
CMS (Centers for Medicare & Medicaid Services), 31
Coagulation cascade, 743
Coagulation tests, 754
Cocci, 770
Code of ethics, AAMA, 3, 4
COLA (Commission on Office Laboratory Accreditation), 646
Collaboration, professionalism, 12
Colles, 608
Collimator, 826
Colonies, 776
Colonoscopy, 446
Colorectal cancer, 450, 451
Color vision deficiency (CVD), 359
Colostomy, 451
Colposcopy, 487
Comminuted, 608
Commission on Accreditation of Allied Health Education Programs (CAAHEP), 13
Commission on Office Laboratory Accreditation (COLA), 646
Communication
  body language, 103
  cycle, 102
  empathy in, 164
  interviewing techniques, 103–105
  nonverbal, 103
  process, 129
  professionalism, 8–9
  screening process, 105–106
  therapeutic, 102–103
Compassion, professionalism, 16
Complementary and alternative medicine (CAM), 530
Complete blood count (CBC), 744
Complete blood count normal values, 751–752
Comprehensivemedical history, 111
Comprehensive medical history
  depression screening, 114
  family medical history, 112–113
  personal medical history, 111–112
  preventive care section, 114–115
  social history, 113–114
Compression, 608
Compulsive overeating, 564
Computed tomography (CT), 836
Computerized provider order entry (CPOE), 653
Computer Physician Order Entry (CPOE), 54
Concentric circles, 259
Conceptually Accurate Signed English (CASE), 133
Conductive hearing loss, 353
Cones, 350
Confidentiality, professionalism, 10
Conjunctiva, 350
Conjunctivitis, 352
Constipation, 452
Constrict, 674
Consumer-mediated exchange, 92
Contact dermatitis, 532
Contaminated gloves, removing, 204–205
Contrast medium, 833
Contrast sensitivity testing, 359–360
Conversion, 884
Corneal abrasion, 352
Coronary artery disease (CAD), 387, 388–389
Correspondence application, 60–61
Cosmetic Dermatologist, 538
Cough etiquette, 159
CPOE (Computerized provider order entry), 54, 653
Crash cart, 949
Credentialing, 13
Crohn's disease, 449
Crutch gaits, 611–616
Cryosurgery, 256

Cryotherapy, 620
Cubic centimeters (cc), 900
Cultural diversity, 126
Culture, 775
Culture and sensitivity (C&S) test, 775
Culture medium, 775
CVA (Cerebrovascular accident), 951
Cystitis, 513
Cystoscopy, 518
Cytologic, 482
Cytology, 482

D

DASH (Dietary Approaches to Stop Hypertension), 563
Debridement, 266, 619
Declining stage, 185
Defibrillation, 387, 950
Dementia, 137
Demographics, and Memory Study (ADAMS), 137
Dentist, 538
Dependability, professionalism, 15
Depolarization, 384
Dermal fillers, 539
Dermatologist, 534, 538
Diabetic coma, 957
Diabetic ketoacidosis, 957
Diabetic teaching and home care, 159–160
Diagnostic imaging
  computed tomography (CT) scan, 836–837
  legal considerations, 826
  medical assistant's role, 827
  radiographic equipment, 826–827
  radiographic films, 830
  radiological procedures outside the office, 832–834
  radiology, 826
  safety precautions, 831–832
  ultrasound/sonography, 837–838
Dialysis, 521–523, 522
Diaphoresis, 949
Diarrhea, 452
Diastole, 304
Diastolic pressure, 304
Diet and nutrition
  digestive process, 552
  healthy diet, 555–558
  life cycle, 554–556
  nutrients, 553–554
  nutrition abbreviations, 552–553
  screening and assessment, 562
  weight maintenance, 560–561
Dietetic Technician, 552
Dietitians, 552
Differential count, 743, 747–748
Differential diagnosis, 643
Digital rectal exam (DRE), 517
Dignity, 3
Dilatation, 521
Dilation, 487
Diluent, 907
Diplomacy, professionalism, 11
Directed exchange, 92
Disinfectants, preparing and storing, 215
Disinfecting solutions, levels of, 215
Disinfection, 183, 214
Disinfection procedures, 214–215
Dislocation, 607, 964
Dispense, 858
Dispose of appropriate PPE, universal or standard precautions, 205–207
Dissect, 223
Distance, professional communication, 9
Diurnal rhythms, 295
Diversity, 126
Dobutamine stress test, 402
Doctor of Osteopathy (D.O.), 540
Documentation
  administration of medication, 93–94
  chief complaints and progress notes, 79–80
  corrections or addendums, 92
  electronic technology, professional correspondence, 92–93
  guidelines for, 75
  in-office procedures, 80, 82
  in-office screening, 108
  laboratory procedures, 80
  for legal success, 75–76
  medical abbreviations, use of, 79
  medications, 82–84
  patient education sessions, 88
  patient's medical record, 76–79
  phone call from patient, 95
  prescriptions, 84–87
  scheduling outside procedures, 90, 91
  telephone calls, 88–89
Domestic violence screening and detection, 165–166
"Do Not Use" abbreviations list, 79
Dosage calculations
  drug dosages, 886–889
  insulin dosages, 889–890
  medication label, 890–891
  medication math fundamentals, 882–886
  medication order, 882
Drawing blood cultures, 690
Dressing, 266, 284–286
Drug, 845
  actions, 855
  administration, 865–867
  ceiling, 854
  classifications, 848–853
  dosage, 882
  dose response, 854
  effects, 856
  interaction, 856
  medicinal uses of, 847–848
  names, 857–858
  origins, 846–847
  regulations and legal classifications of, 858–860
  resources, 864–865
  testing, 811–812
Dry heat sterilization, 216
Dysmenorrhea, 472
Dyspnea, 303, 420
Dysrhythmias, 301
Dysuria, 512

E

Ear
  anatomy, 350–351
  culture, 366
  diseases, 353
  infections, 356
  instillation, 364, 373–374
  irrigation, 364, 375
  medications, 365
Eating disorders, 563–564
Echocardiography, 402
Eclampsia, 495
E. coli, 565
Ectopic, 493
ED (Erectile dysfunction), 514
Educational environment, 201
Educational (coaching) process
  individual diversity, 157
  patient concerns, 157
  resources, 156–157
  self-boundaries, 158
Education, professionalism, 13
Effacement, 492
Effective communication, professionalism, 9–10
Efficacy, 845
Elder abuse, 138
Electrocardiogram (EKG or ECG), 391

Electrocardiograph, 392
Electrocoagulation, 255
Electrodes, 392, 395
Electrodesiccation, 255
Electrofulguration, 255
Electrolytes, 395, 553
Electronic health records (EHRs), 41
 amending information, 44
 application, 51, 58
 bluetooth® capabilities, 58–59
 bluetoothr capabilities, 58–59
 certification of, 44
 computer network provides, 43
 consultation reports, 55
 creating and maintaining, 43–44
 diagnostic reports, 55
 documentation, 81–82
 features of, 43
 flow sheets, 58
 hospital reports, 58
 laboratory documents, 54–55
 living will, 59–60
 nursing home reports, 55
 phone reports, 52–54
 pitfalls of, 43
 push for, 44–45
 responsibilities, 61–62
 therapeutic reports, 55–58
 vital signs, 51–52
Electronic medical records (EMRs), 41
Electrosection, 255
Embolus, 951
Empathy, 164
 in communication, 164
Empathy, professionalism, 16
Endoscopes, 213
Endoscopic retrograde cholangiopancreatogram (ERCP), 835
Endoscopy, 446
Endospores, 180
Engagement, professionalism, 12–15
Enteral, 867
Eosinophils, 743
Epidemiology, 180
Epidermis, 538
Epinephrine, 532
ERCP (Endoscopic retrograde cholangiopancreatogram), 835
Erectile dysfunction (ED), 514
Erosion, 452
Erythrocytes, 741
Erythrocyte sedimentation rate (ESR), 752–753, 759–760
Ethics and morals, 7
Evacuated tube, 674
Examination, 326
Exercises, 621–622
Exhalation, 302
Expiration, 302
Expiration date, 891
Exploitation, 139
Exposure control, 195
Exposure determination
 compliance rules for, 195–196
 employee training, 196
 engineering controls, 196–197
 vaccinations, 196
External controls, 648
Extracorporeal, 521
Extracorporeal shock wave lithotripsy, 512
Extravasation, 920
Exudate, 266
Eye
 anatomy, 350
 contact, professional communication, 9
 diseases, 352–353
 and ear abbreviations, 352
 injuries related to burns, 956
 instillation, 360, 370–371
 irrigation, 360–361, 371–373
 medications, 361

F

Facial expression, professional communication, 8–9
Fahrenheit (F), 296
Faith and Prayer, 542
Fallopian tubes, 471
Familial stature, 575
Family medical history, 112
Fasting blood glucose level, 805
Febrile, 295
Fecal occult blood test, 460–461
Fecal specimen, 458–459
Fee for service model, 30
Fenestrated, 230
Fever, 295
 causes of, 299
 course of, 300
Fiber, 553
Fibrin, 743
Fissures, 453
Fistulas, 449
Flexible sigmoidoscopy, 462–463
Flow sheets, 58, 658
Fluoroscopy, 835
Foley catheters, 518
Fomites, 183
Foodborne ill nesses, 564–555
Foreign body removal, 365
Fovea centralis, 350
Fracture, 607
Frail senior, 136
Frostbite, 961
Fungi, 783

G

Galactosemia, 586
Gas sterilization, 216
Gastritis, 452
Gastroenteritis, 452
Gastroenterologist, 552
Gastroenterology, 456
Gastroesophageal reflux disease (GERD), 449
Gastrointestinal exams and procedures
 fecal occult blood testing, 454–455
 gastroenterology, 456
 gastrointestinal abbreviation, 448
 gastrointestinal diseases, 449–452
 gastrointestinal system, 448
 in-office and telephone screening tips, 448–449
 lab tests, 456–457
 rectal exams, 453–454
Gauge, 675, 900
Generic name, 891
Genogram, 112
GERD (Gastroesophageal reflux disease), 449
Gestation, 489
Gesture, 103
Gestures, professional communication, 9
Glaucoma, 354
Gloving, 188–189
Gluten, 564
Glycemic index (GI), 563
Gram (g, gm), 883
Gram negative, 772
Gram positive, 772
Gram stain, 771
Gravida, 481
Gray (Gy), 831
Greenstick, 608
Grid, 826
Grief, identify common stages of, 164–165
Guide dogs, 132

H

Handle, 220
Handwashing, 159, 188–189
Health care delivery models, 35–36
Health care team dynamics, principles of, 12
Health coach, 155
Health coaching
  hygienic practices, 158–159
  office policies, 158
Health coaching session, 169–171
Health information technology (HIT), 35, 44
Health Information Technology for Economic and Clinical Health (HITECH) Act, 62
Health Insurance Portability and Accountability Act of 1996 (HIPAA), 42
Health maintenance and disease prevention, 159
Heat cramps, 961
Heat exhaustion, 961
Heat stroke, 961
Heat therapy, 619
Hematemesis, 449
Hematochezia, 455
Hematocrit (Hct), 746
Hematoma, 685
Hematopoiesis, 741
Hematuria, 714
Hemoconcentration, 684
Hemodialysis, 521
Hemoglobin, 742, 745
Hemoglobinuria, 714
Hemolysis, 688
Hemorrhaging, 953
Hemorrhoids, 453
Hemostasis, 743
Hernias, 517
Hiatal hernia, 452
High cholesterol teaching, 162
High-complexity testing, 645
High-density lipoprotein (HDL), 803
HIPAA Privacy Rule, 63
HIPAA Security Rule, 63
History of present illness (HPI), 107
HIT (Health information technology), 35
HIV/AIDS
  progression of, 194
  stages of HIV, 193–194
Holter monitor, 400
Home anticoagulation monitoring, 162–163
Home blood sugar monitoring, 160
Home cholesterol monitoring, 162
Home injection therapies, 161
Home monitoring equipment, 163
Homeopathy, 540
Homeostasis, 295, 799
Honesty, professionalism, 16
Human chorionic gonadotropin (hCG), 808
Humoral immunity, 186
Hygiene issues, and physically disabled patient, 141
Hyperbaric oxygen (HBO2) therapy, 269
Hyperglycemia, 804
Hyperopia, 356
Hyperpnea, 304
Hypertension, 307
Hyperthermia, 299
Hypertrophy, 514
Hyperventilation, 304
Hypnosis, 542
Hypodermic, 906
Hypoglycemia, 804
Hypotension, 307
Hypothermia, 300, 962
Hypothyroidism, 586

I

IBS (irritable bowel syndrome), 452
Idiopathic, 449
IIHI (individually identifiable health information), 63
Ileostomy, 451
Immunizations, 581
Immunoglobulins, 187
Immunosuppressed, 182
Immunotherapy, 536
Inanimate, 214
Incisions, 962
Incubation, 776
Incubation stage, 185
Individually identifiable health information (IIHI), 63
Induration, 429
Infant, 574
Infection control
  medical asepsis, 188–189
  surgical asepsis, 189
Infection control standards, 191–192
Infection cycle
  infectious (causative) agents, 180–182
  means of transmission, 183
  portal of entry, 183
  portal of exit, 183
  reservoir, 182
  susceptible host, 182
Infection process, 180
Infection, stages of, 185
Infectious (causative) agents
  bacteria, 180–181
  fungi, 182
  parasites, 182
  protozoa, 181–182
  viruses, 181
Infectious Diseases, 184
Infectious waste, 197
Infertility Specialist, 475
Infiltration, 920
Inflammatory response, 186
Information technology, 35–36
Informed consent, 77
Inhalation, 302
Inhalers, 430
Initiative, professionalism, 12–15
Inoculation, 777
Inspecting instruments, 214
Inspection, 334
Inspiration, 302
Instillation, 349
Institute for Safe Medication Practices (ISMP), 79
Insulin, 552
Insulin shock, 957
Integrative health care, 530, 539
Integrity, professionalism, 15
Intellectual disabilities, 142–143
Internal bleeding, 953–954
Internal controls, 648
International normalized ratio (INR), 754
Interval, 392
Interviewing techniques
  chief complaint and history, 106–107
  common signs and symptoms, 107
  drug allergies, 106
  effective listening techniques, 103, 104, 105
  effective questioning techniques, 103, 104
  greeting stage, 105–106
  ineffective questioning techniques, 103–104
  medication reconciliation, 106
  performance of height, 106
  vital signs, 106
  weight, 106
Intra-articular, 921

Intradermal, 910
Intradermal test, 534
Intramuscular (IM), 912
Intravenous pyelogram (IVP), 519
Invasion and multiplication stage, 185
Irrigation, 349
Irritable bowel syndrome (IBS), 452
Ischemia, 951
Ishihara method, 359
Ishihara test for color vision, 369
ISMP (Institute for Safe Medication Practices), 79
Isoelectric line, 391

J

Jaeger chart, 358
Jaws, 221
Joint Commission (JC), 79

K

Kcalories, 554
Ketones, 713
Kidney transplant, 523
Kinesiology, 540
Korotkoff sounds, 305
Kyphosis, 605

L

Laboratory departments, 646
Laboratory regulations, 644–646
Laboratory report, 656
Laboratory report form, 656
Laboratory, safety in, 651
Laboratory tests, 643
Lab requisition form, 652
Lacerations, 253, 962
Lactose, 564
Lancets, 689
Language development, 579
Laser, 255
Lead, 396
12-lead electrocardiogram, 406–408
Lens, 350
LEP (limited english proficiency), 125
Leukocytes, 743
Licensing, 13
Ligature, 232
Light Therapy, 542
Limited English proficiency (LEP), 125
Lipase, chemistry tests, 807
Lipemia, 688
Lipid profile, 803
Lipoprotein, 803
Liter (L), 883
Lithotomy, 453
Lithotripsy, 521
Local reaction, 856
Lochia, 496
Lot control, 891
Low-density lipoprotein (LDL), 803
Lubricating instruments, 214
Luer-Lok, 900
Lymphocytes, 741

M

Macrocephaly, 577
Macrocyte, 748
Macular degeneration, 352
Magnesium (Mg), chemistry tests, 807
Magnetic resonance imaging (MRI), 836
Malabsorption syndrome, 563
Male reproductive health information, 112
Male reproductive system, 510–511
  diagnostic testing, 518–519
  in-office and telephone screening tips, 512–513
  lab tests, 523–524
  percutaneous suprapubic bladder aspiration, 519
  provider examination, 515–517
  urinary catheterization, 517–518
  urological diseases and conditions, 513–515
  urological treatments and medications, 521–523
Mammography, 487
Manipulation, 334
Mantoux skin test, 429
Mantoux test, 531
Massage, 618
Massage therapist, 540
Massage therapy, 542
Material Safety Data Sheet (MSDS), 215
Mayo stand, 260–261
Meaningful use, 63–66
MEC (minimum effective concentration), 216
Meconium, 496
Medical abbreviation review, 180
Medical asepsis, 187, 188–189, 213
Medical assistant, 263–264
  responsibilities for, 61–62
  role, in history collection, 106–107
Medical history information, tools, 109–111
Medical home, 33–38
Medically aseptic handwashing, 202–203
Medical office emergencies
  identification and response, 944–997
  preparing personnel, 944
Medical office/tray setups
  lasers, or chemicals, 253, 255–256
  no special equipment, 253, 254
Medical records
  administrative information in, 49
  clinical information, 49–61
  confidentiality, 67
  contents, 48–61
  disposal of, 67
  electronic access audit/activity log, 67–68
  formats, 46–48
  important uses of, 45
  laws affect medical records, 62–66
  paper chart creation, 48
  retention of, 67
  sharing protected information, 66–68
Medication dosage, 893
Medication label, 890
Medication order or prescription writing, 860–864, 873–874
Medication tasks, 858
Medicinal, 846
Melanocytes, 538
Melena, 454
Menarche, 472
Menopause, 472, 473–474
Menses, 472
Menstrual cycle, 472
Menstruation, 472
Mensuration, 293, 334
Mental disorders or impairments, 142–143
Mental health, 142
Mental illness, 142
Mental impairment, 142
Mentally challenged, 143
Mentally or emotionally distressed patients, 967
Metabolic syndrome, 563
Metabolism, 296, 554
Meter (m), 882
Metered-Dose Inhalers (MDI), 430
Metric system, 882

Microbiology, 768
bacteria, 769–772
divisions, 769
lab requisition and test report, 785–787
microbiology abbreviation, 769
microorganisms, 769
microscopic techniques, 780–781
parasitology, 781–785
quality control, 785
sensitivity testing, 779–780
specimen collection, 772–775
virology, 781
Microcephaly, 577
Microcyte, 748
Microdermabrasion, 537
Microorganisms, 183–185
Microscope, 658, 666–668
Middle ear infections, 355
Midwife, 475
Milestones, 579
Mindfulness Meditation, 542
Mindfulness, professionalism, 17–19
Minerals, 553
Minimum effective concentration (MEC), 216
Minor surgery
absorbable suture material, 233
anesthetics in, 232
close the skin, 234
nonabsorbable suture material, 233
skin staples, 234–235
solutions in, 229–230
sterile skin closures, 235
supplies in, 230–232
surgical adhesives, 235
surgical glue, 235
suture and staple removal, 236
suture materials in, 232, 233
suture needle, 234
suture sizing, 234
Miscarriages, 489
Modalities, 618
Moderate-complexity tests, 644
Molecular imaging, 838
Monocytes, 743
Morals, 7
Morphology, 743
Motor, 579
Motor development, 579
Multiple allergosorbent test system (MAST), 536
Musculoskeletal system, 602–606
diagnostic tests, 623
in-office and telephone screening tips, 606–607
medications, 623
musculoskeletal abbreviation, 606
orthopedic conditions, 607–611
Mycology, 783–785
Myocardial infarction (MI), 949
Myopia, 356

N

National Association of the Deaf (NAD), 132
National Cancer Institute (NCI), 484–485
National Committee for Quality Assurance (NCQA), 33
National Drug Code (NDC), 891
National Healthcareer Association (NHA), 3
Naturopathic Medicine, 540
NCQA (National Committee for Quality Assurance), 33
NDC (National Drug Code), 891
Near visual acuity (NVA), 358, 368
Nebulizers, 430
Nebulizer treatment, 440
Neglect, 138
Neonate, 574
Neurologist, 606
Neurosensory hearing loss, 353
Neutrophils, 743
Newborn, 574
Newborn screenings, 586
New delivery models, medical assistant's role in, 36
NHA (National Healthcareer Association), 3
Night eating syndrome, 564
Nocturia, 512
Nomogram, 888
Noninvasive heart scan, 403
Nonsteroidal anti-inflammatory drugs (NSAIDs), 452
Nonverbal communication, professionalism, 8–9
Normal flora, 180, 768
Normal sinus rhythm, 386
Normal values, 651
Normocyte, 748
Norovirus, 565
Notice of Privacy Practices (NPP), 63
NPP (Notice of Privacy Practices), 63
NSAIDs (nonsteroidal anti-inflammatory drugs), 452
Nuclear medicine, 838
Nutrient, 553
Nutrition, 551
Nutritionists, 552
NVA (near visual acuity), 358, 368

O

Obama Care. *See* Patient Protection and Affordable Care Act (PPACA)
Obesity, 293, 562–563
OB-GYN, 475
OB-GYN history, 111
Objective impressions, 47
Observations, 335
Obstetrics and gynecology
fallopian tubes, 471
female reproductive system, 470
in-office and telephone screening tips, 476
labor and delivery, 494
lab tests, 488
menopause, 473–474
menstrual cycle, 472
obstetric and gynecologic abbreviation, 476
obstetric and gynecologic diseases, 476–480
obstetric treatments, 494
ovaries, 470–471
postnatal or postpartum period, 497
procedures, 480–487
treatments and medications, 488
uterus, 471–472
Occlusion, 919
Occult, 446
Occupational Safety and Health Administration (OSHA), 179, 194
blood, body fluids, and OPIM, 195
bloodborne pathogen standard, 194–195
exposure control plan, 195–197
exposure determination, 195
regulated waste, 197–199
Occupational therapist (OT), 606
Ocular, 659
Office surgeries
setup procedures, 256–257
surgical suite, 257–262
Oliguria, 512
Opened-container life, 215
Open sterile items, 275–277
Open wounds, 264, 962
Ophthalmic, 360
Ophthalmologist, 534
Ophthalmoscope, 349

Sanguineous, 267
Sanitization, 183, 213
Scatter radiation, 831
Sclera, 350
Scoliosis, 605
Scope of practice, 6
Scrubs, 45
Sebaceous cyst, 253
Secondary dressings, 266
Secondary drug, 907
Secondary sex characteristics, 588
Sediment, 718
Segment, 392
Seizures, 958
Senior abuse, 138
Sensitivity testing, 779
Sensory, 579
Sensory developments, 580
Serology and immunology tests, 807–810
Serosanguineous, 267
Serous, 267
Serrations, 221
Serum, 678, 741, 799
Sexually transmitted diseases (STDs), 479
Sexually transmitted infections (STIs), 479
Shank, 221
Sharps, 190
Shelf life, 215
Shingling, 54
Shock, 959
Side effect, 856
Sievert (Sv), 831
Sighted guide assistance, 130
Sigmoidoscopy, 451
Signed English, 133
Signed Exact English (SEE), 133
Silence, professional communication, 9
Skin closures, procedure, 242–243
Skin prick tests, 534
Skin-prep procedures, 259–260
Sleep apnea, 429
Smoking risks and cessation programs, 162
Snellen chart, 356
Snellen chart visual acuity testing, 366–367
Social history, 113–114
Solutions, in minor surgery, 229–230
Sonogram, 837
Source-oriented medical record (SOMR), 45
Special diets, 563–564, 567–568
Special needs patient
  communication and techniques to overcome, 126–129
  deaf impaired patient, 132–139
  diversity in health care, 126
  hearing impaired patient, 123–124, 132–139
  intellectual disabilities, 142–143
  non-english-speaking patients, 125–126
  pediatric patients, 139–141
  persons with physical disabilities, 125
  physically disabled patients, 141–142
  visually impaired patient, 124, 130–132
Specific gravity, 714
Specimen collection, 663–666
  butterfly method, 685
  microbiology, 772–775
  response and complications, 685
  by syringe method, 684–685
  urinalysis, 708–711
  vacuum tube method, 685
Specimen handling, general guidelines for, 690
Specimen rejection, 687–688
Sphygmomanometer, 306
Spirometer, 425
Spirometry, 425, 434–435
Splint, 607
Splint an arm, 625–626
Sprain, 607
Sputum, 428
Sputum specimen, 438–440
Standard of care, 6
Standard precaution symbols, 192
Standard Precautions and Transmission Based Precautions, 189
Standardization, 398
STDs (sexually transmitted diseases), 479
Stent, 389
Sterile conscience, 252, 252
Sterile solution, 261, 278–280
Sterilization, 185, 216
Sterilization indicators, 218
Stethoscope, 305
STIs (sexually transmitted infections), 479
Stoma, 451
Storing chemical disinfectants, 215
Strain, 607
Streptococcus identification, 778
Stylus, 394
Subatmospheric pressure device, 268
Subcutaneous, 536, 912
Subjective impressions, 47
Subjective information, 106
Subjective, objective, assessment, plan (SOAP), 46
Sublingual, 867
Substance Abuse and Mental Health Services Administration (SAMHSA), 142
Sudden infant death syndrome (SIDS), 587
Supernatant, 718
Supplements, 553
Supplies, in minor surgery, 230–232
Surgical adhesives, 235
Surgical asepsis, 187, 189, 213
Surgical attire, 281–283
Surgical gloves, 270–272
Surgical handwash, 262–263, 270–272
Surgical histories and hospitalizations, 112
Surgical instrument
  categories of, 222
  chemical disinfection, 238
  cutting and dissecting, 223, 224–225
  grasping and clamping, 223, 225–227
  identifying the parts of, 220–221
  sanitization and lubrication, 236–237
  tips of, 221–222
  visualization, 223, 227–229
Surgical procedures, 617
  using one-step scrub, 273–274
Surgical tray, 274–275
Surgical wicks, 231
Suture, 232
Suture and staple removal, 236
Suture materials, in minor surgery, 232, 233
Suture or staple removal procedure, 244–246
Symptoms, 106
Syncope, 961
Systemic reaction, 856
Systole, 304
Systolic pressure, 304

T

Tachycardia, 301
Tachypnea, 304
Tact or tactfulness, professionalism, 11
Taut, 913
Taxonomy, 769
Telecommunications device for the deaf (TDD), 123
Telecommunications Relay Services (TRS), 123
Teletypewriter (TTY), 123
Temperature, 311, 314
  an infant or young child, 591–593

Posture, 335
Practice management, 41
Pre- and post-op care instructions, 164
Precipitate, 905
Precordial leads, 397
Preeclampsia (toxemia), 491, 492
Pregnancy, 491
Prelingual, 133
Prenatal, 489
Prenatal exam, 503–504
Presbyopia, 356
Prescribe, 858
Prescription, 891
Prescriptions, surgical procedure, 258
Primary container, 690
Primary dressings, 266
Primary drug, 907
Primary HIV infection stage, 193
Problem list, 46
Problem-oriented medical record (POMR), 45
Problem-solving, professionalism, 17
Proctoscope, 453
Procurement station, 647
Prodromal stage, 185
Product name, 891
Professional appearance, 17–19
Professional characteristics development, 7–8
Professional communication, 8–9
Professional credentials, 13–15
Professional ethics, 7
Professionalism, 3–24
Professionalism mentor, 20, 31
Professionalism skills development, 20
Proficiency testing, 650
Profile, 643
Progressive Muscle Relaxation, 542
Progress note, 80
Progress notes, 45
Prophylactic, 514, 848
Prostate-specific antigen (PSA), chemistry tests, 807
Prostatitis, 513
Prosthesis, 617
Protected health information (PHI), 63
Proteins, 553
Prothrombin time (PT), 754, 760–762
Provider-performed microscopy (PPM) procedures, 644
Puberty, 574
Puerperium, 488
Pulmonary examinations and procedures
  bronchoscopy, 429
  chest CT, 429
  chest X-ray, 428
  in-office screening and telephone screening tips, 419
  lab tests, 432
  lung anatomy, 417
  magnetic resonance imaging (MRI), 429
  peak flow testing, 426–427
  physiology, 417–418
  pulmonary function testing, 425–426
  pulmonary medical abbreviation, 419–420
  pulse oximetry testing, 427–428
  respiratory diseases, 419–424
  sputum collection, 428
  thoracentesis, 429
  treatments and medications, 430–432
Pulmonary function testing, 425
Pulmonology, 418
Pulse deficit, 302
Pulse pressure, 304
Pulse rate, 300
Pulse rhythm, 301
Pulse volume, 301
Punctures, 963
Pure culture, 776
Purulent, 267
Pyelonephritis, 513

Q

Qualitative, 649
Quality assurance (QA), 648
Quality control (QC), 648, 711
Quantitative, 649
Quantity not sufficient (QNS), 687

R

Radial pulse rate, 315–316
Radiate, 295
Radiation therapy, 839–840. *See also* Diagnostic imaging
Radioallergosorbent test (RAST), 536
Radiographs, 826
Radiologist, 825
Radiolucent, 832
Radiopaque, 832
Radiopharmaceuticals, 838
Random collection, 710
Random collection specimen, 710
Range of motion (ROM), 622
Rapid strep test, 788–789
RAST (radioallergosorbent test), 536
Ratchet, 221
Reagent test strip, 714
Receptors, 853
Rectal vaginal exam, 485
Rectoscope, 453
Red blood cell (RBC)
  count, 744
  indices, 749
  morphology, 748–750
Reduction, 607
Reference ranges, 651
Reflexes, 580
Refractive disorders, 351
Refractometer, 714
Registered Medical Assistant (RMA), 13, 14
Registration, 13
Regulated waste, OSHA'S chemical hygiene plan, 199–201
Rehabilitation, 618
Renal profile, 803
Renal threshold, 708
Repolarization, 384
Resistance, 186
Respect, professionalism, 16–17
Respiration, 302
Respiration rate, 315–316
Responsibility, 3
Reticulocyte, 741
Retin-A (tretinoin), 539
Retina, 350
Retroperitoneal, 510
Reuse life, 215
Reverse chronological order, 45
Rh blood typing, 811
Rhythm strip, 398
RMA (Registered Medical Assistant), 13, 14
Rods, 350
Routes, medication administration, 867–872
Routine urinalysis
  chemical urinalysis, 714–716
  clarity/turbidity, 713–714
  color, 713
  physical examination, 712–713
  specific gravity, 714
Rx Norm, 52

S

Safety Data Sheet (SDS), 215
Salmonella, 565
SAMHSA (Substance Abuse and Mental Health Services Administration), 142

Sanguineous, 267
Sanitization, 183, 213
Scatter radiation, 831
Sclera, 350
Scoliosis, 605
Scope of practice, 6
Scrubs, 45
Sebaceous cyst, 253
Secondary dressings, 266
Secondary drug, 907
Secondary sex characteristics, 588
Sediment, 718
Segment, 392
Seizures, 958
Senior abuse, 138
Sensitivity testing, 779
Sensory, 579
Sensory developments, 580
Serology and immunology tests, 807–810
Serosanguineous, 267
Serous, 267
Serrations, 221
Serum, 678, 741, 799
Sexually transmitted diseases (STDs), 479
Sexually transmitted infections (STIs), 479
Shank, 221
Sharps, 190
Shelf life, 215
Shingling, 54
Shock, 959
Side effect, 856
Sievert (Sv), 831
Sighted guide assistance, 130
Sigmoidoscopy, 451
Signed English, 133
Signed Exact English (SEE), 133
Silence, professional communication, 9
Skin closures, procedure, 242–243
Skin prick tests, 534
Skin-prep procedures, 259–260
Sleep apnea, 429
Smoking risks and cessation programs, 162
Snellen chart, 356
Snellen chart visual acuity testing, 366–367
Social history, 113–114
Solutions, in minor surgery, 229–230
Sonogram, 837
Source-oriented medical record (SOMR), 45
Special diets, 563–564, 567–568
Special needs patient
  communication and techniques to overcome, 126–129
  deaf impaired patient, 132–139
  diversity in health care, 126
  hearing impaired patient, 123–124, 132–139
  intellectual disabilities, 142–143
  non-english-speaking patients, 125–126
  pediatric patients, 139–141
  persons with physical disabilities, 125
  physically disabled patients, 141–142
  visually impaired patient, 124, 130–132
Specific gravity, 714
Specimen collection, 663–666
  butterfly method, 685
  microbiology, 772–775
  response and complications, 685
  by syringe method, 684–685
  urinalysis, 708–711
  vacuum tube method, 685
Specimen handling, general guidelines for, 690
Specimen rejection, 687–688
Sphygmomanometer, 306
Spirometer, 425
Spirometry, 425, 434–435
Splint, 607
Splint an arm, 625–626
Sprain, 607
Sputum, 428
Sputum specimen, 438–440
Standard of care, 6
Standard precaution symbols, 192
Standard Precautions and Transmission Based Precautions, 189
Standardization, 398
STDs (sexually transmitted diseases), 479
Stent, 389
Sterile conscience, 252, 252
Sterile solution, 261, 278–280
Sterilization, 185, 216
Sterilization indicators, 218
Stethoscope, 305
STIs (sexually transmitted infections), 479
Stoma, 451
Storing chemical disinfectants, 215
Strain, 607
Streptococcus identification, 778
Stylus, 394
Subatmospheric pressure device, 268
Subcutaneous, 536, 912
Subjective impressions, 47
Subjective information, 106
Subjective, objective, assessment, plan (SOAP), 46
Sublingual, 867
Substance Abuse and Mental Health Services Administration (SAMHSA), 142
Sudden infant death syndrome (SIDS), 587
Supernatant, 718
Supplements, 553
Supplies, in minor surgery, 230–232
Surgical adhesives, 235
Surgical asepsis, 187, 189, 213
Surgical attire, 281–283
Surgical gloves, 270–272
Surgical handwash, 262–263, 270–272
Surgical histories and hospitalizations, 112
Surgical instrument
  categories of, 222
  chemical disinfection, 238
  cutting and dissecting, 223, 224–225
  grasping and clamping, 223, 225–227
  identifying the parts of, 220–221
  sanitization and lubrication, 236–237
  tips of, 221–222
  visualization, 223, 227–229
Surgical procedures, 617
  using one-step scrub, 273–274
Surgical tray, 274–275
Surgical wicks, 231
Suture, 232
Suture and staple removal, 236
Suture materials, in minor surgery, 232, 233
Suture or staple removal procedure, 244–246
Symptoms, 106
Syncope, 961
Systemic reaction, 856
Systole, 304
Systolic pressure, 304

T

Tachycardia, 301
Tachypnea, 304
Tact or tactfulness, professionalism, 11
Taut, 913
Taxonomy, 769
Telecommunications device for the deaf (TDD), 123
Telecommunications Relay Services (TRS), 123
Teletypewriter (TTY), 123
Temperature, 311, 314
  an infant or young child, 591–593

Microbiology, 768
  bacteria, 769–772
  divisions, 769
  lab requisition and test report, 785–787
  microbiology abbreviation, 769
  microorganisms, 769
  microscopic techniques, 780–781
  parasitology, 781–785
  quality control, 785
  sensitivity testing, 779–780
  specimen collection, 772–775
  virology, 781
Microcephaly, 577
Microcyte, 748
Microdermabrasion, 537
Microorganisms, 183–185
Microscope, 658, 666–668
Middle ear infections, 355
Midwife, 475
Milestones, 579
Mindfulness Meditation, 542
Mindfulness, professionalism, 17–19
Minerals, 553
Minimum effective concentration (MEC), 216
Minor surgery
  absorbable suture material, 233
  anesthetics in, 232
  close the skin, 234
  nonabsorbable suture material, 233
  skin staples, 234–235
  solutions in, 229–230
  sterile skin closures, 235
  supplies in, 230–232
  surgical adhesives, 235
  surgical glue, 235
  suture and staple removal, 236
  suture materials in, 232, 233
  suture needle, 234
  suture sizing, 234
Miscarriages, 489
Modalities, 618
Moderate-complexity tests, 644
Molecular imaging, 838
Monocytes, 743
Morals, 7
Morphology, 743
Motor, 579
Motor development, 579
Multiple allergosorbent test system (MAST), 536
Musculoskeletal system, 602–606
  diagnostic tests, 623
  in-office and telephone screening tips, 606–607
  medications, 623
  musculoskeletal abbreviation, 606
  orthopedic conditions, 607–611
Mycology, 783–785
Myocardial infarction (MI), 949
Myopia, 356

N

National Association of the Deaf (NAD), 132
National Cancer Institute (NCI), 484–485
National Committee for Quality Assurance (NCQA), 33
National Drug Code (NDC), 891
National Healthcareer Association (NHA), 3
Naturopathic Medicine, 540
NCQA (National Committee for Quality Assurance), 33
NDC (National Drug Code), 891
Near visual acuity (NVA), 358, 368
Nebulizers, 430
Nebulizer treatment, 440
Neglect, 138
Neonate, 574
Neurologist, 606
Neurosensory hearing loss, 353
Neutrophils, 743
Newborn, 574
Newborn screenings, 586
New delivery models, medical assistant's role in, 36
NHA (National Healthcareer Association), 3
Night eating syndrome, 564
Nocturia, 512
Nomogram, 888
Noninvasive heart scan, 403
Nonsteroidal anti-inflammatory drugs (NSAIDs), 452
Nonverbal communication, professionalism, 8–9
Normal flora, 180, 768
Normal sinus rhythm, 386
Normal values, 651
Normocyte, 748
Norovirus, 565
Notice of Privacy Practices (NPP), 63
NPP (Notice of Privacy Practices), 63
NSAIDs (nonsteroidal anti-inflammatory drugs), 452
Nuclear medicine, 838
Nutrient, 553
Nutrition, 551
Nutritionists, 552
NVA (near visual acuity), 358, 368

O

Obama Care. *See* Patient Protection and Affordable Care Act (PPACA)
Obesity, 293, 562–563
OB-GYN, 475
OB-GYN history, 111
Objective impressions, 47
Observations, 335
Obstetrics and gynecology
  fallopian tubes, 471
  female reproductive system, 470
  in-office and telephone screening tips, 476
  labor and delivery, 494
  lab tests, 488
  menopause, 473–474
  menstrual cycle, 472
  obstetric and gynecologic abbreviation, 476
  obstetric and gynecologic diseases, 476–480
  obstetric treatments, 494
  ovaries, 470–471
  postnatal or postpartum period, 497
  procedures, 480–487
  treatments and medications, 488
  uterus, 471–472
Occlusion, 919
Occult, 446
Occupational Safety and Health Administration (OSHA), 179, 194
  blood, body fluids, and OPIM, 195
  bloodborne pathogen standard, 194–195
  exposure control plan, 195–197
  exposure determination, 195
  regulated waste, 197–199
Occupational therapist (OT), 606
Ocular, 659
Office surgeries
  setup procedures, 256–257
  surgical suite, 257–262
Oliguria, 512
Opened-container life, 215
Open sterile items, 275–277
Open wounds, 264, 962
Ophthalmic, 360
Ophthalmologist, 534
Ophthalmoscope, 349

Opportunistic infections, 193, 769
Optometrist, 534
Oral food challenge (OFC), 536
Oral glucose tolerance test (OGTT), 805–806
Oral medication, 874–876
Oral medications, 163
Organizational ethics, 7
Orthomolecular Medicine, 542
Orthopedist, 605
Orthopnea, 303
Orthostatic hypotension, 307, 961
Ossicles, 350
Osteopathic Manipulative Therapy (OMT), 542
Osteoporosis, 609
Osteoporosis screening, 164
Other potentially infectious material (OPIM), 189
Otic, 364
Otolaryngologist, 534
Otoscope, 349
Ova and parasite testing, 791–793
Oval window, 350
Ovaries, 470–471
Oxygen administration, 431
Oxygen saturation, 427

P

Pain management specialist, 540
Palpate, 674
Palpation, 334
Pancreatitis, 452
Pap test, 483, 500–502
Para, 481
Parasite, 782
Parasitology, 782–783
Parenteral, 867, 899
Parenteral medications
  equipment and supplies, 899
  general guidelines, 908–910
  immunizations, 915–917
  intravenous therapy, 917–921
  parenteral complications, 915
  routes of administration, 910–915
Participating provider, 90
Parturition, 494
Past health history (PHH), 111
Past history (PH), 111
Patency, 920
Pathogen, 772
Pathogenic, 768
Pathogens, 180
Patient advocate, 166–169
Patient-centered approach, 32
Patient-centered medical home (PCMH), 12, 32–35, 154
Patient mobility equipment and assistive devices, 162
Patient navigator, 166–169
Patient Protection and Affordable Care Act (PPACA), 30–35
  patient-centered approach, 32
  pay for coordination organizations, 32–35
  performance organizations, 31–32
  reforming health care, 30–31
Patient safety considerations, 252
Patients' bill of rights, 7, 22–23
Patient screening
  communication cycle, 102–103
  procedure, 115–117
  therapeutic communication, 103–104
Patients' health care needs, 171–172
Patients' health care needs, 171–172
Patients, professionalism, 3–24
Pay for coordination organizations, 32
Pay for performance organizations, 31
PCMH (patient-centered medical home), 12, 32–35
Peak expiratory flow (PEF), 426
Peak flow meter, 426
Peak flow testing, 435–436
Pediatric, 573
Pediatric development
  language development, 580
  motor development, 579–580
  sensory development, 580
Pediatrician, 574
Pediatric injections, 585–586, 596–597
Pediatric patient
  age-appropriate communication, 574–575
  age classifications, 574
  behavioral and mental health issues, 588–589
  immunizations, 581–585
  infant/toddler measurements, 575–579
  visual and hearing screenings, 581
Pelvic exam, 482
Percentiles, 575
Perception, professional communication, 8
Percussion, 334
Perform pulse oximetry, 437
Perimenopause, 474
Peristalsis, 447
Personal health record (PHR), 41
Personal medical history, 111
Personal morals, 7
Personal protective equipment (PPE), 159, 182
pH, 713
Pharmacodynamics, 853–858
Pharmacokinetics, 856–857
Pharmacology, 845, 846
Phenylketonuria (PKU), 586
Phlebitis, 919
Phlebotomists, 673
Phlebotomy, 673
Phosphorous, chemistry tests, 807
PHR (personal health record), 41
Physiatrist, 606
Physical and chemical urinalysis, 728–730
Physical disability, 141
Physical exam
  age-specific and problem-specific exams, 327
  assist with, 344–345
  examination room, 327–331, 338–340
  patient assessment, 332–337
  patient positioning and draping, 331–332, 340–342
  patient preparation, 331
Physically disabled patient
  general guidelines, 141–142
  hygiene issues, 141
Physical therapist (PT), 606
Physical therapy, 618
Physician's office laboratory (POL), 642, 647
PKU, on Newborn, 594–596
Placebo effect, 540
Plan, 46
Plantar fasciitis, 610
Plasma, 687, 741, 799
Plastic surgeon, 538
Platelet count, 745
Pleural effusion, 429
Podiatrist, 605
Poikilocytosis, 748
Point-of-care testing (POCT), 647
Poisoning, 958
Polyps, 451
Polyuria, 512
POMR (problem-oriented medical record), 45
Population management, 155
Positive attitude, professionalism, 11
Positron emission tomography (PET) scan, 839
Postlingual, 133
Postpartum, 488
Postpartum depression, 497

Terminally ill patients
empathy, 164
Testicular self-examination (TSE), 515
Testosterone, 511
Therapeutic communication, 102–103
Therapeutic effect, 856
Therapeutic index, 854
Therapeutic touch, professional communication, 9
Thermal emergencies, 961
Thermotherapy, 619
Thixotropic separator gel, 678
Thoracentesis, 429
Thrombocytes, 743
Thrombosis, 919
Thrombus, 951
Thyroid panel, 804
TIA (transient ischemic attacks), 952
Time, management principles, 19–20
Toddler, 574
Tonometer, 354
Topical, 871
Tourniquet, 674
Traditional Chinese medicine, 540
Transdermal patches, 871
Transfats, 557
Transient ischemic attacks (TIA), 952
Transition of care, 168
Transmission-based precautions, 191–192
Transrectal ultrasound (TRUS), 520
Transurethral resection of the prostate (TURP), 520
Traumatic brain injury, 966
Traumatic needles, 234
Treadmill stress test, 401
Triage, 944
Triglycerides, 803
Trimesters, 489
Triple Aim Initiative, 35
Trocar, 918
Tuberculosis (TB), 420
Two-hour postprandial blood glucose level, 805
Tympanic membrane (TM), 350
Tympanometer, 363
Tympanostomy, 364–365
Tympany, 334

U

Ulcerative colitis, 449
Ultrasonic cleaner, 213
Ultrasound, 493, 618, 837
Universal Precautions, 189
Urea, 713
Urethritis, 513
Urinalysis
abbreviation, 708
microscopic examination, 718–724
quality control, 711
specimen collection, 708–711
urine, composition of, 708
Urinary catheterization, 732–735
Urinary system, 510
Urine
composition of, 708
pregnancy test, 819
specimen containers, 709
transport system, 730–732
Urochrome, 713
Urological medications, 523
Urology, 509
Urticaria, 531
Usual childhood diseases (UCHD or UCD), 111
Uterus, 471–472

V

Vaccinations, 581
Vaccines type, 187
Vacuum tube, 674
Vaginal/internal exam, 492
Vasectomies, 520
Vasectomy post-op instructions, 521
Vasoconstriction, 295
Vasodilation, 295, 619
Vasography, 520
Vectors, 182
Vegan, 564
Vegetarians, 563
Venipuncture, 674, 691–694
butterfly method, 697–698
capillary puncture, 700–702
vacuum tube method, 694–697
Ventricular fibrillation, 950
Verbal communication, professionalism, 8–9
Vertigo, 331, 961
Vial, 903
ViraPap®, 484
Virology, 781–782
Viruses, identification of, 781–782
Viscosity, 899
Viscosupplementation, 621
Visual acuity, 349
Visual acuity testing, 356–360
Vital capacity (VC), 426
Vital signs and measurements, 292
blood pressure, 304–307
electronic vital signs, 307
height and weight, 293–294, 309–311
pain assessment, 307
patient intake, 293
pulse, 300–302
pulse oximetry, 307
respiration, 302–303
screening the patient, 293
temperature, 295–300
Vitamins, 553
Voiding, 709

W

Waived tests, 644
Walkers, 616, 629–630
Weight loss diets, 563
Wheal, 534, 910
Wheelchairs, 616–617, 631–632
Wheelchairs, assisting patients in, 142
White blood cell count, 744–745
Whole blood, 799
Winged infusion, 680
Withdraw medication, 922–923
Women's health issues. *See* Obstetrics and gynecology
Work practice controls, 196
Wound care
bandage material, 267–268
dressing types, 266–267
stages of wound healing, 264–265
Today's wound care philosophy, 265–266
wound care alternatives, 268–269
Wound specimen, 790–791

X

X-ray, 826

Y

Yoga, 542